Vital Statistics
of the United States
Births, Life Expectancy, Deaths, and Selected Health Data

Fifth Edition, 2012

Vital Statistics
of the United States
Births, Life Expectancy, Deaths, and Selected Health Data

Fifth Edition, 2012

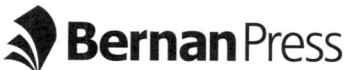

Published in the United States of America
by Bernan Press, a wholly owned subsidiary of
The Rowman & Littlefield Publishing Group, Inc.
4501 Forbes Boulevard, Suite 200
Lanham, Maryland 20706

Bernan Press
800-865-3457
www.bernan.com

Copyright © 2012 by Bernan Press

All rights reserved. No part of this publication may be reproduced, stored in a retrieval system, or transmitted in any form or by any means, electronic, mechanical, photocopying, recording, or otherwise, without the prior permission of the copyright holder. Bernan Press does not claim copyright in U.S. government information.

ISBN-13: 978-1-59888-538-5

ISSN: 1549-8603

∞™ The paper used in this publication meets the minimum requirements of American National Standard for Information Sciences—Permanence of Paper for Printed Library Materials, ANSI/NISO Z39.48-1992.
Manufactured in the United States of America.

CONTENTS

LIST OF TABLES vii

LIST OF FIGURES xv

INTRODUCTION xvii

PART A: BIRTHS **1**
Highlights 3
Notes and Definitions 97

PART B: MORTALITY **99**
Highlights 101
Notes and Definitions 237

PART C: HEALTH **239**
Highlights 241
    Determinants and Measures of Health 241
    Use of Addictive Substances 300
    Ambulatory Care 312
    Inpatient Care 354
    Health Personnel 375
    Health Expenditures 383
    Health Insurance 404
Notes and Definitions 427

INDEX **431**

LIST OF TABLES

PART A: BIRTHS

Table A-1	Selected Characteristics by Race and Hispanic Origin of Mother, Final 2009 and Preliminary 2010	4
Table A-2.	Births and Birth Rates, by Race and Hispanic Origin of Mother, Preliminary 2010 and Final 2000–2009	4
Table A-3.	Births and Birth Rates by Age, Race, and Hispanic Origin of Mother, Final 2009 and Preliminary 2010	5
Table A-4.	Live Births by Age of Mother, Live-Birth Order, and Race and Hispanic Origin of Mother, Preliminary 2010	6
Table A-5.	Birth Rates by Age of Mother, Live-Birth Order, and Race and Hispanic Origin of Mother, Preliminary 2010	7
Table A-6.	Birth Rates for Women Under Age 20 Years, by Age and Race and Hispanic Origin of Mother, Selected Years, 1991–Preliminary 2010	8
Table A-7.	Births to Mothers Under 20 Years of Age by State and Territory, Final 2009 and Preliminary 2010	9
Table A-8.	Number and Percentage of Births to Unmarried Women, by Age, Final 2009 and Preliminary 2010	11
Table A-9.	Live Births by Race and Hispanic Origin of Mother, and Birth and Fertility Rates by State, Preliminary 2010	12
Table A-10.	Selected Characteristics of Births, by Race and Hispanic Origin of Mother, Final 2009 and Preliminary 2010	13
Table A-11.	Low Birthweight Births by State and Territory, Final 2009 and Preliminary 2010	14
Table A-12.	Percentage of Preterm Births, Selected Years, 1990–2010	15
Table A-13.	Preterm and Late Term Births by State and Territory, Final 2009 and Preliminary 2010	16
Table A-14.	Births by Cesarean Delivery by State and Territory, Final 2009 and Preliminary 2010	17
Table A-15.	Birth Rates, by Age and Race and Hispanic Origin of Mother, Final 2000–2009 and Preliminary 2010	18
Table A-16.	Birth Rates by Live-Birth Order and by Race and Hispanic Origin of Mother, 2000–2009 and Preliminary 2010	20
Table A-17.	Births to Unmarried Mothers, by State and Territory, Final 2009 and Preliminary 2010	22
Table A-18.	Total Count of Records and Completeness of Preliminary File of Live Births, by State and Territory, Preliminary 2010	23
Table A-19.	Birth Rates for Teenagers 15–19 Years, by State, Selected Years, 1991–2009	25
Table A-20.	Probability of a First Birth, Ages 15 Through 20 and for Females Aged 15–24, 2002 and 2006–2010	26
Table A-21.	Responses to the Statement "If You Got Pregnant Now or Got a Female Pregnant Now, How Would You Feel?" For Never-Married Females and Males Aged 15–19, 2002 and 2006–2010	27
Table A-22.	Birth Rates for Women Aged 10–19 Years by Age, Race, and Hispanic Origin of Mother, Selected Years, 1991–2009	28
Table A-23.	Mean Age of Mother, by Live-Birth Order and Race and Hispanic Origin of Mother, 1980–2009	29
Table A-24.	Live Births, Birth Rates, and Fertility Rates, by Race, Specified Years, 1940–1955 and Each Year, 1960–2009	30
Table A-25.	Births and Birth Rates, by Hispanic Origin of Mother and by Race for Mothers of Non-Hispanic Origin, 1989–2009	31
Table A-26.	Live Births by Age of Mother, Live-Birth Order, and Race of Mother, 2009	33
Table A-27.	Live Births by Age of Mother, Live-Birth Order, and Hispanic Origin, 2009	34
Table A-28.	Live Births by Race of Mother, by State and Territory, 2009	35
Table A-29.	Live Births by Hispanic Origin of Mother and by Race for Mothers of Non-Hispanic Origin, by State and Territory, 2009	36
Table A-30.	Birth Rates, by Age of Mother, Each State and Territory, 2009	38
Table A-31.	Birth Rates by Age of Mother, Live-Birth Order, and Race of Mother, 2009	39
Table A-32.	Birth Rates by Age and Race of Father, 1980–2009	40
Table A-33.	Total Fertility Rates and Birth Rates by Age of Mother, 1970–2009, and by Age and Race of Mother, 1980–2009	42

Table A-34.	Fertility Rates and Birth Rates, by Age, Live-Birth Order, Specified Hispanic Origin, and Race of Mother, 2009	45
Table A-35.	Total Fertility Rates, Fertility Rates, and Birth Rates by Age and Hispanic Origin of Mother and by Race for Mothers of Non-Hispanic Origin, 1989–2009	47
Table A-36.	Fertility Rates and Birth Rates by Live-Birth Order and by Race and Hispanic Origin of Mother, 1980–2009	51
Table A-37.	Selected Demographic Characteristics of Births by Race of Mother, 2009	53
Table A-38.	Live Births by Day of Week and Index of Occurrence by Method of Delivery, 2009	53
Table A-39.	Live Births and Observed and Seasonally Adjusted Birth and Fertility Rates, by Month, 2009	53
Table A-40.	Number, Rate, and Percentage of Births to Unmarried Women and Birth Rate for Married Women, Selected Years, 1980–2009	55
Table A-41.	Birth Rates for Unmarried Women by Age of Mother, 1970, 1975, and 1980–2009, and by Age, Race, and Hispanic Origin of Mother, 1980–2009	56
Table A-42.	Number, Birth Rate, and Percentage of Births to Unmarried Women by Age, Race, and Hispanic Origin of Mother, 2009	59
Table A-43.	Total Number of Births, Rates (Birth, Fertility, and Total Fertility), and Percentage of Births with Selected Demographic Characteristics, by Hispanic Origin of Mother and by Race for Mothers of Non-Hispanic Origin, 2009	60
Table A-44.	Percentage of Births with Selected Medical or Health Characteristics, by Race of Mother, 2009	60
Table A-45.	Percentage of Births with Selected Medical or Health Characteristics, by Hispanic Origin of Mother and by Race for Mothers of Non-Hispanic Origin, 2009	61
Table A-46.	Number and Percentage of Births to Unmarried Women by Race and Hispanic Origin of Mother, by State and Territory, 2009	62
Table A-47.	Number of Live Births and Percent Distribution, by Weight Gain of Mother During Pregnancy, According to Period of Gestation and Race and Hispanic Origin of Mother, 2009	63
Table A-48.	Number and Rate of Live Births to Mothers with Selected Risk Factors During Pregnancy, Obstetric Procedures, Characteristics of Labor and Delivery, and Congenital Anomalies, by Age, Race, and Hispanic Origin of Mother, 2009	65
Table A-49.	Pregnancy Risk Factors, by Age and Race and Hispanic Origin of Mother, 27 Reporting States, 2008	67
Table A-50	Births Delivered by Forceps or Vacuum Extraction, Selected Years, 1990–2009	68
Table A-51.	Live Births by Method of Delivery and Rates of Cesarean Delivery by Race and Hispanic Origin of Mother, 1989–2009	68
Table A-52.	Number of Live Births, by Method 2009 of Delivery and Rates of Cesarean Delivery by Age and Race and Hispanic Origin of Mother, 2009	69
Table A-53.	Rates of Cesarean Delivery by Race and Hispanic Origin of Mother, by State and Territory, 2009	71
Table A-54.	Live Births by Birthweight and Percentage Very Low and Low Birthweight, by Period of Gestation and Race and Hispanic Origin of Mother, 2009	72
Table A-55.	Percentage of Live Births Very Preterm and Preterm and Percentage of Live Births of Very Low Birthweight and Low Birthweight, by Race and Hispanic Origin of Mother, 1981–2009	74
Table A-56.	Birthweight Distribution in 500 Gram Intervals, Selected Years, 1990–2009	75
Table A-57.	Preterm and Low Birthweight Births, by Age and Race and Hispanic Origin of Mother, 2009	76
Table A-58.	Number and Percentage of Births of Very Low Birthweight, by Race and Hispanic Origin of Mother by State and Territory, 2009	77
Table A-59.	Number and Percentage of Births Delivered Preterm, by Race and Hispanic Origin of Mother by State and Territory, 2009	78
Table A-60.	Number and Percentage of Births of Low Birthweight, by Race and Hispanic Origin of Mother, 2009	79
Table A-61.	Very Low Birthweight Births, by Race and Hispanic Origin of Mother by State and Territory, 2009	80
Table A-62.	Live Births by Plurality of Birth and Ratios, by Age, Race, and Hispanic Origin of Mother, 2009	81
Table A-63.	Numbers and Rates of Twin and Triplet and Higher-Order Multiple Births, by Race and Hispanic Origin of Mother, 1980–2009	82
Table A-64.	Twin and Triplet and Higher Order Multiple Birth Rates by State, 2007–2009	85
Table A-65.	Gestational Age and Birthweight Characteristics by Plurality, 2009	86
Table A-66.	Percent Distribution of Gestational Age for All Births and for Singleton Births Only, Selected Years, 1990–2009	86

Table A-67. Births, by Smoking Status During Pregnancy and Race and Hispanic Origin of Mother, 24 States, 2008 87
Table A-68. Use of Contraception Among Sexually Experienced Females Aged 15–19, by Method of Contraception, 1995, 2002, and 2006–2010 87
Table A-69. Use of Contraception at First Sex Among Females and Males Aged 15–19, by Method Used, Selected Years, 1988–2010 88
Table A-70. Use of Contraception at Last Sex in the Prior 3 Months Among Never-Married Females and Males Aged 15–19, by Method Used, Selected Years, 1988–2010 89
Table A-71. Consistency of Condom Use in the 4 Weeks Prior to the Interview Among Never-Married Females and Males Aged 15–19, 2002 and 2006–2010 90
Table A-72. Number of Live Births by Attendant, Place of Delivery, Race, and Hispanic Origin of Mother, 2009 91
Table A-73. Educational Attainment of Mother, by Age, Hispanic Origin, and Race of Mother: Total of 27 Reporting States, 2008 92
Table A-74. Month Prenatal Care Began, by Age, Race, and Hispanic Origin of Mother, 27 Reporting States, 2008 93
Table A-75. Births, by Educational Attainment, Race, and Hispanic Origin of Mother, 27 Reporting States, 2008 94
Table A-76. Abnormal Conditions of the Newborn, by Age, Race, and Hispanic Origin of Mother, 27 Reporting States, 2008 95
Table A-77. Congenital Anomaly of the Newborn, by Age, Race, and Hispanic Origin of Mother, 27 Reporting States, 2008 96

PART B: MORTALITY

Table B-1. Number of Deaths, Death Rates, and Age-Adjusted Death Rates, by Race and Sex, Selected Years, 1940–2008 102
Table B-2. Number of Deaths, Death Rates, and Age-Adjusted Death Rates, by Hispanic Origin, Race for Non-Hispanic Population, and Sex, 1997–2008 104
Table B-3. Number of Deaths and Death Rates, by Age, Race, and Sex, 2008 105
Table B-4. Number of Deaths and Death Rates by Hispanic Origin, Race for Non-Hispanic Population, Age, and Sex, 2008 106
Table B-5. Number of Deaths and Death Rates by Age, and Age-Adjusted Death Rates, by Specified Hispanic Origin, Race for Non-Hispanic Population, and Sex, 2008 107
Table B-6. Abridged Life Table for the Total Population, 2008 108
Table B-7. Life Expectancy at Birth by Race and Sex, Selected Years, 1940–2008 110
Table B-8. Life Expectancy at Selected Ages by Race, Hispanic Origin, Race for Non-Hispanic Population, and Sex, 2008 112
Table B-9. Life Expectancy at Birth, at 65 Years of Age, and at 75 Years of Age, by Race and Sex, Selected Years, 1900–2009 113
Table B-10. Death Rates by Age and Age-Adjusted Death Rates for the 15 Leading Causes of Death, 1999–2008 115
Table B-11. Number of Deaths from Selected Causes by Age, 2008 119
Table B-12. Death Rates for Selected Causes by Age, 2008 122
Table B-13. Number of Deaths from Selected Causes by Race and Sex, 2008 125
Table B-14. Death Rates for 113 Selected Causes by Race and Sex, 2008 131
Table B-15. Number of Deaths from Selected Causes by Hispanic Origin, Race for Non–Hispanic Population, and Sex, 2008 137
Table B-16. Death Rates from Selected Causes by Hispanic Origin, Race for Non-Hispanic Population, and Sex, 2008 143
Table B-17. Age-Adjusted Death Rates from Selected Causes by Race and Sex, 2008 150
Table B-18. Age-Adjusted Death Rates from Selected Causes by Hispanic Origin, Race for Non-Hispanic Population, and Sex, 2008 156
Table B-19. Age-Adjusted Death Rates, by Race and Hispanic Origin, Average Annual Rates, 1979–1981, 1989–1991, and 2006–2008 162
Table B-20. Age-Adjusted Death Rates for Selected Causes of Death, by Sex, Race, and Hispanic Origin, Selected Years, 1950–2008 163
Table B-21. Number of Deaths, Death Rates, and Age–Adjusted Death Rates for Injury Deaths According to Mechanism and Intent of Death, 2008 166
Table B-22. Leading Causes of Death and Numbers of Death, by Sex, Race, and Hispanic Origin, 1980 and 2008 168

Table B-23. Leading Causes of Death and Numbers of Deaths, by Age, 1980 and 2008 172
Table B-24. Deaths from Selected Occupational Diseases Among Persons 15 Years of Age and Over, Selected Years, 1980–2008 174
Table B-25. Fatal Occupational Injuries, Comparison of 2010 Preliminary and Final Figures, by Selected Characteristics 176
Table B-26. Occupational Fatal Injuries and Rates, by Industry, Sex, Age, Race, and Hispanic Origin, Selected Years, 1995–2009 177
Table B-27. Number of Fatal Work Injuries by Most Frequent Type, 1992–2010 179
Table B-28. Number and Rate of Fatal Occupational Injuries, by Industry Sector and Occupation, 2010 179
Table B-29. Number of Fatal Work Injuries, by State, 2010 180
Table B-30. Years of Potential Life Lost Before Age 75 for Selected Causes of Death, by Sex, Race, and Hispanic Origin, Selected Years, 1980–2007 181
Table B-31. Number of Deaths, Death Rates, and Age–Adjusted Death Rates for Major Causes of Death by State and Territory, 2008 184
Table B-32. Death Rates for All Causes, by Sex, Race, Hispanic Origin, and Age, Selected Years, 1950–2008 190
Table B-33. Death Rates for Diseases of the Heart, by Sex, Race, Hispanic Origin, and Age, Selected Years, 1950–2008 194
Table B-34. Death Rates for Cerebrovascular Diseases, by Sex, Race, Hispanic Origin, and Age, Selected Years, 1950–2008 197
Table B-35. Death Rates for Malignant Neoplasms, by Sex, Race, Hispanic Origin, and Age, Selected Years, 1950–2008 201
Table B-36. Death Rates for Malignant Neoplasm of Breast Among Females, by Race, Hispanic Origin, and Age, Selected Years, 1950–2008 204
Table B-37. Death Rates for Malignant Neoplasms of the Trachea, Bronchus, and Lung, by Sex, Race, Hispanic Origin, and Age, Selected Years, 1950–2008 206
Table B-38. Death Rates for Human Immunodeficiency Virus (HIV) Disease, by Sex, Race, Hispanic Origin, and Age, Selected Years, 1987–2008 209
Table B-39. Death Rates for Drug Poisoning and Drug Poisoning Involving Opioid Analgesics, by Sex, Age, Race, and Hispanic Origin, Selected Years, 1999–2008 211
Table B-40. Unintentional Motor Vehicle Deaths by States, Annual Averages, 2000–2007 213
Table B-41. Death Rates for Motor Vehicle–Related Injuries, by Sex, Race, Hispanic Origin, and Age, Selected Years, 1950–2008 214
Table B-42. Death Rates for Homicide, by Sex, Race, Hispanic Origin, and Age, Selected Years, 1950–2008 218
Table B-43. Death Rates for Suicide, by Sex, Race, Hispanic Origin, and Age, Selected Years, 1950–2008 221
Table B-44. Death Rates for Firearm–Related Injuries, by Sex, Race, Hispanic Origin, and Age, Selected Years, 1970–2008 224
Table B-45. Infant, Neonatal, and Postneonatal Mortality Rates, by Race and Sex, 1940–2008 228
Table B-46. Number of Infant Deaths and Infant Mortality Rates for 130 Selected Causes by Race, 2008 231
Table B-47. Number of Infant and Neonatal Deaths and Mortality Rates, by Race, State, and Territory, 2008 .. 234
Table B-48. Selected Characterisstics of Discharged Hospice Care Patients, 2007 235
Table B-49. Primary Admission Diagnosis of Discharged Hospice Care Patients, 1998 and 2007 235
Table B-50. Services Offered or Provided to Hospice Care Patients' Family Members or Friends, 2007 235
Table B-51. Hospice Care Patients Symptoms at the Last Hospice Care Visit Before Death, 2007 236
Table B-52. Selected Drugs Prescribed to Hospice Care Patients in the Last Week of Life, 2007 236

PART C: HEALTH

DETERMINANTS AND MEASURES OF HEALTH

Table C-1. Nonfatal Occupational Injuries and Illnesses with Days Away from Work, Job Transfer, or Restriction, by Industry, Selected Years, 2005–2009 242
Table C-2. Selected Notifiable Disease Rates and Number of New Cases, Selected Years, 1950–2009 243
Table C-3. Acquired Immunodeficiency Syndrome (AIDS) Cases, by Year of Diagnosis and Selected Characteristics, 2006–2009 245
Table C-4. Age-Adjusted Cancer Incidence Rates for Selected Cancer Sites, by Sex, Race, and Hispanic Origin, Selected Geographic Areas, Selected Years, 1990–2008 and Annual Percent Change (APC), 1990–2008 247
Table C-5. Five-Year Relative Cancer Survival Rates for Selected Cancer Sites, by Race and Sex, Selected Geographic Areas, Selected Years, 1975–1977 through 2001–2007 253
Table C-6 Respondent-Reported Prevalence of Heart Disease, Cancer, and Stroke Among Adults 18 Years of Age and Over, by Selected Characteristics, Selected Years 1997–1998 through 2009–2010 255

Table C-7.	Diabetes Prevalence and Glycemic Control Among Adults 20 Years of Age and Over, by Sex, Age, Race, and Hispanic Origin, Selected Years, 1988–1994 through 2003–2006	261
Table C-8.	End-Stage Renal Disease Patients, by Selected Characteristics, Selected Years, 1980–2008	263
Table C-9.	Severe Headache or Migraine, Low Back Pain, and Neck Pain Among Adults 18 Years of Age and Over, by Selected Characteristics, 1997, 2000, and 2010	266
Table C-10.	Joint Pain Among Adults 18 Years of Age and Over, by Selected Characteristics, Selected Years, 2002–2010	268
Table C-11.	Basic Actions Difficulty and Complex Activity Limitation Among Adults 18 Years of Age and Over, by Selected Characteristics, Selected Years, 1997–2010	272
Table C-12.	Vision and Hearing Limitations Among Adults 18 Years of Age and Over, by Selected Characteristics, Selected Years, 1997–2010	274
Table C-13.	Respondent-Assessed Health Status, by Selected Characteristics, Selected Years, 1991–2010	276
Table C-14.	Selected Measures of Disability and Health Status Among Adults 18–64 Years of Age, by Urbanization Level and Selected Characteristics, Average Annual, 2002–2004 through 2008–2010	278
Table C-15.	Serious Psychological Distress in the Past 30 Days Among Adults 18 Years of Age and Over, by Selected Characteristics, Average Annual, Selected Years, 1997–1998 through 2009–2010	282
Table C-16.	Children Under 18 Years of Age Who Suffer from Asthma, by Selected Characteristics, Average Annual, Selected Years, 1997–1999 through 2008–2010	283
Table C-17.	Hypertension Among Persons 20 Years of Age and Over, by Selected Characteristics, Selected Years, 1988–1994 through 2007–2010	284
Table C-18.	Cholesterol Among Persons 20 Years of Age and Over, by Selected Characteristics, Selected Years, 1988–1994 through 2007–2010	285
Table C-19.	Mean Energy and Macronutrient Intake Among Persons 20 Years of Age and Over, by Sex and Age, Selected Years, 1971–1974 through 2005–2008	287
Table C-20.	Participation in Leisure-Time Aerobic and Muscle-Strengthening Activities that Meet the 2008 Federal Physical Activity Guidelines for Adults 18 Years of Age and Over, by Selected Characteristics, Selected Years, 1998–2010	288
Table C-21.	Healthy Weight, Overweight, and Obesity Among Persons 20 Years of Age and Over, by Selected Characteristics, Selected Years, 1960–1962 through 2007–2010	291
Table C-22.	Obesity Among Children and Adolescents 2–19 Years of Age, by Selected Characteristics, Selected Years, 1963–1965 through 2007–2010	294
Table C-23.	Untreated Dental Caries, by Selected Characteristics, Selected Years, 1971–1974 through 2005–2008	295
Table C-24.	Health-Related Behaviors of Children 6–11 Years of Age, by Selected Characteristics, 2003 and 2007	296
Table C-25.	Selected Health Conditions and Risk Factors, Selected Years, 1988–1994 through 2009–2010	297
Table C-26.	Health Risk Behaviors Among Students in Grades 9–12, by Sex, Grade Level, Race, and Hispanic Origin, Selected Years, 1991–2009	298

USE OF ADDICTIVE SUBSTANCES

Table C-27.	Use of Selected Substances in the Past Month Among Persons 12 Years of Age and Over, by Age, Sex, Race, and Hispanic Origin, Selected Years, 2002–2009	301
Table C-28.	Heavier Drinking and Drinking Five or More Drinks in a Day Among Adults 18 Years of Age and Over, by Selected Characteristics, Selected Years, 1997–2010	303
Table C-29.	Age-Adjusted Prevalence of Current Cigarette Smoking Among Adults 25 Years of Age and Over, by Sex, Race, and Education Level, Selected Years, 1974–2010	305
Table C-30.	Current Cigarette Smoking Among Adults, by Sex, Race, Hispanic Origin, Age, and Education Level, Average Annual, Selected Years, 1990–1992 through 2008–2010	306
Table C-31.	Current Cigarette Smoking Among Adults 18 Years of Age and Over, by Sex, Race, and Age, Selected Years, 1965–2010	308
Table C-32.	Use of Selected Substances Among High School Seniors, 10th Graders, and 8th Graders, by Sex and Race, Selected Years, 1980–2010	310

AMBULATORY CARE

Table C-33.	No Usual Source of Health Care Among Children Under 18 Years of Age, by Selected Characteristics, Average Annual, Selected Years, 1993–1994 through 2009–2010	313
Table C-34.	No Usual Source of Health Care Among Adults 18–64 Years of Age, by Selected Characteristics, Average Annual, Selected Years, 1993–1994 through 2009–2010	314

Table C-35. Reduced Access to Medical Care, Dental Care, and Prescription Drugs During the Past 12 Months Due to Cost, by Selected Characteristics, Selected Years, 1997–2010 316

Table C-36. Reduced Access to Medical Care During the Past 12 Months Due to Cost, by the 25 Largest States, Selected Annual Averages, 1997–1998 through 2009–2010 318

Table C-37. No Health Care Visits to an Office or Clinic Within the Past 12 Months Among Children Under 18 Years of Age, by Selected Characteristics, Selected Annual Averages, 1997–1998 through 2009–2010..319

Table C-38. Health Care Visits to Doctor Offices, Emergency Departments, and Home Visits Within the Past 12 Months, by Selected Characteristics, Selected Years, 2000–2010 320

Table C-39. Vaccination Coverage Among Children 19–35 Months of Age for Selected Diseases, by Race, Hispanic Origin, Poverty Level, and Location of Residence in Metropolitan Statistical Area, Selected Years, 1995–2009..322

Table C-40. Vaccination Coverage Among Children 19–35 Months of Age, by State and Selected Urban Area, Selected Years, 2002–2009 325

Table C-41. Vaccination Coverage Among Adolescents 13–17 Years of Age for Selected Diseases, by Selected Characteristics, 2006–2009 327

Table C-42. Influenza Vaccination Among Adults 18 Years of Age and Over, by Selected Characteristics, Selected Years, 1989–2010 328

Table C-43. Pneumococcal Vaccination Among Adults 18 Years of Age and Over, by Selected Characteristics, Selected Years, 1989–2010 330

Table C-44. Use of Mammography Among Women 40 Years of Age and Over, by Selected Characteristics, Selected Years, 1987–2010 332

Table C-45. Percent of Women 18 Years of Age and Over Who Have Had a Pap Smear Within the Last Three Years, by Selected Characteristics, Selected Years, 1987–2010 334

Table C-46. Use of Colorectal Tests or Procedures Among Adults 50–75 Years of Age, by Selected Characteristics, Selected Years, 2000–2010 336

Table C-47. Emergency Department Visits Within the Past 12 Months Among Children Under 18 Years of Age, by Selected Characteristics, Selected Years, 1997–2010 338

Table C-48. Emergency Department Visits Within the Past 12 Months Among Adults 18 Years of Age and Over, by Selected Characteristics, Selected Years, 1997–2010...341

Table C-49. Initial Injury-Related Visits to Hospital Emergency Departments, by Sex, Age, and Intent and Mechanism of Injury, Selected Annual Averages, 2005–2006 and 2008–2009 343

Table C-50. Visits to Physician Offices, Hospital Outpatient Departments, and Hospital Emergency Departments, by Age, Sex, and Race, Selected Years, 1995–2009 345

Table C-51. Visits to Primary Care Generalist and Specialist Physicians, by Selected Characteristics and Type of Physician, Selected Years, 1980–2009 346

Table C-52. Dental Visits in the Past Year, by Selected Characteristics, Selected Years, 1997–2010 348

Table C-53. Prescription Drug Use in the Past 30 Days, by Sex, Age, Race and Hispanic Origin, Selected Years, 1988–1994 through 2005–2008 349

Table C-54. Selected Prescription Drug Classes Used in the Past 30 Days, by Sex and Age, Selected Years, 1988–1994 through 2005–2008..351

Table C-55. Dietary Supplement Use Among Persons 20 Years of Age and Over, by Selected Characteristics, Selected Years, 1988–1994 through 2005–2008 353

INPATIENT CARE

Table C-56. Persons with Hospital Stays in the Past Year, by Selected Characteristics, Selected Years, 1997–2010..355

Table C-57. Discharges, Days of Care, and Average Length of Stay in Nonfederal Short-Stay Hospitals, by Selected Characteristics, Selected Years, 1980 through 2008–2009 358

Table C-58. Discharges in Nonfederal Short-Stay Hospitals, by Sex, Age, and Selected First-Listed Diagnosis, Selected Years, 1990 through 2008–2009..361

Table C-59. Discharge Rate in Nonfederal Short-Stay Hospitals, by Sex, Age, and Selected First-Listed Diagnosis, Selected Years, 1990 through 2008–2009..364

Table C-60. Average Length of Stay in Nonfederal Short-Stay Hospitals, by Sex, Age, and Selected First-Listed Diagnosis, Selected Years, 1990 through 2008–2009 367

Table C-61. Discharges with at Least One Procedure in Nonfederal Short-Stay Hospitals, by Sex, Age, and Selected Procedures, Selected Years, 1990 through 2009 370

Table C-62. Certified Intermediate Care Facilities and Specialty Hospitals, Number of Facilities and Beds, by State, Selected Years, 1995–2010 373

HEALTH PERSONNEL

Table C-63. Health Care Employment and Wages, by Selected Occupations, Selected Years, 2001–2010 376
Table C-64. Employment and Wages in the Health Care Industry by Occupation, May 2011 377
Table C-65 Employment and Wages for the Highest and Lowest Paying Occupations, May 2011 378
Table C-66. Industries with the Highest Levels of Employment and Highest Concentration of Employment in Health Care and Practitioner and Technical Occupations, May 2011 379
Table C-67. States with the Highest Level of Employment and Highest Concentration of Jobs in Health Care Practitioner and Technical Occupations, May 2011 379
Table C-68. Top Paying Metropolitan Area for Health Care Practitioner and Technical Occupations, May 2011 380
Table C-69. Employers' Costs Per Employee-Hour Worked for Total Compensation, Wages and Salaries, and Health Insurance, by Selected Characteristics, Selected Years, 1991–2011 381

HEALTH EXPENDITURES

Table C-70. Gross Domestic Product, National Health Expenditures, Per Capita Amounts, Percent Distribution, and Average Annual Percent Change, Selected Years, 1960–2009 384
Table C-71. Consumer Price Index and Average Annual Percent Change for All Items, Selected Items, and Medical Care Components, Selected Years, 1960–2010 385
Table C-72. Growth in Personal Health Care Expenditures and Percent Distribution of Factors Affecting Growth, 1960–2009 387
Table C-73. National Health Expenditures for Mental Health Services, Average Annual Percent Change and Percent Distribution, by Type of Expenditure, Selected Years, 1986–2005 388
Table C-74 National Health Expenditures for Substance Abuse Treatment, Average Annual Percent Change and Percent Distribution, by Type of Expenditure, Selected Years, 1986–2005 389
Table C-75. National Health Expenditures, Average Annual Percent Change, and Percent Distribution, by Type of Expenditure, Selected Years, 1960–2009 390
Table C-76. Personal Health Care Expenditures, by Source of Funds and Type of Expenditure, Selected Years, 1960–2009 392
Table C-77. Cost of Hospital Discharges with Common Hospital Operating Room Procedures in Nonfederal Community Hospitals, by Age and Selected Principal Procedure, Selected Years, 2000–2009 395
Table C-78. Expenses for Health Care by Selected Population Characteristics, Selected Years, 1987–2008 397
Table C-79. Percent Distribution of Payment for Health Care, by Selected Population Characteristics, Selected Years, 1987–2008 398
Table C-80. Out-of-Pocket Health Care Expenses Among Persons with Medical Expenses, by Age, Selected Years, 1987–2008 399
Table C-81. Expenditures for Health Services and Supplies and Percent Distribution, by Sponsor, Selected Years, 1987–2009 402
Table C-82. Department of Veterans Affairs Health Care Expenditures and Use, and Persons Treated, by Selected Characteristics, Selected Fiscal Years, 1970–2010 403

HEALTH INSURANCE

Table C-83. Private Health Insurance Coverage Obtained Through the Workplace Among Persons Under 65 Years of Age, by Selected Characteristics, Selected Years, 1984–2010 405
Table C-84. Private Health Insurance Coverage Among Persons Under 65 Years of Age, by Selected Characteristics, Selected Years, 1984–2010 407
Table C-85. No Health Insurance Coverage Among Persons Under 65 Years of Age, by Selected Characteristics, Selected Years, 1984–2010 409
Table C-86. Health Insurance Coverage of Medicare Beneficiaries 65 Years of Age and Over, by Type of Coverage and Selected Characteristics, Selected Years, 1992–2008 411
Table C-87. Persons Without Health Insurance Coverage, by State, Average Annual, Selected Years, 1995–1997 through 2007–2009 413
Table C-88. Change in the Number and Percent of People Without Health Insurance During First Year After a Recession 414
Table C-89. Medicaid Coverage Among Persons Under 65 Years of Age, by Selected Characteristics, Selected Years, 1984–2010 415
Table C-90. Medicaid Beneficiaries and Payments, by Basis of Eligibility, and Race and Hispanic Origin, Selected Fiscal Years, 1999–2009 417
Table C-91. Medicaid Beneficiaries and Payments, by Type of Service, Selected Fiscal Years, 1999–2009 418

Table C-92.	Medicaid Beneficiaries, Beneficiaries in Managed Care, Payments per Beneficiary, and Beneficiaries per 100 Persons Below the Poverty Level, by State, Selected Fiscal Years, 2000–2009	419
Table C-93.	Medicare Enrollees and Expenditures and Percent Distribution, by Medicare Program and Type of Service, Selected Years, 1970–2010	420
Table C-94.	Medicare Enrollees and Program Payments Among Fee-for-Service Medicare Beneficiaries, by Sex and Age, Selected Years, 1994–2009	422
Table C-95.	Medicare Beneficiaries, by Race, Hispanic Origin, and Selected Characteristics, Selected Years, 1992–2007	423
Table C-96.	Medicare Enrollees, Enrollees in Managed Care, Payment per Enrollee, and Short-Stay Hospital Utilization, by State, Selected Years, 1995–2009	425
Table C-97.	Medicare-Certified Providers and Suppliers, Selected Years, 1975–2009	426

LIST OF FIGURES

PART A: BIRTHS

Figure A-1.	Live Births and Fertility Rates, 1930–Preliminary 2010	3
Figure A-2.	Percent of Births by Race and Hispanic Origin, Preliminary 2010	10
Figure A-3.	Percent of Births to Unmarried Women by Race and Hispanic Origin, 2009	10
Figure A-4.	Birth Rates for Teenagers 15–19 Years of Age by Race and Hispanic Origin, 1991 and 2009	24
Figure A-5.	States with the Highest and Lowest Birth Rates for Teenagers 15–19 Years of Age, 2009	24
Figure A-6.	Birth Rates by Age of Mother, 1980–2009	37
Figure A-7.	Birth Rates, by Age of Father, 1980–2009	37
Figure A-8.	Percent of Births to Unmarried Women by Age, 2009	54
Figure A-9.	Birth Rates for Unmarried Women, by Age of Mother, 1980–2009	54
Figure A-10.	Cesarean Delivery Rates by Age of Mother, 1996 and 2009	70
Figure A-11.	Percent of Live Births with Low and Very Low Birthweights: 1986, 1996, 2006 and 2009	70
Figure A-12.	Percent of Preterm Births by Completed Weeks of Gestation and Selected Years, 1990–2010	84
Figure A-13.	Twin and Triplet or Higher Order Birth Rate, 1980–2009	84

PART B: MORTALITY

Figure B-1.	Age-Adjusted Death Rates, by Race, 1940–2008	101
Figure B-2.	Life Expectancy at Selected Ages, by Sex, 2008	109
Figure B-3.	Life Expectancy at Selected Ages, by Race, 2008	109
Figure B-4.	Age-Adjusted Death Rates for Selected Diseases, 2008	149
Figure B-5.	Age-Adjusted Death Rates for Injury Deaths According to Mechanism, 2008	149
Figure B-6.	Number of Fatal Occupational Injuries by Industry and Selected Event or Exposure, 2010	175
Figure B-7.	Number of Fatal Occupational Injuries by Selected Occupations, 2010	175
Figure B-8.	Age-Adjusted Death Rates for Heart Disease by Race and Sex, Selected Years, 1950–2008	200
Figure B-9.	Age-Adjusted Death Rates for Malignant Neoplasms by Race and Sex, Selected Years, 1950–2008	200
Figure B-10.	Death Rates for Homicide by Race and Sex, Selected Years, 1950–2008	217
Figure B-11.	Death Rates for Suicide by Race and Sex, Selected Years, 1950–2008	217
Figure B-12.	Infant Mortality Rates, by Race, 1940–2008	227
Figure B-13.	States with the Highest and Lowest Infant Death Rates, 2008	227

PART C: HEALTH

Figure C-1.	Prevalence of Heart Disease, Cancer, and Stroke Among Persons 18 Years of Age and Over, Age-Adjusted, Selected Years, 1997–1998 through 2009–2010	241
Figure C-2.	Percent Distribution of Men Age 13 Years and Over Diagnosed with AIDS in 2009 by Race	265
Figure C-3.	Percent of Persons Suffering from Severe Headache, Low Back Pain, and Neck Pain, 1997, 2000, and 2010	265
Figure C-4.	Healthy Weight, Overweight, and Obesity Prevalence Among Persons 20–74 Years of Age, Selected Years, 1960–1962 to 2007–2010	290
Figure C-5.	Overweight Children and Adolescents 6–19 Years of Age, Selected Years, 1971–1974 to 2007–2010	290
Figure C-6.	Use of Selected Substances in the Past Month Among Persons 12 Years of Age and Over, 2002, 2005, and 2009	300
Figure C-7.	Cigarette Smoking Among Adults 18 Years of Age and Over, by Sex and Race, 2005–2010	300
Figure C-8.	Influenza Vaccination Among Adults 18 Years of Age and Over, 2005–2010	312
Figure C-9.	Percent of People with Reduced Access to Medical Care by Selected States, 2009–2010	312
Figure C-10.	Percent of Persons with a Hospital Stay in the Past Year, According to Age, 2010	354
Figure C-11.	Average Length of Stay in Non-Federal Short-Stay Hospitals by Sex, Selected Years, 1990–2009	354
Figure C-12.	Wages for Selected Occupations in the Health Care Industry, May 2011	375
Figure C-13.	Median Annual Wages for Selected Specialties in Medicine, May 2011	375
Figure C-14.	Consumer Price Index (CPI), All Items and Medical Care, 1960–2010	383
Figure C-15.	Percent Distribution of Personal Health Care Expenditures by Type, 2009	383
Figure C-16.	Number of People with No Health Insurance, 2005–2010	404
Figure C-17.	Medicaid Coverage Among Persons 65 Years of Age and Under, 2005–2012	404

INTRODUCTION

Bernan Press is pleased to present a comprehensive collection of birth, mortality, and health data in the fifth edition of *Vital Statistics of the United States: Births, Life Expectancy, Deaths, and Selected Health Data*. Similar to previous editions, this volume provides an abundance of information compiled by various government agencies including the center for Disease Control (CDC) and its National Center for Health Statistics (NCHS), the U.S. Census Bureau, and the Bureau of Labor Statistics (BLS).

Until 1993, the federal government published *Vital Statistics of the United States* in several thick-bound volumes. These volumes offered comprehensive data on births, deaths, marriage and divorce, and can be found in libraries now. However, nothing comparable was published shortly afterward although the CDC and NCHS continued to compile much of this information as periodical reports and news releases and provide them electronically on their Web site.

These circumstances gave Bernan Press the motivation to bring together an extensive collection of birth, death, and health statistics into a single volume called *Vital Statistics of the United States*. The first edition was published in 2004. The 2012 volume is the publication's fifth edition.

The fifth edition is presented in a streamlined format similar to the third and fourth editions. There are three parts: births, mortality, and health. Each part is preceded by highlights of salient data and a figure that calls attention to noteworthy trends. Within each part, there are numerous tables and additional figures. Succinct notes and definitions, source information, and references for further guidance are provided at the end of each part.

Part A: Births provides data on many aspects of natality, including birth and fertility rates, number of children, births to unmarried women, maternal health, teenage birth rates, method and place of delivery, contraceptive use, breastfeeding, medical visits by pregnant women, and infant health status. The data were obtained from NCHS.

Part B: Mortality focuses on deaths and death rates, according to a number of medical, demographic, and social characteristics. Especially detailed are the tables on causes of death, which are shown by age, sex, Hispanic origin, race, and (to a lesser extent) state of residence. Death rates are also given by marital status and level of educational attainment, and special tables are provided for infant mortality. These tables were obtained from NCHS.

Part C: Health offers a collection of statistics concerning health and disease. While health is not a traditional component of vital statistics, there are connections between health status and birth and death statistics. For example, a person analyzing death rates from cancer may also be interested in a table on the incidence rate of cancer. This chapter shows selected data on several topics, including determinants and measures of health, use of addictive substances, ambulatory care, inpatient care, health personnel, health expenditures, and health insurance. Data were obtained from different surveys conducted by NCHS, BLS, and the U.S. Census Bureau.

PART A:
BIRTHS

PART A: BIRTHS

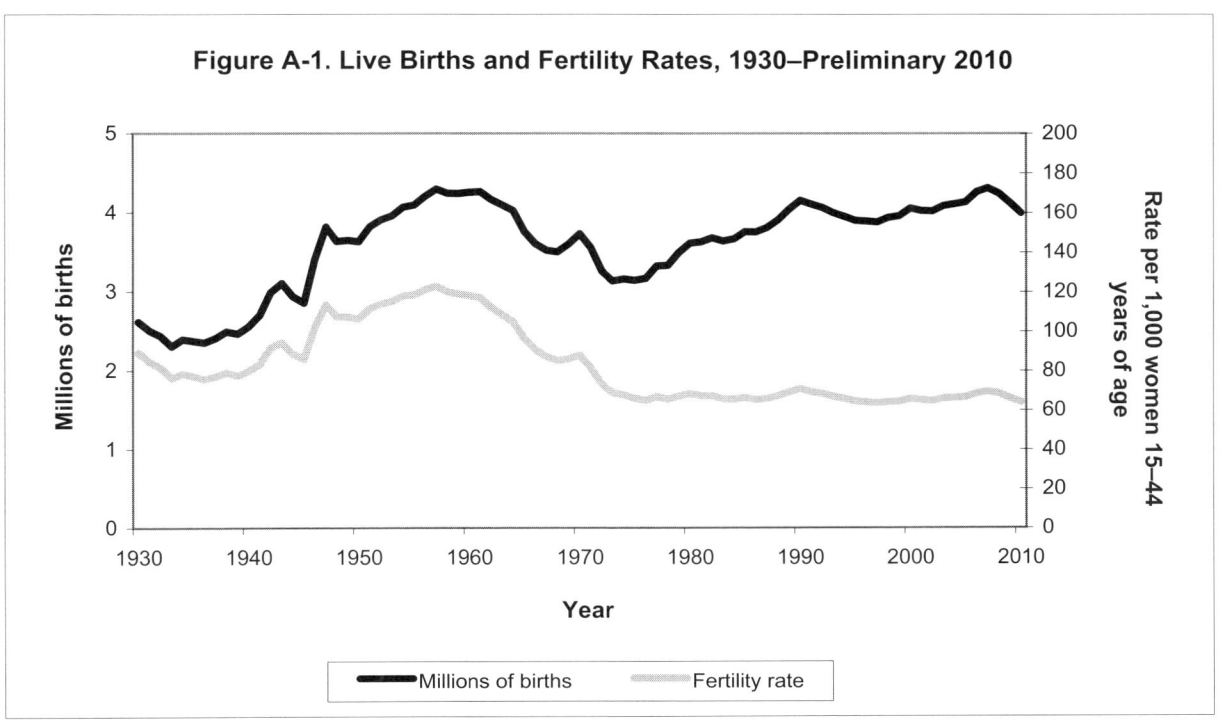

Figure A-1. Live Births and Fertility Rates, 1930–Preliminary 2010

HIGHLIGHTS

- According to preliminary results, there were 4,000,279 births in the United States in 2010, -3.2 percent less than in 2009. While births declined for all racial groups, American Indians and Alaska Natives experienced the greatest decline at 3.9 percent, followed by non-Hispanic Blacks at 3.4 percent. Births declined 2.3 percent for non-Hispanic Whites from 2009 to 2010. (See Table A-1.)

- The birth rate for teenagers aged 15–19 fell to 34.3 births per 1,000 females in 2010, the lowest level ever reported for the United States. From 1991 to 2010, it declined 44 percent. (See Table A-6.)

- In 2009, 41.0 percent of all births were to unmarried women. The numbers varied significantly by state. Utah had the lowest number of births to unmarried woman at 19.4 percent, followed by Colorado at 24.9 percent. The District of Columbia had the highest percentage of births to unmarried women at 55.8 percent followed by Mississippi at 55.3 percent. (See Table A-46.)

- Approximately 98.9 percent of sexually experienced females aged 15–19 have used some method of contraception. The most common methods are the condom (95.9 percent), withdrawal (57.3 percent) and the pill (55.6 percent). (See Table A-68.)

Table A-1. Selected Characteristics by Race and Hispanic Origin of Mother, Final 2009 and Preliminary 2010

(Number, rate.)

Race and Hispanic origin of mother	Number		Birth rate		Fertility rate		Total fertility rate		Percent of births to unmarried women	
	2009	2010	2009	2010	2009	2010	2009	2010	2009	2010
All Races and Origins[1]	4,130,665	4,000,279	13.5	13.0	66.2	64.1	2002.0	1932.0	41.0	40.8
Non-Hispanic White[2]	2,212,552	2,161,669	11.2	10.9	59.6	58.7	1830.0	1791.0	29.0	29.0
Non-Hispanic Black[2]	609,584	589,139	15.7	15.1	68.9	66.6	2045.5	1971.5	72.8	72.5
American Indian or Alaska Native[2,3]	48,665	46,760	11.8	11.0	51.7	48.6	1498.5	1404.0	65.4	65.6
Asian or Pacific Islander[2,3]	251,089	246,915	15.1	14.5	61.3	59.2	1743.0	1689.5	17.2	17.0
Hispanic[4]	999,548	946,000	20.3	18.7	86.5	80.3	2531.5	2352.5	53.2	53.3

[1]Includes births to White Hispanic and Black Hispanic women and births with origin not stated, not shown separately.
[2]Race and Hispanic origin are reported separately on birth certificates.
[3]Includes persons of Hispanic origin according to the mother's reported race.
[4]Persons of Hispanic origin may be of any race.

Table A-2. Births and Birth Rates, by Race and Hispanic Origin of Mother, Preliminary 2010 and Final 2000–2009

(Birth rates are live births per 1,000 population in specified group. Fertility rates are live births per 1,000 women aged 15–44 years in specified group.)

Year	All races and origins[1]	Non-Hispanic White[2]	Non-Hispanic Black[2]	American Indian or Alaska Native[2,3]	Asian or Pacific Islander[2,3]	Hispanic[4]
Number						
2000	4,058,814	2,362,968	604,346	41,668	200,543	815,868
2001	4,025,933	2,326,578	589,917	41,872	200,279	851,851
2002	4,021,726	2,298,156	578,335	42,368	210,907	876,642
2003	4,089,950	2,321,904	576,033	43,052	221,203	912,329
2004	4,112,052	2,296,683	578,772	43,927	229,123	946,349
2005	4,138,349	2,279,768	583,759	44,813	231,108	985,505
2006	4,265,555	2,308,640	617,247	47,721	241,045	1,039,077
2007	4,316,233	2,310,333	627,191	49,443	254,488	1,062,779
2008	4,247,694	2,267,817	623,029	49,537	253,185	1,041,239
2009	4,130,665	2,212,552	609,584	48,665	251,089	999,548
2010	4,000,279	2,161,669	589,139	46,760	246,915	946,000
Birth Rate						
2000	14.4	12.2	17.3	14.0	17.1	23.1
2001	14.1	11.9	16.6	13.6	16.1	22.9
2002	14.0	11.7	16.1	13.3	16.3	22.7
2003	14.1	11.8	15.9	13.0	16.4	22.8
2004	14.0	11.7	15.8	12.8	16.4	22.8
2005	14.0	11.6	15.8	12.6	15.9	22.9
2006	14.3	11.7	16.5	13.0	16.0	23.3
2007	14.3	11.7	16.6	12.9	16.4	23.0
2008	14.0	11.5	16.3	12.5	15.7	21.8
2009	13.5	11.2	15.7	11.8	15.1	20.3
2010	13.0	10.9	15.1	11.0	14.5	18.7
Fertility Rate						
2000	65.9	58.5	71.4	58.7	65.8	95.9
2001	65.1	57.7	69.1	57.0	62.5	95.4
2002	65.0	57.6	67.5	55.8	63.4	94.7
2003	66.1	58.9	67.1	55.0	64.2	95.2
2004	66.4	58.9	67.1	54.3	64.5	95.7
2005	66.7	59.0	67.2	53.6	63.0	96.4
2006	68.6	60.3	70.7	55.4	63.6	98.3
2007	69.3	61.0	71.4	55.6	65.3	97.4
2008	68.1	60.5	70.8	54.1	63.3	92.7
2009	66.2	59.6	68.9	51.7	61.3	86.5
2010	64.1	58.7	66.6	48.6	59.2	80.3

[1]Includes births to White Hispanic and Black Hispanic women and births with origin not stated.
[2]Race and Hispanic origin are reported separately on birth certificates.
[3]Includes persons of Hispanic origin according to the mother's reported race.
[4]Persons of Hispanic origin may be of any race.

Table A-3. Births and Birth Rates by Age, Race, and Hispanic Origin of Mother, Final 2009 and Preliminary 2010

(Number, rates per 1,000 women in specified age-group.)

Age, race, and Hispanic origin of mother	2009 Number	2009 Rate	2010 Number	2010 Rate
All Races and Origins[1]				
Total[2]	4,130,665	66.2	4,000,279	64.1
10–14 years	5,029	0.5	4,500	0.4
15–19 years	409,802	37.9	367,752	34.3
15–17 years	124,247	19.6	109,193	17.3
18–19 years	285,555	64	258,559	58.3
20–24 years	1,005,982	96.2	951,900	90
25–29 years	1,166,787	111.5	1,134,008	108.3
30–34 years	955,246	97.5	962,420	96.6
35–39 years	474,103	46.1	464,943	45.9
40–44 years	105,827	10	107,011	10.2
45–54 years[3]	7,889	0.7	7,744	0.7
Non-Hispanic White[4]				
Total[2]	2,212,552	59.6	2,161,669	58.7
10–14 years	1,053	0.2	967	0.2
15–19 years	159,579	25.7	143,984	23.5
15–17 years	39,975	11	35,433	10
18–19 years	119,604	46.2	108,551	42.6
20–24 years	490,773	79.2	464,645	74.9
25–29 years	657,658	107.1	648,473	105.8
30–34 years	565,026	99.7	574,479	99.9
35–39 years	273,174	44.4	264,044	44.1
40–44 years	60,452	9.1	60,572	9.2
45–54 years[3]	4,837	0.6	4,504	0.6
Non-Hispanic Black[4]				
Total[2]	609,584	68.9	589,139	66.6
10–14 years	1,705	1.1	1,572	1
15–19 years	98,448	56.7	88,142	51.5
15–17 years	31,560	31	27,441	27.4
18–19 years	66,888	93.5	60,701	85.6
20–24 years	194,122	125.9	187,754	119.4
25–29 years	153,210	105.9	147,549	102.5
30–34 years	98,909	73.9	100,697	73.6
35–39 years	50,003	36.1	49,693	36.4
40–44 years	12,314	8.9	12,752	9.2
45–54 years[3]	873	0.6	980	0.7
American Indian or Alaska Native Total[4,5]				
Total[2]	48,665	51.7	46,760	48.6
10–14 years	108	0.6	100	0.5
15–19 years	8,315	43.8	7,409	38.7
15–17 years	2,680	23.7	2,282	20.1
18–19 years	5,635	73.6	5,127	66.1
20–24 years	16,231	96.6	15,746	91
25–29 years	12,634	79.5	12,223	74.4
30–34 years	7,401	50.9	7,310	48.4
35–39 years	3,214	22.7	3,212	22.3
40–44 years	723	5.3	722	5.2
45–54 years[3]	39	0.3	38	0.3
Asian or Pacific Islander Total[4,5]				
Total[2]	251,089	61.3	246,915	59.2
10–14 years	76	0.1	50	0.1
15–19 years	7,053	12.6	6,263	10.9
15–17 years	2,028	6.3	1,685	5.1
18–19 years	5,025	20.9	4,578	18.7
20–24 years	29,436	46.4	27,738	42.7
25–29 years	70,539	94.6	68,379	91.5
30–34 years	85,317	115.1	85,304	113.6
35–39 years	48,100	63.8	48,095	62.8
40–44 years	9,863	14.9	10,315	15.1
45–54 years[3]	705	1.1	770	1.2
Hispanic[6]				
Total[2]	999,548	86.5	946,000	80.3
10–14 years	2,073	1	1,811	0.8
15–19 years	136,263	63.6	121,849	55.7
15–17 years	48,018	37.3	42,310	32.3
18–19 years	88,245	103.3	79,539	90.7
20–24 years	274,726	140.1	254,868	126.2
25–29 years	270,641	134.3	255,236	125.5
30–34 years	195,729	100.8	191,595	96.7
35–39 years	97,261	52.5	97,652	51.8
40–44 years	21,638	13.2	21,793	13
45–54 years[3]	1,217	0.8	1,196	0.8

[1] Includes births to White Hispanic and Black Hispanic women and births with origin not stated, not shown separately.
[2] Includes births to women of all ages, 10–54 years. The rate shown for all ages is the fertility rate, which is defined as the total number of births (regardless of the age of the mother) per 1,000 women aged 15–44 years.
[3] Includes births to women aged 45–54 years. The birth rate for these women is computed by relating the number of births to women aged 45–54 years to the number of births to women aged 45–49 years because most of the births in this group are to women aged 45–49 years.
[4] Race and Hispanic origin are reported separately on birth certificates.
[5] Includes persons of Hispanic origin according to the mother's reported race.
[6] Includes all persons of Hispanic origin of any race. Persons of Hispanic origin may be of any race.

Table A-4. Live Births by Age of Mother, Live-Birth Order, and Race and Hispanic Origin of Mother, Preliminary 2010

(Number.)

Live-birth order, race, and Hispanic origin of mother	All ages	Under 15 years	15–19 years	20–24 years	25–29 years	30–34 years	35–39 years	40–44 years	45–54 years
All Races and Origins[1]	4,000,279	4,500	367,752	951,900	1,134,008	962,420	464,943	107,011	7,744
1st child	1,604,181	4,375	298,160	472,391	420,183	277,963	105,097	23,937	2,075
2nd child	1,248,376	74	57,181	309,206	371,861	328,686	149,453	29,971	1,945
3rd child	654,769	7	8,392	118,836	204,848	194,903	104,573	21,892	1,317
4th child and over	461,280	2	1,158	43,964	128,631	153,525	101,547	30,133	2,319
Not stated	31,673	42	2,861	7,502	8,485	7,344	4,273	1,078	88
Non-Hispanic White[2]	2,161,669	967	143,984	464,645	648,473	574,479	264,044	60,572	4,504
1st child	914,420	953	122,180	252,422	272,912	183,263	66,181	15,298	1,310
2nd child	701,669	10	18,767	146,380	217,359	208,494	90,964	18,494	1,201
3rd child	331,812	-	2,184	49,070	101,903	108,221	57,807	11,866	760
4th child and over	202,496	1	213	14,451	53,353	71,472	47,338	14,477	1,190
Not stated	11,273	3	640	2,322	3,045	3,029	1,754	437	43
Non-Hispanic Black[2]	589,139	1,572	88,142	187,754	147,549	100,697	49,693	12,752	980
1st child	229,266	1,514	69,134	84,294	40,596	21,760	9,316	2,425	226
2nd child	164,237	25	14,627	59,520	44,934	28,724	13,130	3,041	235
3rd child	97,920	4	2,594	27,653	31,218	22,453	11,162	2,652	184
4th child and over	87,841	-	466	13,475	28,326	25,888	15,010	4,359	317
Not stated	9,875	29	1,321	2,811	2,474	1,872	1,075	275	18
American Indian or Alaska Native[2,3]	46,760	100	7,409	15,746	12,223	7,310	3,212	722	38
1st child	16,749	96	5,788	6,392	2,738	1,186	441	101	7
2nd child	12,526	2	1,312	5,319	3,437	1,685	632	131	8
3rd child	8,231	1	253	2,698	2,840	1,629	660	140	10
4th child and over	9,054	-	30	1,278	3,154	2,773	1,458	348	13
Not stated	200	1	26	59	54	37	21	2	-
Asian or Pacific Islander[2,3]	246,915	50	6,263	27,738	68,379	85,304	48,095	10,315	770
1st child	111,448	49	5,118	16,547	37,570	35,003	14,035	2,860	266
2nd child	87,071	1	946	7,690	20,099	34,285	20,124	3,702	224
3rd child	30,238	-	130	2,383	6,639	10,096	8,805	2,062	123
4th child and over	16,430	-	18	932	3,587	5,370	4,762	1,610	151
Not stated	1,727	-	51	186	484	550	369	81	6
Hispanic[4]	946,000	1,811	121,849	254,868	255,236	191,595	97,652	21,793	1,196
1st child	327,923	1,764	95,809	111,907	65,355	35,472	14,381	3,016	218
2nd child	280,511	36	21,615	90,190	85,563	54,616	23,881	4,372	237
3rd child	185,761	2	3,255	37,083	62,188	52,166	25,819	5,058	189
4th child and over	144,475	1	426	13,829	40,112	47,730	32,698	9,139	540
Not stated	7,330	8	744	1,858	2,017	1,610	873	208	12

- = Quantity zero.
[1]Includes births to White Hispanic and Black Hispanic women and births with origin not stated, not shown separately.
[2]Race and Hispanic origin are reported separately on birth certificates.
[3]Includes persons of Hispanic origin according to the mother's reported race.
[4]Persons of Hispanic origin may be of any race.

Table A-5. Birth Rates by Age of Mother, Live-Birth Order, and Race and Hispanic Origin of Mother, Preliminary 2010

(Rates per 1,000 women in specified age groups.)

Live-birth order and race and Hispanic origin of mother	15–44 years[1]	10–14 years	15–19 years	20–24 years	25–29 years	30–34 years	35–39 years	40–44 years	45–49 years[2]
All Races and Origins[3]	64.1	0.4	34.3	90.0	108.3	96.6	45.9	10.2	0.7
1st child	25.9	0.4	28.0	45.0	40.4	28.1	10.5	2.3	0.2
2nd child	20.2	0.0	5.4	29.5	35.8	33.2	14.9	2.9	0.2
3rd child	10.6	*	0.8	11.3	19.7	19.7	10.4	2.1	0.1
4th child and over	7.5	*	0.1	4.2	12.4	15.5	10.1	2.9	0.2
Non-Hispanic White[4]	58.7	0.2	23.5	74.9	105.8	99.9	44.1	9.2	0.6
1st child	25.0	0.2	20.1	40.9	44.7	32.1	11.2	2.3	0.2
2nd child	19.1	*	3.1	23.7	35.6	36.4	15.3	2.8	0.2
3rd child	9.1	*	0.4	8.0	16.7	18.9	9.7	1.8	0.1
4th child and over	5.5	*	0.0	2.3	8.8	12.5	8.0	2.2	0.2
Non-Hispanic Black[4]	66.6	1.0	51.5	119.4	102.5	73.6	36.4	9.2	0.7
1st child	26.4	1.0	41.0	54.5	28.7	16.2	7.0	1.8	0.2
2nd child	18.9	0.0	8.6	38.4	31.7	21.4	9.8	2.2	0.2
3rd child	11.2	*	1.5	17.8	22.0	16.7	8.3	2.0	0.1
4th child and over	10.1	*	0.3	8.7	20.0	19.3	11.2	3.2	0.2
American Indian or Alaska Native Total[4,5]	48.6	0.5	38.7	91.0	74.4	48.4	22.3	5.2	0.3
1st child	17.5	0.5	30.4	37.1	16.7	7.9	3.1	0.7	*
2nd child	13.1	*	6.9	30.8	21.0	11.2	4.4	0.9	*
3rd child	8.6	*	1.3	15.6	17.4	10.8	4.6	1.0	*
4th child and over	9.5	*	0.2	7.4	19.3	18.4	10.2	2.5	*
Asian or Pacific Islander Total[4,5]	59.2	0.1	10.9	42.7	91.5	113.6	62.8	15.1	1.2
1st child	26.9	0.1	9.0	25.6	50.6	46.9	18.5	4.2	0.4
2nd child	21.0	*	1.7	11.9	27.1	45.9	26.5	5.5	0.4
3rd child	7.3	*	0.2	3.7	8.9	13.5	11.6	3.0	0.2
4th child and over	4.0	*	*	1.4	4.8	7.2	6.3	2.4	0.2
Hispanic[6]	80.3	0.8	55.7	126.2	125.5	96.7	51.8	13.0	0.8
1st child	28.0	0.8	44.1	55.8	32.4	18.1	7.7	1.8	0.1
2nd child	24.0	0.0	9.9	45.0	42.4	27.8	12.8	2.6	0.2
3rd child	15.9	*	1.5	18.5	30.8	26.6	13.8	3.0	0.1
4th child and over	12.4	*	0.2	6.9	19.9	24.3	17.5	5.5	0.4

* = Figure does not meet standards of reliability or precision.
0.0 = Quantity more than zero but less than 0.05.
[1] The rate shown is the fertility rate, which is defined as the total number of births, regardless of age of mother, per 1,000 women aged 15–44 years.
[2] The birth rate for ages 45–49 years is computed by relating births to women aged 45–54 years to the number of births to women aged 45–49 years because most of the births in this group are to women aged 45–49 years.
[3] Includes births to White Hispanic and Black Hispanic women and births with origin not stated, not shown separately.
[4] Race and Hispanic origin are reported separately on birth certificates.
[5] Includes persons of Hispanic origin according to the mother's reported race
[6] Persons of Hispanic origin may be of any race.

Table A-6. Birth Rates for Women Under Age 20 Years, by Age and Race and Hispanic Origin of Mother, Selected Years, 1991–Preliminary 2010

(Rates per 1,000 women in specified group.)

Age, race, and Hispanic origin of mother	Year						Percent change			
	1991	2005	2007	2008	2009	2010 Preliminary	1991–2010	2005–2007	2007–2010	2009–2010
10–14 Years										
All races and origins[1]	1.4	0.6	0.6	0.6	0.5	0.4	-71	†	-33	-20
Non-Hispanic White[2]	0.5	0.2	0.2	0.2	0.2	0.2	-60	†	†	†
Non-Hispanic Black[2]	4.9	1.6	1.4	1.4	1.1	1.0	-80	-13	-29	-9
American Indian or Alaska Native total[2,3]	1.6	0.8	0.7	0.7	0.6	0.5	-69	†	-29	†
Asian or Pacific Islander total[2,3]	0.8	0.2	0.2	0.2	0.1	0.1	-88	†	-50	†
Hispanic[4]	2.4	1.3	1.2	1.1	1.0	0.8	-67	-8	-33	-20
15–19 Years										
All races and origins[1]	61.8	39.7	41.5	40.2	37.9	34.3	-44	5	-17	-9
Non-Hispanic White[2]	43.4	26.0	27.2	26.7	25.7	23.5	-46	5	-14	-9
Non-Hispanic Black[2]	118.2	59.4	62.0	60.4	56.7	51.5	-56	4	-17	-9
American Indian or Alaska Native total[2,3]	84.1	46.0	49.4	47.4	43.8	38.7	-54	7	-22	-12
Asian or Pacific Islander total[2,3]	27.3	15.4	14.8	13.8	12.6	10.9	-60	-4	-26	-13
Hispanic[4]	104.6	76.5	75.3	70.3	63.6	55.7	-47	-2	-26	-12
15–17 Years										
All races and origins[1]	38.6	21.1	21.7	21.1	19.6	17.3	-55	3	-20	-12
Non-Hispanic White[2]	23.6	11.5	11.9	11.6	11.0	10.0	-58	3	-16	-9
Non-Hispanic Black[2]	86.1	34.1	34.6	33.6	31.0	27.4	-68	†	-21	-12
American Indian or Alaska Native total[2,3]	51.9	26.3	26.2	25.9	23.7	20.1	-61	†	-23	-15
Asian or Pacific Islander total[2,3]	16.3	7.7	7.4	7.0	6.3	5.1	-69	†	-31	-19
Hispanic[4]	69.2	45.8	44.4	42.2	37.3	32.3	-53	-3	-27	-13
18–19 Years										
All races and origins[1]	94.0	68.4	71.7	68.2	64.0	58.3	-38	5	-19	-9
Non-Hispanic White[2]	70.6	48.0	50.4	48.6	46.2	42.6	-40	5	-15	-8
Non-Hispanic Black[2]	162.2	100.2	105.2	100.0	93.5	85.6	-47	5	-19	-8
American Indian or Alaska Native total[2,3]	134.2	78.1	86.4	80.4	73.6	66.1	-51	11	-23	-10
Asian or Pacific Islander total[2,3]	42.2	26.4	24.9	22.9	20.9	18.7	-56	-6	-25	-11
Hispanic[4]	155.5	124.4	124.7	114.0	103.3	90.7	-42	†	-27	-12

† = Difference not statistically significant.
[1]Includes births to White Hispanic and Black Hispanic women and births with origin not stated, not shown separately.
[2]Race and Hispanic origin are reported separately on birth certificates.
[3]Includes persons of Hispanic origin according to the mother's reported race.
[4]Persons of Hispanic origin may be of any race.

Table A-7. Births to Mothers Under 20 Years of Age by State and Territory, Final 2009 and Preliminary 2010

(Percent.)

Area	2009	2010
United States[1]	10.0	9.3
Alabama	13.4	12.4
Alaska	9.8	8.4
Arizona	11.9	10.8
Arkansas	14.6	13.8
California	9.2	8.5
Colorado	9.1	8.3
Connecticut	6.8	5.9
Delaware	9.5	8.7
District of Columbia	11.7	10.5
Florida	10.1	9.0
Georgia	11.7	10.9
Hawaii	8.3	7.1
Idaho	8.6	8.1
Illinois	9.6	9.1
Indiana	11.1	10.4
Iowa	8.7	7.9
Kansas	10.3	9.6
Kentucky	12.7	12.1
Louisiana	13.1	12.5
Maine	7.8	7.1
Maryland	8.3	7.4
Massachusetts	6.0	5.4
Michigan	10.1	9.6
Minnesota	6.3	5.9
Mississippi	16.5	15.5
Missouri	10.9	10.1
Montana	10.3	9.5
Nebraska	8.3	7.6
Nevada	10.5	9.7
New Hampshire	5.7	5.6
New Jersey	5.9	5.4
New Mexico	15.5	14.1
New York	6.7	6.3
North Carolina	11.3	10.2
North Dakota	7.4	7.3
Ohio	10.8	10.0
Oklahoma	13.8	12.4
Oregon	8.7	7.7
Pennsylvania	8.9	8.5
Rhode Island	9.3	8.0
South Carolina	12.8	11.9
South Dakota	9.2	8.3
Tennessee	12.8	11.8
Texas	13.3	12.6
Utah	6.3	5.9
Vermont	6.5	6.5
Virginia	7.9	7.2
Washington	7.8	7.0
West Virginia	13.5	12.9
Wisconsin	8.3	7.5
Wyoming	10.4	9.6
Puerto Rico	18.2	17.2
Virgin Islands	13.1	—
Guam	11.6	12.3
American Samoa	9.7	9.8
Northern Marianas	9.5	—

— = Data not available.
[1] Excludes data for the territories.

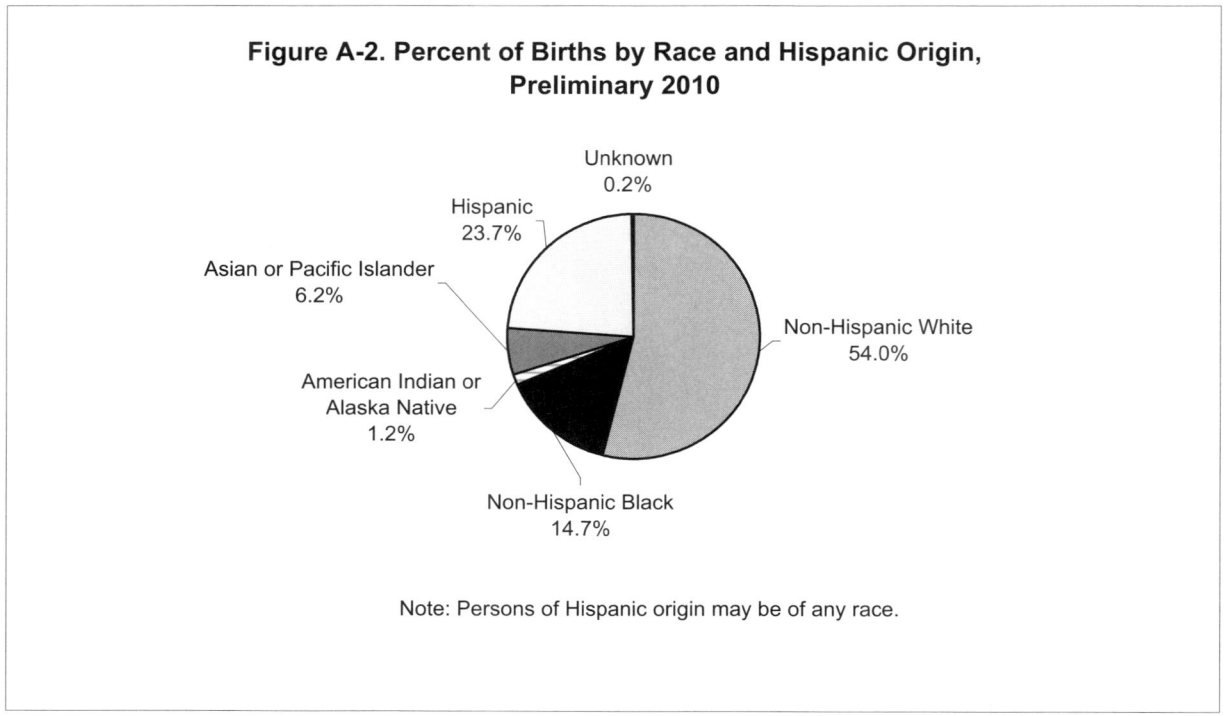

Figure A-2. Percent of Births by Race and Hispanic Origin, Preliminary 2010

Note: Persons of Hispanic origin may be of any race.

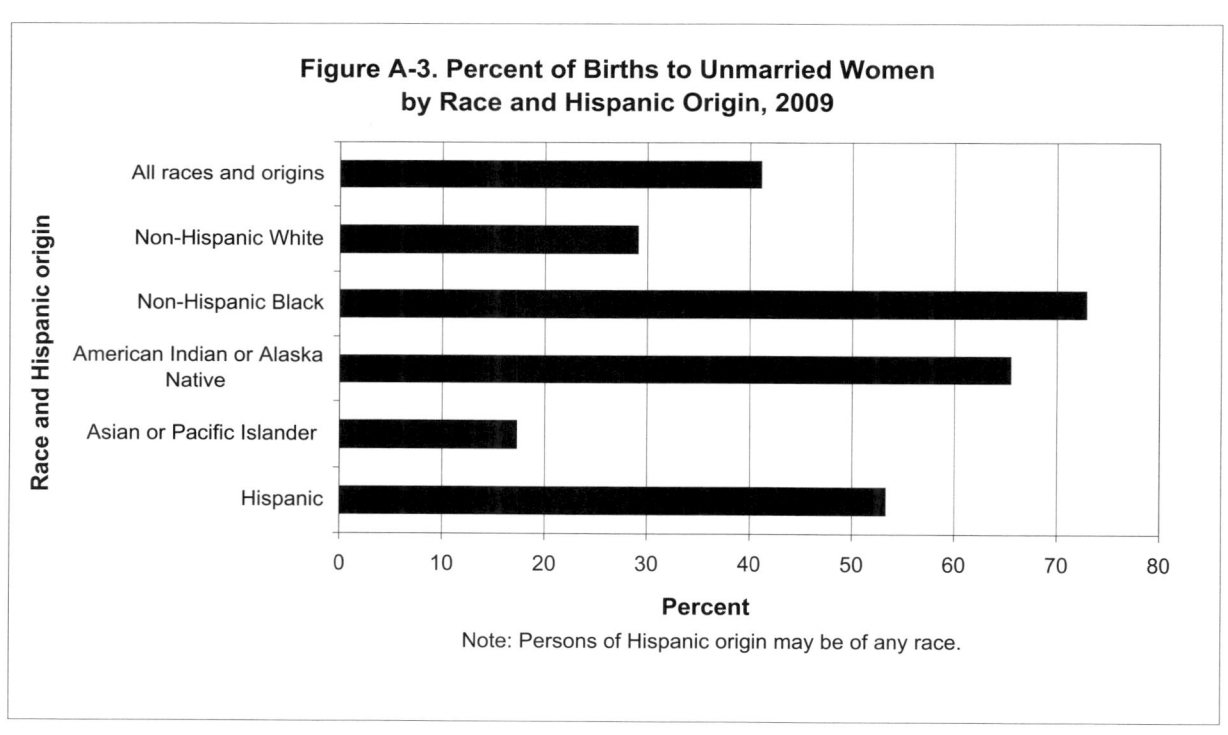

Figure A-3. Percent of Births to Unmarried Women by Race and Hispanic Origin, 2009

Note: Persons of Hispanic origin may be of any race.

Table A-8. Number and Percentage of Births to Unmarried Women, by Age, Final 2009 and Preliminary 2010

(Number, percent.)

Age of mother	Number		Percent	
	2009	2010	2009	2010
All Ages	1,693,658	1,633,785	41.0	40.8
Under 20 years	362,454	328,389	87.4	88.2
Under 15 years	4,980	4,467	99.0	99.3
15–19 years	357,474	323,922	87.2	88.1
15–17 years	117,094	103,776	94.2	95.0
18–19 years	240,380	220,146	84.2	85.1
20–24 years	624,293	600,971	62.1	63.1
25–29 years	394,556	384,955	33.8	33.9
30–34 years	198,168	203,527	20.7	21.1
35–39 years	89,854	91,085	19.0	19.6
40–54 years	24,333	24,858	21.4	21.7

Table A-9. Live Births by Race and Hispanic Origin of Mother, and Birth and Fertility Rates by State, Preliminary 2010

(Birth rates are total births per 1,000, fertility rates are total births per 1,000 women ages 15–44 years.)

Area	All races and origins[1]	Non-Hispanic White[2]	Non-Hispanic Black[2]	American Indian or Alaskan Native[2,3]	Asian or Pacific Islander[2,3]	Hispanic[4]	Birth rate for all races	Fertility rate for all races
UNITED STATES[5]	4,000,279	2,161,669	589,139	46,760	246,915	946,000	13.0	64.1
Alabama	60,053	35,823	18,200	205	978	4,840	12.6	62.5
Alaska	11,466	6,261	409	2,899	1,053	660	16.1	80.1
Arizona	88,905	39,442	4,081	6,135	3,359	36,113	13.9	70.4
Arkansas	38,539	26,112	7,354	285	636	4,047	13.2	67.7
California	509,968	145,835	30,327	3,609	68,915	257,511	13.7	64.7
Colorado	66,344	40,155	3,201	713	2,575	19,457	13.2	64.7
Connecticut	39,441	23,239	4,856	298	2,478	8,522	11.0	57.1
Delaware	11,342	6,326	3,047	14	521	1,427	12.6	63.3
District of Columbia	9,167	2,491	4,874	18	513	1,359	15.2	56.5
Florida	214,552	97,950	49,486	380	7,080	59,596	11.4	60.3
Georgia	133,915	59,682	44,819	335	5,780	21,215	13.8	64.6
Hawaii	18,985	4,756	508	71	12,439	2,967	14.0	72.4
Idaho	23,194	18,612	159	466	444	3,638	14.8	75.7
Illinois	165,194	89,158	28,264	258	9,652	37,359	12.9	62.8
Indiana	83,939	64,303	9,953	127	1,960	7,568	12.9	65.2
Iowa	38,715	32,510	1,840	274	1,118	3,091	12.7	67.1
Kansas	40,640	29,545	3,044	359	1,329	6,428	14.2	73.3
Kentucky	55,790	46,615	5,232	102	1,041	2,858	12.9	65.3
Louisiana	62,383	32,901	24,162	490	1,288	3,586	13.8	67.2
Maine	12,967	12,024	377	112	226	210	9.8	53.6
Maryland	73,776	33,559	24,422	199	5,586	10,260	12.8	61.8
Massachusetts	72,757	48,843	7,048	142	5,950	10,602	11.1	53.9
Michigan	114,523	79,977	22,131	845	3,861	7,807	11.6	59.7
Minnesota	68,605	50,091	6,521	1,583	5,131	5,139	12.9	65.6
Mississippi	40,033	20,342	17,509	269	452	1,426	13.5	66.3
Missouri	76,756	58,467	11,381	407	1,970	4,334	12.8	65.2
Montana	12,060	9,952	64	1,430	139	433	12.2	67.1
Nebraska	25,916	19,203	1,723	553	753	3,943	14.2	73.0
Nevada	35,862	15,703	3,536	436	2,948	13,387	13.3	65.2
New Hampshire	12,867	11,506	224	23	531	528	9.8	51.4
New Jersey	109,249	52,137	16,568	242	11,897	28,218	12.4	62.8
New Mexico	27,769	7,846	486	3,614	540	15,476	13.5	69.7
New York	241,711	116,253	39,115	784	23,136	58,192	12.5	59.7
North Carolina	122,267	68,654	28,982	1,821	4,401	18,716	12.8	62.7
North Dakota	9,100	7,437	193	967	175	304	13.5	70.5
Ohio	139,137	105,366	22,957	285	3,593	6,324	12.1	62.2
Oklahoma	53,234	34,100	4,803	6,332	1,311	6,931	14.2	72.3
Oregon	45,535	31,674	1,141	895	2,744	9,257	11.9	60.4
Pennsylvania	142,325	100,405	20,900	410	6,213	13,669	11.2	58.3
Rhode Island	11,149	6,982	952	164	554	2,433	10.6	51.9
South Carolina	58,293	33,155	18,665	207	1,198	4,945	12.6	62.8
South Dakota	11,809	9,003	260	1,935	152	509	14.5	77.5
Tennessee	79,485	53,912	16,628	218	1,845	7,139	12.5	62.4
Texas	386,096	134,906	44,559	1,179	16,818	189,120	15.4	72.5
Utah	52,232	41,464	585	707	1,634	8,051	18.9	86.7
Vermont	6,223	5,896	112	18	110	77	9.9	52.6
Virginia	102,972	59,705	21,700	173	7,639	12,415	12.9	62.3
Washington	86,530	55,077	4,087	2,217	9,079	16,219	12.9	63.8
West Virginia	20,471	19,234	745	21	189	210	11.0	59.9
Wisconsin	68,483	51,034	6,862	1,238	2,892	6,545	12.0	62.4
Wyoming	7,555	6,047	86	296	88	939	13.4	70.9
Puerto Rico	42,159	1,142	143	—	—	40,846	11.3	54.3
Virgin Islands	—	—	—	—	—	—	—	—
Guam	3,416	208	35	10	3,122	47	18.9	87.1
American Samoa	1,234	—	-	-	1,233	—	18.6	81.8
Northern Marianas	—	—	—	—	—	—	—	—

— = Data not available.
- = Quantity zero.
[1]Includes births to White Hispanic and Black Hispanic women and births with origin not stated, not shown separately.
[2]Race and Hispanic origin are reported separately on birth certificates.
[3]Includes persons of Hispanic origin according to the mother's reported race.
[4]Persons of Hispanic origin may be of any race.
[5]Excludes data for the territories.

Table A-10. Selected Characteristics of Births, by Race and Hispanic Origin of Mother, Final 2009 and Preliminary 2010

(Number, rate.)

Race and Hispanic origin of mother	Number		Cesarean rate[1]		Preterm				Low birthweight			
					Total[2]		Late[3]		Total[4]		Very Low birthweight[5]	
	2009	2010	2009	2010	2009	2010	2009	2010	2009	2010	2009	2010
All Races and Origins[6]	4,130,665	4,000,279	32.9	32.8	12.18	11.99	8.66	8.49	8.16	8.15	1.45	1.45
Non-Hispanic White[7]	2,212,552	2,161,669	32.8	32.6	10.92	10.78	8.00	7.84	7.19	7.14	1.16	1.16
Non-Hispanic Black[7]	609,584	589,139	35.4	35.5	17.47	17.15	11.24	10.99	13.61	13.53	3.06	3.06
American Indian or Alaska Native total[7,8]	48,665	46,760	28.5	28.4	13.45	13.60	9.44	9.62	7.28	7.61	1.31	1.28
Asian or Pacific Islander total[7,8]	251,089	246,915	33.1	33.1	10.85	10.69	8.06	7.84	8.27	8.49	1.13	1.17
Hispanic[9]	999,548	946,000	31.6	31.8	11.97	11.79	8.64	8.52	6.94	6.97	1.19	1.19

[1]All births by cesarean delivery per 100 live births.
[2]Less than 37 completed weeks of gestation.
[3]Born between 34 and 36 completed weeks of gestation.
[4]Less than 2,500 grams (5 lb 8 oz).
[5]Less than 1,500 grams (3 lb 4 oz).
[6]Includes births to White Hispanic and Black Hispanic women and births with origin not stated, not shown separately.
[7]Race and Hispanic origin are reported separately on birth certificates.
[8]Includes persons of Hispanic origin according to the mother's reported race.
[9]Persons of Hispanic origin may be of any race.

Table A-11. Low Birthweight Births by State and Territory, Final 2009 and Preliminary 2010

(Percent.)

Area	2009	2010
United States[1]	8.2	8.1
Alabama	10.3	10.3
Alaska	5.9	5.7
Arizona	7.1	7.1
Arkansas	8.9	8.8
California	6.8	6.8
Colorado	8.8	8.8
Connecticut	8.0	8.0
Delaware	8.6	8.9
District of Columbia	10.3	10.2
Florida	8.7	8.7
Georgia	9.4	9.7
Hawaii	8.4	8.4
Idaho	6.5	6.8
Illinois	8.4	8.3
Indiana	8.3	8.0
Iowa	6.7	7.0
Kansas	7.3	7.1
Kentucky	8.9	9.0
Louisiana	10.6	10.7
Maine	6.3	6.3
Maryland	9.1	8.8
Massachusetts	7.8	7.7
Michigan	8.4	8.4
Minnesota	6.5	6.4
Mississippi	12.2	12.1
Missouri	8.1	8.2
Montana	7.1	7.5
Nebraska	7.1	7.1
Nevada	8.1	8.3
New Hampshire	6.9	6.8
New Jersey	8.3	8.3
New Mexico	8.3	8.7
New York	8.2	8.2
North Carolina	9.0	9.1
North Dakota	6.4	6.7
Ohio	8.6	8.6
Oklahoma	8.4	8.4
Oregon	6.3	6.3
Pennsylvania	8.3	8.3
Rhode Island	8.0	7.7
South Carolina	10.0	9.9
South Dakota	5.8	6.8
Tennessee	9.2	9.0
Texas	8.5	8.4
Utah	7.0	7.0
Vermont	6.7	6.1
Virginia	8.4	8.2
Washington	6.3	6.3
West Virginia	9.2	9.2
Wisconsin	7.1	7.0
Wyoming	8.4	9.0
Puerto Rico	12.4	12.6
Virgin Islands	9.5	—
Guam	7.7	8.6
American Samoa	2.7	3.7
Northern Marianas	8.6	—

— = Data not available.
[1]Excludes data for the territories.

Table A-12. Percentage of Preterm Births, Selected Years, 1990–2010

(Percent.)

Year	Total preterm[1]	Late preterm[2]	Total	Less than 34 weeks	
				32–33 weeks	Less than 32 weeks
1990	10.61	7.30	3.32	1.40	1.92
2000	11.64	8.22	3.42	1.49	1.93
2005	12.73	9.09	3.63	1.60	2.03
2006	12.80	9.14	3.66	1.62	2.04
2007	12.68	9.04	3.64	1.60	2.04
2008	12.33	8.77	3.56	1.57	1.99
2009	12.18	8.66	3.51	1.55	1.97
Preliminary 2010	11.99	8.49	3.50	1.53	1.97

[1] Preterm is less than 37 completed weeks of gestation.
[2] Late preterm is 34–36 completed weeks of gestation.

Table A-13. Preterm and Late Term Births by State and Territory, Final 2009 and Preliminary 2010

(Percent.)

Area	2009		2010	
	Late preterm[2]	Preterm[3]	Late preterm[2]	Preterm[3]
United States[1]	8.7	12.2	8.5	12.0
Alabama	10.7	15.6	10.8	15.6
Alaska	8.1	11.0	7.4	9.7
Arizona	9.5	12.7	9.0	12.1
Arkansas	9.2	13.1	9.3	12.7
California	7.5	10.3	7.2	9.9
Colorado	8.1	11.3	7.7	10.8
Connecticut	7.2	10.2	7.1	10.3
Delaware	8.5	12.5	8.6	12.8
District of Columbia	9.3	14.2	8.5	13.6
Florida	9.6	13.5	9.3	13.3
Georgia	9.9	13.8	9.8	13.8
Hawaii	8.9	12.6	8.7	12.2
Idaho	7.4	10.1	7.6	10.3
Illinois	8.7	12.4	8.5	12.2
Indiana	8.4	11.9	8.4	11.7
Iowa	8.2	11.3	8.2	11.6
Kansas	8.2	11.2	7.6	10.6
Kentucky	9.7	13.6	9.8	13.7
Louisiana	10.2	14.7	10.5	15.1
Maine	7.0	9.9	6.9	9.7
Maryland	8.8	12.7	8.8	12.7
Massachusetts	7.8	10.9	7.6	10.7
Michigan	8.6	12.4	8.5	12.2
Minnesota	7.3	10.1	7.5	10.2
Mississippi	12.6	18.0	12.4	17.6
Missouri	8.7	12.2	8.6	12.1
Montana	7.8	10.9	8.6	12.0
Nebraska	8.4	11.5	8.2	11.4
Nevada	10.0	13.8	10.0	13.9
New Hampshire	7.2	9.9	6.7	9.4
New Jersey	8.2	12.0	7.9	11.7
New Mexico	8.8	12.3	8.7	11.9
New York	8.6	12.2	8.0	11.5
North Carolina	8.9	13.0	8.7	12.7
North Dakota	7.6	10.6	7.8	10.9
Ohio	8.4	12.3	8.4	12.3
Oklahoma	10.0	13.8	10.0	13.9
Oregon	7.3	9.8	7.3	9.9
Pennsylvania	8.0	11.5	7.9	11.4
Rhode Island	7.6	11.4	7.5	10.8
South Carolina	10.0	14.5	9.7	14.2
South Dakota	8.1	10.9	8.0	11.4
Tennessee	9.2	13.0	9.3	12.9
Texas	9.5	13.1	9.5	13.1
Utah	8.7	11.3	8.1	10.9
Vermont	6.6	9.3	5.7	8.4
Virginia	8.0	11.4	8.1	11.6
Washington	7.5	10.3	7.4	10.2
West Virginia	9.6	12.9	8.9	12.1
Wisconsin	7.8	10.9	7.6	10.8
Wyoming	8.1	11.2	7.9	11.0
Puerto Rico	13.5	17.7	12.8	16.7
Virgin Islands	9.7	13.2	—	—
Guam	11.1	16.4	—	—
American Samoa	—	—	—	—
Northern Marianas	12.0	15.6	—	—

* = Figure does not meet standards of reliability or precision.
— = Data not available.
[1] Excludes data for the territories.
[2] Births at 34–36 completed weeks of gestation.
[3] Births of less than 37 completed weeks of gestation.

Table A-14 Births by Cesarean Delivery by State and Territory, Final 2009 and Preliminary 2010

(Percent.)

Area	2009	2010
United States[1]	32.9	32.8
Alabama	35.6	35.5
Alaska	23.8	22.6
Arizona	27.4	27.2
Arkansas	34.6	35.1
California	33.0	33.0
Colorado	26.4	25.9
Connecticut	35.6	35.4
Delaware	35.7	33.8
District of Columbia	32.0	33.0
Florida	38.1	37.8
Georgia	33.6	34.0
Hawaii	27.0	27.4
Idaho	24.5	24.8
Illinois	31.5	31.2
Indiana	30.5	30.3
Iowa	30.3	30.3
Kansas	30.1	30.5
Kentucky	35.9	35.4
Louisiana	39.6	39.7
Maine	29.6	29.9
Maryland	33.5	34.5
Massachusetts	33.4	33.1
Michigan	32.1	32.6
Minnesota	27.4	27.3
Mississippi	37.8	37.2
Missouri	31.7	31.9
Montana	29.6	30.3
Nebraska	31.7	31.1
Nevada	33.7	34.8
New Hampshire	30.8	30.4
New Jersey	39.4	38.7
New Mexico	22.8	22.8
New York	34.9	34.6
North Carolina	31.2	31.0
North Dakota	29.3	27.7
Ohio	31.1	30.8
Oklahoma	34.6	34.7
Oregon	29.4	29.4
Pennsylvania	31.8	31.4
Rhode Island	32.8	33.1
South Carolina	35.3	35.0
South Dakota	26.3	26.6
Tennessee	33.8	34.2
Texas	35.3	35.1
Utah	22.9	23.1
Vermont	27.8	27.5
Virginia	34.3	34.5
Washington	29.2	29.5
West Virginia	36.0	36.3
Wisconsin	25.8	26.0
Wyoming	28.1	27.9
Puerto Rico	48.1	46.3
Virgin Islands	27.1	—
Guam	26.3	24.2
American Samoa	—	—
Northern Marianas	19.2	—

* = Figure does not meet standards of reliability or precision.
— = Data not available.
[1] Excludes data for the territories.

Table A-15. Birth Rates, by Age and Race and Hispanic Origin of Mother, Final 2000–2009 and Preliminary 2010

(Percent.)

State	Total fertility rate	10–14 Years	15–19 years Total	15–17 years	18–19 years	20–24 Years	25–29 Years	30–34 Years	35–39 Years	40–44 Years	45–49 Years[1]
All Races and Origins[2]											
2000	2056.0	0.9	47.7	26.9	78.1	109.7	113.5	91.2	39.7	8.0	0.5
2001	2030.5	0.8	45.0	24.5	75.5	105.6	113.8	91.8	40.5	8.1	0.5
2002	2020.5	0.7	42.6	23.1	72.2	103.1	114.7	92.6	41.6	8.3	0.5
2003	2047.5	0.6	41.1	22.2	69.6	102.3	116.7	95.7	43.9	8.7	0.5
2004	2051.5	0.6	40.5	21.8	68.7	101.5	116.5	96.2	45.5	9.0	0.5
2005	2057.0	0.6	39.7	21.1	68.4	101.8	116.5	96.7	46.4	9.1	0.6
2006	2108.0	0.6	41.1	21.6	71.2	105.5	118.0	98.9	47.5	9.4	0.6
2007	2120.0	0.6	41.5	21.7	71.7	105.4	118.1	100.6	47.6	9.6	0.6
2008	2072.0	0.6	40.2	21.1	68.2	101.8	115.0	99.4	46.8	9.9	0.7
2009	2002.0	0.5	37.9	19.6	64.0	96.2	111.5	97.5	46.1	10.0	0.7
2010	1932.0	0.4	34.3	17.3	58.3	90.0	108.3	96.6	45.9	10.2	0.7
Non-Hispanic White[3]											
2000	1866.0	0.3	32.6	15.8	57.5	91.2	109.4	93.2	38.8	7.3	0.4
2001	1846.0	0.3	30.3	14.0	54.7	87.0	109.6	94.3	39.8	7.5	0.4
2002	1839.5	0.2	28.6	13.1	52.0	84.7	110.3	95.0	40.9	7.7	0.5
2003	1874.5	0.2	27.4	12.4	50.0	84.1	112.7	98.4	43.5	8.1	0.5
2004	1871.0	0.2	26.7	12.0	48.6	83.0	112.1	98.3	45.1	8.3	0.5
2005	1869.0	0.2	26.0	11.5	48.0	82.7	111.7	98.4	46.0	8.3	0.5
2006	1900.5	0.2	26.7	11.8	49.4	85.1	112.2	100.0	46.8	8.5	0.6
2007	1908.0	0.2	27.2	11.9	50.4	85.1	112.0	101.5	46.3	8.7	0.6
2008	1874.5	0.2	26.7	11.6	48.6	82.8	109.7	100.8	45.2	8.9	0.6
2009	1830.0	0.2	25.7	11.0	46.2	79.2	107.1	99.7	44.4	9.1	0.6
2010	1791.0	0.2	23.5	10.0	42.6	74.9	105.8	99.9	44.1	9.2	0.6
Non-Hispanic Black[3]											
2000	2178.5	2.4	79.2	50.1	121.9	145.4	102.8	66.5	31.8	7.2	0.4
2001	2106.5	2.1	73.1	44.8	115.8	137.3	102.7	66.4	32.0	7.3	0.4
2002	2053.0	1.9	67.7	40.6	109.5	131.4	103.1	66.5	32.1	7.5	0.4
2003	2036.5	1.6	63.7	38.2	103.4	128.8	103.9	67.7	33.4	7.7	0.5
2004	2029.0	1.6	61.8	36.4	101.5	127.8	104.9	67.8	33.6	7.8	0.5
2005	2030.5	1.6	59.4	34.1	100.2	127.9	105.5	68.8	34.2	8.2	0.5
2006	2128.5	1.5	61.9	35.2	105.0	134.4	110.0	73.2	35.9	8.3	0.5
2007	2142.0	1.4	62.0	34.6	105.2	134.5	110.5	74.7	36.2	8.5	0.6
2008	2115.0	1.4	60.4	33.6	100.0	131.5	108.8	75.3	36.3	8.7	0.6
2009	2045.5	1.1	56.7	31.0	93.5	125.9	105.9	73.9	36.1	8.9	0.6
2010	1971.5	1.0	51.5	27.4	85.6	119.4	102.5	73.6	36.4	9.2	0.7
American Indian or Alaska Native[3,4]											
2000	1772.5	1.1	58.3	34.1	97.1	117.2	91.8	55.5	24.6	5.7	0.3
2001	1717.0	0.9	54.7	30.3	93.1	114.1	89.4	54.3	24.1	5.6	0.3
2002	1678.5	0.8	51.0	28.9	85.6	110.9	89.1	53.8	24.1	5.7	0.3
2003	1643.5	0.9	49.2	28.0	82.3	107.2	89.5	52.9	23.4	5.2	0.4
2004	1613.5	0.8	47.4	26.7	80.1	105.6	87.2	52.0	23.9	5.6	0.2
2005	1586.5	0.8	46.0	26.3	78.1	103.0	86.6	51.9	23.3	5.4	0.3
2006	1628.0	0.7	47.0	26.0	81.0	106.9	89.2	52.1	24.0	5.4	0.3
2007	1625.5	0.7	49.4	26.2	86.4	106.0	86.4	52.7	24.3	5.3	0.3
2008	1573.5	0.7	47.4	25.9	80.4	103.0	83.4	51.4	23.2	5.3	0.3
2009	1498.5	0.6	43.8	23.7	73.6	96.6	79.5	50.9	22.7	5.3	0.3
2010	1404.0	0.5	38.7	20.1	66.1	91.0	74.4	48.4	22.3	5.2	0.3
Asian or Pacific Islander[3,4]											
2000	1892.0	0.3	20.5	11.6	32.6	60.3	108.4	116.5	59.0	12.6	0.8
2001	1785.5	0.2	19.3	10.1	31.9	56.0	102.4	109.9	56.2	12.2	0.9
2002	1798.5	0.3	17.7	8.8	29.9	55.5	102.4	112.5	57.8	12.6	0.9
2003	1819.0	0.2	16.4	8.5	27.3	54.3	102.7	115.9	60.0	13.4	0.9
2004	1825.0	0.2	16.0	8.4	26.6	53.3	100.4	118.3	62.2	13.6	1.0
2005	1784.5	0.2	15.4	7.7	26.4	52.9	96.6	115.3	61.8	13.7	1.0
2006	1803.0	0.1	15.3	8.2	25.4	53.8	95.7	117.3	63.4	14.0	1.0
2007	1850.0	0.2	14.8	7.4	24.9	53.1	99.2	121.6	65.8	14.2	1.1
2008	1797.0	0.2	13.8	7.0	22.9	50.4	96.6	117.6	64.9	14.7	1.2
2009	1743.0	0.1	12.6	6.3	20.9	46.4	94.6	115.1	63.8	14.9	1.1
2010	1689.5	0.1	10.9	5.1	18.7	42.7	91.5	113.6	62.8	15.1	1.2

Table A-15. Birth Rates, by Age and Race and Hispanic Origin of Mother, Final 2000–2009 and Preliminary 2010—Continued

(Percent.)

State	Total fertility rate	10–14 Years	15–19 years			20–24 Years	25–29 Years	30–34 Years	35–39 Years	40–44 Years	45–49 Years[1]
			Total	15–17 years	18–19 years						
Hispanic[5]											
2000	2730.0	1.7	87.3	55.5	132.6	161.3	139.9	97.1	46.6	11.5	0.6
2001	2726.0	1.5	84.4	51.9	131.3	160.5	140.8	97.8	47.9	11.6	0.7
2002	2711.0	1.4	80.6	49.3	127.1	159.0	141.6	98.3	48.8	11.7	0.8
2003	2736.0	1.3	78.4	47.6	124.8	159.1	144.0	101.5	50.1	12.1	0.7
2004	2759.0	1.2	78.1	47.3	124.8	159.2	144.7	103.4	52.2	12.3	0.7
2005	2792.0	1.3	76.5	45.8	124.4	161.1	147.0	105.6	53.3	12.8	0.8
2006	2856.0	1.2	77.4	45.1	128.7	166.7	149.9	107.5	54.6	13.1	0.8
2007	2840.0	1.2	75.3	44.4	124.7	164.6	149.5	108.5	55.0	13.1	0.8
2008	2706.0	1.1	70.3	42.2	114.0	154.1	142.3	105.3	54.0	13.3	0.8
2009	2531.5	1.0	63.6	37.3	103.3	140.1	134.3	100.8	52.5	13.2	0.8
2010	2352.5	0.8	55.7	32.3	90.7	126.2	125.5	96.7	51.8	13.0	0.8

[1] Rates are computed by relating births to women aged 45 years and over to women aged 45–49.
[2] Includes births to White Hispanic and Black Hispanic women and births with origin not stated.
[3] Race and Hispanic origin are reported separately on birth certificates.
[4] Includes persons of Hispanic origin according to the mother's reported race.
[5] Persons of Hispanic origin may be of any race.

Table A-16. Birth Rates by Live-Birth Order and by Race and Hispanic Origin of Mother, 2000–2009 and Preliminary 2010

(Rates are live births per 1,000 women age 15–44 years.)

Year, race, and Hispanic origin of mother	Fertility rate	Live-birth order			
		1st child	2nd child	3rd child	4th child and over
All Races and Origins[1]					
2000	65.9	26.5	21.4	11.0	7.0
2001	65.1	25.9	21.3	11.0	7.0
2002	65.0	25.8	21.2	10.9	7.0
2003	66.1	26.5	21.4	11.1	7.1
2004	66.4	26.4	21.4	11.2	7.3
2005	66.7	26.5	21.5	11.3	7.4
2006	68.6	27.4	21.9	11.6	7.7
2007	69.3	27.8	22.0	11.7	7.8
2008	68.1	27.5	21.5	11.4	7.8
2009	66.2	26.8	20.8	11.0	7.6
2010	64.1	25.9	20.2	10.6	7.5
Non-Hispanic White[2]					
2000	58.5	24.2	19.8	9.4	5.1
2001	57.7	23.6	19.7	9.4	5.1
2002	57.6	23.6	19.6	9.3	5.1
2003	58.9	24.5	19.8	9.4	5.2
2004	58.9	24.4	19.8	9.5	5.3
2005	59.0	24.4	19.8	9.5	5.3
2006	60.3	25.1	20.0	9.6	5.5
2007	61.0	25.6	20.1	9.7	5.6
2008	60.5	25.5	19.8	9.5	5.6
2009	59.6	25.3	19.5	9.2	5.6
2010	58.7	25.0	19.1	9.1	5.5
Non-Hispanic Black[2]					
2000	71.4	26.7	21.2	12.8	10.8
2001	69.1	25.9	20.4	12.4	10.5
2002	67.5	25.4	19.7	12.1	10.4
2003	67.1	25.4	19.6	11.9	10.3
2004	67.1	25.5	19.4	11.9	10.3
2005	67.2	25.8	19.3	11.8	10.3
2006	70.7	27.5	20.3	12.3	10.6
2007	71.4	27.9	20.4	12.3	10.8
2008	70.8	28.1	20.0	12.1	10.7
2009	68.9	27.3	19.4	11.7	10.5
2010	66.6	26.4	18.9	11.2	10.1
American Indian or Alaska Native[2,3]					
2000	58.7	20.6	16.5	10.4	11.2
2001	57.0	20.0	15.9	10.3	10.7
2002	55.8	19.6	15.6	10.0	10.6
2003	55.0	19.5	15.1	9.9	10.4
2004	54.3	19.0	15.0	9.8	10.6
2005	53.6	18.8	14.5	9.8	10.5
2006	55.4	19.5	15.1	10.2	10.6
2007	55.6	19.9	15.1	10.0	10.6
2008	54.1	19.4	14.7	9.6	10.4
2009	51.7	18.7	13.9	9.2	10.0
2010	48.6	17.5	13.1	8.6	9.5
Asian or Pacific Islander[2,3]					
2000	65.8	30.6	22.4	8.1	4.6
2001	62.5	29.4	21.2	7.7	4.3
2002	63.4	29.8	21.8	7.7	4.1
2003	64.2	30.2	22.2	7.7	4.1
2004	64.5	29.9	22.5	8.0	4.2
2005	63.0	29.0	22.1	7.8	4.1
2006	63.6	29.3	22.4	7.8	4.1
2007	65.3	29.9	23.0	8.1	4.2
2008	63.3	29.0	22.2	7.8	4.2
2009	61.3	27.8	21.8	7.6	4.0
2010	59.2	26.9	21.0	7.3	4.0

Table A-16. Birth Rates by Live-Birth Order and by Race and Hispanic Origin of Mother, 2000–2009 and Preliminary 2010—Continued

(Rates are live births per 1,000 women age 15–44 years.)

Year, race, and Hispanic origin of mother	Fertility rate	Live-birth order			
		1st child	2nd child	3rd child	4th child and over
Hispanic[4]					
2000	95.9	35.8	29.2	18.0	12.9
2001	95.4	35.2	29.3	18.0	12.9
2002	94.7	34.7	29.1	18.0	12.9
2003	95.2	34.5	29.4	18.3	13.0
2004	95.7	34.4	29.3	18.7	13.4
2005	96.4	34.4	29.6	19.0	13.5
2006	98.3	35.1	29.9	19.3	14.0
2007	97.4	34.7	29.4	19.3	14.1
2008	92.7	33.0	27.8	18.3	13.6
2009	86.5	30.6	25.9	17.0	13.0
2010	80.3	28.0	24.0	15.9	12.4

[1]Includes births to White Hispanic and Black Hispanic women and births with origin not stated.
[2]Race and Hispanic origin are reported separately on birth certificates.
[3]Includes persons of Hispanic origin according to the mother's reported race.
[4]Persons of Hispanic origin may be of any race.

Table A-17. Births to Unmarried Mothers, by State and Territory, Final 2009 and Preliminary 2010

(Percent.)

Area	2009	2010
United States[1]	41.0	40.8
Alabama	41.0	41.9
Alaska	38.0	37.6
Arizona	45.4	44.9
Arkansas	45.5	45.3
California	40.6	40.5
Colorado	24.9	23.9
Connecticut	37.5	36.5
Delaware	47.7	47.6
District of Columbia	55.8	54.8
Florida	47.7	47.5
Georgia	45.5	45.8
Hawaii	37.9	37.8
Idaho	25.7	26.5
Illinois	40.8	40.5
Indiana	43.8	43.0
Iowa	35.2	34.2
Kansas	37.9	37.8
Kentucky	41.3	41.2
Louisiana	53.6	53.3
Maine	40.6	41.2
Maryland	42.7	41.9
Massachusetts	34.7	34.7
Michigan	41.3	41.8
Minnesota	33.6	33.2
Mississippi	55.3	54.8
Missouri	40.9	40.2
Montana	36.3	36.4
Nebraska	34.5	33.6
Nevada	43.4	44.3
New Hampshire	33.4	33.2
New Jersey	35.3	35.0
New Mexico	53.5	52.3
New York	41.5	42.0
North Carolina	42.3	42.0
North Dakota	32.7	32.7
Ohio	44.1	43.8
Oklahoma	42.0	41.8
Oregon	35.4	35.7
Pennsylvania	41.0	41.7
Rhode Island	44.7	45.0
South Carolina	47.6	47.5
South Dakota	38.4	37.6
Tennessee	44.5	44.1
Texas	42.4	42.4
Utah	19.4	19.2
Vermont	39.5	39.2
Virginia	35.8	35.5
Washington	33.6	33.0
West Virginia	43.6	44.0
Wisconsin	37.0	36.7
Wyoming	34.0	34.0
Puerto Rico	64.3	65.4
Virgin Islands	73.9	—
Guam	57.9	59.7
American Samoa	38.8	35.4
Northern Marianas	56.7	—

— = Data not available.
[1] Excludes data for the territories.

PART A: BIRTHS

Table A-18. Total Count of Records and Completeness of Preliminary File of Live Births, by State and Territory, Preliminary 2010

(By place of occurrence.)

Area	Live Births	
	Count of Records	Percent Completeness
United States[1]	4,006,978	100.00
Alabama	58,783	100.00
Alaska	11,365	100.00
Arizona	88,090	100.00
Arkansas	37,537	100.00
California	510,982	100.00
Colorado	66,822	100.00
Connecticut	38,538	100.00
Delaware	11,682	100.00
District of Columbia	13,789	100.00
Florida	214,959	100.00
Georgia	135,392	100.00
Hawaii	18,948	100.00
Idaho	22,799	100.00
Illinois	161,760	100.00
Indiana	84,795	100.00
Iowa	38,574	100.00
Kansas	41,598	100.00
Kentucky	53,565	100.00
Louisiana	62,535	100.00
Maine	12,814	100.00
Maryland	71,739	100.00
Massachusetts	73,267	100.00
Michigan	113,509	100.00
Minnesota	68,269	100.00
Mississippi	39,177	100.00
Missouri	77,588	100.00
Montana	12,066	100.00
Nebraska	26,242	100.00
Nevada	35,660	100.00
New Hampshire	13,032	100.00
New Jersey	103,932	100.00
New Mexico	27,028	100.00
New York	246,058	100.00
New York excluding New York City	121,267	100.00
New York City	124,791	100.00
North Carolina	123,403	100.00
North Dakota	10,470	100.00
Ohio	139,861	100.00
Oklahoma	52,347	100.00
Oregon	45,899	99.99
Pennsylvania	142,710	100.00
Rhode Island	11,841	100.00
South Carolina	55,602	100.00
South Dakota	12,382	100.00
Tennessee	84,533	100.00
Texas	392,768	100.00
Utah	53,396	100.00
Vermont	5,775	100.00
Virginia	101,202	100.00
Washington	86,507	100.00
West Virginia	20,755	99.99
Wisconsin	67,719	100.00
Wyoming	6,914	100.00

[1] Excludes data for the territories.

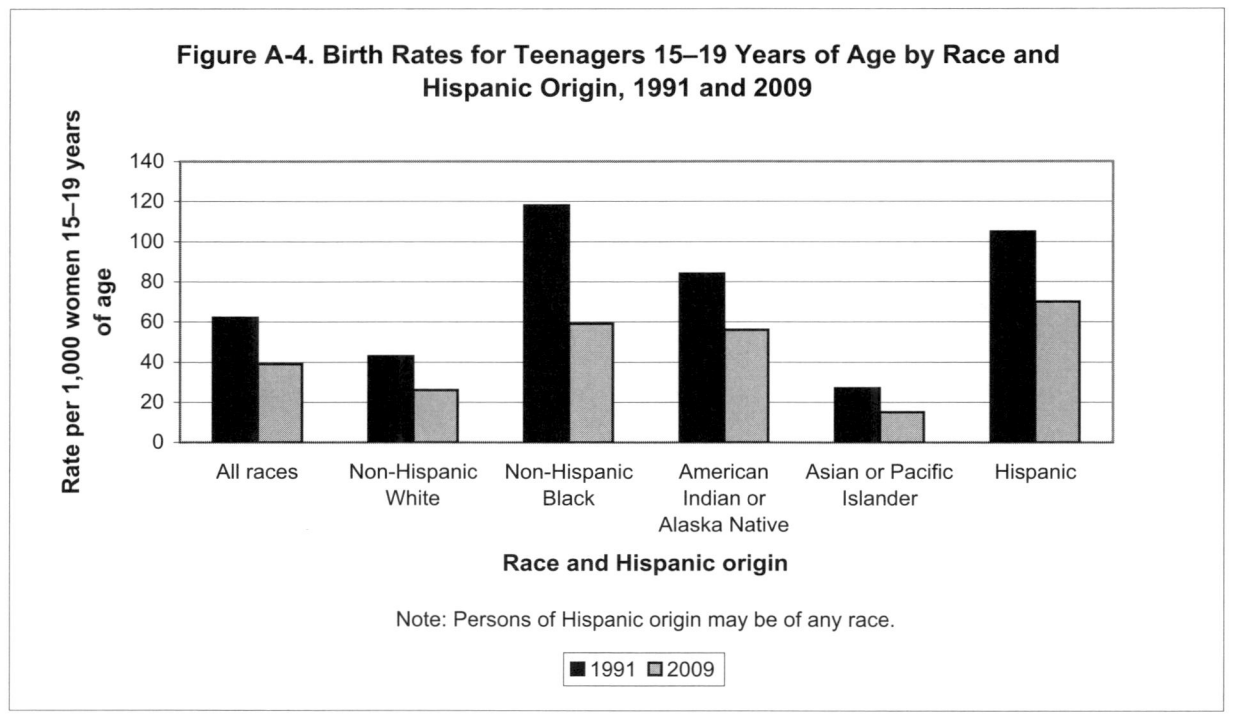

Figure A-4. Birth Rates for Teenagers 15–19 Years of Age by Race and Hispanic Origin, 1991 and 2009

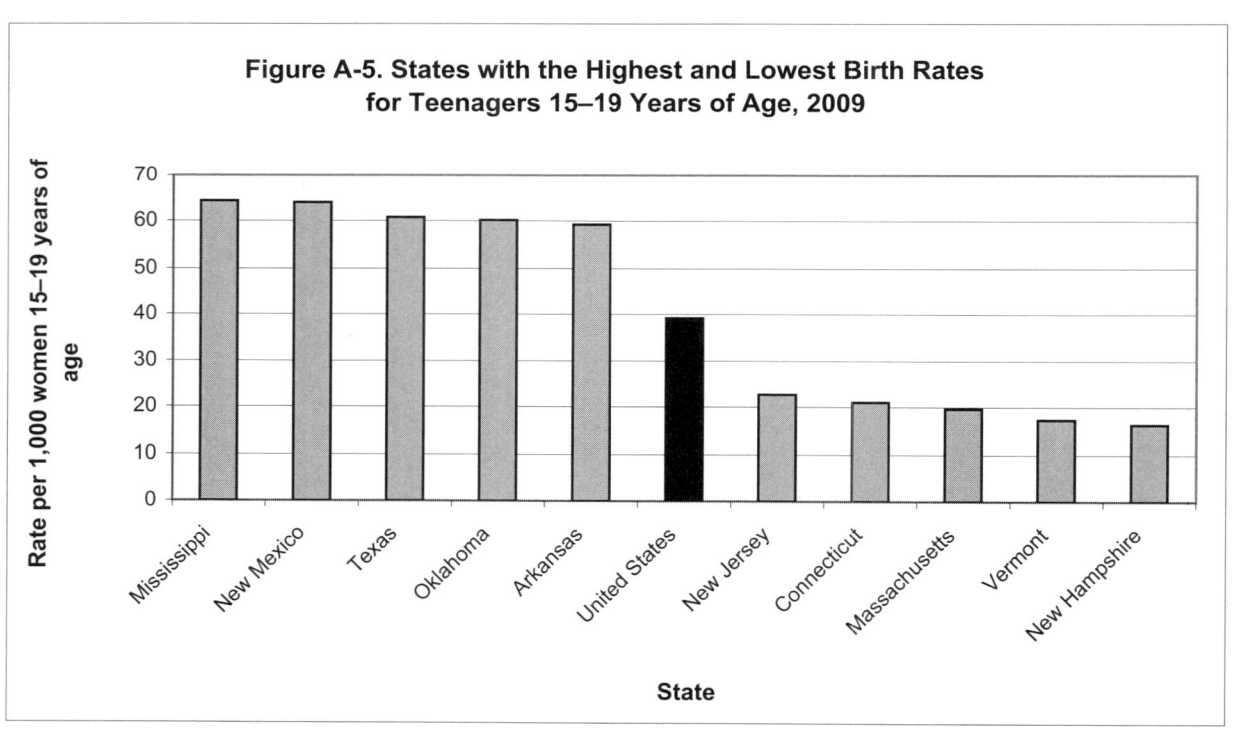

Figure A-5. States with the Highest and Lowest Birth Rates for Teenagers 15–19 Years of Age, 2009

Table A-19. Birth Rates for Teenagers 15–19 Years, by State, Selected Years, 1991–2009

(Birth rates per 1,000 estimated female population aged 15–19 years in each area.)

State	1991	2005	2006	2007	2008	2009	Percent change (1991–2005)	Percent change (2005–2007)	Percent change (2007–2009)	Percent change (2008–2009)
UNITED STATES[1]	61.8	40.5	41.9	42.5	41.5	39.1	-34	5	-8	-6
Alabama	73.6	49.7	53.5	54.1	53.0	50.7	-32	9	-6	-4
Alaska	66.0	37.3	44.3	44.7	46.8	44.5	-43	20	†	†
Arizona	79.7	58.2	62.0	61.2	56.2	50.6	-27	5	-17	-10
Arkansas	79.5	59.1	62.3	61.7	61.8	59.2	-26	4	-4	-4
California	73.8	38.8	39.9	39.7	38.4	36.6	-47	2	-8	-5
Colorado	58.3	42.6	43.8	43.4	42.5	38.5	-27	†	-11	-9
Connecticut	40.1	23.3	235.0	23.1	22.9	21.0	-42	†	-9	-8
Delaware	60.4	44.0	41.9	40.6	40.4	35.3	-27	-8	-13	-13
District of Columbia	109.6	63.4	48.4	49.9	50.9	47.7	-42	-21	†	†
Florida	67.9	42.4	45.2	45.5	42.8	39.0	-38	7	-14	-9
Georgia	76.0	52.7	54.2	54.9	51.8	47.7	-31	4	-13	-8
Hawaii	59.2	36.2	40.5	41.3	42.1	40.9	-39	14	†	†
Idaho	53.9	37.7	39.2	41.4	41.2	35.9	-30	10	-13	-13
Illinois	64.5	38.6	39.5	40.0	38.1	36.1	-40	4	-10	-5
Indiana	60.4	43.2	43.5	45.2	43.7	42.5	-28	5	-6	†
Iowa	42.5	32.6	32.9	33.2	33.9	32.1	-23	†	†	-5
Kansas	55.4	41.4	42.0	43.7	45.6	43.8	-25	6	†	†
Kentucky	68.8	49.1	54.6	55.1	55.6	51.3	-29	12	-7	-8
Louisiana	76.0	49.1	53.9	55.9	54.1	52.7	-35	14	-6	†
Maine	43.5	24.4	25.8	26.9	26.1	24.4	-44	10	-9	†
Maryland	54.1	31.8	33.6	34.4	32.8	31.3	-41	8	-9	-5
Massachusetts	37.5	21.8	21.3	22.1	20.1	19.6	-42	†	-11	†
Michigan	58.9	32.5	33.8	34.2	33.2	32.7	-45	5	-4	†
Minnesota	37.3	26.1	27.9	28.6	27.2	24.3	-30	10	-15	-11
Mississippi	85.3	60.5	68.4	71.9	65.7	64.2	-29	19	-11	†
Missouri	64.4	42.5	45.7	45.7	45.5	41.6	-34	8	-9	-9
Montana	46.8	35.2	39.6	36.8	40.7	38.5	-25	†	†	†
Nebraska	42.4	34.2	33.4	36.1	36.5	34.6	-19	†	†	†
Nevada	74.5	50.1	55.8	55.3	53.5	47.4	-33	10	-14	-11
New Hampshire	33.1	17.9	18	20.0	19.8	16.4	-46	12	-18	-17
New Jersey	41.3	23.4	24.9	25.2	24.5	22.7	-43	8	-10	-7
New Mexico	79.5	61.6	64.1	66.1	64.1	63.9	-23	7	†	†
New York	45.5	26.5	25.7	25.8	25.2	24.4	-42	-3	-5	-3
North Carolina	70.0	48.5	49.7	49.9	49.4	44.9	-31	3	-10	-9
North Dakota	35.5	29.7	26.5	29.3	28.6	27.9	-16	†	†	†
Ohio	60.5	38.9	40	41.3	41.0	38.9	-36	6	-6	-5
Oklahoma	72.1	54.2	59.6	61.5	61.6	60.1	-25	13	†	†
Oregon	54.8	33.0	35.7	35.9	37.2	33.1	-40	9	-8	-11
Pennsylvania	46.7	30.4	31	31.5	31.5	29.3	-35	4	-7	-7
Rhode Island	44.7	31.4	27.8	30.0	28.5	26.8	-30	†	-11	†
South Carolina	72.5	51.0	53	53.6	53.1	49.1	-30	5	-8	-8
South Dakota	47.6	37.5	40.2	42.2	40.0	38.4	-21	13	-9	†
Tennessee	74.8	54.9	54.7	56.2	55.6	50.6	-27	†	-10	-9
Texas	78.4	61.6	63.1	64.2	63.4	60.7	-21	4	-5	-4
Utah	48.0	33.4	34	36.1	35.1	30.7	-30	8	-15	-13
Vermont	39.2	18.6	20.8	22.0	21.3	17.4	-53	18	-21	-18
Virginia	53.4	34.4	35.2	35.1	33.5	31.0	-36	†	-12	-7
Washington	53.7	31.1	33.4	34.8	34.6	31.9	-42	12	-8	-8
West Virginia	58.0	43.4	44.9	47.4	48.8	49.8	-25	9	†	†
Wisconsin	43.7	30.3	30.9	32.2	31.3	29.4	-31	6	-9	-6
Wyoming	54.3	43.2	47.3	51.9	49.2	45.0	-20	20	-13	†
Puerto Rico	72.4	61.2	60	57.1	54.9	54.7	-15	-7	-4	†
Virgin Islands	77.9	50.0	49.6	51.5	51.1	51.5	-36	†	†	†
Guam	95.7	59.2	58.7	60.0	55.0	50.8	-38	†	-15	†
America Samoa	—	34.2	37.1	28.9	37.1	35.2	—	†	†	†
Northern Marinas	—	30.4	31.6	35.1	42.3	50.2	—	†	43	†

— = Data not available.
† = Difference not statistically significant.
[1]Excludes data for the territories.

Table A-20. Probability of a First Birth, Ages 15 Through 20 and for Females Aged 15–24, 2002 and 2006–2010

(Percent.)

Characteristic	Probability of a First Birth by Age					
	15	16	17	18	19	20
Total 2002	0.01	0.02	0.04	0.09	0.13	0.18
Total 2006–2010[1]	0.00	0.01	0.04	0.08	0.13	0.18
2006–2010						
Hispanic Origin and Race						
Hispanic or Latina	0.01	0.03	0.09	0.16	0.23	0.30
Non-Hispanic White	0.00	0.01	0.03	0.05	0.09	0.14
Non-Hispanic Black	0.00	0.01	0.04	0.10	0.17	0.26
Contraceptive Use at First Sex						
Used contraception at first sex	0.00	0.01	0.03	0.09	0.13	0.20
Used more than one method at first sex	0.00	0.00	0.01	0.02	0.06	0.07
Did not use contraception at first sex	0.02	0.05	0.12	0.18	0.32	0.37
Mother's Age at First Birth						
Under 20 years	0.01	0.02	0.07	0.14	0.22	0.29
20 years or over	0.00	0.01	0.02	0.05	0.09	0.14
Mother's Education						
No high school diploma or GED	0.01	0.04	0.11	0.18	0.28	0.37
High school diploma or GED	0.00	0.01	0.04	0.09	0.14	0.19
Some college or higher	0.00	0.01	0.01	0.04	0.07	0.12
Family Structure at Age 14						
Both biological or adoptive parents	0.00	0.01	0.02	0.04	0.07	0.11
Biological mom and step father	0.01	0.02	0.06	0.14	0.23	0.30
Other[2]	0.01	0.02	0.06	0.13	0.23	0.29

0.0 Quantity more than zero but less than 0.01.
[1]Includes persons of other or unknown origin and race groups, those with a mother-figure who had no births, and those who reported no mother-figure, not shown separately.
[2]Refers to anything other than two biological or adoptive parents or biological mother and stepfather, including one biological parent and no other parents(s)/parent-figures or no parent(s)/parent figures.

NOTE: GED is General Educational Development high school equivalency diploma.

Table A-21. Responses to the Statement "If You Got Pregnant Now or Got a Female Pregnant Now, How Would You Feel?" For Never-Married Females and Males Aged 15–19, 2002 and 2006–2010

(Number in thousands, percent.)

Characteristic	Number in thousands	Total	Very upset		A little upset		A little pleased		Very pleased	
			Percent	Standard error	Percent	Standard error	Percent	Standard error	Percent	Standard error
Total 2002	9,598	100.0	60.2	1.8	26.7	1.6	8.0	0.9	4.7	0.8
Total 2006–2010[1]	10,361	100.0	57.5	1.5	29.1	1.3	8.2	0.8	4.8	0.7
Hispanic Origin and Race										
Hispanic or Latina	1,849	100.0	47.7	3.0	32.5	3.0	13.2	2.5	6.0	1.3
Non-Hispanic White	6,150	100.0	63.1	2.0	28.2	1.9	5.4	1.0	3.2	0.8
Non-Hispanic Black	1,691	100.0	48.9	3.0	30.6	2.4	9.9	1.6	9.5	1.7
Age										
15–17 years	5,820	100.0	63.3	1.9	28.6	1.6	5.7	1.0	2.2	0.5
18–19 years	4,541	100.0	50.0	2.3	29.7	2.1	11.5	1.1	8.3	1.4
Ever Had Sex										
Yes	4,417	100.0	44.2	2.1	33.9	1.9	12.7	1.4	8.6	1.4
No	5,944	100.0	67.3	2.0	25.5	1.8	4.9	0.9	2.1	0.6
Family Structure at Age 14										
Both biological or adoptive parents	6,317	100.0	63.7	2.0	25.2	1.8	7.1	1.0	3.8	0.8
Other[2]	4,044	100.0	47.7	2.1	35.2	1.8	10.1	1.3	6.6	1.1
Male										
Total 2002	10,139	100.0	51.4	2.0	33.4	1.8	11.0	1.4	3.7	0.6
Total 2006–2010[1]	10,766	100.0	46.4	1.8	34.0	1.5	14.3	1.2	4.3	0.5
Male, 2006–2010										
Hispanic origin and race:										
Hispanic or Latino	2,000	100.0	26.6	2.9	37.8	2.6	23.3	3.2	11.7	2.2
Non-Hispanic White	6,405	100.0	56.0	2.1	32.1	2.0	9.7	1.2	1.5	0.5
Non-Hispanic Black	1,673	100.0	29.9	3.3	40.0	3.3	22.4	2.4	6.5	1.3
Age										
15–17 years	6,623	100.0	53.1	2.2	32.3	2.0	11.1	1.4	2.8	0.5
18–19 years	4,143	100.0	35.8	2.4	36.9	2.0	19.2	1.9	6.8	1.1
Ever Had Sex										
Yes	4,501	100.0	32.8	2.0	37.5	1.8	21.1	2.2	6.9	1.0
No	6,266	100.0	56.2	2.2	31.5	2.1	9.3	1.1	2.5	0.6
Family Structure at Age 14										
Both biological or adoptive parents	6,737	100.0	52.0	2.1	32.5	1.6	11.5	1.3	3.3	0.6
Other[2]	4,029	100.0	37.1	2.0	36.7	2.3	18.9	1.8	6.0	0.8

[1]Includes persons of other or unknown origin and race groups, not shown separately.
[2]Refers to anything other than two biological or adoptive parents or biological mother and stepfather, including one biological parent and no other parents(s)/parent-figures or no parent(s)/parent figures.

NOTE: Percentages may not add to 100 because responses of "would not care" (coded only if respondent insisted) are not shown separately.

Table A-22. Birth Rates for Women Aged 10–19 Years by Age, Race, and Hispanic Origin of Mother, Selected Years, 1991–2009

(Rates per 1,000 women in specified age, race, and Hispanic origin group.)

Age, race, and Hispanic origin of mother	1991	2005	2007	2008	2009	Percent change 1991–2009	Percent change 2005–2007	Percent change 2007–2009	Percent change 2008–2009
10–14 Years									
All races and origins[1]	1.4	0.7	0.6	0.6	0.5	-64	-14	-17	-17
Non-Hispanic White[2]	0.5	0.2	0.2	0.2	0.2	-60	†	†	†
Non-Hispanic Black[2]	4.9	1.7	1.5	1.4	1.2	-76	-12	-20	-14
American Indian or Alaska Native total[2,3]	1.6	0.9	0.9	0.9	0.8	-50	†	†	†
Asian or Pacific Islander total[2,3]	0.8	0.2	0.2	0.2	0.2	-75	†	†	†
Hispanic[4]	2.4	1.3	1.2	1.2	1.0	-58	-8	†	†
15–19 Years									
All races and origins[1]	61.8	40.5	42.5	41.5	39.1	-37	5	-8	-6
Non-Hispanic White[2]	43.4	25.9	27.2	26.7	25.6	-41	5	-6	-4
Non-Hispanic Black[2]	118.2	60.9	64.2	62.8	59.0	-50	5	-8	-6
American Indian or Alaska Native total[2,3]	84.1	52.7	59.3	58.4	55.5	-34	13	-6	-5
Asian or Pacific Islander total[2,3]	27.3	17.0	16.9	16.2	14.7	-46	†	-13	-9
Hispanic[4]	104.6	81.7	81.8	77.5	70.1	-33	†	-14	-10
15–17 Years									
All races and origins[1]	38.6	21.4	22.1	21.7	20.1	-48	3	-9	-7
Non-Hispanic White[2]	23.6	11.5	11.8	11.5	11.0	-53	3	-7	-4
Non-Hispanic Black[2]	86.1	34.9	35.8	34.8	32.1	-63	3	-10	-8
American Indian or Alaska Native total[2,3]	51.9	30.5	31.8	32.5	30.6	-41	†	†	-6
Asian or Pacific Islander total[2,3]	16.3	8.2	8.2	7.9	7.1	-56	†	-13	-10
Hispanic[4]	69.2	48.5	47.9	46.1	41.0	-41	-1	-14	-11
18–19 Years									
All races and origins[1]	94.0	69.9	73.9	70.6	66.2	-30	6	-10	-6
Non-Hispanic White[2]	70.6	48.0	50.4	48.5	46.1	-35	5	-9	-5
Non-Hispanic Black[2]	162.2	103.0	109.3	104.6	97.5	-40	6	-11	-7
American Indian or Alaska Native total[2,3]	134.2	87.6	101.6	96.6	90.5	-33	16	-11	-6
Asian or Pacific Islander total[2,3]	42.2	30.1	29.9	28.4	25.8	-39	†	-14	-9
Hispanic[4]	155.5	134.6	137.2	127.2	114.0	-27	2	-17	-10

† = Difference not statistically significant.
[1]Includes births to White Hispanic and Black Hispanic women and births with origin not stated, not shown separately.
[2]Race and Hispanic origin are reported separately on birth certificates.
[3]Includes persons of Hispanic origin according to the mother's reported race.
[4]Persons of Hispanic origin may be of any race.

Table A-23. Mean Age of Mother, by Live-Birth Order and Race and Hispanic Origin of Mother, 1980–2009

(The arithmetic average of the age of mothers at the time of birth.)

Year, race, and Hispanic origin of mother	Total	Live-birth order							
		1	2	3	4	5	6 and 7	8 and over	Unknown or not stated
All Races[1]									
1980[2]	25.0	22.7	25.4	27.3	29.0	30.6	32.7	36.0	23.9
1985	25.8	23.7	26.3	27.9	29.3	30.6	32.5	35.7	26.1
1990	26.4	24.2	26.9	28.3	29.4	30.6	32.1	35.1	27.4
1995	26.9	24.5	27.5	29.1	30.1	31.2	32.6	35.4	27.1
2000	27.2	24.9	27.7	29.2	30.3	31.4	32.9	35.8	27.4
2001	27.3	25.0	27.8	29.2	30.3	31.4	32.9	35.9	27.0
2002	27.3	25.1	27.9	29.2	30.3	31.4	32.9	35.9	27.7
2003	27.4	25.2	28.0	29.3	30.4	31.4	33.0	35.8	27.9
2004	27.5	25.2	28.0	29.4	30.4	31.4	32.9	35.9	27.6
2005	27.4	25.2	28.0	29.4	30.4	31.4	32.9	35.9	28.0
2006	27.4	25.0	27.9	29.3	30.4	31.4	33.0	35.8	28.0
2007	27.4	25.0	27.9	29.3	30.4	31.5	32.9	35.7	27.9
2008	27.4	25.1	27.9	29.4	30.5	31.5	32.9	35.7	27.7
2009	27.5	25.2	28.0	29.5	30.6	31.6	32.9	35.7	27.6
Non-Hispanic White[3]									
1990[4]	27.1	25.0	27.6	29.1	30.3	31.6	33.2	36.2	28.5
1995	27.6	25.4	28.3	29.9	31.2	32.4	33.9	36.7	28.5
2000	28.0	25.9	28.6	30.0	31.3	32.4	34.0	37.0	28.9
2001	28.1	26.0	28.6	30.1	31.3	32.4	33.9	37.0	28.2
2002	28.2	26.1	28.7	30.1	31.2	32.3	33.9	37.1	28.6
2003	28.2	26.2	28.8	30.1	31.2	32.3	33.9	37.0	28.8
2004	28.2	26.2	28.8	30.2	31.2	32.2	33.8	36.9	28.7
2005	28.2	26.2	28.8	30.1	31.2	32.2	33.8	36.9	29.1
2006	28.1	26.0	28.8	30.1	31.1	32.1	33.7	36.7	29.1
2007	28.1	26.0	28.7	30.0	31.1	32.1	33.7	36.7	28.8
2008	28.1	26.0	28.7	30.1	31.1	32.1	33.6	36.7	28.7
2009	28.1	26.1	28.8	30.1	31.1	32.1	33.6	36.7	28.6
Non-Hispanic Black[3]									
1990[4]	24.4	21.7	24.6	26.3	27.4	28.7	30.3	33.3	26.0
1995	24.8	21.9	25.3	27.0	28.0	29.3	30.8	33.2	25.4
2000	25.2	22.3	25.5	27.1	28.2	29.5	31.0	33.9	26.0
2001	25.3	22.4	25.7	27.2	28.3	29.6	31.2	34.1	26.4
2002	25.4	22.6	25.8	27.3	28.5	29.6	31.2	34.1	26.5
2003	25.6	22.7	25.9	27.5	28.6	29.7	31.3	34.0	26.3
2004	25.6	22.7	25.9	27.5	28.6	29.8	31.2	34.1	25.7
2005	25.6	22.7	26.0	27.6	28.8	29.8	31.3	34.2	25.8
2006	25.6	22.7	26.0	27.7	28.8	29.9	31.4	34.1	25.9
2007	25.6	22.7	26.0	27.7	28.9	30	31.4	34.2	26.1
2008	25.6	22.8	26.0	27.8	29.0	30	31.5	34.2	26.2
2009	25.7	22.9	26.1	27.9	29.1	30.2	31.5	34.3	26.2
Hispanic[5]									
1990[4]	25.3	22.4	25.2	27.4	29.1	30.6	32.3	35.3	26.1
1995	25.4	22.4	25.5	27.8	29.6	31.1	32.8	35.5	24.2
2000	25.7	22.7	25.8	28.1	29.8	31.3	33.0	35.5	24.2
2001	25.9	22.8	25.9	28.2	29.9	31.4	33.1	35.7	24.4
2002	26.0	23.0	26.0	28.3	29.9	31.4	33.1	35.7	25.7
2003	26.1	23.1	26.1	28.4	30.0	31.4	33.1	35.4	25.8
2004	26.2	23.1	26.2	28.5	30.1	31.5	33.1	35.5	25.8
2005	26.2	23.1	26.2	28.5	30.1	31.4	33.2	35.6	26.5
2006	26.2	23.1	26.2	28.6	30.2	31.5	33.2	35.5	26.6
2007	26.3	23.1	26.3	28.6	30.3	31.6	33.1	35.3	26.7
2008	26.4	23.1	26.4	28.7	30.4	31.6	33.2	35.3	26.7
2009	26.5	23.3	26.5	28.9	30.5	31.8	33.1	35.3	26.8

[1]Includes races other than White and Black and origin not stated.
[2]Based on 100 percent of births in selected states and on a 50-percent sample of births in all other states.
[3]Race and Hispanic origin are reported separately on birth certificates. Persons of Hispanic origin may be of any race.
[4]Excludes data for New Hampshire and Oklahoma, which did not report Hispanic origin.
[5]Persons of Hispanic origin may be of any race.

Table A-24. Live Births, Birth Rates, and Fertility Rates, by Race, Specified Years, 1940–1955 and Each Year, 1960–2009

(Number, rate per 1,000 live population in specified group.)

Year	Number					Birth rate					Fertility rate				
	All races[1]	White	Black	American Indian or Alaska Native	Asian or Pacific Islander	All races[1]	White	Black	American Indian or Alaska Native	Asian or Pacific Islander	All races[1]	White	Black	American Indian or Alaska Native	Asian or Pacific Islander
Race of Mother															
1980[2]	3,612,258	2,936,351	568,080	29,389	74,355	15.9	15.1	21.3	20.7	19.9	68.4	65.6	84.7	82.7	73.2
1981[2]	3,629,238	2,947,679	564,955	29,688	84,553	15.8	15.0	20.8	20.0	20.1	67.3	64.8	82.0	79.6	73.7
1982[2]	3,680,537	2,984,817	568,506	32,436	93,193	15.9	15.1	20.7	21.1	20.3	67.3	64.8	80.9	83.6	74.8
1983[2]	3,638,933	2,946,468	562,624	32,881	95,713	15.6	14.8	20.2	20.6	19.5	65.7	63.4	78.7	81.8	71.7
1984[2]	3,669,141	2,967,100	568,138	33,256	98,926	15.6	14.8	20.1	20.1	18.8	65.5	63.2	78.2	79.8	69.2
1985	3,760,561	3,037,913	581,824	34,037	104,606	15.8	15.0	20.4	19.8	18.7	66.3	64.1	78.8	78.6	68.4
1986	3,756,547	3,019,175	592,910	34,169	107,797	15.6	14.8	20.5	19.2	18.0	65.4	63.1	78.9	75.9	66.0
1987	3,809,394	3,043,828	611,173	35,322	116,560	15.7	14.9	20.8	19.1	18.4	65.8	63.3	80.1	75.6	67.1
1988	3,909,510	3,102,083	638,562	37,088	129,035	16.0	15.0	21.5	19.3	19.2	67.3	64.5	82.6	76.8	70.2
1989	4,040,958	3,192,355	673,124	39,478	133,075	16.4	15.4	22.3	19.7	18.7	69.2	66.4	86.2	79.0	68.2
1990	4,158,212	3,290,273	684,336	39,051	141,635	16.7	15.8	22.4	18.9	19.0	70.9	68.3	86.8	76.2	69.6
1991	4,110,907	3,241,273	682,602	38,841	145,372	16.2	15.3	21.8	18.3	18.3	69.3	66.7	84.8	73.9	67.1
1992	4,065,014	3,201,678	673,633	39,453	150,250	15.8	15.0	21.1	17.9	17.9	68.4	66.1	82.4	73.1	66.1
1993	4,000,240	3,149,833	658,875	38,732	152,800	15.4	14.6	20.2	17.0	17.3	67.0	64.9	79.6	69.7	64.3
1994	3,952,767	3,121,004	636,391	37,740	157,632	15.0	14.3	19.1	16.0	17.1	65.9	64.2	75.9	65.8	63.9
1995	3,899,589	3,098,885	603,139	37,278	160,287	14.6	14.1	17.8	15.3	16.7	64.6	63.6	71.0	63.0	62.6
1996	3,891,494	3,093,057	594,781	37,880	165,776	14.4	13.9	17.3	14.9	16.5	64.1	63.3	69.2	61.8	62.3
1997	3,880,894	3,072,640	599,913	38,572	169,769	14.2	13.7	17.1	14.7	16.2	63.6	62.8	69.0	60.8	61.3
1998	3,941,553	3,118,727	609,902	40,272	172,652	14.3	13.8	17.1	14.8	15.9	64.3	63.6	69.4	61.3	60.1
1999	3,959,417	3,132,501	605,970	40,170	180,776	14.2	13.7	16.8	14.2	15.9	64.4	64.0	68.5	59.0	60.9
2000	4,058,814	3,194,005	622,598	41,668	200,543	14.4	13.9	17.0	14.0	17.1	65.9	65.3	70.0	58.7	65.8
2001	4,025,933	3,177,626	606,156	41,872	200,279	14.1	13.7	16.3	13.7	16.4	65.3	65.0	67.6	58.1	64.2
2002	4,021,726	3,174,760	593,691	42,368	210,907	13.9	13.5	15.7	13.8	16.5	64.8	64.8	65.8	58.0	64.1
2003	4,089,950	3,225,848	599,847	43,052	221,203	14.1	13.6	15.7	13.8	16.8	66.1	66.1	66.3	58.4	66.3
2004	4,112,052	3,222,928	616,074	43,927	229,123	14.0	13.5	16.0	14.0	16.8	66.3	66.1	67.6	58.9	67.1
2005	4,138,349	3,229,294	633,134	44,813	231,108	14.0	13.4	16.2	14.2	16.5	66.7	66.3	69.0	59.9	66.6
2006	4,265,555	3,310,308	666,481	47,721	241,045	14.2	13.7	16.8	14.9	16.6	68.5	68.0	72.1	63.1	67.5
2007	4,316,233	3,336,626	675,676	49,443	254,488	14.3	13.7	16.9	15.3	17.2	69.5	68.8	72.7	64.9	71.3
2008	4,247,694	3,274,163	670,809	49,537	253,185	14.0	13.4	16.6	14.5	16.8	68.6	67.8	71.9	64.6	71.3
2009	4,130,665	3,173,293	657,618	48,665	251,089	13.5	12.8	16.0	13.9	16.2	66.7	66.0	69.9	62.8	68.7
Race of Child															
1960[3]	4,257,850	3,600,744	602,264	21,114	—	-23.7	22.7	31.9	—	—	118.0	113.2	153.5	—	—
1961[3]	4,268,326	3,600,864	611,072	21,464	—	-23.3	22.2	—	—	—	-117.1	112.3	—	—	—
1962[3,4]	4,167,362	3,394,068	584,610	21,968	—	-22.4	21.4	—	—	—	-112.0	107.5	—	—	—
1963[3,4]	4,098,020	3,326,344	580,658	22,358	—	-21.7	20.7	—	—	—	-108.3	103.6	—	—	—
1964[2]	4,027,490	3,369,160	607,556	24,382	—	-21.1	20	29.5	—	—	104.7	99.8	142.6	—	—
1965[3]	3,760,358	3,123,860	581,126	24,066	—	-19.4	18.3	27.7	—	—	96.3	91.3	133.2	—	—
1966[3]	3,606,274	2,993,230	558,244	23,014	—	-18.4	17.4	26.2	—	—	90.8	86.2	124.7	—	—
1967[5]	3,520,959	2,922,502	543,976	22,665	—	-17.8	16.8	25.1	—	—	87.2	82.8	118.5	—	—
1968[3]	3,501,564	2,912,224	531,152	24,156	—	-17.6	16.6	24.2	—	—	85.2	81.3	112.7	—	—
1969[3]	3,600,206	2,993,614	543,132	24,008	—	-17.9	16.9	24.4	—	—	86.1	82.2	112.1	—	—
1970[3]	3,731,386	3,091,264	572,362	25,864	—	-18.4	17.4	25.3	—	—	87.9	84.1	115.4	—	—
1971[3]	3,555,970	2,919,746	564,960	27,148	—	-17.2	16.1	24.4	—	—	81.6	77.3	109.7	—	—
1972[2]	3,258,411	2,655,558	531,329	27,368	—	-15.6	14.5	22.5	—	—	73.1	68.9	99.9	—	—
1973[2]	3,136,965	2,551,030	512,597	26,464	—	-14.8	13.8	21.4	—	—	68.8	64.9	93.6	—	—
1974[2]	3,159,958	2,575,792	507,162	26,631	—	-14.8	13.9	20.8	—	—	67.8	64.2	89.7	—	—
1975[2]	3,144,198	2,551,996	511,581	27,546	—	-14.6	13.6	20.7	—	—	66.0	62.5	87.9	—	—
1976[2]	3,167,788	2,567,614	514,479	29,009	—	-14.6	13.6	20.5	—	—	65.0	61.5	85.8	—	—
1977[2]	3,326,632	2,691,070	544,221	30,500	—	-15.1	14.1	21.4	—	—	66.8	63.2	88.1	—	—
1978[2]	3,333,279	2,681,116	551,540	33,160	—	-15	14	21.3	—	—	65.5	61.7	86.7	—	—
1979[2]	3,494,398	2,808,420	577,855	34,269	—	-15.6	14.5	22	—	—	67.2	63.4	88.3	—	—
1980[2]	3,612,258	2,898,732	589,616	36,797	—	-15.9	14.9	22.1	—	—	68.4	64.7	88.1	—	—
Births adjusted for underregistration															
Race of Child															
1940	2,559,000	2,199,000	—	—	—	19.4	18.6	—	—	—	79.9	77.1	—	—	—
1945	2,858,000	2,471,000	—	—	—	20.4	19.7	—	—	—	85.9	83.4	—	—	—
1950	3,632,000	3,108,000	—	—	—	24.1	23.0	—	—	—	106.2	102.3	—	—	—
1955	4,097,000	3,485,000	—	—	—	25.0	23.8	—	—	—	118.3	113.7	—	—	—

— = Data not available.
[1] Data for 1960–1991 includes births to races not shown. For 1992 and later years, unknown race of mother is imputed.
[2] Based on 100 percent of births in selected states and on a 50-percent sample of births in all other states.
[3] Figures by race exclude New Jersey.
[4] Based on a 50-percent sample of births.
[5] Based on a 20-to 50-percent sample of births.

PART A: BIRTHS 31

Table A-25. Births and Birth Rates, by Hispanic Origin of Mother and by Race for Mothers of Non-Hispanic Origin, 1989–2009

(Birth rates are live births per 1,000 population in specified group. Fertility rates are live births per 1,000 women aged 15–44 years in specified group.)

Measure and year	All origins[1]	Hispanic						Non-Hispanic		
		Total	Mexican	Puerto Rican	Cuban	Central and South American	Other and unknown Hispanic	Total[2]	White	Black
Number										
1989[3]	3,903,012	532,249	327,233	56,229	10,842	72,443	65,502	3,297,493	2,526,367	611,269
1990[4]	4,092,994	595,073	385,640	58,807	11,311	83,008	56,307	3,457,417	2,626,500	661,701
1991[5]	4,094,566	623,085	411,233	59,833	11,058	86,908	54,053	3,434,464	2,589,878	666,758
1992[5]	4,049,024	643,271	432,047	59,569	11,472	89,031	51,152	3,365,862	2,527,207	657,450
1993	4,000,240	654,418	443,733	58,102	11,916	92,371	48,296	3,295,345	2,472,031	641,273
1994	3,952,767	665,026	454,536	57,240	11,889	93,485	47,876	3,245,115	2,438,855	619,198
1995	3,899,589	679,768	469,615	54,824	12,473	94,996	47,860	3,160,495	2,382,638	587,781
1996	3,891,494	701,339	489,666	54,863	12,613	97,888	46,309	3,133,484	2,358,989	578,099
1997	3,880,894	709,767	499,024	55,450	12,887	97,405	45,001	3,115,174	2,333,363	581,431
1998	3,941,553	734,661	516,011	57,349	13,226	98,226	49,849	3,158,975	2,361,462	593,127
1999	3,959,417	764,339	540,674	57,138	13,088	103,307	50,132	3,147,580	2,346,450	588,981
2000	4,058,814	815,868	581,915	58,124	13,429	113,344	49,056	3,199,994	2,362,968	604,346
2001	4,025,933	851,851	611,000	57,568	14,017	121,365	47,901	3,149,572	2,326,578	589,917
2002	4,021,726	876,642	627,505	57,465	14,232	125,981	51,459	3,119,944	2,298,156	578,335
2003	4,089,950	912,329	654,504	58,400	14,867	135,586	48,972	3,149,034	2,321,904	576,033
2004	4,112,052	946,349	677,621	61,221	14,943	143,520	49,044	3,133,125	2,296,683	578,772
2005	4,138,349	985,505	693,197	63,340	16,064	151,201	61,703	3,123,005	2,279,768	583,759
2006	4,265,555	1,039,077	718,146	66,932	16,936	165,321	71,742	3,196,082	2,308,640	617,247
2007	4,316,233	1,062,779	722,055	68,488	16,981	169,851	85,404	3,222,460	2,310,333	627,191
2008	4,247,694	1,041,239	684,883	69,015	16,718	155,578	115,045	3,173,629	2,267,817	623,029
2009	4,130,665	999,548	645,297	68,486	16,641	148,647	120,477	3,101,330	2,212,552	609,584
Birth Rate										
1989[3,6]	16.3	26.2	25.7	23.7	10.0	28.3	(6)	15.4	14.2	22.8
1990[4,6]	16.7	26.7	28.7	21.6	10.9	27.5	(6)	15.7	14.4	23.0
1991[5,6]	16.2	26.5	27.6	23.3	9.8	28.3	(6)	15.2	13.9	22.4
1992[5,6]	15.8	26.1	27.4	22.9	10.1	27.5	(6)	14.8	13.4	21.6
1993[6]	15.4	25.4	26.8	21.5	10.5	26.3	(6)	14.3	13.1	20.7
1994[6]	15.0	24.7	26.1	20.8	10.7	24.9	(6)	13.9	12.8	19.5
1995[6]	14.6	24.1	25.8	19.0	10.8	24.2	(6)	13.5	12.5	18.2
1996[6]	14.4	23.8	26.2	17.2	10.6	22.5	(6)	13.3	12.3	17.6
1997[6]	14.2	23.0	25.3	17.2	10.0	21.3	(6)	13.1	12.2	17.4
1998[6]	14.3	22.7	24.6	17.9	9.7	21.7	(6)	13.2	12.2	17.5
1999[6]	14.2	22.5	24.2	18.0	9.4	21.7	(6)	13.0	12.1	17.1
2000[6]	14.4	23.1	25.0	18.1	9.7	21.8	(6)	13.2	12.2	17.3
2001[6]	14.1	23.0	24.8	17.8	10.3	21.8	(6)	12.8	11.8	16.6
2002[6]	13.9	22.6	24.2	16.5	10.0	22.4	(6)	12.6	11.7	16.1
2003[6]	14.1	22.9	24.7	15.1	9.9	23.0	(6)	12.7	11.8	15.9
2004[6]	14.0	22.9	24.9	16.1	9.3	22.2	(6)	12.5	11.6	15.8
2005[6]	14.0	23.1	24.7	17.2	10.2	22.8	(6)	12.4	11.5	15.7
2006[6]	14.2	23.4	24.8	17.6	10.4	23.9	(6)	12.6	11.6	16.5
2007[6]	14.3	23.4	24.3	17.4	10.2	25.0	(6)	12.7	11.6	16.6
2008[6]	14.0	22.2	22.1	16.7	10.2	26.6	(6)	12.5	11.3	16.4
2009[6]	13.5	20.6	20.1	15.8	9.6	26.0	(6)	12.1	11.0	15.8
Fertility Rate										
1989[3,6]	69.2	104.9	106.6	86.6	49.8	95.8	(6)	65.7	60.5	84.8
1990[4,6]	71.0	107.7	118.9	82.9	52.6	102.7	(6)	67.1	62.8	89.0
1991[5,6]	69.3	106.9	114.9	87.9	47.6	105.5	(6)	65.2	60.9	87.0
1992[5,6]	68.4	106.1	113.3	87.9	49.4	104.7	(6)	64.2	60.0	84.5
1993[6]	67.0	103.3	110.9	79.8	53.9	101.5	(6)	62.7	58.9	81.5
1994[6]	65.9	100.7	109.9	78.2	53.6	93.2	(6)	61.6	58.2	77.5
1995[6]	64.6	98.8	109.9	71.3	52.2	89.1	(6)	60.2	57.5	72.8
1996[6]	64.1	97.5	110.7	66.5	55.1	84.2	(6)	59.6	57.1	70.7
1997[6]	63.6	94.2	106.6	65.8	53.1	80.6	(6)	59.3	56.8	70.3
1998[6]	64.3	93.2	103.2	69.7	46.5	83.5	(6)	60.0	57.6	70.9
1999[6]	64.4	93.0	101.5	71.1	47.0	84.8	(6)	60.0	57.7	69.9

Table A-25. Births and Birth Rates, by Hispanic Origin of Mother and by Race for Mothers of Non-Hispanic Origin, 1989–2009—Continued

(Birth rates are live births per 1,000 population in specified group. Fertility rates are live births per 1,000 women aged 15–44 years in specified group.)

Measure and year	All origins[1]	Hispanic						Non-Hispanic		
		Total	Mexican	Puerto Rican	Cuban	Central and South American	Other and unknown Hispanic	Total[2]	White	Black
2000[6]	65.9	95.9	105.1	73.5	49.3	85.1	(6)	61.1	58.5	71.4
2001[6]	65.3	96.0	105.7	72.2	56.7	82.7	(6)	60.1	57.7	69.1
2002[6]	64.8	94.4	102.8	65.4	59.0	86.1	(6)	59.6	57.4	67.4
2003[6]	66.1	96.9	105.5	61.6	61.7	91.2	(6)	60.5	58.5	67.1
2004[6]	66.3	97.8	106.8	68.4	53.2	89.3	(6)	60.5	58.4	67.0
2005[6]	66.7	99.4	107.7	72.1	50.4	93.2	(6)	60.4	58.3	67.2
2006[6]	68.5	101.5	109.0	74.0	49.3	98.6	(6)	62.0	59.5	70.6
2007[6]	69.5	102.2	107.8	73.6	49.7	104.9	(6)	62.9	60.1	71.6
2008[6]	68.6	98.8	98.9	71.5	53.3	116.1	(6)	62.4	59.4	71.1
2009[6]	66.7	93.3	91.4	68.7	49.5	115.7	(6)	61.1	58.4	68.9

[1]Includes origin not stated.
[2]Includes races other than White and Black.
[3]Excludes data for Louisiana, New Hampshire, and Oklahoma, which did not report Hispanic origin.
[4]Excludes data for New Hampshire and Oklahoma, which did not report Hispanic origin.
[5]Excludes data for New Hampshire, which did not report Hispanic origin.
[6]Rates for the Central and South American population includes other and unknown Hispanic.

PART A: BIRTHS 33

Table A-26. Live Births by Age of Mother, Live-Birth Order, and Race of Mother, 2009

(Number of children born alive to mother.)

| Live birth order and race of mother | All ages | Under 15 years | Total | 15–19 years ||||| 20–24 years | 25–29 years | 30–34 years | 35–39 years | 40–44 years | 45–49 years | 50–54 years |
				15 years	16 years	17 years	18 years	19 years							
All Races	4,130,665	5,029	409,802	15,641	37,802	70,804	117,444	168,111	1,005,982	1,166,787	955,246	474,103	105,827	7,320	569
1st child	1,660,231	4,920	330,500	15,026	35,086	61,931	94,841	123,616	493,851	426,362	272,219	106,971	23,330	1,906	172
2nd child	1,291,074	70	65,700	497	2,388	7,737	19,168	35,910	330,327	383,678	326,908	152,565	29,803	1,888	135
3rd child	679,135	2	9,736	20	102	649	2,465	6,500	127,290	214,724	196,272	107,931	21,851	1,242	87
4th child	284,086	1	1,167	-	9	54	241	863	36,621	87,584	90,349	54,420	13,078	809	57
5th child	107,131	-	118	-	1	6	24	87	8,634	30,879	35,712	24,270	7,018	458	42
6th child	43,743	-	18	-	3	4	1	10	1,907	10,799	15,443	11,440	3,813	300	23
7th child	19,385	-	8	-	-	-	4	4	417	3,661	6,993	5,849	2,237	203	17
8th child and over	19,308	-	6	-	-	-	1	5	236	1,806	5,446	7,457	3,880	453	24
Not stated	26,572	36	2,549	98	213	423	699	1,116	6,699	7,294	5,904	3,200	817	61	12
White	3,173,293	3,022	288,709	10,163	25,811	49,611	82,823	120,301	751,430	917,877	755,396	368,753	81,904	5,758	444
1st child	1,271,317	2,955	235,339	9,804	24,097	43,739	67,648	90,051	376,517	340,180	214,124	82,385	18,159	1,528	130
2nd child	1,005,320	50	45,157	296	1,550	5,197	13,145	24,969	249,948	308,427	259,638	117,526	22,971	1,490	113
3rd child	529,304	1	6,144	13	50	412	1,514	4,155	90,815	168,984	159,615	85,827	16,836	973	73
4th child	216,041	-	645	-	8	33	139	465	23,732	65,038	72,131	43,606	10,218	627	44
5th child	77,708	-	62	-	1	4	9	48	5,076	20,878	26,959	18,927	5,430	344	32
6th child	30,512	-	9	-	-	4	-	5	1,004	6,611	10,960	8,721	2,957	230	20
7th child	13,029	-	6	-	-	-	3	3	205	2,038	4,592	4,269	1,743	163	13
8th child and over	13,101	-	5	-	-	-	1	4	144	941	3,330	5,284	3,026	359	12
Not stated	16,961	16	1,342	50	105	222	364	601	3,989	4,780	4,011	2,208	564	44	7
Black	657,618	1,823	105,725	4,815	10,571	18,568	30,278	41,493	208,885	165,737	107,132	54,036	13,337	882	61
1st child	258,075	1,782	82,860	4,588	9,667	15,899	23,707	28,999	93,302	44,755	22,543	10,125	2,506	185	17
2nd child	183,934	20	18,031	178	748	2,249	5,321	9,535	66,779	50,682	30,548	14,450	3,221	193	10
3rd child	110,239	1	3,192	7	49	211	834	2,091	31,145	35,894	24,584	12,436	2,821	161	5
4th child	53,174	1	481	-	1	19	93	368	11,088	18,487	13,827	7,285	1,888	111	6
5th child	23,420	-	53	-	-	2	15	36	3,083	8,238	6,895	3,961	1,107	77	6
6th child	10,684	-	8	-	2	-	1	5	809	3,521	3,608	2,082	604	49	3
7th child	5,128	-	2	-	-	-	1	1	194	1,375	1,949	1,232	346	28	2
8th child and over	5,012	-	1	-	-	-	-	1	81	753	1,735	1,705	661	67	9
Not stated	7,952	19	1,097	42	104	188	306	457	2,404	2,032	1,443	760	183	11	3
American Indian or Alaska Native	48,665	108	8,315	390	791	1,499	2,369	3,266	16,231	12,634	7,401	3,214	723	36	3
1st child	17,445	108	6,524	370	736	1,304	1,872	2,242	6,500	2,687	1,145	402	75	3	1
2nd child	13,030	-	1,464	17	53	178	399	817	5,549	3,545	1,741	622	105	4	-
3rd child	8,570	-	256	-	2	11	85	158	2,744	3,068	1,688	691	119	3	1
4th child	4,753	-	27	-	-	1	5	21	1,036	1,791	1,192	566	132	8	1
5th child	2,419	-	2	-	-	-	-	2	267	911	753	369	113	4	-
6th child	1,103	-	-	-	-	-	-	-	48	346	430	219	57	3	-
7th child	566	-	-	-	-	-	-	-	8	147	226	129	51	5	-
8th child and over	506	-	-	-	-	-	-	-	3	57	176	201	64	5	-
Not stated	273	-	42	3	-	5	8	26	76	82	50	15	7	1	-
Asian or Pacific Islander	251,089	76	7,053	273	629	1,126	1,974	3,051	29,436	70,539	85,317	48,100	9,863	644	61
1st child	113,394	75	5,777	264	586	989	1,614	2,324	17,532	38,740	34,407	14,059	2,590	190	24
2nd child	88,790	-	1,048	6	37	113	303	589	8,051	21,024	34,981	19,967	3,506	201	12
3rd child	31,022	-	144	-	1	15	32	96	2,586	6,778	10,349	8,977	2,075	105	8
4th child	10,118	-	14	-	-	1	4	9	765	2,268	3,199	2,963	840	63	6
5th child	3,584	-	1	-	-	-	-	1	208	852	1,105	1,013	368	33	4
6th child	1,444	-	1	-	-	1	-	-	46	321	445	418	195	18	-
7th child	662	-	-	-	-	-	-	-	10	101	226	219	97	7	2
8th child and over	689	-	-	-	-	-	-	-	8	55	205	267	129	22	3
Not stated	1,386	1	68	3	4	8	21	32	230	400	400	217	63	5	2

- = Quantity zero.

Table A-27. Live Births by Age of Mother, Live-Birth Order, and Hispanic Origin, 2009

(Number of children born alive to mother, includes births with stated origin of mother only.)

Live-birth order and origin of mother	All ages	Under 15 years	Total	15 years	16 years	17 years	18 years	19 years	20–24 years	25–29 years	30–34 years	35–39 years	40–44 years	45–49 years	50–54 years
HISPANIC[1]															
Total	999,548	2,073	136,263	6,638	15,369	26,011	38,306	49,939	274,726	270,641	195,729	97,261	21,638	1,168	49
1st child	351,023	2,022	106,312	6,338	14,115	22,107	29,374	34,378	120,025	68,735	36,142	14,413	3,152	209	13
2nd child	297,931	40	24,898	247	1,147	3,447	7,595	12,462	97,700	91,236	55,578	23,807	4,432	229	11
3rd child	195,062	-	3,838	10	37	296	1,029	2,466	40,160	66,346	53,837	25,827	4,848	198	8
4th child	92,216	-	431	-	5	20	96	310	11,732	28,539	29,924	17,422	3,958	200	10
5th child	34,771	-	45	-	-	3	6	36	2,698	9,494	11,632	8,430	2,343	124	5
6th child	13,374	-	8	-	1	3	-	4	575	3,136	4,525	3,710	1,338	81	1
7th child	5,303	-	3	-	-	-	2	1	123	1,019	1,762	1,625	723	48	-
8th child and over	3,772	-	-	-	-	-	-	-	47	433	1,123	1,388	710	71	-
Not stated	6,096	11	728	43	64	135	204	282	1,666	1,703	1,206	639	134	8	1
Mexican	645,297	1,425	91,992	4,683	10,668	17,852	25,892	32,897	179,938	174,816	123,341	60,360	12,805	605	15
1st child	211,864	1,392	71,248	4,472	9,791	15,124	19,628	22,233	74,100	38,769	18,083	6,794	1,409	66	3
2nd child	189,133	27	17,372	177	811	2,430	5,362	8,592	66,457	58,650	32,040	12,394	2,109	80	4
3rd child	133,853	-	2,645	6	26	210	729	1,674	27,959	46,426	37,036	16,894	2,791	100	2
4th child	66,216	-	305	-	4	16	64	221	8,172	20,179	21,901	12,808	2,723	125	3
5th child	25,029	-	32	-	-	3	3	26	1,867	6,658	8,388	6,292	1,700	90	2
6th child	9,494	-	4	-	-	2	-	2	383	2,189	3,200	2,683	976	58	1
7th child	3,788	-	1	-	-	-	1	-	82	707	1,256	1,188	523	31	-
8th child and over	2,614	-	-	-	-	-	-	-	34	295	748	969	514	54	-
Not stated	3,306	6	385	28	36	67	105	149	884	943	689	338	60	1	-
Puerto Rican	68,486	141	11,162	467	1,143	2,006	3,159	4,387	21,320	17,457	11,611	5,440	1,273	79	3
1st child	27,781	135	8,909	450	1,063	1,734	2,496	3,166	9,714	4,921	2,687	1,111	285	18	1
2nd child	20,326	4	1,875	15	76	247	572	965	7,218	5,682	3,587	1,621	314	24	1
3rd child	11,474	-	276	-	2	9	67	198	3,004	3,891	2,716	1,279	291	17	-
4th child	5,047	-	30	-	-	-	8	22	956	1,760	1,422	688	184	6	1
5th child	2,008	-	3	-	-	-	1	2	243	708	623	353	73	5	-
6th child	847	-	1	-	-	-	-	1	56	266	293	173	53	5	-
7th child	330	-	1	-	-	-	1	-	7	94	110	88	29	1	-
8th child and over	280	-	-	-	-	-	-	-	-	37	115	90	35	3	-
Not stated	393	2	67	2	2	16	14	33	122	98	58	37	9	-	-
Cuban	16,641	4	1,153	29	90	165	330	539	3,960	4,292	4,079	2,536	569	44	4
1st child	7,775	4	966	28	84	139	285	430	2,423	2,022	1,497	706	141	16	-
2nd child	5,795	-	159	1	6	23	37	92	1,149	1,482	1,669	1,110	215	11	-
3rd child	2,087	-	13	-	-	1	4	8	267	542	633	497	124	10	1
4th child	580	-	2	-	-	-	-	2	79	141	174	131	48	3	2
5th child	181	-	1	-	-	-	-	1	16	51	41	46	23	2	1
6th child	66	-	-	-	-	-	-	-	3	15	22	16	10	-	-
7th child	20	-	-	-	-	-	-	-	1	2	7	8	2	-	-
8th child and over	23	-	-	-	-	-	-	-	-	2	8	10	3	-	-
Not stated	114	-	12	-	-	2	4	6	22	35	28	12	3	2	-
Central and South American	148,647	175	11,488	441	1,128	2,032	3,237	4,650	33,950	42,788	36,269	18,892	4,766	308	11
1st child	54,578	174	9,210	413	1,045	1,741	2,598	3,413	17,303	13,832	9,168	3,918	896	71	6
2nd child	47,913	-	1,879	19	71	246	533	1,010	11,334	15,423	12,111	5,845	1,241	78	2
3rd child	26,817	-	263	2	2	23	68	168	3,843	8,547	8,434	4,580	1,097	52	1
4th child	11,285	-	26	-	1	2	9	14	947	3,292	3,885	2,385	701	48	1
5th child	4,110	-	2	-	-	-	-	2	175	966	1,501	1,081	365	20	-
6th child	1,621	-	-	-	-	-	-	-	27	260	586	531	202	15	-
7th child	608	-	1	-	-	-	-	1	6	69	196	211	112	13	-
8th child and over	453	-	-	-	-	-	-	-	5	30	117	184	108	9	-
Not stated	1,262	1	107	7	9	20	29	42	310	369	271	157	44	2	1
Other and Unknown Hispanic	120,477	328	20,468	1,018	2,340	3,956	5,688	7,466	35,558	31,288	20,429	10,033	2,225	132	16
1st child	49,025	317	15,979	975	2,132	3,369	4,367	5,136	16,485	9,191	4,707	1,884	421	38	3
2nd child	34,764	9	3,613	35	183	501	1,091	1,803	11,542	9,999	6,171	2,837	553	36	4
3rd child	20,831	-	641	2	7	53	161	418	5,087	6,940	5,018	2,577	545	19	4
4th child	9,088	-	68	-	-	2	15	51	1,578	3,167	2,542	1,410	302	18	3
5th child	3,443	-	7	-	-	-	2	5	397	1,111	1,079	658	182	7	2
6th child	1,346	-	3	-	1	1	-	1	106	406	424	307	97	3	-
7th child	557	-	-	-	-	-	-	-	27	147	193	130	57	3	-
8th child and over	402	-	-	-	-	-	-	-	8	69	135	135	50	5	-
Not stated	1,021	2	157	6	17	30	52	52	328	258	160	95	18	3	-

– = Quantity zero.
[1] Persons of Hispanic origin may be of any race.

Table A-28. Live Births by Race of Mother, by State and Territory, 2009

(Number.)

Area	All races	White	Black	American Indian or Alaska Native	Asian or Pacific Islander
UNITED STATES[1]	4,130,665	3,173,293	657,618	48,665	251,089
Alabama	62,475	41,975	19,294	217	989
Alaska	11,324	6,935	479	2,960	950
Arizona	92,798	78,582	4,505	6,269	3,442
Arkansas	39,808	31,207	7,718	214	669
California	527,020	418,252	33,622	3,669	71,477
Colorado	68,628	61,883	3,430	771	2,544
Connecticut	38,896	30,929	5,460	275	2,232
Delaware	11,559	7,785	3,235	22	517
District of Columbia	9,040	3,284	5,325	28	403
Florida	221,394	157,327	55,994	644	7,429
Georgia	141,377	83,455	51,570	360	5,992
Hawaii	18,887	5,679	501	105	12,602
Idaho	23,737	22,660	198	458	421
Illinois	171,163	131,016	30,267	269	9,611
Indiana	86,673	74,109	10,437	130	1,997
Iowa	39,701	36,322	2,063	256	1,060
Kansas	41,396	36,384	3,270	375	1,367
Kentucky	57,551	50,726	5,668	82	1,075
Louisiana	64,973	37,936	25,322	452	1,263
Maine	13,470	12,706	403	125	236
Maryland	75,059	43,410	26,061	201	5,387
Massachusetts	75,016	59,228	9,580	173	6,035
Michigan	117,294	89,803	22,576	824	4,091
Minnesota	70,646	56,720	6,858	1,755	5,313
Mississippi	42,901	22,943	19,115	339	504
Missouri	78,905	64,369	12,133	375	2,028
Montana	12,257	10,509	76	1,537	135
Nebraska	26,936	23,491	2,025	598	822
Nevada	37,612	30,168	3,785	515	3,144
New Hampshire	13,377	12,512	265	23	577
New Jersey	110,331	78,136	20,350	178	11,667
New Mexico	29,000	23,854	649	3,999	498
New York	248,110	174,867	49,213	756	23,274
North Carolina	126,845	90,339	30,571	1,828	4,107
North Dakota	9,001	7,622	185	1,035	159
Ohio	144,841	115,804	25,206	288	3,543
Oklahoma	54,553	41,523	5,275	6,391	1,364
Oregon	47,132	42,238	1,244	919	2,731
Pennsylvania	146,434	113,170	26,429	413	6,422
Rhode Island	11,442	9,233	1,369	178	662
South Carolina	60,620	38,740	20,439	206	1,235
South Dakota	11,934	9,510	253	2,018	153
Tennessee	82,211	61,386	18,399	319	2,107
Texas	401,977	334,634	49,212	1,175	16,956
Utah	53,887	50,800	687	764	1,636
Vermont	6,110	5,897	85	17	111
Virginia	105,059	73,563	23,533	179	7,784
Washington	89,313	72,794	4,962	2,407	9,150
West Virginia	21,268	20,261	841	20	146
Wisconsin	70,843	59,205	7,410	1,258	2,970
Wyoming	7,881	7,412	71	296	102
Puerto Rico	44,773	39,740	5,025	—	—
Virgin Islands	1,687	469	1,193	6	19
Guam	3,417	256	34	3	3,124
American Samoa	1,340	4	-	1	1,335
Northern Marianas	1,109	12	-	-	1,097

— = Data not available.
- = Quantity zero.
[1] Excludes data for the territories.

Table A-29. Live Births by Hispanic Origin of Mother and by Race for Mothers of Non-Hispanic Origin, by State and Territory, 2009

(Number.)

Area	All origins	Total	Hispanic[1]					Non-Hispanic			Not stated
			Mexican	Puerto Rican	Cuban	Central and South American	Other and unknown Hispanic	Total	White	Black	
UNITED STATES[2]	4,130,665	999,548	645,297	68,486	16,641	148,647	120,477	3,101,330	2,212,552	609,584	29,787
Alabama	62,475	5,134	3,467	162	34	1,357	114	57,316	36,902	19,230	25
Alaska	11,324	695	334	85	13	94	169	10,230	6,018	408	399
Arizona	92,798	39,168	36,750	353	81	987	997	52,963	40,037	4,135	667
Arkansas	39,808	4,202	3,318	60	16	725	83	35,477	26,973	7,635	129
California	527,020	270,236	219,865	1,987	696	23,733	23,955	247,640	146,402	31,090	9,144
Colorado	68,628	20,681	14,359	353	83	1,055	4,831	47,192	41,169	3,120	755
Connecticut	38,896	8,588	1,141	4,586	86	2,573	202	30,242	22,800	4,970	66
Delaware	11,559	1,647	801	356	12	413	65	9,891	6,183	3,176	21
District of Columbia	9,040	1,514	170	32	11	1,124	177	7,341	2,337	4,718	185
Florida	221,394	61,988	14,558	11,736	11,342	21,387	2,965	158,552	100,577	50,723	854
Georgia	141,377	24,594	16,299	1,011	266	4,420	2,598	113,375	61,727	46,235	3,408
Hawaii	18,887	3,135	669	871	9	173	1,413	15,725	4,603	411	27
Idaho	23,737	3,680	3,038	42	7	159	434	19,894	19,053	137	163
Illinois	171,163	40,394	33,481	2,574	187	1,617	2,535	130,683	90,930	29,925	86
Indiana	86,673	8,078	6,445	352	37	657	587	78,407	66,325	10,077	188
Iowa	39,701	3,210	2,461	73	12	487	177	36,484	33,382	1,907	7
Kansas	41,396	6,795	4,975	158	27	857	778	34,508	29,856	3,063	93
Kentucky	57,551	2,986	1,998	187	135	467	199	54,527	48,054	5,436	38
Louisiana	64,973	3,557	1,651	164	108	1,468	166	61,405	34,583	25,144	11
Maine	13,470	198	42	26	3	46	81	13,250	12,504	392	22
Maryland	75,059	10,612	1,984	447	73	7,469	639	64,295	34,012	24,986	152
Massachusetts	75,016	11,009	490	4,842	60	5,448	169	63,753	50,345	7,227	254
Michigan	117,294	7,913	5,242	440	91	711	1,429	108,999	82,093	22,145	382
Minnesota	70,646	5,625	3,845	128	39	962	651	64,110	51,288	6,475	911
Mississippi	42,901	1,513	739	23	8	324	419	41,361	21,428	19,096	27
Missouri	78,905	4,289	2,992	165	59	579	494	74,519	60,170	12,026	97
Montana	12,257	425	282	16	1	29	97	11,486	9,996	65	346
Nebraska	26,936	4,265	3,144	62	26	737	296	22,664	19,782	1,759	7
Nevada	37,612	14,347	11,428	302	241	1,669	707	22,971	15,934	3,599	294
New Hampshire	13,377	552	99	142	10	134	167	12,737	11,954	217	88
New Jersey	110,331	29,004	6,380	6,718	738	12,873	2,295	80,976	52,163	17,135	351
New Mexico	29,000	16,158	6,717	97	46	313	8,985	12,641	8,080	513	201
New York	248,110	59,801	11,675	14,792	522	17,845	14,967	183,906	119,526	40,970	4,403
North Carolina	126,845	20,169	13,845	1,159	247	4,648	270	106,621	70,430	30,314	55
North Dakota	9,001	312	213	23	5	19	52	8,578	7,319	162	111
Ohio	144,841	6,895	3,495	1,283	70	1,113	934	137,203	109,760	23,837	743
Oklahoma	54,553	7,270	6,075	175	21	634	365	47,189	34,720	5,083	94
Oregon	47,132	9,701	8,491	130	56	538	486	37,304	32,788	1,143	127
Pennsylvania	146,434	14,113	2,793	6,906	185	1,678	2,551	130,773	103,297	21,480	1,548
Rhode Island	11,442	2,508	136	674	23	777	898	8,521	6,978	906	413
South Carolina	60,620	5,562	3,577	401	76	1,107	401	54,689	33,978	19,478	369
South Dakota	11,934	476	292	28	3	95	58	11,449	9,117	247	9
Tennessee	82,211	7,433	4,830	310	93	1,563	637	74,716	55,444	17,405	62
Texas	401,977	201,227	150,989	1,700	508	12,418	35,612	200,100	137,594	45,482	650
Utah	53,887	8,773	6,547	135	22	1,102	967	45,109	42,386	548	5
Vermont	6,110	94	25	22	1	22	24	6,005	5,803	76	11
Virginia	105,059	13,688	3,174	911	99	8,441	1,063	91,144	60,405	23,019	227
Washington	89,313	17,189	13,630	413	89	1,113	1,944	70,851	56,567	4,084	1,273
West Virginia	21,268	231	87	35	4	45	60	20,960	19,965	831	77
Wisconsin	70,843	6,934	5,594	818	57	387	78	63,860	52,462	7,288	49
Wyoming	7,881	980	665	21	3	55	236	6,738	6,353	56	163
Puerto Rico	44,773	43,295	53	41,973	38	234	997	1,463	1,283	172	15
Virgin Islands	1,687	390	6	105	-	116	163	1,245	154	1,072	52
Guam	3,417	48	36	3	1	4	4	3,366	214	33	3
American Samoa	1,340	—	—	—	—	—	—	—	—	—	1,340
Northern Marianas	1,109	—	—	—	—	—	—	—	—	—	1,109

— = Data not available.
- = Quantity zero.
[1]Persons of Hispanic origin may be of any race.
[2]Excludes data for the territories.

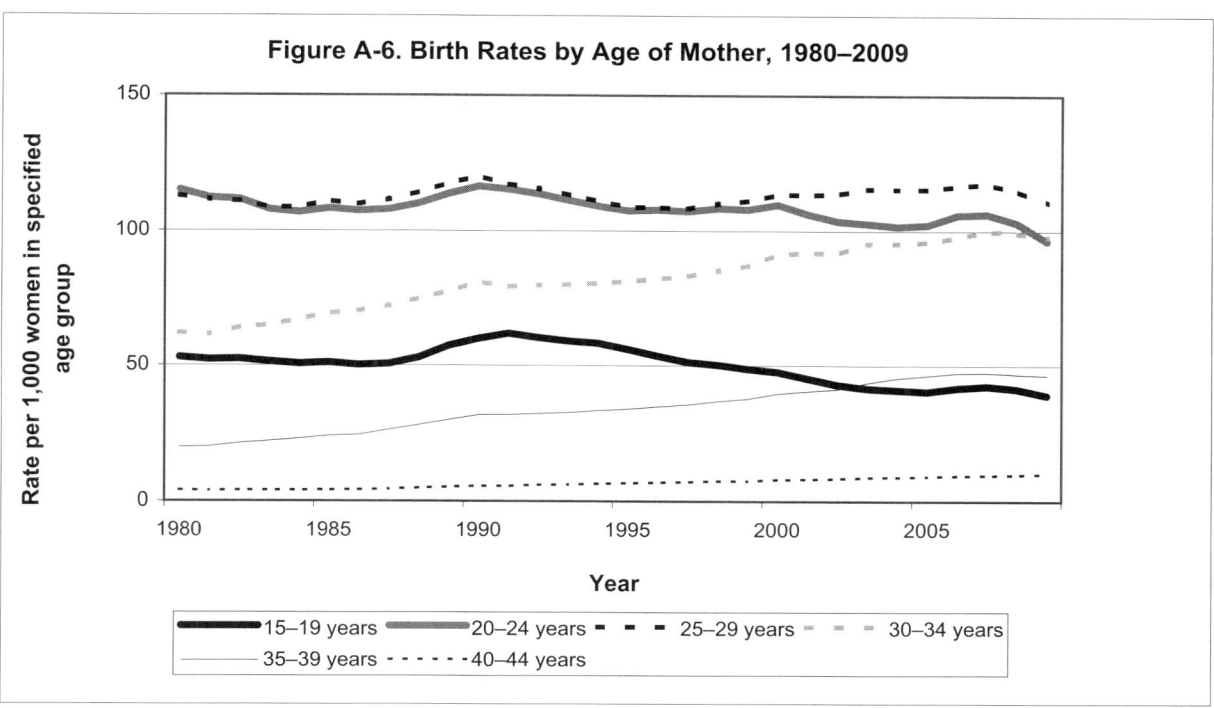

Figure A-6. Birth Rates by Age of Mother, 1980–2009

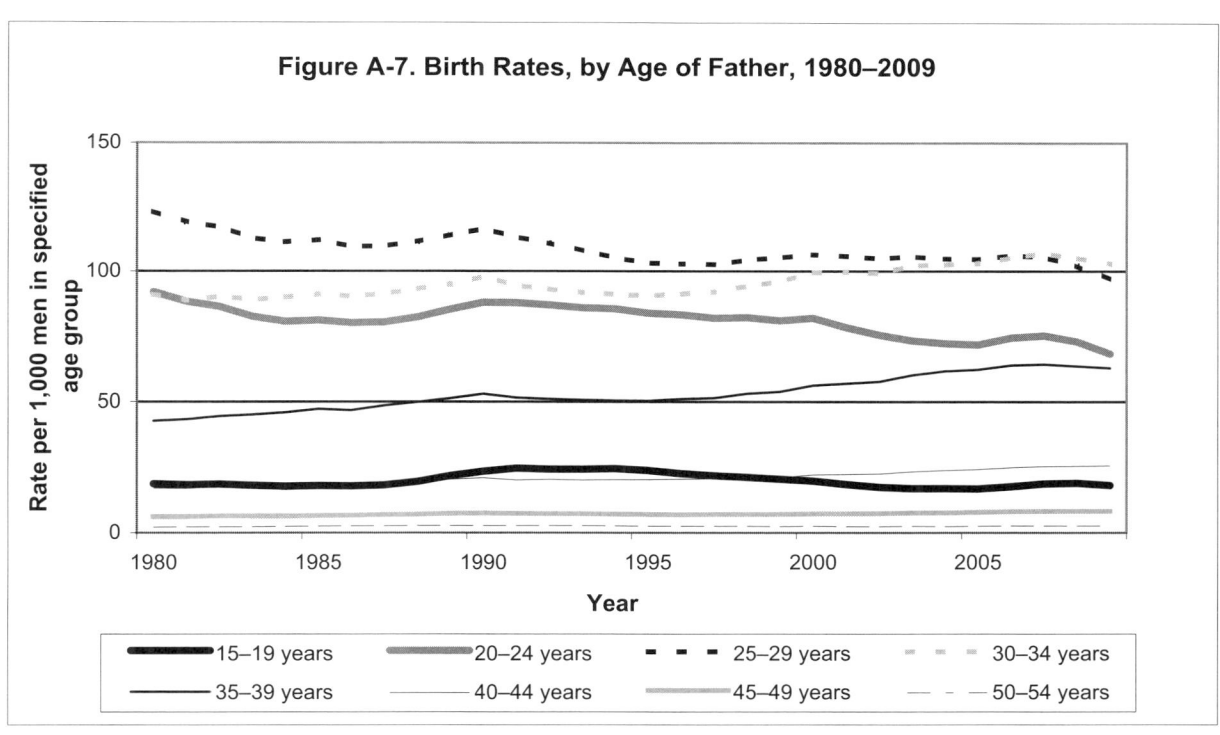

Figure A-7. Birth Rates, by Age of Father, 1980–2009

Table A-30. Birth Rates, by Age of Mother, Each State and Territory, 2009

(By place of residence. Fertility rates are births per 1,000 women aged 15–44 years estimated in each area; total fertility rates are sums of birth rates for 5-year age groups multiplied by 5; birth rates by age are births per 1,000 women in specified age group estimated in each area.)

Area	Birth rate	Fertility rate	Total fertility rate	10–14 years	15–19 years Total	15–17 years	18–19 years	20–24 years	25–29 years	30–34 years	35–39 years	40–44 years	45–49 years
United States[2]	13.5	66.7	2007.0	0.5	39.1	20.1	66.2	96.3	110.5	97.7	46.5	10.1	0.7
Alabama	13.3	65.7	1958.5	1.1	50.7	26.2	85.7	115.4	111.3	77.7	29.5	5.7	0.3
Alaska	16.2	78.3	2279.0	*	44.5	19.0	84.1	120.8	125.5	101.7	51.3	10.9	0.8
Arizona	14.1	71.5	2117.5	0.6	50.6	26.6	89.2	115.4	112.6	90.2	43.8	9.6	0.7
Arkansas	13.8	70.0	2077.0	0.8	59.2	29.3	102.7	138.0	113.4	71.4	27.5	4.9	0.2
California	14.3	68.5	2056.0	0.5	36.6	19.7	61.7	89.9	106.0	103.9	58.7	14.4	1.2
Colorado	13.7	66.8	1982.5	0.5	38.5	20.6	64.5	88.8	103.9	101.5	51.3	11.3	0.7
Connecticut	11.1	56.5	1801.0	0.2	21.0	10.6	35.3	60.4	97.0	111.6	56.6	12.4	1.0
Delaware	13.1	65.4	1997.0	*	35.3	18.3	57.7	102.6	113.0	93.6	44.5	8.9	0.8
District of Columbia	15.1	59.9	1736.5	1.9	47.7	38.4	55.0	67.6	63.4	83.6	64.0	17.3	1.8
Florida	11.9	63.6	1926.5	0.5	39.0	18.7	69.2	98.0	103.8	89.6	44.1	9.7	0.6
Georgia	14.4	67.7	2053.5	0.6	47.7	23.6	84.0	113.0	109.8	88.9	41.4	8.7	0.6
Hawaii	14.6	75.8	2232.5	*	40.9	18.4	75.3	108.6	112.5	105.3	63.0	15.0	0.9
Idaho	15.4	77.5	2273.5	*	35.9	16.9	61.5	125.5	138.9	102.9	42.0	8.5	0.7
Illinois	13.3	64.7	1942.5	0.4	36.1	19.1	60.3	81.1	104.2	105.2	50.0	10.8	0.7
Indiana	13.5	67.6	2028.0	0.4	42.5	20.9	73.2	108.0	122.9	89.8	34.6	6.9	0.5
Iowa	13.2	68.7	2072.5	0.3	32.1	15.8	53.1	88.0	138.6	108.3	39.4	7.3	0.5
Kansas	14.7	74.7	2192.0	0.4	43.8	20.7	76.3	105.4	131.9	106.9	41.2	8.4	0.4
Kentucky	13.3	66.6	2000.0	0.6	51.3	24.7	90.7	118.9	112.0	80.4	30.6	5.8	0.4
Louisiana	14.5	69.8	2022.0	0.8	52.7	27.1	88.9	120.1	112.0	79.2	32.6	6.7	0.3
Maine	10.2	54.8	1725.5	*	24.4	10.0	44.4	87.0	104.7	84.8	37.0	6.7	*
Maryland	13.2	63.8	1959.0	0.5	31.3	16.3	52.8	83.3	103.3	105.5	55.0	12.0	0.9
Massachusetts	11.4	55.3	1712.0	0.3	19.6	10.6	30.4	52.3	85.4	111.3	60.4	12.3	0.8
Michigan	11.8	59.8	1851.5	0.4	32.7	16.0	56.3	83.4	112.6	95.8	37.4	7.6	0.4
Minnesota	13.4	67.5	2044.5	0.2	24.3	11.5	41.8	76.4	127.9	119.2	50.2	10.1	0.6
Mississippi	14.5	70.9	2069.0	1.4	64.2	35.2	105.9	130.3	111.8	72.3	28.1	5.4	0.3
Missouri	13.2	66.2	1968.0	0.4	41.6	19.5	74.1	105.6	114.2	89.0	35.9	6.6	0.3
Montana	12.6	67.2	1982.0	*	38.5	18.8	65.8	92.6	118.3	99.3	39.6	7.6	*
Nebraska	15.0	76.4	2270.0	0.5	34.6	17.4	57.3	93.8	144.7	122.8	48.2	8.9	0.5
Nevada	14.2	71.2	2128.5	0.6	47.4	24.5	87.6	116.7	111.4	91.2	46.6	11.1	0.7
New Hampshire	10.1	51.9	1674.0	*	16.4	7.1	28.5	62.0	102.5	102.4	43.2	7.9	*
New Jersey	12.7	64.5	2000.5	0.3	22.7	11.1	41.4	71.2	106.3	123.0	62.4	13.3	0.9
New Mexico	14.4	73.4	2141.0	0.8	63.9	36.1	104.1	124.4	112.4	78.8	38.3	9.0	0.6
New York	12.7	61.7	1871.0	0.4	24.4	12.2	41.3	74.4	97.7	104.5	57.8	13.9	1.1
North Carolina	13.5	66.3	2016.5	0.6	44.9	23.1	74.8	107.5	110.7	90.8	40.3	8.1	0.4
North Dakota	13.9	70.8	2124.5	*	27.9	13.2	43.4	74.5	145.9	121.6	46.3	8.4	*
Ohio	12.5	63.8	1938.0	0.5	38.9	18.7	68.3	101.9	112.7	88.9	37.1	7.1	0.5
Oklahoma	14.8	74.8	2157.5	0.8	60.1	30.0	103.8	125.9	122.6	82.0	33.5	5.2	0.4
Oregon	12.3	62.4	1847.0	0.3	33.1	16.1	57.6	84.8	102.4	93.6	45.0	9.6	0.6
Pennsylvania	11.6	60.1	1856.0	0.4	29.3	15.6	47.4	79.8	107.7	99.7	44.9	8.9	0.5
Rhode Island	10.9	53.6	1670.0	*	26.8	17.9	36.7	66.5	93.5	90.9	45.3	10.1	0.6
South Carolina	13.3	66.3	1994.0	0.6	49.1	24.6	82.8	114.6	109.3	82.0	36.0	6.8	0.4
South Dakota	14.7	77.7	2289.5	*	38.4	18.5	65.7	105.2	146.0	116.2	42.7	8.6	*
Tennessee	13.1	64.7	1952.5	0.6	50.6	24.0	90.8	117.1	106.3	76.6	32.8	6.1	0.4
Texas	16.2	77.6	2299.5	1.0	60.7	34.3	100.5	123.9	120.7	97.3	45.7	10.0	0.6
Utah	19.4	88.4	2474.0	0.3	30.7	16.2	49.3	110.5	163.4	127.2	51.7	10.2	0.8
Vermont	9.8	50.8	1620.0	*	17.4	6.7	29.8	60.9	96.9	97.4	41.9	8.7	*
Virginia	13.3	64.4	1947.5	0.4	31.0	14.6	52.6	86.7	105.0	104.2	50.7	10.7	0.8
Washington	13.4	66.4	1970.5	0.3	31.9	14.5	58.7	92.2	107.7	100.5	49.3	11.4	0.8
West Virginia	11.7	61.7	1863.5	0.4	49.8	24.7	84.2	113.2	107.2	70.6	26.5	4.6	0.4
Wisconsin	12.5	63.7	1953.0	0.3	29.4	14.3	49.5	77.5	123.8	108.8	42.4	7.9	0.5
Wyoming	14.5	75.0	2142.5	*	45.0	19.5	81.2	115.5	129.0	94.8	35.4	8.3	*
Puerto Rico	11.3	53.3	1592.5	1.1	54.7	33.8	85.9	106.5	79.0	49.9	22.5	4.6	0.2
Virgin Islands	15.4	75.7	2381.0	*	51.5	22.2	98.9	135.8	133.7	93.0	50.7	10.0	*
Guam	19.2	87.9	2666.0	*	50.8	28.4	85.4	142.9	148.0	113.3	60.1	16.8	*
American Samoa	20.4	90.4	2860.5	*	35.2	13.2	74.3	136.2	148.5	147.3	80.4	24.5	*
Northern Marianas	21.5	77.1	2267.5	*	50.2	31.9	78.9	89.1	76.8	106.8	94.5	34.0	*

* = Figure does not meet standards of reliability or percision; birth rates based on fewer than 20 births.
[1] Rates computed by relating births to women aged 45 and over to women aged 45–49.
[2] Excludes data for the territories.

Table A-31. Birth Rates by Age of Mother, Live-Birth Order, and Race of Mother, 2009

(Live births per 1,000 women in specified age and racial group.)

Live-birth order and race of mother	15–44 years	10–14 Years	Age of mother 15–19 years			20–24 years	25–29 years	30–34 years	35–39 years	40–44 years	45–49 years[1]
			Total	15–17 years	18–19 years						
All Races	66.7	0.5	39.1	20.1	66.2	96.3	110.5	97.7	46.5	10.1	0.7
1st child	27.0	0.5	31.7	18.3	51.0	47.6	40.6	28.0	10.6	2.2	0.2
2nd child	21.0	0.0	6.3	1.7	12.8	31.8	36.6	33.6	15.1	2.9	0.2
3rd child	11.0	*	0.9	0.1	2.1	12.3	20.5	20.2	10.7	2.1	0.1
4th child	4.6	*	0.1	0.0	0.3	3.5	8.3	9.3	5.4	1.3	0.1
5th child	1.7	*	0.0	*	0.0	0.8	2.9	3.7	2.4	0.7	0.0
6th and 7th child	1.0	*	0.0	*	*	0.2	1.4	2.3	1.7	0.6	0.0
8th child and over	0.3	*	*	*	*	0.0	0.2	0.6	0.7	0.4	0.0
White	66.0	0.4	35.7	18.0	61.0	92.5	112.1	100.3	46.7	9.9	0.7
1st child	26.6	0.4	29.3	16.4	47.6	46.6	41.8	28.6	10.5	2.2	0.2
2nd child	21.0	0.0	5.6	1.5	11.5	30.9	37.9	34.7	15.0	2.8	0.2
3rd child	11.1	*	0.8	0.1	1.7	11.2	20.7	21.3	10.9	2.0	0.1
4th child	4.5	*	0.1	0.0	0.2	2.9	8.0	9.6	5.6	1.2	0.1
5th child	1.6	*	0.0	*	0.0	0.6	2.6	3.6	2.4	0.7	0.0
6th and 7th child	0.9	*	*	*	*	0.1	1.1	2.1	1.7	0.6	0.0
8th child and over	0.3	*	*	*	*	0.0	0.1	0.4	0.7	0.4	0.0
Black	69.9	1.2	59.5	32.4	98.5	125.9	103.8	74.1	36.9	9.1	0.6
1st child	27.8	1.1	47.1	29.1	73.1	56.9	28.4	15.8	7.0	1.7	0.1
2nd child	19.8	0.0	10.3	3.1	20.6	40.7	32.1	21.4	10.0	2.2	0.1
3rd child	11.9	*	1.8	0.3	4.1	19.0	22.8	17.2	8.6	2.0	0.1
4th child	5.7	*	0.3	0.0	0.6	6.8	11.7	9.7	5.0	1.3	0.1
5th child	2.5	*	0.0	*	0.1	1.9	5.2	4.8	2.7	0.8	0.1
6th and 7th child	1.7	*	*	*	*	0.6	3.1	3.9	2.3	0.7	0.1
8th child and over	0.5	*	*	*	*	0.0	0.5	1.2	1.2	0.5	0.1
American Indian or Alaska Native	62.8	0.8	55.5	30.6	90.5	109.1	90.8	63.9	29.0	6.5	0.3
1st child	22.6	*	43.8	27.6	66.5	43.9	19.4	10	3.6	0.7	*
2nd child	16.9	*	9.8	2.8	19.6	37.5	25.6	15.1	5.6	1	*
3rd child	11.1	*	1.7	*	3.9	18.5	22.2	14.7	6.3	1.1	*
4th child	6.2	*	0.2	*	0.4	7	13	10.4	5.1	1.2	*
5th child	3.1	*	*	*	*	1.8	6.6	6.5	3.3	1	*
6th and 7th child	2.2	*	*	*	*	0.4	3.6	5.7	3.2	1	*
8th child and over	0.7	*	*	*	*	*	0.4	1.5	1.8	0.6	*
Asian or Pacific Islander	68.7	0.2	14.7	7.1	25.8	57.5	110.5	123.3	68.1	15.8	1.2
1st child	31.2	0.2	12.1	6.5	20.4	34.5	61.1	50.0	20.0	4.2	0.4
2nd child	24.4	*	2.2	0.5	4.6	15.9	33.1	50.8	28.4	5.6	0.4
3rd child	8.5	*	0.3	*	0.7	5.1	10.7	15.0	12.8	3.3	0.2
4th child	2.8	*	*	*	*	1.5	3.6	4.6	4.2	1.4	0.1
5th child	1.0	*	*	*	*	0.4	1.3	1.6	1.4	0.6	0.1
6th and 7th child	0.6	*	*	*	*	0.1	0.7	1.0	0.9	0.5	0.0
8th child and over	0.2	*	*	*	*	*	0.1	0.3	0.4	0.2	0.0

* = Figure does not meet standards of reliability or precision.
0.0 = Quantity more than zero but less than 0.05.
[1]Birth rates computed by relating births to women aged 45–54 years to women aged 45–49 years.

Table A-32. Birth Rates by Age and Race of Father, 1980–2009

(Rates are live births per 1,000 men in specified group.)

Year and race of father	Total, 15–54 years[1]	Age of father								
		15–19 years[2]	20–24 years	25–29 years	30–34 years	35–39 years	40–44 years	45–49 years	50–54 years	55 years and over
All Races[3]										
1980[4]	57.0	18.8	92.0	123.1	91.0	42.8	17.1	6.1	2.2	0.3
1981[4]	56.3	18.4	88.4	119.1	88.7	43.3	17.0	6.2	2.3	0.4
1982[4]	56.4	18.6	86.5	117.3	90.3	44.5	17.5	6.4	2.3	0.4
1983[4]	55.1	18.2	82.6	113.0	89.1	45.2	17.4	6.4	2.3	0.4
1984[4]	55.0	17.8	80.7	111.4	89.9	46.0	17.8	6.3	2.4	0.4
1985	55.6	18.0	81.2	112.3	91.1	47.3	18.1	6.6	2.5	0.4
1986	54.8	17.9	80.3	109.6	90.3	46.8	18.3	6.7	2.6	0.4
1987	55.0	18.3	80.5	109.9	91.2	48.6	19.0	6.9	2.6	0.4
1988	55.8	19.6	82.4	111.6	93.2	49.9	19.9	7.1	2.7	0.4
1989	57.2	21.9	85.4	114.3	94.8	51.3	20.4	7.4	2.7	0.6
1990	58.4	23.5	88.0	116.4	97.8	53.0	21.0	7.5	2.8	0.4
1991	56.8	24.7	87.9	113.5	94.3	51.6	20.2	7.4	2.7	0.4
1992	55.3	24.4	87.1	111.1	93.0	51.1	20.4	7.3	2.7	0.4
1993	53.7	24.4	86.0	108.1	91.7	50.7	20.2	7.3	2.7	0.4
1994	52.4	24.6	85.6	105.3	91.1	50.5	20.3	7.2	2.6	0.3
1995	51.0	23.9	83.9	103.2	90.7	50.4	20.3	7.0	2.5	0.3
1996	50.2	22.7	83.4	102.8	91.3	51.1	20.5	6.9	2.5	0.3
1997	49.4	21.9	82.1	102.6	92.0	51.5	20.7	7.0	2.5	0.3
1998	49.6	21.3	82.3	104.4	94.4	53.1	21.0	7.1	2.5	0.3
1999	49.2	20.6	81.1	105.3	95.9	53.9	21.1	7.0	2.4	0.3
2000	50.0	19.8	82.1	106.5	99.5	56.3	22.2	7.3	2.5	0.3
2001	49.0	18.5	78.5	105.8	99.6	57.0	22.3	7.3	2.4	0.3
2002	48.4	17.4	75.6	105.0	99.1	57.7	22.6	7.4	2.4	0.3
2003	48.9	16.9	73.5	105.7	102.2	60.2	23.4	7.6	2.5	0.3
2004	48.8	17.0	72.4	104.9	102.5	61.7	23.9	7.7	2.4	0.3
2005	48.7	16.8	71.9	104.7	103.1	62.4	24.2	7.9	2.5	0.3
2006	49.9	17.7	74.5	106.2	105.3	64.0	25.0	8.1	2.6	0.2
2007	50.3	18.7	75.3	105.6	107.0	64.4	25.4	8.2	2.6	0.4
2008	49.4	19.0	73.1	102.2	105.2	63.6	25.5	8.3	2.6	0.4
2009	47.9	18.2	68.4	96.9	102.8	62.9	25.7	8.2	2.6	0.3
White										
1980[4]	53.4	15.4	84.9	119.4	87.8	39.7	15.0	5.1	1.8	0.3
1981[4]	52.9	15.0	81.7	115.8	85.8	40.3	15.0	5.2	1.8	0.3
1982[4]	53.1	14.9	80.1	114.2	87.5	41.7	15.6	5.3	1.9	0.3
1983[4]	52.0	14.4	76.3	110.2	86.8	42.6	15.5	5.3	1.8	0.3
1984[4]	51.8	14.0	74.3	108.8	87.9	43.5	16.0	5.3	1.9	0.3
1985	52.6	14.0	74.7	109.9	89.5	44.8	16.3	5.6	1.9	0.3
1986	51.7	13.8	73.3	107.0	88.7	44.4	16.6	5.7	2.0	0.3
1987	51.6	13.9	72.8	107.0	89.5	46.2	17.3	5.9	2.0	0.3
1988	52.2	14.8	73.7	108.3	91.2	47.6	18.1	6.1	2.1	0.3
1989	53.3	16.7	75.9	110.8	93.0	49.1	18.7	6.3	2.1	0.4
1990	54.6	18.1	78.3	113.2	96.1	50.9	19.2	6.5	2.2	0.3
1991	53.1	19.0	78.4	110.2	92.8	49.6	18.5	6.5	2.2	0.3
1992	51.8	18.8	77.8	108.2	91.9	49.1	18.8	6.4	2.2	0.3
1993	50.3	18.9	77.2	105.5	90.7	48.9	18.7	6.4	2.2	0.2
1994	49.3	19.5	77.4	103.1	90.4	48.9	18.9	6.3	2.2	0.3
1995	48.4	19.4	77.0	101.7	90.4	49.1	19.1	6.2	2.1	0.2
1996	47.7	18.7	76.7	101.4	91.1	49.9	19.2	6.1	2.1	0.2
1997	46.8	18.0	75.3	100.9	91.7	50.2	19.3	6.2	2.1	0.3
1998	47.1	17.7	75.6	102.7	94.3	51.9	19.6	6.3	2.1	0.3
1999	46.9	17.3	74.7	104.1	96.2	52.7	19.8	6.3	2.1	0.3
2000	47.6	16.6	75.8	105.4	99.5	54.7	20.7	6.5	2.1	0.3
2001	46.9	15.5	73.1	105.4	99.9	55.7	20.8	6.5	2.0	0.3
2002	46.4	14.8	70.8	104.8	99.4	56.4	21.0	6.6	2.0	0.3
2003	47.1	14.3	69.2	106.1	102.8	58.9	21.9	6.7	2.1	0.3
2004	46.7	14.3	67.7	105.0	102.5	60.2	22.2	6.8	2.0	0.2
2005	46.6	14.2	66.9	104.6	103.1	60.7	22.5	6.8	2.1	0.2
2006	47.5	14.8	69.0	106.0	105.0	62.0	23.1	7.0	2.1	0.1
2007	47.8	15.7	69.5	105.3	106.5	62.1	23.4	7.1	2.1	0.3
2008	46.8	15.9	67.1	101.7	104.7	61.0	23.4	7.1	2.1	0.3
2009	45.4	15.4	62.4	96.6	102.5	60.3	23.5	7.0	2.1	0.3

Table A-32. Birth Rates by Age and Race of Father, 1980–2009—Continued

(Rates are live births per 1,000 men in specified group.)

Year and race of father	Total, 15–54 years[1]	Age of father								
		15–19 years[2]	20–24 years	25–29 years	30–34 years	35–39 years	40–44 years	45–49 years	50–54 years	55 years and over
Black										
1980[4]	83.0	40.1	145.3	152.8	109.6	62.0	31.2	13.6	5.9	1.1
1981[4]	80.4	38.9	138.4	145.6	104.3	61.3	29.7	13.3	5.7	1.2
1982[4]	79.5	40.3	133.4	141.2	103.6	61.1	29.6	13.9	6.0	1.2
1983[4]	77.2	40.7	129.1	134.4	99.0	59.6	29.6	13.5	6.0	1.2
1984[4]	76.7	40.9	128.0	132.2	98.3	58.4	29.3	13.3	6.1	1.2
1985	77.2	41.8	129.5	132.7	97.3	59.4	29.5	13.3	6.5	1.2
1986	77.2	42.6	131.4	131.6	97.4	58.0	29.1	13.5	6.7	1.3
1987	78.3	44.6	136.1	133.9	97.4	58.0	30.0	13.8	6.6	1.3
1988	80.7	48.1	144.1	137.9	100.0	58.0	30.6	14.3	6.9	1.4
1989	84.1	52.9	153.4	143.5	101.4	59.9	31.1	14.9	6.9	2.7
1990	84.9	55.2	158.2	144.9	103.2	60.4	31.1	15.0	7.1	1.4
1991	83.0	57.8	158.5	142.0	99.2	58.5	29.4	14.1	6.7	1.4
1992	80.4	57.0	157.1	138.6	95.8	56.7	28.4	13.7	6.1	1.4
1993	77.6	56.2	152.7	134.2	94.0	56.3	27.7	13.4	6.3	1.3
1994	74.0	54.1	149.1	129.6	91.4	53.8	26.4	12.8	5.8	1.1
1995	69.1	49.9	139.2	123.9	87.7	52.0	25.7	11.9	5.4	1.1
1996	67.2	46.7	137.6	123.9	87.0	51.8	25.7	11.3	5.3	1.1
1997	66.7	45.1	136.3	126.3	88.8	52.6	26.1	11.4	5.2	1.0
1998	66.8	42.8	137.0	130.3	90.9	54.0	26.7	11.6	5.0	1.0
1999	65.4	41.0	133.8	129.6	91.6	54.3	26.5	11.2	4.9	1.0
2000	66.2	39.6	135.5	131.0	95.2	56.9	28.4	11.7	5.0	1.0
2001	63.3	36.5	124.5	125.9	95.6	57.1	28.2	11.8	4.7	1.0
2002	61.2	33.3	116.2	123.6	94.0	57.8	28.5	12.0	4.7	0.9
2003	61.0	32.5	111.9	122.3	96.2	59.9	29.6	12.4	4.9	0.9
2004	61.7	32.7	111.6	122.7	98.7	61.8	30.4	12.7	4.9	0.8
2005	62.5	32.2	112.1	123.6	101.0	64.1	31.5	13.6	5.2	0.7
2006	65.0	34.3	117.0	126.7	105.3	67.6	32.9	14.1	5.5	0.6
2007	65.4	35.5	118.2	123.9	106.1	68.2	33.5	14.0	5.8	1.0
2008	64.4	35.8	115.8	119.0	103.5	68.3	34.0	14.4	5.7	1.0
2009	62.2	34.0	110.0	111.7	99.8	66.6	34.3	14.5	5.9	1.0

[1]Rates computed by relating total births, regardless of age of father, to men aged 15–54 years.
[2]Rates computed by relating births of fathers under 20 years of age to men aged 15–19 years.
[3]Includes races other than White and Black.
[4]Based on 100 percent of births in selected states and on a 50-percent sample of births in all other states.

NOTE: Race and Hispanic origin are reported separately on birth certificates.

Table A-33. Total Fertility Rates and Birth Rates by Age of Mother, 1970–2009, and by Age and Race of Mother, 1980–2009

(Live births per 1,000 women in specified group.)

Year and race	Total fertility rate	Age of mother									
		10–14 years	15–19 years			20–24 years	25–29 years	30–34 years	35–39 years	40–44 years	45–49 years[1]
			Total	15–17 years	18–19 years						
All Races[2]											
1970[3]	2,480.0	1.2	68.3	38.8	114.7	167.8	145.1	73.3	31.7	8.1	0.5
1971[3]	2,266.5	1.1	64.5	38.2	105.3	150.1	134.1	67.3	28.7	7.1	0.4
1972[4]	2,010.0	1.2	61.7	39.0	96.9	130.2	117.7	59.8	24.8	6.2	0.4
1973[4]	1,879.0	1.2	59.3	38.5	91.2	119.7	112.2	55.6	22.1	5.4	0.3
1974[4]	1,835.0	1.2	57.5	37.3	88.7	117.7	111.5	53.8	20.2	4.8	0.3
1975[4]	1,774.0	1.3	55.6	36.1	85.0	113.0	108.2	52.3	19.5	4.6	0.3
1976[4]	1,738.0	1.2	52.8	34.1	80.5	110.3	106.2	53.6	19.0	4.3	0.2
1977[4]	1,789.5	1.2	52.8	33.9	80.9	112.9	111.0	56.4	19.2	4.2	0.2
1978[4]	1,760.0	1.2	51.5	32.2	79.8	109.9	108.5	57.8	19.0	3.9	0.2
1979[4]	1,808.0	1.2	52.3	32.3	81.3	112.8	111.4	60.3	19.5	3.9	0.2
1980[4]	1,839.5	1.1	53.0	32.5	82.1	115.1	112.9	61.9	19.8	3.9	0.2
1981[4]	1,812.0	1.1	52.2	32.0	80.0	112.2	111.5	61.4	20.0	3.8	0.2
1982[4]	1,827.5	1.1	52.4	32.3	79.4	111.6	111.0	64.1	21.2	3.9	0.2
1983[4]	1,799.0	1.1	51.4	31.8	77.4	107.8	108.5	64.9	22.0	3.9	0.2
1984[4]	1,806.5	1.2	50.6	31.0	77.4	106.8	108.7	67.0	22.9	3.9	0.2
1985	1,844.0	1.2	51.0	31.0	79.6	108.3	111.0	69.1	24.0	4.0	0.2
1986	1,837.5	1.3	50.2	30.5	79.6	107.4	109.8	70.1	24.4	4.1	0.2
1987	1,872.0	1.3	50.6	31.7	78.5	107.9	111.6	72.1	26.3	4.4	0.2
1988	1,934.0	1.3	53.0	33.6	79.9	110.2	114.4	74.8	28.1	4.8	0.2
1989	2,014.0	1.4	57.3	36.4	84.2	113.8	117.6	77.4	29.9	5.2	0.2
1990	2,081.0	1.4	59.9	37.5	88.6	116.5	120.2	80.8	31.7	5.5	0.2
1991	2,062.5	1.4	61.8	38.6	94.0	115.3	117.2	79.2	31.9	5.5	0.2
1992	2,046.0	1.4	60.3	37.6	93.6	113.7	115.7	79.6	32.3	5.9	0.3
1993	2,019.5	1.4	59.0	37.5	91.1	111.3	113.2	79.9	32.7	6.1	0.3
1994	2,001.5	1.4	58.2	37.2	90.2	109.2	111.0	80.4	33.4	6.4	0.3
1995	1,978.0	1.3	56.0	35.5	87.7	107.5	108.8	81.1	34.0	6.6	0.3
1996	1,976.0	1.2	53.5	33.3	84.7	107.8	108.6	82.1	34.9	6.8	0.3
1997	1,971.0	1.1	51.3	31.4	82.1	107.3	108.3	83.0	35.7	7.1	0.4
1998	1,999.0	1.0	50.3	29.9	80.9	108.4	110.2	85.2	36.9	7.4	0.4
1999	2,007.5	0.9	48.8	28.2	79.1	107.9	111.2	87.1	37.8	7.4	0.4
2000	2,056.0	0.9	47.7	26.9	78.1	109.7	113.5	91.2	39.7	8.0	0.5
2001	2,034.0	0.8	45.3	24.7	76.1	106.2	113.4	91.9	40.6	8.1	0.5
2002	2,013.0	0.7	43.0	23.2	72.8	103.6	113.6	91.5	41.4	8.3	0.5
2003	2,042.5	0.6	41.6	22.4	70.7	102.6	115.6	95.1	43.8	8.7	0.5
2004	2,045.5	0.7	41.1	22.1	70.0	101.7	115.5	95.3	45.4	8.9	0.5
2005	2,053.5	0.7	40.5	21.4	69.9	102.2	115.5	95.8	46.3	9.1	0.6
2006	2,100.5	0.6	41.9	22.0	73.0	105.9	116.7	97.7	47.3	9.4	0.6
2007	2,122.0	0.6	42.5	22.1	73.9	106.3	117.5	99.9	47.5	9.5	0.6
2008	2,084.5	0.6	41.5	21.7	70.6	103.0	115.1	99.3	46.9	9.8	0.7
2009	2,007.0	0.5	39.1	20.1	66.2	96.3	110.5	97.7	46.5	10.1	0.7
White											
1980[4]	1,773.0	0.6	45.4	25.5	73.2	111.1	113.8	61.2	18.8	3.5	0.2
1981[4]	1,748.0	0.5	44.9	25.4	71.5	108.3	112.3	61.0	19.0	3.4	0.2
1982[4]	1,767.0	0.6	45.0	25.5	70.8	107.7	111.9	64.0	20.4	3.6	0.2
1983[4]	1,740.5	0.6	43.9	25.0	68.8	103.8	109.4	65.3	21.3	3.6	0.2
1984[4]	1,748.5	0.6	42.9	24.3	68.4	102.7	109.8	67.7	22.2	3.6	0.2
1985	1,787.0	0.6	43.3	24.4	70.4	104.1	112.3	69.9	23.3	3.7	0.2
1986	1,776.0	0.6	42.3	23.8	70.1	102.7	110.8	70.9	23.9	3.8	0.2
1987	1,804.5	0.6	42.5	24.6	68.9	102.3	112.3	73.0	25.9	4.1	0.2
1988	1,856.5	0.6	44.4	26.0	69.6	103.7	114.8	75.4	27.7	4.5	0.2
1989	1,931.0	0.7	47.9	28.1	72.9	106.9	117.8	78.1	29.7	4.9	0.2
1990	2,003.0	0.7	50.8	29.5	78.0	109.8	120.7	81.7	31.5	5.2	0.2
1991	1,988.0	0.8	52.6	30.5	83.3	108.8	118.0	80.2	31.8	5.2	0.2
1992	1,978.0	0.8	51.4	29.9	83.2	107.7	116.9	80.8	32.1	5.7	0.2
1993	1,961.5	0.8	50.6	30.0	81.5	106.1	114.7	81.3	32.6	5.9	0.3
1994	1,957.5	0.8	50.5	30.4	81.2	105.0	113.0	82.2	33.5	6.2	0.3

Table A-33. Total Fertility Rates and Birth Rates by Age of Mother, 1970–2009, and by Age and Race of Mother, 1980–2009—Continued

(Live births per 1,000 women in specified group.)

Year and race	Total fertility rate	Age of mother									
		10–14 years	15–19 years			20–24 years	25–29 years	30–34 years	35–39 years	40–44 years	45–49 years[1]
			Total	15–17 years	18–19 years						
1995	1,954.5	0.8	49.5	29.6	80.2	104.7	111.7	83.3	34.2	6.4	0.3
1996	1,960.5	0.7	47.5	28.0	77.6	105.3	111.7	84.6	35.3	6.7	0.3
1997	1,955.0	0.7	45.5	26.6	75.0	104.5	111.3	85.7	36.1	6.9	0.3
1998	1,991.0	0.6	44.9	25.6	74.1	105.4	113.6	88.5	37.5	7.3	0.4
1999	2,007.5	0.6	44.0	24.4	73.0	105.0	114.9	90.7	38.5	7.4	0.4
2000	2,051.0	0.6	43.2	23.3	72.3	106.6	116.7	94.6	40.2	7.9	0.4
2001	2,040.0	0.5	41.2	21.4	70.8	103.7	117.0	95.8	41.3	8.0	0.5
2002	2,027.5	0.5	39.4	20.5	68.0	101.6	117.4	95.5	42.4	8.2	0.5
2003	2,061.0	0.5	38.3	19.8	66.2	100.6	119.5	99.3	44.8	8.7	0.5
2004	2,054.5	0.5	37.7	19.5	65.0	99.2	118.6	99.1	46.4	8.9	0.5
2005	2,056.0	0.5	37.0	18.9	64.7	99.2	118.3	99.3	47.3	9.0	0.6
2006	2,096.0	0.5	38.2	19.4	67.5	102.5	119.1	100.9	48.2	9.2	0.6
2007	2,111.5	0.5	38.8	19.7	68.1	102.8	119.4	102.7	48.1	9.4	0.6
2008	2,066.5	0.4	37.8	19.3	65.0	99.2	116.6	101.8	47.2	9.7	0.6
2009	1,991.5	0.4	35.7	18.0	61.0	92.5	112.1	100.3	46.7	9.9	0.7
Black											
1980[4]	2,176.5	4.3	97.8	72.5	135.1	140.0	103.9	59.9	23.5	5.6	0.3
1981[4]	2,117.5	4.0	94.5	69.3	131.0	136.5	102.3	57.4	23.1	5.4	0.3
1982[4]	2,106.5	4.0	94.3	69.7	128.9	135.4	101.3	57.5	23.3	5.1	0.4
1983[4]	2,066.0	4.1	93.9	69.6	127.1	131.9	98.4	56.2	23.3	5.1	0.3
1984[4]	2,070.5	4.4	94.1	69.2	128.1	132.2	98.4	56.7	23.3	4.8	0.2
1985	2,109.0	4.5	95.4	69.3	132.4	135.0	100.2	57.9	23.9	4.6	0.3
1986	2,135.5	4.7	95.8	69.3	135.1	137.3	101.1	59.3	23.8	4.8	0.3
1987	2,198.0	4.8	97.6	72.1	135.8	142.7	104.3	60.6	24.6	4.8	0.2
1988	2,298.0	4.9	102.7	75.7	142.7	149.7	108.2	63.1	25.6	5.1	0.3
1989	2,432.5	5.1	111.5	81.9	151.9	156.8	114.4	66.3	26.7	5.4	0.3
1990	2,480.0	4.9	112.8	82.3	152.9	160.2	115.5	68.7	28.1	5.5	0.3
1991	2,462.0	4.7	114.8	83.5	157.6	159.7	112.0	67.3	28.2	5.5	0.2
1992	2,416.0	4.6	111.3	80.5	156.3	156.2	109.7	67.0	28.6	5.6	0.2
1993	2,351.0	4.5	107.3	78.9	150.2	150.2	106.4	66.6	29.0	5.9	0.3
1994	2,258.5	4.5	102.9	75.1	146.2	142.9	101.5	65.0	28.7	5.9	0.3
1995	2,127.5	4.1	94.4	68.5	135.0	133.7	95.6	63.0	28.4	6.0	0.3
1996	2,088.5	3.5	89.6	63.3	130.5	133.2	94.3	62.0	28.7	6.1	0.3
1997	2,091.5	3.1	86.3	59.3	127.7	135.2	95.0	62.6	29.3	6.5	0.3
1998	2,111.5	2.8	83.5	55.4	124.8	138.4	97.5	63.2	30.0	6.6	0.3
1999	2,082.5	2.5	79.1	50.5	120.6	137.9	97.3	62.7	30.2	6.5	0.3
2000	2,129.0	2.3	77.4	49.0	118.8	141.3	100.3	65.4	31.5	7.2	0.4
2001	2,051.0	2.0	71.8	43.9	114.0	133.2	99.2	64.8	31.6	7.2	0.4
2002	1,991.0	1.8	66.6	40.0	107.6	127.1	99.0	64.4	31.5	7.4	0.4
2003	1,999.0	1.6	63.8	38.2	103.7	126.1	100.4	66.5	33.2	7.7	0.5
2004	2,032.5	1.6	63.3	37.2	104.4	127.7	103.6	67.9	34.0	7.9	0.5
2005	2,070.5	1.7	62.0	35.5	104.9	129.9	105.9	70.3	35.3	8.5	0.5
2006	2,154.5	1.5	64.6	36.6	110.2	135.8	109.4	74.0	36.6	8.5	0.5
2007	2,168.0	1.5	64.9	36.1	110.7	135.9	109.6	75.4	36.9	8.8	0.6
2008	2,132.0	1.4	63.4	35.2	105.6	132.3	107.2	75.6	37.0	8.9	0.6
2009	2,055.5	1.2	59.5	32.4	98.5	125.9	103.8	74.1	36.9	9.1	0.6
American Indian or Alaska Native											
1980[4]	2,165.0	1.9	82.2	51.5	129.5	143.7	106.6	61.8	28.1	8.2	*
1981[4]	2,092.5	2.1	78.4	49.7	121.5	141.2	105.6	58.9	25.2	6.6	*
1982[4]	2,215.0	1.4	83.5	52.6	127.6	148.1	115.8	60.9	26.9	6.0	*
1983[4]	2,182.0	1.9	84.2	55.2	121.4	145.5	113.7	58.9	25.5	6.4	*
1984[4]	2,137.5	1.7	81.5	50.7	124.7	142.4	109.2	60.5	26.3	5.6	*
1985	2,129.5	1.7	79.2	47.7	124.1	139.1	109.6	62.6	27.4	6.0	*
1986	2,083.0	1.8	78.1	48.7	125.3	138.8	107.9	60.7	23.8	5.3	*
1987	2,100.5	1.7	77.2	48.8	122.2	140.0	107.9	63.0	24.4	5.6	*
1988	2,155.0	1.7	77.5	49.7	121.1	145.2	110.9	64.5	25.6	5.3	*
1989	2,248.5	1.5	82.7	51.6	128.9	152.4	114.2	64.8	27.4	6.4	*

Table A-33. Total Fertility Rates and Birth Rates by Age of Mother, 1970–2009, and by Age and Race of Mother, 1980–2009—*Continued*

(Live births per 1,000 women in specified group.)

Year and race	Total fertility rate	Age of mother									
		10–14 years	15–19 years			20–24 years	25–29 years	30–34 years	35–39 years	40–44 years	45–49 years[1]
			Total	15–17 years	18–19 years						
1990	2,184.5	1.6	81.1	48.5	129.3	148.7	110.3	61.5	27.5	5.9	*
1991	2,142.5	1.6	84.1	51.9	134.2	143.8	105.6	60.8	26.4	5.8	0.4
1992	2,135.5	1.6	82.4	52.3	130.5	142.3	107.0	61.0	26.7	5.9	*
1993	2,048.5	1.4	79.8	51.5	126.3	134.2	103.5	59.5	25.5	5.6	*
1994	1,950.0	1.8	76.4	48.4	123.7	126.5	98.2	56.6	24.8	5.4	0.3
1995	1,878.5	1.6	72.9	44.6	122.2	123.1	91.6	56.5	24.3	5.5	*
1996	1,855.0	1.6	68.2	42.7	113.3	123.5	91.1	56.5	24.4	5.5	*
1997	1,834.5	1.5	65.2	41.0	107.1	122.5	91.6	56.0	24.4	5.4	0.3
1998	1,851.0	1.5	64.7	39.7	106.9	125.1	92.0	56.8	24.6	5.3	*
1999	1,783.5	1.4	59.9	36.5	98.0	120.7	90.6	53.8	24.3	5.7	0.3
2000	1,772.5	1.1	58.3	34.1	97.1	117.2	91.8	55.5	24.6	5.7	0.3
2001	1,746.5	1.0	56.3	31.4	94.8	115.0	90.4	55.9	24.7	5.7	0.3
2002	1,735.0	0.9	53.8	30.7	89.2	112.6	91.8	56.4	25.4	5.8	0.3
2003	1,731.5	1.0	53.1	30.6	87.3	110.0	93.5	57.4	25.4	5.5	0.4
2004	1,734.5	0.9	52.5	30.0	87.0	109.7	92.8	58.0	26.8	6.0	0.2
2005	1,750.0	0.9	52.7	30.5	87.6	109.2	93.8	60.1	27.0	6.0	0.3
2006	1,829.0	0.9	55.0	30.7	93.0	115.4	97.8	61.8	28.4	6.1	0.4
2007	1,866.5	0.9	59.3	31.8	101.6	116.8	96.4	64.0	29.5	6.1	0.3
2008	1,843.5	0.9	58.4	32.5	96.6	115.6	94.4	63.8	28.8	6.4	0.4
2009	1,779.5	0.8	55.5	30.6	90.5	109.1	90.8	63.9	29.0	6.5	0.3
Asian or Other Pacific Islander											
1980[4]	1,953.5	0.3	26.2	12.0	46.2	93.3	127.4	96.0	38.3	8.5	0.7
1981[4]	1,976.0	0.3	28.5	13.4	49.5	96.4	129.1	93.4	38.0	8.6	0.9
1982[4]	2,015.5	0.4	29.4	14.0	50.8	98.9	130.9	94.4	39.2	8.8	1.1
1983[4]	1,943.5	0.5	26.1	12.9	44.5	94.0	126.2	93.3	39.4	8.2	1.0
1984[4]	1,892.0	0.5	24.2	12.6	40.7	86.7	124.3	92.4	40.6	8.7	1.0
1985	1,885.0	0.4	23.8	12.5	40.8	83.6	123.0	93.6	42.7	8.7	1.2
1986	1,836.0	0.5	22.8	12.1	38.8	79.2	119.9	92.6	41.9	9.3	1.0
1987	1,886.0	0.6	22.4	12.6	37.0	79.7	122.7	97.0	44.2	9.5	1.1
1988	1,983.5	0.6	24.2	13.6	39.6	80.7	128.0	104.4	47.5	10.3	1.0
1989	1,947.5	0.6	25.6	15.0	40.4	78.8	124.0	102.3	47.0	10.2	1.0
1990	2,002.5	0.7	26.4	16.0	40.2	79.2	126.3	106.5	49.6	10.7	1.1
1991	1,928.0	0.8	27.3	16.3	42.2	73.8	118.9	103.3	49.2	11.2	1.1
1992	1,894.5	0.7	26.5	15.4	41.9	71.7	114.6	102.7	50.7	11.1	0.9
1993	1,841.5	0.7	26.5	16.1	41.2	68.1	110.3	101.2	49.4	11.2	0.9
1994	1,834.0	0.7	26.6	16.3	41.3	66.4	108.0	102.2	50.4	11.5	1.0
1995	1,795.5	0.7	25.5	15.6	40.1	64.2	103.7	102.3	50.1	11.8	0.8
1996	1,787.0	0.6	23.5	14.7	36.8	63.5	102.8	104.1	50.2	11.9	0.8
1997	1,757.5	0.5	22.3	14.0	34.9	61.2	101.6	102.5	51.0	11.5	0.9
1998	1,731.5	0.5	22.2	13.8	34.5	59.2	98.7	101.6	51.4	11.8	0.9
1999	1,754.5	0.4	21.4	12.4	33.9	58.9	100.8	104.3	52.9	11.3	0.9
2000	1,892.0	0.3	20.5	11.6	32.6	60.3	108.4	116.5	59.0	12.6	0.8
2001	1,840.0	0.2	19.8	10.3	32.8	59.1	106.4	112.6	56.7	12.3	0.9
2002	1,819.5	0.3	18.3	9.0	31.5	60.4	105.4	109.6	56.5	12.5	0.9
2003	1,873.0	0.2	17.4	8.8	29.8	59.6	108.5	114.6	59.9	13.5	0.9
2004	1,897.5	0.2	17.3	8.9	29.6	59.8	108.6	116.9	62.1	13.6	1.0
2005	1,889.0	0.2	17.0	8.2	30.1	61.1	107.9	115.0	61.8	13.8	1.0
2006	1,919.0	0.2	17.0	8.8	29.5	63.2	108.4	116.9	63.0	14.1	1.0
2007	2,039.0	0.2	16.9	8.2	29.9	65.5	118.0	125.4	66.3	14.4	1.1
2008	2,054.5	0.2	16.2	7.9	28.4	64.4	120.1	126.8	66.8	15.2	1.2
2009	1,956.5	0.2	14.7	7.1	25.8	57.5	110.5	123.3	68.1	15.8	1.2

* = Figure does not meet standards of reliability or precision.
[1]Beginning 1997, rates computed by relating births to women aged 45–54 years to women aged 45–49 years.
[2]For 1970–1991 includes births to races not shown separately. For 1992 and later years, unknown race of mother is imputed.
[3]Based on a 50-percent sample of births.
[4]Based on 100-percent of births in selected states and on a 50-percent sample of births in all other states.

Table A-34. Fertility Rates and Birth Rates, by Age, Live-Birth Order, Specified Hispanic Origin, and Race of Mother, 2009

(Live births per 1,000 women in specified age and race groups.)

Live-birth order and race of mother	15–44[1] years	Age of mother									
		10–14 years	15–19 years			20–24 years	25–29 years	30–34 years	35–39 years	40–44 years	45–49 years[2]
			Total	15–17 years	18–19 years						
HISPANIC											
Total	93.3	1.0	70.1	41.0	114.0	151.2	145.0	108.2	56.1	14.0	0.9
1st child	33.0	1.0	55.0	36.5	82.8	66.5	37.1	20.1	8.4	2.0	0.2
2nd child	28.0	0.0	12.9	4.2	26.0	54.1	49.2	30.9	13.8	2.9	0.2
3rd child	18.3	*	2.0	0.3	4.5	22.2	35.8	30	15	3.1	0.1
4th child	8.7	*	0.2	0.0	0.5	6.5	15.4	16.7	10.1	2.6	0.2
5th child	3.3	*	0.0	*	0.1	1.5	5.1	6.5	4.9	1.5	0.1
6th and 7th child	1.8	*	*	*	*	0.4	2.2	3.5	3.1	1.3	0.1
8th child and over	0.4	*	*	*	*	0.0	0.2	0.6	0.8	0.5	0.1
Mexican	91.4	1.0	69.2	41.5	110.9	145.9	139.3	103.1	54.2	13.8	0.8
1st child	30.2	1.0	53.8	36.9	79.3	60.4	31.1	15.2	6.1	1.5	0.1
2nd child	26.9	0.0	13.1	4.3	26.4	54.1	47.0	26.9	11.2	2.3	0.1
3rd child	19.1	*	2.0	0.3	4.6	22.8	37.2	31.1	15.3	3.0	0.1
4th child	9.4	*	0.2	0.0	0.5	6.7	16.2	18.4	11.6	2.9	0.2
5th child	3.6	*	0.0	*	0.1	1.5	5.3	7.1	5.7	1.8	0.1
6th and 7th child	1.9	*	*	*	*	0.4	2.3	3.7	3.5	1.6	0.1
8th child and over	0.4	*	*	*	*	0.0	0.2	0.6	0.9	0.6	0.1
Puerto Rican	68.7	0.7	55.9	31.0	90.9	128.4	115.1	71.8	34.9	7.8	0.6
1st child	28.0	0.7	44.9	28.0	68.7	58.8	32.6	16.7	7.2	1.8	*
2nd child	20.5	*	9.5	2.9	18.6	43.7	37.7	22.3	10.5	1.9	0.2
3rd child	11.6	*	1.4	*	3.2	18.2	25.8	16.9	8.3	1.8	*
4th child	5.1	*	0.2	*	0.4	5.8	11.7	8.8	4.4	1.1	*
5th child	2.0	*	*	*	*	1.5	4.7	3.9	2.3	0.5	*
6th and 7th child	1.2	*	*	*	*	0.4	2.4	2.5	1.7	0.5	*
8th child and over	0.3	*	*	*	*	*	0.2	0.7	0.6	0.2	*
Cuban	49.5	*	*	*	*	*	*	*	*	*	*
1st child	23.3	*	*	*	*	*	*	*	*	*	*
2nd child	17.4	*	*	*	*	*	*	*	*	*	*
3rd child	6.3	*	*	*	*	*	*	*	*	*	*
4th child	1.7	*	*	*	*	*	*	*	*	*	*
5th child	0.5	*	*	*	*	*	*	*	*	*	*
6th and 7th child	0.3	*	*	*	*	*	*	*	*	*	*
8th child and over	0.1	*	*	*	*	*	*	*	*	*	*
Other Hispanic[3]	115.7	1.4	86.3	48.5	144.9	195.6	182.9	143.4	73.1	17.3	1.2
1st child	44.9	1.3	68.6	43.4	107.8	96.0	57.3	35.4	14.8	3.3	0.3
2nd child	35.8	*	15.0	4.7	30.8	65.0	63.3	46.6	22.1	4.5	0.3
3rd child	20.7	*	2.5	0.4	5.7	25.4	38.6	34.3	18.2	4.1	0.2
4th child	8.8	*	0.3	*	0.6	7.2	16.1	16.4	9.7	2.5	0.2
5th child	3.3	*	*	*	*	1.6	5.2	6.6	4.4	1.4	0.1
6th and 7th child	1.8	*	*	*	*	0.5	2.2	3.6	3	1.2	0.1
8th child and over	0.4	*	*	*	*	*	0.2	0.6	0.8	0.4	*
NON-HISPANIC[4]											
Total[5]	61.1	0.4	32.0	15.2	55.7	84.7	103.1	95.3	44.6	9.4	0.7
1st child	25.7	0.4	26.4	14.0	44.0	43.6	41.4	29.8	11	2.3	0.2
2nd child	19.5	0.0	4.8	1.2	10.0	27.1	33.8	34.2	15.3	2.9	0.2
3rd child	9.5	*	0.7	0.1	1.6	10.2	17.2	18	9.8	1.9	0.1
4th child	3.8	*	0.1	0.0	0.2	2.9	6.8	7.6	4.4	1.0	0.1
5th child	1.4	*	0.0	*	0.0	0.7	2.5	3	1.9	0.5	0.0
6th and 7th child	0.9	*	*	*	*	0.2	1.2	2	1.4	0.4	0.0
8th child and over	0.3	*	*	*	*	0.0	0.2	0.5	0.7	0.4	0.0
White	58.4	0.2	25.6	11.0	46.1	76.7	102.6	97.4	43.9	9.0	0.6
1st child	24.8	0.2	21.7	10.3	37.7	41.3	42.9	30.9	11.0	2.2	0.2
2nd child	19.1	*	3.5	0.7	7.4	24.6	34.6	35.6	15.2	2.8	0.2
3rd child	9.1	*	0.4	0.0	0.9	8.3	16.5	18.6	9.8	1.8	0.1
4th child	3.4	*	0.0	*	0.1	2.0	5.9	7.5	4.3	0.9	0.1
5th child	1.2	*	0.0	*	0.0	0.4	1.9	2.7	1.7	0.5	0.0
6th and 7th child	0.7	*	*	*	*	0.1	0.7	1.7	1.3	0.4	0.0
8th child and over	0.3	*	*	*	*	0.0	0.1	0.4	0.6	0.3	0.0

Table A-34. Fertility Rates and Birth Rates, by Age, Live-Birth Order, Specified Hispanic Origin, and Race of Mother, 2009—Continued

(Live births per 1,000 women in specified age and race groups.)

Live-birth order and race of mother	15–44[1] years	Age of mother									
		10–14 years	15–19 years			20–24 years	25–29 years	30–34 years	35–39 years	40–44 years	45–49 years[2]
			Total	15–17 years	18–19 years						
Black	68.9	1.2	59.0	32.1	97.5	123.8	101.9	73.2	36.5	9.0	0.6
1st child	27.3	1.1	46.7	28.8	72.3	55.7	27.7	15.7	7.0	1.7	0.1
2nd child	19.4	*	10.2	3.0	20.4	40.0	31.3	21.0	9.9	2.2	0.1
3rd child	11.7	*	1.8	0.3	4.0	18.8	22.3	16.8	8.4	1.9	0.1
4th child	5.7	*	0.3	0.0	0.7	6.8	11.6	9.6	5.0	1.3	0.1
5th child	2.5	*	0.0	*	0.1	1.9	5.2	4.9	2.7	0.8	0.1
6th and 7th child	1.7	*	*	*	*	0.6	3.1	3.9	2.3	0.6	0.1
8th child and over	0.6	*	*	*	*	0.1	0.5	1.3	1.2	0.5	0.0

* = Figure does not meet standards of reliability or precision.
0.0 = Quantity more than zero but less than 0.05.
[1]Fertility rates computed by relating total births, regardless of age of mother, to women aged 15–44 years.
[2]Birth rates computed by relating births to women aged 45–54 years to women aged 45–49 years.
[3]Includes Central and South American and other and unknown Hispanic.
[4]Includes origin not stated.
[5]Includes races other than White and Black.

Table A-35. Total Fertility Rates, Fertility Rates, and Birth Rates by Age and Hispanic Origin of Mother and by Race for Mothers of Non-Hispanic Origin, 1989–2009

(Fertility rates are live births per 1,000 women aged 15–44 years in specified racial group and birth rates are live births per 1,000 women in specified age group.)

Year, origin, and race of mother	Total fertlity rate	Fertility rate[1]	Age of mother									
			10–14 years	15–19 years			20–24 years	25–29 years	30–34 years	35–39 years	40–44 years	45–49 years[2]
				Total	15–17 years	18–19 years						
All Origins												
1989	2,014.0	69.2	1.4	57.3	36.4	84.2	113.8	117.6	77.4	29.9	5.2	0.2
1990	2,081.0	70.9	1.4	59.9	37.5	88.6	116.5	120.2	80.8	31.7	5.5	0.2
1991	2,062.5	69.3	1.4	61.8	38.6	94.0	115.3	117.2	79.2	31.9	5.5	0.2
1992	2,046.0	68.4	1.4	60.3	37.6	93.6	113.7	115.7	79.6	32.3	5.9	0.3
1993	2,019.5	67.0	1.4	59.0	37.5	91.1	111.3	113.2	79.9	32.7	6.1	0.3
1994	2,001.5	65.9	1.4	58.2	37.2	90.2	109.2	111.0	80.4	33.4	6.4	0.3
1995	1,978.0	64.6	1.3	56.0	35.5	87.7	107.5	108.8	81.1	34.0	6.6	0.3
1996	1,976.0	64.1	1.2	53.5	33.3	84.7	107.8	108.6	82.1	34.9	6.8	0.3
1997	1,971.0	63.6	1.1	51.3	31.4	82.1	107.3	108.3	83.0	35.7	7.1	0.4
1998	1,999.0	64.3	1.0	50.3	29.9	80.9	108.4	110.2	85.2	36.9	7.4	0.4
1999	2,007.5	64.4	0.9	48.8	28.2	79.1	107.9	111.2	87.1	37.8	7.4	0.4
2000	2,056.0	65.9	0.9	47.7	26.9	78.1	109.7	113.5	91.2	39.7	8.0	0.5
2001	2,034.0	65.3	0.8	45.3	24.7	76.1	106.2	113.4	91.9	40.6	8.1	0.5
2002	2,013.0	64.8	0.7	43.0	23.2	72.8	103.6	113.6	91.5	41.4	8.3	0.5
2003	2,042.5	66.1	0.6	41.6	22.4	70.7	102.6	115.6	95.1	43.8	8.7	0.5
2004	2,045.5	66.3	0.7	41.1	22.1	70.0	101.7	115.5	95.3	45.4	8.9	0.5
2005	2,053.5	66.7	0.7	40.5	21.4	69.9	102.2	115.5	95.8	46.3	9.1	0.6
2006	2,100.5	68.5	0.6	41.9	22.0	73.0	105.9	116.7	97.7	47.3	9.4	0.6
2007	2,122.0	69.5	0.6	42.5	22.1	73.9	106.3	117.5	99.9	47.5	9.5	0.6
2008	2,084.5	68.6	0.6	41.5	21.7	70.6	103.0	115.1	99.3	46.9	9.8	0.7
2009	2,007.0	66.7	0.5	39.1	20.1	66.2	96.3	110.5	97.7	46.5	10.1	0.7
HISPANIC[3]												
Total												
1989[4]	2,903.5	104.9	2.3	100.8	—	—	184.4	146.6	92.1	43.5	10.4	0.6
1990[5]	2,959.5	107.7	2.4	100.3	65.9	147.7	181.0	153.0	98.3	45.3	10.9	0.7
1991[6]	2,963.5	106.9	2.4	104.6	69.2	155.5	184.6	150.0	95.1	44.7	10.7	0.6
1992[6]	2,957.5	106.1	2.5	103.3	68.9	153.9	185.2	148.8	94.8	45.3	11.0	0.6
1993	2,894.5	103.3	2.6	101.8	68.5	151.1	180.0	146.0	93.2	44.1	10.6	0.6
1994	2,839.0	100.7	2.6	101.3	69.9	147.5	175.7	142.4	91.1	43.4	10.7	0.6
1995	2,798.5	98.8	2.6	99.3	68.3	145.4	171.9	140.4	90.5	43.7	10.7	0.6
1996	2,772.5	97.5	2.4	94.6	64.2	140.0	170.2	140.7	91.3	43.9	10.7	0.6
1997	2,680.5	94.2	2.1	89.6	61.1	132.4	162.6	137.5	89.6	43.4	10.7	0.6
1998	2,652.5	93.2	1.9	87.9	58.5	131.5	159.3	136.1	90.5	43.4	10.8	0.6
1999	2,649.0	93.0	1.9	86.8	56.9	129.5	157.3	135.8	92.3	44.5	10.6	0.6
2000	2,730.0	95.9	1.7	87.3	55.5	132.6	161.3	139.9	97.1	46.6	11.5	0.6
2001	2,748.5	96.0	1.6	86.4	52.8	135.5	163.5	140.4	97.6	47.9	11.6	0.7
2002	2,718.0	94.4	1.4	83.4	50.7	133.0	164.3	139.4	95.1	47.8	11.5	0.7
2003	2,785.5	96.9	1.3	82.3	49.7	132.0	163.4	144.4	102.0	50.8	12.2	0.7
2004	2,824.5	97.8	1.3	82.6	49.7	133.5	165.3	145.6	104.1	52.9	12.4	0.7
2005	2,885.0	99.4	1.3	81.7	48.5	134.6	170.0	149.2	106.8	54.2	13.0	0.8
2006	2,959.5	101.5	1.3	83.0	47.9	139.7	177.0	152.4	108.5	55.6	13.3	0.8
2007	2,995.0	102.2	1.2	81.8	47.9	137.2	178.6	155.7	111.0	56.5	13.4	0.8
2008	2,911.5	98.8	1.2	77.5	46.1	127.2	170.7	152.6	109.6	56.1	13.7	0.9
2009	2,732.5	93.3	1.0	70.1	41.0	114.0	151.2	145.0	108.2	56.1	14.0	0.9
Mexican												
1989[4]	2,916.5	106.6	2.0	94.5	—	—	184.3	153.7	96.1	41.0	11.1	0.6
1990[5]	3,214.0	118.9	2.5	108.0	69.7	162.2	200.3	165.3	104.4	49.1	12.4	0.8
1991[6]	3,103.5	114.9	2.5	108.3	70.0	164.7	192.4	156.1	99.7	49.1	11.9	0.7
1992[6]	3,107.0	113.3	2.4	105.1	—	—	196.6	160.2	97.1	47.4	11.8	0.8
1993	3,041.5	110.9	2.5	103.6	68.4	156.6	187.9	159.5	97.2	45.5	11.3	0.8
1994	3,024.0	109.9	2.7	109.2	73.6	163.3	189.1	153.6	92.5	45.3	11.7	0.7
1995	3,033.5	109.9	2.7	115.9	79.1	170.7	190.4	146.6	93.0	45.5	11.9	0.7
1996	3,052.0	110.7	2.6	112.2	77.7	161.6	185.3	154.7	96.5	46.4	12.0	0.7
1997	2,957.0	106.6	2.3	103.4	71.3	151.6	180.9	150.0	95.3	47.4	11.5	0.6
1998	2,878.0	103.2	2.1	96.4	62.9	149.2	176.5	147.4	94.9	46.9	10.8	0.6
1999	2,823.0	101.5	2.1	94.3	60.8	145.6	170.8	141.4	97.4	47.2	10.7	0.7

Table A-35. Total Fertility Rates, Fertility Rates, and Birth Rates by Age and Hispanic Origin of Mother and by Race for Mothers of Non-Hispanic Origin, 1989–2009—Continued

(Fertility rates are live births per 1,000 women aged 15–44 years in specified racial group and birth rates are live births per 1,000 women in specified age group.)

Year, origin, and race of mother	Total fertlity rate	Fertility rate[1]	Age of mother									
			10–14 years	15–19 years			20–24 years	25–29 years	30–34 years	35–39 years	40–44 years	45–49 years[2]
				Total	15–17 years	18–19 years						
2000	2,906.5	105.1	1.9	95.4	60.6	146.7	174.9	144.7	102.3	49.2	12.2	0.7
2001	2,928.5	105.7	1.7	95.4	59.3	147.0	177.0	146.4	101.9	50.0	12.6	0.7
2002	2,879.5	102.8	1.5	94.5	58.6	147.5	176.9	144.5	97.9	47.5	12.3	0.8
2003	2,957.5	105.5	1.5	93.2	56.9	148.8	176.9	151.5	104.7	50.2	12.8	0.7
2004	3,021.0	106.8	1.4	95.5	58.4	152.4	180.0	153.5	106.2	54.3	12.6	0.7
2005	3,055.5	107.7	1.4	93.4	55.4	156.3	183.2	154.4	108.3	56.3	13.3	0.8
2006	3,107.5	109.0	1.4	92.9	53.9	157.8	191.4	154.8	109.9	56.5	13.8	0.8
2007	3,107.5	107.8	1.3	88.7	53.8	143.8	191.0	156.5	112.5	56.9	13.8	0.8
2008	2,866.5	98.9	1.2	78.7	48.5	124.6	170.9	148.3	106.0	53.5	13.9	0.8
2009	2,636.5	91.4	1.0	69.2	41.5	110.9	145.9	139.3	103.1	54.2	13.8	0.8
Puerto Rico												
1989[4]	2,421.0	86.6	3.8	112.7	—	—	171.0	98.0	65.2	26.9	6.3	*
1990[5]	2,301.0	82.9	2.9	101.6	71.6	141.6	150.1	109.9	62.8	26.2	6.2	0.5
1991[6]	2,573.5	87.9	2.7	111.0	*	*	193.3	108.9	68.1	23.9	6.5	*
1992[6]	2,568.5	87.9	3.4	106.5	—	—	199.1	102.6	65.3	29.9	6.6	*
1993	2,416.0	79.8	3.1	104.9	70.1	*	184.6	102.8	54.4	26.7	6.2	*
1994	2,341.5	78.2	3.1	99.6	68.8	*	169.0	103.8	59.5	27.5	5.6	0.2
1995	2,078.0	71.3	2.9	82.8	57.3	*	138.1	97.9	61.2	26.9	5.5	0.3
1996	1,965.0	66.5	1.9	76.5	48.6	*	133.7	95.6	54.3	25.2	5.5	*
1997	1,931.5	65.8	1.7	68.9	45.0	*	136.0	92.9	54.1	26.1	6.2	0.4
1998	2,043.5	69.7	1.8	76.2	51.7	*	146.7	88.7	61.9	25.8	7.2	0.4
1999	2,104.5	71.1	1.6	74.0	49.4	*	146.0	106.5	58.0	27.3	7.2	0.3
2000	2,178.5	73.5	1.7	82.9	54.7	120.4	149.5	101.6	61.1	32.0	6.6	0.3
2001	2,165.0	72.2	1.7	82.2	*	*	147.2	93.6	70.5	30.7	6.7	0.4
2002	1,947.5	65.4	1.4	61.4	39.7	*	136.5	90.6	61.5	31.3	6.3	0.5
2003	1,841.0	61.6	1.0	60.8	35.9	*	127.9	86.6	55.6	29.5	6.4	0.4
2004	2,056.5	68.4	0.9	62.6	38.9	*	139.1	102.2	66.4	32.8	6.8	0.5
2005	2,137.5	72.1	1.0	63.3	37.2	*	131.0	110.4	77.5	36.0	7.9	0.4
2006	2,167.0	74.0	1.0	69.3	38.1	*	138.7	102.4	72.9	39.9	8.6	0.6
2007	2,222.5	73.6	0.9	67.1	35.4	*	151.0	110.3	66.5	40.9	7.4	0.4
2008	2,160.0	71.5	0.8	61.7	31.5	*	132.1	122.5	68.6	38.8	7.1	0.4
2009	2,076.0	68.7	0.7	55.9	31.0	90.9	128.4	115.1	71.8	34.9	7.8	0.6
Cuban												
1989[4]	1,479.0	49.8	*	*	—	—	*	*	*	*	*	*
1990[5]	1,459.5	52.6	*	30.3	18.2	46.1	64.6	95.4	67.6	28.2	4.9	*
1991[6]	1,352.5	47.6	*	*	*	*	*	*	*	*	*	*
1992[6]	1,453.5	49.4	*	*	—	—	*	*	*	*	*	*
1993	1,570.0	53.9	*	*	*	*	*	*	*	*	*	*
1994	1,587.0	53.6	*	*	*	*	*	*	*	*	*	*
1995	1,584.0	52.2	*	*	*	*	*	*	*	*	*	*
1996	1,617.0	55.1	*	*	*	*	*	*	*	*	*	*
1997	1,619.5	53.1	*	*	*	*	*	*	*	*	*	*
1998	1,402.5	46.5	*	*	*	*	*	*	*	*	*	*
1999	1,388.5	47.0	*	*	*	*	*	*	*	*	*	*
2000	1,528.0	49.3	*	23.5	14.2	43.4	64.2	104.0	68.1	37.3	7.9	*
2001	1,792.5	56.7	*	*	*	*	*	*	*	*	*	*
2002	1,940.5	59.0	*	*	*	*	*	*	*	*	*	*
2003	2,059.5	61.7	*	*	*	*	*	*	*	*	*	*
2004	1,732.5	53.2	*	*	*	*	*	*	*	*	*	*
2005	1,583.0	50.4	*	*	*	*	*	*	*	*	*	*
2006	1,601.5	49.3	*	*	*	*	*	*	*	*	6.9	*
2007	1,615.5	49.7	*	*	*	*	*	*	*	*	6.6	*
2008	1,643.0	53.3	*	*	*	*	*	*	*	*	*	*
2009	1,457.0	49.5	*	*	*	*	*	*	*	*	*	*

Table A-35. Total Fertility Rates, Fertility Rates, and Birth Rates by Age and Hispanic Origin of Mother and by Race for Mothers of Non-Hispanic Origin, 1989–2009—Continued

(Fertility rates are live births per 1,000 women aged 15–44 years in specified racial group and birth rates are live births per 1,000 women in specified age group.)

Year, origin, and race of mother	Total fertlity rate	Fertility rate[1]	Age of mother									
			10–14 years	15–19 years			20–24 years	25–29 years	30–34 years	35–39 years	40–44 years	45–49 years[2]
				Total	15–17 years	18–19 years						
Other Hispanic[7]												
1989[4]	2,683.0	95.8	1.7	66.4	—	—	159.2	150.4	85.1	60.3	12.7	0.8
1990[5]	2,877.0	102.7	2.1	86.0	57.2	123.8	162.9	155.8	106.9	49.4	11.6	0.7
1991[6]	3,064.5	105.5	2.2	100.7	67.3	145.6	184.1	164.5	100.2	49.2	11.4	0.6
1992[6]	2,989.0	104.7	2.4	108.2	—	—	168.0	151.9	104.4	49.9	12.5	0.5
1993	2,914.5	101.5	2.6	102.0	74.7	134.6	167.5	139.4	106.7	51.7	12.5	0.5
1994	2,693.0	93.2	2.5	82.6	62.7	105.0	151.2	137.0	104.4	48.4	11.9	0.6
1995	2,629.5	89.1	2.3	72.1	51.3	99.4	144.3	147.7	97.9	49.4	11.6	0.6
1996	2,516.5	84.2	2.2	64.8	43.4	95.6	149.6	127.9	98.0	49.1	11.0	0.7
1997	2,376.5	80.6	1.8	66.4	44.5	98.0	129.3	125.8	95.6	43.9	11.8	0.7
1998	2,448.5	83.5	1.8	75.0	53.3	100.3	122.7	133.6	97.8	45.4	12.8	0.6
1999	2,517.0	84.8	1.5	75.5	53.1	100.5	130.2	138.4	98.3	46.5	12.3	0.7
2000	2,563.5	85.1	1.2	69.9	44.4	102.0	133.2	143.9	103.6	47.7	12.5	0.7
2001	2,519.5	82.7	1.1	65.3	35.6	115.2	136.0	143.3	95.4	50.3	11.6	0.9
2002	2,610.5	86.1	1.1	63.0	34.7	110.3	143.3	147.2	98.4	56.1	12.2	0.8
2003	2,733.0	91.2	1.0	60.4	36.4	93.1	142.2	152.8	112.3	63.2	13.9	0.8
2004	2,648.0	89.3	1.1	57.7	32.7	96.4	136.2	144.4	114.2	60.0	15.2	0.8
2005	2,822.5	93.2	1.1	62.2	37.1	97.6	156.3	154.6	116.3	58.7	14.5	0.8
2006	3,014.0	98.6	1.2	67.0	38.6	108.3	163.8	175.5	119.1	60.3	14.9	1.0
2007	3,151.0	104.9	1.3	74.0	41.8	124.7	167.6	180.6	126.9	62.4	16.3	1.1
2008	3,523.0	116.1	1.5	88.7	52.3	144.3	200.0	183.5	141.4	71.8	16.6	1.1
2009	3,506.0	115.7	1.4	86.3	48.5	144.9	195.6	182.9	143.4	73.1	17.3	1.2
NON-HISPANIC[8]												
Total[9]												
1989[4]	1,921.0	65.7	1.3	53.4	—	—	107.8	113.4	74.7	28.6	4.8	0.2
1990[5]	1,979.5	67.1	1.3	54.8	33.8	81.4	108.1	116.5	79.2	30.7	5.1	0.2
1991[6]	1,953.0	65.2	1.3	56.1	34.4	86.1	106.5	113.1	77.5	30.8	5.1	0.2
1992[6]	1,929.0	64.2	1.2	54.3	33.2	85.3	104.3	111.4	77.9	31.1	5.4	0.2
1993	1,901.5	62.7	1.2	52.7	32.9	82.3	101.7	108.7	78.4	31.6	5.7	0.3
1994	1,883.5	61.6	1.2	51.7	32.3	81.4	99.5	106.5	79.1	32.4	6.0	0.3
1995	1,856.5	60.2	1.1	49.3	30.5	78.6	97.4	104.1	79.9	33.0	6.2	0.3
1996	1,852.0	59.6	1.0	47.0	28.4	75.8	97.3	103.6	80.8	33.9	6.5	0.3
1997	1,853.0	59.3	0.9	45.0	26.7	73.7	97.4	103.5	82.0	34.8	6.7	0.3
1998	1,887.5	60.0	0.8	44.0	25.2	72.4	98.9	105.8	84.4	36.2	7.0	0.4
1999	1,894.0	60.0	0.8	42.2	23.3	70.2	98.4	106.7	86.2	37.0	7.1	0.4
2000	1,931.5	61.1	0.7	40.7	21.9	68.2	99.5	108.4	90.2	38.8	7.6	0.4
2001	1,898.5	60.1	0.6	37.9	19.6	65.2	94.9	107.7	90.9	39.5	7.7	0.5
2002	1,877.0	59.6	0.6	35.5	18.2	61.8	91.8	107.9	90.8	40.4	7.9	0.5
2003	1,897.5	60.5	0.5	34.1	17.3	59.4	90.5	109.2	93.8	42.6	8.3	0.5
2004	1,891.0	60.5	0.5	33.3	16.7	58.1	89.0	108.7	93.6	44.1	8.5	0.5
2005	1,885.5	60.4	0.5	32.4	16.0	57.6	88.7	108.0	93.4	44.9	8.6	0.6
2006	1,925.0	62.0	0.5	33.6	16.6	59.8	91.6	108.8	95.3	45.8	8.8	0.6
2007	1,942.0	62.9	0.5	34.3	16.6	61.1	91.7	109.2	97.4	45.8	8.9	0.6
2008	1,910.0	62.4	0.4	33.6	16.2	59.0	89.3	107.0	96.8	45.1	9.2	0.6
2009	1,851.0	61.1	0.4	32.0	15.2	55.7	84.7	103.1	95.3	44.6	9.4	0.7
White												
1989[4]	1,770.0	60.5	0.4	39.9	—	—	94.7	111.7	75.0	27.8	4.3	0.2
1990[5]	1,850.5	62.8	0.5	42.5	23.2	66.6	97.5	115.3	79.4	30.0	4.7	0.2
1991[6]	1,822.5	60.9	0.5	43.4	23.6	70.6	95.7	112.1	77.7	30.2	4.7	0.2
1992[6]	1,803.5	60.0	0.5	41.7	22.7	69.8	93.9	110.6	78.3	30.4	5.1	0.2
1993	1,786.0	53.9	0.5	40.7	22.7	67.7	92.2	108.2	79.0	31.0	5.4	0.2
1994	1,782.5	53.2	0.5	40.4	22.7	67.6	90.9	106.6	80.2	32.0	5.7	0.2

Table A-35. Total Fertility Rates, Fertility Rates, and Birth Rates by Age and Hispanic Origin of Mother and by Race for Mothers of Non-Hispanic Origin, 1989–2009—Continued

(Fertility rates are live births per 1,000 women aged 15–44 years in specified racial group and birth rates are live births per 1,000 women in specified age group.)

Year, origin, and race of mother	Total fertlity rate	Fertility rate[1]	Age of mother									
			10–14 years	15–19 years			20–24 years	25–29 years	30–34 years	35–39 years	40–44 years	45–49 years[2]
				Total	15–17 years	18–19 years						
1995	1,777.5	57.5	0.4	39.3	22.0	66.2	90.2	105.1	81.5	32.8	5.9	0.3
1996	1,781.0	57.1	0.4	37.6	20.6	64.0	90.1	104.9	82.8	33.9	6.2	0.3
1997	1,785.5	56.8	0.4	36.0	19.3	62.1	90.0	104.8	84.3	34.8	6.5	0.3
1998	1,825.0	57.6	0.3	35.3	18.3	60.9	91.2	107.4	87.2	36.4	6.8	0.4
1999	1,838.5	57.7	0.3	34.1	17.1	59.4	90.6	108.6	89.5	37.3	6.9	0.4
2000	1,866.0	58.5	0.3	32.6	15.8	57.5	91.2	109.4	93.2	38.8	7.3	0.4
2001	1,843.0	57.7	0.3	30.3	14.0	54.8	87.1	108.9	94.3	39.8	7.5	0.4
2002	1,828.5	57.4	0.2	28.5	13.1	51.9	84.3	109.3	94.4	40.9	7.6	0.5
2003	1,856.5	58.5	0.2	27.4	12.4	50.0	83.5	110.8	97.6	43.2	8.1	0.5
2004	1,847.0	58.4	0.2	26.7	12.0	48.7	81.9	110.0	97.1	44.8	8.2	0.5
2005	1,839.5	58.3	0.2	25.9	11.5	48.0	81.4	109.1	96.9	45.6	8.3	0.5
2006	1,863.5	59.5	0.2	26.6	11.8	49.3	83.4	109.1	98.1	46.3	8.4	0.6
2007	1,868.5	60.1	0.2	27.2	11.8	50.4	83.2	108.6	99.5	45.8	8.6	0.6
2008	1,832.0	59.4	0.2	26.7	11.5	48.5	80.7	106.0	98.7	44.7	8.8	0.6
2009	1,780.0	58.4	0.2	25.6	11.0	46.1	76.7	102.6	97.4	43.9	9.0	0.6
Black												
1989[4]	2,424.0	84.8	5.2	111.9	—	—	156.3	113.8	65.7	26.3	5.3	0.3
1990[5]	2,547.5	89.0	5.0	116.2	84.9	157.5	165.1	118.4	70.2	28.7	5.6	0.3
1991[6]	2,532.0	87.0	4.9	118.2	86.1	162.2	164.8	115.1	68.9	28.7	5.6	0.2
1992[6]	2,482.5	84.5	4.8	114.7	82.9	161.1	160.8	112.8	68.4	29.1	5.7	0.2
1993	2,412.5	81.5	4.6	110.5	81.1	154.6	154.5	109.2	68.1	29.4	5.9	0.3
1994	2,314.5	77.5	4.6	105.7	77.0	150.4	146.8	104.1	66.3	29.1	6.0	0.3
1995	2,186.5	72.8	4.2	97.2	70.4	139.2	137.8	98.5	64.4	28.8	6.1	0.3
1996	2,140.0	70.7	3.6	91.9	64.8	134.1	137.0	96.7	63.2	29.1	6.2	0.3
1997	2,137.5	70.3	3.2	88.3	60.7	131.0	138.8	97.2	63.6	29.6	6.5	0.3
1998	2,164.0	70.9	2.9	85.7	56.8	128.2	142.5	99.9	64.4	30.4	6.7	0.3
1999	2,134.0	69.9	2.6	81.0	51.7	123.9	142.1	99.8	63.9	30.6	6.5	0.3
2000	2,178.5	71.4	2.4	79.2	50.1	121.9	145.4	102.8	66.5	31.8	7.2	0.4
2001	2,104.5	69.1	2.1	73.5	44.9	116.7	137.2	102.1	66.2	32.1	7.3	0.4
2002	2,047.0	67.4	1.9	68.3	41.0	110.3	131.0	102.1	66.1	32.1	7.5	0.4
2003	2,027.5	67.1	1.6	64.7	38.7	105.3	128.1	102.1	67.4	33.4	7.7	0.5
2004	2,020.0	67.0	1.6	63.1	37.1	103.9	126.9	103.0	67.4	33.7	7.8	0.5
2005	2,019.0	67.2	1.7	60.9	34.9	103.0	126.8	103.0	68.4	34.3	8.2	0.5
2006	2,115.0	70.6	1.6	63.7	36.2	108.4	133.2	107.1	72.6	36.0	8.3	0.5
2007	2,133.5	71.6	1.5	64.2	35.8	109.3	133.6	107.5	74.3	36.4	8.6	0.6
2008	2,107.5	71.1	1.4	62.8	34.8	104.6	130.6	105.7	74.9	36.7	8.8	0.6
2009	2,026.0	68.9	1.2	59.0	32.1	97.5	123.8	101.9	73.2	36.5	9.0	0.6

— = Data not available.
* = Figure does not meet standards of reliability or precision.
[1] Fertility rates computed by relating total births, regardless of age of mother, to women 15–44 years.
[2] Beginning 1997, rates computed by relating births to women aged 45–54 years to women aged 45–49 years.
[3] Persons of Hispanic origin may be of any race.
[4] Excludes data for Louisiana, New Hampshire, and Oklahoma, which did not report Hispanic origin.
[5] Excludes data for New Hampshire and Oklahoma, which did not report Hispanic origin.
[6] Excludes data for New Hampshire, which did not report Hispanic origin.
[7] Includes Central and South American and other and unknown Hispanic.
[8] Includes origin not stated.
[9] Includes races other than White and Black.

PART A: BIRTHS

Table A-36. Fertility Rates and Birth Rates by Live-Birth Order and by Race and Hispanic Origin of Mother, 1980–2009

(Rates are live births per 1,000 women age 15–44 years.)

Year, race, and Hispanic origin of mother	Fertility rate	Live-birth order						
		1	2	3	4	5	6 and 7	8 and over
All Races[1,2]								
1980[3]	68.4	29.5	21.8	10.3	3.9	1.5	1.0	0.4
1981[3]	67.3	29.0	21.6	10.1	3.8	1.5	0.9	0.4
1982[3]	67.3	28.6	22.0	10.2	3.8	1.4	0.9	0.3
1983[3]	65.7	27.8	21.5	10.1	3.7	1.4	0.9	0.3
1984[3]	65.5	27.4	21.7	10.1	3.7	1.4	0.9	0.3
1985	66.3	27.6	22.0	10.4	3.8	1.4	0.8	0.3
1986	65.4	27.2	21.6	10.3	3.8	1.4	0.8	0.3
1987	65.8	27.2	21.6	10.5	3.9	1.4	0.8	0.3
1988	67.3	27.6	22.0	10.9	4.1	1.5	0.9	0.3
1989	69.2	28.4	22.4	11.3	4.3	1.6	0.9	0.3
1990	70.9	29.0	22.8	11.7	4.5	1.7	1.0	0.3
1991	69.3	28.2	22.3	11.4	4.4	1.7	1.0	0.3
1992	68.4	27.6	22.2	11.2	4.4	1.7	1.0	0.3
1993	67.0	27.3	21.7	10.9	4.3	1.6	1.0	0.3
1994	65.9	27.1	21.2	10.6	4.1	1.6	0.9	0.3
1995	64.6	26.9	20.7	10.3	4.0	1.5	0.9	0.3
1996	64.1	26.3	20.7	10.4	4.0	1.5	0.9	0.3
1997	63.6	25.9	20.7	10.4	4.0	1.5	0.9	0.3
1998	64.3	25.9	21.0	10.6	4.1	1.5	0.9	0.3
1999	64.4	26.0	21.0	10.7	4.1	1.5	0.9	0.3
2000	65.9	26.5	21.4	11.0	4.2	1.6	0.9	0.3
2001	65.3	26.0	21.3	11.0	4.3	1.6	0.9	0.3
2002	64.8	25.8	21.1	10.9	4.3	1.5	0.9	0.3
2003	66.1	26.5	21.4	11.1	4.3	1.6	0.9	0.3
2004	66.3	26.4	21.4	11.2	4.4	1.6	0.9	0.3
2005	66.7	26.5	21.5	11.3	4.5	1.6	0.9	0.3
2006	68.5	27.4	21.9	11.6	4.7	1.7	1.0	0.3
2007	69.5	27.9	22.1	11.7	4.8	1.8	1.0	0.3
2008	68.6	27.7	21.6	11.5	4.7	1.8	1.0	0.3
2009	66.7	27.0	21.0	11.0	4.6	1.7	1.0	0.3
Non-Hispanic White[2,4]								
1990[5]	62.8	26.7	21.2	9.9	3.3	1.1	0.5	0.2
1991[6]	60.9	25.8	20.6	9.6	3.2	1.0	0.5	0.2
1992[6]	60.0	25.1	20.5	9.5	3.2	1.0	0.5	0.2
1993	58.9	24.8	20.1	9.2	3.1	1.0	0.5	0.2
1994	58.2	24.6	19.7	9.1	3.1	1.0	0.5	0.2
1995	57.5	24.5	19.3	8.9	3.0	1.0	0.5	0.2
1996	57.1	24.1	19.3	8.9	3.0	1.0	0.5	0.2
1997	56.8	23.8	19.3	8.9	3.0	1.0	0.5	0.2
1998	57.6	23.8	19.7	9.2	3.1	1.0	0.6	0.2
1999	57.7	24.0	19.6	9.2	3.2	1.0	0.6	0.2
2000	58.5	24.2	19.8	9.4	3.3	1.1	0.6	0.2
2001	57.7	23.6	19.7	9.3	3.3	1.1	0.6	0.2
2002	57.4	23.5	19.5	9.3	3.3	1.1	0.6	0.2
2003	58.5	24.3	19.7	9.4	3.3	1.1	0.6	0.2
2004	58.4	24.1	19.6	9.4	3.3	1.1	0.6	0.2
2005	58.3	24.1	19.5	9.4	3.3	1.1	0.6	0.2
2006	59.5	24.8	19.7	9.5	3.4	1.1	0.6	0.2
2007	60.1	25.2	19.8	9.5	3.5	1.2	0.7	0.2
2008	59.4	25.1	19.5	9.3	3.4	1.2	0.7	0.2
2009	58.4	24.8	19.1	9.1	3.4	1.2	0.7	0.3
Non-Hispanic Black[2,4]								
1990[5]	89.0	33.2	26.3	16.0	7.6	3.3	2.0	0.6
1991[6]	87.0	32.1	25.5	15.7	7.5	3.4	2.2	0.6
1992[6]	84.5	31.1	24.8	15.2	7.3	3.4	2.2	0.6
1993	81.5	30.5	23.6	14.3	7.0	3.2	2.2	0.7
1994	77.5	30.0	22.4	13.2	6.3	2.9	2.0	0.6
1995	72.8	28.9	20.9	12.1	5.8	2.7	1.9	0.6
1996	70.7	27.6	20.5	12.0	5.6	2.6	1.8	0.6
1997	70.3	27.2	20.6	12.0	5.7	2.5	1.8	0.6
1998	70.9	27.0	21.0	12.3	5.7	2.6	1.8	0.6
1999	69.9	26.4	20.8	12.3	5.7	2.5	1.7	0.6

Table A-36. Fertility Rates and Birth Rates by Live-Birth Order and by Race and Hispanic Origin of Mother, 1980–2009—Continued

(Rates are live births per 1,000 women age 15–44 years.)

Year, race, and Hispanic origin of mother	Fertility rate	Live-birth order						
		1	2	3	4	5	6 and 7	8 and over
2000	71.4	26.7	21.2	12.8	5.9	2.6	1.8	0.6
2001	69.1	25.9	20.4	12.4	5.8	2.5	1.7	0.6
2002	67.4	25.3	19.7	12.0	5.6	2.5	1.7	0.5
2003	67.1	25.4	19.6	11.9	5.6	2.5	1.6	0.5
2004	67.0	25.5	19.4	11.9	5.6	2.5	1.7	0.5
2005	67.2	25.8	19.3	11.8	5.6	2.5	1.7	0.5
2006	70.6	27.5	20.2	12.3	5.8	2.5	1.7	0.5
2007	71.6	28.0	20.4	12.3	5.9	2.6	1.7	0.5
2008	71.1	28.2	20.1	12.1	5.9	2.6	1.7	0.5
2009	68.9	27.3	19.4	11.7	5.7	2.5	1.7	0.6
Hispanic[7]								
1990[5]	107.7	40.7	30.9	19.5	9.3	4.0	2.6	0.8
1991[6]	106.9	40.8	30.6	19.2	9.2	3.9	2.5	0.7
1992[6]	106.1	40.1	30.9	19.0	9.1	3.9	2.5	0.7
1993	103.3	39.3	30.4	18.3	8.6	3.7	2.3	0.6
1994	100.7	39.0	29.7	17.6	8.2	3.4	2.1	0.6
1995	98.8	38.4	29.3	17.4	7.8	3.3	2.0	0.6
1996	97.5	37.2	29.4	17.4	7.8	3.2	1.9	0.5
1997	94.2	35.6	28.6	17.1	7.6	3.0	1.8	0.5
1998	93.2	34.8	28.5	17.2	7.6	3.0	1.7	0.4
1999	93.0	34.6	28.5	17.3	7.5	2.9	1.7	0.4
2000	95.9	35.8	29.2	18.0	7.7	3.0	1.7	0.4
2001	96.0	35.4	29.5	18.1	7.9	3.0	1.7	0.4
2002	94.4	34.6	29.0	17.9	7.9	3.0	1.6	0.4
2003	96.9	35.2	29.9	18.7	8.1	3.1	1.6	0.4
2004	97.8	35.1	29.9	19.1	8.4	3.2	1.7	0.4
2005	99.4	35.5	30.5	19.5	8.6	3.2	1.7	0.4
2006	101.5	36.3	30.9	19.9	9.0	3.4	1.8	0.4
2007	102.2	36.4	30.8	20.2	9.2	3.4	1.8	0.4
2008	98.8	35.2	29.6	19.5	9.0	3.4	1.8	0.4
2009	93.3	33.0	28.0	18.3	8.7	3.3	1.8	0.4

[1] Includes races other than White and Black.
[2] Includes origin not stated.
[3] Based on 100 percent of births in selected states and on a 50-percent sample of births in all other states.
[4] Race and Hispanic origin are reported separately on birth certificates. Persons of Hispanic origin may be of any race.
[5] Excludes data for New Hampshire and Oklahoma, which did not report Hispanic origin.
[6] Excludes data for New Hampshire, which did not report Hispanic origin.
[7] Persons of Hispanic origin may be of any race.

Table A-37. Selected Demographic Characteristics of Births by Race of Mother, 2009

(Number, rates are live births per 1,000 population, percent.)

Characteristic	All races	White	Black	American Indian or Alaska Native	Asian or Pacific Islander
Number					
Births	4,130,665	3,173,293	657,618	48,665	251,089
Rate					
Birth rate	13.5	12.8	16.0	13.9	16.2
Fertility rate	66.7	66.0	69.9	62.8	68.7
Total fertility rate	2,007.0	1,991.5	2,055.50	1,779.5	1,956.5
Sex ratio[1]	1,048	1,050	1,033	1,035	1,066
Percent					
Births to mothers under 20 years	10.0	9.2	16.4	17.3	2.8
4th and higher-order births[2]	11.5	11.1	15.0	19.3	6.6
Births to unmarried mothers	41.0	36.0	72.3	65.4	17.2
Mothers born in the 50 states and D.C.	76.1	78.4	84.7	92.9	21.1
Mean					
Age of mother at first birth	25.2	25.4	22.9	22	28.8

[1]Male live births per 1,000 female live births.
[2]Based on live-birth order.

Table A-38. Live Births by Day of Week and Index of Occurence by Method of Delivery, 2009

(Number, ratio.)

Day of the week	Average number of births	Index of occurrence[1]		
		Total[2]	Method of delivery	
			Vaginal	Cesarean
TOTAL	11,317	100.0	100.0	100.0
Sunday	7,298	64.5	73.4	46.4
Monday	12,087	106.8	102.5	115.5
Tuesday	13,336	117.8	113.8	126.0
Wednesday	13,034	115.2	112.3	120.9
Thursday	12,765	112.8	110.4	117.8
Friday	12,364	109.3	105.0	117.9
Saturday	8,308	73.4	82.4	55.2

[1]Index is the ratio of the average number of births by a specified method of delivery on a given day of the week to the average daily number of births by a specified method of delivery for the year, multiplied by 100.
[2]Includes method of delivery not stated.

Table A-39. Live Births and Observed and Seasonally Adjusted Birth and Fertility Rates, by Month, 2009

(Rates on an annual basis per 1,000 population for specified month. Birth rates are live births per 1,000 total population.)

Month	Number	Observed		Seasonally adjusted	
		Birth rate	Fertility rate	Birth rate	Fertility rate
TOTAL	4,130,665	13.5	66.7	X	X
January	337,980	13.0	64.2	13.7	67.4
February	316,641	13.5	66.6	13.7	67.5
March	347,803	13.4	66.1	13.6	67.0
April	337,272	13.4	66.2	13.6	67.1
May	345,257	13.3	65.6	13.5	66.9
June	346,971	13.8	68.1	13.5	66.9
July	368,450	14.1	70.0	13.5	67.2
August	359,554	13.8	68.3	13.3	66.1
September	361,922	14.3	71.1	13.5	66.9
October	347,625	13.3	66.1	13.3	66.0
November	320,195	12.6	62.9	13.1	65.6
December	340,995	13.0	64.8	13.2	65.7

X = Category not applicable.

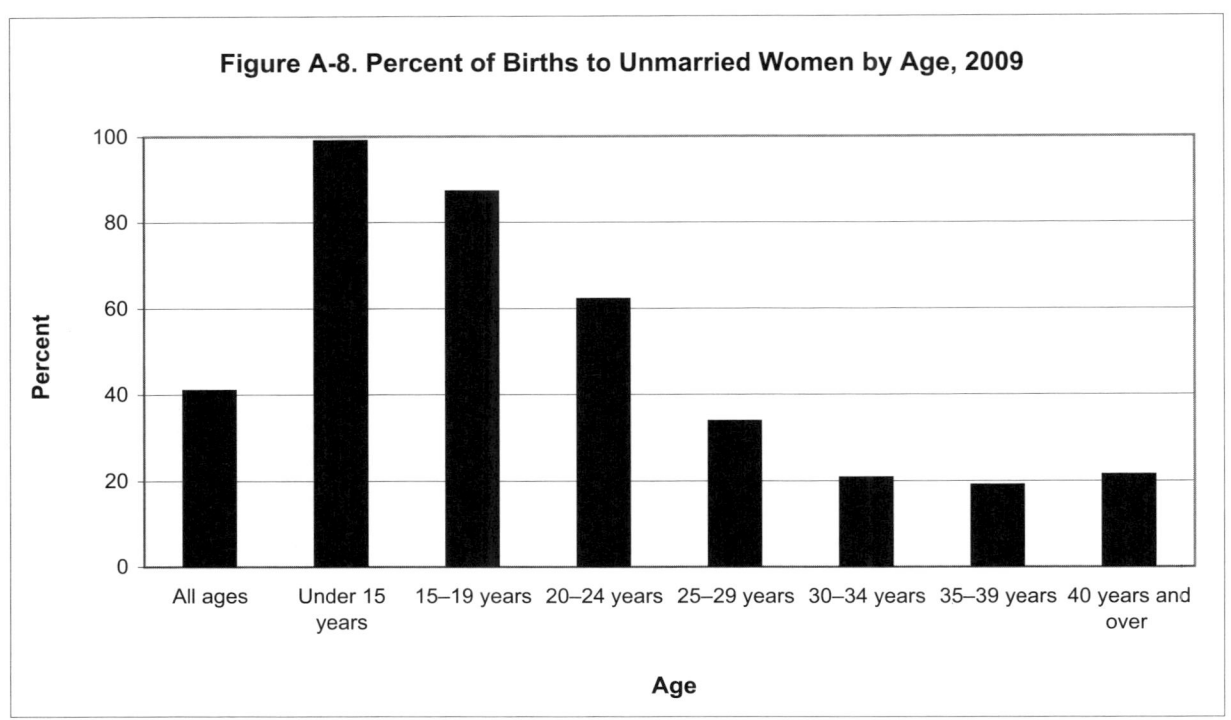

Figure A-8. Percent of Births to Unmarried Women by Age, 2009

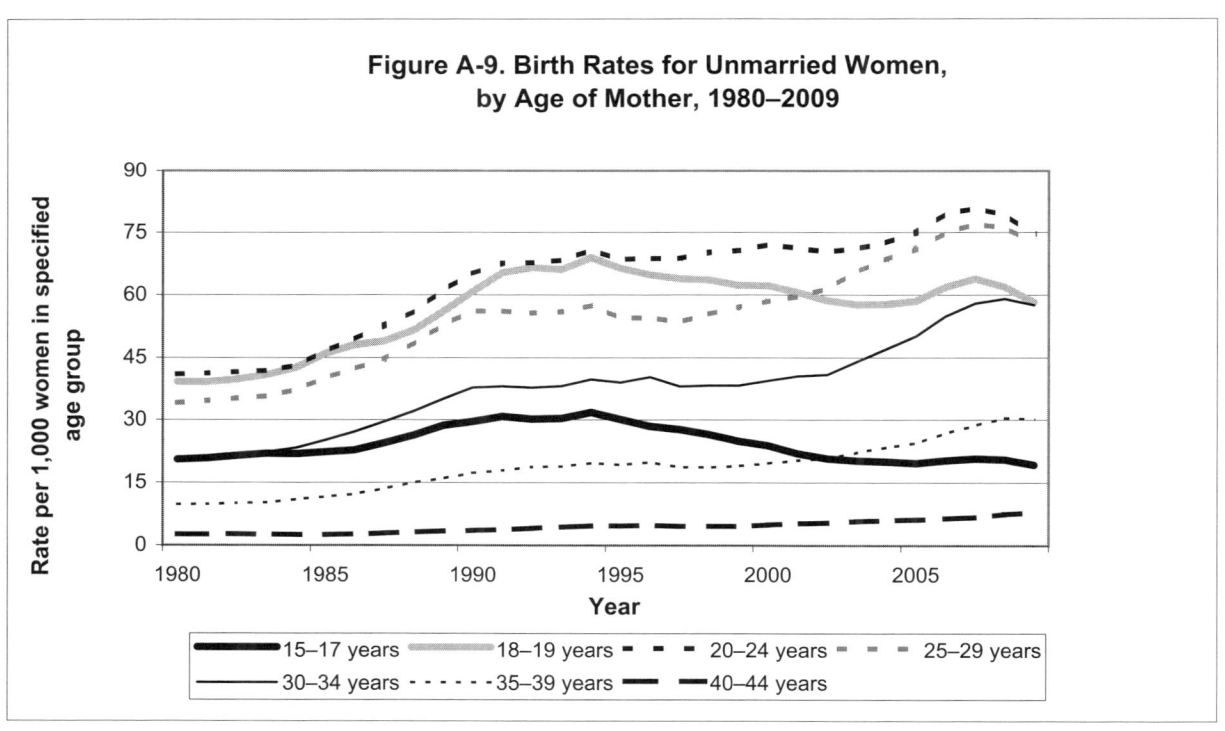

Figure A-9. Birth Rates for Unmarried Women, by Age of Mother, 1980–2009

Table A-40. Number, Rate, and Percentage of Births to Unmarried Women and Birth Rate for Married Women, Selected Years, 1980–2009

(Number, rate per 1,000 women aged 15–44 years, percent.)

Year	Births to unmarried women			Birth rate for married women[3]
	Number	Rate[1]	Percent[2]	
1980	665,747	29.4	18.4	97.0
1985	828,174	32.8	22.0	93.3
1986	878,477	34.2	23.4	90.7
1987	933,013	36.0	24.5	90.0
1988	1,005,299	38.5	25.7	90.8
1989	1,094,169	41.6	27.1	91.9
1990	1,165,384	43.8	28.0	93.2
1991	1,213,769	45.0	29.5	89.6
1992	1,224,876	44.9	30.1	88.5
1993	1,240,172	44.8	31.0	86.1
1994	1,289,592	46.2	32.6	82.9
1995	1,253,976	44.3	32.2	82.6
1996	1,260,306	43.8	32.4	82.3
1997	1,257,444	42.9	32.4	82.7
1998	1,293,567	43.3	32.8	84.2
1999	1,308,560	43.3	33.0	84.8
2000	1,347,043	44.1	33.2	87.4
2001	1,349,249	43.8	33.5	86.7
2002	1,365,966	43.7	34.0	86.3
2003	1,415,995	44.9	34.6	88.1
2004	1,470,189	46.1	35.8	87.6
2005	1,527,034	47.5	36.9	87.3
2006	1,641,946	50.6	38.5	88.0
2007	1,715,047	52.3	39.7	88.7
2008	1,726,566	52.5	40.6	86.8
2009	1,693,658	50.5	41.0	85.7

[1]Births to unmarried women per 1,000 unmarried women aged 15–44 years.
[2]Percentage of all births to unmarried women.
[3]Births to married women per 1,000 married women aged 15–44 years.

Table A-41. Birth Rates for Unmarried Women by Age of Mother, 1970, 1975, and 1980–2009, and by Age, Race, and Hispanic Origin of Mother, 1980–2009

(Rates are live births to unmarried women per 1,000 unmarried women. Populations estimated as of July 1 for all years.)

All Races	15–44 years[1]	Age of mother			20–24 years	25–29 years	30–34 years	35–39 years	40–44 years[2]
		15–19 years							
		Total	15–17 years	18–19 years					
All Races[3]									
1970[4,5]	26.4	22.4	17.1	32.9	38.4	37.0	27.1	13.6	3.5
1975[4,6]	24.5	23.9	19.3	32.5	31.2	27.5	17.9	9.1	2.6
1980[6,7]	29.4	27.6	20.6	39.0	40.9	34.0	21.1	9.7	2.6
1980[4,6]	28.4	27.5	20.7	38.7	39.7	31.4	18.5	8.4	2.3
1981[6,7]	29.5	27.9	20.9	39.0	41.1	34.5	20.8	9.8	2.6
1982[6,7]	30.0	28.7	21.5	39.6	41.5	35.1	21.9	10.0	2.7
1983[6,7]	30.3	29.5	22.0	40.7	41.8	35.5	22.4	10.2	2.6
1984[6,7]	31.0	30.0	21.9	42.5	43.0	37.1	23.3	10.9	2.5
1985[7]	32.8	31.4	22.4	45.9	46.5	39.9	25.2	11.6	2.5
1986[7]	34.2	32.3	22.8	48.0	49.3	42.2	27.2	12.2	2.7
1987[7]	36.0	33.8	24.5	48.9	52.6	44.5	29.6	13.5	2.9
1988[7]	38.5	36.4	26.4	51.5	56.0	48.5	32.0	15.0	3.2
1989[7]	41.6	40.1	28.7	56.0	61.2	52.8	34.9	16.0	3.4
1990[7]	43.8	42.5	29.6	60.7	65.1	56.0	37.6	17.3	3.6
1991[7]	45.0	44.6	30.8	65.4	67.8	56.0	37.9	17.9	3.8
1992[7]	44.9	44.2	30.2	67.9	67.9	55.6	37.6	18.8	4.1
1993[7]	44.8	44.0	30.3	66.2	68.5	55.9	38.0	18.9	4.4
1994[7]	46.2	45.8	31.7	69.1	70.9	57.4	39.6	19.7	4.7
1995[7]	44.3	43.8	30.1	66.5	68.7	54.3	38.9	19.3	4.7
1996[7]	43.8	42.2	28.5	64.9	68.9	54.5	40.2	19.9	4.8
1997[7]	42.9	41.4	27.7	63.9	68.9	53.4	37.9	18.7	4.6
1998[7]	43.3	40.9	26.5	63.6	70.4	55.4	38.1	18.7	4.6
1999[7]	43.3	39.7	25.0	62.3	70.8	56.9	38.1	19.0	4.6
2000[7]	44.1	39.0	23.9	62.2	72.2	58.5	39.3	19.7	5.0
2001[7]	43.8	37.0	22.0	60.6	71.3	59.5	40.4	20.4	5.3
2002[7]	43.7	35.4	20.8	58.6	70.5	61.5	40.8	20.8	5.4
2003[7]	44.9	34.8	20.3	57.6	71.2	65.7	44.0	22.3	5.8
2004[7]	46.1	34.7	20.1	57.7	72.5	68.6	47.0	23.5	6.0
2005[7]	47.5	34.5	19.7	58.4	74.9	71.1	50.0	24.5	6.2
2006[7]	50.6	36.2	20.4	61.8	79.5	74.9	54.8	26.8	6.5
2007[7]	52.3	37.4	20.8	63.9	80.6	76.9	57.9	28.7	6.8
2008[7]	52.5	37.0	20.6	61.9	79.2	76.1	59.0	30.4	7.5
2009[7]	50.5	35.0	19.3	58.2	74.6	72.7	57.5	30.2	7.9
White									
1980[6,7]	18.1	16.5	12.0	24.1	25.1	21.5	14.1	7.1	1.8
1981[6,7]	18.6	17.2	12.6	24.6	25.8	22.3	14.2	7.2	1.9
1982[6,7]	19.3	18.0	13.1	25.3	26.5	23.1	15.3	7.4	2.1
1983[6,7]	19.8	18.7	13.6	26.4	27.1	23.8	15.9	7.8	2.0
1984[6,7]	20.6	19.3	13.7	27.9	28.5	25.5	16.8	8.4	2.0
1985[7]	22.5	20.8	14.5	31.2	31.7	28.5	18.4	9.0	2.0
1986[7]	23.9	21.8	14.9	33.5	34.2	30.5	20.1	9.7	2.2
1987[7]	25.3	23.2	16.2	34.5	36.6	32.0	22.3	10.7	2.4
1988[7]	27.4	25.3	17.6	36.8	39.2	35.4	24.2	12.1	2.7
1989[7]	30.2	28.0	19.3	40.2	43.8	39.1	26.8	13.1	2.9
1990[7]	32.9	30.6	20.4	44.9	48.2	43.0	29.9	14.5	3.2
1991[7]	34.5	32.7	21.7	49.4	51.4	44.3	30.9	15.2	3.2
1992[7]	35.0	32.7	21.4	51.2	52.4	44.8	31.3	16.1	3.6
1993[7]	35.6	33.3	21.9	52.0	53.8	46.0	31.9	16.3	3.9
1994[7]	37.8	35.8	23.9	55.8	57.5	48.6	33.8	17.2	4.3
1995[7]	37.0	35.0	23.3	54.7	57.2	47.4	33.7	16.8	4.2
1996[7]	37.0	34.0	22.3	53.5	57.9	48.1	35.4	17.7	4.3
1997[7]	36.3	33.6	22.0	52.9	57.9	47.0	33.6	16.6	3.9
1998[7]	36.9	33.6	21.5	53.1	59.5	48.6	34.1	16.9	4.1
1999[7]	37.4	33.2	20.6	52.9	60.2	50.8	34.9	17.4	4.1
2000[7]	38.2	32.7	19.7	53.1	61.7	52.9	35.9	17.9	4.5
2001[7]	38.5	31.3	18.1	52.1	61.8	54.6	37.2	18.6	4.9
2002[7]	38.9	30.4	17.5	51.0	61.6	56.8	38.3	19.4	5.0
2003[7]	40.4	30.1	17.2	50.4	63.0	60.8	42.0	21.2	5.5
2004[7]	41.6	30.1	17.1	50.4	64.1	63.9	45.7	22.6	5.6

PART A: BIRTHS

Table A-41. Birth Rates for Unmarried Women by Age of Mother, 1970, 1975, and 1980–2009, and by Age, Race, and Hispanic Origin of Mother, 1980–2009—Continued

(Rates are live births to unmarried women per 1,000 unmarried women. Populations estimated as of July 1 for all years.)

All Races		Age of mother							
	15–44 years[1]	15–19 years			20–24 years	25–29 years	30–34 years	35–39 years	40–44 years[2]
		Total	15–17 years	18–19 years					
2005[7]	43.0	29.9	16.8	50.9	66.6	66.3	49.1	23.8	5.8
2006[7]	46.1	31.4	17.4	53.9	71.0	70.6	54.5	26.4	6.2
2007[7]	48.1	32.6	18.0	55.9	72.1	72.7	58.5	28.8	6.4
2008[7]	48.2	32.3	18.0	54.2	70.6	71.7	59.2	30.9	7.3
2009[7]	46.3	30.8	16.9	51.1	66.1	68.0	57.1	30.6	7.8
Non-Hispanic White									
1990[7,8]	24.4	25.0	16.2	37.0	36.4	30.3	20.5	6.1	—
1991[7]	—	—	—	—	—	—	—	—	—
1992[7]	—	—	—	—	—	—	—	—	—
1993[7]	—	—	—	—	—	—	—	—	—
1994[7]	28.4	28.1	17.9	45.0	43.8	34.7	24.6	12.8	3.1
1995[7]	28.1	27.7	17.6	44.6	43.9	34.4	25.1	12.9	3.2
1996[7]	28.2	27.0	16.9	43.9	44.5	35.0	26.4	13.8	3.3
1997[7]	27.5	26.4	16.2	43.3	44.8	34.4	24.9	12.7	2.9
1998[7]	27.9	26.2	15.5	43.1	46.3	35.4	25.0	13.1	3.1
1999[7]	27.9	25.6	14.6	42.7	46.3	36.2	24.8	13.0	3.1
2000[7]	28.0	24.7	13.6	42.1	47.0	36.9	24.8	12.9	3.3
2001[7]	27.8	23.1	12.1	40.3	46.4	37.5	25.4	13.2	3.6
2002[7]	27.8	22.1	11.5	38.8	46.1	38.5	26.0	13.5	3.7
2003[7]	28.6	21.5	11.0	37.9	47.2	40.8	27.8	14.7	4.1
2004[7]	29.4	21.2	10.7	37.5	48.0	43.3	29.6	15.6	4.1
2005[7]	30.1	20.9	10.3	37.4	49.1	45.0	31.2	16.0	4.2
2006[7]	32.0	21.6	10.7	38.8	51.6	47.7	34.4	17.7	4.4
2007[7]	33.3	22.6	10.9	40.7	52.3	49.2	36.5	19.0	4.6
2008[7]	33.7	22.4	10.7	39.7	51.6	49.1	37.6	20.1	5.1
2009[7]	33.0	21.7	10.3	38.1	49.8	47.2	37.0	19.8	5.5
Black									
1980[6,7]	81.1	87.9	68.8	118.2	112.3	81.4	46.7	19.0	5.5
1981[6,7]	79.4	85.0	65.9	114.2	110.7	83.1	45.5	19.6	5.6
1982[6,7]	77.9	85.1	66.3	112.7	109.3	82.7	44.1	19.5	5.2
1983[6,7]	76.2	85.5	66.8	111.9	107.2	79.7	43.8	19.4	4.8
1984[6,7]	75.2	86.1	66.5	113.6	107.9	77.8	43.8	19.4	4.3
1985[7]	77.0	87.6	66.8	117.9	113.1	79.3	47.5	20.4	4.3
1986[7]	79.0	88.5	67.0	121.1	118.0	84.6	50.0	20.6	4.4
1987[7]	82.6	90.9	69.9	123.0	126.1	91.6	53.1	22.4	4.7
1988[7]	86.5	96.1	73.5	130.5	133.6	97.2	57.4	24.1	5.0
1989[7]	90.7	104.5	78.9	140.9	142.4	102.9	60.5	24.9	5.0
1990[7]	90.5	106.0	78.8	143.7	144.8	105.3	61.5	25.5	5.1
1991[7]	89.0	107.8	79.9	147.7	146.4	100.0	59.8	25.5	5.4
1992[7]	85.7	104.8	77.2	146.4	142.6	96.8	57.3	25.6	5.4
1993[7]	83.0	101.2	75.9	140.0	139.9	92.8	56.7	25.7	5.8
1994[7]	80.3	99.3	73.9	139.6	135.2	91.3	56.5	26.0	5.9
1995[7]	74.5	91.2	67.4	129.2	124.6	82.3	53.3	25.3	6.0
1996[7]	72.8	87.5	62.6	127.2	122.6	81.2	53.4	25.2	6.1
1997[7]	71.5	84.5	59.0	124.8	124.2	81.4	51.0	24.3	6.5
1998[7]	71.6	81.5	55.0	121.5	127.8	86.5	50.5	24.3	6.0
1999[7]	69.7	76.5	50.0	115.8	126.8	85.5	49.0	24.2	5.8
2000[7]	70.5	75.0	48.3	115.0	129.0	85.9	50.2	25.4	6.3
2001[7]	68.1	69.9	43.8	110.2	122.8	84.1	51.1	25.4	6.3
2002[7]	66.2	64.8	39.9	104.1	119.2	85.9	49.9	24.9	6.3
2003[7]	66.3	62.2	38.1	100.4	118.0	90.4	51.2	25.3	6.5
2004[7]	67.2	61.7	37.0	100.9	119.8	91.8	52.0	25.8	6.8
2005[7]	67.8	60.6	35.4	101.6	120.7	93.8	54.0	26.1	7.1
2006[7]	71.5	63.5	36.6	107.8	126.0	96.9	58.6	27.6	7.2
2007[7]	72.6	64.1	36.3	109.1	126.5	98.3	60.3	28.4	7.5
2008[7]	72.5	63.0	35.5	104.4	125.6	96.3	61.7	28.9	7.7
2009[7]	69.9	58.9	32.6	96.8	120.2	94.3	60.8	29.0	7.8

Table A-41. Birth Rates for Unmarried Women by Age of Mother, 1970, 1975, and 1980–2009, and by Age, Race, and Hispanic Origin of Mother, 1980–2009—Continued

(Rates are live births to unmarried women per 1,000 unmarried women. Populations estimated as of July 1 for all years.)

All Races		Age of mother							
	15–44 years[1]	15–19 years			20–24 years	25–29 years	30–34 years	35–39 years	40–44 years[2]
		Total	15–17 years	18–19 years					
Asian or Pacific Islander Total									
2000[7]	20.9	15.2	9.6	23.2	24.2	25.4	29.7	18.4	6.9
2001[7]	21.2	14.6	8.7	23.0	25.2	26.7	29.4	19.7	6.3
2002[7]	21.3	13.4	7.5	22.2	26.5	27.5	28.6	18.7	6.8
2003[7]	22.2	13.1	7.5	21.4	26.6	30.7	31.5	19.8	7.9
2004[7]	23.6	13.3	7.7	21.6	27.9	33.2	35.4	20.7	8.6
2005[7]	24.9	13.1	7.3	22.1	29.7	35.1	36.6	24.7	9.4
2006[7]	25.9	13.4	7.8	21.9	31.4	34.5	37.5	29.5	9.4
2007[7]	27.3	13.6	7.4	23.1	33.4	38.5	38.0	29.1	10.0
2008[7]	28.2	13.3	7.1	22.7	33.8	41.6	40.8	31.2	11.2
2009[7]	27.4	12.4	6.7	21.1	31.4	42.2	42.0	29.2	10.4
Hispanic[9]									
1990[7,8]	89.6	65.9	45.9	98.9	129.8	131.7	88.1	50.8	13.7
1991[7]	92.5	71.0	49.5	107.5	134.2	135.1	88.2	47.6	14.1
1992[7]	92.8	70.3	49.2	106.6	138.2	133.4	89.9	47.8	14.6
1993[7]	91.4	71.1	49.6	108.8	134.3	130.4	87.8	47.1	14.1
1994[7]	95.8	77.7	55.7	115.4	144.5	131.7	91.2	47.4	13.9
1995[7]	88.8	73.2	52.8	108.6	135.8	122.3	84.1	42.2	12.1
1996[7]	86.2	69.3	49.7	102.3	131.6	122.0	84.6	41.2	12.3
1997[7]	83.2	69.2	50.7	100.6	122.8	114.8	78.8	40.5	12.1
1998[7]	82.8	69.3	49.8	101.2	120.6	115.9	78.2	38.8	12.0
1999[7]	84.9	68.6	48.7	99.9	126.1	119.6	84.2	42.4	11.2
2000[7]	87.2	68.5	47.0	102.2	130.5	121.6	89.4	46.1	12.2
2001[7]	87.8	67.1	44.2	104.3	132.3	120.7	91.4	49.7	12.2
2002[7]	87.9	66.1	43.0	105.3	131.4	123.1	88.1	51.3	12.6
2003[7]	92.2	66.6	43.0	107.0	133.7	136.0	99.2	54.7	13.3
2004[7]	95.7	67.9	43.3	110.1	138.6	143.4	109.6	56.8	13.8
2005[7]	100.3	68.0	42.7	112.4	150.4	153.5	118.1	59.2	14.3
2006[7]	106.1	70.6	43.1	119.7	164.7	163.3	124.0	62.4	15.0
2007[7]	108.4	71.0	43.8	120.2	166.8	167.8	129.9	66.7	15.3
2008[7]	105.1	68.8	43.1	112.8	156.2	162.0	126.5	69.5	16.8
2009[7]	96.8	62.5	38.8	100.3	135.3	150.5	120.8	68.2	18.1

— = Data not available.
[1] Rates computed by relating total births to unmarried mothers, regardless of age of mother, to unmarried women aged 15–44 years.
[2] Rates computed by relating births to unmarried mothers aged 40 years and over to unmarried women aged 40–44 years.
[3] Includes races other than White, Black, and Asian or other Pacific Islander.
[4] Births to unmarried women are estimated for the United States from data for registration areas in which marital status of mother was reported.
[5] Based on a 50-percent sample of births.
[6] Based on 100 percent of births in selected states and on a 50-percent sample of births in all other states.
[7] Data for states in which marital status was not reported have been inferred and included with data from the remaining states.
[8] Rates based on data for 48 states and the District of Columbia that reported Hispanic origin on the birth certificate. Rate for age group 35–39 years are based on births to unmarried women aged 35–44 years.
[9] Persons of Hispanic origin may be of any race.

NOTE: Race and Hispanic origin are reported separately on birth certificates.

PART A: BIRTHS

Table A-42. Number, Birth Rate, and Percentage of Births to Unmarried Women by Age, Race, and Hispanic Origin of Mother, 2009

(Number, rate, percent.)

Measure and age of mother	All races[1]	White		Black		American Indian or Alaska Native	Asian or Pacific Islander[2]	Hispanic[3]
		Total[2]	Non-Hispanic	Total[2]	Non-Hispanic			
Number								
All ages	1,693,658	1,142,871	641,252	475,718	444,044	31,812	43,257	531,445
Under 15 years	4,980	2,981	1,035	1,821	1,703	105	73	2,048
15–19 years	357,474	241,568	132,030	102,664	95,973	7,519	5,723	116,011
15 years	15,398	9,949	3,812	4,802	4,486	379	268	6,481
16 years	36,101	24,249	10,567	10,507	9,766	766	579	14,390
17 years	65,595	44,818	22,558	18,360	17,098	1,425	992	23,507
18 years	103,092	69,836	39,188	29,501	27,626	2,145	1,610	32,426
19 years	137,288	92,716	55,905	39,494	36,997	2,804	2,274	39,207
20–24 years	624,293	419,174	253,757	180,128	168,818	11,902	13,089	176,486
25–29 years	394,556	266,157	147,026	109,131	101,690	7,141	12,127	126,112
30–34 years	198,168	134,133	66,761	53,532	49,620	3,445	7,058	70,993
35–39 years	89,854	61,737	31,048	22,681	20,971	1,399	4,037	32,017
40 years and over	24,333	17,121	9,595	5,761	5,269	301	1,150	7,778
Rate per 1,000 Unmarried Women in Specified Group								
15–44 years[4]	50.5	46.3	33.0	69.9	—	—	27.4	96.8
15–19 years	35.0	30.8	21.7	58.9	—	—	12.4	62.5
15–17 years	19.3	16.9	10.3	32.6	—	—	6.7	38.8
18–19 years	58.2	51.1	38.1	96.8	—	—	21.1	100.3
20–24 years	74.6	66.1	49.8	120.2	—	—	31.4	135.3
25–29 years	72.7	68.0	47.2	94.3	—	—	42.2	150.5
30–34 years	57.5	57.1	37.0	60.8	—	—	42.0	120.8
35–39 years	30.2	30.6	19.8	29.0	—	—	29.2	68.2
40–44 years[5]	7.9	7.8	5.5	7.8	—	—	10.4	18.1
Percent of Births to Unmarried Women								
All ages	41.0	36.0	29.0	72.3	72.8	65.4	17.2	53.2
Under 15 years	99.0	98.6	98.3	99.9	99.9	97.2	96.1	98.8
15–19 years	87.2	83.7	82.7	97.1	97.5	90.4	81.1	85.1
15 years	98.4	97.9	98.2	99.7	99.8	97.2	98.2	97.6
16 years	95.5	93.9	94.5	99.4	99.6	96.8	92.1	93.6
17 years	92.6	90.3	90.6	98.9	99.1	95.1	88.1	90.4
18 years	87.8	84.3	84.3	97.4	97.8	90.5	81.6	84.6
19 years	81.7	77.1	76.5	95.2	95.7	85.9	74.5	78.5
20–24 years	62.1	55.8	51.7	86.2	87.0	73.3	44.5	64.2
25–29 years	33.8	29.0	22.4	65.8	66.4	56.5	17.2	46.6
30–34 years	20.7	17.8	11.8	50.0	50.2	46.5	8.3	36.3
35–39 years	19.0	16.7	11.4	42.0	41.9	43.5	8.4	32.9
40 years and over	21.4	19.4	14.7	40.3	40.0	39.5	10.9	34.0

— = Data not available.
[1] Includes races other than White and Black and origin not stated.
[2] Race and Hispanic origin are reported separately on birth certificates.
[3] Persons of Hispanic origin may be of any race.
[4] Birth rates computed by relating total births to unmarried mothers, regardless of age of mother, to unmarried women aged 15–44 years.
[5] Birth rates computed by relating births to unmarried mothers aged 40 years and over to unmarried women aged 40–44 years.

Table A-43. Total Number of Births, Rates (Birth, Fertility, and Total Fertility), and Percentage of Births with Selected Demographic Characteristics, by Hispanic Origin of Mother and by Race for Mothers of Non-Hispanic Origin, 2009

(Birth rates are live births per 1,000 population. Fertility rates are computed by relating total births, regardless of age of mother, to women aged 15–44 years.)

Characteristic	All origins[1]	Hispanic[2]						Non-Hispanic		
		Total	Mexican	Puerto Rican	Cuban	Central and South American	Other and unknown Hispanic	Total[3]	White	Black
Number										
Births	4,130,665	999,548	645,297	68,486	16,641	148,647	120,477	3,101,330	2,212,552	609,584
Rate										
Birth rate[4]	13.5	20.6	20.1	15.8	9.6	26.0	(4)	12.1	11.0	15.8
Fertility rate[4]	66.7	93.3	91.4	68.7	49.5	115.7	(4)	61.1	58.4	68.9
Total fertility rate[4]	2,007.0	2,732.5	2,636.5	2,076.0	1,457.0	3,506.0	(4)	1,851.0	1,780.0	2,026.0
Sex ratio[5]	1,048	1,044	1,042	1,053	1,038	1,044	1,048	1,050	1,053	1,033
Percent										
Births to mothers under 20 years	10.0	13.8	14.5	16.5	7.0	7.8	17.3	8.8	7.3	16.4
4th and higher-order births[6]	11.5	15.0	16.7	12.5	5.3	12.3	12.4	10.4	9.4	15.2
Births to unmarried mothers	41.0	53.2	51.8	65.2	46.0	52.4	55.8	37.1	29.0	72.8
Mothers born in the 50 states and D.C.	76.1	42.5	40.0	74.1	48.6	14.1	71.9	87.0	93.9	87.2
Mean										
Age of mother at first birth	25.2	23.3	22.7	23.0	26.4	25.5	23.0	25.7	26.1	22.9

[1]Includes origin not stated.
[2]Persons of Hispanic origin may be of any race.
[3]Includes races other than White and Black.
[4]Rates for Central and South American include other and unknown Hispanic.
[5]Male live births per 1,000 female live births.
[6]Based on live-birth order.

Table A-44. Percentage of Births with Selected Medical or Health Characteristics, by Race of Mother, 2009

(Percent.)

Characteristic	All races	White	Black	American Indian or Alaska Native	Asian or Pacific Islander
ALL BIRTHS					
Mother					
Diabetes during pregancy	4.8	4.6	4.2	6.6	8.2
Weight gain of less than 11 lbs	8.0	7.3	12.5	11.1	5.6
Weight gain of more than 40 lbs	20.8	21.3	20.5	20.9	15.3
Induction of labor	23.2	24.1	21.0	21.9	17.2
CNM delivery[1]	7.6	7.7	7.1	17.2	6.1
Cesarean delivery	32.9	32.4	35.2	28.5	33.1
Infant					
Gestational Age					
Preterm[2]	12.2	11.2	17.2	13.5	10.8
Early preterm[3]	3.5	3.0	6.1	4.0	2.8
Late Preterm[4]	8.7	8.2	11.1	9.4	8.1
Birthweight					
Very low birthweight[5]	1.5	1.2	3.0	1.3	1.1
Low birthweight[6]	8.2	7.1	13.3	7.3	8.3
4,000 grams or more[7]	7.6	8.5	4.2	9.7	4.6
Low 5 minute Apgar[8]	1.8	1.6	2.9	2.2	1.2
Twin birth[9]	33.2	32.8	37.1	23.5	30.6
Triplet or higher order birth[10]	153.5	166.1	110.6	*	129.8

* = Figure does not meet standards of reliability or precision.
[1]Births delivered by certified nurse midwives.
[2]Born prior to 37 completed weeks of gestation.
[3]Born prior to 34 completed weeks of gestation.
[4]Born between 34 and 36 completed weeks of gestation.
[5]Birthweight of less than 1,500 grams (3 lb 4 oz).
[6]Birthweight of less than 2,500 grams (5 lb 8 oz).
[7]Equivalent to 8 lb 14 oz.
[8]Score of less than 7 on a 10 point scale.
[9]Live births in twin deliveries per 1,000 live births.
[10]Live births in triplet and other higher order multiple deliveries per 100,000 live births.

Table A-45. Percentage of Births with Selected Medical or Health Characteristics, by Hispanic Origin of Mother and by Race for Mothers of Non-Hispanic Origin, 2009

(Percent.)

Characteristic	All origins[1]	Hispanic						Non-Hispanic		
		Total	Mexican	Puerto Rican	Cuban	Central and South American	Other and unknown Hispanic	Total[2]	White	Black
Mother										
Diabetes during pregancy	4.8	5.0	5.1	5.5	4.9	4.7	4.2	4.7	4.4	4.2
Weight gain of less than 11 lbs	8.0	9.2	9.5	8.9	5.5	8.2	9.1	7.7	6.5	12.6
Weight gain of more than 40 lbs	20.8	16.1	15.0	22.0	24.5	14.5	19.8	22.2	23.5	20.5
Induction of labor	23.2	17.5	16.9	20.2	19.5	15.7	20.6	25	27	21.1
CNM delivery[3]	7.6	8.1	7.8	9.8	4.1	9.6	7.4	7.4	7.5	6.9
Cesarean delivery	32.9	31.6	30.3	34.3	48.8	32.6	33.2	33.3	32.8	35.4
Infant										
Gestational Age										
Preterm[4]	12.2	12.0	11.5	13.8	13.2	12	13.4	12.2	10.9	17.5
Early preterm[5]	3.5	3.3	3.1	4.3	3.7	3.2	3.9	3.6	2.9	6.2
Late Preterm[6]	8.7	8.6	8.3	9.5	9.5	8.8	9.5	8.7	8	11.2
Birthweight										
Very low birthweight[7]	1.5	1.2	1.1	1.9	1.5	1.1	1.4	1.5	1.2	3.1
Low birthweight[8]	8.2	6.9	6.5	9.6	7.5	6.6	8.3	8.5	7.2	13.6
4,000 grams or more[9]	7.6	7.1	7.5	5.8	6.9	6.9	5.8	7.8	9.1	4.1
Low 5 minute Apgar[10]	1.8	1.3	1.3	1.5	1.4	1.1	1.7	1.9	1.7	3.0
Twin birth[11]	33.2	22.5	20.6	29.6	34.8	23.4	25.5	36.5	37.0	38.0
Triplet or higher order birth[12]	153.5	83.5	67.9	127.0	162.2	85.4	129.5	174.8	201.4	105.6

[1]Includes origin not stated.
[2]Includes races other than White and Black.
[3]Births delivered by certified nurse midwives.
[4]Born prior to 37 completed weeks of gestation.
[5]Born prior to 34 completed weeks of gestation.
[6]Born between 34 and 36 completed weeks of gestation.
[7]Birthweight of less than 1,500 grams (3 lb 4 oz).
[8]Birthweight of less than 2,500 grams (5 lb 8 oz).
[9]Equivalent to 8 lb 14 oz.
[10]Score of less than 7 on a 10 point scale.
[11]Live births in twin deliveries per 1,000 live births.
[12]Live births in triplet and other higher order multiple deliveries per 100,000 live births.

Table A-46. Number and Percentage of Births to Unmarried Women by Race and Hispanic Origin of Mother, by State and Territory, 2009

(Number, percent.)

Area	Births to unmarried women				Percent unmarried			
	All races[1]	Non-Hispanic		Hispanic[3]	All races[1]	Non-Hispanic		Hispanic[3]
		White[2]	Black[2]			White[2]	Black[2]	
UNITED STATES[4]	1,693,658	641,252	444,044	531,445	41.0	29.0	72.8	53.2
Alabama	25,592	9,832	14,154	1,357	41.0	26.6	73.6	26.4
Alaska	4,303	1,462	195	256	38.0	24.3	47.8	36.8
Arizona	42,161	12,008	2,560	22,260	45.4	30.0	61.9	56.8
Arkansas	18,104	9,503	6,221	2,115	45.5	35.2	81.5	50.3
California	213,905	35,295	21,396	142,019	40.6	24.1	68.8	52.6
Colorado	17,074	7,380	1,526	7,436	24.9	17.9	48.9	36.0
Connecticut	14,605	5,299	3,382	5,668	37.5	23.2	68.0	66.0
Delaware	5,513	2,107	2,277	1,069	47.7	34.1	71.7	64.9
District of Columbia	5,047	129	3,731	1,016	55.8	5.5	79.1	67.1
Florida	105,647	36,243	36,057	31,638	47.7	36.0	71.1	51.0
Georgia	64,290	16,408	32,686	12,676	45.5	26.6	70.7	51.5
Hawaii	7,154	1,169	106	1,558	37.9	25.4	25.8	49.7
Idaho	6,092	4,147	43	1,603	25.7	21.8	31.4	43.6
Illinois	69,783	23,760	24,081	21,040	40.8	26.1	80.5	52.1
Indiana	38,001	24,817	8,117	4,688	43.8	37.4	80.5	58.0
Iowa	13,977	10,590	1,414	1,655	35.2	31.7	74.1	51.6
Kansas	15,692	9,317	2,276	3,667	37.9	31.2	74.3	54.0
Kentucky	23,757	17,742	4,207	1,625	41.3	36.9	77.4	54.4
Louisiana	34,809	12,175	20,043	2,078	53.6	35.2	79.7	58.4
Maine	5,466	5,111	134	94	40.6	40.9	34.2	47.5
Maryland	32,077	9,330	16,168	6,017	42.7	27.4	64.7	56.7
Massachusetts	26,058	13,258	4,277	7,438	34.7	26.3	59.2	67.6
Michigan	48,405	25,724	17,669	4,067	41.3	31.3	79.8	51.4
Minnesota	23,702	13,362	3,982	3,277	33.6	26.1	61.5	58.3
Mississippi	23,710	6,896	15,584	858	55.3	32.2	81.6	56.7
Missouri	32,255	19,914	9,567	2,267	40.9	33.1	79.6	52.9
Montana	4,444	2,984	31	214	36.3	29.9	47.7	50.4
Nebraska	9,284	5,448	1,249	2,155	34.5	27.5	71.0	50.5
Nevada	16,324	4,866	2,586	7,593	43.4	30.5	71.9	52.9
New Hampshire	4,463	4,008	98	272	33.4	33.5	45.2	49.3
New Jersey	38,898	9,234	11,778	17,147	35.3	17.7	68.7	59.1
New Mexico	15,510	2,560	307	9,642	53.5	31.7	59.8	59.7
New York	103,050	29,574	28,569	39,277	41.5	24.7	69.7	65.7
North Carolina	53,665	18,888	22,259	10,816	42.3	26.8	73.4	53.6
North Dakota	2,943	1,914	53	137	32.7	26.2	32.7	43.9
Ohio	63,939	39,553	19,038	4,315	44.1	36.0	79.9	62.6
Oklahoma	22,918	12,109	3,851	3,325	42.0	34.9	75.8	45.7
Oregon	16,678	10,315	738	4,647	35.4	31.5	64.6	47.9
Pennsylvania	60,033	32,014	16,762	9,318	41.0	31.0	78.0	66.0
Rhode Island	5,120	2,471	609	1,629	44.7	35.4	67.2	65.0
South Carolina	28,871	10,468	15,247	2,625	47.6	30.8	78.3	47.2
South Dakota	4,580	2,555	134	277	38.4	28.0	54.3	58.2
Tennessee	36,596	18,581	13,675	3,997	44.5	33.5	78.6	53.8
Texas	170,509	37,459	30,475	100,284	42.4	27.2	67.0	49.8
Utah	10,452	5,642	260	3,943	19.4	13.3	47.4	44.9
Vermont	2,415	2,296	32	49	39.5	39.6	42.1	52.1
Virginia	37,628	14,430	15,406	7,075	35.8	23.9	66.9	51.7
Washington	29,974	15,841	2,150	8,782	33.6	28.0	52.6	51.1
West Virginia	9,279	8,451	647	107	43.6	42.3	77.9	46.3
Wisconsin	26,227	14,719	6,210	3,869	37.0	28.1	85.2	55.8
Wyoming	2,679	1,894	27	508	34.0	29.8	48.2	51.8
Puerto Rico	28,774	804	121	27,833	64.3	62.7	70.3	64.3
Virgin Islands	1,247	49	846	310	73.9	31.8	78.9	79.5
Guam	1,978	23	4	8	57.9	10.7	*	*
American Samoa	520	—	—	—	38.8	—	—	—
Northern Marianas	629	—	—	—	56.7	—	—	—

— = Data not available.
* = Figure does not meet standards of reliability or precision.
[1]Includes races other than White and Black and origin not stated.
[2]Race and Hispanic origin are reported separately on birth certificates. Persons of Hispanic origin may be of any race.
[3]Includes all persons of Hispanic origin of any race.
[4]Excludes data for the territories.

Table A-47. Number of Live Births and Percent Distribution, by Weight Gain of Mother During Pregnancy, According to Period of Gestation and Race and Hispanic Origin of Mother, 2009

(Number, percent distribution.)

Period of gestation[1], race, and Hispanic origin of mother	All births	Less than 11 pounds	11–20 pounds	21–30 pounds	31–40 pounds	41–98 pounds	Not stated
NUMBER							
All Pluralities							
All Gestation Periods[2]							
All races[3]	4,130,665	313,101	638,349	1,148,654	992,014	811,096	227,451
Non-Hispanic White[4]	2,212,552	137,605	287,613	610,583	584,478	497,455	94,818
Non-Hispanic Black[4]	609,584	71,275	106,583	151,215	120,030	115,687	44,794
Hispanic[5]	999,548	85,524	196,057	291,228	210,393	150,793	65,553
Under 37 Weeks							
All races[3]	502,306	55,764	97,207	132,707	97,335	84,168	35,125
Non-Hispanic White[4]	241,301	21,398	40,758	64,995	52,399	48,510	13,241
Non-Hispanic Black[4]	106,316	16,950	22,134	25,272	17,007	15,609	9,344
Hispanic[5]	119,507	14,177	27,509	32,276	21,012	15317	9,216
37 Weeks and Over							
All races[3]	3,623,074	256,809	540,721	1,015,398	894,271	726,541	189,334
Non-Hispanic White[4]	1,968,901	115,962	246,658	545,323	531,853	448,727	80,378
Non-Hispanic Black[4]	502,401	54,188	84,363	125,842	102,963	100,010	35,035
Hispanic[5]	878,854	71,246	168,442	258,820	189,298	135,409	55,639
Live Births in Singleton Deliveries							
All Gestation Periods[2]							
All races[3]	3,987,108	305,063	624,006	1,121,227	959,049	759,357	218,406
Non-Hispanic White[4]	2,126,141	133,891	280,558	594,932	563,989	462,497	90,274
Non-Hispanic Black[4]	585,781	68,773	103,319	146,566	115,388	108,905	42,830
Hispanic[5]	976,232	84,089	193,002	286,223	205,025	143,993	63,900
Under 37 Weeks							
All races[3]	415,735	50,051	87,173	114,732	77,790	56,633	29,356
Non-Hispanic White[4]	189,412	18,755	35,714	54,620	40,049	29,884	10,390
Non-Hispanic Black[4]	91,137	15,133	19,840	22,095	14,239	11,838	7,992
Hispanic[5]	105,787	13,198	25,472	29,191	17,954	11,760	8,212
37 Weeks and Over							
All races[3]	3,566,272	254,504	536,425	1,005,954	880,863	702,348	186,178
Non-Hispanic White[4]	1,934,482	114,900	244,654	540,049	523,721	432,401	78,757
Non-Hispanic Black[4]	493,815	53,510	83,395	124,376	101,092	97,001	34,441
Hispanic[5]	869,275	70,793	167,426	256,900	186,990	132,167	54,999
PERCENT DISTRIBUTION							
All Pluralities							
All Gestation Periods[2]							
All races[3]	100.0	8.0	16.4	29.4	25.4	20.8	X
Non-Hispanic White[4]	100.0	6.5	13.6	28.8	27.6	23.5	X
Non-Hispanic Black[4]	100.0	12.6	18.9	26.8	21.3	20.5	X
Hispanic[5]	100.0	9.2	21.0	31.2	22.5	16.1	X
Under 37 Weeks							
All races[3]	100.0	11.9	20.8	28.4	20.8	18.0	X
Non-Hispanic White[4]	100.0	9.4	17.9	28.5	23.0	21.3	X
Non-Hispanic Black[4]	100.0	17.5	22.8	26.1	17.5	16.1	X
Hispanic[5]	100.0	12.9	24.9	29.3	19.1	13.9	X
37 Weeks and Over							
All races[3]	100.0	7.5	15.7	29.6	26.0	21.2	X
Non-Hispanic White[4]	100.0	6.1	13.1	28.9	28.2	23.8	X
Non-Hispanic Black[4]	100.0	11.6	18.1	26.9	22.0	21.4	X
Hispanic[5]	100.0	8.7	20.5	31.4	23.0	16.4	X
Live Births in Singleton Deliveries							
All Gestation Periods[2]							
All races[3]	100.0	8.1	16.6	29.8	25.4	20.1	X
Non-Hispanic White[4]	100.0	6.6	13.8	29.2	27.7	22.7	X
Non-Hispanic Black[4]	100.0	12.7	19.0	27.0	21.3	20.1	X
Hispanic[5]	100.0	9.2	21.2	31.4	22.5	15.8	X

Table A-47. Number of Live Births and Percent Distribution, by Weight Gain of Mother During Pregnancy, According to Period of Gestation and Race and Hispanic Origin of Mother, 2009—*Continued*

(Number, percent distribution.)

Period of gestation[1], race, and Hispanic origin of mother	All births	Less than 11 pounds	11–20 pounds	21–30 pounds	31–40 pounds	41–98 pounds	Not stated
Under 37 Weeks							
All races[3]	100.0	13.0	22.6	29.7	20.1	14.7	X
Non-Hispanic White[4]	100.0	10.5	19.9	30.5	22.4	16.7	X
Non-Hispanic Black[4]	100.0	18.2	23.9	26.6	17.1	14.2	X
Hispanic[5]	100.0	13.5	26.1	29.9	18.4	12.1	X
37 Weeks and Over							
All races[3]	100.0	7.5	15.9	29.8	26.1	20.8	X
Non-Hispanic White[4]	100.0	6.2	13.2	29.1	28.2	23.3	X
Non-Hispanic Black[4]	100.0	11.6	18.2	27.1	22.0	21.1	X
Hispanic[5]	100.0	8.7	20.6	31.5	23.0	16.2	X

X = Category not applicable.
[1]Expressed in completed weeks.
[2]Includes births with period of gestation not stated.
[3]Includes races other than White and Black and origin not stated.
[4]Race and Hispanic origin are reported separately on birth certificates.
[5]Persons of Hispanic origin may be of any race.

NOTE: Excludes data for California, which did not require reporting of weight gain during pregnancy.

Table A-48. Number and Rate of Live Births to Mothers with Selected Risk Factors During Pregnancy, Obstetric Procedures, Characteristics of Labor and Delivery, and Congenital Anomalies, by Age, Race, and Hispanic Origin of Mother, 2009

(Rates are number of live births with specified risk factors, procedures, or anomaly per 1,000 live births in specified group; congenital anomalies are per 100,000 live births.)

Risk factor, procedure, characteristic, and anomaly	All births[1]	Factor reported	All ages	Under 20 years	20–24 years	25–29 years	30–34 years	35–39 years	40–54 years	Not stated[2]
ALL RACES[3]										
Risk factors in This Pregnancy										
Diabetes	4,130,665	195,757	47.6	14.6	27.0	44.2	62.1	84.8	108.3	18,442
Hypertension, pregnancy-associated	4,130,665	169,351	41.2	43.3	40.7	40.5	39.2	42.9	54.9	18,442
Hypertension, chronic	4,130,665	52,067	12.7	4.4	7.6	11.2	15.5	23.0	35.6	18,442
Obstetric Procedures and Characteristics of Labor or Delivery										
Induction of labor	4,130,665	953,346	231.7	254.2	244.9	237.1	219.3	203.7	199.1	16,255
Tocolysis[4]	4,101,665	54,397	13.3	15.3	14.3	13.0	12.4	12.3	13.7	25,371
Meconium, moderate/heavy	4,130,665	188,690	45.9	51.8	47.5	45.6	43.8	42.7	43.1	16,172
Breech/malpresentation	4,130,665	216,838	53.7	42.8	45.2	51.3	58.8	69.1	84.6	89,414
Precipitous labor	4,130,665	96,860	23.6	15.3	21.1	24.5	26.5	27.1	27.2	25,098
Congenital Anomalies[4]										
Anencephaly	4,130,665	466	11.4	12.4	12.5	11.5	10.4	10.9	*	39,260
Meningomyelocele/Spina Bifida	4,130,665	740	18.1	16.6	20.3	17.7	17.2	16.8	20.4	39,260
Omphalocele/Gastroschisis	4,130,665	1,630	39.8	111.0	61.6	27.2	15.7	15.1	23.1	39,260
Cleft lip/palate	4,130,665	2,976	72.7	73.5	75.7	71.8	67.4	74.3	91.5	39,260
Down syndrome	4,130,665	1,994	48.7	23.4	27.4	28.4	41.2	112.0	338.6	39,260
NON-HISPANIC WHITE[5]										
Risk factors in This Pregnancy										
Diabetes	2,212,552	97,511	44.2	17.1	28.1	40.3	52.5	70.7	89.7	8,530
Hypertension, pregnancy-associated	2,212,552	101,540	46.1	48.5	47.1	46.6	43.1	45.0	57.1	8,530
Hypertension, chronic	2,212,552	27,041	12.3	4.3	7.6	10.9	14.4	20.2	29.5	8,530
Obstetric Procedures and Characteristics of Labor or Delivery										
Induction of labor	2,212,552	595,696	270.2	323.2	296.5	277.3	249.1	229.8	222.3	7,713
Tocolysis[4]	2,204,472	30,802	14.0	17.4	15.3	13.8	13.0	12.6	14.0	11,931
Meconium, moderate/heavy	2,212,552	89,763	40.7	44.0	41.5	40.8	39.7	39.3	39.7	7,745
Breech/malpresentation	2,212,552	118,924	54.5	43.1	45.0	52.0	58.7	68.4	84.8	29,984
Precipitous labor	2,212,552	52,487	23.9	13.9	20.2	24.1	27.1	28.0	28.3	11,918
Congenital Anomalies[4]										
Anencephaly	2,212,552	245	11.2	15.1	12.5	10.7	9.6	10.7	*	19,746
Meningomyelocele/Spina Bifida	2,212,552	450	20.5	20.7	22.6	20.5	18.9	19.6	*	19,746
Omphalocele/Gastroschisis	2,212,552	976	44.5	141.4	79.0	30.2	18.4	18.1	*	19,746
Cleft lip/palate	2,212,552	1,904	86.8	96.8	97.5	84.8	76.4	85.4	99.1	19,746
Down syndrome	2,212,552	1,243	56.7	28.3	33.3	30.8	47.3	124.5	360.7	19,746
NON-HISPANIC BLACK[5]										
Risk factors in This Pregnancy										
Diabetes	609,584	25,129	41.6	12.6	23.4	44.7	67.8	90.6	110.9	5,560
Hypertension, pregnancy-associated	609,584	30,336	50.2	51.0	46.3	49.1	52.0	59.4	67.0	5,560
Hypertension, chronic	609,584	15,514	25.7	7.3	13.5	25.4	41.3	63.3	87.1	5,560
Obstetric Procedures and Characteristics of Labor or Delivery										
Induction of labor	609,584	127,685	211.1	231.1	214.7	209.1	200.3	191.8	184.3	4,681
Tocolysis[4]	609,071	11,638	19.3	21.6	20.5	19.1	17.2	16.7	14.5	7,460
Meconium, moderate/heavy	609,584	35,109	58.0	62.6	56.8	57.4	58.0	55.6	58.8	4,756
Breech/malpresentation	609,584	29,120	48.9	36.4	42.1	49.7	59.2	70.2	79.7	14,502
Precipitous labor	609,584	14,822	24.6	18.5	23.3	27.1	27.5	28.0	27.2	7,347
Congenital Anomalies										
Anencephaly	609,584	57	9.5	*	10.5	*	*	*	*	10,057
Meningomyelocele/Spina Bifida	609,584	96	16.0	*	19.9	13.3	*	*	*	10,057
Omphalocele/Gastroschisis	609,584	211	35.2	69.1	38.2	28.5	*	*	*	10,057
Cleft lip/palate	609,584	258	43.0	39.6	40.8	43.8	47.3	*	*	10,057
Down syndrome	609,584	187	31.2	*	21.5	19.2	25.7	81.4	262.3	10,057

Table A-48. **Number and Rate of Live Births to Mothers with Selected Risk Factors During Pregnancy, Obstetric Procedures, Characteristics of Labor and Delivery, and Congenital Anomalies, by Age, Race, and Hispanic Origin of Mother, 2009**—*Continued*

(Rates are number of live births with specified risk factors, procedures, or anomaly per 1,000 live births in specified group; congenital anomalies are per 100,000 live births.)

Risk factor, procedure, characteristic, and anomaly	All births[1]	Factor reported	All ages	Under 20 years	20–24 years	25–29 years	30–34 years	35–39 years	40–54 years	Not stated[2]
HISPANIC[6]										
Risk factors in This Pregnancy										
Diabetes	999,548	49,369	49.5	12.8	25.7	46.5	74.5	105.7	140.3	2,727
Hypertension, pregnancy-associated	999,548	28,814	28.9	31.8	26.9	25.9	28.7	34.9	47.0	2,727
Hypertension, chronic	999,548	6,740	6.8	2.6	3.7	5.7	9.1	14.7	28.0	2,727
Obstetric Procedures and Characteristics of Labor or Delivery										
Induction of labor	999,548	174,197	174.7	196.7	182.7	169.3	164.8	159.1	159.6	2,410
Tocolysis[4]	983,390	8,566	8.7	8.4	8.5	8.4	9.0	9.6	12.2	3,612
Meconium, moderate/heavy	999,548	49,409	49.5	53.2	51.0	49.2	47.7	45.8	45.2	2,232
Breech/malpresentation	999,548	52,626	54.7	47.6	48.1	52.1	60.5	71.5	84.9	36,909
Precipitous labor	999,548	21,303	21.4	14.1	20.5	23.4	23.9	23.1	22.7	3,538
Congenital Anomalies										
Anencephaly	999,548	129	13.0	*	12.4	16.4	14.9	*	*	5,683
Meningomyelocele/Spina Bifida	999,548	157	15.8	*	17.6	16.4	16.4	*	*	5,683
Omphalocele/Gastroschisis	999,548	356	35.8	100.2	46.5	20.4	11.3	*	*	5,683
Cleft lip/palate	999,548	575	57.9	62.5	58.9	53.9	55.0	60.0	*	5,683
Down syndrome	999,548	451	45.4	24.0	20.9	32.3	36.5	113.7	409.3	5,683

* = Figure does not meet standards of reliability or precision.
[1]Total number of births to residents of areas reporting risk factors, procedure or anomaly.
[2]No response reported for specific item.
[3]Includes races not shown.
[4]Excludes data for New Mexico, which did not report congenital anomalies.
[5]Race and Hispanic origin are reported separately on birth certificates.
[6]Persons of Hispanic origin may be of any race.

PART A: BIRTHS

Table A-49. Pregnancy Risk Factors, by Age and Race and Hispanic Origin of Mother, 27 Reporting States, 2008

(Number, Rates per 1,000 live births in specified group.)

Risk factor and race and Hispanic origin of mother	All births[1]	Factor reported	All ages	Under 20 years	20–24 years	25–29 years	30–34 years	35–39 years	40–54 years	Not stated[2]
All Races[3]										
Diabetes										
Prepregnancy (diagnosis prior to this pregnancy)	2,748,302	17,688	6.5	2.3	4.2	6.1	8.3	11.3	14.9	38,770
Gestational (diagnosis in this pregnancy)	2,748,302	110,140	40.6	12.7	23.7	38.5	54.2	70.6	88.6	38,770
Hypertension										
Prepregnancy (chronic)	2,748,302	29,989	11.1	4.5	6.8	10.0	13.6	19.4	30.6	38,770
Gestational (PIH, preeclampsia)	2,748,302	104,850	38.7	41.3	38.0	37.8	37.0	40.7	50.2	38,770
Eclampsia[4]	2,128,437	3,818	1.8	2.6	1.9	1.6	1.6	1.8	2.2	30,752
Previous preterm birth	2,748,302	50,575	18.7	6.4	17.1	20.6	21.0	23.0	23.5	38,770
Other previous poor pregnancy outcome	2,748,302	50,811	18.8	6.7	15.1	19.2	22.1	27.0	32.5	38,770
Mother had a previous cesarean delivery[5]	1,782,194	346,180	196.4	117.8	163.4	184.0	214.8	247.5	254.7	19,811
White[6]										
Diabetes										
Prepregnancy (diagnosis prior to this pregnancy)	1,366,527	7,979	5.9	2.3	4.3	5.6	6.9	8.5	10.4	8,697
Gestational (diagnosis in this pregnancy)	1,366,527	53,107	39.1	15.0	25.3	36.6	47.3	60.7	74.6	8,697
Hypertension										
Prepregnancy (chronic)	1,366,527	15,902	11.7	5.1	7.5	10.7	13.8	18.3	27.0	8,697
Gestational (PIH, preeclampsia)	1,366,527	59,692	44.0	47.2	45.0	44.6	40.7	43.2	52.5	8,697
Eclampsia[4]	947,743	1,905	2.0	2.7	2.2	1.9	1.8	2.0	2.4	6,995
Previous preterm birth	1,366,527	28,742	21.2	7.0	19.2	22.3	23.1	25.6	26.6	8,697
Other previous poor pregnancy outcome	1,366,527	31,636	23.3	8.5	18.4	22.6	26.3	32.9	40.5	8,697
Mother had a previous cesarean delivery[5]	871,960	165,349	190.4	105.2	153.0	172.2	206.3	242.8	252.6	3,396
Black[6]										
Diabetes										
Prepregnancy (diagnosis prior to this pregnancy)	349,243	3,139	9.2	2.8	5.5	9.2	14.0	21.9	26.4	8,702
Gestational (diagnosis in this pregnancy)	349,243	11,892	34.9	11.5	20.9	37.7	54.9	72.2	88.1	8,702
Hypertension										
Prepregnancy (chronic)	349,243	7,749	22.8	7.5	11.8	22.2	36.0	54.2	81.3	8,702
Gestational (PIH, preeclampsia)	349,243	16,738	49.2	48.9	44.7	47.5	54.1	57.5	64.9	8,702
Eclampsia[4]	259,004	761	3.0	3.9	2.9	2.6	2.8	3.5	3.8	8,292
Previous preterm birth	349,243	9,599	28.2	9.0	24.7	35.2	36.6	39.4	35.4	8,702
Other previous poor pregnancy outcome	349,243	8,064	23.7	9.0	20.6	27.8	31.5	33.6	35.2	8,702
Mother had a previous cesarean delivery[5]	228,425	44,549	198.1	125.4	176.4	198.8	219.0	249.6	248.8	3,523
Hispanic[7]										
Diabetes										
Prepregnancy (diagnosis prior to this pregnancy)	787,484	5,003	6.4	1.8	3.3	5.7	10.0	14.0	20.4	5,195
Gestational (diagnosis in this pregnancy)	787,484	31,442	40.2	11.1	22.0	38.6	61.4	84.1	110.2	5,195
Hypertension										
Prepregnancy (chronic)	787,484	4,588	5.9	2.6	3.6	4.9	8.1	12.0	22.2	5,195
Gestational (PIH, preeclampsia)	787,484	22,350	28.6	32.3	26.5	24.9	28.7	34.9	46.2	5,195
Eclampsia[4]	721,835	942	1.3	2.0	1.3	1.0	1.2	1.5	1.5	4,736
Previous preterm birth	787,484	9,136	11.7	4.4	10.7	13.4	14.3	14.8	15.4	5,195
Other previous poor pregnancy outcome	787,484	7,933	10.1	3.7	8.1	11.0	13.0	16.1	17.4	5,195
Mother had a previous cesarean delivery[5]	533,199	109,848	207.0	127.0	174.2	201.2	233.6	260.7	266.2	2,618

[1]Refers to total number of births to residents of areas reporting specified pregnancy risk factor.
[2]No response reported for pregnancy risk factor.
[3]Includes other races not shown and origin not stated.
[4]Excludes data for Idaho, Kentucky, Michigan, Nebraska, New York City, Pennsylvania, South Carolina, Tennessee, and Washington, which did not report eclampsia.
[5]Excludes women who have not had a previous pregnancy and for whom total birth order is unknown.
[6]Race and Hispanic origin are reported separately on the birth certificate.
[7]Persons of Hispanic origin may be of any race.

NOTE: PIH is pregnancy-induced hypertension. Includes California, Colorado, Delaware, Florida, Georgia, Idaho, Indiana, Iowa, Kansas, Kentucky, Michigan, Montana, Nebraska, New Hampshire, New Mexico, New York, North Dakota, Ohio, Oregon, Pennsylvania, South Carolina, South Dakota, Tennessee, Texas, Vermont, Washington, and Wyoming. Births to residents of states using the 2003 U.S. Standard Certificate of Live Birth occurring in states using the 1989 Standard Certificate of Live Birth (0.6 percent) are included in the "not stated" category.

Table A-50 Births Delivered by Forceps or Vacuum Extraction, Selected Years, 1990–2009

(Percent.)

Year and type of birth	Forceps	Vacuum extraction	Forceps or vacuum
All Births			
1990[1]	5.1	3.9	9.0
1995	3.5	5.9	9.4
2000	2.1	4.9	7.0
2005	0.9	3.9	4.8
2007	0.8	3.5	4.3
2008	0.7	3.2	3.9
2009	0.7	3.0	3.7
Vaginal Births Only			
1990[1]	6.6	5.0	11.7
1995	4.4	7.5	11.9
2000	2.7	6.3	9.0
2005	1.3	5.6	6.9
2007	1.1	5.1	6.2
2008	1.1	4.8	5.8
2009	1.0	4.5	5.5

[1]Excludes data for Oklahoma, which did not report method of delivery.

Table A-51. Live Births by Method of Delivery and Rates of Cesarean Delivery by Race and Hispanic Origin of Mother, 1989–2009

(Number, rate.)

Year	All births	Vaginal				Cesarean							
		Number				Number				Percentage of all live births by cesarean delivery			
		Total[1]	Non-Hispanic White[2]	Non-Hispanic Black[2]	Hispanic[3]	Total[1]	Non-Hispanic White[2]	Non-Hispanic Black[2]	Hispanic[3]	Total[1]	Non-Hispanic White[2]	Non-Hispanic Black[2]	Hispanic[3]
1989[4]	3,798,734	2,793,463	1,806,753	440,310	385,462	826,955	556,585	125,290	105,268	22.8	23.6	22.2	21.5
1990[5]	4,110,563	3,111,421	1,972,754	503,720	458,242	914,096	603,467	142,838	122,969	22.7	23.4	22.1	21.2
1991[6]	4,110,907	3,100,891	1,941,726	507,522	472,126	905,077	587,802	142,417	129,752	22.6	23.2	21.9	21.6
1992[6]	4,065,014	3,100,710	1,916,414	502,669	494,338	888,622	566,788	143,153	133,369	22.3	22.8	22.2	21.2
1993	4,000,240	3,098,796	1,902,433	496,333	514,493	861,987	542,013	139,702	136,279	21.8	22.2	22.0	20.9
1994	3,952,767	3,087,576	1,896,609	480,551	525,928	830,517	518,021	134,526	135,569	21.2	21.5	21.9	20.5
1995	3,899,589	3,063,724	1,867,024	457,104	539,731	806,722	496,103	127,171	136,640	20.8	21.0	21.8	20.2
1996	3,891,494	3,061,092	1,851,058	449,544	558,105	797,119	485,530	124,836	139,554	20.7	20.8	21.7	20.0
1997	3,880,894	3,046,621	1,829,213	451,744	563,114	799,033	481,982	126,138	142,907	20.8	20.9	21.8	20.2
1998	3,941,553	3,078,537	1,842,420	457,186	580,143	825,870	495,550	131,999	150,317	21.2	21.2	22.4	20.6
1999	3,959,417	3,063,870	1,810,682	449,580	599,118	862,086	514,051	135,508	161,035	22.0	22.1	23.2	21.2
2000	4,058,814	3,108,188	1,804,550	454,736	633,220	923,991	540,794	146,042	179,583	22.9	23.1	24.3	22.1
2001	4,025,933	3,027,993	1,746,551	435,455	648,821	978,411	567,488	151,908	199,874	24.4	24.5	25.9	23.6
2002	4,021,726	2,958,423	1,687,144	416,516	653,516	1,043,846	598,682	159,297	219,777	26.1	26.2	27.7	25.2
2003	4,089,950	2,949,853	1,671,414	405,671	667,656	1,119,388	637,482	167,506	241,159	27.5	27.6	29.2	26.5
2004	4,112,052	2,903,341	1,617,994	397,877	679,118	1,190,210	667,836	178,461	263,454	29.1	29.2	31.0	28.0
2005	4,138,349	2,873,918	1,579,613	392,064	698,089	1,248,815	690,260	189,287	285,376	30.3	30.4	32.6	29.0
2006	4,265,555	2,929,590	1,580,794	411,097	728,854	1,321,054	718,960	203,723	307,981	31.1	31.3	33.1	29.7
2007	4,316,233	2,933,056	1,565,555	413,088	737,478	1,367,340	735,744	211,615	322,554	31.8	32.0	33.9	30.4
2008	4,247,694	2,864,343	1,527,340	406,379	716,811	1,369,273	732,641	214,416	321,859	32.3	32.4	34.5	31.0
2009	4,130,665	2,764,285	1,481,660	392,715	682,512	1,353,572	723,687	214,810	315,025	32.9	32.8	35.4	31.6

[1]Includes races other than White and Black and origin not stated.
[2]Race and Hispanic origin are reported separately on birth certificates.
[3]Persons of Hispanic origin may be of any race.
[4]Excludes data for Louisiana, Maryland, Nebraska, Nevada, and Oklahoma, which did not report method of delivery on the birth certificate; data by Hispanic origin also excludes New Hampshire, which did not report Hispanic origin.
[5]Excludes data for New Hampshire and Oklahoma, which did not report data by Hispanic origin. Oklahoma did not report method of delivery.
[6]Excludes data for New Hampshire, which did not report Hispanic origin.

Table A-52. Number of Live Births, by Method 2009 of Delivery and Rates of Cesarean Delivery by Age and Race and Hispanic Origin of Mother, 2009

(Number, rate.)

Age, race, and Hispanic origin of mother	Number				Cesarean delivery rate[1]
	All births	Vaginal	Cesarean	Not stated	
All Races[2]	4,130,665	2,764,285	1,353,572	12,808	32.9
Under 20 years	414,831	318,124	95,802	905	23.1
20–24 years	1,005,982	717,208	285,906	2,868	28.5
25–29 years	1,166,787	794,512	368,707	3,568	31.7
30–34 years	955,246	606,937	345,157	3,152	36.3
35–39 years	474,103	270,359	201,936	1,808	42.8
40–54 years	113,716	57,145	56,064	507	49.5
Non-Hispanic White[3]	2,212,552	1,481,660	723,687	7,205	32.8
Under 20 years	160,632	122,630	37,575	427	23.5
20–24 years	490,773	351,635	137,665	1,473	28.1
25–29 years	657,658	452,686	202,951	2,021	31.0
30–34 years	565,026	363,549	199,554	1,923	35.4
35–39 years	273,174	157,872	114,226	1,076	42.1
40–54 years	65,289	33,288	31,716	285	48.8
Non-Hispanic Black[3]	609,584	392,715	214,810	2,059	35.4
Under 20 years	100,153	74,551	25,371	231	25.4
20–24 years	194,122	131,135	62,373	614	32.2
25–29 years	153,210	97,077	55,615	518	36.4
30–34 years	98,909	57,933	40,603	373	41.2
35–39 years	50,003	25,983	23,775	245	47.8
40–54 years	13,187	6,036	7,073	78	54.0
Hispanic[4]	999,548	682,512	315,025	2,011	31.6
Under 20 years	138,336	108,301	29,854	181	21.6
20–24 years	274,726	199,511	74,694	521	27.2
25–29 years	270,641	184,918	85,167	556	31.5
30–34 years	195,729	123,175	72,104	450	36.9
35–39 years	97,261	55,041	41,981	239	43.3
40–54 years	22,855	11,566	11,225	64	49.3

[1]Percentage of all live births by cesarean delivery.
[2]Includes races other than White and Black and origin not stated.
[3]Race and Hispanic origin are reported separately on birth certificates.
[4]Persons of Hispanic origin may be of any race.

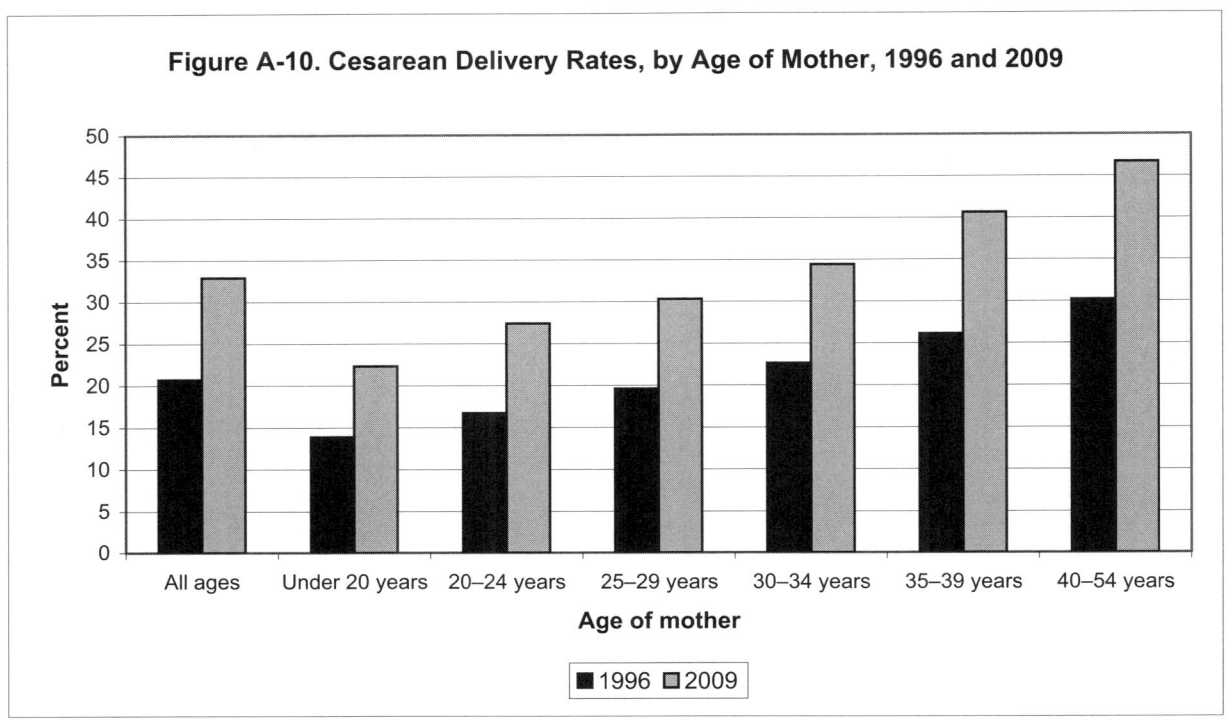

Figure A-10. Cesarean Delivery Rates, by Age of Mother, 1996 and 2009

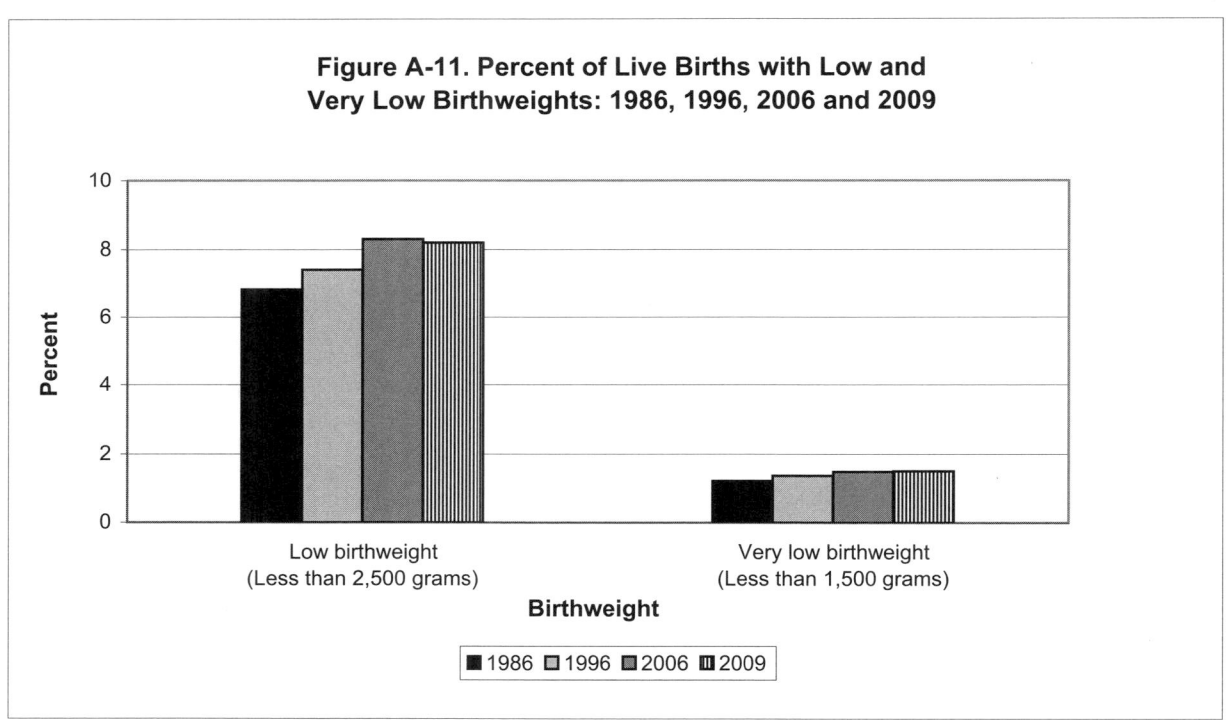

Figure A-11. Percent of Live Births with Low and Very Low Birthweights: 1986, 1996, 2006 and 2009

Table A-53. Rates of Cesarean Delivery by Race and Hispanic Origin of Mother, by State and Territory, 2009

(Rate.)

Area	Total cesarean delivery rate[1]			
	All races[2]	Non-Hispanic		Hispanic[4]
		White[3]	Black	
UNITED STATES[5]	32.9	32.8	35.4	31.6
Alabama	35.6	36.3	36.9	26.5
Alaska	23.8	27.0	31.1	30.3
Arizona	27.4	29.2	30.4	25.5
Arkansas	34.6	34.6	36.8	30.8
California	33.0	33.0	36.8	32.5
Colorado	26.4	27.8	28.2	23.1
Connecticut	35.6	36.6	36.2	32.2
Delaware	35.7	35.3	37.5	32.2
District of Columbia	32.0	33.9	32.7	27.6
Florida	38.1	36.1	38.5	41.2
Georgia	33.6	34.6	35.5	27.4
Hawaii	27.0	27.2	32.8	26.8
Idaho	24.5	23.8	32.4	26.8
Illinois	31.5	32.5	31.4	28.4
Indiana	30.5	30.3	33.4	28.3
Iowa	30.3	30.3	32.5	29.9
Kansas	30.1	30.7	31.6	26.5
Kentucky	35.9	36.4	35.7	29.4
Louisiana	39.6	41.0	38.4	35.7
Maine	29.6	29.7	24.2	35.4
Maryland	33.5	33.0	36.5	28.6
Massachusetts	33.4	34.7	33.4	29.2
Michigan	32.1	32.1	32.3	30.2
Minnesota	27.4	28.2	28.2	24.5
Mississippi	37.8	38.3	38.2	28.2
Missouri	31.7	31.9	32.3	27.2
Montana	29.6	29.0	33.8	33.7
Nebraska	31.7	32.7	32.4	27.4
Nevada	33.7	34.8	41.1	30.0
New Hampshire	30.8	30.8	27.6	30.6
New Jersey	39.4	39.9	40.7	36.9
New Mexico	22.8	23.7	26.9	22.8
New York	34.9	34.7	37.5	34.1
North Carolina	31.2	32.2	32.9	25.1
North Dakota	29.3	29.0	25.3	27.9
Ohio	31.1	31.1	31.7	28.9
Oklahoma	34.6	35.6	35.3	29.7
Oregon	29.4	29.2	33.9	28.2
Pennsylvania	31.8	32.1	31.6	30.6
Rhode Island	32.8	35.3	31.8	26.5
South Carolina	35.3	36.3	35.5	29.2
South Dakota	26.3	25.9	28.3	26.1
Tennessee	33.8	34.3	33.9	28.4
Texas	35.3	36.6	38.4	33.5
Utah	22.9	22.2	25.2	25.3
Vermont	27.8	27.7	*	38.3
Virginia	34.3	33.9	35.8	31.0
Washington	29.2	29.2	33.1	26.7
West Virginia	36.0	35.9	39.1	31.1
Wisconsin	25.8	26.8	23.3	24.2
Wyoming	28.1	27.2	35.7	31.2
Puerto Rico	48.1	48.6	49.4	48.1
Virgin Islands	27.1	29.5	26.9	27.9
Guam	26.3	19.7	*	*
American Samoa	—	—	—	—
Northern Marianas	19.2	—	—	—

— = Data not available.
* = Figure does not meet standards of reliability or precision.
[1] Percent of all live births by cesarean delivery.
[2] Includes races other than White and Black and origin not stated.
[3] Race and Hispanic origin are reported separately on birth certificates. Persons of Hispanic origin may be of any race.
[4] Includes all persons of Hispanic origin of any race.
[5] Excludes data for the territories.

Table A-54. Live Births by Birthweight and Percentage Very Low and Low Birthweight, by Period of Gestation and Race and Hispanic Origin of Mother, 2009

(Number, percent.)

Birthweight[1], race, and Hispanic origin of mother	All births	Period of gestation[2]								Postterm (42 weeks and over)	Not stated
		Preterm					Term				
		Total under 37 weeks	Under 28 weeks	28–31 weeks	32–33 weeks	34–36 weeks	Total 37–41 weeks	37–38 weeks	39 weeks	40–41 weeks		
ALL RACES[3]												
Total	4,130,665	502,306	30,642	50,543	63,776	357,345	3,394,486	1,138,029	1,133,391	1,123,066	228,588	5,285
Less than 500 grams	6,331	6,270	6,036	204	12	18	13	5	4	4	5	43
500–999 grams	22,696	22,436	16,774	5,127	337	198	175	62	59	54	22	63
1,000–1,499 grams	30,890	29,052	4,136	16,790	5,127	2,999	1,560	746	394	420	227	51
1,500–1,999 grams	65,603	55,409	908	12,203	19,492	22,806	9,258	6,178	1,624	1,456	816	120
2,000–2,499 grams	211,227	109,474	651	4,184	17,491	87,148	96,590	63,266	19,156	14,168	4,856	307
2,500–2,999 grams	767,266	134,745	1,159	4,259	8,943	120,384	599,289	297,535	174,326	127,428	32,248	984
3,000–3,499 grams	1,618,454	97,917	-	5,080	7,985	84,852	1,427,439	482,072	496,313	449,054	91,582	1,516
3,500–3,999 grams	1,090,696	37,418	-	2,596	3,528	31,294	978,743	233,666	346,769	398,308	73,579	956
4,000–4,499 grams	271,307	6,958	-	-	655	6,303	242,799	46,395	82,245	114,159	21,305	245
4,500–4,999 grams	37,909	1,048	-	-	107	941	33,365	6,662	10,763	15,940	3,458	38
5,000 grams or more	4,258	175	-	-	27	148	3,712	942	1,229	1,541	364	7
Not stated	4,028	1,404	978	100	72	254	1,543	500	509	534	126	955
Percent												
Very low birthweight[4]	1.5	11.5	90.8	43.9	8.6	0.9	0.1	0.1	0.0	0.0	0.1	3.6
Low birthweight[5]	8.2	44.4	96.1	76.3	66.6	31.7	3.2	6.2	1.9	1.4	2.6	13.5
NON-HISPANIC WHITE[6]												
Total	2,212,552	241,301	11,856	22,949	29,620	176,876	1,843,476	590,838	626,414	626,224	125,425	2,350
Less than 500 grams	2,339	2,318	2,214	91	3	10	5	1	1	3	1	15
500–999 grams	9,000	8,880	6,423	2,210	157	90	80	28	23	29	15	25
1,000–1,499 grams	14,336	13,499	1,837	7,870	2,406	1,386	701	332	166	203	116	20
1,500–1,999 grams	31,709	26,990	332	6,007	9,610	11,041	4,277	2,892	728	657	388	54
2,000–2,499 grams	101,570	54,662	239	1,694	8,963	43,766	44,393	29,405	8,625	6,363	2,393	122
2,500–2,999 grams	359,371	66,344	458	1,574	3,565	60,747	277,539	139,144	80,223	58,172	15,103	385
3,000–3,499 grams	843,903	46,024	-	2,157	3,012	40,855	749,503	250,587	264,194	234,722	47,716	660
3,500–3,999 grams	647,282	17,929	-	1,292	1,525	15,112	585,453	135,575	210,689	239,189	43,415	485
4,000–4,499 grams	174,177	3,525	-	-	302	3,223	156,859	28,224	53,709	74,926	13,661	132
4,500–4,999 grams	24,540	492	-	-	40	452	21,702	3,923	7,054	10,725	2,318	28
5,000 grams or more	2,491	75	-	-	8	67	2,179	485	738	956	233	4
Not stated	1,834	563	353	54	29	127	785	242	264	279	66	420
Percent												
Very low birthweight[4]	1.2	10.3	91.1	44.4	8.7	0.8	0.0	0.1	0.0	0.0	0.1	3.1
Low birthweight[5]	7.2	44.2	96	78.1	71.4	31.8	2.7	5.5	1.5	1.2	2.3	12.2
NON-HISPANIC BLACK[6]												
Total	609,584	106,316	10,607	12,934	14,326	68,449	471,889	177,717	152,020	142,152	30,512	867
Less than 500 grams	2,372	2,347	2,275	60	6	6	6	3	3	-	3	16
500–999 grams	7,752	7,680	5,955	1,584	92	49	48	15	23	10	2	22
1,000–1,499 grams	8,475	8,039	1,207	4,606	1,408	818	367	186	102	79	50	19
1,500–1,999 grams	15,924	13,393	270	2,820	4,722	5,581	2,299	1,527	409	363	193	39
2,000–2,499 grams	48,338	23,949	224	1,128	3,523	19,074	23,153	14,996	4,670	3,487	1,157	79
2,500–2,999 grams	154,872	26,515	335	1,143	2,123	22,914	121,519	60,417	35,497	25,605	6,621	217
3,000–3,499 grams	235,951	17,409	-	1,145	1,726	14,538	204,773	70,738	70,183	63,852	13,517	252
3,500–3,999 grams	110,264	5,512	-	429	601	4,482	97,436	24,688	33,750	38,998	7,198	118
4,000–4,499 grams	21,452	891	-	-	84	807	19,046	4,242	6,333	8,471	1,501	14
4,500–4,999 grams	2,882	117	-	-	12	105	2,547	672	826	1,049	216	2
5,000 grams or more	376	22	-	-	4	18	329	99	102	128	25	-
Not stated	926	442	341	19	25	57	366	134	122	110	29	89
Percent												
Very low birthweight[4]	3.1	17.1	91.9	48.4	10.5	1.3	0.1	0.1	0.1	0.1	0.2	7.3
Low birthweight[5]	13.6	52.3	96.7	79	68.2	37.3	5.5	9.4	3.4	2.8	4.6	22.5

Table A-54. Live Births by Birthweight and Percentage Very Low and Low Birthweight, by Period of Gestation and Race and Hispanic Origin of Mother, 2009—Continued

(Number, percent.)

Birthweight[1], race, and Hispanic origin of mother	All births	Period of gestation[2]									Postterm (42 weeks and over)	Not stated
		Preterm					Term					
		Total under 37 weeks	Under 28 weeks	28–31 weeks	32–33 weeks	34–36 weeks	Total 37–41 weeks	37–38 weeks	39 weeks	40–41 weeks		
HISPANIC[7]												
Total	999,548	119,507	6,272	11,411	15,520	86,304	820,908	282,462	267,487	270,959	57,946	1,187
Less than 500 grams	1,197	1,188	1,143	40	3	2	2	1	-	1	1	6
500–999 grams	4,574	4,531	3,396	1,022	66	47	31	16	9	6	3	9
1,000–1,499 grams	6,069	5,642	864	3,239	951	588	369	168	94	107	48	10
1,500–1,999 grams	13,250	11,086	251	2,616	3,822	4,397	1,967	1,266	371	330	179	18
2,000–2,499 grams	44,266	22,696	154	1,070	3,888	17,584	20,512	13,111	4,173	3,228	992	66
2,500–2,999 grams	184,327	32,025	275	1,232	2,628	27,890	143,924	70,923	41,483	31,518	8,121	257
3,000–3,499 grams	411,536	27,974	-	1,459	2,737	23,778	359,062	124,369	121,071	113,622	24,071	429
3,500–3,999 grams	263,252	11,595	-	720	1,148	9,727	232,727	59,072	79,816	93,839	18,688	242
4,000–4,499 grams	61,020	2,111	-	-	214	1,897	53,847	11,470	17,800	24,577	5,001	61
4,500–4,999 grams	8,382	352	-	-	43	309	7,276	1,701	2,277	3,298	751	3
5,000 grams or more	1,086	55	-	-	6	49	955	284	319	352	74	2
Not stated	589	252	189	13	14	36	236	81	734	81	17	84
Percent												
Very low birthweight[4]	1.2	9.5	88.8	37.7	6.6	0.7	0.0	0.1	0.0	0.0	0.1	2.3
Low birthweight[5]	6.9	37.9	95.5	70.1	56.3	26.2	2.8	5.2	1.7	1.4	2.1	9.9

– = Quantity zero.
0.0 = Quantity more than zero but less than 0.05.
[1]Equivalent of the gram weights in pounds and ounces are shown in the notes and definitions at the end of the chapter.
[2]Expressed in completed weeks.
[3]Includes races other than White and Black and origin not stated.
[4]Birthweight of less than 1,500 grams (3 lb 4 oz).
[5]Birthweight of less than 2,500 grams (5 lb 8 oz).
[6]Race and Hispanic origin are reported separately on the birth certificate.
[7]Persons of Hispanic origin may be of any race.

Table A-55. Percentage of Live Births Very Preterm and Preterm and Percentage of Live Births of Very Low Birthweight and Low Birthweight, by Race and Hispanic Origin of Mother, 1981–2009

(Percent.)

Year	Very preterm[1]				Preterm[2]			
	All races[3]	Non-Hispanic		Hispanic[5]	All races[3]	Non-Hispanic		Hispanic[5]
		White[4]	Black[4]			White[4]	Black[4]	
1981	1.81	—	—	—	9.44	—	—	—
1982	1.84	—	—	—	9.50	—	—	—
1983	1.86	—	—	—	9.61	—	—	—
1984	1.83	—	—	—	9.40	—	—	—
1985	1.88	—	—	—	9.76	—	—	—
1986	1.90	—	—	—	9.97	—	—	—
1987	1.96	—	—	—	10.20	—	—	—
1988	1.96	—	—	—	10.22	—	—	—
1989[6]	1.95	1.34	4.68	1.76	10.58	8.40	19.05	11.10
1990[7]	1.92	1.33	4.63	1.69	10.62	8.50	18.89	10.96
1991[8]	1.94	1.35	4.65	1.65	10.82	8.73	19.00	10.96
1992[8]	1.91	1.33	4.50	1.64	10.69	8.72	18.49	10.75
1993	1.93	1.39	4.45	1.67	10.99	9.08	18.58	10.98
1994	1.91	1.39	4.36	1.67	11.02	9.27	18.18	10.94
1995	1.89	1.41	4.29	1.66	10.99	9.40	17.77	10.91
1996	1.89	1.43	4.17	1.66	10.99	9.50	17.51	10.89
1997	1.94	1.49	4.19	1.68	11.36	9.94	17.61	11.20
1998	1.96	1.52	4.15	1.72	11.69	10.24	17.60	11.43
1999	1.96	1.54	4.18	1.68	11.77	10.52	17.63	11.43
2000	1.93	1.51	4.09	1.69	11.64	10.43	17.41	11.24
2001	1.95	1.55	4.05	1.69	11.95	10.81	17.63	11.45
2002	1.96	1.56	4.04	1.72	12.08	10.98	17.66	11.61
2003	1.97	1.60	3.99	1.73	12.33	11.30	17.83	11.87
2004	2.01	1.63	4.05	1.77	12.49	11.50	17.91	12.00
2005	2.03	1.64	4.17	1.79	12.73	11.69	18.43	12.13
2006	2.04	1.66	4.08	1.80	12.80	11.70	18.46	12.25
2007	2.04	1.64	4.08	1.82	12.68	11.50	18.29	12.29
2008	1.99	1.60	3.84	1.80	12.33	11.14	17.54	12.10
2009	1.97	1.57	3.87	1.77	12.18	10.92	17.47	11.97

Table A-55. Percentage of Live Births Very Preterm and Preterm and Percentage of Live Births of Very Low Birthweight and Low Birthweight, by Race and Hispanic Origin of Mother, 1981–2009—Continued

(Percent.)

Year	Very low birthweight[9]				Low birthweight[10]			
	All races[3]	Non-Hispanic		Hispanic[5]	All races[3]	Non-Hispanic		Hispanic[5]
		White[4]	Black[4]			White[4]	Black[4]	
1981	1.16	—	—	—	6.81	—	—	—
1982	1.18	—	—	—	6.75	—	—	—
1983	1.19	—	—	—	6.82	—	—	—
1984	1.19	—	—	—	6.72	—	—	—
1985	1.21	—	—	—	6.75	—	—	—
1986	1.21	—	—	—	6.81	—	—	—
1987	1.24	—	—	—	6.90	—	—	—
1988	1.24	—	—	—	6.93	—	—	—
1989[6]	1.28	0.93	2.97	1.05	7.05	5.62	13.61	6.18
1990[7]	1.27	0.93	2.93	1.03	6.97	5.61	13.32	6.06
1991[8]	1.29	0.94	2.97	1.02	7.12	5.72	13.62	6.15
1992[8]	1.29	0.94	2.97	1.04	7.08	5.73	13.40	6.10
1993	1.33	1.00	2.99	1.06	7.22	5.92	13.43	6.24
1994	1.33	1.01	2.99	1.08	7.28	6.06	13.34	6.25
1995	1.35	1.04	2.98	1.11	7.32	6.20	13.21	6.29
1996	1.37	1.08	3.02	1.12	7.39	6.36	13.12	6.28
1997	1.42	1.12	3.05	1.13	7.51	6.47	13.11	6.42
1998	1.45	1.15	3.11	1.15	7.57	6.55	13.17	6.44
1999	1.45	1.15	3.18	1.14	7.62	6.64	13.23	6.38
2000	1.43	1.14	3.10	1.14	7.57	6.60	13.13	6.41
2001	1.44	1.17	3.08	1.14	7.68	6.76	13.07	6.47
2002	1.46	1.17	3.15	1.17	7.82	6.91	13.39	6.55
2003	1.45	1.18	3.12	1.16	7.93	7.04	13.55	6.69
2004	1.48	1.20	3.15	1.20	8.08	7.20	13.74	6.79
2005	1.49	1.21	3.27	1.20	8.19	7.29	14.02	6.88
2006	1.49	1.20	3.15	1.19	8.26	7.32	13.97	6.99
2007	1.49	1.19	3.20	1.21	8.22	7.28	13.90	6.93
2008	1.46	1.18	3.01	1.20	8.18	7.22	13.71	6.96
2009	1.45	1.16	3.06	1.19	8.16	7.19	13.61	6.94

— = Data not available.
[1]Births of less than 32 completed weeks of gestation.
[2]Births of less than 37 completed weeks of gestation.
[3]Includes races other than White and Black and origin not stated.
[4]Race and Hispanic origin are reported separately on birth certificates.
[5]Includes all persons of Hispanic origin of any race.
[6]Data by Hispanic origin exclude New Hampshire, Oklahoma, and Louisiana, which did not report Hispanic origin.
[7]Data by Hispanic origin exclude New Hampshire and Oklahoma, which did not report Hispanic origin.
[8]Data by Hispanic origin exclude New Hampshire, which did not report Hispanic origin.
[9]Less than 1,500 grams (3 lb. 4 oz.).
[10]Less than 2,500 grams (5 lb. 8 oz.).

Table A-56. Birthweight Distribution in 500 Gram Intervals, Selected Years, 1990–2009

(Percent.)

Weight	All births				Percent change		
	1990	2006	2008	2009	1990–2006	1990–2009	2006–2009
Total <1,000	0.63	0.72	0.70	0.70	14	11	-3
1,000–1,499 grams	0.65	0.76	0.75	0.75	17	15	-2
1,500–1,999 grams	1.33	1.63	1.58	1.59	23	20	-2
2,000–2,499 grams	4.37	5.15	5.14	5.12	18	17	-1
2,500–2,999 grams	16.03	18.44	18.57	18.59	15	16	1
3,000–3,499 grams	36.71	38.87	39.20	39.22	6	7	1
3,500–3,999 grams	29.40	26.61	26.41	26.43	-9	-10	-1
4,000–4,499 grams	9.10	6.75	6.60	6.57	-26	-28	-3
4,500–4,999 grams	1.59	0.96	0.92	0.92	-40	-42	-4
5,000 grams or more	0.19	0.11	0.10	0.10	-42	-46	-6

Table A-57. Preterm and Low Birthweight Births, by Age and Race and Hispanic Origin of Mother, 2009

(Percent, number.)

Age, race, and Hispanic origin of mother	Preterm[1]							Low birthweight[2]						
	Percent			Number				Percent			Number			
	Total	Early[3]	Late[4]	Total	Early[3]	Late[4]	Unknown	Total	Very[5]	Moderately[6]	Total	Very[5]	Moderately[6]	Unknown
All Races[7]														
All ages	12.2	3.5	8.7	502,306	144,961	357,345	5,285	8.2	1.5	6.7	336,747	59,917	276,830	4,028
Under 15 years	20.5	7.7	12.8	1,028	384	644	17	12.3	2.7	9.6	618	137	481	10
15–19 years	13.6	4.4	9.2	55,625	18,063	37,562	603	9.6	1.7	7.9	39,335	6,996	32,339	408
15 years	16.8	6.1	10.7	2,626	952	1,674	32	10.7	1.9	8.8	1,668	300	1,368	16
16 years	15.7	5.5	10.2	5,924	2,063	3,861	70	10.3	1.9	8.4	3,897	730	3,167	48
17 years	14.1	4.6	9.5	9,980	3,263	6,717	102	9.8	1.7	8.0	6,904	1,229	5,675	66
18 years	13.6	4.5	9.1	15,911	5,225	10,686	180	9.8	1.8	8.0	11,485	2,061	9,424	125
19 years	12.6	3.9	8.7	21,184	6,560	14,624	219	9.2	1.6	7.6	15,381	2,676	12,705	153
20–24 years	12.1	3.5	8.5	121,073	35,471	85,602	1,301	8.3	1.4	6.8	82,946	14,192	68,754	996
25–29 years	11.2	3.1	8.0	129,958	36,188	93,770	1,450	7.4	1.3	6.1	86,268	15,255	71,013	1,146
30–34 years	11.6	3.2	8.4	110,552	30,585	79,967	1,074	7.6	1.4	6.2	72,319	12,947	59,372	862
35–39 years	13.7	3.9	9.8	64,648	18,473	46,175	629	8.9	1.7	7.2	41,990	7,925	34,065	479
40–44 years	16.4	4.8	11.6	17,313	5,066	12,247	191	11.0	2.0	8.9	11,584	2,146	9,438	118
45–54 years	26.8	9.3	17.5	2,109	731	1,378	20	21.4	4.0	17.4	1,687	319	1,368	9
Non-Hispanic White[8]														
All ages	10.9	2.9	8.0	241,301	64,425	176,876	2,350	7.2	1.2	6.0	158,954	25,675	133,279	1,834
Under 15 years	18.2	6.8	11.4	191	71	120	3	10.5	2.3	8.3	111	24	87	0
15–19 years	11.8	3.7	8.2	18,869	5,825	13,044	188	8.5	1.5	7.0	13,540	2,403	11,137	131
15 years	15.0	5.5	9.5	582	214	368	6	9.5	1.8	7.7	367	68	299	4
16 years	14.0	4.8	9.1	1,559	539	1,020	14	9.4	1.8	7.6	1,053	202	851	9
17 years	12.0	3.8	8.3	2,988	933	2,055	34	8.5	1.6	7.0	2,119	387	1,732	16
18 years	12.2	3.9	8.3	5,660	1,792	3,868	50	8.9	1.6	7.3	4,121	749	3,372	35
19 years	11.1	3.2	7.8	8,080	2,347	5,733	84	8.0	1.4	6.7	5,880	997	4,883	67
20–24 years	10.7	2.9	7.7	52,320	14,374	37,946	551	7.2	1.1	6.1	35,538	5,599	29,939	415
25–29 years	10.1	2.6	7.5	66,044	16,984	49,060	606	6.5	1.0	5.5	42,982	6,840	36,142	502
30–34 years	10.5	2.7	7.8	59,385	15,187	44,198	533	6.7	1.1	5.7	37,945	6,028	31,917	455
35–39 years	12.5	3.3	9.2	33,987	8,999	24,988	355	8.0	1.3	6.6	21,704	3,623	18,081	255
40–44 years	15.3	4.2	11.1	9,228	2,550	6,678	98	10.1	1.6	8.5	6,100	982	5,118	71
45–54 years	26.5	9.0	17.5	1,277	435	842	16	21.4	3.6	17.8	1,034	176	858	5
Non-Hispanic Black[8]														
All ages	17.5	6.2	11.2	106,316	37,867	68,449	867	13.6	3.1	10.6	82,861	18,599	64,262	926
Under 15 years	23.9	9.9	14.0	405	168	237	9	15.5	3.6	11.9	264	61	203	5
15–19 years	17.5	6.4	11.2	17,223	6,261	10,962	177	13.9	2.7	11.2	13,675	2,677	10,998	142
15 years	20.6	8.1	12.5	923	362	561	8	14.0	2.5	11.4	627	113	514	5
16 years	19.7	7.7	12.0	1,931	757	1,174	30	14.4	3.0	11.4	1,409	295	1,114	13
17 years	17.9	6.5	11.4	3,089	1,123	1,966	26	13.9	2.6	11.3	2,399	453	1,946	28
18 years	17.3	6.4	10.9	4,873	1,798	3,075	59	14.0	2.8	11.2	3,943	797	3,146	46
19 years	16.6	5.8	10.8	6,407	2,221	4,186	54	13.7	2.6	11.1	5,297	1,019	4,278	50
20–24 years	16.7	5.8	10.9	32,363	11,231	21,132	255	13.3	2.7	10.6	25,863	5,306	20,557	289
25–29 years	16.8	6.0	10.8	25,673	9,108	16,565	217	13.0	3.1	10.0	19,926	4,689	15,237	238
30–34 years	17.8	6.4	11.4	17,607	6,363	11,244	129	13.5	3.3	10.1	13,300	3,307	9,993	159
35–39 years	20.2	7.4	12.8	10,108	3,720	6,388	57	15.2	4.0	11.2	7,609	2,019	5,590	79
40–44 years	21.8	7.5	14.3	2,685	926	1,759	22	16.5	4.0	12.5	2,028	492	1,536	12
45–54 years	28.9	10.3	18.6	252	90	162	1	22.5	5.5	17.0	196	48	148	2
Hispanic[9]														
All ages	12.0	3.3	8.6	119,507	33,203	86,304	1,187	6.9	1.2	5.8	69,356	11,840	57,516	589
Under 15 years	19.4	6.4	13.0	401	132	269	4	10.6	2.4	8.2	219	49	170	4
15–19 years	12.7	3.8	8.9	17,291	5,203	12,088	191	7.9	1.2	6.6	10,696	1,661	9,035	98
15 years	15.2	5.0	10.2	1,005	329	676	16	9.0	1.6	7.4	600	107	493	5
16 years	14.4	4.5	9.8	2,206	695	1,511	22	8.4	1.4	7.0	1,291	214	1,077	19
17 years	13.3	4.0	9.4	3,461	1,027	2,434	36	8.2	1.3	6.9	2,121	326	1,795	19
18 years	12.5	3.8	8.7	4,785	1,440	3,345	54	8.0	1.2	6.8	3,044	451	2,593	32
19 years	11.7	3.4	8.3	5,834	1,712	4,122	63	7.3	1.1	6.2	3,640	563	3,077	23
20–24 years	11.3	3.1	8.2	30,969	8,385	22,584	334	6.5	1.0	5.5	17,925	2,741	15,184	159
25–29 years	11.0	2.9	8.1	29,730	7,910	21,820	309	6.3	1.1	5.2	16,967	2,854	14,113	160
30–34 years	12.0	3.3	8.7	23,545	6,443	17,102	213	6.9	1.3	5.6	13,469	2,513	10,956	106
35–39 years	14.1	4.1	10.0	13,677	3,937	9,740	107	7.9	1.6	6.4	7,703	1,529	6,174	56
40–44 years	16.6	5.0	11.6	3,583	1,080	2,503	28	9.9	2.1	7.8	2,143	450	1,693	4
45–54 years	25.6	9.3	16.3	311	113	198	1	19.3	3.5	15.7	234	43	191	2

[1] Less than 37 completed weeks of gestation.
[2] Less than 2,500 grams.
[3] Less than 34 completed weeks of gestation.
[4] 34–36 completed weeks of gestation.
[5] Less than 1,500 grams.
[6] 1,500–2,499 grams.
[7] Includes races other than White and Black and origin not stated.
[8] Race and Hispanic origin are reported separately on birth certificates.
[9] Persons of Hispanic origin of any race.

PART A: BIRTHS

Table A-58. Number and Percentage of Births of Very Low Birthweight, by Race and Hispanic Origin of Mother by State and Territory, 2009

(Number, percent.)

Area	Number				Percent			
	All races[1]	Non-Hispanic		Hispanic[3]	All races[1]	Non-Hispanic		Hispanic[3]
		White[2]	Black[2]			White[2]	Black[2]	
UNITED STATES[4]	59,917	25,675	18,599	11,840	1.5	1.2	3.1	1.2
Alabama	1,195	482	648	44	1.9	1.3	3.4	0.9
Alaska	113	54	5	8	1.0	0.9	*	*
Arizona	1,084	421	116	440	1.2	1.1	2.8	1.1
Arkansas	642	347	247	35	1.6	1.3	3.2	0.8
California	6,064	1,430	813	2,890	1.2	1.0	2.6	1.1
Colorado	829	463	68	247	1.2	1.1	2.2	1.2
Connecticut	555	239	157	135	1.4	1.0	3.2	1.6
Delaware	214	73	110	20	1.9	1.2	3.5	1.2
District of Columbia	187	19	140	24	2.1	*	3.0	1.6
Florida	3,498	1,093	1,535	764	1.6	1.1	3.0	1.2
Georgia	2,414	712	1,344	247	1.7	1.2	2.9	1.0
Hawaii	264	59	10	53	1.4	1.3	*	1.7
Idaho	248	186	4	47	1.0	1.0	*	1.3
Illinois	2,588	1,054	946	454	1.5	1.2	3.2	1.1
Indiana	1,263	800	305	122	1.5	1.2	3.0	1.5
Iowa	435	352	46	31	1.1	1.1	2.4	1.0
Kansas	567	355	95	89	1.4	1.2	3.1	1.3
Kentucky	858	633	168	46	1.5	1.3	3.1	1.5
Louisiana	1,308	450	812	35	2.0	1.3	3.2	1.0
Maine	129	121	1	4	1.0	1.0	*	*
Maryland	1,339	370	763	134	1.8	1.1	3.1	1.3
Massachusetts	1,006	587	168	181	1.3	1.2	2.3	1.7
Michigan	1,890	987	740	87	1.6	1.2	3.3	1.1
Minnesota	792	509	149	59	1.1	1.0	2.3	1.0
Mississippi	898	264	608	18	2.1	1.2	3.2	*
Missouri	1,222	761	384	48	1.5	1.3	3.2	1.1
Montana	125	91	1	5	1.0	0.9	*	*
Nebraska	315	209	51	38	1.2	1.1	2.9	0.9
Nevada	477	191	86	147	1.3	1.2	2.4	1.0
New Hampshire	147	125	4	7	1.1	1.0	*	*
New Jersey	1,667	592	548	398	1.5	1.1	3.2	1.4
New Mexico	355	105	20	176	1.2	1.3	3.9	1.1
New York	3,767	1,398	1,242	830	1.5	1.2	3.0	1.4
North Carolina	2,263	905	1,032	231	1.8	1.3	3.4	1.1
North Dakota	112	86	-	7	1.2	1.2	*	*
Ohio	2,331	1,432	740	94	1.6	1.3	3.1	1.4
Oklahoma	799	456	157	92	1.5	1.3	3.1	1.3
Oregon	479	328	16	98	1.0	1.0	*	1.0
Pennsylvania	2,347	1,242	704	244	1.6	1.2	3.3	1.7
Rhode Island	193	110	22	39	1.7	1.6	2.4	1.6
South Carolina	1,104	419	610	60	1.8	1.2	3.1	1.1
South Dakota	129	86	4	7	1.1	0.9	*	*
Tennessee	1,364	722	547	70	1.7	1.3	3.1	0.9
Texas	5,906	1,771	1,398	2,502	1.5	1.3	3.1	1.2
Utah	550	395	13	105	1.0	0.9	*	1.2
Vermont	67	64	1	1	1.1	1.1	*	*
Virginia	1,703	724	717	157	1.6	1.2	3.1	1.1
Washington	862	514	73	176	1.0	0.9	1.8	1.0
West Virginia	313	285	24	1	1.5	1.4	2.9	*
Wisconsin	850	534	207	78	1.2	1.0	2.8	1.1
Wyoming	90	70	-	15	1.1	1.1	*	*
Puerto Rico	641	18	3	617	1.4	*	*	1.4
Virgin Islands	21	1	15	5	1.3	*	*	*
Guam	39	4	-	-	1.1	*	*	*
American Samoa	2	—	—	—	*	—	—	—
Northern Marianas	4	—	—	—	*	—	—	—

— = Data not available.
– = Quantity zero.
* = Figure does not meet standards of reliability or precision.
[1]Includes races other than White and Black and origin not stated.
[2]Race and Hispanic origin are reported separately on birth certificates.
[3]Persons of Hispanic origin may be of any race.
[4]Excludes data for the territories.

Table A-59. Number and Percentage of Births Delivered Preterm, by Race and Hispanic Origin of Mother by State and Territory, 2009

(Number, percent.)

Area	Number				Percent			
	All races[1]	Non-Hispanic		Hispanic[3]	All races[1]	Non-Hispanic		Hispanic[3]
		White[2]	Black[2]			White[2]	Black[2]	
UNITED STATES[4]	502,306	241,301	106,316	119,507	12.2	10.9	17.5	12.0
Alabama	9,712	4,818	3,961	769	15.6	13.1	20.6	15.0
Alaska	1,240	529	72	79	11.0	8.8	17.8	11.4
Arizona	11,821	4,758	758	4,997	12.7	11.9	18.3	12.8
Arkansas	5,189	3,193	1,390	475	13.1	11.9	18.3	11.3
California	53,956	13,637	4,449	27,794	10.3	9.3	14.3	10.3
Colorado	7,730	4,366	463	2,454	11.3	10.6	14.8	11.9
Connecticut	3,973	2,099	660	959	10.2	9.2	13.3	11.2
Delaware	1,445	612	561	207	12.5	9.9	17.7	12.6
District of Columbia	1,280	201	820	205	14.2	8.7	17.4	13.6
Florida	29,975	11,494	9,204	8,243	13.5	11.4	18.2	13.3
Georgia	19,407	7,157	8,165	2,948	13.8	11.6	17.7	12.0
Hawaii	2,367	459	60	402	12.6	10.0	14.6	12.8
Idaho	2,394	1,796	17	482	10.1	9.4	*	13.1
Illinois	21,168	9,942	5,348	4,809	12.4	10.9	17.9	12.0
Indiana	10,316	7,388	1,715	957	11.9	11.1	17.0	11.8
Iowa	4,467	3,649	324	361	11.3	10.9	17.0	11.2
Kansas	4,609	3,157	508	735	11.2	10.6	16.6	10.9
Kentucky	7,849	6,334	991	404	13.6	13.2	18.2	13.5
Louisiana	9,572	4,132	4,841	394	14.7	12.0	19.3	11.1
Maine	1,334	1,237	44	19	9.9	9.9	11.2	*
Maryland	9,550	3,566	4,089	1,316	12.7	10.5	16.4	12.4
Massachusetts	8,099	5,153	1,013	1,265	10.9	10.3	14.0	11.5
Michigan	14,564	9,119	3,987	868	12.4	11.1	18.0	11.0
Minnesota	7,084	4,989	787	537	10.1	9.8	12.2	9.6
Mississippi	7,712	3,104	4,260	214	18.0	14.5	22.3	14.2
Missouri	9,578	6,537	2,220	561	12.2	10.9	18.5	13.1
Montana	1,331	1,050	9	39	10.9	10.5	*	9.2
Nebraska	3,096	2,130	294	536	11.5	10.8	16.7	12.6
Nevada	5,133	1,920	694	1,944	13.8	12.2	19.4	13.6
New Hampshire	1,323	1,159	40	60	9.9	9.7	18.5	10.9
New Jersey	13,188	5,546	2,866	3,570	12.0	10.6	16.7	12.3
New Mexico	3,572	839	97	2,031	12.3	10.4	18.9	12.6
New York	30,229	12,467	6,898	7,815	12.2	10.4	16.8	13.1
North Carolina	16,494	7,987	5,338	2,436	13.0	11.3	17.6	12.1
North Dakota	952	730	22	31	10.6	10.0	13.6	9.9
Ohio	17,824	12,206	4,251	876	12.3	11.1	17.9	12.7
Oklahoma	7,512	4,570	978	964	13.8	13.2	19.3	13.3
Oregon	4,624	3,134	132	1,003	9.8	9.6	11.6	10.3
Pennsylvania	16,754	10,633	3,444	1,833	11.5	10.3	16.1	13.0
Rhode Island	1,305	712	140	308	11.4	10.2	15.5	12.3
South Carolina	8,806	4,210	3,697	687	14.5	12.4	19.0	12.4
South Dakota	1,302	907	46	64	10.9	10.0	18.6	13.4
Tennessee	10,630	6,479	3,053	865	13.0	11.7	17.6	11.7
Texas	52,650	16,281	7,988	26,365	13.1	11.8	17.6	13.1
Utah	6,092	4,503	93	1,189	11.3	10.6	17.0	13.6
Vermont	570	535	8	12	9.3	9.2	*	*
Virginia	12,002	6,049	3,548	1,533	11.4	10.0	15.4	11.2
Washington	9,180	5,396	542	1,929	10.3	9.5	13.3	11.2
West Virginia	2,739	2,537	155	20	12.9	12.7	18.7	8.7
Wisconsin	7,724	5,215	1,272	815	10.9	9.9	17.5	11.8
Wyoming	883	680	4	128	11.2	10.7	*	13.1
Puerto Rico	7,895	236	33	7,621	17.7	18.4	19.2	17.6
Virgin Islands	221	17	148	49	13.2	*	13.9	12.6
Guam	560	20	3	1	16.4	9.3	*	*
American Samoa	—	—	—	—	—	—	—	—
Northern Marianas	173	—	—	—	15.6	—	—	—

— = Data not available
* = Figure does not meet standards of reliability or precision.
[1]Includes races other than White and Black and origin not stated.
[2]Race and Hispanic origin are reported separately on birth certificates.
[3]Includes all persons of Hispanic origin of any race.
[4]Excludes data for the territories.

Table A-60. Number and Percentage of Births of Low Birthweight, by Race and Hispanic Origin of Mother, 2009

(Number, percent.)

Area	Number				Percent			
	All races[1]	Non-Hispanic		Hispanic[3]	All races[1]	Non-Hispanic		Hispanic[3]
		White[2]	Black[2]			White[2]	Black[2]	
UNITED STATES[4]	336,747	158,954	82,861	69,356	8.2	7.2	13.6	6.9
Alabama	6,454	3,088	2,942	310	10.3	8.4	15.3	6.0
Alaska	666	306	53	43	5.9	5.1	13.0	6.2
Arizona	6,575	2,751	521	2,618	7.1	6.9	12.6	6.7
Arkansas	3,546	2,060	1,132	259	8.9	7.6	14.8	6.2
California	35,802	9,101	3,666	16,637	6.8	6.2	11.8	6.2
Colorado	6,007	3,471	422	1,738	8.8	8.4	13.5	8.4
Connecticut	3,127	1,588	590	727	8.0	7.0	11.9	8.5
Delaware	994	420	422	100	8.6	6.8	13.3	6.1
District of Columbia	929	163	613	114	10.3	7.0	13.0	7.5
Florida	19,247	7,354	6,793	4,379	8.7	7.3	13.4	7.1
Georgia	13,190	4,601	6,199	1,561	9.4	7.5	13.5	6.4
Hawaii	1,592	315	52	287	8.4	6.8	12.7	9.2
Idaho	1,541	1,160	11	302	6.5	6.1	*	8.2
Illinois	14,316	6,444	4,224	2,727	8.4	7.1	14.1	6.8
Indiana	7,225	5,088	1,389	550	8.3	7.7	13.8	6.8
Iowa	2,671	2,161	236	190	6.7	6.5	12.4	5.9
Kansas	3,011	2,028	394	437	7.3	6.8	12.9	6.4
Kentucky	5,141	4,079	756	217	8.9	8.5	13.9	7.3
Louisiana	6,915	2,826	3,683	250	10.6	8.2	14.7	7.0
Maine	851	791	17	21	6.3	6.3	*	10.6
Maryland	6,836	2,427	3,232	702	9.1	7.1	13.0	6.6
Massachusetts	5,802	3,590	784	941	7.8	7.2	10.9	8.6
Michigan	9,799	5,766	3,059	513	8.4	7.0	13.8	6.5
Minnesota	4,604	3,080	651	325	6.5	6.0	10.1	5.8
Mississippi	5,249	1,945	3,129	104	12.2	9.1	16.4	6.9
Missouri	6,393	4,206	1,705	297	8.1	7.0	14.2	6.9
Montana	865	715	2	27	7.1	7.2	*	6.4
Nebraska	1,922	1,284	232	297	7.1	6.5	13.2	7.0
Nevada	3,046	1,229	500	965	8.1	7.7	13.9	6.7
New Hampshire	925	806	20	49	6.9	6.7	9.2	8.9
New Jersey	9,137	3,767	2,243	2,069	8.3	7.2	13.1	7.1
New Mexico	2,416	627	86	1,357	8.3	7.8	16.8	8.4
New York	20,341	8,250	5,270	4,640	8.2	6.9	12.9	7.8
North Carolina	11,454	5,275	4,336	1,281	9.0	7.5	14.3	6.4
North Dakota	572	445	8	21	6.4	6.1	*	6.7
Ohio	12,378	8,174	3,319	509	8.6	7.5	14.0	7.4
Oklahoma	4,558	2,795	731	483	8.4	8.1	14.4	6.7
Oregon	2,955	1,988	114	603	6.3	6.1	10.0	6.2
Pennsylvania	12,187	7,374	2,844	1,277	8.3	7.2	13.3	9.1
Rhode Island	913	519	95	195	8.0	7.4	10.5	7.8
South Carolina	6,047	2,678	2,853	367	10.0	7.9	14.7	6.6
South Dakota	696	514	30	28	5.8	5.6	12.2	5.9
Tennessee	7,539	4,474	2,402	479	9.2	8.1	13.8	6.4
Texas	34,137	10,798	6,448	15,284	8.5	7.8	14.2	7.6
Utah	3,766	2,851	50	669	7.0	6.7	9.1	7.6
Vermont	411	389	2	6	6.7	6.7	*	*
Virginia	8,779	4,288	3,018	844	8.4	7.1	13.1	6.2
Washington	5,580	3,315	421	1,018	6.3	5.9	10.3	5.9
West Virginia	1,952	1,797	122	14	9.2	9.0	14.7	*
Wisconsin	5,027	3,293	1,032	423	7.1	6.3	14.2	6.1
Wyoming	661	500	8	102	8.4	7.9	*	10.4
Puerto Rico	5,525	155	18	5,348	12.4	12.1	*	12.4
Virgin Islands	159	14	100	39	9.5	*	9.4	10.1
Guam	261	11	-	-	7.7	*	*	*
American Samoa	36	—	—	—	2.7	—	—	—
Northern Marianas	95	—	—	—	8.6	—	—	—

— = Data not available
 - = Quantity zero.
* = Figure does not meet standards of reliability or precision.
[1]Includes races other than White and Black and origin not stated.
[2]Race and Hispanic origin are reported separately on birth certificates. Persons of Hispanic origin may be of any race.
[3]Includes all persons of Hispanic origin of any race.
[4]Excludes data for the territories.

Table A-61. Very Low Birthweight Births, by Race and Hispanic Origin of Mother by State and Territory, 2009

(Number, percent.)

Area	Number				Percent			
	All races[1]	White[2]	Black[2]	Hispanic[3]	All races[1]	White[2]	Black[2]	Hispanic[3]
United States[4]	59,917	25,675	18,599	11,840	1.5	1.2	3.1	1.2
Alabama	1,195	482	648	44	1.9	1.3	3.4	0.9
Alaska	113	54	5	8	1.0	0.9	*	*
Arizona	1,084	421	116	440	1.2	1.1	2.8	1.1
Arkansas	642	347	247	35	1.6	1.3	3.2	0.8
California	6,064	1,430	813	2,890	1.2	1.0	2.6	1.1
Colorado	829	463	68	247	1.2	1.1	2.2	1.2
Connecticut	555	239	157	135	1.4	1.0	3.2	1.6
Delaware	214	73	110	20	1.9	1.2	3.5	1.2
District of Columbia	187	19	140	24	2.1	*	3.0	1.6
Florida	3,498	1,093	1,535	764	1.6	1.1	3.0	1.2
Georgia	2,414	712	1,344	247	1.7	1.2	2.9	1.0
Hawaii	264	59	10	53	1.4	1.3	*	1.7
Idaho	248	186	4	47	1.0	1.0	*	1.3
Illinois	2,588	1,054	946	454	1.5	1.2	3.2	1.1
Indiana	1,263	800	305	122	1.5	1.2	3.0	1.5
Iowa	435	352	46	31	1.1	1.1	2.4	1.0
Kansas	567	355	95	89	1.4	1.2	3.1	1.3
Kentucky	858	633	168	46	1.5	1.3	3.1	1.5
Louisiana	1,308	450	812	35	2.0	1.3	3.2	1.0
Maine	129	121	1	4	1.0	1.0	*	*
Maryland	1,339	370	763	134	1.8	1.1	3.1	1.3
Massachusetts	1,006	587	168	181	1.3	1.2	2.3	1.7
Michigan	1,890	987	740	87	1.6	1.2	3.3	1.1
Minnesota	792	509	149	59	1.1	1.0	2.3	1.0
Mississippi	898	264	608	18	2.1	1.2	3.2	*
Missouri	1,222	761	384	48	1.5	1.3	3.2	1.1
Montana	125	91	1	5	1.0	0.9	*	*
Nebraska	315	209	51	38	1.2	1.1	2.9	0.9
Nevada	477	191	86	147	1.3	1.2	2.4	1.0
New Hampshire	147	125	4	7	1.1	1.0	*	*
New Jersey	1,667	592	548	398	1.5	1.1	3.2	1.4
New Mexico	355	105	20	176	1.2	1.3	3.9	1.1
New York	3,767	1,398	1,242	830	1.5	1.2	3.0	1.4
North Carolina	2,263	905	1,032	231	1.8	1.3	3.4	1.1
North Dakota	112	86	–	7	1.2	1.2	*	*
Ohio	2,331	1,432	740	94	1.6	1.3	3.1	1.4
Oklahoma	799	456	157	92	1.5	1.3	3.1	1.3
Oregon	479	328	16	98	1.0	1.0	*	1.0
Pennsylvania	2,347	1,242	704	244	1.6	1.2	3.3	1.7
Rhode Island	193	110	22	39	1.7	1.6	2.4	1.6
South Carolina	1,104	419	610	60	1.8	1.2	3.1	1.1
South Dakota	129	86	4	7	1.1	0.9	*	*
Tennessee	1,364	722	547	70	1.7	1.3	3.1	0.9
Texas	5,906	1,771	1,398	2,502	1.5	1.3	3.1	1.2
Utah	550	395	13	105	1.0	0.9	*	1.2
Vermont	67	64	1	1	1.1	1.1	*	*
Virginia	1,703	724	717	157	1.6	1.2	3.1	1.1
Washington	862	514	73	176	1.0	0.9	1.8	1.0
West Virginia	313	285	24	1	1.5	1.4	2.9	*
Wisconsin	850	534	207	78	1.2	1.0	2.8	1.1
Wyoming	90	70	–	15	1.1	1.1	*	*
Puerto Rico	641	18	3	617	1.4	*	*	1.4
Virgin Islands	21	1	15	5	1.3	*	*	*
Guam	39	4	–	–	1.1	*	*	*
American Samoa	2	—	—	—	*	—	—	—
Northern Marianas	4	—	—	—	*	—	—	—

— = Data not available.
* = Figure does not meet standards of reliability or precision.
– = Quantity zero.
[1]Includes races other than white and black and origin not stated.
[2]Race and Hispanic origin are reported separately on birth certificates.
[3]Persons of Hispanic origin may be of any race.
[4]Excludes data for the territories.

Table A-62. Live Births by Plurality of Birth and Ratios, by Age, Race, and Hispanic Origin of Mother, 2009

(Number, ratio per 1,000 live births.)

Plurality, race, and Hispanic origin of mother	All ages	Age of Mother									
		Under 15 years	15–19 years			20–24 years	25–29 years	30–34 years	35–39 years	40–44 years	45–54 years
			Total	15–17 years	18–19 years						
	Number										
All Live Births											
All races[1]	4,130,665	5,029	409,802	124,247	285,555	1,005,982	1,166,787	955,246	474,103	105,827	7,889
Non-Hispanic White[2]	2,212,552	1,053	159,579	39,975	119,604	490,773	657,658	565,026	273,174	60,452	4,837
Non-Hispanic Black[2]	609,584	1,705	98,448	31,560	66,888	194,122	153,210	98,909	50,003	12,314	873
Hispanic[3]	999,548	2,073	136,263	48,018	88,245	274,726	270,641	195,729	97,261	21,638	1,217
Live Births in Single Deliveries											
All races[1]	3,987,108	4,982	403,003	122,484	280,519	982,052	1,129,444	913,550	448,878	99,182	6,017
Non-Hispanic White[2]	2,126,141	1,038	157,074	39,429	117,645	479,576	635,206	537,402	256,510	55,819	3,516
Non-Hispanic Black[2]	585,781	1,701	96,158	30,980	65,178	187,233	146,540	94,216	47,397	11,781	755
Hispanic[3]	976,232	2,045	134,447	47,438	87,009	269,798	264,434	189,731	93,864	20,889	1,024
Live Births in Twin Deliveries											
All races[1]	137,217	47	6,721	1,739	4,982	23,427	35,762	39,532	23,675	6,298	1,755
Non-Hispanic White[2]	81,954	15	2,481	543	1,938	10,905	21,296	26,047	15,582	4,384	1,244
Non-Hispanic Black[2]	23,159	4	2,260	571	1,689	6,777	6,492	4,526	2,482	506	112
Hispanic[3]	22,481	28	1,792	568	1,224	4,852	6,019	5,685	3,217	716	172
Live Births in Triplet and Higher Order Multiple Births[4]											
All races[1]	6,340	-	78	24	54	503	1,581	2,164	1,550	347	117
Non-Hispanic White[2]	4,457	-	24	3	21	292	1,156	1,577	1,082	249	77
Non-Hispanic Black[2]	644	-	30	9	21	112	178	167	124	27	6
Hispanic[3]	835	-	24	12	12	76	188	313	180	33	21
	Ratio per 1,000 live births										
All Multiple Births											
All races[1]	34.8	9.3	16.6	14.2	17.6	23.8	32.0	43.6	53.2	62.8	237.3
Non-Hispanic White[2]	39.1	*	15.7	13.7	16.4	22.8	34.1	48.9	61.0	76.6	273.1
Non-Hispanic Black[2]	39.0	*	23.3	18.4	25.6	35.5	43.5	47.4	52.1	43.3	135.2
Hispanic[3]	23.3	13.5	13.3	12.1	14.0	17.9	22.9	30.6	34.9	34.6	158.6
Twin Births											
All races[1]	33.2	9.3	16.4	14.0	17.4	23.3	30.6	41.4	49.9	59.5	222.5
Non-Hispanic White[2]	37.0	*	15.5	13.6	16.2	22.2	32.4	46.1	57.0	72.5	257.2
Non-Hispanic Black[2]	38.0	*	23.0	18.1	25.3	34.9	42.4	45.8	49.6	41.1	128.3
Hispanic[3]	22.5	13.5	13.2	11.8	13.9	17.7	22.2	29.0	33.1	33.1	141.3
	Ratio per 1,000 live births										
Triplet and Higher Order Multiple Births[4]											
All races[1]	153.5	*	19.0	19.3	18.9	50.0	135.5	226.5	326.9	327.9	1,483.1
Non-Hispanic White[2]	201.4	*	15.0	*	17.6	59.5	175.8	279.1	396.1	411.9	1,591.9
Non-Hispanic Black[2]	105.6	*	30.5	*	31.4	57.7	116.2	168.8	248.0	219.3	*
Hispanic[3]	83.5	*	17.6	*	*	27.7	69.5	159.9	185.1	152.5	1,725.6

- = Quantity zero.
* = Figure does not meet standards of reliability or precision.
[1]Includes races other than White and Black and origin not stated.
[2]Race and Hispanic origin are reported separately on birth certificates.
[3]Persons of Hispanic origin may be of any race.
[4]Triplet, quadruplet, quintuplet, and higher order multiple deliveries.

Table A-63. Numbers and Rates of Twin and Triplet and Higher-Order Multiple Births, by Race and Hispanic Origin of Mother, 1980–2009

(Number, rate per 1,000 live births; rate per 100,000 live births.)

Year, race, and Hispanic origin of mother	Total births	Twin births	Triplet and higher order births	Twin birth rate[1]	Multiple birth rate[2]	Triplet or higher order birth rate[3]
All Races[4]						
1980	3,612,258	68,339	1,337	18.9	19.3	37.0
1981	3,629,238	70,049	1,385	19.3	19.7	38.2
1982	3,680,537	71,631	1,484	19.5	19.9	40.3
1983	3,638,933	72,287	1,575	19.9	20.3	43.3
1984	3,669,141	72,949	1,653	19.9	20.3	45.1
1985	3,760,561	77,102	1,925	20.5	21.0	51.2
1986	3,756,547	79,485	1,814	21.2	21.6	48.3
1987	3,809,394	81,778	2,139	21.5	22.0	56.2
1988	3,909,510	85,315	2,385	21.8	22.4	61.0
1989	4,040,958	90,118	2,798	22.3	23.0	69.2
1990	4,158,212	93,865	3,028	22.6	23.3	72.8
1991	4,110,907	94,779	3,346	23.1	23.9	81.4
1992	4,065,014	95,372	3,883	23.5	24.4	95.5
1993	4,000,240	96,445	4,168	24.1	25.2	104.2
1994	3,952,767	97,064	4,594	24.6	25.7	116.2
1995	3,899,589	96,736	4,973	24.8	26.1	127.5
1996	3,891,494	100,750	5,939	25.9	27.4	152.6
1997	3,880,894	104,137	6,737	26.8	28.6	173.6
1998	3,941,553	110,670	7,625	28.1	30.0	193.5
1999	3,959,417	114,307	7,321	28.9	30.7	184.9
2000	4,058,814	118,916	7,325	29.3	31.1	180.5
2001	4,025,933	121,246	7,471	30.1	32.0	185.6
2002	4,021,726	125,134	7,401	31.1	33.0	184.0
2003	4,089,950	128,665	7,663	31.5	33.3	187.4
2004	4,112,052	132,219	7,275	32.2	33.9	176.9
2005	4,138,349	133,122	6,694	32.2	33.8	161.8
2006	4,265,555	137,085	6,540	32.1	33.7	153.3
2007	4,316,233	138,961	6,427	32.2	33.7	148.9
2008	4,247,694	138,660	6,268	32.6	34.1	147.6
2009	4,130,665	137,217	6,340	33.2	34.8	153.5
Non-Hispanic White[5]						
1990[6]	2,626,500	60,210	2,358	22.9	23.8	89.8
1991[7]	2,589,878	60,904	2,612	23.5	24.5	100.9
1992[7]	2,527,207	60,640	3,115	24.0	25.2	123.3
1993	2,472,031	61,525	3,360	24.9	26.2	135.9
1994	2,438,855	62,476	3,721	25.6	27.1	152.6
1995	2,382,638	62,370	4,050	26.2	27.9	170.0
1996	2,358,989	65,523	4,885	27.8	29.8	207.1
1997	2,333,363	67,191	5,386	28.8	31.1	230.8
1998	2,283,986	71,270	6,206	30.2	32.8	262.8
1999	2,346,450	73,964	5,909	31.5	34.0	251.8
2000	2,362,968	76,018	5,821	32.2	34.6	246.3
2001	2,326,578	77,882	5,894	33.5	36.0	253.3
2002	2,298,156	79,949	5,754	34.8	37.3	250.4
2003	2,321,904	81,691	5,922	35.2	37.7	255.0
2004	2,296,683	83,346	5,590	36.3	38.7	243.4
2005	2,279,768	82,223	4,966	36.1	38.2	217.8
2006	2,308,640	83,108	4,805	36.0	38.1	208.1
2007	2,310,333	83,632	4,559	36.2	38.2	197.3
2008	2,267,817	82,903	4,493	36.6	38.5	198.1
2009	2,212,552	81,954	4,457	37.0	39.1	201.4
Non-Hispanic Black[5]						
1990[6]	661,701	17,646	306	26.7	27.1	46.2
1991[7]	666,758	18,243	367	27.4	27.9	55.0
1992[7]	657,450	18,294	346	27.8	28.4	52.6
1993	641,273	18,115	314	28.2	28.7	49.0
1994	619,198	17,934	357	29.0	29.5	57.7
1995	587,781	16,622	340	28.3	28.9	57.8
1996	578,099	16,873	425	29.2	29.9	73.5
1997	581,431	17,472	523	30.0	30.9	90.0
1998	593,127	18,589	518	31.3	32.2	87.3
1999	588,981	18,920	561	32.1	33.1	95.2

PART A: BIRTHS

Table A-63. Numbers and Rates of Twin and Triplet and Higher-Order Multiple Births, by Race and Hispanic Origin of Mother, 1980–2009—*Continued*

(Number, rate per 1,000 live births; rate per 100,000 live births.)

Year, race, and Hispanic origin of mother	Total births	Twin births	Triplet and higher order births	Twin birth rate[1]	Multiple birth rate[2]	Triplet or higher order birth rate[3]
2000	604,346	20,173	506	33.4	34.2	83.7
2001	589,917	19,974	531	33.9	34.8	90.0
2002	578,335	20,064	591	34.7	35.7	102.2
2003	576,033	20,010	631	34.7	35.8	109.5
2004	578,772	20,605	577	35.6	36.6	99.7
2005	583,759	21,254	616	36.4	37.5	105.5
2006	617,247	22,702	580	36.8	37.7	94.0
2007	627,191	23,101	612	36.8	37.8	97.6
2008	623,029	22,924	569	36.8	37.7	91.3
2009	609,584	23,159	644	38.0	39.0	105.6
Hispanic[8]						
1990[6]	595,073	10,713	235	18.0	18.4	39.5
1991[7]	623,085	11,356	235	18.2	18.6	37.7
1992[7]	643,271	11,932	239	18.5	18.9	37.2
1993	654,418	12,294	321	18.8	19.3	49.1
1994	665,026	12,206	348	18.4	18.9	52.3
1995	679,768	12,685	355	18.7	19.2	52.2
1996	701,339	13,014	409	18.6	19.1	58.3
1997	709,767	13,821	516	19.5	20.2	72.7
1998	734,661	15,015	553	20.4	21.2	75.3
1999	764,339	15,388	583	20.1	20.9	76.3
2000	815,868	16,470	659	20.2	21.0	80.8
2001	851,851	17,257	710	20.3	21.1	83.3
2002	876,642	18,128	737	20.7	21.5	84.1
2003	912,329	19,472	784	21.3	22.2	85.9
2004	946,349	20,351	723	21.5	22.3	76.4
2005	985,505	21,723	761	22.0	22.8	77.2
2006	1,039,077	22,698	787	21.8	22.6	75.7
2007	1,062,779	23,405	857	22.0	22.8	80.6
2008	1,041,239	23,266	834	22.3	23.1	80.1
2009	999,548	22,481	835	22.5	23.3	83.5

[1]The number of live births in twin deliveries per 1,000 live births.
[2]The number of live births in all multiple deliveries per 1,000 live births.
[3]The number of live births in triplet and other higher-order deliveries per 100,000 live births.
[4]Includes races other than White and Black and origin not stated.
[5]Race and Hispanic origin are reported separately on birth certificates.
[6]Excludes data for New Hampshire and Oklahoma, which did not report Hispanic origin.
[7]Excludes data for New Hampshire, which did not report Hispanic origin.
[8]Persons of Hispanic origin may be of any race.

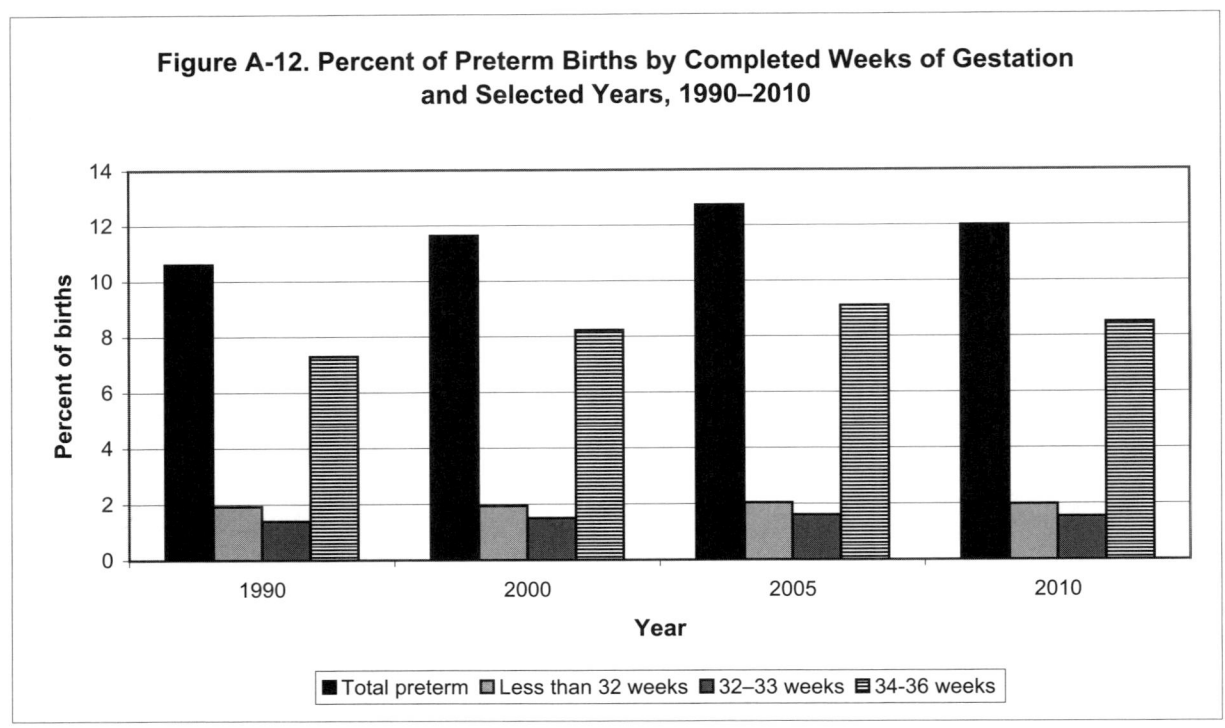

Figure A-12. Percent of Preterm Births by Completed Weeks of Gestation and Selected Years, 1990–2010

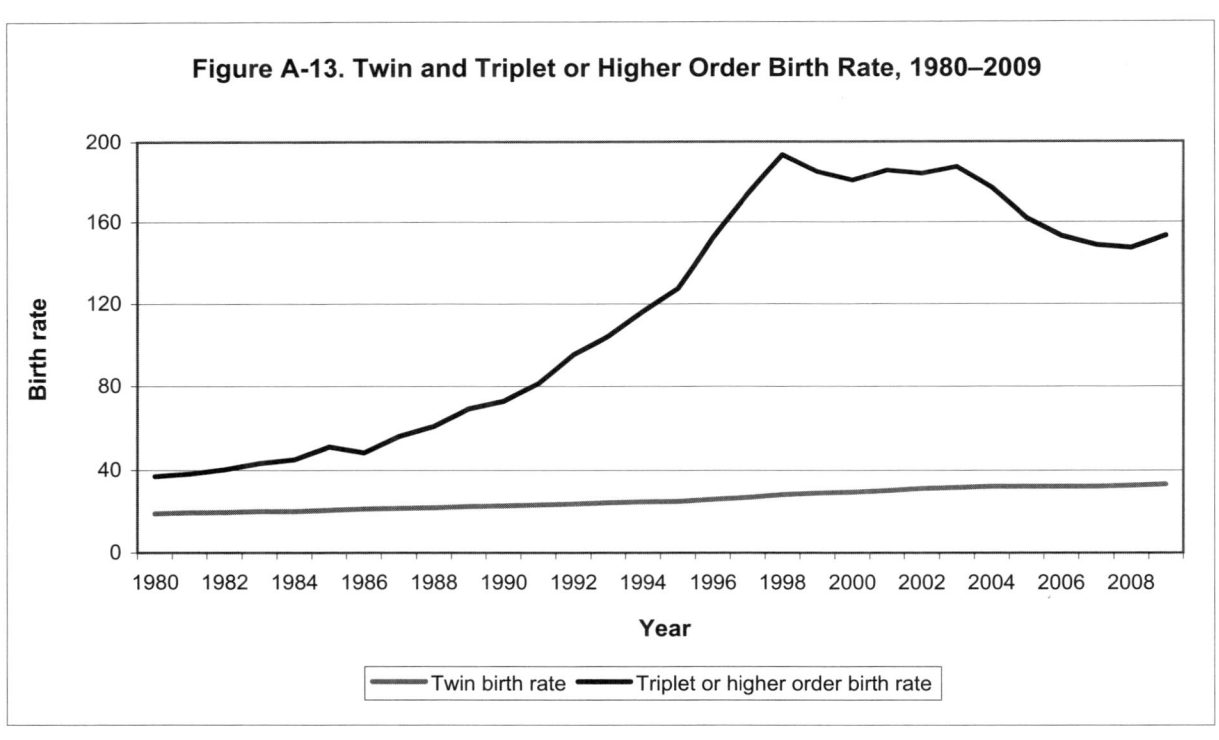

Figure A-13. Twin and Triplet or Higher Order Birth Rate, 1980–2009

Table A-64. Twin and Triplet and Higher Order Multiple Birth Rates by State, 2007–2009

(Number, rate per 1,000 live births.)

Area	Twin		Triplet or higher order[1]	
	Number	Rate per 1,000 live births	Number	Rate per 100,000 live births
UNITED STATES	414,838	32.7	19,035	149.9
Alabama	6,279	32.7	281	146.5
Alaska	993	29.4	25	73.9
Arizona	7,838	26.5	449	152.1
Arkansas	3,653	30.0	101	82.9
California	49,507	30.1	2,190	133.1
Colorado	6,612	31.6	325	155.2
Connecticut	5,297	43.8	245	202.6
Delaware	1,160	32.4	51	142.4
District of Columbia	992	36.7	24	88.8
Florida	21,366	30.9	888	128.3
Georgia	14,462	32.9	510	116.1
Hawaii	1,669	29.0	65	113
Idaho	2,107	28.5	98	132.6
Illinois	19,107	36.1	958	181.2
Indiana	8,313	31.3	513	193.4
Iowa	4,131	34.2	202	167.2
Kansas	3,765	30.1	178	142.1
Kentucky	5,317	30.3	237	135.2
Louisiana	6,333	32.2	263	133.8
Maine	1,299	31.5	30	72.8
Maryland	8,758	38.0	311	135
Massachusetts	10,081	43.8	412	179.1
Michigan	12,479	34.3	679	186.7
Minnesota	7,378	34.0	335	154.5
Mississippi	4,460	33.2	142	105.7
Missouri	7,675	31.7	492	203.5
Montana	1,130	30.3	25	67
Nebraska	2,791	34.5	175	216.4
Nevada	3,382	28.6	161	136.1
New Hampshire	1,601	38.8	52	126.1
New Jersey	14,812	43.7	812	239.5
New Mexico	2,159	24.0	78	86.9
New York	28,279	37.6	1,510	200.8
North Carolina	12,683	32.6	608	156.4
North Dakota	852	31.8	55	205.4
Ohio	14,917	33.6	805	181.1
Oklahoma	4,609	28.0	177	107.7
Oregon	4,402	30.2	151	103.7
Pennsylvania	15,497	34.7	730	163.5
Rhode Island	1,292	36.0	62	172.9
South Carolina	6,212	33.3	232	124.4
South Dakota	1,061	29.3	45	124.1
Tennessee	7,748	30.4	332	130.5
Texas	36,053	29.7	1,732	142.5
Utah	4,841	29.4	168	102
Vermont	606	32.0	18	*
Virginia	11,246	35.1	442	137.9
Washington	8,352	31.1	270	100.5
West Virginia	1,955	30.2	51	78.7
Wisconsin	6,637	30.7	316	146.4
Wyoming	690	29.0	24	100.8

* = Figure does not meet standards of reliability or precision.
[1]Includes triplet and quadruplet and other higher order multiple births.

Table A-65. Gestational Age and Birthweight Characteristics by Plurality, 2009

(Number, percent.)

Characteristic	All births	Singletons	Twins	Triplets	Quadruplets	Quintuplets and higher order multiples[1]
Number of Births	4,130,665	3,987,108	137,217	5,905	355	80
Percent, very preterm[2]	2.0	1.6	11.4	36.8	64.5	95.0
Percent, preterm[3]	12.2	10.4	58.8	94.4	98.3	96.3
Mean gestational age in weeks (standard deviation)	38.6 (2.5)	38.7 (2.4)	35.3 (3.6)	31.9 (3.9)	29.5 (4.0)	26.6 (4.6)
Percent, very low birthweight[4]	1.5	1.1	9.9	35.0	68.1	86.5
Percent, low birthweight[5]	8.2	6.4	56.6	95.1	98.6	94.6
Mean birthweight in grams (standard deviation)	3,262 (591)	3,296 (560)	2,336 (626)	1,660 (558)	1,291 (520)	1,002 (672)

[1]Quintuplets, sextuplets, and higher order multiple births are not differentiated in the national data set.
[2]Very preterm is less than 32 completed weeks of gestation.
[3]Preterm is less than 37 completed weeks of gestation.
[4]Very low birthweight is less than 1,500 grams.
[5]Low birthweight is less than 2,500 grams.

Table A-66. Percent Distribution of Gestational Age for All Births and for Singleton Births Only, Selected Years, 1990–2009

(Percent.)

Gestational age	All births						
	1990	2000	2005	2006	2007	2008	2009
Under 28 weeks	0.71	0.72	0.77	0.76	0.77	0.74	0.74
28–31 weeks	1.21	1.21	1.26	1.29	1.27	1.24	1.23
32–33 weeks	1.40	1.49	1.60	1.62	1.60	1.57	1.55
Total under 34 weeks	3.32	3.42	3.63	3.66	3.64	3.56	3.51
34–36 weeks	7.30	8.22	9.09	9.15	9.04	8.77	8.66
Total under 37 weeks	10.62	11.64	12.73	12.80	12.68	12.33	12.18
37–38 weeks	19.66	24.50	28.29	28.89	28.60	27.85	27.59
39 weeks	21.72	24.32	25.25	25.43	25.85	26.62	27.47
40–41 weeks	36.68	32.26	27.90	27.20	27.24	27.52	27.22
42 weeks and higher	11.33	7.28	5.84	5.67	5.62	5.68	5.54
	Singleton births						
Under 28 weeks	0.61	0.59	0.61	0.61	0.62	0.60	0.60
28–31 weeks	1.08	0.99	1.02	1.04	1.03	1.00	0.99
32–33 weeks	1.24	1.22	1.28	1.31	1.29	1.27	1.24
Total under 34 weeks	2.93	2.80	2.91	2.96	2.95	2.87	2.82
34–36 weeks	6.77	7.33	8.09	8.14	8.03	7.76	7.62
Total under 37 weeks	9.70	10.12	11.00	11.09	10.98	10.63	10.44
37–38 weeks	19.43	24.38	28.30	28.91	28.59	27.79	27.50
39 weeks	21.98	24.89	25.96	26.15	26.59	27.38	28.29
40–41 weeks	37.35	33.15	28.75	28.03	28.07	28.37	28.08
42 weeks and higher	11.53	7.46	5.99	5.83	5.77	5.83	5.69

PART A: BIRTHS

Table A-67. Births, by Smoking Status During Pregnancy and Race and Hispanic Origin of Mother, 24 States, 2008

(Number, percent.)

Number, percent, and type of birth	All births	Smoker[1]	Quit smoking[2]
All Races and Origins[3]	2,249,127	9.7	19.8
Non-Hispanic			
White[4]	1,116,123	15.5	18.3
Black[4]	228,759	8.7	21.8
American Indian or Alaska Native[4]	15,405	19.2	26.0
Asian[4]	131,675	1.0	40.2
Hispanic[5]	686,729	2.1	31.6
Mexican	490,296	1.4	34.1
Puerto Rican	29,926	9.2	26.9
Cuban	2,715	6.5	31.8
Central and South American	70,061	0.7	43.5

[1] Includes smoking during any trimester of pregnancy.
[2] Includes women who quit smoking in the first or second trimester of pregnancy.
[3] Includes other races not shown separately and origin not stated.
[4] Race and Hispanic origin are reported separately on the birth certificate.
[5] Includes all persons of Hispanic origin of any race and of other Hispanic groups.

NOTE: Includes California, Colorado, Delaware, Idaho, Indiana, Iowa, Kansas, Kentucky, Montana, Nebraska, New Hampshire, New Mexico, New York, North Dakota, Ohio, Oregon, Pennsylvania, South Carolina, South Dakota, Tennessee, Texas, Vermont, Washington, and Wyoming.

Table A-68. Use of Contraception Among Sexually Experienced Females Aged 15–19, by Method of Contraception, 1995, 2002, and 2006–2010

(Number in thousands, percent.)

Method	1995	2002	2006–2010
Percent Who Ever Used Method of Birth Contol			
Any method	96.2	97.7	98.9
Pill	51.6	61.4	55.6
Injectable	9.7	20.7	20.3
Emergency contraception	*	8.1	13.7
Contraceptive patch	—	1.5	10.3
Contraceptive ring	—		5.2
Condom	93.5	93.7	95.9
Female condom	1.1	1.7	1.5
Periodic abstinence-calendar	13.2	10.8	15
Withdrawal	42.3	55.0	57.3
Other methods	14.5	9.9	7.1

* = Figure does not meet standards of reliability or precision.
— = Data not available.

Table A-69. Use of Contraception at First Sex Among Females and Males Aged 15–19, by Method Used, Selected Years, 1988–2010

(Number in thousands, percent.)

Characteristic	Number	Any method	No method	Pill (at all)	Other hormonal[1]	Condom	All other methods[2]	Dual methods (hormonal and condom)
Female								
1988	4,410	66.9	33.1	8.0	X	50.4	10.0	1.8
2002	4,598	74.5	25.5	16.5	2.1	66.4	2.6	13.1
Total 2006–2010[3]	4,532	78.3	21.7	15.7	6.1	68.0	3.4	14.8
Hispanic Origin and Race								
Hispanic or Latina	833	74.0	26.0	7.2	5.8	65.4	1.3	5.7
Non-Hispanic White	2,633	82.3	17.7	21.8	6.3	70.7	4.3	20.8
Non-Hispanic Black	785	71.1	28.9	8.9	6.6	64.1	*	9.5
Age at First Sex								
14 years or under	1,244	59.1	40.9	7.1	2.4	53.5	2.3	6.3
5–16 years	2,108	83.1	16.9	16.7	9.0	69.6	3.6	15.8
17–19 years	1,180	90.1	9.9	22.8	4.7	80.5	4.2	22.0
Age Difference Between Female and First Male Partner								
Male partner same age or younger	1,252	82.9	17.1	17.3	7.6	71.8	1.0	14.7
Male partner 1 year older	1,222	78.7	21.3	14.4	6.5	71.0	4.5	17.6
Male partner 2–3 years older	1,326	81.7	18.3	16.6	5.3	68.3	5.6	14.0
Male partner 4 or more years older	732	63.7	36.3	13.4	4.2	56.3	1.7	11.7
Male								
Total 1988	5,379	71.4	28.6	9.5	X	55.0	10.6	2.6
Total 1995	4,989	75.7	24.3	10.3	0.4	69.3	4.4	6.8
Total 2002	4,697	82.0	18.0	14.9	2.1	70.9	4.7	10.4
Total 2006–2010[3]	4,551	85.4	14.6	17.9	1.4	79.6	2.7	16.2
MALE: 2006–2010								
Hispanic Origin and Race								
Hispanic or Latino	931	84.1	15.9	9.1	*	78.5	4.5	8.3
Non-Hispanic White	2,387	88.5	11.5	24.8	2.4	80.9	2.6	22.3
Non-Hispanic Black	977	81.7	18.3	11.7	*	79.6	*	11.1
Age at First Sex								
14 years or under	1,513	74.9	25.1	8.0	*	71.0	3.3	9.0
15–16 years	1,994	89.3	10.7	19.8	1.8	82.2	3.5	18.0
17–19 years	1,044	93.3	6.7	28.7	*	86.9	*	23.2
Age Difference Between Male and First Female Partner								
Female partner younger	723	88.3	11.7	14.5	*	79.6	5.0	15.1
Female partner same age	2,034	89.4	10.6	16.1	1.3	85.2	1.9	15.1
Female partner 1 year older	1,011	83.2	16.8	22.4	*	78.5	*	19.1
Female partner 2 or more years older	783	75.4	24.6	20.1	–	66.4	5.1	16.2

X = Category not applicable.
– = Quantity zero.
* = Figure does not meet standards of reliability or precision.

[1] Includes Lunelle injectable, emergency contraception, and contraceptive patch in 2002; adds contraceptive ring (Nuva-Ring) and Implanon implant in 2006–2010.
[2] Excludes condom and hormonal methods. Thus, if other method was combined with condom or hormonal method, it is not counted. Other methods include withdrawal, sterilization, IUD, female condom, diaphragm, cervical cap, spermicidal foam, jelly, cream or suppository, sponge, calendar rhythm method, and "other" methods.
[3] Includes persons of other or unknown origin and race groups.

NOTES: Statistics for condom "at all," pill "at all," and other hormonal reflect use of that method regardless of whether it was used alone or in combination with another method. Statistics not available for females in 1995 because of differences in the universe of respondents asked the questions.

Table A-70. Use of Contraception at Last Sex in the Prior 3 Months Among Never-Married Females and Males Aged 15–19, by Method Used, Selected Years, 1988–2010

(Number in thousands, percent.)

Characteristic	Number	Any method	No method	Pill (at all)	Other hormonal[1]	Condom (at all)	All other methods[2]	Dual methods (hormonal and condom)
Female								
1988	3,521	79.9	20.1	42.7	X	31.3	9.3	3.3
1995	3,225	70.7	29.3	25.0	7.0	38.2	9.6	8.4
2002	3,304	83.2	16.8	34.2	9.1	54.3	5.1	19.5
Total 2006–2010[3]	3,175	85.6	14.4	30.5	12.2	52.0	11.0	20.1
FEMALE: 2006–2010								
Hispanic Origin and Race								
Hispanic or Latina	539	79.5	20.5	17.2	18.0	47.7	10.6	14.0
Non-Hispanic White	1,873	89.3	10.7	38.6	10.5	52.4	12.3	24.4
Non-Hispanic Black	564	81.1	18.9	14.4	16.2	57.6	5.7	12.8
Age at First Sex								
14 years or under	835	73.0	27.0	18.0	11.6	38.3	16.7	11.7
15–16 years	1,528	88.7	11.3	33.5	12.9	50.1	10.9	18.7
17–19 years	812	92.8	7.2	37.9	11.3	69.6	5.5	31.4
Male								
Total 1988	3,847	84.2	15.8	37.4	X	53.3	13.6	15.2
Total 1995	3,416	81.8	18.2	28.2	2.8	63.9	10.0	16.5
Total 2002	3,165	90.7	9.3	31.0	6.3	70.7	2.0	23.9
Total 2006–2010[3]	2,970	92.5	7.5	39.0	9.3	74.7	3.4	33.9
MALE: 2006–2010								
Hispanic Origin and Race								
Hispanic or Latino	593	86.2	13.8	29.4	6.8	65.5	4.3	19.6
Non-Hispanic White	1,567	96.8	3.2	49.6	11.0	76.8	2.9	43.4
Non-Hispanic Black	638	91.6	8.4	25.6	9.8	79.0	4.1	26.9
Age at First Sex								
14 years or under	1,009	85.3	14.7	31.1	11.1	68.0	5.0	29.7
15–16 years	1,363	95.3	4.7	41.3	10.1	74.4	3.6	34.2
17–19 years	598	98.1	*	47.2	4.5	86.3	*	40.2

X = Category not applicable.
* = Figure does not meet standards of reliability or precision.
[1]Includes Depo-Provera injectible and Norplant implants in 1995; adds Lunelle injectable, emergency contraception, and contraceptive patch in 2002; adds contraceptive ring (Nuva-Ring) and Implanon implant in 2006–2010.
[2]Excludes condom and hormonal methods. Thus, if other method was combined with condom or hormonal method, it is not counted. Other methods include withdrawal, sterilization, IUD, female condom, diaphragm, cervical cap, spermicidal foam, jelly, cream or suppository, sponge, calendar rhythm method, and "other" methods.
[3]Includes persons of other or unknown origin and race groups.

NOTE: Statistics for condom "at all," pill "at all," and other hormonal reflect use of that method regardless of whether it was used alone or in combination with another method.

Table A-71. Consistency of Condom Use in the 4 Weeks Prior to the Interview Among Never-Married Females and Males Aged 15–19, 2002 and 2006–2010

(Number in thousands, percent.)

Characteristic	Number	Total	Percent of times a condom was used		
			0	Some	100
Female					
Total 2002	2,552	100	42.8	15.7	41.4
Total 2006–2010[1]	2,646	100	39.2	11.9	49
Hispanic Origin and Race					
Hispanic or Latina	437	100	42.9	13.8	43.3
Non-Hispanic White	1,555	100	41.0	10.2	48.7
Non-Hispanic Black	483	100	31.9	16.8	51.2
Number of Partners in the Past 12 Months					
1 partner	1,542	100	44.9	7.0	48.1
2 or more partners	1,085	100	31.1	18.7	50.2
MALE					
Total 2002	2,525	100	26.5	5.3	68.2
Total 2006–2010[1]	2,312	100	22.7	10.8	66.5
Hispanic Origin and Race					
Hispanic or Latino	432	100	30.9	11.4	57.6
Non-Hispanic White	1,247	100	21.0	12.3	66.7
Non-Hispanic Black	490	100	15.8	9.1	75.1
Number of Partners in the Past 12 Months					
1 partner	976	100	22.1	11.2	66.7
2 or more partners	1,336	100	23.1	10.5	66.4

[1]Includes persons of other or unknown origin and race groups, not shown separately.

NOTE: Numbers and percentages reflect heterosexual vaginal sexual intercourse only, not other types of sexual activity. Percentages may not add to 100 due to rounding.

Table A-72. Number of Live Births by Attendant, Place of Delivery, Race, and Hispanic Origin of Mother, 2009

(Number.)

Place of delivery and race and Hispanic origin of mother	All births	Physician			Midwife			Other	Unspecified
		Total	Doctor of medicine	Doctor of osteopathy	Total	Certified nurse midwife	Other midwife		
ALL RACES[1]									
Total	4,130,665	3,766,578	3,545,597	220,981	335,303	313,516	21,787	26,670	2,114
In hospital[2]	4,086,289	3,763,781	3,543,125	220,656	305,665	301,270	4,395	15,637	1,206
Not in hospital	44,121	2,742	2,419	323	29,553	12,181	17,372	10,993	833
Freestanding birthing center	12,169	679	528	151	11,108	6,346	4,762	369	13
Clinic or doctor's office	399	213	187	26	156	102	54	29	1
Residence	29,650	1,402	1,285	117	18,056	5,636	12,420	9,522	670
Other	1,903	448	419	29	233	97	136	1,073	149
Not specified	255	55	53	2	85	65	20	40	75
NON-HISPANIC WHITE[3]									
Total	2,212,552	2,013,414	1,871,046	142,368	183,533	166,090	17,443	14,867	738
In hospital[2]	2,177,158	2,011,661	1,869,572	142,089	158,051	155,902	2,149	7,087	359
Not in hospital	35,286	1,728	1,450	278	25,416	10,137	15,279	7,771	371
Freestanding birthing center	10,042	611	461	150	9,109	5,128	3,981	312	10
Clinic or doctor's office	299	151	126	25	130	80	50	17	1
Residence	24,118	778	692	86	15,990	4,866	11,124	7,036	314
Other	827	188	171	17	187	63	124	406	46
Not specified	108	25	24	1	66	51	15	9	8
NON-HISPANIC BLACK[3]									
Total	609,584	562,186	538,953	23,233	42,871	42,190	681	4,032	495
In hospital[2]	606,700	561,629	538,413	23,216	41,982	41,680	302	2,716	373
Not in hospital	2,870	552	535	17	886	508	378	1,310	122
Freestanding birthing center	532	16	16	-	504	325	179	12	-
Clinic or doctor's office	32	19	19	-	11	10	1	2	-
Residence	1,875	385	371	14	353	158	195	1,039	98
Other	431	132	129	3	18	15	3	257	24
Not specified	14	5	5	-	3	2	1	6	-
HISPANIC[4]									
Total	999,548	909,563	865,189	44,374	83,865	81,109	2,756	5,473	647
In hospital[2]	995,751	909,259	864,905	44,354	81,694	80,106	1,588	4,397	401
Not in hospital	3,759	287	268	19	2,162	996	1,166	1,068	242
Freestanding birthing center	1,224	44	44	-	1,147	689	458	31	2
Clinic or doctor's office	26	12	12	-	11	8	3	3	-
Residence	2,129	150	139	11	988	289	699	803	188
Other	380	81	73	8	16	10	6	231	52
Not specified	38	17	16	1	9	7	2	8	4

– = Quantity zero.
[1]Includes races other than White and Black and origin not stated.
[2]Includes births occurring en route to or on arrival at hospital.
[3]Race and Hispanic origin are reported separately on birth certificates.
[4]Persons of Hispanic origin may be of any race.

Table A-73. Educational Attainment of Mother, by Age, Hispanic Origin, and Race of Mother: Total of 27 Reporting States, 2008

(Number, rates per 100,000 in specified group; age-adjusted rates per 100,000 U.S. standard population.)

Education level and sex	All ages	Under 20	20–24 years	25–29 years	30–34 years	35–39 years	40–54 years
ALL RACES[1]	100.0	100.0	100.0	100.0	100.0	100.0	100.0
12 grade or less with no diploma	22.2	57.5	25.6	17.3	13.5	13.1	14.7
High school graduate[2]	27.0	33.7	39.5	25.6	17.8	16.7	17.8
Some college credit, but no degree	19.6	8.5	25.8	22.2	17.0	15.5	15.5
Associate's degree[3]	6.8	0.3	4.7	8.9	8.5	8.5	8.2
Bachelor's degree[4]	16.3	0.0	4.1	19.4	26.9	27.5	25.8
Master's degree[5]	6.4	*	0.3	5.6	12.8	13.9	12.6
Doctorate or professional degree[6]	1.8	*	0.0	1.0	3.5	4.8	5.3
All births	2,748,302	289,202	684,971	769,935	613,235	316,488	74,471
Not stated[7]	52,906	4,488	11,131	14,108	12,984	7,736	2,459
White[8]	100.0	100.0	100.0	100.0	100.0	100.0	100.0
12 grade or less with no diploma	11.3	50.0	17.2	7.2	3.7	3.2	3.7
High school graduate[2]	24.7	39.1	40.7	23.0	14.3	13.4	14.7
Some college credit, but no degree	21.4	10.5	29.5	23.9	17.5	16.1	16.4
Associate's degree[3]	8.7	0.4	6.4	11.2	10.0	9.6	9.3
Bachelor's degree[4]	22.5	*	5.7	26.1	34.0	34.0	32.7
Master's degree[5]	9.1	*	0.4	7.4	16.5	17.9	16.5
Doctorate or professional degree[6]	2.3	–	0.0	1.3	4.0	5.7	6.7
All births	1,366,527	103,622	313,625	404,436	333,446	171,589	39,809
Not stated[7]	9,276	707	1,851	2,443	2,358	1,446	471
Black[8]	100.0	100.0	100.0	100.0	100.0	100.0	100.0
12 grade or less with no diploma	22.7	55.4	20.5	15.3	12.0	11.4	13.9
High school graduate[2]	34.7	34.9	42.9	32.5	27.4	25.7	27.1
Some college credit, but no degree	24.6	9.4	29.7	28.9	25.5	22.4	20.8
Associate's degree[3]	5.9	0.2	3.7	8.0	9.6	10.2	10.0
Bachelor's degree[4]	8.4	*	3.0	11.7	16.3	18.4	16.7
Master's degree[5]	3.1	*	0.2	3.1	7.5	9.5	9.2
Doctorate or professional degree[6]	0.6	*	0.0	0.5	1.6	2.4	2.4
All births	349,243	58,110	109,188	88,153	56,649	29,446	7,697
Not stated[7]	4,175	627	1,136	1,035	787	456	134
Hispanic[9]	100.0	100.0	100.0	100.0	100.0	100.0	100.0
12 grade or less with no diploma	43.7	65.9	40.8	39.4	39.2	40.1	43.3
High school graduate[2]	29.2	27.9	36.2	29.0	24.1	22.4	21.9
Some college credit, but no degree	14.9	6.0	18.2	17.2	14.7	13.2	12.8
Associate's degree[3]	3.8	0.2	2.8	5.1	5.5	5.4	5.0
Bachelor's degree[4]	6.1	0.0	1.8	7.5	11.5	12.5	11.0
Master's degree[5]	1.7	*	0.1	1.5	3.9	4.9	4.3
Doctorate or professional degree[6]	0.5	*	0.0	0.3	1.1	1.6	1.8
All births	787,484	112,705	221,920	210,785	150,512	74,250	17,312
Not stated[7]	12,437	1,555	3,260	3,366	2,549	1,331	376

0.0 = Quantity more than zero but less than 0.5.
* = Figure does not meet standards of reliability or precision
– = Quantity zero
[1]Includes other races not shown and origin not stated.
[2]Includes General Educational Development.
[3]Includes Associate in Arts and Associate in Science.
[4]Includes Bachelor of Arts and Bachelor of Science.
[5]Includes Master of Arts and Master of Science.
[6]Includes Doctor of Philosophy, Doctor of Education, Doctor of Medicine, Doctor of Dental Surgery, Doctor of Veterinary Medicine, Doctor of Laws, and Juris Doctor.
[7]No response reported for education attainment of mother item.
[8]Race and Hispanic origin are reported separately on the birth certificate.
[9]Persons of Hispanic origin may be of any race.

NOTES: Includes California, Colorado, Delaware, Florida, Georgia, Idaho, Indiana, Iowa, Kansas, Kentucky, Michigan, Montana, Nebraska, New Hampshire, New Mexico, New York, North Dakota, Ohio, Oregon, Pennsylvania, South Carolina, South Dakota, Tennessee, Texas, Vermont, Washington, and Wyoming.

Table A-74. Month Prenatal Care Began, by Age, Race, and Hispanic Origin of Mother, 27 Reporting States, 2008

(Percent, Number.)

Month care began and race and Hispanic origin of mother	All ages	Under 20 years	20–24 years	25–29 years	30–34 years	35–39 years	40–54 years
All Races[1]							
1st trimester	71.0	54.0	63.2	73.9	79.1	79.2	76.2
2nd trimester	22.0	34.0	27.7	20.0	16.1	16.1	18.3
Late or no care	7.0	12.0	9.1	6.1	4.8	4.7	5.5
3rd trimester	5.1	8.9	6.7	4.4	3.4	3.3	3.9
No care	1.9	3.0	2.4	1.7	1.4	1.4	1.6
Total	2,748,302	289,202	684,971	769,935	613,235	316,488	74,471
Not stated[2]	178,325	20,067	44,692	47,717	39,013	21,586	5,250
White[3]							
1st trimester	76.7	59.3	67.5	79.0	84.0	83.8	80.5
2nd trimester	18.5	32.0	25.6	16.7	12.9	13.0	15.4
Late or no care	4.8	8.7	6.9	4.3	3.2	3.2	4.1
3rd trimester	3.7	7.0	5.5	3.2	2.3	2.3	3.0
No care	1.1	1.7	1.5	1.0	0.8	0.9	1.2
Total	1,366,527	103,622	313,625	404,436	333,446	171,589	39,809
Not stated[2]	62,119	4,687	13,807	17,117	15,573	8,781	2,154
Black[3]							
1st trimester	60.2	47.7	56.4	64.8	68.3	68.4	65.0
2nd trimester	28.4	37.2	31.3	25.3	22.4	22.4	24.6
Late or no care	11.3	5.1	12.2	9.9	9.3	9.2	10.4
3rd trimester	7.7	10.6	8.2	6.7	6.3	5.9	6.5
No care	3.7	4.5	4.0	3.2	3.0	3.3	4.0
Total	349,243	58,110	109,188	88,153	56,649	29,446	7,697
Not stated[2]	36,838	6,464	11,455	9,003	5,929	3,175	812
Hispanic[4]							
1st trimester	64.7	52.6	60.7	67.6	71.3	71.4	69.7
2nd trimester	26.1	34.1	28.7	24.3	21.7	21.5	23.1
Late or no care	9.2	13.3	10.6	8.1	7.0	7.0	7.2
3rd trimester	6.6	9.7	7.6	5.7	4.9	4.9	5.2
No care	2.7	3.6	3.0	2.4	2.1	2.1	2.0
Total	787,484	112,705	221,920	210,785	150,512	74,250	17,312
Not stated[2]	50,508	7,057	14,368	13,554	9,423	4,946	1,160

[1]Includes other races not shown and origin not stated.
[2]No response reported for timing of prenatal care.
[3]Race and Hispanic origin are reported separately on the birth certificate.
[4]Persons of Hispanic origin may be of any race.

NOTE: Includes California, Colorado, Delaware, Florida, Georgia, Idaho, Indiana, Iowa, Kansas, Kentucky, Michigan, Montana, Nebraska, New Hampshire, New Mexico, New York, North Dakota, Ohio, Oregon, Pennsylvania, South Carolina, South Dakota, Tennessee, Texas, Vermont, Washington, and Wyoming.

Table A-75. Births, by Educational Attainment, Race, and Hispanic Origin of Mother, 27 Reporting States, 2008

(Number, percent.)

Number, percent, and type of birth	All births	High school diploma or higher[1]	Bachelor's degree of higher[2]
All Races and Origins[3]	2,748,302	77.8	24.5
Non-Hispanic			
White[4]	1,366,527	88.7	33.9
Black[4]	349,243	77.3	12.2
American Indian or Alaska Native[4]	16,494	69.8	6.0
Asian[4]	147,132	90.9	55.2
Hispanic[5]	787,484	56.3	8.3
Mexican	529,677	51.1	5.8
Puerto Rican	43,484	72.2	12.6
Cuban	14,627	88.5	24.2
Central and South American	98,171	59.0	14.6

[1] Includes General Educational Development (GED).
[2] Includes Bachelor of Arts, Bachelor of Science, Master of Arts, Master of Science, Doctor of Philosophy, Doctor of Education, Doctor of Medicine, Doctor of Dental Surgery, Doctor of Education, Doctor of Veterinary Medicine, Doctor of Laws, and Juris Doctor.
[3] Includes other races not shown separately and origin not stated.
[4] Race and Hispanic origin are reported separately on the birth certificate.
[5] Persons of Hispanic origin may be of any race.

NOTE: Includes California, Colorado, Delaware, Florida, Georgia, Idaho, Indiana, Iowa, Kansas, Kentucky, Michigan, Montana, Nebraska, New Hampshire, New Mexico, New York, North Dakota, Ohio, Oregon, Pennsylvania, South Carolina, South Dakota, Tennessee, Texas, Vermont, Washington, and Wyoming.

Table A-76. Abnormal Conditions of the Newborn, by Age, Race, and Hispanic Origin of Mother, 27 Reporting States, 2008

(Number, Rates per 1,000 live births in specified group.)

Abnormal condition and race and Hispanic origin of mother	All birth[1]	Condition reported	All ages	Under 20 years	20–24 years	25–29 years	30–34 years	35–39 years	40–54 years	Not stated[2]
All Races[3]										
Assisted ventilation required immediately following delivery	2,748,302	110,715	41.0	44.2	40.1	39.2	40.5	43.1	49.1	45,689
Assisted ventilation required for more than 6 hours	2,748,302	23,697	8.8	9.8	8.5	8.3	8.5	9.2	11.9	45,689
NICU admission	2,748,302	180,274	66.7	68.4	62.6	62.6	66.1	77.3	100.1	45,689
Surfactant replacement therapy given to newborn	2,748,302	9,139	3.4	3.7	3.2	3.2	3.3	3.6	4.8	45,689
Antibiotics received by newborn for suspected neonatal sepsis	2,748,302	46,874	17.3	21.0	18.2	16.4	15.9	16.7	19.9	45,689
Seizure or serious neurologic dysfunction	2,748,302	754	0.3	0.3	0.3	0.2	0.3	0.3	0.4	45,689
Significant birth injury	2,748,302	1,881	0.7	0.7	0.7	0.7	0.6	0.7	1.0	45,689
White[4]										
Assisted ventilation required immediately following delivery	1,366,527	61,396	45.3	49.7	44.3	43.7	44.8	47.4	54.0	12,072
Assisted ventilation required for more than 6 hours	1,366,527	13,479	10.0	11.7	9.9	9.6	9.5	10.0	13.1	12,072
NICU admission	1,366,527	89,207	65.9	66.1	61.5	62.4	65.0	75.7	99.3	12,072
Surfactant replacement therapy given to newborn	1,366,527	5,606	4.1	5.0	4.0	4.0	3.9	4.3	5.5	12,072
Antibiotics received by newborn for suspected neonatal sepsis	1,366,527	25,987	19.2	24.1	20.8	18.5	17.2	18.1	22.2	12,072
Seizure or serious neurologic dysfunction	1,366,527	481	0.4	0.4	0.4	0.3	0.3	0.3	*	12,072
Significant birth injury	1,366,527	998	0.7	0.9	0.8	0.7	0.6	0.6	1.0	12,072
Black[4]										
Assisted ventilation required immediately following delivery	349,243	17,584	51.9	52.2	49.2	50.3	54.2	58.3	62.8	10,184
Assisted ventilation required for more than 6 hours	349,243	4,071	12.0	12.0	11.3	11.3	13.0	13.8	16.9	10,184
NICU admission	349,243	31,483	92.9	87.2	85.5	87.6	100.9	120.7	133.8	10,184
Surfactant replacement therapy given to newborn	349,243	1,576	4.6	4.7	4.3	4.2	5.1	6.1	5.6	10,184
Antibiotics received by newborn for suspected neonatal sepsis	349,243	6,887	20.3	21.9	20.6	18.0	20.8	22.1	20.9	10,184
Seizure or serious neurologic dysfunction	349,243	77	0.2	0.4	*	*	0.4	*	*	10,184
Significant birth injury	349,243	160	0.5	0.6	0.4	0.4	0.6	*	*	10,184
Hispanic[5]										
Assisted ventilation required immediately following delivery	787,484	24,601	31.5	35.3	30.8	28.9	31.4	33.9	38.5	6,835
Assisted ventilation required for more than 6 hours	787,484	4,674	6.0	7.1	5.6	5.4	5.8	7.0	8.2	6,835
NICU admission	787,484	44,993	57.6	60.3	53.1	53.2	59.2	69.3	88.4	6,835
Surfactant replacement therapy given to newborn	787,484	1,397	1.8	2.0	1.8	1.5	1.8	1.9	3.6	6,835
Antibiotics received by newborn for suspected neonatal sepsis	787,484	10,476	13.4	17.4	13.6	12.0	12.2	13.0	15.6	6,835
Seizure or serious neurologic dysfunction	787,484	144	0.2	0.2	0.2	0.2	0.2	*	*	6,835
Significant birth injury	787,484	471	0.6	0.6	0.6	0.6	0.6	0.6	*	6,835

* = Figure does not meet standards of reliability or precision.
[1] Refers to total number of births to residents of areas reporting specified abnormal condition.
[2] No response reported for abnormal conditions of the newborn item; includes births to residents of states using the 2003 U.S. Standard Certificate of Live Birth occurring in states using the 1989 U.S. Standard Certificate of Live Birth.
[3] Includes other races not shown and origin not stated.
[4] Race and Hispanic origin are reported separately on the birth certificate.
[5] Persons of Hispanic origin may be of any race.

NOTE: Includes California, Colorado, Delaware, Florida, Georgia, Idaho, Indiana, Iowa, Kansas, Kentucky, Michigan, Montana, Nebraska, New Hampshire, New Mexico, New York, North Dakota, Ohio, Oregon, Pennsylvania, South Carolina, South Dakota, Tennessee, Texas, Vermont, Washington, and Wyoming.

Table A-77. Congenital Anomaly of the Newborn, by Age, Race, and Hispanic Origin of Mother, 27 Reporting States, 2008

(Number, Rates per 100,000 live births in specified group.)

Congenital anomaly	All birth[1]	Condition reported	All ages	Under 20 years	20–24 years	25–29 years	30–34 years	35–39 years	40–54 years	Not stated[2]
All Races[3]										
Anencephaly	2,748,302	372	13.8	16.5	13.2	17.1	10.6	11.6	*	50,501
Menigomyelocele or spina bifida	2,748,302	402	14.9	16.5	14.9	14.8	15.3	12.6	*	50,501
Cyanotic congenital heart disease	2,748,302	1,225	45.4	38.0	38.5	42.9	45.5	60.3	100.1	50,501
Congenital diaphragmatic hernia	2,748,302	293	10.9	10.6	11.0	12.0	9.8	10.6	*	50,501
Omphalocele	2,748,302	193	7.2	7.7	6.8	5.7	5.8	11.0	*	50,501
Gastroschisis	2,748,302	790	29.3	95.0	52.2	15.5	5.3	*	*	50,501
Limb reduction defect	2,748,302	438	16.2	18.3	20.2	16.5	12.5	13.5	*	50,501
Cleft lip with or without cleft palate	2,748,302	1,396	51.7	59.1	55.0	52.8	44.2	52.2	42.5	50,501
Cleft palate alone	2,748,302	596	22.1	23.6	25.1	20.8	18.3	23.8	*	50,501
Down syndrome	2,748,302	1,298	48.1	28.2	22.0	22.8	44.2	119.2	359.3	50,501
Suspected chromosomal disorder	2,748,302	1,093	40.5	36.6	37.6	31.8	37.4	51.2	153.6	50,501
Hypospadias[3]	2,748,302	1,434	53.2	46.1	52.6	56.1	54.5	54.8	37.0	50,501
Males only[4]	1,406,875	1,434	103.8	89.8	103.0	109.6	106.3	106.9	72.2	25,868

* = Figure does not meet standards of reliability or precision.
[1]Refers to total number of births to residents of areas reporting specified abnormal condition.
[2]No response reported for congenital anomaly of the newborn item.
[3]Denominator includes both male and female births.
[4]Denominator includes male only.

NOTE: Includes California, Colorado, Delaware, Florida, Georgia, Idaho, Indiana, Iowa, Kansas, Kentucky, Michigan, Montana, Nebraska, New Hampshire, New Mexico, New York, North Dakota, Ohio, Oregon, Pennsylvania, South Carolina, South Dakota, Tennessee, Texas, Vermont, Washington, and Wyoming.

NOTES AND DEFINITIONS

SOURCES OF DATA

All of the tables in Part A are from the National Center for Health Statistics (NCHS), a component of the Centers for Disease Control and Prevention (CDC). Four different publications were used to obtain the data.

Most of the tables found in Part A were obtained from: Martin JA, Hamilton BE, Ventura SJ, et al. *Births: Final Data for 2009*. National Vital Statistics Reports: Volume 60, No 1. Hyattsville, MD: National Center for Health Statistics. 2011.

Data for Tables A-1 through A-18 were obtained from: Hamilton BE, Martin JA, Ventura SJ. *Births: Preliminary Data for 2010*. National Vital Statistics Reports: Volume 60, No 2. Hyattsville, MD: National Center for Health Statistics. 2011.

The data for Tables A-49, A-67, and A-73 through A-77 are from Osterman MJK, Martin JA, Mathews TJ, Hamilton BE. *Expanded Data From The New Birth Certificate, 2008*. National Vital Statistics Reports: Volume 59, No 7. Hyattsville, MD: National Center for Health Statistics. July, 2011.

Data for Tables A-20, A-21, and A-68 through A-70 were obtained from Martinez G, Copen CE, Abma JC. *Teenagers in the United States: Sexual Activity, Contraceptive Use, and Childbearing, 2006–2010 National Survey of Family Growth*. National Center for Health Statistics. Vital Health Stat 23 (31). 2011.

NOTES ON THE DATA

Preliminary data for 2010 are based on all births for that year. Preliminary data for 2010 are based on a continuous receipt and processing of statistical records through August 31, 2011. Final data for 2009 are based on 100 percent of the birth certificates filed in all states and the District of Columbia.

CONCEPTS AND DEFINITIONS

Anencephaly—a congenital anomaly that consists of a partial or complete absence of the brain and skull.

Apgar score—has been employed for over 50 years to assess the physical condition and short term prognosis of newborns. Historically, the score has been measured at 1 minute, 5 minutes, and if needed, at additional 5-minute intervals after delivery. Information on the 5 minute score is included in national birth certificate data. The Apgar score measures five easily identifiable characteristics of newborns. A 5-minute score of 0 to 3 indicates an infant in immediate need of resuscitation; 4 to 6 is considered intermediate, and 7 to 10 is considered normal. The Apgar score is a useful clinical indicator for reporting overall status of the neonate and need for, and response to resuscitation efforts.

Birth cohort—consists of all persons born within a given period of time, such as a calendar year.

Birthweight—the first weight of the newborn obtained after birth. Low birthweight is defined as less than 2,500 grams or 5 pounds 8 ounces. Very low birthweight is defined as less than 1,500 grams or 3 pounds 4 ounces. Before 1979, low birthweight was defined as weighing 2,500 grams or less, and very low birthweight was defined as 1,500 grams or less. Equivalents of the gram weights in terms of pounds and ounces are as follows:

Less than 500 grams = 1 lb 1 oz or less
500–999 grams = 1 lb 2 oz–2 lb 3 oz
1,000–1,499 grams = 2 lb 4 oz–3 lb 4 oz
1,500–1,999 grams = 3 lb 5 oz–4 lb 6 oz
2,000–2,499 grams = 4 lb 7 oz–5 lb 8 oz
2,500–2,999 grams = 5 lb 9 oz–6 lb 9 oz
3,000–3,499 grams = 6 lb 10 oz–7 lb 11 oz
3,500–3,999 grams = 7 lb 12 oz–8 lb 13 oz
4,000–4,499 grams = 8 lb 14 oz–9 lb 14 oz
4,500–4,999 grams = 9 lb 15 oz–11 lb 0 oz
5,000 grams or more = 11 lb 1 oz or more

Birth rate—calculated by dividing the number of live births in a population in a year by the midyear resident population. Birth rates are expressed as the number of live births per 1,000 population. The rate may be restricted to births to women of specific age, race, marital status, or geographic location (specific rate), or it may be related to the entire population (crude rate).

Breech/Malpresentation—presenting part of the fetus listed as breech, complete breech, frank breech, footling breech.

Cervical cerclage—circumferential banding or suture of the cervix to prevent or treat early dilation of the cervix (e.g., incompetent cervix) in an attempt to avoid premature delivery.

Cleft lip/palate—incomplete closure of the lip. May be unilateral, bilateral, or median. Cleft palate is incomplete fusion of the palatal shelves. May be limited to the soft palate, or may extend into the hard palate.

Contraception—The National Survey of Family Growth collects information on contraceptive use reported by women 15–44 years old. For current contraceptive use, women were asked about contraceptive use during the month of interview. Women were classified by whether they reported using any of the 19 methods of contraception at any time in the month of interview.

Cyanotic heart disease—congenital heart defects resulting in lack of oxygen that cause cyanosis.

Down syndrome—the most common chromosomal defect (trisomy 21).

Fertility rate—total number of live births per 1,000 women of reproductive age (defined as women age 15–44 years).

Gestation—the time period between the first day of the last normal menstrual period and the day of birth or day of termination of pregnancy according to the National Vital Statistics System and the CDC's Abortion Surveillance.

Hispanic origin—includes persons of Mexican, Puerto Rican, Cuban, Central and South American, and other or unknown Latin American or Spanish origins. Persons of Hispanic origin may be of any race.

Hypertension, chronic—diagnosis prior to the onset of this pregnancy of elevated blood pressure above normal for age, gender, and physiological condition.

Hypertension, pregnancy-associated—diagnosis in pregnancy of elevated blood pressure above normal for age, gender, and physiological condition.

Induction of labor—initiation of uterine contractions by medical and/or surgical means for the purpose of delivery before the spontaneous onset of labor.

Meconium, moderate/heavy—staining of the amniotic fluid caused by passage of fetal bowel contents during labor and/or at delivery that is more than enough to cause a greenish color change of an otherwise clear fluid.

Meningomyecele/Spina bifida—meningomyelocele is herniation of meninges and spinal cord tissue. Meningocele (herniation of meninges without spinal cord tissue) should also be included in this category. Both open and closed (covered with skin) lesions should be included. Spina bifida is herniation of the meninges and/or spinal cord tissue through a bony defect of spine closure.

Nonvertex presentation—includes any nonvertex fetal presentation, that is, presentation of a part of the infant's body other than the upper and back part of the infant's head.

Omphalocele/Gastroschisis—omphalocele is a defect in the anterior abdominal wall, accompanied by herniation of some abdominal organs through a widened umbilical ring into the umbilical stalk. Gastroschisis is an abnormality of the anterior abdominal wall, lateral to the umbilicus, resulting in herniation of the abdominal contents directly into the amniotic cavity.

Precipitous labor—labor lasting less than 3 hours.

Prenatal care—medical care provided to a pregnant woman to prevent complications and decrease the incidence of maternal and prenatal mortality. Information on when pregnancy care began is recorded on the birth certificate. Between 1970 and 1980, the reporting area for prenatal care expanded. In 1970, 39 states and the District of Columbia (D.C.) reported prenatal care on the birth certificate. Data were not available from Alabama, Alaska, Arkansas, Connecticut, Delaware, Georgia, Idaho, Massachusetts, New Mexico, Pennsylvania, and Virginia. In 1975, these data were available from three additional states—Connecticut, Delaware, and Georgia—increasing the number of states reporting prenatal care to 42 and D.C. During 1980–2002, prenatal care information was available for the entire United States.

Suspected chromosomal disorder—includes any constellation of congenital malformations resulting from, or compatible with, known syndromes caused by detectable defects in chromosome structure.

Tocolysis—administration of any agent with the intent to inhibit preterm uterine contractions to extend the length of the pregnancy.

PART B:
MORTALITY

MORTALITY

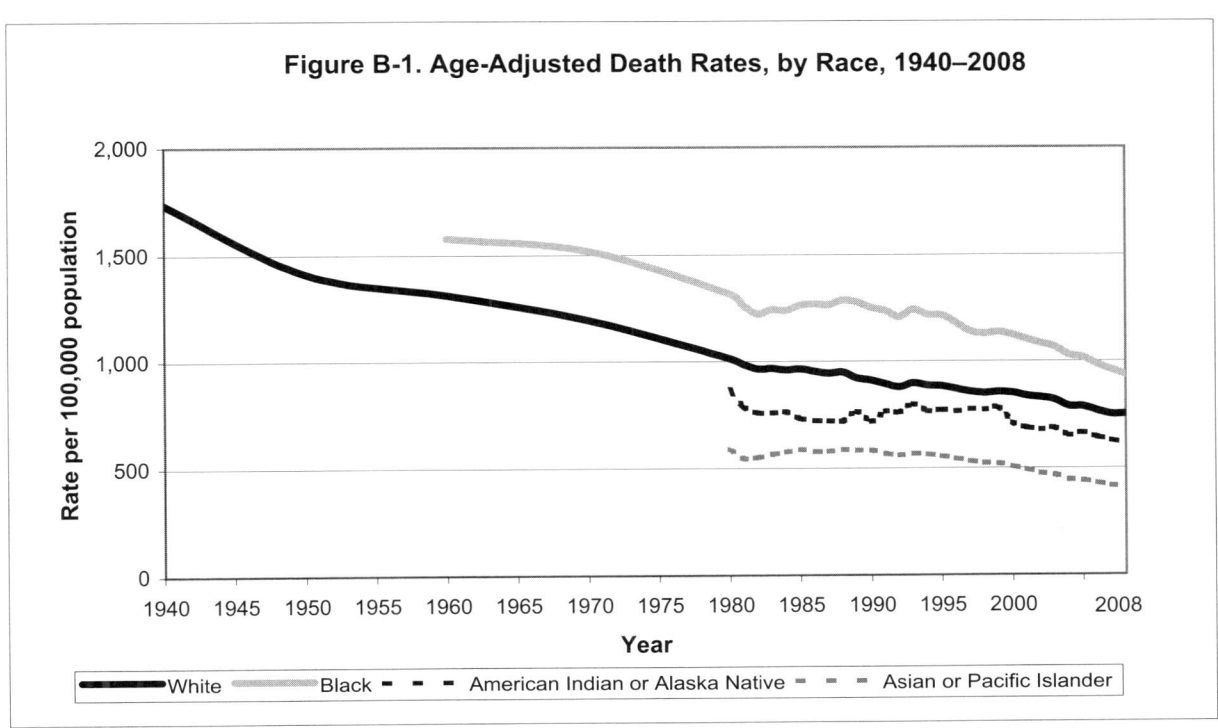

HIGHLIGHTS

- In 2008, there was a total of 2,471,984 registered deaths in the United States. The age-adjusted death rate declined to a record low at 758.3 per 100,000 standard population. Among all states, West Virginia has the highest age-adjusted death rate at 958.5 while Hawaii had the lowest at 590.6. (See Tables B-1 and B-31.)

- Hispanics had the highest life expectancy among all races and ethnic origins at 81.0 years in 2008. Life expectancy increased for the entire population from 77.9 years in 2007 to 78.1 years in 2008. (See Table B-7.)

- While age-adjusted death rates declined for six out of the 15 leading causes of deaths including heart disease, cancer, and cerebrovascular disease; death rates increased for chronic lower respiratory disease, Alzheimer's disease, kidney disease, and suicide in 2008. (See Table B-10.)

- The infant mortality rate declined to a record-low in 2008—dropping to 6.61 deaths per 1,000 live births after increasing in 2007. The neonatal and postneonatal mortality rates also declined. The neonatal rate fell 2.9 percent in 2008 while the postneonatal rate dropped 0.9 percent. (See Table B-45.)

- The leading cause of infant deaths in 2008 were congenital malformations, deformations, and chromosomal abnormalities followed by disorders related to length of gestation and fetal malnutrition. (See Table B-46.)

Table B-1. Number of Deaths, Death Rates, and Age-Adjusted Death Rates, by Race and Sex, Selected Years, 1940–2008

(Number, rate per 100,000 population.)

Year	All races[1]			White[2]			Black[2]			American Indian or Alaskan Native[2,3]			Asian or Pacific Islander[2,4]		
	Both sexes	Male	Female	Both sexes	Male	Female	Both sexes	Male	Female	Both sexes	Male	Female	Both sexes	Male	Female
Number															
1940	1,417,269	791,003	626,266	1,231,223	690,901	540,322	178,743	95,517	83,226	4,791	2,527	2,264	—	—	—
1950	1,452,454	827,749	624,705	1,276,085	731,366	544,719	169,606	92,004	77,602	4,440	2,497	1,943	—	—	—
1960	1,711,982	975,648	736,334	1,505,335	860,857	644,478	196,010	107,701	88,309	4,528	2,658	1,870	—	—	—
1970	1,921,031	1,078,478	842,553	1,682,096	942,437	739,659	225,647	127,540	98,107	5,675	3,391	2,284	—	—	—
1980	1,989,841	1,075,078	914,763	1,738,607	933,878	804,729	233,135	130,138	102,997	6,923	4,193	2,730	11,071	6,809	4,262
1981	1,977,981	1,063,772	914,209	1,731,233	925,490	805,743	228,560	127,296	101,264	6,608	4,016	2,592	11,475	6,908	4,567
1982	1,974,797	1,056,440	918,357	1,729,085	919,239	809,846	226,513	125,610	100,903	6,679	3,974	2,705	12,430	7,564	4,866
1983	2,019,201	1,071,923	947,278	1,765,582	931,779	833,803	233,124	127,911	105,213	6,839	4,064	2,775	13,554	8,126	5,428
1984	2,039,369	1,076,514	962,855	1,781,897	934,529	847,368	235,884	129,147	106,737	6,949	4,117	2,832	14,483	8,627	5,856
1985	2,086,440	1,097,758	988,682	1,819,054	950,455	868,599	244,207	133,610	110,597	7,154	4,181	2,973	15,887	9,441	6,446
1986	2,105,361	1,104,005	1,001,356	1,831,083	952,554	878,529	250,326	137,214	113,112	7,301	4,365	2,936	16,514	9,795	6,719
1987	2,123,323	1,107,958	1,015,365	1,843,067	953,382	889,685	254,814	139,551	115,263	7,602	4,432	3,170	17,689	10,496	7,193
1988	2,167,999	1,125,540	1,042,459	1,876,906	965,419	911,487	264,019	144,228	119,791	7,917	4,617	3,300	18,963	11,155	7,808
1989	2,150,466	1,114,190	1,036,276	1,853,841	950,852	902,989	267,642	146,393	121,249	8,614	5,066	3,548	20,042	11,688	8,354
1990	2,148,463	1,113,417	1,035,046	1,853,254	950,812	902,442	265,498	145,359	120,139	8,316	4,877	3,439	21,127	12,211	8,916
1991	2,169,518	1,121,665	1,047,853	1,868,904	956,497	912,407	269,525	147,331	122,194	8,621	4,948	3,673	22,173	12,727	9,446
1992	2,175,613	1,122,336	1,053,277	1,873,781	956,957	916,824	269,219	146,630	122,589	8,953	5,181	3,772	23,660	13,568	10,092
1993	2,268,553	1,161,797	1,106,756	1,951,437	988,329	963,108	282,151	153,502	128,649	9,579	5,434	4,145	25,386	14,532	10,854
1994	2,278,994	1,162,747	1,116,247	1,959,875	988,823	971,052	282,379	153,019	129,360	9,637	5,497	4,140	27,103	15,408	11,695
1995	2,312,132	1,172,959	1,139,173	1,987,437	997,277	990,160	286,401	154,175	132,226	9,997	5,574	4,423	28,297	15,933	12,364
1996	2,314,690	1,163,569	1,151,121	1,992,966	991,984	1,000,982	282,089	149,472	132,617	10,127	5,563	4,564	29,508	16,550	12,958
1997	2,314,245	1,154,039	1,160,206	1,996,393	986,884	1,009,509	276,520	144,110	132,410	10,576	5,985	4,591	30,756	17,060	13,696
1998	2,337,256	1,157,260	1,179,996	2,015,984	990,190	1,025,794	278,440	143,417	135,023	10,845	5,994	4,851	31,987	17,659	14,328
1999	2,391,399	1,175,460	1,215,939	2,061,348	1,005,335	1,056,013	285,064	145,703	139,361	11,312	6,092	5,220	33,675	18,330	15,345
2000	2,403,351	1,177,578	1,225,773	2,071,287	1,007,191	1,064,096	285,826	145,184	140,642	11,363	6,185	5,178	34,875	19,018	15,857
2001	2,416,425	1,183,421	1,233,004	2,079,691	1,011,218	1,068,473	287,709	145,908	141,801	11,977	6,466	5,511	37,048	19,829	17,219
2002	2,443,387	1,199,264	1,244,123	2,102,589	1,025,196	1,077,393	290,051	146,835	143,216	12,415	6,750	5,665	38,332	20,483	17,849
2003	2,448,288	1,201,964	1,246,324	2,103,714	1,025,650	1,078,064	291,300	148,022	143,278	13,147	7,106	6,041	40,127	21,186	18,941
2004	2,397,615	1,181,668	1,215,947	2,056,643	1,007,266	1,049,377	287,315	145,970	141,345	13,124	7,134	5,990	40,533	21,298	19,235
2005	2,448,017	1,207,675	1,240,342	2,098,097	1,028,152	1,069,945	292,808	149,108	143,700	13,918	7,607	6,311	43194	22808	20386
2006	2,426,264	1,201,942	1,224,322	2,077,549	1,022,328	1,055,221	289,971	148,602	141,369	14,037	7,630	6,407	44707	23382	21325
2007	2,423,712	1,203,968	1,219,744	2,074,151	1,023,951	1,050,200	289,585	148,309	141,276	14,367	7,885	6,482	45609	23823	21786
2008	2,471,984	1,226,197	1,245,787	2,120,233	1,046,183	1,074,050	289,072	147,143	141,929	14,776	8,163	6,613	47903	24708	23195
Death Rate															
1940	1076.4	1197.4	954.6	1041.5	1162.2	919.4	—	—	—	—	—	—	—	—	—
1950	963.8	1106.1	823.5	945.7	1089.5	803.3	—	—	—	—	—	—	—	—	—
1960	954.7	1104.5	809.2	947.8	1098.5	800.9	1038.6	1181.7	905.0	—	—	—	—	—	—
1970	945.3	1090.3	807.8	946.3	1086.7	812.6	999.3	1186.6	829.2	—	—	—	—	—	—
1980	878.3	976.9	785.3	892.5	983.3	806.1	875.4	1034.1	733.3	487.4	597.1	380.1	296.9	375.3	222.5
1981	862.0	954.0	775.0	880.4	965.2	799.8	842.4	992.6	707.7	445.6	547.9	345.6	272.3	336.2	211.5
1982	852.4	938.4	771.2	873.1	951.8	798.2	823.4	966.2	695.5	434.5	522.9	348.1	271.3	338.3	207.4
1983	863.7	943.2	788.4	885.4	957.7	816.4	836.6	971.2	715.9	428.5	515.1	343.9	276.1	339.1	216.1
1984	864.8	938.8	794.7	887.8	954.1	824.6	836.1	968.5	717.4	419.6	502.7	338.4	275.9	336.5	218.1
1985	876.9	948.6	809.1	900.4	963.6	840.1	854.8	989.3	734.2	416.4	492.5	342.5	283.4	344.6	224.9
1986	876.7	944.7	812.3	900.1	958.6	844.3	864.9	1002.6	741.5	409.5	494.9	325.9	276.2	335.1	219.9
1987	876.4	939.3	816.7	900.1	952.7	849.8	868.9	1006.2	745.7	410.7	483.8	339.0	278.9	338.3	222.0
1988	886.7	945.1	831.2	910.5	957.9	865.3	888.3	1026.1	764.6	411.7	485.0	339.9	282.0	339.0	227.4
1989	871.3	926.3	818.9	893.2	936.5	851.8	887.9	1026.7	763.2	430.5	510.7	351.3	280.9	334.5	229.4
1990	863.8	918.4	812.0	888.0	930.9	846.9	871.0	1008.0	747.9	402.8	476.4	330.4	283.3	334.3	234.3
1991	857.6	908.8	808.7	883.2	922.7	845.2	861.4	994.8	741.4	405.3	468.9	342.7	278.7	326.9	232.4
1992	848.1	896.1	802.4	875.8	912.2	840.8	841.8	967.6	728.6	406.6	474.1	340.0	282.1	331.1	235.3
1993	872.8	915.0	832.5	902.7	931.8	874.6	864.6	992.2	749.6	419.8	479.6	360.7	288.0	338.1	240.3
1994	866.1	904.2	829.7	897.8	922.6	873.8	849.0	970.2	739.7	408.2	468.8	348.3	294.6	344.0	247.7
1995	868.3	900.8	837.2	901.8	921.0	883.2	846.2	960.2	743.2	409.4	459.4	360.1	294.6	341.4	250.4
1996	859.2	882.8	836.7	896.0	907.1	885.3	819.7	915.3	733.3	399.5	441.5	358.0	294.4	340.2	251.1
1997	848.8	864.6	833.6	889.1	893.3	885.0	789.9	867.1	720.1	402.7	458.2	347.7	294.1	336.8	253.9
1998	847.3	856.4	838.5	889.5	887.3	891.6	782.3	848.2	722.6	397.8	441.9	354.2	293.8	335.4	254.9
1999	857.0	859.2	854.9	901.4	892.1	910.4	788.1	847.4	734.3	399.3	431.8	367.1	296.8	333.2	262.5

Table B-1. **Number of Deaths, Death Rates, and Age-Adjusted Death Rates, by Race and Sex, Selected Years, 1940–2008**—*Continued*

(Number, rate per 100,000 population.)

Year	All races[1]			White[2]			Black[2]			American Indian or Alaskan native[2,3]			Asian or Pacific Islander[2,4]		
	Both sexes	Male	Female	Both sexes	Male	Female	Both sexes	Male	Female	Both sexes	Male	Female	Both sexes	Male	Female
2000	854.0	853.0	855.0	900.2	887.8	912.3	781.1	834.1	733.0	380.8	415.6	346.1	296.6	332.9	262.3
2001	848.5	846.4	850.4	895.1	881.9	907.9	773.5	823.9	727.7	392.1	424.2	360.2	303.8	335.0	274.4
2002	847.3	846.6	848.0	895.7	884.0	907.0	768.4	816.7	724.4	403.6	439.6	367.7	299.5	331.4	269.7
2003	841.9	840.3	843.4	890.1	877.6	902.3	763.6	813.7	717.9	422.6	457.6	387.7	303.9	330.0	279.2
2004	816.5	817.6	815.4	863.2	854.2	871.9	744.3	792.6	700.3	416.8	453.8	380.0	297.2	321.1	274.6
2005	825.9	827.2	824.6	873.7	864.5	882.8	749.4	799.2	703.9	440.3	481.9	398.8	307.7	333.9	282.8
2006	810.4	814.8	806.1	858.1	852.3	863.9	733.0	786.7	684.0	438.5	477.1	399.9	307.4	330.6	285.6
2007	803.6	809.9	797.4	851.5	848.1	854.9	723.4	775.6	675.7	444.0	488.2	400.0	308.7	331.4	287.2
2008	813.0	817.9	808.2	864.6	860.3	868.7	716.1	762.7	673.5	431.8	477.6	386.1	318.7	337.7	300.7
Age-Adjusted Death Rate															
1940	1785.0	1976.0	1599.4	1735.3	1925.2	1550.4	—	—	—	—	—	—	—	—	—
1950	1446.0	1674.2	1236.0	1410.8	1642.5	1198.0	—	—	—	—	—	—	—	—	—
1960	1339.2	1609.0	1105.3	1311.3	1586.0	1074.4	1577.5	1811.1	1369.7	—	—	—	—	—	—
1970	1222.6	1542.1	971.4	1193.3	1513.7	944.0	1518.1	1873.9	1228.7	—	—	—	—	—	—
1980	1039.1	1348.1	817.9	1012.7	1317.6	796.1	1314.8	1697.8	1033.3	867.0	1111.5	662.4	589.9	786.5	425.9
1981	1007.1	1308.2	792.7	984.0	1282.2	773.6	1258.4	1626.6	986.6	784.6	1030.2	588.0	544.7	710.3	405.3
1982	985.0	1279.9	776.6	963.6	1255.9	758.7	1221.3	1580.4	960.1	757.0	940.1	604.4	550.4	738.2	410.3
1983	990.0	1284.5	783.3	967.3	1259.4	763.9	1240.5	1600.7	980.7	757.3	945.0	605.5	565.1	718.8	428.8
1984	982.5	1271.4	779.8	959.7	1245.9	760.7	1236.7	1600.8	976.9	761.7	946.0	567.9	574.4	724.7	443.1
1985	988.1	1278.1	784.5	963.6	1249.8	764.3	1261.2	1634.5	994.4	731.7	926.1	577.2	586.5	755.4	456.7
1986	978.6	1261.7	778.7	952.8	1230.5	758.1	1266.7	1650.1	994.4	720.8	926.7	549.3	576.4	730.5	445.4
1987	970.0	1246.1	774.2	943.4	1213.4	753.3	1263.1	1650.3	989.7	719.8	899.3	583.7	577.3	732.4	448.1
1988	975.7	1250.7	781.0	947.6	1215.9	759.1	1284.3	1677.6	1006.8	718.6	917.4	563.6	584.2	732.0	451.0
1989	950.5	1215.0	761.8	920.2	1176.6	738.8	1275.5	1670.1	998.1	761.6	999.8	586.3	581.3	729.6	458.4
1990	938.7	1202.8	750.9	909.8	1165.9	728.8	1250.3	1644.5	975.1	716.3	916.2	561.8	582.0	716.4	469.3
1991	922.3	1180.5	738.2	893.2	1143.1	716.1	1235.4	1626.1	963.3	763.9	970.6	608.3	566.2	703.4	453.2
1992	905.6	1158.3	725.5	877.7	1122.4	704.1	1206.7	1587.8	942.5	759.0	970.4	599.4	558.5	697.3	445.8
1993	926.1	1177.3	745.9	897.0	1138.9	724.1	1241.2	1632.2	969.5	796.4	1006.3	641.6	565.8	709.9	450.4
1994	913.5	1155.5	738.6	885.6	1118.7	717.5	1216.9	1592.8	954.6	764.8	953.3	618.8	562.7	702.5	452.1
1995	909.8	1143.9	739.4	882.3	1107.5	718.7	1213.9	1585.7	955.9	771.2	932.0	643.9	554.8	693.4	446.7
1996	894.1	1115.7	733.0	869.0	1082.9	713.6	1178.4	1524.2	940.3	763.6	924.8	641.7	543.2	676.1	439.6
1997	878.1	1088.1	725.6	855.7	1059.1	707.8	1139.8	1458.8	922.1	774.0	974.8	625.3	531.8	660.2	432.6
1998	870.6	1069.4	724.7	849.3	1042.0	707.3	1127.8	1430.5	921.6	770.4	943.9	640.5	522.4	646.9	426.7
1999	875.6	1067.0	734.0	854.6	1040.0	716.6	1135.7	1432.6	933.6	780.9	925.9	668.2	519.7	641.2	427.5
2000	869.0	1053.8	731.4	849.8	1029.4	715.3	1121.4	1403.5	927.6	709.3	841.5	604.5	506.4	624.2	416.8
2001	854.5	1029.1	721.8	836.5	1006.1	706.7	1101.2	1375.0	912.5	686.7	798.9	594.0	492.1	597.4	412.0
2002	845.3	1013.7	715.2	829.0	992.9	701.3	1083.3	1341.4	901.8	677.4	794.2	581.1	474.4	578.4	395.9
2003	832.7	994.3	706.2	817.0	973.9	693.1	1065.9	1319.1	885.6	685.0	797.0	592.1	465.7	562.7	392.7
2004	800.8	955.7	679.2	786.3	936.9	666.9	1027.3	1269.4	855.3	650.0	758.1	557.9	443.9	534.7	375.5
2005	798.8	951.1	677.6	785.3	933.2	666.5	1016.5	1252.9	845.7	663.4	775.3	567.7	440.2	534.4	369.3
2006	776.5	924.8	657.8	764.4	908.2	648.2	982.0	1215.6	813.0	642.1	739.9	555.7	428.6	516.0	362.6
2007	760.2	905.6	643.4	749.4	890.5	634.8	958.0	1184.4	793.8	627.2	736.7	533.2	415.0	499.2	350.6
2008	758.3	900.6	643.4	750.3	889.2	636.9	934.9	1150.4	778.4	610.1	717.3	515.1	413.7	492.8	353.1

—- = Data not available.
[1]For 1940–1991, data includes deaths among races not shown separately; beginning in 1992, records coded as "other races" and records for which race was unknown, not stated, or not classifiable were assigned to the race of previous record.
[2]Multiple-race data were reported by 34 states and the District of Columbia in 2008, by 27 states and the District of Columbia in 2007, by 25 states and the District of Columbia in 2006, by 21 states and the District of Columbia in 2005, by 15 states in 2004, and by 7 states in 2003.
[3]Includes Aleuts and Eskimos.
[4]Includes Chinese, Filipino, Hawaiian, Japanese, and Other Asian or Pacific Islander.

Table B-2. Number of Deaths, Death Rates, and Age-Adjusted Death Rates, by Hispanic Origin, Race for Non-Hispanic Population, and Sex, 1997–2008

(Number, rate per 100,000.)

Year	All origins[1]			Hispanic			Non-Hispanic[2]			Non-Hispanic White[3]			Non-Hispanic Black[3]		
	Both sexes	Male	Female	Both sexes	Male	Female	Both sexes	Male	Female	Both sexes	Male	Female	Both sexes	Male	Female
Number															
1997	2,314,245	1,154,039	1,160,206	95,460	54,348	41,112	2,209,450	1,094,541	1,114,909	1,895,461	929,703	965,758	273,381	142,241	131,140
1998	2,337,256	1,157,260	1,179,996	98,406	55,821	42,585	2,230,127	1,096,677	1,133,450	1,912,802	931,844	980,958	275,264	141,627	133,637
1999	2,391,399	1,175,460	1,215,939	103,740	57,991	45,749	2,279,325	1,112,718	1,166,607	1,953,197	944,913	1,008,284	281,979	143,883	138,096
2000	2,403,351	1,177,578	1,225,773	107,254	60,172	47,082	2,287,846	1,112,704	1,175,142	1,959,919	944,781	1,015,138	282,676	143,297	139,379
2001	2,416,425	1,183,421	1,233,004	113,413	63,317	50,096	2,295,244	1,115,683	1,179,561	1,962,810	945,967	1,016,843	284,343	143,971	140,372
2002	2,443,387	1,199,264	1,244,123	117,135	65,703	51,432	2,318,269	1,129,090	1,189,179	1,981,973	957,645	1,024,328	286,573	144,802	141,771
2003	2,448,288	1,201,964	1,246,324	122,026	68,119	53,907	2,319,476	1,129,927	1,189,549	1,979,465	956,194	1,023,271	287,968	145,136	141,832
2004	2,397,615	1,181,668	1,215,947	122,416	68,544	53,872	2,269,583	1,109,848	1,159,735	1,933,382	938,143	995,239	283,859	144,022	139,837
2005	2,448,017	1,207,675	1,240,342	131,161	73,788	57,373	2,312,028	1,131,013	1,181,015	1,967,142	954,402	1,012,740	289,163	147,010	142,153
2006	2,426,264	1,201,942	1,224,322	133,004	74,250	58,754	2,288,424	1,124,813	1,163,611	1,944,617	947,966	996,651	286,581	146,729	139,852
2007	2,423,712	1,203,968	1,219,744	135,519	75,708	59,811	2,284,446	1,125,974	1,158,472	1,939,606	948,662	990,944	286,366	146,474	139,892
2008	2,471,984	1,226,197	1,245,787	139,241	76,861	62,380	2,327,636	1,146,394	1,181,242	1,981,034	969,288	1,011,746	285,522	145,168	140,354
Death Rate															
1997	848.8	864.6	833.6	309	343.2	272.9	913.9	930.4	898.3	967.4	970.6	964.3	813.5	892.9	741.9
1998	847.3	856.4	838.5	303.9	336.0	270.0	916.0	925.3	907.1	972.9	969.2	976.5	805.6	873.7	744.1
1999	857.0	859.2	854.9	305.7	332.6	277.2	929.9	932.2	927.8	990.7	979.6	1001.3	812.1	872.8	757.3
2000	854.0	853.0	855.0	303.8	331.3	274.6	929.6	928.1	931.0	993.2	978.5	1007.3	805.5	859.5	756.7
2001	848.5	846.4	850.4	306.8	332.9	279.0	926.2	923.6	928.6	991.1	975.6	1006.1	798.1	849.7	751.2
2002	847.3	846.6	848.0	302.2	328.7	274.0	928.8	928.0	929.5	997.5	983.9	1010.6	792.8	842.3	748.0
2003	841.9	840.3	843.4	305.8	330.7	279.3	924.4	922.9	925.9	993.6	979.1	1007.6	788.8	840.6	741.6
2004	816.5	817.6	815.4	296.2	321.1	269.7	899.4	900.9	898.0	967.8	957.4	977.7	768.8	818.7	723.4
2005	825.9	827.2	824.6	307.3	334.4	278.2	911.2	912.6	910.0	981.8	970.6	992.6	774.4	825.7	727.6
2006	810.4	814.8	806.1	300.1	323.9	274.6	897.1	902.8	891.7	968.5	962.0	974.7	759.1	815.3	708.0
2007	803.6	809.9	797.4	297.8	321.8	272.1	892.0	899.8	884.5	964.1	960.4	967.6	750.7	805.1	701.0
2008	813.0	817.9	808.2	296.6	316.9	274.9	905.3	912.2	898.7	982.0	978.2	985.5	745.2	794.3	700.5
Age-Adjusted Death Rate															
1997	878.1	1088.1	725.6	669.3	840.5	538.8	885.3	1096.4	732.6	859.7	1063.2	712.5	1154.3	1476.7	934.2
1998	870.6	1,069.40	724.7	665.4	833.6	536.9	878.4	1,078.20	732.4	854.1	1,046.70	712.8	1,141.80	1,448.20	932.9
1999	875.6	1067.0	734.0	676.4	830.5	555.9	883.9	1076.4	741.9	859.8	1045.5	722.3	1150.1	1449.4	946.0
2000	869.0	1053.8	731.4	665.7	818.1	546.0	877.9	1063.8	740.0	855.5	1035.4	721.5	1137.0	1422.0	941.2
2001	854.5	1029.1	721.8	658.7	802.5	544.2	864.0	1039.8	730.9	842.9	1012.8	713.5	1116.5	1393.7	925.5
2002	845.3	1013.7	715.2	629.3	766.7	518.3	856.5	1026.5	725.8	837.5	1002.2	709.9	1099.2	1360.6	915.3
2003	832.7	994.3	706.2	621.2	748.1	515.8	844.5	1008.0	717.2	826.1	984.0	702.1	1083.2	1341.1	899.8
2004	800.8	955.7	679.2	586.7	706.8	485.9	814.1	971.1	691.4	797.1	949.0	677.5	1044.7	1291.5	869.4
2005	798.8	951.1	677.6	590.7	717.0	485.3	812.5	966.7	690.3	796.6	945.4	677.7	1034.5	1275.3	860.5
2006	776.5	924.8	657.8	564.0	675.6	468.6	791.4	942.6	671.1	777.0	922.8	660.0	1001.4	1241.0	828.4
2007	760.2	905.6	643.4	546.1	654.5	452.7	776.3	924.9	657.7	763.3	906.8	647.7	978.6	1210.9	810.4
2008	758.3	900.6	643.4	532.2	630.7	445.7	775.8	922.2	658.5	766.2	908.5	650.8	955.2	1176.6	794.8

[1]Figures for origin not stated are included in "All origins" but are not distributed among specified origins.
[2]Includes races other than White and Black.
[3]Multiple-race data were reported by 34 states and the District of Columbia in 2008, by 27 states and the District of Columbia in 2007, by 25 states and the District of Columbia in 2006, by 21 states and the District of Columbia in 2005, by 15 states in 2004, and by 7 states in 2003.

Table B-3. Number of Deaths and Death Rates, by Age, Race, and Sex, 2008

(Number, rate per 100,000.)

Year	All races			White[1]			Black[1]			American Indian[1,2] or Alaska Native			Asian or Pacific Islander[1,3]		
	Both sexes	Male	Female	Both sexes	Male	Female	Both sexes	Male	Female	Both sexes	Male	Female	Both sexes	Male	Female
Number															
All ages	2,471,984	1,226,197	1,245,787	2,120,233	1,046,183	1,074,050	289,072	147,143	141,929	14,776	8,163	6,613	47,903	24,708	23,195
Under 1 year	28,059	15,669	12,390	18,164	10,151	8,013	8,543	4,748	3,795	403	234	169	949	536	413
1–4 years	4,730	2,693	2,037	3,349	1,919	1,430	1,118	647	471	100	50	50	163	77	86
5–9 years	2,502	1,396	1,106	1,787	979	808	576	347	229	40	21	19	99	49	50
10–14 years	3,149	1,884	1,265	2,276	1,359	917	709	420	289	57	31	26	107	74	33
15–19 years	12,407	8,958	3,449	9,014	6,416	2,598	2,856	2,175	681	264	174	90	273	193	80
20–24 years	19,791	15,069	4,722	14,611	11,137	3,474	4,361	3,338	1023	371	288	83	448	306	142
25–29 years	20,786	15,000	5,786	15,302	11,147	4,155	4,562	3,268	1,294	380	259	121	542	326	216
30–34 years	21,489	14,635	6,854	15,810	10,917	4,893	4,704	3,095	1,609	392	269	123	583	354	229
35–39 years	29,864	19,104	10,760	22,323	14,536	7,787	6,251	3,771	2,480	524	314	210	766	483	283
40–44 years	46,506	28,582	17,924	35,286	22,128	13,158	9,527	5,417	4,110	692	413	279	1,001	624	377
45–49 years	77,417	47,339	30,078	59,992	37,399	22,593	14,944	8,396	6,548	963	617	346	1,518	927	591
50–54 years	109,125	67,699	41,426	84,784	53,419	31,365	21,016	12,288	8,728	1,124	700	424	2,201	1,292	909
55–59 years	134,708	83,423	51,285	106,166	66,337	39,829	24,523	14,728	9,795	1,185	715	470	2,834	1,643	1,191
60–64 years	161,474	96,127	65,347	132,749	79,561	53,188	24,189	13,936	10,253	1,256	723	533	3,280	1,907	1,373
65–69 years	183,450	105,403	78,047	153,212	88,436	64,776	25,229	14,089	11,140	1,291	735	556	3,718	2,143	1,575
70–74 years	218,129	119,997	98,132	185,485	102,806	82,679	26,538	13,884	12,654	1,378	729	649	4,728	2,578	2,150
75–79 years	287,370	149,204	138,166	251,323	131,606	119,717	28,994	14,054	14,940	1,318	681	637	5,735	2,863	2,872
80–84 years	366,190	172,692	193,498	328,103	155,817	172,286	30,136	13,019	17,117	1,269	588	681	6,682	3,268	3,414
85 years and over	744,691	261,221	483,470	680,379	240,030	440,349	50,273	15,506	34,767	1,766	622	1,144	12,273	5,063	7,210
Not stated	147	102	45	118	83	35	23	17	6	3	-	3	3	2	1
Rate															
All ages[4]	813.0	817.9	808.2	864.6	860.3	868.7	716.1	762.7	673.5	431.8	477.6	386.1	318.7	337.7	300.7
Under 1 year[5]	650.5	709.7	588.5	549.8	600.2	496.9	1,194.9	1,298.7	1,086.3	579.1	659.7	495.3	421.9	464.2	377.2
1–4 years	28.3	31.5	25.0	26.0	29.1	22.8	41.6	47.3	35.7	38.9	38.4	39.5	18.6	17.1	20.1
5–9 years	12.5	13.6	11.3	11.4	12.2	10.6	18.2	21.6	14.7	14.2	14.7	*	10.0	9.7	10.2
10–14 years	15.7	18.4	12.9	14.6	17.0	12.1	21.8	25.4	18.1	20.9	22.4	19.4	11.2	15.3	7.0
15–19 years	57.7	81.2	32.9	54.1	75.0	32.1	79.6	119.5	38.5	86.5	112.7	59.7	28.4	39.0	17.2
20–24 years	94.0	138.9	46.2	88.4	130.3	43.5	134.2	202.9	63.7	124.8	189.4	57.1	45.4	60.7	29.5
25–29 years	97.4	137.1	55.7	91.3	128.7	51.4	146.2	211.7	82.1	136.2	178.7	90.3	45.9	55.5	36.4
30–34 years	109.6	147.0	71.1	103.0	138.1	65.7	174.9	240.7	114.6	167.7	221.6	109.5	44.1	54.7	33.9
35–39 years	142.3	180.8	103.2	134.7	172.0	95.8	223.7	285.8	168.1	230.0	269.6	188.7	54.9	70.9	39.7
40–44 years	216.2	266.0	166.6	204.6	253.8	154.3	337.3	408.9	274.0	304.8	363.4	246.1	82.8	106.1	60.7
45–49 years	338.4	418.4	260.1	321.2	400.4	242.0	522.1	631.5	427.2	414.7	543.2	291.6	137.0	174.6	102.4
50–54 years	507.7	642.4	378.2	477.6	606.6	350.6	825.0	1,050.0	633.9	545.9	702.9	398.8	222.6	278.1	173.4
55–59 years	724.9	925.4	536.0	683.7	870.1	504.0	1,193.1	1,591.2	866.9	714.2	895.9	545.8	339.5	426.5	265.0
60–64 years	1,069.2	1,328.5	830.7	1,029.1	1,273.5	799.6	1,653.7	2,164.0	1,252.2	1,022.2	1,230.7	831.2	530.8	667.9	413.0
65–69 years	1,616.5	1,986.4	1,291.6	1,571.8	1,920.2	1,259.8	2,359.3	3,107.6	1,808.5	1,526.8	1,840.6	1,245.9	831.1	1,033.8	656.1
70–74 years	2,486.0	3,031.2	2,037.8	2,457.9	2,987.3	2,014.1	3,215.1	4,116.2	2,592.4	2,294.0	2,647.2	1,995.1	1,381.5	1,691.7	1,132.5
75–79 years	3,950.0	4,818.0	3,306.7	3,948.6	4,801.0	3,303.8	4,745.0	6,078.4	3,933.3	3,097.3	3,622.9	2,681.4	2,234.0	2,711.3	1,900.5
80–84 years	6,368.7	7,711.2	5,512.2	6,421.9	7,759.8	5,555.6	6,915.8	8,679.9	5,989.9	4,462.3	4,991.5	4,088.1	3,785.5	4,687.3	3,196.7
85 years and over	13,015.1	14,017.3	12,531.0	13,283.8	14,354.0	12,765.0	12,061.1	12,528.3	11,863.8	6,169.4	6,513.8	5,997.1	7,946.9	8,724.9	7,478.6

- = Quantity zero.
* = Figure does not meet standards of reliability or precision.
[1]Race categories are consistent with the 1977 Office of Management and Budget (OMB) standards.
[2]Includes Aleuts and Eskimos.
[3]Includes Chinese, Filipino, Hawaiian, Japanese, and Other Asian or Pacific Islander.
[4]Figures for age not stated are included in "All ages" but not distributed among age groups.
[5]Death rates for "Under 1 year" (based on population estimates) differ from infant mortality rates (based on live births).

Table B-4. Number of Deaths and Death Rates by Hispanic Origin, Race for Non-Hispanic Population, Age, and Sex, 2008

(Number, rate per 100,000.)

Age	All origins[1]			Hispanic			Non-Hispanic[2]			Non-Hispanic White[3]			Non-Hispanic Black[3]		
	Both sexes	Male	Female	Both sexes	Male	Female	Both sexes	Male	Female	Both sexes	Male	Female	Both sexes	Male	Female
Number															
All ages	2,471,984	1,226,197	1,245,787	139,241	76,861	62,380	2,327,636	1,146,394	1,181,242	1,981,034	969,288	1,011,746	285,522	145,168	140,354
Under 1 year	28,059	15,669	12,390	5,890	3,279	2,611	21,937	12,260	9,677	12,519	7,022	5,497	8,187	4,546	3,641
1–4 years	4,730	2,693	2,037	1,029	587	442	3,685	2,101	1,584	2,373	1,365	1,008	1,076	619	457
5–9 years	2,502	1,396	1,106	480	253	227	2,018	1,140	878	1,325	737	588	560	336	224
10–14 years	3,149	1,884	1,265	540	295	245	2,601	1,584	1,017	1,745	1,069	676	698	414	284
15–19 years	12,407	8,958	3,449	2,035	1,519	516	10,347	7,422	2,925	7,046	4,940	2,106	2,806	2,144	662
20–24 years	19,791	15,069	4,722	3,168	2,560	608	16,568	12,469	4,099	11,514	8,635	2,879	4,286	3,279	1007
25–29 years	20,786	15,000	5,786	3,218	2,483	735	17,513	12,475	5,038	12,154	8,718	3,436	4,490	3,211	1,279
30–34 years	21,489	14,635	6,854	3,178	2,356	822	18,260	12,244	6,016	12,698	8,612	4,086	4,626	3,037	1,589
35–39 years	29,864	19,104	10,760	3,672	2,571	1,101	26,122	16,493	9,629	18,699	11,998	6,701	6,176	3,727	2,449
40–44 years	46,506	28,582	17,924	4,949	3,353	1,596	41,431	25,151	16,280	30,392	18,812	11,580	9,403	5,343	4,060
45–49 years	77,417	47,339	30,078	6,548	4,353	2,195	70,590	42,803	27,787	53,459	33,044	20,415	14,751	8,279	6,472
50–54 years	109,125	67,699	41,426	7,822	5,116	2,706	100,954	62,336	38,618	76,964	48,287	28,677	20,776	12,125	8,651
55–59 years	134,708	83,423	51,285	9,012	5,731	3,281	125,290	77,412	47,878	97,100	60,557	36,543	24,278	14,563	9,715
60–64 years	161,474	96,127	65,347	9,490	5,730	3,760	151,524	90,071	61,453	123,155	73,733	49,422	23,950	13,781	10,169
65–69 years	183,450	105,403	78,047	10,117	5,895	4,222	172,923	99,239	73,684	143,045	82,493	60,552	24,971	13,935	11,036
70–74 years	218,129	119,997	98,132	11,826	6,526	5,300	205,858	113,190	92,668	173,637	96,237	77,400	26,249	13,718	12,531
75–79 years	287,370	149,204	138,166	14,455	7,390	7,065	272,397	141,525	130,872	236,819	124,175	112,644	28,665	13,885	14,780
80–84 years	366,190	172,692	193,498	15,807	7,461	8,346	349,893	164,976	184,917	312,267	148,307	163,960	29,816	12,876	16,940
85 years and over	744,691	261,221	483,470	25,996	9,394	16,602	717,622	251,435	466,187	654,044	230,495	423,549	49,738	15,336	34,402
Not stated	147	102	45	9	9	-	103	68	35	79	52	27	20	14	6
Rate															
All ages[4]	813.0	817.9	808.2	296.6	316.9	274.9	905.3	912.2	898.7	982.0	978.2	985.5	745.2	794.3	700.5
Under 1 year[5]	650.5	709.7	588.5	531.4	578.5	482.2	684.5	747.2	618.8	542.8	594.4	488.6	1,270.8	1,380.7	1,155.9
1–4 years	28.3	31.5	25.0	24.6	27.5	21.6	29.4	32.8	25.9	26.1	29.3	22.7	44.2	50.0	38.2
5–9 years	12.5	13.6	11.3	10.8	11.1	10.4	12.9	14.3	11.5	11.5	12.5	10.5	19.0	22.4	15.4
10–14 years	15.7	18.4	12.9	13.5	14.4	12.6	16.2	19.3	13.0	14.7	17.5	11.7	22.8	26.6	18.8
15–19 years	57.7	81.2	32.9	52.9	76.7	27.6	58.6	82.0	33.9	53.7	73.4	33.0	82.3	124.1	39.4
20–24 years	94.0	138.9	46.2	86.5	131.6	35.4	95.2	140.1	48.2	87.7	128.1	45.0	138.4	209.5	65.8
25–29 years	97.4	137.1	55.7	77.7	108.1	39.9	101.9	144.3	58.9	94.2	133.8	53.9	151.8	220.0	85.4
30–34 years	109.6	147.0	71.1	78.6	106.3	45.0	117.4	158.1	77.0	109.7	147.9	71.1	182.4	251.1	119.8
35–39 years	142.3	180.8	103.2	98.4	128.7	63.5	151.3	192.4	110.8	142.8	182.4	102.9	233.1	298.1	175.0
40–44 years	216.2	266.0	166.6	150.9	193.6	103.2	227.3	279.0	176.7	214.2	265.1	163.3	349.0	423.4	283.4
45–49 years	338.4	418.4	260.1	234.3	302.0	162.1	351.5	433.5	272.1	332.6	413.5	252.7	536.1	648.4	438.9
50–54 years	507.7	642.4	378.2	357.6	464.8	249.0	522.9	660.5	391.4	489.8	620.9	361.3	845.3	1,074.9	650.5
55–59 years	724.9	925.4	536.0	546.0	709.9	389.1	739.9	943.2	548.7	694.1	881.4	513.3	1,221.3	1,629.3	887.9
60–64 years	1,069.2	1,328.5	830.7	788.5	1,003.0	594.7	1,090.2	1,351.5	849.4	1,046.1	1,290.7	815.5	1,691.2	2,213.3	1,281.6
65–69 years	1,616.5	1,986.4	1,291.6	1,186.0	1,506.5	914.4	1,647.6	2,019.1	1,320.3	1,599.0	1,946.7	1,286.1	2,408.1	3,174.3	1,845.6
70–74 years	2,486.0	3,031.2	2,037.8	1,812.1	2,261.4	1,455.9	2,534.7	3,084.1	2,081.7	2,504.8	3,036.5	2,057.0	3,277.9	4,197.5	2,643.8
75–79 years	3,950.0	4,818.0	3,306.7	2,912.1	3,524.8	2,464.2	4,018.4	4,901.9	3,362.9	4,016.9	4,883.7	3,359.6	4,829.1	6,192.9	4,001.3
80–84 years	6,368.7	7,711.2	5,512.2	4,567.6	5,381.9	4,023.4	6,475.0	7,852.8	5,598.6	6,531.6	7,905.2	5,644.5	7,030.3	8,835.8	6,085.2
85 years and over	13,015.1	14,017.3	12,531.0	8,299.3	8,379.0	8,254.9	13,268.3	14,355.8	12,747.5	13,556.7	14,721.8	12,996.9	12,239.0	12,742.6	12,027.1

— = Quantity zero.
[1]Figures for origin not stated are included in "All origins" but not distributed among specified origins.
[2]Includes races other than White and Black.
[3]Race categories are consistent with the 1977 Office of Management and Budget (OMB) standards.
[4]Figures for age not stated are included in "All ages" but not distributed among age groups.
[5]Death rates for "Under 1 year" (based on population estimates) differ from infant mortality rates (based on live births).

Table B-5. Number of Deaths and Death Rates by Age, and Age-Adjusted Death Rates, by Specified Hispanic Origin, Race for Non-Hispanic Population, and Sex, 2008

(Number, rate per 100,000.)

Origin, race, and sex	All ages	Under 1 year[1]	1–4 years	5–14 years	15–24 years	25–34 years	35–44 years	45–54 years	55–64 years	65–74 years	75–84 years	85 years and over	Age not stated	Age-adjusted rate
NUMBER														
All Origins	2,471,984	28,059	4,730	5,651	32,198	42,275	76,370	186,542	296,182	401,579	653,560	744,691	147	X
Male	1,226,197	15,669	2,693	3,280	24,027	29,635	47,686	115,038	179,550	225,400	321,896	261,221	102	X
Female	1,245,787	12,390	2,037	2,371	8,171	12,640	28,684	71,504	116,632	176,179	331,664	483,470	45	X
Hispanic[2]	139,241	5,890	1,029	1,020	5,203	6,396	8,621	14,370	18,502	21,943	30,262	25,996	9	X
Male	76,861	3,279	587	548	4,079	4,839	5,924	9,469	11,461	12,421	14,851	9,394	9	X
Female	62,380	2,611	442	472	1,124	1,557	2,697	4,901	7,041	9,522	15,411	16,602	-	X
Mexican	78,495	4,104	724	719	3,549	4,112	5,270	8,451	10,643	12,067	16,237	12,614	5	X
Male	44,689	2,272	402	391	2,828	3,170	3,661	5,609	6,610	6,753	8,076	4,912	5	X
Female	33,806	1,832	322	328	721	942	1,609	2,842	4,033	5,314	8,161	7,702	-	X
Puerto Rican	17,554	544	88	83	405	662	1,081	1,966	2,886	3,197	3,652	2,988	2	X
Male	9,537	308	52	42	297	470	709	1,296	1,794	1,807	1,741	1019	2	X
Female	8,017	236	36	41	108	192	372	670	1092	1,390	1,911	1,969	-	X
Cuban	13,549	79	14	13	106	135	306	738	1,053	2,185	4,207	4,713	-	X
Male	6,955	46	11	8	82	92	215	506	739	1,387	2,213	1,656	-	X
Female	6,594	33	3	5	24	43	91	232	314	798	1,994	3,057	-	X
Central and South American	12,398	487	80	82	597	851	978	1,393	1,618	1,813	2,332	2,166	1	X
Male	6,512	270	45	39	475	651	692	884	924	925	991	615	1	X
Female	5,886	217	35	43	122	200	286	509	694	888	1,341	1,551	-	X
Other and unknown Hispanic	17,245	676	123	123	546	636	986	1,822	2,302	2,681	3,834	3,515	1	X
Male	9,168	383	77	68	397	456	647	1,174	1,394	1,549	1,830	1,192	1	X
Female	8,077	293	46	55	149	180	339	648	908	1132	2,004	2,323	-	X
Non-Hispanic[3]	2,327,636	21,937	3,685	4,619	26,915	35,773	67,553	171,544	276,814	378,781	622,290	717,622	103	X
Male	1,146,394	12,260	2,101	2,724	19,891	24,719	41,644	105,139	167,483	212,429	306,501	251,435	68	X
Female	1,181,242	9,677	1,584	1,895	7,024	11,054	25,909	66,405	109,331	166,352	315,789	466,187	35	X
White	1,981,034	12,519	2,373	3,070	18,560	24,852	49,091	130,423	220,255	316,682	549,086	654,044	79	X
Male	969,288	7,022	1,365	1,806	13,575	17,330	30,810	81,331	134,290	178,730	272,482	230,495	52	X
Female	1,011,746	5,497	1,008	1,264	4,985	7,522	18,281	49,092	85,965	137,952	276,604	423,549	27	X
Black	285,522	8,187	1,076	1,258	7,092	9,116	15,579	35,527	48,228	51,220	58,481	49,738	20	X
Male	145,168	4,546	619	750	5,423	6,248	9,070	20,404	28,344	27,653	26,761	15,336	14	X
Female	140,354	3,641	457	508	1,669	2,868	6,509	15,123	19,884	23,567	31,720	34,402	6	X
Origin Not Stated[4]	5,107	232	16	12	80	106	196	628	866	855	1008	1073	35	X
Male	2,942	130	5	8	57	77	118	430	606	550	544	392	25	X
Female	2,165	102	11	4	23	29	78	198	260	305	464	681	10	X
RATE														
All Origins	813.0	650.5	28.3	14.1	75.6	103.3	179.7	420.4	879.2	1,995.6	5,017.7	13,015.1	X	758.3
Male	817.9	709.7	31.5	16.0	109.8	141.8	223.7	526.4	1,104.9	2,432.8	6,032.2	14,017.3	X	900.6
Female	808.2	588.5	25.0	12.1	39.5	63.1	135.4	317.5	668.9	1,622.6	4,313.7	12,531.0	X	643.4
Hispanic	296.6	531.4	24.6	12.1	69.3	78.2	123.0	288.4	648.3	1,457.4	3,592.2	8,299.3	X	532.2
Male	316.9	578.5	27.5	12.7	103.9	107.2	158.9	372.5	831.3	1,826.9	4,264.0	8,379.0	X	630.7
Female	274.9	482.2	21.6	11.4	31.3	42.4	82.2	200.8	477.2	1,153.1	3,118.7	8,254.9	X	445.7
Mexican	253.4	512.2	23.7	12.0	70.2	74.8	116.3	280.8	650.1	1,411.1	3,902.8	9,146.0	X	553.5
Male	275.7	547.5	25.7	12.9	107.1	104.2	147.8	352.5	805.6	1,679.0	4,382.4	10,074.0	X	645.3
Female	228.9	474.1	21.5	11.1	29.8	38.4	78.3	200.3	493.9	1,173.3	3,521.4	8,638.5	X	470.9
Puerto Rican	425.0	605.0	28.2	11.2	56.9	105.8	185.8	410.6	956.2	2,010.9	4,682.4	6,047.8	X	639.3
Male	470.1	*	30.7	10.9	82.9	148.4	253.6	575.7	1,381.6	2,473.3	*	*	X	799.2
Female	381.5	*	25.3	11.6	30.5	62.2	123.0	264.1	635.0	1,617.6	3,887.5	*	X	517.2
Cuban	823.9	*	*	*	54.7	62.4	120.8	335.5	614.9	1,498.9	3,409.5	*	X	565.3
Male	833.9	*	*	*	85.6	78.0	158.2	449.2	820.3	1,983.2	*	*	X	641.6
Female	813.7	*	*	*	*	43.7	77.5	216.1	386.8	1,052.3	2,631.7	*	X	516.3
Central and South American	155.9	326.9	14.3	7.0	49.7	55.2	73.7	139.3	292.2	735.3	1,575.6	4,111.5	X	259.9
Male	160.1	344.6	16.5	6.4	72.8	73.8	101.8	180.8	376.6	1,040.6	1,764.4	*	X	319.0
Female	151.6	307.3	12.1	7.7	22.2	30.3	44.2	99.6	225.0	563.2	1,460.2	*	X	217.5
Other and unknown Hispanic	770.6	1,353.1	70.3	32.6	156.7	211.5	311.8	666.3	1,210.8	2,702.5	4,978.3	*	X	904.8
Male	823.4	*	81.3	33.1	222.3	295.0	413.5	947.4	1,502.1	*	*	*	X	1,164.5
Female	718.3	*	*	31.9	87.8	123.2	212.3	433.4	933.0	2,120.0	*	*	X	719.2

Table B-5. Number of Deaths and Death Rates by Age, and Age-Adjusted Death Rates, by Specified Hispanic Origin, Race for Non-Hispanic Population, and Sex, 2008—Continued

(Number, rate per 100,000.)

Origin, race, and sex	All ages	Under 1 year[1]	1–4 years	5–14 years	15–24 years	25–34 years	35–44 years	45–54 years	55–64 years	65–74 years	75–84 years	85 years and over	Age not stated	Age-adjusted rate
Non-Hispanic	905.3	684.5	29.4	14.6	76.8	109.2	190.3	435.5	897.8	2,034.6	5,108.0	13,268.3	X	775.8
Male	912.2	747.2	32.8	16.8	110.8	150.9	236.8	544.5	1,126.2	2,474.4	6,144.7	14,355.8	X	922.2
Female	898.7	618.8	25.9	12.3	41.0	67.6	144.7	330.7	685.0	1,658.2	4,389.3	12,747.5	X	658.5
White	982.0	542.8	26.1	13.1	70.7	101.6	180.0	410.3	855.0	1,994.4	5,143.0	13,556.7	X	766.2
Male	978.2	594.4	29.3	15.0	100.8	140.4	225.3	515.8	1,067.2	2,413.0	6,166.5	14,721.8	X	908.5
Female	985.5	488.6	22.7	11.1	39.0	62.0	134.4	306.5	652.3	1,628.5	4,420.2	12,996.9	X	650.8
Black	745.2	1,270.8	44.2	20.9	109.0	166.0	291.5	682.0	1,416.8	2,787.1	5,746.4	12,239.0	X	955.2
Male	794.3	1,380.7	50.0	24.5	164.7	234.1	361.1	848.5	1,869.1	3,610.9	7,234.0	12,742.6	X	1,176.6
Female	700.5	1,155.9	38.2	17.1	52.0	101.6	229.8	539.2	1,053.4	2,198.5	4,896.9	12,027.1	X	794.8

X = Category not applicable.
– = Quantity zero.
* = Figure does not meet standards of reliability or precision.
[1]Death rates for "Under 1 year" (based on population estimates) differ from infant mortality rates (based on live births).
[2]Persons of Hispanic origin may be of any race.
[3]Includes races other than White and Black.
[4]Includes deaths for which Hispanic origin was not reported on the death certificate.

Table B–6. Abridged Life Table for the Total Population, 2008

(Number.)

Age	Probability of dying between ages x to $x+n$	Number surviving to age x	Number dying between ages x to $x+n$	Person-years lived between ages x to $x+n$	Total number of person-years lived above age x	Expectancy of life at age x
	$_nq_x$	l_x	$_nd_x$	$_nL_x$	T_x	e_x
0–1	0.006593	100,000	659	99,425	7,812,637	78.1
1–5	0.001132	99,341	112	397,092	7,713,212	77.6
5–10	0.000623	99,228	62	495,972	7,316,120	73.7
10–15	0.000779	99,167	77	495,692	6,820,148	68.8
15–20	0.002875	99,089	285	494,821	6,324,456	63.8
20–25	0.004689	98,804	463	492,902	5,829,635	59
25–30	0.004861	98,341	478	490,514	5,336,734	54.3
30–35	0.005466	97,863	535	488,017	4,846,220	49.5
35–40	0.007077	97,328	689	485,012	4,358,203	44.8
40–45	0.010733	96,639	1,037	480,795	3,873,191	40.1
45–50	0.016773	95,602	1,604	474,262	3,392,396	35.5
50–55	0.025150	93,999	2,364	464,410	2,918,134	31
55–60	0.035784	91,635	3,279	450,415	2,453,723	26.8
60–65	0.052463	88,356	4,635	430,823	2,003,308	22.7
65–70	0.078443	83,720	6,567	403,086	1,572,485	18.8
70–75	0.118559	77,153	9,147	364,140	1,169,400	15.2
75–80	0.182982	68,006	12,444	310,338	805,259	11.8
80–85	0.283728	55,562	15,764	239,561	494,921	8.9
85–90	0.437742	39,797	17,421	155,398	255,360	6.4
90–95	0.628312	22,376	14,059	74,153	99,961	4.5
95–100	0.797864	8,317	6,636	22,079	25,808	3.1
100 and over	1.000000	1,681	1,681	3,729	3,729	2.2

PART B: MORTALITY 109

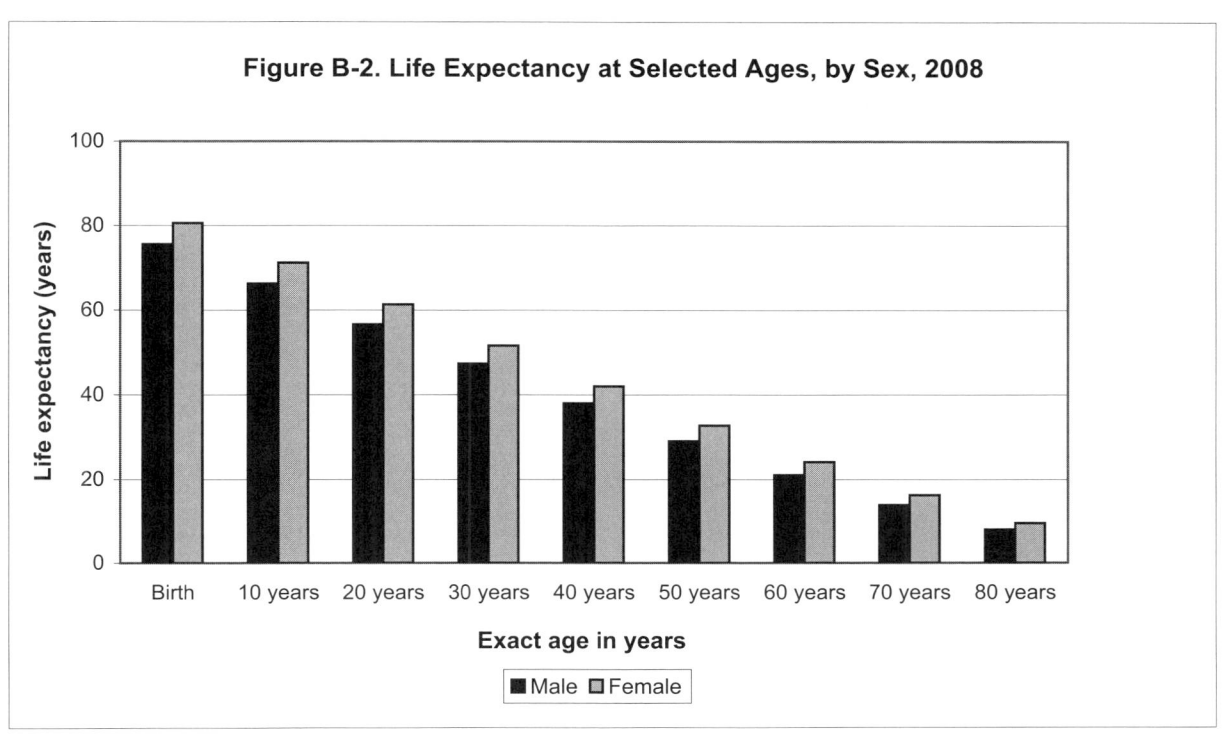

Figure B-2. Life Expectancy at Selected Ages, by Sex, 2008

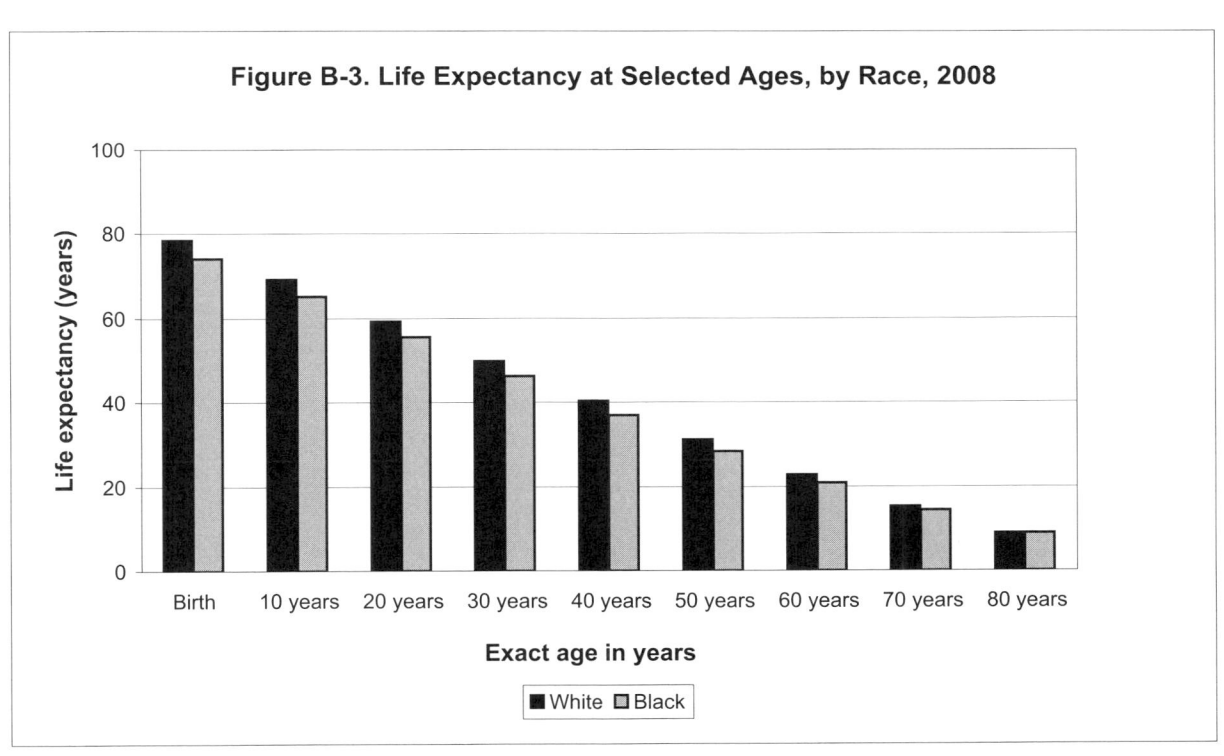

Figure B-3. Life Expectancy at Selected Ages, by Race, 2008

Table B-7. Life Expectancy at Birth by Race and Sex, Selected Years, 1940–2008

(Number.)

Year	All races[1]			White			Black		
	Both sexes	Male	Female	Both sexes	Male	Female	Both sexes	Male	Female
1940	62.9	60.8	65.2	64.2	62.1	66.6	—	—	—
1950	68.2	65.6	71.1	69.1	66.5	72.2	—	—	—
1960	69.7	66.6	73.1	70.6	67.4	74.1	—	—	—
1970	70.8	67.1	74.7	71.7	68.0	75.6	64.1	60.0	68.3
1975	72.6	68.8	76.6	73.4	69.5	77.3	66.8	62.4	71.3
1976	72.9	69.1	76.8	73.6	69.9	77.5	67.2	62.9	71.6
1977	73.3	69.5	77.2	74.0	70.2	77.9	67.7	63.4	72.0
1978	73.5	69.6	77.3	74.1	70.4	78.0	68.1	63.7	72.4
1979	73.9	70.0	77.8	74.6	70.8	78.4	68.5	64.0	72.9
1980	73.7	70.0	77.4	74.4	70.7	78.1	68.1	63.8	72.5
1981	74.1	70.4	77.8	74.8	71.1	78.4	68.9	64.5	73.2
1982	74.5	70.8	78.1	75.1	71.5	78.7	69.4	65.1	73.6
1983	74.6	71.0	78.1	75.2	71.6	78.7	69.4	65.2	73.5
1984	74.7	71.1	78.2	75.3	71.8	78.7	69.5	65.3	73.6
1985	74.7	71.1	78.2	75.3	71.8	78.7	69.3	65.0	73.4
1986	74.7	71.2	78.2	75.4	71.9	78.8	69.1	64.8	73.4
1987	74.9	71.4	78.3	75.6	72.1	78.9	69.1	64.7	73.4
1988	74.9	71.4	78.3	75.6	72.2	78.9	68.9	64.4	73.2
1989	75.1	71.7	78.5	75.9	72.5	79.2	68.8	64.3	73.3
1990	75.4	71.8	78.8	76.1	72.7	79.4	69.1	64.5	73.6
1991	75.5	72.0	78.9	76.3	72.9	79.6	69.3	64.6	73.8
1992	75.8	72.3	79.1	76.5	73.2	79.8	69.6	65.0	73.9
1993	75.5	72.2	78.8	76.3	73.1	79.5	69.2	64.6	73.7
1994	75.7	72.4	79.0	76.5	73.3	79.6	69.5	64.9	73.9
1995	75.8	72.5	78.9	76.5	73.4	79.6	69.6	65.2	73.9
1996	76.1	73.1	79.1	76.8	73.9	79.7	70.2	66.1	74.2
1997	76.5	73.6	79.4	77.1	74.3	79.9	71.1	67.2	74.7
1998	76.7	73.8	79.5	77.3	74.5	80.0	71.3	67.6	74.8
1999	76.7	73.9	79.4	77.3	74.6	79.9	71.4	67.8	74.7
2000	76.8	74.1	79.3	77.3	74.7	79.9	71.8	68.2	75.1
2001	76.9	74.2	79.4	77.4	74.8	79.9	72.0	68.4	75.2
2002	76.9	74.3	79.5	77.4	74.9	79.9	72.1	68.6	75.4
2003	77.1	74.5	79.6	77.6	75.0	80.0	72.3	68.8	75.6
2004	77.5	74.9	79.9	77.9	75.4	80.4	72.8	69.3	76.0
2005	77.4	74.9	79.9	77.9	75.4	80.4	72.8	69.3	76.1
2006	77.7	75.1	80.2	78.2	75.7	80.6	73.2	69.7	76.5
2007	77.9	75.4	80.4	78.4	75.9	80.8	73.6	70.0	76.8
2008	78.1	75.6	80.6	78.5	76.1	80.9	74.0	70.6	77.2

Table B-7. Life Expectancy at Birth by Race and Sex, Selected Years, 1940–2008—*Continued*

(Number.)

Year	Hispanic			Non-Hispanic White			Non-Hispanic Black		
	Both sexes	Male	Female	Both sexes	Male	Female	Both sexes	Male	Female
1940	—	—	—	—	—	—	—	—	—
1950	—	—	—	—	—	—	—	—	—
1960	—	—	—	—	—	—	—	—	—
1970	—	—	—	—	—	—	—	—	—
1975	—	—	—	—	—	—	—	—	—
1976	—	—	—	—	—	—	—	—	—
1977	—	—	—	—	—	—	—	—	—
1978	—	—	—	—	—	—	—	—	—
1979	—	—	—	—	—	—	—	—	—
1980	—	—	—	—	—	—	—	—	—
1981	—	—	—	—	—	—	—	—	—
1982	—	—	—	—	—	—	—	—	—
1983	—	—	—	—	—	—	—	—	—
1984	—	—	—	—	—	—	—	—	—
1985	—	—	—	—	—	—	—	—	—
1986	—	—	—	—	—	—	—	—	—
1987	—	—	—	—	—	—	—	—	—
1988	—	—	—	—	—	—	—	—	—
1989	—	—	—	—	—	—	—	—	—
1990	—	—	—	—	—	—	—	—	—
1991	—	—	—	—	—	—	—	—	—
1992	—	—	—	—	—	—	—	—	—
1993	—	—	—	—	—	—	—	—	—
1994	—	—	—	—	—	—	—	—	—
1995	—	—	—	—	—	—	—	—	—
1996	—	—	—	—	—	—	—	—	—
1997	—	—	—	—	—	—	—	—	—
1998	—	—	—	—	—	—	—	—	—
1999	—	—	—	—	—	—	—	—	—
2000	—	—	—	—	—	—	—	—	—
2001	—	—	—	—	—	—	—	—	—
2002	—	—	—	—	—	—	—	—	—
2003	—	—	—	—	—	—	—	—	—
2004	—	—	—	—	—	—	—	—	—
2005	—	—	—	—	—	—	—	—	—
2006	80.6	77.9	83.1	78.1	75.6	80.4	72.9	69.2	76.2
2007	80.9	78.2	83.4	78.2	75.8	80.6	73.2	69.6	76.5
2008	81.0	78.4	83.3	78.4	75.9	80.8	73.7	70.2	76.9

— = Data not available.
[1]Includes races other than White and Black.

Table B-8. Life Expectancy at Selected Ages by Race, Hispanic Origin, Race for Non-Hispanic Population, and Sex, 2008

(Number.)

Exact age in years	All races[1]			White			Black		
	Both sexes	Male	Female	Both sexes	Male	Female	Both sexes	Male	Female
0	78.1	75.6	80.6	78.5	76.1	80.9	74.0	70.6	77.2
1	77.6	75.1	80.1	77.9	75.5	80.3	74.0	70.6	77.1
5	73.7	71.2	76.1	74.0	71.6	76.4	70.1	66.7	73.2
10	68.8	66.3	71.2	69.1	66.6	71.4	65.2	61.8	68.2
15	63.8	61.3	66.2	64.1	61.7	66.5	60.2	56.8	63.3
20	59.0	56.6	61.3	59.3	56.9	61.6	55.5	52.2	58.4
25	54.3	52.0	56.5	54.5	52.3	56.7	50.8	47.7	53.6
30	49.5	47.3	51.6	49.8	47.6	51.8	46.2	43.1	48.8
35	44.8	42.6	46.8	45.0	42.9	47.0	41.6	38.6	44.1
40	40.1	38.0	42.0	40.3	38.3	42.2	37.0	34.2	39.4
45	35.5	33.5	37.3	35.7	33.7	37.5	32.6	29.8	34.9
50	31.0	29.1	32.8	31.2	29.3	32.9	28.4	25.7	30.6
55	26.8	25.0	28.4	26.9	25.2	28.5	24.5	21.9	26.5
60	22.7	21.0	24.1	22.8	21.2	24.1	20.8	18.5	22.6
65	18.8	17.3	20.0	18.8	17.4	20.0	17.4	15.4	18.9
70	15.2	13.9	16.2	15.2	13.9	16.2	14.3	12.6	15.4
75	11.8	10.7	12.6	11.8	10.7	12.6	11.3	9.9	12.3
80	8.9	8.0	9.5	8.9	8.0	9.4	8.8	7.6	9.4
85	6.4	5.7	6.8	6.4	5.7	6.7	6.7	5.8	7.0
90	4.5	4.0	4.7	4.4	3.9	4.6	5.0	4.4	5.2
95	3.1	2.8	3.2	3.0	2.8	3.1	3.7	3.3	3.8
100	2.2	2.0	2.2	2.2	2.0	2.2	2.8	2.5	2.8

Exact age in years	Hispanic[2]			Non-Hispanic White			Non-Hispanic Black		
	Both sexes	Male	Female	Both sexes	Male	Female	Both sexes	Male	Female
0	81.0	78.4	83.3	78.4	75.9	80.8	73.7	70.2	76.9
1	80.4	77.9	82.8	77.8	75.4	80.2	73.6	70.2	76.8
5	76.5	74.0	78.8	73.9	71.5	76.2	69.8	66.3	72.9
10	71.5	69.0	73.9	68.9	66.5	71.3	64.8	61.4	68.0
15	66.6	64.0	68.9	64.0	61.6	66.3	59.9	56.5	63.0
20	61.8	59.3	64.0	59.1	56.8	61.4	55.1	51.8	58.2
25	57.0	54.6	59.1	54.4	52.1	56.5	50.5	47.3	53.3
30	52.2	49.9	54.2	49.6	47.5	51.7	45.9	42.8	48.6
35	47.4	45.2	49.3	44.9	42.8	46.9	41.3	38.3	43.8
40	42.7	40.5	44.5	40.2	38.2	42.1	36.7	33.9	39.2
45	38.0	35.9	39.7	35.6	33.6	37.4	32.3	29.5	34.7
50	33.4	31.4	35.1	31.1	29.3	32.9	28.2	25.4	30.4
55	29.0	27.1	30.5	26.8	25.1	28.4	24.3	21.7	26.3
60	24.8	23.0	26.1	22.7	21.1	24.1	20.7	18.4	22.4
65	20.7	19.1	21.8	18.8	17.3	20.0	17.3	15.3	18.8
70	16.9	15.5	17.8	15.1	13.9	16.1	14.2	12.5	15.4
75	13.4	12.2	14.0	11.8	10.7	12.6	11.3	9.8	12.2
80	10.2	9.2	10.6	8.9	8.0	9.4	8.8	7.6	9.4
85	7.4	6.6	7.7	6.4	5.7	6.7	6.6	5.8	7.0
90	5.2	4.7	5.3	4.4	3.9	4.6	4.9	4.3	5.2
95	3.7	3.3	3.7	3.0	2.8	3.1	3.7	3.3	3.8
100	2.6	2.4	2.6	2.2	2.0	2.2	2.8	2.5	2.8

[1]Includes races other than White and Black.
[2]Persons of Hispanic origin may be of any race.

Table B-9. Life Expectancy at Birth, at 65 Years of Age, and at 75 Years of Age, by Race and Sex, Selected Years, 1900–2009

(Number.)

Specified age and year	All races			White			Black or African American[1]		
	Both sexes	Male	Female	Both sexes	Male	Female	Both sexes	Male	Female
	Remaining life expectancy in years								
At Birth									
1900[2,3]	47.3	46.3	48.3	47.6	46.6	48.7	33.0	32.5	33.5
1950[3]	68.2	65.6	71.1	69.1	66.5	72.2	60.8	59.1	62.9
1960[3]	69.7	66.6	73.1	70.6	67.4	74.1	63.6	61.1	66.3
1970	70.8	67.1	74.7	71.7	68.0	75.6	64.1	60.0	68.3
1975	72.6	68.8	76.6	73.4	69.5	77.3	66.8	62.4	71.3
1980	73.7	70.0	77.4	74.4	70.7	78.1	68.1	63.8	72.5
1981	74.1	70.4	77.8	74.8	71.1	78.4	68.9	64.5	73.2
1982	74.5	70.8	78.1	75.1	71.5	78.7	69.4	65.1	73.6
1983	74.6	71.0	78.1	75.2	71.6	78.7	69.4	65.2	73.5
1984	74.7	71.1	78.2	75.3	71.8	78.7	69.5	65.3	73.6
1985	74.7	71.1	78.2	75.3	71.8	78.7	69.3	65.0	73.4
1986	74.7	71.2	78.2	75.4	71.9	78.8	69.1	64.8	73.4
1987	74.9	71.4	78.3	75.6	72.1	78.9	69.1	64.7	73.4
1988	74.9	71.4	78.3	75.6	72.2	78.9	68.9	64.4	73.2
1989	75.1	71.7	78.5	75.9	72.5	79.2	68.8	64.3	73.3
1990	75.4	71.8	78.8	76.1	72.7	79.4	69.1	64.5	73.6
1991	75.5	72.0	78.9	76.3	72.9	79.6	69.3	64.6	73.8
1992	75.8	72.3	79.1	76.5	73.2	79.8	69.6	65.0	73.9
1993	75.5	72.2	78.8	76.3	73.1	79.5	69.2	64.6	73.7
1994	75.7	72.4	79.0	76.5	73.3	79.6	69.5	64.9	73.9
1995	75.8	72.5	78.9	76.5	73.4	79.6	69.6	65.2	73.9
1996	76.1	73.1	79.1	76.8	73.9	79.7	70.2	66.1	74.2
1997	76.5	73.6	79.4	77.1	74.3	79.9	71.1	67.2	74.7
1998	76.7	73.8	79.5	77.3	74.5	80.0	71.3	67.6	74.8
1999	76.7	73.9	79.4	77.3	74.6	79.9	71.4	67.8	74.7
2000	76.8	74.1	79.3	77.3	74.7	79.9	71.8	68.2	75.1
2001	76.9	74.2	79.4	77.4	74.8	79.9	72.0	68.4	75.2
2002	76.9	74.3	79.5	77.4	74.9	79.9	72.1	68.6	75.4
2003	77.1	74.5	79.6	77.6	75.0	80.0	72.3	68.8	75.6
2004	77.5	74.9	79.9	77.9	75.4	80.4	72.8	69.3	76.0
2005	77.4	74.9	79.9	77.9	75.4	80.4	72.8	69.3	76.1
2006	77.7	75.1	80.2	78.2	75.7	80.6	73.2	69.7	76.5
2007	77.9	75.4	80.4	78.4	75.9	80.8	73.6	70.0	76.8
2008	78.1	75.6	80.6	78.5	76.1	80.9	74.0	70.6	77.2
2009	78.5	76.0	80.9	78.8	76.4	81.2	74.5	71.1	77.6
At 65 Years									
1950[3]	13.9	12.8	15.0	14.1	12.8	15.1	13.9	12.9	14.9
1960[3]	14.3	12.8	15.8	14.4	12.9	15.9	13.9	12.7	15.1
1970	15.2	13.1	17.0	15.2	13.1	17.1	14.2	12.5	15.7
1975	16.1	13.8	18.1	16.1	13.8	18.2	15.0	13.1	16.7
1980	16.4	14.1	18.3	16.5	14.2	18.4	15.1	13.0	16.8
1981	16.6	14.3	18.6	16.7	14.4	18.7	15.5	13.4	17.2
1982	16.8	14.5	18.7	16.9	14.5	18.8	15.7	13.5	17.5
1983	16.7	14.4	18.6	16.8	14.5	18.7	15.4	13.2	17.2
1984	16.8	14.5	18.6	16.8	14.6	18.7	15.4	13.2	17.2
1985	16.7	14.5	18.5	16.8	14.5	18.7	15.2	13.0	16.9
1986	16.8	14.6	18.6	16.9	14.7	18.7	15.2	13.0	17.0
1987	16.9	14.7	18.7	17.0	14.8	18.8	15.2	13.0	17.0
1988	16.9	14.7	18.6	17.0	14.8	18.7	15.1	12.9	16.9
1989	17.1	15.0	18.8	17.2	15.1	18.9	15.2	13.0	16.9
1990	17.2	15.1	18.9	17.3	15.2	19.1	15.4	13.2	17.2
1991	17.4	15.3	19.1	17.5	15.4	19.2	15.5	13.4	17.2
1992	17.5	15.4	19.2	17.6	15.5	19.3	15.7	13.5	17.4
1993	17.3	15.3	18.9	17.4	15.4	19.0	15.5	13.4	17.1
1994	17.4	15.5	19.0	17.5	15.6	19.1	15.7	13.6	17.2
1995	17.4	15.6	18.9	17.6	15.7	19.1	15.6	13.6	17.1
1996	17.5	15.7	19.0	17.6	15.8	19.1	15.8	13.9	17.2
1997	17.7	15.9	19.2	17.8	16.0	19.3	16.1	14.2	17.6
1998	17.8	16.0	19.2	17.8	16.1	19.3	16.1	14.3	17.4
1999	17.7	16.1	19.1	17.8	16.1	19.2	16.0	14.3	17.3
2000	17.6	16.0	19.0	17.7	16.1	19.1	16.1	14.1	17.5
2001	17.7	16.2	19.0	17.8	16.3	19.1	16.2	14.2	17.6
2002	17.8	16.2	19.1	17.9	16.3	19.2	16.3	14.4	17.7
2003	17.9	16.4	19.2	18.0	16.5	19.3	16.4	14.5	17.9
2004	18.2	16.7	19.5	18.3	16.8	19.5	16.7	14.8	18.2

Table B-9. Life Expectancy at Birth, at 65 Years of Age, and at 75 Years of Age, by Race and Sex, Selected Years, 1900–2009—Continued

(Number.)

Specified age and year	All races			White			Black or African American[1]		
	Both sexes	Male	Female	Both sexes	Male	Female	Both sexes	Male	Female
2005	18.2	16.8	19.5	18.3	16.9	19.5	16.8	14.9	18.2
2006	18.5	17.0	19.7	18.6	17.1	19.8	17.1	15.1	18.6
2007	18.6	17.2	19.9	18.7	17.3	19.9	17.2	15.2	18.7
2008	18.8	17.3	20.0	18.8	17.4	20.0	17.4	15.4	18.9
2009	19.2	17.6	20.3	19.1	17.7	20.4	17.8	15.8	19.3
At 75 Years									
1980	10.4	8.8	11.5	10.4	8.8	11.5	9.7	8.3	10.7
1981	10.6	9.0	11.7	10.6	9.0	11.7	10.4	9.0	11.4
1982	10.7	9.1	11.9	10.7	9.0	11.9	10.6	9.1	11.6
1983	10.6	9.0	11.7	10.6	8.9	11.7	10.3	8.9	11.4
1984	10.7	9.0	11.8	10.7	9.0	11.8	10.3	8.9	11.4
1985	10.6	9.0	11.7	10.6	9.0	11.7	10.1	8.7	11.1
1986	10.7	9.1	11.7	10.7	9.1	11.8	10.1	8.6	11.1
1987	10.7	9.1	11.8	10.7	9.1	11.8	10.1	8.6	11.1
1988	10.6	9.1	11.7	10.7	9.1	11.7	10.0	8.5	11.0
1989	10.9	9.3	11.9	10.9	9.3	11.9	10.1	8.6	11.0
1990	10.9	9.4	12.0	11.0	9.4	12.0	10.2	8.6	11.2
1991	11.1	9.5	12.1	11.1	9.5	12.1	10.2	8.7	11.2
1992	11.2	9.6	12.2	11.2	9.6	12.2	10.4	8.9	11.4
1993	10.9	9.5	11.9	11.0	9.5	12.0	10.2	8.7	11.1
1994	11.0	9.6	12.0	11.1	9.6	12.0	10.3	8.9	11.2
1995	11.0	9.7	11.9	11.1	9.7	12.0	10.2	8.8	11.1
1996	11.1	9.8	12.0	11.1	9.8	12.0	10.3	9.0	11.2
1997	11.2	9.9	12.1	11.2	9.9	12.1	10.7	9.3	11.5
1998	11.3	10.0	12.2	11.3	10.0	12.2	10.5	9.2	11.3
1999	11.2	10.0	12.1	11.2	10.0	12.1	10.4	9.2	11.1
2000	11.0	9.8	11.8	11.0	9.8	11.9	10.4	9.0	11.3
2001	11.1	9.9	11.9	11.1	9.9	11.9	10.5	9.1	11.4
2002	11.0	9.9	11.9	11.1	9.9	11.9	10.5	9.2	11.4
2003	11.1	10.0	11.9	11.1	10.0	11.9	10.6	9.3	11.5
2004	11.4	10.3	12.2	11.4	10.3	12.2	10.8	9.5	11.7
2005	11.3	10.2	12.1	11.4	10.3	12.1	10.8	9.5	11.7
2006	11.6	10.5	12.3	11.5	10.5	12.3	11.1	9.8	12.0
2007	11.7	10.6	12.5	11.7	10.6	12.4	11.2	9.9	12.1
2008	11.8	10.7	12.6	11.8	10.7	12.6	11.3	9.9	12.3
2009	12.2	11.0	12.9	12.1	11.0	12.9	11.7	10.3	12.6

— =Data not available.
[1]Data shown for 1900–1960 are for the nonwhite population.
[2]Death registration area only. The death registration area increased from 10 states and the District of Columbia (D.C.) in 1900 to the coterminous United States in 1933.
[3]Includes deaths of persons who were not residents of the 50 states and D.C.

PART B: MORTALITY

Table B-10. Death Rates by Age and Age-Adjusted Death Rates for the 15 Leading Causes of Death, 1999–2008

(Rate per 100,000 population in specified group; age-adjusted rates per 100,000 U.S. standard population.)

Cause of death (based on ICD–10, 2004) and year	Age											Age-adjusted rate
	All ages[1]	Under 1 year[2]	1–4 years	5–14 years	15–24 years	25–34 years	35–44 years	45–54 years	55–64 years	65–74 years	75–84 years	85 years and over	
All Causes													
1999	857.0	736.0	34.2	18.6	79.3	102.2	198.0	418.2	1005.0	2457.3	5714.5	15554.6	875.6
2000	854.0	736.7	32.4	18.0	79.9	101.4	198.9	425.6	992.2	2399.1	5666.5	15524.4	869.0
2001	848.5	683.4	33.3	17.3	80.7	105.2	203.6	428.9	964.6	2353.3	5582.4	15112.8	854.5
2002	847.3	695.0	31.2	17.4	81.4	103.6	202.9	430.1	952.4	2314.7	5556.9	14828.3	845.3
2003	841.9	700.0	31.5	17.0	81.5	103.6	201.6	433.2	940.9	2255.0	5463.1	14593.3	832.7
2004	816.5	685.2	29.9	16.8	80.1	102.1	193.5	427.0	910.3	2164.6	5275.1	13823.5	800.8
2005	825.9	692.5	29.4	16.3	81.4	104.4	193.3	432.0	906.9	2137.1	5260.0	13798.6	798.8
2006	810.4	690.7	28.4	15.2	82.2	106.3	190.2	427.5	890.9	2062.1	5115.0	13253.1	776.5
2007	803.6	684.5	28.6	15.3	79.9	104.9	184.4	420.9	877.7	2011.3	5011.6	12946.5	760.2
2008	813.0	650.5	28.3	14.1	75.6	103.3	179.7	420.4	879.2	1995.6	5017.7	13015.1	758.3
Diseases of Heart (I00–I09, I11, I13, I20–I51)													
1999	259.9	13.8	1.2	0.7	2.8	7.6	30.2	95.7	269.9	701.7	1849.9	6063.0	266.5
2000	252.6	13.0	1.2	0.7	2.6	7.4	29.2	94.2	261.2	665.6	1780.3	5926.1	257.6
2001	245.8	11.9	1.5	0.7	2.5	8.0	29.6	92.9	246.9	635.1	1725.7	5664.2	247.8
2002	241.7	12.4	1.1	0.6	2.5	7.9	30.5	93.7	241.5	615.9	1677.2	5466.8	240.8
2003	235.6	11.0	1.2	0.6	2.7	8.2	30.7	92.5	233.2	585.0	1611.1	5278.4	232.3
2004	222.2	10.3	1.2	0.6	2.5	7.9	29.3	90.2	218.8	541.6	1506.3	4895.9	217.0
2005	220.0	8.7	0.9	0.6	2.7	8.1	28.9	89.7	214.8	518.9	1460.8	4778.4	211.1
2006	211.0	8.4	1.0	0.6	2.5	8.2	28.3	88.0	207.3	490.3	1383.1	4480.8	200.2
2007	204.3	10.0	1.1	0.6	2.6	7.9	27.4	85.3	200.3	462.9	1315.0	4267.7	190.9
2008	202.9	9.2	1.1	0.6	2.5	7.9	26.7	85.4	198.0	449.8	1276.7	4175.7	186.5
Malignant Neoplasms (C00-C97)													
1999	197.0	1.8	2.7	2.5	4.5	10.0	37.1	127.6	374.6	827.1	1331.5	1805.8	200.8
2000	196.5	2.4	2.7	2.5	4.4	9.8	36.6	127.5	366.7	816.3	1335.6	1819.4	199.6
2001	194.4	1.6	2.7	2.5	4.3	10.1	36.8	126.5	356.5	802.8	1315.8	1765.6	196.0
2002	193.2	1.8	2.6	2.6	4.3	9.7	35.8	123.8	351.1	792.1	1311.9	1723.9	193.5
2003	191.5	1.9	2.5	2.6	4.0	9.4	35.0	122.2	343.0	770.3	1302.5	1698.2	190.1
2004	188.6	1.8	2.5	2.5	4.1	9.1	33.4	119.0	333.4	755.1	1280.4	1653.3	185.8
2005	188.7	1.8	2.3	2.5	4.1	9.0	33.2	118.6	326.9	742.7	1274.8	1637.7	183.8
2006	187.0	1.8	2.3	2.2	3.9	9.0	31.9	116.3	321.2	727.2	1263.8	1606.1	180.7
2007	186.6	1.7	2.2	2.4	3.9	8.5	30.8	114.3	315.4	715.5	1256.3	1590.2	178.4
2008	186.0	1.6	2.4	2.2	3.9	8.6	29.9	113.6	309.0	701.5	1235.8	1566.1	175.3
Chronic Lower Respiratory Disease (J40-J47)													
1999	44.5	0.9	0.4	0.3	0.5	0.8	2.0	8.5	47.5	177.2	397.8	646.0	45.4
2000	43.4	0.9	0.3	0.3	0.5	0.7	2.1	8.6	44.2	169.4	386.1	648.6	44.2
2001	43.2	1.0	0.3	0.3	0.4	0.7	2.2	8.5	44.1	167.9	379.8	644.7	43.7
2002	43.3	1.0	0.4	0.3	0.5	0.8	2.2	8.7	42.4	163.0	386.7	637.6	43.5
2003	43.5	0.8	0.3	0.3	0.5	0.7	2.1	8.7	43.3	163.2	383.0	635.1	43.3
2004	41.5	0.9	0.3	0.3	0.4	0.6	2.0	8.4	40.4	153.8	366.7	601.7	41.1
2005	44.2	0.8	0.3	0.3	0.4	0.6	2.0	9.4	42.0	160.5	385.6	637.2	43.2
2006	41.6	0.7	0.3	0.3	0.4	0.6	1.9	9.1	39.2	149.3	363.4	589.1	40.5
2007	42.4	1.0	0.3	0.3	0.4	0.6	1.8	9.5	39.1	148.1	368.9	596.1	40.8
2008	46.4	0.7	0.3	0.3	0.4	0.6	1.9	9.9	41.7	158.9	396.9	656.2	44.0
Cerebrovascular Diseases (I60–I69)													
1999	60.0	2.7	0.3	0.2	0.5	1.4	5.7	15.2	40.6	130.8	469.8	1614.8	61.6
2000	59.6	3.3	0.3	0.2	0.5	1.5	5.8	16.0	41.0	128.6	461.3	1589.2	60.9
2001	57.4	2.7	0.4	0.2	0.5	1.5	5.5	15.1	38.0	123.4	443.9	1500.2	57.9
2002	56.4	2.9	0.3	0.2	0.4	1.4	5.4	15.1	37.2	120.3	431.0	1445.9	56.2
2003	54.2	2.5	0.3	0.2	0.5	1.5	5.5	15.0	35.6	112.9	410.7	1370.1	53.5
2004	51.1	3.1	0.3	0.2	0.5	1.4	5.4	14.9	34.3	107.8	386.2	1245.9	50.0
2005	48.4	3.1	0.4	0.2	0.5	1.4	5.2	15.0	33.0	101.1	359.0	1141.8	46.6
2006	45.8	3.4	0.3	0.2	0.5	1.3	5.1	14.7	33.3	96.3	335.1	1039.6	43.6
2007	45.1	3.1	0.3	0.2	0.5	1.2	4.9	14.6	32.1	93.0	322.3	1015.5	42.2
2008	44.1	3.3	0.4	0.2	0.4	1.3	4.8	13.8	31.0	88.9	314.5	972.6	40.7

Table B-10. Death Rates by Age and Age-Adjusted Death Rates for the 15 Leading Causes of Death, 1999–2008—Continued

(Rate per 100,000 population in specified group; age-adjusted rates per 100,000 U.S. standard population.)

Cause of death (based on ICD-10, 2004) and year	All ages[1]	Age											Age-adjusted rate
		Under 1 year[2]	1–4 years	5–14 years	15–24 years	25–34 years	35–44 years	45–54 years	55–64 years	65–74 years	75–84 years	85 years and over	
Accidents (Unintentional Injuries) (V01–X59, Y85–Y86)													
1999	35.1	22.3	12.4	7.6	35.3	29.6	33.8	31.8	30.6	44.6	100.5	282.4	35.3
2000	34.8	23.1	11.9	7.3	36.0	29.5	34.1	32.6	30.9	41.9	95.1	273.5	34.9
2001	35.7	24.2	11.2	6.9	36.1	29.9	35.4	34.1	30.3	42.8	100.9	276.4	35.7
2002	37.0	23.5	10.5	6.6	38.0	31.5	37.2	36.6	31.4	44.2	101.3	275.4	36.9
2003	37.6	23.6	10.9	6.4	37.1	31.5	37.8	38.8	32.9	44.1	101.9	278.9	37.3
2004	38.1	25.8	10.3	6.5	37.0	32.6	37.3	40.7	33.2	44.0	103.7	276.7	37.7
2005	39.7	26.4	10.3	6.0	37.4	34.9	38.6	43.2	35.8	46.3	106.1	279.5	39.1
2006	40.6	27.8	9.9	5.6	38.2	37.0	40.2	45.5	36.2	44.5	105.1	274.9	39.8
2007	41.0	30.2	9.6	5.5	37.4	36.9	39.2	46.3	37.3	45.2	105.5	286.7	40.0
2008	40.1	30.5	8.8	4.6	33.1	35.6	37.8	45.9	37.9	44.7	106.2	289.0	38.8
Alzheimer's Disease (G30)													
1999	16.0	*	*	*	*	*	*	0.2	1.9	17.4	129.5	601.3	16.5
2000	17.6	*	*	*	*	*	*	0.2	2.0	18.7	139.6	667.7	18.1
2001	18.9	*	*	*	*	*	*	0.2	2.1	18.7	147.5	710.3	19.1
2002	20.4	*	*	*	*	*	*	0.1	1.9	19.7	158.1	752.3	20.2
2003	21.8	*	*	*	*	*	*	0.2	2.0	20.9	164.4	802.4	21.4
2004	22.5	*	*	*	*	*	*	0.2	1.9	19.7	168.7	818.8	21.8
2005	24.2	*	*	*	*	*	*	0.2	2.1	20.5	177.3	861.6	22.9
2006	24.2	*	*	*	*	*	*	0.2	2.1	20.2	175.6	848.3	22.6
2007	24.7	*	*	*	*	*	*	0.2	2.2	20.6	176.7	849.1	22.7
2008	27.1	*	*	*	*	*	*	0.2	2.2	21.5	193.3	910.1	24.4
Diabetes Mellitus (E10–E14)													
1999	24.5	*	*	0.1	0.4	1.4	4.3	12.9	38.3	91.8	178.0	317.2	25.0
2000	24.6	*	*	0.1	0.4	1.6	4.3	13.1	37.8	90.7	179.5	319.7	25.0
2001	25.1	*	*	0.1	0.4	1.5	4.3	13.6	37.8	91.4	181.4	321.8	25.3
2002	25.4	*	*	0.1	0.4	1.6	4.8	13.7	37.7	91.4	182.8	320.6	25.4
2003	25.5	*	*	0.1	0.4	1.6	4.6	13.9	38.5	90.8	181.1	317.5	25.3
2004	24.9	*	*	0.1	0.4	1.5	4.6	13.4	37.1	87.2	176.9	307.0	24.5
2005	25.3	*	*	0.1	0.5	1.5	4.7	13.4	37.2	86.8	177.2	312.1	24.6
2006	24.2	*	*	0.1	0.4	1.7	4.8	13.2	36.2	81.8	166.8	285.2	23.3
2007	23.7	*	*	0.1	0.4	1.5	4.6	13.1	34.6	78.1	162.7	276.2	22.5
2008	23.2	*	*	0.1	0.5	1.4	4.4	12.7	33.8	76.1	153.8	271.4	21.8
Influenza and Pneumonia (J09–J18)													
1999	22.8	8.4	0.8	0.2	0.5	0.8	2.4	4.6	11.0	37.2	157.0	751.8	23.5
2000	23.2	7.6	0.7	0.2	0.5	0.9	2.4	4.7	11.9	39.1	160.3	744.1	23.7
2001	21.8	7.4	0.7	0.2	0.5	0.9	2.2	4.6	10.7	36.3	148.5	685.6	22.0
2002	22.8	6.5	0.7	0.2	0.4	0.9	2.2	4.8	11.2	37.5	156.9	696.6	22.6
2003	22.4	8.0	1.0	0.4	0.5	0.9	2.2	5.2	11.2	37.3	151.1	661.7	22.0
2004	20.3	6.7	0.7	0.2	0.4	0.8	2.0	4.6	10.8	34.6	139.3	582.6	19.8
2005	21.3	6.5	0.7	0.3	0.4	0.9	2.1	5.1	11.3	35.5	142.2	593.9	20.3
2006	18.8	6.4	0.8	0.2	0.4	0.8	1.9	4.6	10.0	32.0	127.8	502.5	17.8
2007	17.5	5.2	0.7	0.3	0.4	0.8	1.8	4.4	9.6	28.7	114.1	463.2	16.2
2008	18.5	5.2	0.9	0.2	0.5	0.9	2.1	5.1	11.1	31.1	119.1	465.2	16.9
Nephritis, Nephrotic Syndrome and Nephrosis (N00–N07, N17–N19, N25–N27)													
1999	12.7	4.4	*	0.1	0.2	0.6	1.6	4.0	12.0	37.1	97.6	268.9	13.0
2000	13.2	4.3	*	0.1	0.2	0.6	1.6	4.4	12.8	38.0	100.8	277.8	13.5
2001	13.9	3.3	*	0.0	0.2	0.6	1.7	4.6	13.0	40.2	104.2	287.7	14.0
2002	14.2	4.3	*	0.1	0.2	0.7	1.7	4.7	13.0	39.2	109.1	288.6	14.2
2003	14.6	4.5	*	0.1	0.2	0.7	1.8	4.9	13.6	40.1	109.5	293.1	14.4
2004	14.5	4.3	*	0.1	0.2	0.6	1.8	5.0	13.6	38.6	108.4	286.6	14.2
2005	14.8	3.9	*	0.1	0.2	0.7	1.7	4.8	13.6	39.3	110.3	288.3	14.3
2006	15.1	3.9	*	*	0.2	0.7	1.8	5.2	13.8	39.4	111.4	290.5	14.5
2007	15.4	3.4	0.1	0.1	0.2	0.6	1.7	5.1	13.6	40.1	113.0	290.6	14.5
2008	15.9	3.3	*	*	0.2	0.6	1.8	5.0	14.3	40.7	113.8	295.7	14.8

Table B-10. Death Rates by Age and Age-Adjusted Death Rates for the 15 Leading Causes of Death, 1999–2008—Continued

(Rate per 100,000 population in specified group; age-adjusted rates per 100,000 U.S. standard population.)

Cause of death (based on ICD–10, 2004) and year	Age											Age-adjusted rate
	All ages[1]	Under 1 year[2]	1–4 years	5–14 years	15–24 years	25–34 years	35–44 years	45–54 years	55–64 years	65–74 years	75–84 years	85 years and over	
Intentional Self–Harm (Suicide) (*U03, X60–X84, Y87.0)													
1999	10.5	*	*	0.6	10.1	12.7	14.3	13.9	12.2	13.4	18.1	19.3	10.5
2000	10.4	*	*	0.7	10.2	12.0	14.5	14.4	12.1	12.5	17.6	19.6	10.4
2001[4]	10.8	*	*	0.7	9.9	12.8	14.7	15.2	13.1	13.3	17.4	17.5	10.7
2002	11.0	*	*	0.6	9.9	12.6	15.3	15.7	13.6	13.5	17.7	18.0	10.9
2003	10.8	*	*	0.6	9.7	12.7	14.9	15.9	13.8	12.7	16.4	16.9	10.8
2004	11.0	*	*	0.7	10.3	12.7	15.0	16.6	13.8	12.3	16.3	16.4	10.9
2005	11.0	*	*	0.7	10.0	12.4	14.9	16.5	13.9	12.6	16.9	16.9	10.9
2006	11.1	*	*	0.5	9.9	12.3	15.1	17.2	14.5	12.6	15.9	15.9	10.9
2007	11.5	*	*	0.5	9.7	13.0	15.6	17.7	15.5	12.6	16.3	15.6	11.3
2008	11.9	*	*	0.6	10.1	12.9	15.8	18.7	16.2	13.9	16.2	14.9	11.6
Septicemia (A40–A41)													
1999	11.0	7.5	0.6	0.2	0.3	0.7	1.8	4.6	11.4	31.2	79.4	220.7	11.3
2000	11.1	7.2	0.6	0.2	0.3	0.7	1.9	4.9	11.9	31.0	80.4	215.7	11.3
2001	11.3	7.7	0.7	0.2	0.3	0.7	1.8	5.0	12.3	32.8	82.3	205.9	11.4
2002	11.7	7.3	0.5	0.2	0.3	0.8	1.9	5.2	12.6	34.7	86.5	203.0	11.7
2003	11.7	6.9	0.5	0.2	0.4	0.8	2.1	5.3	13.1	32.6	85.0	202.5	11.6
2004	11.4	6.6	0.5	0.2	0.3	0.8	1.9	5.4	12.9	32.4	81.6	186.7	11.2
2005	11.5	7.4	0.5	0.2	0.4	0.8	1.9	5.2	12.9	32.6	81.4	187.3	11.2
2006	11.4	6.5	0.5	0.2	0.3	0.7	2.0	5.2	12.8	32.1	82.4	177.3	11.0
2007	11.5	6.6	0.5	0.2	0.4	0.7	2.1	5.5	12.9	32.8	79.9	174.4	11.0
2008	11.8	6.7	0.6	0.2	0.3	0.9	2.1	5.7	13.5	32.0	82.3	172.4	11.1
Chronic Liver Disease and Cirrhosis (K70, K73–K74)													
1999	9.4	*	*	*	0.1	1.0	7.3	17.4	23.7	30.6	31.9	23.2	9.6
2000	9.4	*	*	*	0.1	1.0	7.5	17.7	23.8	29.8	31.0	23.1	9.5
2001	9.5	*	*	*	0.1	1.0	7.4	18.5	22.7	30.0	30.2	22.2	9.5
2002	9.5	*	*	*	0.1	0.9	7.0	18.0	22.9	29.4	31.4	21.4	9.4
2003	9.5	*	*	*	*	0.9	6.8	18.3	23.0	29.5	30.0	20.1	9.3
2004	9.2	*	*	*	*	0.8	6.3	18.0	22.6	27.7	28.8	19.7	9.0
2005	9.3	*	*	*	0.1	0.8	6.1	17.7	23.5	27.2	29.0	19.7	9.0
2006	9.2	*	*	*	0.1	0.8	5.8	17.8	22.8	26.0	29.0	19.4	8.8
2007	9.7	*	*	*	0.1	0.9	6.0	18.7	24.5	26.7	28.4	19.8	9.1
2008	9.9	*	*	*	0.1	1.0	6.0	18.5	25.3	26.8	28.1	19.9	9.2
Essential Hypertension and Hypertensive Renal Disease (I10, I12, I15)													
1999	6.1	*	*	*	*	0.2	0.7	2.2	5.5	15.2	43.6	152.1	6.2
2000	6.4	*	*	*	*	0.2	0.8	2.3	5.9	15.1	45.5	162.9	6.5
2001	6.8	*	*	*	0.1	0.3	0.7	2.4	5.8	15.5	47.7	171.9	6.8
2002	7.0	*	*	*	0.1	0.2	0.8	2.3	5.7	16.0	48.2	180.4	7.0
2003	7.5	*	*	*	0.1	0.2	0.8	2.5	6.3	16.9	51.7	188.9	7.4
2004	7.9	*	*	*	0.1	0.3	0.8	2.7	6.3	17.1	52.6	198.5	7.7
2005	8.4	*	*	*	0.1	0.2	0.9	2.7	6.4	17.7	55.6	210.0	8.0
2006	8.0	*	*	*	0.0	0.3	0.9	3.0	6.9	16.8	51.0	189.4	7.5
2007	7.9	*	*	*	0.1	0.2	0.9	2.8	6.5	16.2	49.5	191.1	7.4
2008	8.5	*	*	*	0.1	0.3	1.0	3.0	7.3	16.8	52.1	195.6	7.7
Parkinson's Disease (G20–G21)													
1999	5.2	*	*	*	*	*	*	0.1	1.0	11.0	58.2	124.4	5.4
2000	5.6	*	*	*	*	*	*	0.1	1.1	11.5	61.9	131.9	5.7
2001	5.8	*	*	*	*	*	*	0.1	1.2	11.7	64.6	134.2	5.9
2002	5.9	*	*	*	*	*	*	0.1	1.2	12.2	63.9	135.2	5.9
2003	6.2	*	*	*	*	*	*	0.2	1.3	12.7	67.8	138.2	6.2
2004	6.1	*	*	*	*	*	*	0.2	1.2	12.0	67.5	135.8	6.1
2005	6.6	*	*	*	*	*	*	0.2	1.4	13.0	71.2	143.7	6.4
2006	6.5	*	*	*	*	*	*	0.2	1.3	12.2	69.8	144.8	6.3
2007	6.7	*	*	*	*	*	*	0.1	1.2	11.9	71.9	143.5	6.4
2008	6.7	*	*	*	*	*	*	0.2	1.2	12.5	71.4	142.9	6.4

Table B-10. Death Rates by Age and Age-Adjusted Death Rates for the 15 Leading Causes of Death, 1999–2008—*Continued*

(Rate per 100,000 population in specified group; age-adjusted rates per 100,000 U.S. standard population.)

Cause of death (based on ICD-10, 2004) and year	All ages[1]	Under 1 year[2]	Age									Age-adjusted rate
			1–4 years	5–14 years	15–24 years	25–34 years	35–44 years	45–54 years	55–64 years	65–74 years	75–84 years	85 years and over	
Assault (Homicide) (*U01–*U02, X85–Y09, Y87.1)													
1999	6.1	8.7	2.5	1.1	12.9	10.5	7.1	4.6	3.0	2.6	2.5	2.4	6.0
2000	6.0	9.2	2.3	0.9	12.6	10.4	7.1	4.7	3.0	2.4	2.4	2.4	5.9
2001[3]	7.1	8.2	2.7	0.8	13.3	13.1	9.5	6.3	4.0	2.9	2.5	2.4	7.1
2002	6.1	7.5	2.7	0.9	12.9	11.2	7.2	4.8	3.2	2.3	2.3	2.1	6.1
2003	6.1	8.5	2.4	0.8	13.0	11.3	7.0	4.9	2.8	2.4	2.5	2.2	6.0
2004	5.9	8.0	2.4	0.8	12.2	11.2	6.8	4.8	3.0	2.4	2.2	2.1	5.9
2005	6.1	7.5	2.3	0.8	13.0	11.8	7.1	4.8	2.8	2.4	2.2	2.1	6.1
2006	6.2	8.1	2.2	1.0	13.5	11.7	6.9	5.1	3.2	2.1	2.1	1.9	6.2
2007	6.1	8.3	2.4	0.9	13.1	11.7	7.1	4.9	3.0	2.1	2.1	1.5	6.1
2008	5.9	7.9	2.5	0.8	12.4	11.3	6.8	4.8	2.9	2.3	1.8	2.1	5.9

X = Category not applicable.
* = Figure does not meet standards of reliability or precision.
[1] Figures for age not stated included in "All ages" but not distributed among age groups.
[2] Death rates for "Under 1 year" (based on population estimates) differ from infant mortality rates (based on live births).
[3] Figures include September 11, 2001 related deaths for which death certificates were filed as of October 24, 2002.

PART B: MORTALITY   119

Table B-11. Number of Deaths from Selected Causes by Age, 2008

(Number.)

Cause of death (based on ICD-10, 2004)	All ages	Under 1 year	1–4 years	5–14 years	15–24 years	25–34 years	35–44 years	45–54 years	55–64 years	65–74 years	75–84 years	85 years and over	Not stated
ALL CAUSES	2,471,984	28,059	4,730	5,651	32,198	42,275	76,370	186,542	296,182	401,579	653,560	744,691	147
Salmonella infections (A01-A02)	44	4	2	1	2	1	1	3	3	8	8	11	-
Shigellosis and amebiasis (A03, A06)	6	-	-	-	-	-	1	-	3	1	1	-	-
Certain other intestinal infections (A04, A07-A09)	7,876	8	6	-	4	15	39	142	435	1003	2,791	3,432	1
Tuberculosis (A16-A19)	585	-	2	3	6	14	26	80	90	114	145	105	-
Respiratory tuberculosis (A16)	449	-	2	1	5	8	15	58	69	85	121	85	-
Other tuberculosis (A17-A19)	136	-	-	2	1	6	11	22	21	29	24	20	-
Whooping cough (A37)	20	18	-	-	-	-	1	-	-	-	-	1	-
Scarlet fever and erysipelas (A38, A46)	3	-	-	-	-	1	-	-	-	1	-	1	-
Meningococcal infection (A39)	102	9	11	8	19	11	11	8	6	8	6	5	-
Septicemia (A40-A41)	35,927	289	93	61	139	359	892	2,514	4,552	6,448	10,717	9,863	-
Syphilis (A50-A53)	34	-	-	-	1	-	2	3	5	3	7	13	-
Acute poliomyelitis (A80)	-	-	-	-	-	-	-	-	-	-	-	-	-
Arthropod-borne viral encephalitis (A83-A84, A85.2)	2	-	-	-	1	-	-	-	-	-	-	-	-
Measles (B05)	-	-	-	-	-	-	-	-	-	-	1	-	-
Viral hepatitis (B15-B19)	7,629	2	-	2	9	51	447	2,732	2,751	882	600	153	-
Human immunodeficiency virus (HIV) disease (B20-B24)	10,285	-	2	1	168	975	2,838	3,730	1,908	516	116	31	-
Malaria (B50-B54)	5	-	-	-	-	1	-	2	1	-	1	-	-
Other and unspecified infectious and parasitic diseases and their sequelae (A00, A05, A20-A36, A42-A44, A48- A49, A54-A79, A81-A82, A85.0-A85.1, A85.8, A86-B04, B06-B09, B25-B49, B55-B99)	5,914	148	66	46	78	107	219	507	912	1,129	1,557	1,145	-
Malignant neoplasms (C00-C97)	565,469	70	394	890	1,663	3,521	12,699	50,403	104,091	141,159	160,960	89,610	9
Malignant neoplasms of lip, oral cavity and pharynx (C00-C14)	8,019	-	-	2	17	53	236	1,144	1,995	1,941	1,633	998	-
Malignant neoplasm of esophagus (C15)	13,714	-	-	3	3	29	236	1,441	3,304	3,838	3,443	1,417	-
Malignant neoplasm of stomach (C16)	11,352	-	-	1	20	129	407	1,182	1,978	2,558	3,059	2,018	-
Malignant neoplasms of colon, rectum and anus (C18-C21)	53,321	1	-	1	52	314	1,419	4,802	9,076	11,770	14,936	10,948	2
Malignant neoplasms of liver and intrahepatic bile ducts (C22)	18,213	1	20	17	38	81	335	2,480	4,737	4,105	4,465	1,934	-
Malignant neoplasm of pancreas (C25)	35,236	1	-	1	7	53	506	2,840	6,681	9,115	10,414	5,616	2
Malignant neoplasm of larynx (C32)	3,760	-	-	-	-	3	52	411	973	1136	853	332	-
Malignant neoplasms of trachea, bronchus and lung (C33-C34)	158,656	4	3	5	29	145	1,604	12,532	30,796	48,293	47,948	17,297	-
Malignant melanoma of skin (C43)	8,623	2	1	-	40	188	412	1,104	1,742	1,897	2,123	1,114	-
Malignant neoplasm of breast (C50)	41,026	-	-	-	13	331	2,148	5,962	8,797	8,441	8,820	6,514	-
Malignant neoplasm of cervix uteri (C53)	4,008	-	-	-	13	152	609	977	880	653	473	251	-
Malignant neoplasms of corpus uteri and uterus, part unspecified (C54-C55)	7,675	-	-	-	6	30	147	612	1,702	2,032	1,896	1,250	-
Malignant neoplasm of ovary (C56)	14,362	-	-	3	12	94	379	1,539	2,921	3,609	3,783	2,022	-
Malignant neoplasm of prostate (C61)	28,472	-	1	-	-	1	23	458	2,385	5,645	10,721	9,237	1
Malignant neoplasms of kidney and renal pelvis (C64-C65)	12,895	1	12	33	24	49	225	1,268	2,679	3,211	3,436	1,957	-
Malignant neoplasm of bladder (C67)	14,036	1	-	-	3	14	95	592	1,600	2,952	4,932	3,847	-
Malignant neoplasms of meninges, brain and other parts of central nervous system (C70-C72)	13724	11	119	299	220	362	844	2016	3161	3139	2587	966	-
Malignant neoplasms of lymphoid, hematopoietic and related tissue (C81-C96)	54954	28	127	287	594	813	1320	3555	7859	12329	17591	10449	2
Hodgkin's disease (C81)	1171	-	-	1	56	94	117	146	177	210	256	114	-
Non-Hodgkin's lymphoma (C82-C85)	20369	1	4	34	127	221	469	1290	2910	4413	6791	4108	1
Leukemia (C91-C95)	22335	27	123	252	410	490	621	1436	2956	4798	6840	4381	1
Multiple myeloma and immunoproliferative neoplasms (C88, C90)	11020	-	-	-	1	8	112	679	1811	2898	3676	1835	-
Other and unspecified malignant neoplasms of lymphoid, hematopoietic and related tissue (C96)	59	-	-	-	-	-	1	4	5	10	28	11	-
All other and unspecified malignant neoplasms (C17, C23-C24, C26-C31, C37-C41, C44-C49, C51- C52, C57-C60, C62-C63, C66, C68-C69, C73-C80, C97)	63423	20	111	238	572	680	1702	5488	10825	14495	17847	11443	2
In situ neoplasms, benign neoplasms and neoplasms of uncertain or unknown behavior (D00-D48)	14470	61	46	88	95	152	306	714	1379	2517	4724	4388	-
Anemias (D50-D64)	5018	15	34	38	102	155	211	244	366	562	1276	2015	-
Diabetes mellitus (E10-E14)	70553	4	5	36	204	574	1854	5622	11370	15315	20037	15531	1
Nutritional deficiencies (E40-E64)	2976	10	2	2	6	13	46	124	214	369	808	1382	-
Malnutrition (E40-E46)	2760	8	2	1	6	11	43	113	197	350	760	1269	-
Other nutritional deficiencies (E50-E64)	216	2	-	1	-	2	3	11	17	19	48	113	-
Meningitis (G00, G03)	633	68	11	16	24	46	52	110	105	85	76	40	-
Parkinson's disease (G20-G21)	20483	1	-	-	4	4	13	68	398	2512	9304	8179	-
Alzheimer's disease (G30)	82435	-	-	-	-	1	8	107	745	4326	25172	52075	1
Major cardiovascular diseases (I00-I78)	804483	571	256	337	1333	4058	14226	46432	82009	116296	222494	316436	35
Diseases of heart (I00-I09, I11, I13, I20-I51)	616828	396	186	229	1065	3254	11336	37892	66711	90520	166286	238924	29
Acute rheumatic fever and chronic rheumatic heart diseases (I00-I09)	3141	2	4	-	10	34	55	188	340	548	992	968	-
Hypertensive heart disease (I11)	32391	1	-	1	53	353	1390	3895	4837	4251	6416	11189	5
Hypertensive heart and renal disease (I13)	2872	-	-	1	6	24	93	198	287	380	692	1191	-
Ischemic heart diseases (I20-I25)	405309	12	4	21	144	1045	5952	24359	46665	63623	112397	151064	23

Table B-11. Number of Deaths from Selected Causes by Age, 2008—Continued

(Number.)

Cause of death (based on ICD-10, 2004)	All ages	Under 1 year	1–4 years	5–14 years	15–24 years	25–34 years	35–44 years	45–54 years	55–64 years	65–74 years	75–84 years	85 years and over	Not stated
Acute myocardial infarction (I21-I22)	133958	4	2	5	57	416	2250	9511	18164	23410	37190	42945	4
Other acute ischemic heart diseases (I24)	4252	2	-	2	3	21	104	435	663	725	1008	1289	-
Other forms of chronic ischemic heart disease (I20, I25)	267099	6	2	14	84	608	3598	14413	27838	39488	74199	106830	19
Atherosclerotic cardiovascular disease, so described (I25.0)	58625	1	-	3	21	217	1351	5803	10009	10078	13553	17576	13
All other forms of chronic ischemic heart disease (I20, I25.1-I25.9)	208474	5	2	11	63	391	2247	8610	17829	29410	60646	89254	6
Other heart diseases (I26-I51)	173115	381	178	206	852	1798	3846	9252	14582	21718	45789	74512	1
Acute and subacute endocarditis (I33)	1180	2	2	-	16	37	70	161	214	262	268	148	-
Diseases of pericardium and acute myocarditis (I30-I31, I40)	827	25	29	13	30	61	74	111	130	109	143	102	-
Heart failure (I50)	56830	23	8	10	36	99	294	1166	2765	5627	15396	31406	-
All other forms of heart disease (I26-I28, I34-I38, I42-I49, I51)	114278	331	139	183	770	1601	3408	7814	11473	15720	29982	42856	1
Essential hypertension and hypertensive renal disease (I10, I12, I15)	25742	7	3	1	22	126	438	1322	2464	3387	6783	11189	-
Cerebrovascular diseases (I60-I69)	134148	141	63	97	189	539	2035	6112	10459	17897	40963	55648	5
Atherosclerosis (I70)	7836	4	-	1	-	3	21	131	372	769	2103	4431	1
Other diseases of circulatory system (I71-I78)	19929	23	4	9	57	136	396	975	2003	3723	6359	6244	-
Aortic aneurysm and dissection (I71)	11079	1	-	5	39	99	284	638	1159	2228	3742	2884	-
Other diseases of arteries, arterioles and capillaries (I72-I78)	8850	22	4	4	18	37	112	337	844	1495	2617	3360	-
Other disorders of circulatory system (I80-I99)	4042	23	2	3	53	138	315	564	581	594	850	919	-
Influenza and pneumonia (J09-J18)[1]	56284	226	142	89	206	371	880	2253	3734	6252	15512	26618	1
Influenza (J09-J11)[1]	1722	16	24	32	20	29	44	77	122	129	413	816	-
Pneumonia (J12-J18)	54562	210	118	57	186	342	836	2176	3612	6123	15099	25802	1
Other acute lower respiratory infections (J20-J22, U04)[2]	284	43	23	3	2	5	7	22	20	20	43	96	-
Acute bronchitis and bronchiolitis (J20-J21)	235	43	23	3	2	5	6	20	17	13	32	71	-
Other and unspecified acute lower respiratory infections (J22, U04)[2,3]	49	-	-	-	-	-	1	2	3	7	11	25	-
Chronic lower respiratory diseases (J40-J47)	141090	32	54	119	163	252	812	4392	14042	31975	51700	37548	1
Bronchitis, chronic and unspecified (J40-J42)	731	23	15	2	5	13	13	29	61	97	175	298	-
Emphysema (J43)	12448	1	-	-	1	4	69	502	1485	3260	4585	2541	-
Asthma (J45-J46)	3397	6	37	112	141	182	308	497	470	438	547	659	-
Other chronic lower respiratory diseases (J44, J47)	124514	2	2	5	16	53	422	3364	12026	28180	46393	34050	1
Pneumoconioses and chemical effects (J60-J66, J68)	908	-	-	-	-	2	3	18	60	176	361	288	-
Pneumonitis due to solids and liquids (J69)	16608	11	10	5	41	81	158	467	923	1683	5031	8198	-
Other diseases of respiratory system (J00-J06, J30-J39, J67, J70-J98)	29925	266	100	61	136	204	489	1442	3192	5806	10050	8179	-
Peptic ulcer (K25-K28)	3073	1	3	1	6	13	72	268	434	479	874	922	-
Diseases of appendix (K35-K38)	418	2	4	10	9	13	21	40	59	65	105	90	-
Hernia (K40-K46)	1674	17	2	2	4	11	36	104	168	212	491	627	-
Chronic liver disease and cirrhosis (K70, K73-K74)	29963	10	-	1	24	423	2562	8220	8526	5395	3664	1137	1
Alcoholic liver disease (K70)	14864	-	-	-	18	318	1827	5180	4576	2060	759	126	-
Other chronic liver disease and cirrhosis (K73-K74)	15099	10	-	1	6	105	735	3040	3950	3335	2905	1011	1
Cholelithiasis and other disorders of gallbladder (K80-K82)	3417	-	-	1	7	29	51	141	273	509	1057	1349	-
Nephritis, nephrotic syndrome and nephrosis (N00-N07, N17-N19, N25-N27)	48237	143	12	17	80	258	780	2220	4803	8182	14819	16920	3
Acute and rapidly progressive nephritic and nephrotic syndrome (N00-N01, N04)	160	4	2	-	3	2	5	11	14	28	49	42	-
Chronic glomerulonephritis, nephritis and nephropathy not specified as acute or chronic, and renal sclerosis unspecified (N02-N03, N05-N07, N26)	4109	-	2	1	7	19	39	130	310	529	1187	1884	1
Renal failure (N17-N19)	43935	139	8	16	69	236	736	2074	4474	7619	13574	14988	2
Other disorders of kidney (N25, N27)	33	-	-	-	1	1	-	5	5	6	9	6	-
Infections of kidney (N10-N12, N13.6, N15.1)	627	4	1	2	6	6	25	62	68	81	180	192	-
Hyperplasia of prostate (N40)	502	-	-	-	-	-	-	1	12	47	165	277	-
Inflammatory diseases of female pelvic organs (N70-N76)	136	1	-	-	2	5	7	9	14	20	40	38	-
Pregnancy, childbirth and the puerperium (O00-O99)	795	X	X	X	169	352	202	67	3	1	1	-	-
Pregnancy with abortive outcome (O00-O07)	34	X	X	X	11	13	10	-	-	-	-	-	-
Other complications of pregnancy, childbirth and the puerperium (O10-O99)	761	X	X	X	158	339	192	67	3	1	1	-	-
Certain conditions originating in the perinatal period (P00-P96)	13933	13800	51	32	20	9	6	5	5	1	2	1	1
Congenital malformations, deformations and chromosomal abnormalities (Q00-Q99)	10288	5638	521	331	467	379	450	720	762	379	344	297	-
Symptoms, signs and abnormal clinical and laboratory findings, not elsewhere classified (R00-R99)	38522	3546	273	146	670	1046	1688	2855	2856	3039	6703	15655	45
All other diseases (Residual)	252490	1245	620	816	1989	3134	6945	16645	23972	30451	63816	102849	8
Accidents (unintentional injuries) (V01-X59, Y85-Y86)	121902	1315	1469	1859	14089	14588	16065	20354	12782	8994	13827	16538	22
Transport accidents (V01-V99, Y85)	42709	104	489	1090	9297	6930	6164	6766	4840	3110	2655	1258	6
Motor vehicle accidents (V02-V04, V09.0, V09.2, V12-V14, V19.0-V19.2, V19.4-V19.6, V20-V79, V80.3-V80.5, V81.0-V81.1, V82.0-V82.1, V83-V86, V87.0-V87.8, V88.0-V88.8, V89.0, V89.2)	39790	103	463	1027	8946	6570	5672	6101	4356	2826	2515	1208	3

Table B-11. Number of Deaths from Selected Causes by Age, 2008—*Continued*

(Number.)

Cause of death (based on ICD-10, 2004)	All ages	Under 1 year	1–4 years	5–14 years	15–24 years	25–34 years	35–44 years	45–54 years	55–64 years	65–74 years	75–84 years	85 years and over	Not stated
Other land transport accidents (V01,V05-V06, V09.1, V09.3-V09.9, V10-V11, V15-V18, V19.3, V19.8-V19.9, V80.0-V80.2, V80.6-V80.9, V81.2- V81.9, V82.2-V82.9, V87.9, V88.9, V89.1, V89.3, V89.9)	1140	-	20	30	189	146	173	250	147	99	56	27	3
Water, air and space, and other and unspecified transport accidents and their sequelae (V90-V99, Y85)	1779	1	6	33	162	214	319	415	337	185	84	23	-
Nontransport accidents (W00-X59, Y86)	79193	1211	980	769	4792	7658	9901	13588	7942	5884	11172	15280	16
Falls (W00-W19)	24013	13	38	40	233	297	540	1300	1809	2745	7007	9990	1
Accidental discharge of firearms (W32-W34)	592	-	21	41	132	89	85	99	57	37	22	9	-
Accidental drowning and submersion (W65-W74)	3548	41	443	261	569	429	406	510	356	210	217	103	3
Accidental exposure to smoke, fire and flames (X00-X09)	2912	20	166	175	146	151	248	468	464	427	405	240	2
Accidental poisoning and exposure to noxious substances (X40-X49)	31116	11	35	48	3188	5946	7545	9496	3547	725	375	196	4
Other and unspecified nontransport accidents and their sequelae (W20-W31, W35-W64, W75-W99, X10-X39, X50-X59, Y86)	17012	1126	277	204	524	746	1077	1715	1709	1740	3146	4742	6
Intentional self-harm (suicide) (*U03, X60-X84, Y87.0)	36035	X	X	222	4298	5300	6703	8287	5465	2796	2108	851	5
Intentional self-harm (suicide) by discharge of firearms (X72-X74)	18223	X	X	50	2009	2357	2796	3789	3079	1933	1607	603	-
Intentional self-harm (suicide) by other and unspecified means and their sequelae (*U03, X60-X71, X75-X84, Y87.0)	17812	X	X	172	2289	2943	3907	4498	2386	863	501	248	5
Assault (homicide) (*U01-*U02, X85-Y09, Y87.1)	17826	340	421	320	5275	4610	2906	2137	987	466	235	122	7
Assault (homicide) by discharge of firearms (*U01.4, X93-X95)	12179	9	56	187	4394	3612	1966	1146	489	196	88	34	2
Assault (homicide) by other and unspecified means and their sequelae (*U01.0-*U01.3, *U01.5-*U01.9, *U02, X85-X92, X96-Y09, Y87.1)	5,647	331	365	133	881	998	940	991	498	270	147	88	5
Legal intervention (Y35, Y89.0)	381	-	-	-	85	108	94	67	18	7	1	1	-
Events of undetermined intent (Y10-Y34, Y87.2,Y89.9)	5,051	94	74	60	500	823	1,079	1,403	669	167	104	72	6
Discharge of firearms, undetermined intent (Y22-Y24)	273	-	2	10	70	53	36	40	32	18	8	2	2
Other and unspecified events of undetermined intent and their sequelae (Y10-Y21, Y25-Y34, Y87.2, Y89.9)	4,778	94	72	50	430	770	1,043	1,363	637	149	96	70	4
Operations of war and their sequelae (Y36, Y89.1)	31	-	-	1	3	2	2	1	4	3	11	4	-
Complications of medical and surgical care (Y40-Y84, Y88)	2,590	24	18	21	36	54	120	233	407	525	665	487	-
Enterocolitis due to Clostridium difficile (A04.7)	7,476	3	1	-	3	12	35	128	411	968	2,673	3,241	1
Drug-induced deaths[2]	38,649	21	55	56	3592	7002	9377	11921	4774	1068	518	261	4
Alcohol-induced deaths[2]	24,189	1	-	2	189	811	3207	8254	7080	3144	1,230	269	2
Injury by firearms[2]	31,593	9	79	288	6685	6202	4959	5127	3674	2191	1,726	649	4

X = Category not applicable.
– = Quantity zero
[1]Included in certain other intestinal infections (A04, A07–A09)
[2]Included in selected categories above.

NOTE: Complete confirmation of deaths from selected causes of death, considered to be of public health concern, were not provided by the following states—Massachusetts, North Carolina, and West Virginia.

Table B-12. Death Rates for Selected Causes by Age, 2008

(Rate per 100,000 population in specified group.)

Cause of death (based on ICD-10, 2004)	All ages[1]	Under 1 year[2]	1–4 years	5–14 years	15–24 years	25–34 years	35–44 years	45–54 years	55–64 years	65–74 years	75–84 years	85 years and over
ALL CAUSES	813.0	650.5	28.3	14.1	75.6	103.3	179.7	420.4	879.2	1995.6	5017.7	13015.1
Salmonella infections (A01-A02)	0.0	*	*	*	*	*	*	*	*	*	*	*
Shigellosis and amebiasis (A03, A06)	*	*	*	*	*	*	*	*	*	*	*	*
Certain other intestinal infections (A04, A07-A09)	2.6	*	*	*	*	*	0.1	0.3	1.3	5.0	21.4	60.0
Tuberculosis (A16-A19)	0.2	*	*	*	*	*	0.1	0.2	0.3	0.6	1.1	1.8
Respiratory tuberculosis (A16)	0.1	*	*	*	*	*	*	0.1	0.2	0.4	0.9	1.5
Other tuberculosis (A17-A19)	0.0	*	*	*	*	*	*	0.0	0.1	0.1	0.2	0.3
Whooping cough (A37)	0.0	*	*	*	*	*	*	*	*	*	*	*
Scarlet fever and erysipelas (A38, A46)	*	*	*	*	*	*	*	*	*	*	*	*
Meningococcal infection (A39)	0.0	*	*	*	*	*	*	*	*	*	*	*
Septicemia (A40-A41)	11.8	6.7	0.6	0.2	0.3	0.9	2.1	5.7	13.5	32.0	82.3	172.4
Syphilis (A50-A53)	0.0	*	*	*	*	*	*	*	*	*	*	*
Acute poliomyelitis (A80)	*	*	*	*	*	*	*	*	*	*	*	*
Arthropod-borne viral encephalitis (A83-A84, A85.2)	*	*	*	*	*	*	*	*	*	*	*	*
Measles (B05)	*	*	*	*	*	*	*	*	*	*	*	*
Viral hepatitis (B15-B19)	2.5	*	*	*	*	0.1	1.1	6.2	8.2	4.4	4.6	2.7
Human immunodeficiency virus (HIV) disease (B20-B24)	3.4	*	*	*	0.4	2.4	6.7	8.4	5.7	2.6	0.9	0.5
Malaria (B50-B54)	*	*	*	*	*	*	*	*	*	*	*	*
Other and unspecified infectious and parasitic diseases and their sequelae (A00, A05, A20-A36, A42-A44, A48- A49, A54-A79, A81-A82, A85.0-A85.1, A85.8, A86-B04, B06-B09, B25-B49, B55-B99)	1.9	3.4	0.4	0.1	0.2	0.3	0.5	1.1	2.7	5.6	12.0	20.0
Malignant neoplasms (C00-C97)	186.0	1.6	2.4	2.2	3.9	8.6	29.9	113.6	309.0	701.5	1235.8	1566.1
Malignant neoplasms of lip, oral cavity and pharynx (C00-C14)	2.6	*	*	*	*	0.1	0.6	2.6	5.9	9.6	12.5	17.4
Malignant neoplasm of esophagus (C15)	4.5	*	*	*	*	0.1	0.6	3.2	9.8	19.1	26.4	24.8
Malignant neoplasm of stomach (C16)	3.7	*	*	*	0.0	0.3	1.0	2.7	5.9	12.7	23.5	35.3
Malignant neoplasms of colon, rectum and anus (C18-C21)	17.5	*	*	*	0.1	0.8	3.3	10.8	26.9	58.5	114.7	191.3
Malignant neoplasms of liver and intrahepatic bileducts (C22)	6.0	*	0.1	*	0.1	0.2	0.8	5.6	14.1	20.4	34.3	33.8
Malignant neoplasm of pancreas (C25)	11.6	*	*	*	*	0.1	1.2	6.4	19.8	45.3	80.0	98.2
Malignant neoplasm of larynx (C32)	1.2	*	*	*	*	*	0.1	0.9	2.9	5.6	6.5	5.8
Malignant neoplasms of trachea, bronchus and lung (C33-C34)	52.2	*	*	*	0.1	0.4	3.8	28.2	91.4	240.0	368.1	302.3
Malignant melanoma of skin (C43)	2.8	*	*	*	0.1	0.5	1.0	2.5	5.2	9.4	16.3	19.5
Malignant neoplasm of breast (C50)	13.5	*	*	*	*	0.8	5.1	13.4	26.1	41.9	67.7	113.8
Malignant neoplasm of cervix uteri (C53)	1.3	*	*	*	*	0.4	1.4	2.2	2.6	3.2	3.6	4.4
Malignant neoplasms of corpus uteri and uterus, part unspecified (C54-C55)	2.5	*	*	*	*	0.1	0.3	1.4	5.1	10.1	14.6	21.8
Malignant neoplasm of ovary (C56)	4.7	*	*	*	*	0.2	0.9	3.5	8.7	17.9	29.0	35.3
Malignant neoplasm of prostate (C61)	9.4	*	*	*	*	*	0.1	1.0	7.1	28.1	82.3	161.4
Malignant neoplasms of kidney and renal pelvis (C64-C65)	4.2	*	*	*	0.1	0.1	0.5	2.9	8.0	16.0	26.4	34.2
Malignant neoplasm of bladder (C67)	4.6	*	*	*	*	*	0.2	1.3	4.7	14.7	37.9	67.2
Malignant neoplasms of meninges, brain and other parts of central nervous system (C70-C72)	4.5	*	0.7	0.7	0.5	0.9	2.0	4.5	9.4	15.6	19.9	16.9
Malignant neoplasms of lymphoid, hematopoietic and related tissue (C81-C96)	18.1	0.6	0.8	0.7	1.4	2.0	3.1	8.0	23.3	61.3	135.1	182.6
Hodgkin's disease (C81)	0.4	*	*	*	0.1	0.2	0.3	0.3	0.5	1.0	2.0	2.0
Non-Hodgkin's lymphoma (C82-C85)	6.7	*	*	0.1	0.3	0.5	1.1	2.9	8.6	21.9	52.1	71.8
Leukemia (C91-C95)	7.3	0.6	0.7	0.6	1.0	1.2	1.5	3.2	8.8	23.8	52.5	76.6
Multiple myeloma and immunoproliferative neoplasms (C88, C90)	3.6	*	*	*	*	*	0.3	1.5	5.4	14.4	28.2	32.1
Other and unspecified malignant neoplasms of lymphoid, hematopoietic and related tissue (C96)	0.0	*	*	*	*	*	*	*	*	*	0.2	*
All other and unspecified malignant neoplasms (C17, C23-C24, C26-C31, C37-C41, C44-C49, C51- C52, C57-C60, C62-C63, C66, C68-C69, C73-C80, C97)	20.9	0.5	0.7	0.6	1.3	1.7	4.0	12.4	32.1	72.0	137.0	200.0
In situ neoplasms, benign neoplasms and neoplasms of uncertain or unknown behavior (D00-D48)	4.8	1.4	0.3	0.2	0.2	0.4	0.7	1.6	4.1	12.5	36.3	76.7
Anemias (D50-D64)	1.7	*	0.2	0.1	0.2	0.4	0.5	0.5	1.1	2.8	9.8	35.2
Diabetes mellitus (E10-E14)	23.2	*	*	0.1	0.5	1.4	4.4	12.7	33.8	76.1	153.8	271.4
Nutritional deficiencies (E40-E64)	1.0	*	*	*	*	*	0.1	0.3	0.6	1.8	6.2	24.2
Malnutrition (E40-E46)	0.9	*	*	*	*	*	0.1	0.3	0.6	1.7	5.8	22.2
Other nutritional deficiencies (E50-E64)	0.1	*	*	*	*	*	*	*	*	*	0.4	2.0
Meningitis (G00, G03)	0.2	1.6	*	*	0.1	0.1	0.1	0.2	0.3	0.4	0.6	0.7
Parkinson's disease (G20-G21)	6.7	*	*	*	*	*	*	0.2	1.2	12.5	71.4	142.9
Alzheimer's disease (G30)	27.1	*	*	*	*	*	*	0.2	2.2	21.5	193.3	910.1
Major cardiovascular diseases (I00-I78)	264.6	13.2	1.5	0.8	3.1	9.9	33.5	104.6	243.4	577.9	1708.2	5530.4
Diseases of heart (I00-I09, I11, I13, I20-I51)	202.9	9.2	1.1	0.6	2.5	7.9	26.7	85.4	198.0	449.8	1276.7	4175.7
Acute rheumatic fever and chronic rheumatic heart diseases (I00-I09)	1.0	*	*	*	*	0.1	0.1	0.4	1.0	2.7	7.6	16.9
Hypertensive heart disease (I11)	10.7	*	*	*	0.1	0.9	3.3	8.8	14.4	21.1	49.3	195.6
Hypertensive heart and renal disease (I13)	0.9	*	*	*	*	0.1	0.2	0.4	0.9	1.9	5.3	20.8
Ischemic heart diseases (I20-I25)	133.3	*	*	0.1	0.3	2.6	14.0	54.9	138.5	316.2	862.9	2640.2
Acute myocardial infarction (I21-I22)	44.1	*	*	*	0.1	1.0	5.3	21.4	53.9	116.3	285.5	750.6
Other acute ischemic heart diseases (I24)	1.4	*	*	*	*	0.1	0.2	1.0	2.0	3.6	7.7	22.5
Other forms of chronic ischemic heart disease (I20, I25)	87.8	*	*	*	0.2	1.5	8.5	32.5	82.6	196.2	569.7	1867.1
Atherosclerotic cardiovascular disease, so described (I25.0)	19.3	*	*	*	0.0	0.5	3.2	13.1	29.7	50.1	104.1	307.2
All other forms of chronic ischemic heart disease (I20, I25.1-I25.9)	68.6	*	*	*	0.1	1.0	5.3	19.4	52.9	146.2	465.6	1559.9

Table B-12. Death Rates for Selected Causes by Age, 2008—Continued

(Rate per 100,000 population in specified group.)

Cause of death (based on ICD-10, 2004)	All ages[1]	Under 1 year[2]	1–4 years	5–14 years	15–24 years	25–34 years	35–44 years	45–54 years	55–64 years	65–74 years	75–84 years	85 years and over
Other heart diseases (I26-I51)	56.9	8.8	1.1	0.5	2.0	4.4	9.0	20.9	43.3	107.9	351.5	1,302.3
Acute and subacute endocarditis (I33)	0.4	*	*	*	*	0.1	0.2	0.4	0.6	1.3	2.1	2.6
Diseases of pericardium and acute myocarditis (I30-I31, I40)	0.3	0.6	0.2	*	0.1	0.1	0.2	0.3	0.4	0.5	1.1	1.8
Heart failure (I50)	18.7	0.5	*	*	0.1	0.2	0.7	2.6	8.2	28.0	118.2	548.9
All other forms of heart disease (I26-I28, I34-I38, I42-I49, I51)	37.6	7.7	0.8	0.5	1.8	3.9	8.0	17.6	34.1	78.1	230.2	749.0
Essential hypertension and hypertensive renal disease (I10, I12, I15)	8.5	*	*	*	0.1	0.3	1.0	3.0	7.3	16.8	52.1	195.6
Cerebrovascular diseases (I60-I69)	44.1	3.3	0.4	0.2	0.4	1.3	4.8	13.8	31.0	88.9	314.5	972.6
Atherosclerosis (I70)	2.6	*	*	*	*	*	0.0	0.3	1.1	3.8	16.1	77.4
Other diseases of circulatory system (I71-I78)	6.6	0.5	*	*	0.1	0.3	0.9	2.2	5.9	18.5	48.8	109.1
Aortic aneurysm and dissection (I71)	3.6	*	*	*	0.1	0.2	0.7	1.4	3.4	11.1	28.7	50.4
Other diseases of arteries, arterioles and capillaries (I72-I78)	2.9	0.5	*	*	*	0.1	0.3	0.8	2.5	7.4	20.1	58.7
Other disorders of circulatory system (I80-I99)	1.3	0.5	*	*	0.1	0.3	0.7	1.3	1.7	3.0	6.5	16.1
Influenza and pneumonia (J09-J18)[3]	18.5	5.2	0.9	0.2	0.5	0.9	2.1	5.1	11.1	31.1	119.1	465.2
Influenza (J09-J11)[3]	0.6	*	0.1	0.1	0.0	0.1	0.1	0.2	0.4	0.6	3.2	14.3
Pneumonia (J12-J18)	17.9	4.9	0.7	0.1	0.4	0.8	2.0	4.9	10.7	30.4	115.9	450.9
Other acute lower respiratory infections (J20-J22, U04)[4]	0.1	1.0	0.1	*	*	*	*	0.0	0.1	0.1	0.3	1.7
Acute bronchitis and bronchiolitis (J20-J21)	0.1	1.0	0.1	*	*	*	*	0.0	*	*	0.2	1.2
Other and unspecified acute lower respiratory infections (J22, U04)[4,5]	0.0	*	*	*	*	*	*	*	*	*	*	0.4
Chronic lower respiratory diseases (J40-J47)	46.4	0.7	0.3	0.3	0.4	0.6	1.9	9.9	41.7	158.9	396.9	656.2
Bronchitis, chronic and unspecified (J40-J42)	0.2	0.5	*	*	*	*	*	0.1	0.2	0.5	1.3	5.2
Emphysema (J43)	4.1	*	*	*	*	*	0.2	1.1	4.4	16.2	35.2	44.4
Asthma (J45-J46)	1.1	*	0.2	0.3	0.3	0.4	0.7	1.1	1.4	2.2	4.2	11.5
Other chronic lower respiratory diseases (J44, J47)	41.0	*	*	*	*	0.1	1.0	7.6	35.7	140.0	356.2	595.1
Pneumoconioses and chemical effects (J60-J66, J68)	0.3	*	*	*	*	*	*	*	0.2	0.9	2.8	5.0
Pneumonitis due to solids and liquids (J69)	5.5	*	*	*	0.1	0.2	0.4	1.1	2.7	8.4	38.6	143.3
Other diseases of respiratory system (J00-J06, J30-J39, J67, J70-J98)	9.8	6.2	0.6	0.2	0.3	0.5	1.2	3.2	9.5	28.9	77.2	142.9
Peptic ulcer (K25-K28)	1.0	*	*	*	*	*	0.2	0.6	1.3	2.4	6.7	16.1
Diseases of appendix (K35-K38)	0.1	*	*	*	*	*	0.0	0.1	0.2	0.3	0.8	1.6
Hernia (K40-K46)	0.6	*	*	*	*	*	0.1	0.2	0.5	1.1	3.8	11.0
Chronic liver disease and cirrhosis (K70, K73-K74)	9.9	*	*	*	0.1	1.0	6.0	18.5	25.3	26.8	28.1	19.9
Alcoholic liver disease (K70)	4.9	*	*	*	*	0.8	4.3	11.7	13.6	10.2	5.8	2.2
Other chronic liver disease and cirrhosis (K73-K74)	5.0	*	*	*	*	0.3	1.7	6.9	11.7	16.6	22.3	17.7
Cholelithiasis and other disorders of gallbladder (K80-K82)	1.1	*	*	*	*	0.1	0.1	0.3	0.8	2.5	8.1	23.6
Nephritis, nephrotic syndrome and nephrosis (N00-N07, N17-N19, N25-N27)	15.9	3.3	*	*	0.2	0.6	1.8	5.0	14.3	40.7	113.8	295.7
Acute and rapidly progressive nephritic and nephrotic syndrome (N00-N01, N04)	0.1	*	*	*	*	*	*	*	*	0.1	0.4	0.7
Chronic glomerulonephritis, nephritis and nephropathy not specified as acute or chronic, and renal sclerosis unspecified (N02-N03, N05-N07, N26)	1.4	*	*	*	*	*	0.1	0.3	0.9	2.6	9.1	32.9
Renal failure (N17-N19)	14.4	3.2	*	*	0.2	0.6	1.7	4.7	13.3	37.9	104.2	261.9
Other disorders of kidney (N25, N27)	0.0	*	*	*	*	*	*	*	*	*	*	*
Infections of kidney (N10-N12, N13.6, N15.1)	0.2	*	*	*	*	*	0.1	0.1	0.2	0.4	1.4	3.4
Hyperplasia of prostate (N40)	0.2	*	*	*	*	*	*	*	*	0.2	1.3	4.8
Inflammatory diseases of female pelvic organs (N70-N76)	0.0	*	*	*	*	*	*	*	*	0.1	0.3	0.7
Pregnancy, childbirth and the puerperium (O00-O99)	0.3	X	X	*	0.4	0.9	0.5	0.2	*	*	*	*
Pregnancy with abortive outcome (O00-O07)	0.0	X	X	*	*	*	*	*	*	*	*	*
Other complications of pregnancy, childbirth and the puerperium (O10-O99)	0.3	X	X	*	0.4	0.8	0.5	0.2	*	*	*	*
Certain conditions originating in the perinatal period (P00-P96)	4.6	320.0	0.3	0.1	0.0	*	*	*	*	*	*	*
Congenital malformations, deformations and chromosomal abnormalities (Q00-Q99)	3.4	130.7	3.1	0.8	1.1	0.9	1.1	1.6	2.3	1.9	2.6	5.2
Symptoms, signs and abnormal clinical and laboratory findings, not elsewhere classified (R00-R99)	12.7	82.2	1.6	0.4	1.6	2.6	4.0	6.4	8.5	15.1	51.5	273.6
All other diseases (Residual)	83.0	28.9	3.7	2.0	4.7	7.7	16.3	37.5	71.2	151.3	489.9	1,797.5
Accidents (unintentional injuries) (V01-X59, Y85-Y86)	40.1	30.5	8.8	4.6	33.1	35.6	37.8	45.9	37.9	44.7	106.2	289.0
Transport accidents (V01-V99, Y85)	14.0	2.4	2.9	2.7	21.8	16.9	14.5	15.2	14.4	15.5	20.4	22.0
Motor vehicle accidents (V02-V04, V09.0, V09.2, V12-V14, V19.0-V19.2, V19.4-V19.6, V20-V79, V80.3-V80.5, V81.0-V81.1,V82.0-V82.1, V83- V86, V87.0-V87.8, V88.0-V88.8, V89.0, V89.2)	13.1	2.4	2.8	2.6	21.0	16.1	13.3	13.7	12.9	14.0	19.3	21.1
Other land transport accidents (V01,V05-V06, V09.1, V09.3-V09.9, V10-V11, V15-V18, V19.3, V19.8-V19.9, V80.0-V80.2, V80.6-V80.9, V81.2- V81.9, V82.2-V82.9, V87.9, V88.9, V89.1, V89.3, V89.9)	0.4	*	0.1	0.1	0.4	0.4	0.4	0.6	0.4	0.5	0.4	0.5
Water, air and space, and other and unspecified transport accidents and their sequelae (V90-V99, Y85)	0.6	*	*	0.1	0.4	0.5	0.8	0.9	1.0	0.9	0.6	0.4
Nontransport accidents (W00-X59, Y86)	26.0	28.1	5.9	1.9	11.3	18.7	23.3	30.6	23.6	29.2	85.8	267.1
Falls (W00-W19)	7.9	*	0.2	0.1	0.5	0.7	1.3	2.9	5.4	13.6	53.8	174.6
Accidental discharge of firearms (W32-W34)	0.2	*	0.1	0.1	0.3	0.2	0.2	0.2	0.2	0.2	0.2	*
Accidental drowning and submersion (W65-W74)	1.2	1.0	2.7	0.7	1.3	1.0	1.0	1.1	1.1	1.0	1.7	1.8
Accidental exposure to smoke, fire and flames (X00-X09)	1.0	0.5	1.0	0.4	0.3	0.4	0.6	1.1	1.4	2.1	3.1	4.2
Accidental poisoning and exposure to noxious substances (X40-X49)	10.2	*	0.2	0.1	7.5	14.5	17.8	21.4	10.5	3.6	2.9	3.4

Table B-12. Death Rates for Selected Causes by Age, 2008—Continued

(Rate per 100,000 population in specified group.)

Cause of death (based on ICD-10, 2004)	All ages[1]	Under 1 year[2]	1–4 years	5–14 years	15–24 years	25–34 years	35–44 years	45–54 years	55–64 years	65–74 years	75–84 years	85 years and over
Other and unspecified nontransport accidents and their sequelae (W20-W31, W35-W64, W75-W99, X10-X39, X50-X59, Y86)	5.6	26.1	1.7	0.5	1.2	1.8	2.5	3.9	5.1	8.6	24.2	82.9
Intentional self-harm (suicide) (*U03, X60-X84, Y87.0)	11.9	X	X	0.6	10.1	12.9	15.8	18.7	16.2	13.9	16.2	14.9
Intentional self-harm (suicide) by discharge of firearms (X72-X74)	6.0	X	X	0.1	4.7	5.8	6.6	8.5	9.1	9.6	12.3	10.5
Intentional self-harm (suicide) by other and unspecified means and their sequelae (*U03, X60-X71, X75-X84, Y87.0)	5.9	X	X	0.4	5.4	7.2	9.2	10.1	7.1	4.3	3.8	4.3
Assault (homicide) (*U01-*U02, X85-Y09, Y87.1)	5.9	7.9	2.5	0.8	12.4	11.3	6.8	4.8	2.9	2.3	1.8	2.1
Assault (homicide) by discharge of firearms (*U01.4, X93-X95)	4.0	*	0.3	0.5	10.3	8.8	4.6	2.6	1.5	1.0	0.7	0.6
Assault (homicide) by other and unspecified means and their sequelae (*U01.0-*U01.3, *U01.5-*U01.9, *U02,X85-X92, X96-Y09, Y87.1)	1.9	7.7	2.2	0.3	2.1	2.4	2.2	2.2	1.5	1.3	1.1	1.5
Legal intervention (Y35, Y89.0)	0.1	*	*	*	0.2	0.3	0.2	0.2	*	*	*	*
Events of undetermined intent (Y10-Y34, Y87.2, Y89.9)	1.7	2.2	0.4	0.1	1.2	2.0	2.5	3.2	2.0	0.8	0.8	1.3
Discharge of firearms, undetermined intent (Y22-Y24)	0.1	*	*	*	0.2	0.1	0.1	0.1	0.1	*	*	*
Other and unspecified events of undetermined intent and their sequelae (Y10-Y21, Y25-Y34, Y87.2, Y89.9)	1.6	2.2	0.4	0.1	1.0	1.9	2.5	3.1	1.9	0.7	0.7	1.2
Operations of war and their sequelae (Y36, Y89.1)	0.0	*	*	*	*	*	*	*	*	*	*	*
Complications of medical and surgical care (Y40-Y84, Y88)	0.9	0.6	*	0.1	0.1	0.1	0.3	0.5	1.2	2.6	5.1	8.5
Enterocolitis due to Clostridium difficile (A04.7)[3]	2.5	*	*	*	*	*	0.1	0.3	1.2	4.8	20.5	56.6
Drug-induced deaths[4]	12.7	0.5	0.3	0.1	8.4	17.1	22.1	26.9	14.2	5.3	4.0	4.6
Alcohol-induced deaths[4]	8.0	*	*	*	0.4	2.0	7.5	18.6	21.0	15.6	9.4	4.7
Injury by firearms[4]	10.4	*	0.5	0.7	15.7	15.2	11.7	11.6	10.9	10.9	13.3	11.3

X = Category not applicable
* = Figure does not meet standards of reliability or precision.
0.0 = Quantity more than zero but less than 0.05.
[1]Figures for age not stated included in "All ages" but not distributed among age groups.
[2]Death rates for "Under 1 year" (based on population estimates) differ from infant mortality rates (based on live births).
[3]Included in certain other intestinal infections (A04, A07–A09).
[4]Included in selected categories above.

NOTE: Complete confirmation of deaths from selected causes of death, considered to be of public health concern, were not provided by the following states—Massachusetts, North Carolina, and West Virginia.

PART B: MORTALITY

Table B-13. Number of Deaths from Selected Causes by Race and Sex, 2008

(Number.)

Cause of death (based on ICD–10, 2004)	All races			White[1]			Black[1]		
	Both sexes	Male	Female	Both sexes	Male	Female	Both sexes	Male	Female
ALL CAUSES	2,471,984	1,226,197	1,245,787	2,120,233	1,046,183	1,074,050	289,072	147,143	141,929
Salmonella infections (A01-A02)	44	24	20	32	20	12	9	2	7
Shigellosis and amebiasis (A03, A06)	6	4	2	5	3	2	-	-	-
Certain other intestinal infections (A04, A07-A09)	7,876	2,996	4,880	7,268	2,749	4,519	467	178	289
Tuberculosis (A16-A19)	585	375	210	332	210	122	136	87	49
Respiratory tuberculosis (A16)	449	294	155	246	154	92	106	73	33
Other tuberculosis (A17-A19)	136	81	55	86	56	30	30	14	16
Whooping cough (A37)	20	9	11	18	7	11	-	-	-
Scarlet fever and erysipelas (A38, A46)	3	2	1	2	1	1	-	-	-
Meningococcal infection (A39)	102	56	46	75	42	33	25	13	12
Septicemia (A40-A41)	35,927	16,328	19,599	28,697	13,066	15,631	6,426	2,877	3,549
Syphilis (A50-A53)	34	23	11	13	11	2	19	10	9
Acute poliomyelitis (A80)	-	-	-	-	-	-	-	-	-
Arthropod-borne viral encephalitis (A83-A84, A85.2)	2	1	1	2	1	1	-	-	-
Measles (B05)	-	-	-	-	-	-	-	-	-
Viral hepatitis (B15-B19)	7,629	5,019	2,610	6,111	4,064	2,047	1,115	728	387
Human immunodeficiency virus (HIV) disease (B20-B24)	10,285	7,406	2,879	4,339	3,489	850	5,780	3,790	1,990
Malaria (B50-B54)	5	4	1	2	2	-	3	2	1
Other and unspecified infectious and parasitic diseases and their sequelae (A00, A05, A20-A36, A42-A44, A48- A49, A54-A79, A81-A82, A85.0-A85.1, A85.8, A86-B04, B06-B09, B25-B49, B55-B99)	5,914	2,979	2,935	4,952	2,458	2,494	738	408	330
Malignant neoplasms (C00-C97)	565,469	295,259	270,210	485,893	254,124	231,769	63,954	33,019	30,935
Malignant neoplasms of lip, oral cavity and pharynx (C00-C14)	8,019	5,488	2,531	6,712	4,551	2,161	1,002	730	272
Malignant neoplasm of esophagus (C15)	13,714	10,847	2,867	12,019	9,629	2,390	1,432	1,016	416
Malignant neoplasm of stomach (C16)	11,352	6,735	4,617	8,469	5,064	3,405	2,057	1,196	861
Malignant neoplasms of colon, rectum and anus (C18-C21)	53,321	27,094	26,227	44,751	22,741	22,010	6,908	3,508	3,400
Malignant neoplasms of liver and intrahepatic bile ducts (C22)	18,213	12,302	5,911	14,377	9,631	4,746	2,466	1,748	718
Malignant neoplasm of pancreas (C25)	35,236	17,515	17,721	30,124	15,125	14,999	4,109	1,894	2,215
Malignant neoplasm of larynx (C32)	3,760	2,949	811	3,059	2,399	660	645	503	142
Malignant neoplasms of trachea, bronchus and lung (C33-C34)	158,656	88,586	70,070	138,715	76,761	61,954	16,250	9,638	6,612
Malignant melanoma of skin (C43)	8,623	5,672	2,951	8,450	5,586	2,864	120	57	63
Malignant neoplasm of breast (C50)	41,026	437	40,589	34,055	350	33,705	5,928	77	5,851
Malignant neoplasm of cervix uteri (C53)	4,008	X	4,008	3,018	X	3,018	799	X	799
Malignant neoplasms of corpus uteri and uterus, part unspecified (C54-C55)	7,675	X	7,675	6,176	X	6,176	1,286	X	1,286
Malignant neoplasm of ovary (C56)	14,362	X	14,362	12,725	X	12,725	1,200	X	1,200
Malignant neoplasm of prostate (C61)	28,472	28,472	X	23,362	23,362	X	4,588	4,588	X
Malignant neoplasms of kidney and renal pelvis (C64-C65)	12,895	8,206	4,689	11,352	7,241	4,111	1,203	743	460
Malignant neoplasm of bladder (C67)	14,036	9,791	4,245	12,853	9,107	3,746	950	516	434
Malignant neoplasms of meninges, brain and other parts of central nervous system (C70-C72)	13,724	7,686	6,038	12,568	7,049	5,519	840	455	385
Malignant neoplasms of lymphoid, hematopoietic and related tissue (C81-C96)	54,954	30,449	24,505	48,348	26,927	21,421	5,269	2,804	2,465
Hodgkin's disease (C81)	1,171	639	532	1,026	559	467	119	64	55
Non-Hodgkin's lymphoma (C82-C85)	20,369	11,004	9,365	18,476	9,984	8,492	1,360	736	624
Leukemia (C91-C95)	22,335	12,711	9,624	19,894	11,374	8,520	1,903	1,057	846
Multiple myeloma and immunoproliferative neoplasms (C88, C90)	11,020	6,057	4,963	8,900	4,978	3,922	1,882	943	939
Other and unspecified malignant neoplasms of lymphoid, hematopoietic and related tissue (C96)	59	38	21	52	32	20	5	4	1
All other and unspecified malignant neoplasms (C17, C23-C24, C26-C31, C37-C41, C44-C49, C51- C52, C57-C60, C62-C63, C66, C68-C69, C73-C80, C97)	63,423	33,030	30,393	54,760	28,601	26,159	6,902	3,546	3,356
In situ neoplasms, benign neoplasms and neoplasms of uncertain or unknown behavior (D00-D48)	14,470	7,461	7,009	12,944	6,727	6,217	1,157	554	603
Anemias (D50-D64)	5,018	2,052	2,966	3,879	1,551	2,328	1,015	451	564
Diabetes mellitus (E10-E14)	70,553	35,346	35,207	55,893	28,598	27,295	12,064	5,457	6,607
Nutritional deficiencies (E40-E64)	2,976	1,138	1,838	2,528	934	1,594	374	176	198
Malnutrition (E40-E46)	2,760	1,058	1,702	2,335	866	1,469	356	167	189
Other nutritional deficiencies (E50-E64)	216	80	136	193	68	125	18	9	9
Meningitis (G00,G03)	633	341	292	483	261	222	119	63	56
Parkinson's disease (G20-G21)	20,483	11,960	8,523	19,330	11,325	8,005	745	399	346
Alzheimer's disease (G30)	82,435	24,516	57,919	76,263	22,752	53,511	5,075	1,412	3,663
Major cardiovascular diseases (I00-I78)	804,483	388,514	415,969	689,805	332,360	357,445	95,273	46,119	49,154
Diseases of heart (I00-I09, I11, I13, I20-I51)	616,828	311,201	305,627	532,304	268,317	263,987	70,731	35,387	35,344

Table B-13. Number of Deaths from Selected Causes by Race and Sex, 2008—Continued

(Number.)

Cause of death (based on ICD-10, 2004)	American Indian and Alaskan Native[1,2]			Asian or Pacific Islander[1,3]		
	Both sexes	Male	Female	Both sexes	Male	Female
ALL CAUSES	14,776	8,163	6,613	47,903	24,708	23,195
Salmonella infections (A01-A02)	-	-	-	3	2	1
Shigellosis and amebiasis (A03, A06)	-	-	-	1	1	-
Certain other intestinal infections (A04, A07-A09)	30	16	14	111	53	58
Tuberculosis (A16-A19)	18	8	10	99	70	29
Respiratory tuberculosis (A16)	13	5	8	84	62	22
Other tuberculosis (A17-A19)	5	3	2	15	8	7
Whooping cough (A37)	2	2	-	-	-	-
Scarlet fever and erysipelas (A38, A46)	-	-	-	1	1	-
Meningococcal infection (A39)	1	1	-	1	-	1
Septicemia (A40-A41)	244	117	127	560	268	292
Syphilis (A50-A53)	-	-	-	2	2	-
Acute poliomyelitis (A80)	-	-	-	-	-	-
Arthropod-borne viral encephalitis (A83-A84, A85.2)	-	-	-	-	-	-
Measles (B05)	-	-	-	-	-	-
Viral hepatitis (B15-B19)	100	61	39	303	166	137
Human immunodeficiency virus (HIV) disease (B20-B24)	66	50	16	100	77	23
Malaria (B50-B54)	-	-	-	-	-	-
Other and unspecified infectious and parasitic diseases and their sequelae (A00, A05, A20-A36, A42-A44, A48- A49, A54-A79, A81-A82, A85.0-A85.1, A85.8, A86-B04, B06-B09, B25-B49, B55-B99)	54	26	28	170	87	83
Malignant neoplasms (C00-C97)	2,727	1,452	1,275	12,895	6,664	6,231
Malignant neoplasms of lip, oral cavity and pharynx (C00-C14)	49	39	10	256	168	88
Malignant neoplasm of esophagus (C15)	63	54	9	200	148	52
Malignant neoplasm of stomach (C16)	71	45	26	755	430	325
Malignant neoplasms of colon, rectum and anus (C18-C21)	313	157	156	1,349	688	661
Malignant neoplasms of liver and intrahepatic bile ducts (C22)	151	103	48	1,219	820	399
Malignant neoplasm of pancreas (C25)	130	67	63	873	429	444
Malignant neoplasm of larynx (C32)	18	15	3	38	32	6
Malignant neoplasms of trachea, bronchus and lung (C33-C34)	730	415	315	2,961	1,772	1,189
Malignant melanoma of skin (C43)	13	3	10	40	26	14
Malignant neoplasm of breast (C50)	173	3	170	870	7	863
Malignant neoplasm of cervix uteri (C53)	49	X	49	142	X	142
Malignant neoplasms of corpus uteri and uterus, part unspecified (C54-C55)	32	X	32	181	X	181
Malignant neoplasm of ovary (C56)	66	X	66	371	X	371
Malignant neoplasm of prostate (C61)	133	133	X	389	389	X
Malignant neoplasms of kidney and renal pelvis (C64-C65)	115	72	43	225	150	75
Malignant neoplasm of bladder (C67)	48	30	18	185	138	47
Malignant neoplasms of meninges, brain and other parts of central nervous system (C70-C72)	63	33	30	253	149	104
Malignant neoplasms of lymphoid, hematopoietic and related tissue (C81-C96)	198	114	84	1,139	604	535
Hodgkin's disease (C81)	3	3	-	23	13	10
Non-Hodgkin's lymphoma (C82-C85)	67	35	32	466	249	217
Leukemia (C91-C95)	83	47	36	455	233	222
Multiple myeloma and immunoproliferative neoplasms (C88, C90)	45	29	16	193	107	86
Other and unspecified malignant neoplasms of lymphoid, hematopoietic and related tissue (C96)	-	-	-	2	2	-
All other and unspecified malignant neoplasms (C17, C23-C24, C26-C31, C37-C41, C44-C49, C51- C52, C57-C60, C62-C63, C66, C68-C69, C73-C80, C97)	312	169	143	1,449	714	735
In situ neoplasms, benign neoplasms and neoplasms of uncertain or unknown behavior (D00-D48)	56	28	28	313	152	161
Anemias (D50-D64)	27	11	16	97	39	58
Diabetes mellitus (E10-E14)	779	388	391	1,817	903	914
Nutritional deficiencies (E40-E64)	22	7	15	52	21	31
Malnutrition (E40-E46)	21	6	15	48	19	29
Other nutritional deficiencies (E50-E64)	1	1	-	4	2	2
Meningitis (G00,G03)	11	6	5	20	11	9
Parkinson's disease (G20-G21)	69	39	30	339	197	142
Alzheimer's disease (G30)	204	62	142	893	290	603
Major cardiovascular diseases (I00-I78)	3,398	1,873	1,525	16,007	8,162	7,845
Diseases of heart (I00-I09, I11, I13, I20-I51)	2,657	1,527	1,130	11,136	5,970	5,166

Table B-13. Number of Deaths from Selected Causes by Race and Sex, 2008—*Continued*

(Number.)

Cause of death (based on ICD–10, 2004)	All races			White[1]			Black[1]		
	Both sexes	Male	Female	Both sexes	Male	Female	Both sexes	Male	Female
Acute rheumatic fever and chronic rheumatic heart diseases (I00-I09)	3,141	1,025	2,116	2,755	882	1,873	263	97	166
Hypertensive heart disease (I11)	32,391	15,201	17,190	24,115	10,996	13,119	7,471	3,786	3,685
Hypertensive heart and renal disease (I13)	2,872	1,250	1,622	1,945	834	1,111	835	375	460
Ischemic heart diseases (I20-I25)	405,309	216,248	189,061	353,839	189,354	164,485	41,898	21,407	20,491
Acute myocardial infarction (I21-I22)	133,958	72,447	61,511	117,118	63,842	53,276	13,791	6,883	6,908
Other acute ischemic heart diseases (I24)	4,252	2,219	2,033	3,580	1,859	1,721	565	302	263
Other forms of chronic ischemic heart disease (I20, I25)	267,099	141,582	125,517	233,141	123,653	109,488	27,542	14,222	13,320
Atherosclerotic cardiovascular disease, so described (I25.0)	58,625	33,341	25,284	48,490	27,425	21,065	8,608	4,952	3,656
All other forms of chronic ischemic heart disease (I20,I25.1-I25.9)	208,474	108,241	100,233	184,651	96,228	88,423	18,934	9,270	9,664
Other heart diseases (I26-I51)	173,115	77,477	95,638	149,650	66,251	83,399	20,264	9,722	10,542
Acute and subacute endocarditis (I33)	1,180	662	518	946	542	404	207	108	99
Diseases of pericardium and acute myocarditis (I30-I31, I40)	827	406	421	650	318	332	146	70	76
Heart failure (I50)	56,830	23,017	33,813	50,522	20,278	30,244	5,459	2,391	3,068
All other forms of heart disease (I26-I28, I34-I38, I42-I49, I51)	114,278	53,392	60,886	97,532	45,113	52,419	14,452	7,153	7,299
Essential hypertension and hypertensive renal disease (I10, I12, I15)	25,742	10,325	15,417	19,858	7,746	12,112	5,066	2,209	2,857
Cerebrovascular diseases (I60-I69)	134,148	53,525	80,623	113,244	44,457	68,787	16,710	7,222	9,488
Atherosclerosis (I70)	7,836	3,012	4,824	7,063	2,673	4,390	651	277	374
Other diseases of circulatory system (I71-I78)	19,929	10,451	9,478	17,336	9,167	8,169	2,115	1,024	1,091
Aortic aneurysm and dissection (I71)	11,079	6,502	4,577	9,834	5,797	4,037	924	512	412
Other diseases of arteries, arterioles and capillaries (I72-I78)	8,850	3,949	4,901	7,502	3,370	4,132	1,191	512	679
Other disorders of circulatory system (I80-I99)	4,042	1,857	2,185	3,220	1,460	1,760	760	365	395
Influenza and pneumonia (J09-J18)[1]	56,284	25,571	30,713	48,941	22,048	26,893	5,456	2,572	2,884
Influenza (J09-J11)[1]	1,722	690	1,032	1,596	630	966	83	37	46
Pneumonia (J12-J18)	54,562	24,881	29,681	47,345	21,418	25,927	5,373	2,535	2,838
Other acute lower respiratory infections (J20-J22, U04)[2]	284	126	158	237	100	137	36	19	17
Acute bronchitis and bronchiolitis (J20-J21)	235	106	129	193	81	112	31	18	13
Other and unspecified acute lower respiratory infections (J22, U04)[2,3]	49	20	29	44	19	25	5	1	4
Chronic lower respiratory diseases (J40-J47)	141,090	67,122	73,968	130,221	61,383	68,838	8,766	4,548	4,218
Bronchitis, chronic and unspecified (J40-J42)	731	311	420	658	269	389	62	37	25
Emphysema (J43)	12,448	6,467	5,981	11,595	5,945	5,650	677	404	273
Asthma (J45-J46)	3,397	1,186	2,211	2,342	755	1,587	902	375	527
Other chronic lower respiratory diseases (J44, J47)	124,514	59,158	65,356	115,626	54,414	61,212	7,125	3,732	3,393
Pneumoconioses and chemical effects (J60-J66, J68)	908	859	49	865	820	45	37	34	3
Pneumonitis due to solids and liquids (J69)	16,608	8,650	7,958	14,776	7,702	7,074	1,478	754	724
Other diseases of respiratory system (J00-J06, J30-J39, J67, J70-J98)	29,925	14,916	15,009	26,368	13,199	13,169	2,786	1,311	1,475
Peptic ulcer (K25-K28)	3,073	1,551	1,522	2,646	1,305	1,341	309	188	121
Diseases of appendix (K35-K38)	418	242	176	347	197	150	56	37	19
Hernia (K40-K46)	1,674	717	957	1,502	634	868	146	73	73
Chronic liver disease and cirrhosis (K70, K73-K74)	29,963	19,646	10,317	26,275	17,288	8,987	2,506	1,680	826
Alcoholic liver disease (K70)	14,864	10,817	4,047	12,955	9,551	3,404	1,200	820	380
Other chronic liver disease and cirrhosis (K73-K74)	15,099	8,829	6,270	13,320	7,737	5,583	1,306	860	446
Cholelithiasis and other disorders of gall bladder (K80-K82)	3,417	1,585	1,832	2,990	1,381	1,609	308	143	165
Nephritis, nephrotic syndrome and nephrosis (N00-N07, N17-N19, N25-N27)	48,237	23,533	24,704	38,352	18,992	19,360	8,619	3,919	4,700
Acute and rapidly progressive nephritic and nephrotic syndrome (N00-N01,N04)	160	73	87	129	61	68	28	9	19
Chronic glomerulonephritis, nephritis and nephropathy not specified as acute or chronic, and renal sclerosis unspecified (N02-N03, N05-N07, N26)	4,109	1,970	2,139	3,312	1,608	1,704	686	310	376
Renal failure (N17-N19)	43,935	21,477	22,458	34,884	17,313	17,571	7,900	3,598	4,302
Other disorders of kidney (N25, N27)	33	13	20	27	10	17	5	2	3
Infections of kidney (N10-N12,N13.6,N15.1)	627	179	448	533	147	386	67	24	43
Hyperplasia of prostate (N40)	502	502	X	458	458	X	37	37	X
Inflammatory diseases of female pelvic organs (N70-N76)	136	X	136	112	X	112	19	X	19
Pregnancy, childbirth and the puerperium (O00-O99)	795	X	795	499	X	499	252	X	252
Pregnancy with abortive outcome (O00-O07)	34	X	34	18	X	18	15	X	15
Other complications of pregnancy, childbirth and the puerperium (O10-O99)	761	X	761	481	X	481	237	X	237
Certain conditions originating in the perinatal period (P00-P96)	13,933	7,919	6,014	8,455	4,831	3,624	4,844	2,731	2,113
Congenital malformations, deformations and chromosomal abnormalities (Q00-Q99)	10,288	5,395	4,893	8,156	4,271	3,885	1,689	881	808
Symptoms, signs and abnormal clinical and laboratory findings, not elsewhere classified (R00-R99)	38,522	16,803	21,719	32,544	13,783	18,761	5,235	2,640	2,595
All other diseases (Residual)	252,490	101,521	150,969	219,962	87,775	132,187	27,092	11,315	15,777

Table B-13. Number of Deaths from Selected Causes by Race and Sex, 2008—Continued

(Number.)

Cause of death (based on ICD–10, 2004)	American Indian and Alaskan Native[1,2]			Asian or Pacific Islander[1,3]		
	Both sexes	Male	Female	Both sexes	Male	Female
Acute rheumatic fever and chronic rheumatic heart diseases (I00-I09)	20	12	8	103	34	69
Hypertensive heart disease (I11)	139	83	56	666	336	330
Hypertensive heart and renal disease (I13)	13	6	7	79	35	44
Ischemic heart diseases (I20-I25)	1,739	1,058	681	7,833	4,429	3,404
Acute myocardial infarction (I21-I22)	601	377	224	2,448	1,345	1,103
Other acute ischemic heart diseases (I24)	59	36	23	48	22	26
Other forms of chronic ischemic heart disease (I20, I25)	1,079	645	434	5,337	3,062	2,275
Atherosclerotic cardiovascular disease, so described (I25.0)	331	214	117	1,196	750	446
All other forms of chronic ischemic heart disease (I20,I25.1-I25.9)	748	431	317	4,141	2,312	1,829
Other heart diseases (I26-I51)	746	368	378	2,455	1,136	1,319
Acute and subacute endocarditis (I33)	12	5	7	15	7	8
Diseases of pericardium and acute myocarditis (I30-I31, I40)	8	5	3	23	13	10
Heart failure (I50)	235	97	138	614	251	363
All other forms of heart disease (I26-I28, I34-I38, I42-I49, I51)	491	261	230	1,803	865	938
Essential hypertension and hypertensive renal disease (I10, I12, I15)	111	56	55	707	314	393
Cerebrovascular diseases (I60-I69)	517	234	283	3,677	1,612	2,065
Atherosclerosis (I70)	33	15	18	89	47	42
Other diseases of circulatory system (I71-I78)	80	41	39	398	219	179
Aortic aneurysm and dissection (I71)	42	23	19	279	170	109
Other diseases of arteries, arterioles and capillaries (I72-I78)	38	18	20	119	49	70
Other disorders of circulatory system (I80-I99)	21	12	9	41	20	21
Influenza and pneumonia (J09-J18)[1]	379	186	193	1,508	765	743
Influenza (J09-J11)[1]	16	9	7	27	14	13
Pneumonia (J12-J18)	363	177	186	1,481	751	730
Other acute lower respiratory infections (J20-J22, U04)[2]	3	1	2	8	6	2
Acute bronchitis and bronchiolitis (J20-J21)	3	1	2	8	6	2
Other and unspecified acute lower respiratory infections (J22, U04)[2,3]	-	-	-	-	-	-
Chronic lower respiratory diseases (J40-J47)	619	308	311	1,484	883	601
Bronchitis, chronic and unspecified (J40-J42)	3	2	1	8	3	5
Emphysema (J43)	55	31	24	121	87	34
Asthma (J45-J46)	22	10	12	131	46	85
Other chronic lower respiratory diseases (J44, J47)	539	265	274	1,224	747	477
Pneumoconioses and chemical effects (J60-J66, J68)	3	2	1	3	3	-
Pneumonitis due to solids and liquids (J69)	76	39	37	278	155	123
Other diseases of respiratory system (J00-J06, J30-J39, J67, J70-J98)	209	111	98	562	295	267
Peptic ulcer (K25-K28)	25	14	11	93	44	49
Diseases of appendix (K35-K38)	6	5	1	9	3	6
Hernia (K40-K46)	11	3	8	15	7	8
Chronic liver disease and cirrhosis (K70, K73-K74)	742	406	336	440	272	168
Alcoholic liver disease (K70)	527	295	232	182	151	31
Other chronic liver disease and cirrhosis (K73-K74)	215	111	104	258	121	137
Cholelithiasis and other disorders of gallbladder (K80-K82)	26	9	17	93	52	41
Nephritis, nephrotic syndrome and nephrosis (N00-N07, N17-N19, N25-N27)	338	155	183	928	467	461
Acute and rapidly progressive nephritic and nephrotic syndrome (N00-N01,N04)	1	1	-	2	2	-
Chronic glomerulonephritis, nephritis and nephropathy not specified as acute or chronic, and renal sclerosis unspecified (N02-N03, N05-N07, N26)	21	10	11	90	42	48
Renal failure (N17-N19)	315	143	172	836	423	413
Other disorders of kidney (N25, N27)	1	1	-	-	-	-
Infections of kidney (N10-N12,N13.6,N15.1)	7	2	5	20	6	14
Hyperplasia of prostate (N40)	1	1	X	6	6	X
Inflammatory diseases of female pelvic organs (N70-N76)	2	X	2	3	X	3
Pregnancy, childbirth and the puerperium (O00-O99)	10	X	10	34	X	34
Pregnancy with abortive outcome (O00-O07)	-	X	-	1	X	1
Other complications of pregnancy, childbirth and the puerperium (O10-O99)	10	X	10	33	X	33
Certain conditions originating in the perinatal period(P00-P96)	139	79	60	495	278	217
Congenital malformations, deformations andchromosomal abnormalities (Q00-Q99)	117	69	48	326	174	152
Symptoms, signs and abnormal clinical and laboratory findings, not elsewhere classified (R00-R99)	258	136	122	485	244	241
All other diseases (Residual)	1,536	752	784	3,900	1,679	2,221

Table B-13. Number of Deaths from Selected Causes by Race and Sex, 2008—Continued

(Number.)

Cause of death (based on ICD–10, 2004)	All races			White[1]			Black[1]		
	Both sexes	Male	Female	Both sexes	Male	Female	Both sexes	Male	Female
Accidents (unintentional injuries) (V01-X59, Y85-Y86)	121,902	78,378	43,524	105,715	67,471	38,244	12,447	8,453	3,994
Transport accidents (V01-V99, Y85)	42,709	30,650	12,059	35,772	25,732	10,040	5,206	3,789	1,417
Motor vehicle accidents (V02-V04, V09.0, V09.2, V12-V14, V19.0-V19.2, V19.4-V19.6, V20-V79, V80.3-V80.5, V81.0-V81.1, V82.0-V82.1,V83-V86, V87.0-V87.8, V88.0-V88.8, V89.0, V89.2)	39,790	28,291	11,499	33,293	23,721	9,572	4,872	3,521	1,351
Other land transport accidents (V01,V05-V06, V09.1, V09.3-V09.9, V10-V11, V15-V18, V19.3, V19.8-V19.9, V80.0-V80.2, V80.6-V80.9, V81.2-V81.9, V82.2-V82.9, V87.9, V88.9, V89.1, V89.3, V89.9)	1,140	907	233	925	739	186	173	137	36
Water, air and space, and other and unspecified transport accidents and their sequelae (V90-V99, Y85)	1,779	1,452	327	1,554	1,272	282	161	131	30
Nontransport accidents (W00-X59, Y86)	79,193	47,728	31,465	69,943	41,739	28,204	7,241	4,664	2,577
Falls (W00-W19)	24,013	12,318	11,695	22,351	11,335	11,016	1,036	603	433
Accidental discharge of firearms (W32-W34)	592	510	82	479	411	68	94	85	9
Accidental drowning and submersion (W65-W74)	3,548	2,726	822	2,808	2,149	659	548	433	115
Accidental exposure to smoke, fire and flames (X00-X09)	2,912	1,705	1,207	2,231	1,303	928	611	362	249
Accidental poisoning and exposure to noxious substances (X40-X49)	31,116	20,533	10,583	27,430	18,063	9,367	3,001	1,995	1,006
Other and unspecified nontransport accidents and their sequelae (W20-W31, W35-W64, W75-W99, X10-X39, X50-X59, Y86)	17,012	9,936	7,076	14,644	8,478	6,166	1,951	1,186	765
Intentional self-harm (suicide) (*U03, X60-X84, Y87.0)	36,035	28,450	7,585	32,644	25,801	6,843	2,106	1,759	347
Intentional self-harm (suicide) by discharge of firearms (X72-X74)	18,223	15,931	2,292	16,840	14,683	2,157	1,049	952	97
Intentional self-harm (suicide) by other and unspecified means and their sequelae (*U03, X60-X71, X75-X84, Y87.0)	17,812	12,519	5,293	15,804	11,118	4,686	1,057	807	250
Assault (homicide) (*U01-*U02, X85-Y09, Y87.1)	17,826	14,135	3,691	8,893	6,556	2,337	8,335	7,148	1,187
Assault (homicide) by discharge of firearms (*U01.4, X93-X95)	12,179	10,361	1,818	5,305	4,198	1,107	6,569	5,925	644
Assault (homicide) by other and unspecified means and their sequelae (*U01.0-*U01.3, *U01.5-*U01.9, *U02, X85-X92, X96-Y09, Y87.1)	5,647	3,774	1,873	3,588	2,358	1,230	1,766	1,223	543
Legal intervention (Y35, Y89.0)	381	369	12	245	237	8	120	118	2
Events of undetermined intent (Y10-Y34, Y87.2,Y89.9)	5,051	3,144	1,907	4,237	2,594	1,643	669	454	215
Discharge of firearms, undetermined intent (Y22-Y24)	273	220	53	225	179	46	41	34	7
Other and unspecified events of undetermined intent and their sequelae (Y10-Y21, Y25-Y34, Y87.2, Y89.9)	4,778	2,924	1,854	4,012	2,415	1,597	628	420	208
Operations of war and their sequelae (Y36, Y89.1)	31	31	-	25	25	-	4	4	-
Complications of medical and surgical care (Y40-Y84, Y88)	2,590	1,183	1,407	2,149	970	1,179	399	191	208
Enterocolitis due to Clostridium difficile (A04.7)[4]	7,476	2,847	4,629	6,899	2,619	4,280	445	165	280
Drug-induced deaths[5,6]	38,649	23,928	14,721	34,237	21,093	13,144	3,662	2,381	1,281
Alcohol-induced deaths[5,7]	24,189	18,152	6,037	20,783	15,689	5,094	2,279	1,692	587
Injury by firearms[5,8]	31,593	27,336	4,257	23,065	19,679	3,386	7,847	7,088	759

Table B-13. Number of Deaths from Selected Causes by Race and Sex, 2008—Continued

(Number.)

Cause of death (based on ICD-10, 2004)	American Indian and Alaskan Native[1,2]			Asian or Pacific Islander[1,3]		
	Both sexes	Male	Female	Both sexes	Male	Female
Accidents (unintentional injuries) (V01-X59, Y85-Y86)	1,682	1,158	524	2,058	1,296	762
Transport accidents (V01-V99, Y85)	759	508	251	972	621	351
Motor vehicle accidents (V02-V04, V09.0, V09.2, V12-V14, V19.0-V19.2, V19.4-V19.6, V20-V79, V80.3-V80.5, V81.0-V81.1, V82.0-V82.1,V83- V86, V87.0-V87.8, V88.0-V88.8, V89.0, V89.2)	716	470	246	909	579	330
Other land transport accidents (V01,V05-V06, V09.1, V09.3-V09.9, V10-V11, V15-V18, V19.3, V19.8-V19.9, V80.0-V80.2, V80.6-V80.9, V81.2- V81.9, V82.2-V82.9, V87.9, V88.9, V89.1, V89.3, V89.9)	22	19	3	20	12	8
Water, air and space, and other and unspecified transport accidents and their sequelae (V90-V99, Y85)	21	19	2	43	30	13
Nontransport accidents (W00-X59, Y86)	923	650	273	1,086	675	411
Falls (W00-W19)	142	93	49	484	287	197
Accidental discharge of firearms (W32-W34)	16	11	5	3	3	-
Accidental drowning and submersion (W65-W74)	64	53	11	128	91	37
Accidental exposure to smoke, fire and flames (X00-X09)	36	23	13	34	17	17
Accidental poisoning and exposure to noxious substances (X40-X49)	470	325	145	215	150	65
Other and unspecified nontransport accidents and their sequelae (W20-W31, W35-W64, W75-W99, X10-X39, X50-X59, Y86)	195	145	50	222	127	95
Intentional self-harm (suicide) (*U03, X60-X84, Y87.0)	409	308	101	876	582	294
Intentional self-harm (suicide) by discharge of firearms (X72-X74)	153	136	17	181	160	21
Intentional self-harm (suicide) by other and unspecified means and their sequelae (*U03, X60-X71, X75-X84, Y87.0)	256	172	84	695	422	273
Assault (homicide) (*U01-*U02, X85-Y09, Y87.1)	255	192	63	343	239	104
Assault (homicide) by discharge of firearms (*U01.4, X93-X95)	97	74	23	208	164	44
Assault (homicide) by other and unspecified means and their sequelae (*U01.0-*U01.3, *U01.5-*U01.9, *U02, X85-X92, X96-Y09, Y87.1)	158	118	40	135	75	60
Legal intervention (Y35, Y89.0)	10	9	1	6	5	1
Events of undetermined intent (Y10-Y34, Y87.2,Y89.9)	70	51	19	75	45	30
Discharge of firearms, undetermined intent (Y22-Y24)	3	3	-	4	4	-
Other and unspecified events of undetermined intent and their sequelae (Y10-Y21, Y25-Y34, Y87.2, Y89.9)	67	48	19	71	41	30
Operations of war and their sequelae (Y36, Y89.1)	-	-	-	2	2	-
Complications of medical and surgical care (Y40-Y84, Y88)	14	8	6	28	14	14
Enterocolitis due to Clostridium difficile (A04.7)[4]	28	14	14	104	49	55
Drug-induced deaths[5,6]	451	273	178	299	181	118
Alcohol-induced deaths[5,7]	853	542	311	274	229	45
Injury by firearms[5,8]	279	233	46	402	336	66

X = Category not applicable.
- = Quantity zero.
[1]Race categories are consistent with the 1977 Office of Management and Budget (OMB) standards.
[2]Includes Aleuts and Eskimos.
[3]Includes Chinese, Filipino, Hawaiian, Japanese, and Other Asian and Pacific Islander.
[4]Included in certain other intestinal infections (A04, A07–A09).
[5]Included in selected categories above.
[6]Includes ICD-10 codes D52.1,D59.0,D59.2,D61.1,D64.2,E06.4,E16.0,E23.1,E24.2,E27.3,E66.1,F11.0-F11.5,F11.7-F11.9,F12.0-F12.5,F12.7-F12.9,F13.0-F13.5,F13.7-F13.9,F14.0-F14.5,F14.7-F14.9,F15.0-F15.5,F15.7-F15.9,F16.0-F16.5,F16.7F16.9,F17.0,F17.3-F17.5,F17.7-F17.9,F18.0-F18.5,F18.7-F18.9,F19.0-F19.5,F19.7-F19.9,G21.1,G24.0,G25.1,G25.4,G25.6,G44.4, G62.0,G72.0,I95.2,J70.2-J70.4,K85.3,L10.5,L27.0-L27.1,M10.2,M32.0,M80.4,M81.4,M83.5,M87.1,R50.2,R78.1-R78.5,X40X44,X60-X64,X85, and Y10-Y14.
[7]Includes ICD-10 codes E24.4,F10,G31.2,G62.1,G72.1,I42.6,K29.2,K70,K85.2,K86.0,R78.0,X45,X65, and Y15.
[8]Includes ICD-10 codes *U01.4,W32-W34,X72-X74,X93-X95,Y22-Y24, and Y35.0.

NOTE: Complete confirmation of deaths from selected causes of death, considered to be of public health concern, were not provided by the following states—Massachusetts, North Carolina, and West Virginia.

Table B-14. Death Rates for 113 Selected Causes by Race and Sex, 2008

(Rates per 100,000 population in specified group.)

Cause of death (based on ICD–10, 2004)	All races			White			Black		
	Both sexes	Male	Female	Both sexes	Male	Female	Both sexes	Male	Female
ALL CAUSES	813.0	817.9	808.2	864.6	860.3	868.7	716.1	762.7	673.5
Salmonella infections (A01-A02)	0.0	0.0	0.0	0.0	0.0	*	*	*	*
Shigellosis and amebiasis (A03, A06)	*	*	*	*	*	*	*	*	*
Certain other intestinal infections (A04, A07-A09)	2.6	2.0	3.2	3.0	2.3	3.7	1.2	0.9	1.4
Tuberculosis (A16-A19)	0.2	0.3	0.1	0.1	0.2	0.1	0.3	0.5	0.2
Respiratory tuberculosis (A16)	0.1	0.2	0.1	0.1	0.1	0.1	0.3	0.4	0.2
Other tuberculosis (A17-A19)	0.0	0.1	0.0	0.0	0.0	0.0	0.1	*	*
Whooping cough (A37)	0.0	*	*	*	*	*	*	*	*
Scarlet fever and erysipelas (A38, A46)	*	*	*	*	*	*	*	*	*
Meningococcal infection (A39)	0.0	0.0	0.0	0.0	0.0	0.0	0.1	*	*
Septicemia (A40-A41)	11.8	10.9	12.7	11.7	10.7	12.6	15.9	14.9	16.8
Syphilis (A50-A53)	0.0	0.0	*	*	*	*	*	*	*
Acute poliomyelitis (A80)	*	*	*	*	*	*	*	*	*
Arthropod-borne viral encephalitis (A83-A84, A85.2)	*	*	*	*	*	*	*	*	*
Measles (B05)	*	*	*	*	*	*	*	*	*
Viral hepatitis (B15-B19)	2.5	3.3	1.7	2.5	3.3	1.7	2.8	3.8	1.8
Human immunodeficiency virus (HIV) disease (B20-B24)	3.4	4.9	1.9	1.8	2.9	0.7	14.3	19.6	9.4
Malaria (B50-B54)	*	*	*	*	*	*	*	*	*
Other and unspecified infectious and parasitic diseases and their sequelae (A00, A05, A20-A36, A42-A44, A48- A49, A54-A79, A81-A82, A85.0-A85.1, A85.8, A86-B04, B06-B09, B25-B49, B55-B99)	1.9	2.0	1.9	2.0	2.0	2.0	1.8	2.1	1.6
Malignant neoplasms (C00-C97)	186.0	196.9	175.3	198.1	209.0	187.5	158.4	171.1	146.8
Malignant neoplasms of lip, oral cavity and pharynx (C00-C14)	2.6	3.7	1.6	2.7	3.7	1.7	2.5	3.8	1.3
Malignant neoplasm of esophagus (C15)	4.5	7.2	1.9	4.9	7.9	1.9	3.5	5.3	2.0
Malignant neoplasm of stomach (C16)	3.7	4.5	3.0	3.5	4.2	2.8	5.1	6.2	4.1
Malignant neoplasms of colon, rectum and anus (C18-C21)	17.5	18.1	17.0	18.2	18.7	17.8	17.1	18.2	16.1
Malignant neoplasms of liver and intrahepatic bileducts (C22)	6.0	8.2	3.8	5.9	7.9	3.8	6.1	9.1	3.4
Malignant neoplasm of pancreas (C25)	11.6	11.7	11.5	12.3	12.4	12.1	10.2	9.8	10.5
Malignant neoplasm of larynx (C32)	1.2	2.0	0.5	1.2	2.0	0.5	1.6	2.6	0.7
Malignant neoplasms of trachea, bronchus and lung (C33-C34)	52.2	59.1	45.5	56.6	63.1	50.1	40.3	50.0	31.4
Malignant melanoma of skin (C43)	2.8	3.8	1.9	3.4	4.6	2.3	0.3	0.3	0.3
Malignant neoplasm of breast (C50)	13.5	0.3	26.3	13.9	0.3	27.3	14.7	0.4	27.8
Malignant neoplasm of cervix uteri (C53)	1.3	X	2.6	1.2	X	2.4	2.0	X	3.8
Malignant neoplasms of corpus uteri and uterus, part unspecified (C54-C55)	2.5	X	5.0	2.5	X	5.0	3.2	X	6.1
Malignant neoplasm of ovary (C56)	4.7	X	9.3	5.2	X	10.3	3.0	X	5.7
Malignant neoplasm of prostate (C61)	9.4	19.0	X	9.5	19.2	X	11.4	23.8	X
Malignant neoplasms of kidney and renal pelvis (C64-C65)	4.2	5.5	3.0	4.6	6.0	3.3	3.0	3.9	2.2
Malignant neoplasm of bladder (C67)	4.6	6.5	2.8	5.2	7.5	3.0	2.4	2.7	2.1
Malignant neoplasms of meninges, brain and other parts of central nervous system (C70-C72)	4.5	5.1	3.9	5.1	5.8	4.5	2.1	2.4	1.8
Malignant neoplasms of lymphoid, hematopoietic and related tissue (C81-C96)	18.1	20.3	15.9	19.7	22.1	17.3	13.1	14.5	11.7
Hodgkin's disease (C81)	0.4	0.4	0.3	0.4	0.5	0.4	0.3	0.3	0.3
Non-Hodgkin's lymphoma (C82-C85)	6.7	7.3	6.1	7.5	8.2	6.9	3.4	3.8	3.0
Leukemia (C91-C95)	7.3	8.5	6.2	8.1	9.4	6.9	4.7	5.5	4.0
Multiple myeloma and immunoproliferative neoplasms (C88, C90)	3.6	4.0	3.2	3.6	4.1	3.2	4.7	4.9	4.5
Other and unspecified malignant neoplasms of lymphoid, hematopoietic and related tissue (C96)	0.0	0.0	0.0	0.0	0.0	0.0	*	*	*
All other and unspecified malignant neoplasms (C17, C23-C24, C26-C31, C37-C41, C44-C49, C51- C52, C57-C60, C62-C63, C66, C68-C69, C73-C80, C97)	20.9	22.0	19.7	22.3	23.5	21.2	17.1	18.4	15.9
In situ neoplasms, benign neoplasms and neoplasms of uncertain or unknown behavior (D00-D48)	4.8	5.0	4.5	5.3	5.5	5.0	2.9	2.9	2.9
Anemias (D50-D64)	1.7	1.4	1.9	1.6	1.3	1.9	2.5	2.3	2.7
Diabetes mellitus (E10-E14)	23.2	23.6	22.8	22.8	23.5	22.1	29.9	28.3	31.4
Nutritional deficiencies (E40-E64)	1.0	0.8	1.2	1.0	0.8	1.3	0.9	0.9	0.9
Malnutrition (E40-E46)	0.9	0.7	1.1	1.0	0.7	1.2	0.9	0.9	0.9
Other nutritional deficiencies (E50-E64)	0.1	0.1	0.1	0.1	0.1	0.1	*	*	*
Meningitis (G00,G03)	0.2	0.2	0.2	0.2	0.2	0.2	0.3	0.3	0.3
Parkinson's disease (G20-G21)	6.7	8.0	5.5	7.9	9.3	6.5	1.8	2.1	1.6
Alzheimer's disease (G30)	27.1	16.4	37.6	31.1	18.7	43.3	12.6	7.3	17.4

Table B-14. Death Rates for 113 Selected Causes by Race and Sex, 2008—Continued

(Rates per 100,000 population in specified group.)

Cause of death (based on ICD-10, 2004)	American Indian and Alaskan Native[1]			Asian or Pacific Islander[2]		
	Both sexes	Male	Female	Both sexes	Male	Female
ALL CAUSES	431.8	477.6	386.1	318.7	337.7	300.7
Salmonella infections (A01-A02)	*	*	*	*	*	*
Shigellosis and amebiasis (A03, A06)	*	*	*	*	*	*
Certain other intestinal infections (A04, A07-A09)	0.9	*	*	0.7	0.7	0.8
Tuberculosis (A16-A19)	*	*	*	0.7	1.0	0.4
Respiratory tuberculosis (A16)	*	*	*	0.6	0.8	0.3
Other tuberculosis (A17-A19)	*	*	*	*	*	*
Whooping cough (A37)	*	*	*	*	*	*
Scarlet fever and erysipelas (A38, A46)	*	*	*	*	*	*
Meningococcal infection (A39)	*	*	*	*	*	*
Septicemia (A40-A41)	7.1	6.8	7.4	3.7	3.7	3.8
Syphilis (A50-A53)	*	*	*	*	*	*
Acute poliomyelitis (A80)	*	*	*	*	*	*
Arthropod-borne viral encephalitis (A83-A84, A85.2)	*	*	*	*	*	*
Measles (B05)	*	*	*	*	*	*
Viral hepatitis (B15-B19)	2.9	3.6	2.3	2.0	2.3	1.8
Human immunodeficiency virus (HIV) disease (B20-B24)	1.9	2.9	*	0.7	1.1	0.3
Malaria (B50-B54)	*	*	*	*	*	*
Other and unspecified infectious and parasitic diseases and their sequelae (A00, A05, A20-A36, A42-A44, A48- A49, A54-A79, A81-A82, A85.0-A85.1, A85.8, A86-B04, B06-B09, B25-B49, B55-B99)	1.6	1.5	1.6	1.1	1.2	1.1
Malignant neoplasms (C00-C97)	79.7	84.9	74.4	85.8	91.1	80.8
Malignant neoplasms of lip, oral cavity and pharynx (C00-C14)	1.4	2.3	*	1.7	2.3	1.1
Malignant neoplasm of esophagus (C15)	1.8	3.2	*	1.3	2.0	0.7
Malignant neoplasm of stomach (C16)	2.1	2.6	1.5	5.0	5.9	4.2
Malignant neoplasms of colon, rectum and anus (C18-C21)	9.1	9.2	9.1	9.0	9.4	8.6
Malignant neoplasms of liver and intrahepatic bileducts (C22)	4.4	6.0	2.8	8.1	11.2	5.2
Malignant neoplasm of pancreas (C25)	3.8	3.9	3.7	5.8	5.9	5.8
Malignant neoplasm of larynx (C32)	*	*	*	0.3	0.4	*
Malignant neoplasms of trachea, bronchus and lung (C33-C34)	21.3	24.3	18.4	19.7	24.2	15.4
Malignant melanoma of skin (C43)	*	*	*	0.3	0.4	*
Malignant neoplasm of breast (C50)	5.1	*	9.9	5.8	*	11.2
Malignant neoplasm of cervix uteri (C53)	1.4	X	2.9	0.9	X	1.8
Malignant neoplasms of corpus uteri and uterus, part unspecified (C54-C55)	0.9	X	1.9	1.2	X	2.3
Malignant neoplasm of ovary (C56)	1.9	X	3.9	2.5	X	4.8
Malignant neoplasm of prostate (C61)	3.9	7.8	X	2.6	5.3	X
Malignant neoplasms of kidney and renal pelvis (C64-C65)	3.4	4.2	2.5	1.5	2.0	1.0
Malignant neoplasm of bladder (C67)	1.4	1.8	*	1.2	1.9	0.6
Malignant neoplasms of meninges, brain and other parts of central nervous system (C70-C72)	1.8	1.9	1.8	1.7	2.0	1.3
Malignant neoplasms of lymphoid, hematopoietic and related tissue (C81-C96)	5.8	6.7	4.9	7.6	8.3	6.9
Hodgkin's disease (C81)	*	*	*	0.2	*	*
Non-Hodgkin's lymphoma (C82-C85)	2.0	2.0	1.9	3.1	3.4	2.8
Leukemia (C91-C95)	2.4	2.7	2.1	3.0	3.2	2.9
Multiple myeloma and immunoproliferative neoplasms (C88, C90)	1.3	1.7	*	1.3	1.5	1.1
Other and unspecified malignant neoplasms of lymphoid, hematopoietic and related tissue (C96)	*	*	*	*	*	*
All other and unspecified malignant neoplasms (C17, C23-C24, C26-C31, C37-C41, C44-C49, C51- C52, C57-C60, C62-C63, C66, C68-C69, C73-C80, C97)	9.1	9.9	8.3	9.6	9.8	9.5
In situ neoplasms, benign neoplasms and neoplasms of uncertain or unknown behavior (D00-D48)	1.6	1.6	1.6	2.1	2.1	2.1
Anemias (D50-D64)	0.8	*	*	0.6	0.5	0.8
Diabetes mellitus (E10-E14)	22.8	22.7	22.8	12.1	12.3	11.8
Nutritional deficiencies (E40-E64)	0.6	*	*	0.3	0.3	0.4
Malnutrition (E40-E46)	0.6	*	*	0.3	*	0.4
Other nutritional deficiencies (E50-E64)	*	*	*	*	*	*
Meningitis (G00,G03)	*	*	*	0.1	*	*
Parkinson's disease (G20-G21)	2.0	2.3	1.8	2.3	2.7	1.8
Alzheimer's disease (G30)	6.0	3.6	8.3	5.9	4.0	7.8

Table B-14. Death Rates for 113 Selected Causes by Race and Sex, 2008—*Continued*

(Rates per 100,000 population in specified group.)

Cause of death (based on ICD–10, 2004)	All races			White			Black		
	Both sexes	Male	Female	Both sexes	Male	Female	Both sexes	Male	Female
Major cardiovascular diseases (I00-I78)	264.6	259.1	269.9	281.3	273.3	289.1	236.0	239.1	233.2
Diseases of heart (I00-I09, I11, I13, I20-I51)	202.9	207.6	198.3	217.1	220.6	213.5	175.2	183.4	167.7
Acute rheumatic fever and chronic rheumatic heart diseases (I00-I09)	1.0	0.7	1.4	1.1	0.7	1.5	0.7	0.5	0.8
Hypertensive heart disease (I11)	10.7	10.1	11.2	9.8	9.0	10.6	18.5	19.6	17.5
Hypertensive heart and renal disease (I13)	0.9	0.8	1.1	0.8	0.7	0.9	2.1	1.9	2.2
Ischemic heart diseases (I20-I25)	133.3	144.2	122.7	144.3	155.7	133.0	103.8	111.0	97.2
Acute myocardial infarction (I21-I22)	44.1	48.3	39.9	47.8	52.5	43.1	34.2	35.7	32.8
Other acute ischemic heart diseases (I24)	1.4	1.5	1.3	1.5	1.5	1.4	1.4	1.6	1.2
Other forms of chronic ischemic heart disease (I20, I25)	87.8	94.4	81.4	95.1	101.7	88.6	68.2	73.7	63.2
Atherosclerotic cardiovascular disease, so described (I25.0)	19.3	22.2	16.4	19.8	22.6	17.0	21.3	25.7	17.3
All other forms of chronic ischemic heart disease (I20,I25.1-I25.9)	68.6	72.2	65.0	75.3	79.1	71.5	46.9	48.0	45.9
Other heart diseases (I26-I51)	56.9	51.7	62.0	61.0	54.5	67.5	50.2	50.4	50.0
Acute and subacute endocarditis (I33)	0.4	0.4	0.3	0.4	0.4	0.3	0.5	0.6	0.5
Diseases of pericardium and acute myocarditis (I30-I31, I40)	0.3	0.3	0.3	0.3	0.3	0.3	0.4	0.4	0.4
Heart failure (I50)	18.7	15.4	21.9	20.6	16.7	24.5	13.5	12.4	14.6
All other forms of heart disease (I26-I28, I34-I38, I42-I49, I51)	37.6	35.6	39.5	39.8	37.1	42.4	35.8	37.1	34.6
Essential hypertension and hypertensive renal disease (I10, I12, I15)	8.5	6.9	10.0	8.1	6.4	9.8	12.6	11.5	13.6
Cerebrovascular diseases (I60-I69)	44.1	35.7	52.3	46.2	36.6	55.6	41.4	37.4	45.0
Atherosclerosis (I70)	2.6	2.0	3.1	2.9	2.2	3.6	1.6	1.4	1.8
Other diseases of circulatory system (I71-I78)	6.6	7.0	6.1	7.1	7.5	6.6	5.2	5.3	5.2
Aortic aneurysm and dissection (I71)	3.6	4.3	3.0	4.0	4.8	3.3	2.3	2.7	2.0
Other diseases of arteries, arterioles and capillaries (I72-I78)	2.9	2.6	3.2	3.1	2.8	3.3	3.0	2.7	3.2
Other disorders of circulatory system (I80-I99)	1.3	1.2	1.4	1.3	1.2	1.4	1.9	1.9	1.9
Influenza and pneumonia (J09-J18)[1]	18.5	17.1	19.9	20.0	18.1	21.8	13.5	13.3	13.7
Influenza (J09-J11)[1]	0.6	0.5	0.7	0.7	0.5	0.8	0.2	0.2	0.2
Pneumonia (J12-J18)	17.9	16.6	19.3	19.3	17.6	21.0	13.3	13.1	13.5
Other acute lower respiratory infections (J20-J22, U04)[2]	0.1	0.1	0.1	0.1	0.1	0.1	0.1	*	*
Acute bronchitis and bronchiolitis (J20-J21)	0.1	0.1	0.1	0.1	0.1	0.1	0.1	*	*
Other and unspecified acute lower respiratory infections (J22, U04)[2,3]	0.0	0.0	0.0	0.0	*	0.0	*	*	*
Chronic lower respiratory diseases (J40-J47)	46.4	44.8	48.0	53.1	50.5	55.7	21.7	23.6	20.0
Bronchitis, chronic and unspecified (J40-J42)	0.2	0.2	0.3	0.3	0.2	0.3	0.2	0.2	0.1
Emphysema (J43)	4.1	4.3	3.9	4.7	4.9	4.6	1.7	2.1	1.3
Asthma (J45-J46)	1.1	0.8	1.4	1.0	0.6	1.3	2.2	1.9	2.5
Other chronic lower respiratory diseases (J44, J47)	41.0	39.5	42.4	47.1	44.7	49.5	17.7	19.3	16.1
Pneumoconioses and chemical effects (J60-J66, J68)	0.3	0.6	0.0	0.4	0.7	0.0	0.1	0.2	*
Pneumonitis due to solids and liquids (J69)	5.5	5.8	5.2	6.0	6.3	5.7	3.7	3.9	3.4
Other diseases of respiratory system (J00-J06, J30-J39, J67, J70-J98)	9.8	9.9	9.7	10.8	10.9	10.7	6.9	6.8	7.0
Peptic ulcer (K25-K28)	1.0	1.0	1.0	1.1	1.1	1.1	0.8	1.0	0.6
Diseases of appendix (K35-K38)	0.1	0.2	0.1	0.1	0.2	0.1	0.1	0.2	*
Hernia (K40-K46)	0.6	0.5	0.6	0.6	0.5	0.7	0.4	0.4	0.3
Chronic liver disease and cirrhosis (K70, K73-K74)	9.9	13.1	6.7	10.7	14.2	7.3	6.2	8.7	3.9
Alcoholic liver disease (K70)	4.9	7.2	2.6	5.3	7.9	2.8	3.0	4.3	1.8
Other chronic liver disease and cirrhosis (K73-K74)	5.0	5.9	4.1	5.4	6.4	4.5	3.2	4.5	2.1
Cholelithiasis and other disorders of gallbladder (K80-K82)	1.1	1.1	1.2	1.2	1.1	1.3	0.8	0.7	0.8
Nephritis, nephrotic syndrome and nephrosis (N00-N07, N17-N19, N25-N27)	15.9	15.7	16.0	15.6	15.6	15.7	21.4	20.3	22.3
Acute and rapidly progressive nephritic and nephrotic syndrome (N00-N01,N04)	0.1	0.0	0.1	0.1	0.1	0.1	0.1	*	*
Chronic glomerulonephritis, nephritis and nephropathy not specified as acute or chronic, and renal sclerosis unspecified (N02-N03, N05-N07, N26)	1.4	1.3	1.4	1.4	1.3	1.4	1.7	1.6	1.8
Renal failure (N17-N19)	14.4	14.3	14.6	14.2	14.2	14.2	19.6	18.6	20.4
Other disorders of kidney (N25, N27)	0.0	*	0.0	0.0	*	*	*	*	*
Infections of kidney (N10-N12,N13.6,N15.1)	0.2	0.1	0.3	0.2	0.1	0.3	0.2	0.1	0.2
Hyperplasia of prostate (N40)	0.2	0.3	X	0.2	0.4	X	0.1	0.2	X
Inflammatory diseases of female pelvic organs (N70-N76)	0.0	X	0.1	0.0	X	0.1	*	X	*

PART B: MORTALITY 133

Table B-14. Death Rates for 113 Selected Causes by Race and Sex, 2008—Continued

(Rates per 100,000 population in specified group.)

Cause of death (based on ICD–10, 2004)	American Indian and Alaskan Native[1]			Asian or Pacific Islander[2]		
	Both sexes	Male	Female	Both sexes	Male	Female
Major cardiovascular diseases (I00-I78)	99.3	109.6	89.0	106.5	111.5	101.7
Diseases of heart (I00-I09, I11, I13, I20-I51)	77.6	89.3	66.0	74.1	81.6	67.0
Acute rheumatic fever and chronic rheumatic heart diseases (I00-I09)	0.6	*	*	0.7	0.5	0.9
Hypertensive heart disease (I11)	4.1	4.9	3.3	4.4	4.6	4.3
Hypertensive heart and renal disease (I13)	*	*	*	0.5	0.5	0.6
Ischemic heart diseases (I20-I25)	50.8	61.9	39.8	52.1	60.5	44.1
Acute myocardial infarction (I21-I22)	17.6	22.1	13.1	16.3	18.4	14.3
Other acute ischemic heart diseases (I24)	1.7	2.1	1.3	0.3	0.3	0.3
Other forms of chronic ischemic heart disease (I20, I25)	31.5	37.7	25.3	35.5	41.8	29.5
Atherosclerotic cardiovascular disease, so described (I25.0)	9.7	12.5	6.8	8.0	10.2	5.8
All other forms of chronic ischemic heart disease (I20,I25.1-I25.9)	21.9	25.2	18.5	27.5	31.6	23.7
Other heart diseases (I26-I51)	21.8	21.5	22.1	16.3	15.5	17.1
Acute and subacute endocarditis (I33)	*	*	*	*	*	*
Diseases of pericardium and acute myocarditis (I30-I31, I40)	*	*	*	0.2	*	*
Heart failure (I50)	6.9	5.7	8.1	4.1	3.4	4.7
All other forms of heart disease (I26-I28, I34-I38, I42-I49, I51)	14.3	15.3	13.4	12.0	11.8	12.2
Essential hypertension and hypertensive renal disease (I10, I12, I15)	3.2	3.3	3.2	4.7	4.3	5.1
Cerebrovascular diseases (I60-I69)	15.1	13.7	16.5	24.5	22.0	26.8
Atherosclerosis (I70)	1.0	*	*	0.6	0.6	0.5
Other diseases of circulatory system (I71-I78)	2.3	2.4	2.3	2.6	3.0	2.3
Aortic aneurysm and dissection (I71)	1.2	1.3	*	1.9	2.3	1.4
Other diseases of arteries, arterioles and capillaries (I72-I78)	1.1	*	1.2	0.8	0.7	0.9
Other disorders of circulatory system (I80-I99)	0.6	*	*	0.3	0.3	0.3
Influenza and pneumonia (J09-J18)[1]	11.1	10.9	11.3	10.0	10.5	9.6
Influenza (J09-J11)[1]	*	*	*	0.2	*	*
Pneumonia (J12-J18)	10.6	10.4	10.9	9.9	10.3	9.5
Other acute lower respiratory infections (J20-J22, U04)[2]	*	*	*	*	*	*
Acute bronchitis and bronchiolitis (J20-J21)	*	*	*	*	*	*
Other and unspecified acute lower respiratory infections (J22, U04)[2,3]	*	*	*	*	*	*
Chronic lower respiratory diseases (J40-J47)	18.1	18.0	18.2	9.9	12.1	7.8
Bronchitis, chronic and unspecified (J40-J42)	*	*	*	*	*	*
Emphysema (J43)	1.6	1.8	1.4	0.8	1.2	0.4
Asthma (J45-J46)	0.6	*	*	0.9	0.6	1.1
Other chronic lower respiratory diseases (J44, J47)	15.8	15.5	16.0	8.1	10.2	6.2
Pneumoconioses and chemical effects (J60-J66, J68)	*	*	*	*	*	*
Pneumonitis due to solids and liquids (J69)	2.2	2.3	2.2	1.8	2.1	1.6
Other diseases of respiratory system (J00-J06, J30-J39, J67, J70-J98)	6.1	6.5	5.7	3.7	4.0	3.5
Peptic ulcer (K25-K28)	0.7	*	*	0.6	0.6	0.6
Diseases of appendix (K35-K38)	*	*	*	*	*	*
Hernia (K40-K46)	*	*	*	*	*	*
Chronic liver disease and cirrhosis (K70, K73-K74)	21.7	23.8	19.6	2.9	3.7	2.2
Alcoholic liver disease (K70)	15.4	17.3	13.5	1.2	2.1	0.4
Other chronic liver disease and cirrhosis (K73-K74)	6.3	6.5	6.1	1.7	1.7	1.8
Cholelithiasis and other disorders of gall bladder (K80-K82)	0.8	*	*	0.6	0.7	0.5
Nephritis, nephrotic syndrome and nephrosis (N00-N07, N17-N19, N25-N27)	9.9	9.1	10.7	6.2	6.4	6.0
Acute and rapidly progressive nephritic and nephrotic syndrome (N00-N01,N04)	*	*	*	*	*	*
Chronic glomerulonephritis, nephritis and nephropathy not specified as acute or chronic, and renal sclerosis unspecified (N02-N03, N05-N07, N26)	0.6	*	*	0.6	0.6	0.6
Renal failure (N17-N19)	9.2	8.4	10.0	5.6	5.8	5.4
Other disorders of kidney (N25, N27)	*	*	*	*	*	*
Infections of kidney (N10-N12,N13.6,N15.1)	*	*	*	0.1	*	*
Hyperplasia of prostate (N40)	*	*	X	*	*	X
Inflammatory diseases of female pelvic organs (N70-N76)	*	X	*	*	X	*

Table B-14. Death Rates for 113 Selected Causes by Race and Sex, 2008—*Continued*

(Rates per 100,000 population in specified group.)

Cause of death (based on ICD–10, 2004)	All races			White			Black		
	Both sexes	Male	Female	Both sexes	Male	Female	Both sexes	Male	Female
Pregnancy, childbirth and the puerperium (O00-O99)	0.3	X	0.5	0.2	X	0.4	0.6	X	1.2
Pregnancy with abortive outcome (O00-O07)	0.0	X	0.0	*	X	*	*	X	*
Other complications of pregnancy, childbirth and the puerperium (O10-O99)	0.3	X	0.5	0.2	X	0.4	0.6	X	1.1
Certain conditions originating in the perinatal period (P00-P96)	4.6	5.3	3.9	3.4	4.0	2.9	12.0	14.2	10.0
Congenital malformations, deformations and chromosomal abnormalities (Q00-Q99)	3.4	3.6	3.2	3.3	3.5	3.1	4.2	4.6	3.8
Symptoms, signs and abnormal clinical and laboratory findings, not elsewhere classified (R00-R99)	12.7	11.2	14.1	13.3	11.3	15.2	13.0	13.7	12.3
All other diseases (Residual)	83.0	67.7	97.9	89.7	72.2	106.9	67.1	58.6	74.9
Accidents (unintentional injuries) (V01-X59, Y85-Y86)	40.1	52.3	28.2	43.1	55.5	30.9	30.8	43.8	19.0
Transport accidents (V01-V99, Y85)	14.0	20.4	7.8	14.6	21.2	8.1	12.9	19.6	6.7
Motor vehicle accidents (V02-V04, V09.0, V09.2, V12-V14, V19.0-V19.2, V19.4-V19.6, V20-V79, V80.3-V80.5, V81.0-V81.1, V82.0-V82.1, V83-V86, V87.0-V87.8, V88.0-V88.8, V89.0, V89.2)	13.1	18.9	7.5	13.6	19.5	7.7	12.1	18.3	6.4
Other land transport accidents (V01,V05-V06, V09.1, V09.3-V09.9, V10-V11, V15-V18, V19.3, V19.8-V19.9, V80.0-V80.2, V80.6-V80.9, V81.2- V81.9, V82.2-V82.9, V87.9, V88.9, V89.1, V89.3, V89.9)	0.4	0.6	0.2	0.4	0.6	0.2	0.4	0.7	0.2
Water, air and space, and other and unspecified transport accidents and their sequelae (V90-V99, Y85)	0.6	1.0	0.2	0.6	1.0	0.2	0.4	0.7	0.1
Nontransport accidents (W00-X59, Y86)	26.0	31.8	20.4	28.5	34.3	22.8	17.9	24.2	12.2
Falls (W00-W19)	7.9	8.2	7.6	9.1	9.3	8.9	2.6	3.1	2.1
Accidental discharge of firearms (W32-W34)	0.2	0.3	0.1	0.2	0.3	0.1	0.2	0.4	*
Accidental drowning and submersion (W65-W74)	1.2	1.8	0.5	1.1	1.8	0.5	1.4	2.2	0.5
Accidental exposure to smoke, fire and flames (X00-X09)	1.0	1.1	0.8	0.9	1.1	0.8	1.5	1.9	1.2
Accidental poisoning and exposure to noxious substances (X40-X49)	10.2	13.7	6.9	11.2	14.9	7.6	7.4	10.3	4.8
Other and unspecified nontransport accidents and their sequelae (W20-W31, W35-W64, W75-W99, X10-X39, X50-X59, Y86)	5.6	6.6	4.6	6.0	7.0	5.0	4.8	6.1	3.6
Intentional self-harm (suicide) (*U03, X60-X84, Y87.0)	11.9	19.0	4.9	13.3	21.03	5.5	5.2	9.1	1.6
Intentional self-harm (suicide) by discharge of firearms (X72-X74)	6.0	10.6	1.5	6.9	12.1	1.7	2.6	4.9	0.5
Intentional self-harm (suicide) by other and unspecified means and their sequelae (*U03, X60-X71, X75-X84, Y87.0)	5.9	8.4	3.4	6.4	9.1	3.8	2.6	4.2	1.2
Assault (homicide) (*U01-*U02, X85-Y09, Y87.1)	5.9	9.4	2.4	3.6	5.4	1.9	20.6	37.1	5.6
Assault (homicide) by discharge of firearms (*U01.4, X93-X95)	4.0	6.9	1.2	2.2	3.5	0.9	16.3	30.7	3.1
Assault (homicide) by other and unspecified means and their sequelae (*U01.0-*U01.3, *U01.5-*U01.9, *U02, X85-X92, X96-Y09, Y87.1)	1.9	2.5	1.2	1.5	1.9	1.0	4.4	6.3	2.6
Legal intervention (Y35, Y89.0)	0.1	0.2	*	0.1	0.2	*	0.3	0.6	*
Events of undetermined intent (Y10-Y34, Y87.2,Y89.9)	1.7	2.1	1.2	1.7	2.1	1.3	1.7	2.4	1.0
Discharge of firearms, undetermined intent (Y22-Y24)	0.1	0.1	0.0	0.1	0.1	0.0	0.1	0.2	*
Other and unspecified events of undetermined intent and their sequelae (Y10-Y21, Y25-Y34, Y87.2, Y89.9)	1.6	2.0	1.2	1.6	2.0	1.3	1.6	2.2	1.0
Operations of war and their sequelae (Y36, Y89.1)	0.0	0.0	*	0.0	0.0	*	*	*	*
Complications of medical and surgical care (Y40-Y84, Y88)	0.9	0.8	0.9	0.9	0.8	1.0	1.0	1.0	1.0
Enterocolitis due to Clostridium difficile (A04.7)[4]	2.5	1.9	3.0	2.8	2.2	3.5	1.1	0.9	1.3
Drug-induced deaths[5]	12.7	16.0	9.6	14.0	17.3	10.6	9.1	12.3	6.1
Alcohol-induced deaths[5]	8.0	12.1	3.9	8.5	12.9	4.1	5.6	8.8	2.8
Injury by firearms[5]	10.4	18.2	2.8	9.4	16.2	2.7	19.4	36.7	3.6

Table B-14. Death Rates for 113 Selected Causes by Race and Sex, 2008—*Continued*

(Rates per 100,000 population in specified group.)

Cause of death (based on ICD–10, 2004)	American Indian and Alaskan Native[1]			Asian or Pacific Islander[2]		
	Both sexes	Male	Female	Both sexes	Male	Female
Pregnancy, childbirth and the puerperium (O00-O99)	*	X	*	0.2	X	0.4
Pregnancy with abortive outcome (O00-O07)	*	X	*	*	X	*
Other complications of pregnancy, childbirth and the puerperium (O10-O99)	*	X	*	0.2	X	0.4
Certain conditions originating in the perinatal period (P00-P96)	4.1	4.6	3.5	3.3	3.8	2.8
Congenital malformations, deformations andchromosomal abnormalities (Q00-Q99)	3.4	4.0	2.8	2.2	2.4	2.0
Symptoms, signs and abnormal clinical and laboratory findings, not elsewhere classified (R00-R99)	7.5	8.0	7.1	3.2	3.3	3.1
All other diseases (Residual)	44.9	44.0	45.8	25.9	22.9	28.8
Accidents (unintentional injuries) (V01-X59, Y85-Y86)	49.2	67.7	30.6	13.7	17.7	9.9
Transport accidents (V01-V99, Y85)	22.2	29.7	14.7	6.5	8.5	4.6
Motor vehicle accidents (V02-V04, V09.0, V09.2, V12-V14, V19.0-V19.2, V19.4-V19.6, V20-V79, V80.3-V80.5, V81.0-V81.1, V82.0-V82.1, V83- V86, V87.0-V87.8, V88.0-V88.8, V89.0, V89.2)	20.9	27.5	14.4	6.0	7.9	4.3
Other land transport accidents (V01,V05-V06, V09.1, V09.3-V09.9, V10-V11, V15-V18, V19.3, V19.8-V19.9, V80.0-V80.2, V80.6-V80.9, V81.2- V81.9, V82.2-V82.9, V87.9, V88.9, V89.1, V89.3, V89.9)	0.6	*	*	0.1	*	*
Water, air and space, and other and unspecified transport accidents and their sequelae (V90-V99, Y85)	0.6	*	*	0.3	0.4	*
Nontransport accidents (W00-X59, Y86)	27.0	38.0	15.9	7.2	9.2	5.3
Falls (W00-W19)	4.1	5.4	2.9	3.2	3.9	2.6
Accidental discharge of firearms (W32-W34)	*	*	*	*	*	*
Accidental drowning and submersion (W65-W74)	1.9	3.1	*	0.9	1.2	0.5
Accidental exposure to smoke, fire and flames (X00-X09)	1.1	1.3	*	0.2	*	*
Accidental poisoning and exposure to noxious substances (X40-X49)	13.7	19.0	8.5	1.4	2.0	0.8
Other and unspecified nontransport accidents and their sequelae (W20-W31, W35-W64, W75-W99, X10-X39, X50-X59, Y86)	5.7	8.5	2.9	1.5	1.7	1.2
Intentional self-harm (suicide) (*U03, X60-X84, Y87.0)	12.0	18.0	5.9	5.8	8.0	3.8
Intentional self-harm (suicide) by discharge of firearms (X72-X74)	4.5	8.0	*	1.2	2.2	0.3
Intentional self-harm (suicide) by other and unspecified means and their sequelae (*U03, X60-X71, X75-X84, Y87.0)	7.5	10.1	4.9	4.6	5.8	3.5
Assault (homicide) (*U01-*U02, X85-Y09, Y87.1)	7.5	11.2	3.7	2.3	3.3	1.3
Assault (homicide) by discharge of firearms (*U01.4, X93-X95)	2.8	4.3	1.3	1.4	2.2	0.6
Assault (homicide) by other and unspecified means and their sequelae (*U01.0-*U01.3, *U01.5-*U01.9, *U02, X85-X92, X96-Y09, Y87.1)	4.6	6.9	2.3	0.9	1.0	0.8
Legal intervention (Y35, Y89.0)	*	*	*	*	*	*
Events of undetermined intent (Y10-Y34, Y87.2,Y89.9)	2.0	3.0	*	0.5	0.6	0.4
Discharge of firearms, undetermined intent (Y22-Y24)	*	*	*	*	*	*
Other and unspecified events of undetermined intent and their sequelae (Y10-Y21, Y25-Y34, Y87.2, Y89.9)	2.0	2.8	*	0.5	0.6	0.4
Operations of war and their sequelae (Y36, Y89.1)	*	*	*	*	*	*
Complications of medical and surgical care (Y40-Y84, Y88)	*	*	*	0.2	*	*
Enterocolitis due to Clostridium difficile (A04.7)[4]	0.8	*	*	0.7	0.7	0.7
Drug-induced deaths[5]	13.2	16.0	10.4	2.0	2.5	1.5
Alcohol-induced deaths[5]	24.9	31.7	18.2	1.8	3.1	0.6
Injury by firearms[5]	8.2	13.6	2.7	2.7	4.6	0.9

X = Category not applicable.
* = Figure does not meet standards of reliability or precision.
0.0 = Quantity more than zero but less than 0.05.
[2]Includes Aleuts and Eskimos.
[3]Includes Chinese, Filipino, Hawaiian, Japanese, and Other Asian and Pacific Islander.
[4]Included in certain other intestinal infections (A04, A07–A09).
[5]Included in selected categories above.

Table B-15. Number of Deaths from Selected Causes by Hispanic Origin, Race for Non–Hispanic Population, and Sex, 2008

(Number.)

Cause of death (based on ICD–10, 2004)	All origins			Hispanic[1]			Non–Hispanic[2]		
	Both sexes	Male	Female	Both sexes	Male	Female	Both sexes	Male	Female
ALL CAUSES	2,471,984	1,226,197	1,245,787	139,241	76,861	62,380	2,327,636	1,146,394	1,181,242
Salmonella infections (A01-A02)	44	24	20	4	4	-	40	20	20
Shigellosis and amebiasis (A03, A06)	6	4	2	1	-	1	5	4	1
Certain other intestinal infections (A04, A07-A09)	7,876	2,996	4,880	373	150	223	7,493	2,841	4,652
Tuberculosis (A16-A19)	585	375	210	103	77	26	480	296	184
Respiratory tuberculosis (A16)	449	294	155	74	54	20	373	238	135
Other tuberculosis (A17-A19)	136	81	55	29	23	6	107	58	49
Whooping cough (A37)	20	9	11	9	4	5	11	5	6
Scarlet fever and erysipelas (A38, A46)	3	2	1	-	-	-	3	2	1
Meningococcal infection (A39)	102	56	46	17	11	6	85	45	40
Septicemia (A40-A41)	35,927	16,328	19,599	2,004	973	1031	33,839	15,310	18,529
Syphilis (A50-A53)	34	23	11	3	1	2	31	22	9
Acute poliomyelitis (A80)	-	-	-	-	-	-	-	-	-
Arthropod-borne viral encephalitis (A83-A84, A85.2)	2	1	1	2	1	1	-	-	-
Measles (B05)	-	-	-	-	-	-	-	-	-
Viral hepatitis (B15-B19)	7,629	5,019	2,610	1,189	774	415	6,422	4,232	2,190
Human immunodeficiency virus (HIV) disease (B20-B24)	10,285	7,406	2,879	1,365	1,037	328	8,846	6,314	2,532
Malaria (B50-B54)	5	4	1	-	-	-	5	4	1
Other and unspecified infectious and parasitic diseases and their sequelae (A00, A05, A20-A36, A42-A44, A48- A49, A54-A79, A81-A82, A85.0-A85.1, A85.8, A86-B04, B06-B09, B25-B49, B55-B99)	5,914	2,979	2,935	441	242	199	5,462	2,732	2,730
Malignant neoplasms (C00-C97)	565,469	295,259	270,210	28,851	15,283	13,568	535,675	279,433	256,242
Malignant neoplasms of lip, oral cavity and pharynx (C00-C14)	8,019	5,488	2,531	357	264	93	7,645	5,211	2,434
Malignant neoplasm of esophagus (C15)	13,714	10,847	2,867	565	461	104	13,127	10,366	2,761
Malignant neoplasm of stomach (C16)	11,352	6,735	4,617	1,398	804	594	9,934	5,918	4,016
Malignant neoplasms of colon, rectum and anus (C18-C21)	53,321	27,094	26,227	2,954	1,658	1,296	50,273	25,390	24,883
Malignant neoplasms of liver and intrahepatic bile ducts (C22)	18,213	12,302	5,911	2,071	1,391	680	16,108	10,885	5,223
Malignant neoplasm of pancreas (C25)	35,236	17,515	17,721	1,942	1011	931	33,240	16,471	16,769
Malignant neoplasm of larynx (C32)	3,760	2,949	811	191	164	27	3,558	2,775	783
Malignant neoplasms of trachea, bronchus and lung (C33-C34)	158,656	88,586	70,070	4,804	3,007	1,797	153,586	85,415	68,171
Malignant melanoma of skin (C43)	8,623	5,672	2,951	185	116	69	8,429	5,550	2,879
Malignant neoplasm of breast (C50)	41,026	437	40,589	2,151	11	2,140	38,815	423	38,392
Malignant neoplasm of cervix uteri (C53)	4,008	X	4,008	472	X	472	3,530	X	3,530
Malignant neoplasms of corpus uteri and uterus, part unspecified (C54-C55)	7,675	X	7,675	472	X	472	7,193	X	7,193
Malignant neoplasm of ovary (C56)	14,362	X	14,362	783	X	783	13,562	X	13,562
Malignant neoplasm of prostate (C61)	28,472	28,472	X	1,436	1,436	X	26,980	26,980	X
Malignant neoplasms of kidney and renal pelvis (C64-C65)	12,895	8,206	4,689	841	525	316	12,040	7,671	4,369
Malignant neoplasm of bladder (C67)	14,036	9,791	4,245	463	308	155	13,552	9,468	4,084
Malignant neoplasms of meninges, brain and other parts of central nervous system (C70-C72)	13,724	7,686	6,038	857	466	391	12,844	7,207	5,637
Malignant neoplasms of lymphoid, hematopoietic and related tissue (C81-C96)	54,954	30,449	24,505	3,295	1,833	1,462	51,569	28,567	23,002
Hodgkin's disease (C81)	1,171	639	532	118	63	55	1,051	574	477
Non-Hodgkin's lymphoma (C82-C85)	20,369	11,004	9,365	1,213	670	543	19,132	10,318	8,814
Leukemia (C91-C95)	22,335	12,711	9,624	1,360	770	590	20,927	11,917	9,010
Multiple myeloma and immunoproliferative neoplasms (C88, C90)	11,020	6,057	4,963	601	328	273	10,403	5,722	4,681
Other and unspecified malignant neoplasms of lymphoid, hematopoietic and related tissue (C96)	59	38	21	3	2	1	56	36	20
All other and unspecified malignant neoplasms (C17, C23-C24, C26-C31, C37-C41, C44-C49, C51- C52, C57-C60, C62-C63, C66, C68-C69, C73-C80, C97)	63,423	33,030	30,393	3,614	1,828	1,786	59,690	31,136	28,554
In situ neoplasms, benign neoplasms and neoplasms of uncertain or unknown behavior (D00-D48)	14,470	7,461	7,009	697	338	359	13,764	7,120	6,644
Anemias (D50-D64)	5,018	2,052	2,966	236	120	116	4,772	1,926	2,846
Diabetes mellitus (E10-E14)	70,553	35,346	35,207	6,544	3,314	3,230	63,848	31,938	31,910
Nutritional deficiencies (E40-E64)	2,976	1,138	1,838	150	68	82	2,824	1,069	1,755
Malnutrition (E40-E46)	2,760	1058	1,702	143	66	77	2,615	991	1,624
Other nutritional deficiencies (E50-E64)	216	80	136	7	2	5	209	78	131
Meningitis (G00,G03)	633	341	292	86	47	39	545	292	253
Parkinson's disease (G20-G21)	20,483	11,960	8,523	842	473	369	19,617	11,473	8,144
Alzheimer's disease (G30)	82,435	24,516	57,919	3,005	966	2,039	79,323	23,519	55,804

Table B-15. Number of Deaths from Selected Causes by Hispanic Origin, Race for Non–Hispanic Population, and Sex, 2008—Continued

(Number.)

Cause of death (based on ICD–10, 2004)	Non–Hispanic White			Non–Hispanic Black			Orgin not stated[3]		
	Both sexes	Male	Female	Both sexes	Male	Female	Both sexes	Male	Female
ALL CAUSES	1,981,034	969,288	1,011,746	285,522	145,168	140,354	5,107	2,942	2,165
Salmonella infections (A01-A02)	28	16	12	9	2	7	-	-	-
Shigellosis and amebiasis (A03, A06)	4	3	1	-	-	-	-	-	-
Certain other intestinal infections (A04, A07-A09)	6,890	2,595	4,295	464	177	287	10	5	5
Tuberculosis (A16-A19)	231	134	97	134	85	49	2	2	-
Respiratory tuberculosis (A16)	174	101	73	104	71	33	2	2	-
Other tuberculosis (A17-A19)	57	33	24	30	14	16	-	-	-
Whooping cough (A37)	9	3	6	-	-	-	-	-	-
Scarlet fever and erysipelas (A38, A46)	2	1	1	-	-	-	-	-	-
Meningococcal infection (A39)	58	31	27	25	13	12	-	-	-
Septicemia (A40-A41)	26,692	12,092	14,600	6,359	2,841	3,518	84	45	39
Syphilis (A50-A53)	11	10	1	18	10	8	-	-	-
Acute poliomyelitis (A80)	-	-	-	-	-	-	-	-	-
Arthropod-borne viral encephalitis (A83-A84, A85.2)	-	-	-	-	-	-	-	-	-
Measles (B05)	-	-	-	-	-	-	-	-	-
Viral hepatitis (B15-B19)	4,935	3,295	1,640	1,103	721	382	18	13	5
Human immunodeficiency virus (HIV) disease (B20-B24)	3,003	2,471	532	5,686	3,724	1,962	74	55	19
Malaria (B50-B54)	2	2	-	3	2	1	-	-	-
Other and unspecified infectious and parasitic diseases and their sequelae (A00, A05, A20-A36, A42-A44, A48- A49, A54-A79, A81-A82, A85.0-A85.1, A85.8, A86-B04, B06-B09, B25-B49, B55-B99)	4,518	2,219	2,299	725	402	323	11	5	6
Malignant neoplasms (C00-C97)	457,084	238,846	218,238	63,279	32,654	30,625	943	543	400
Malignant neoplasms of lip, oral cavity and pharynx (C00-C14)	6,353	4,282	2,071	992	724	268	17	13	4
Malignant neoplasm of esophagus (C15)	11,458	9,167	2,291	1,415	1,004	411	22	20	2
Malignant neoplasm of stomach (C16)	7,085	4,269	2,816	2,029	1,180	849	20	13	7
Malignant neoplasms of colon, rectum and anus (C18-C21)	41,812	21,090	20,722	6,833	3,473	3,360	94	46	48
Malignant neoplasms of liver and intrahepatic bile ducts (C22)	12,321	8,250	4,071	2,444	1,735	709	34	26	8
Malignant neoplasm of pancreas (C25)	28,191	14,112	14,079	4,062	1,870	2,192	54	33	21
Malignant neoplasm of larynx (C32)	2,869	2,234	635	635	496	139	11	10	1
Malignant neoplasms of trachea, bronchus and lung (C33-C34)	133,866	73,732	60,134	16,101	9,542	6,559	266	164	102
Malignant melanoma of skin (C43)	8,260	5,468	2,792	118	55	63	9	6	3
Malignant neoplasm of breast (C50)	31,903	338	31,565	5,883	75	5,808	60	3	57
Malignant neoplasm of cervix uteri (C53)	2,551	X	2,551	793	X	793	6	X	6
Malignant neoplasms of corpus uteri and uterus, part unspecified (C54-C55)	5,712	X	5,712	1,275	X	1,275	10	X	10
Malignant neoplasm of ovary (C56)	11,951	X	11,951	1,184	X	1,184	17	X	17
Malignant neoplasm of prostate (C61)	21,951	21,951	X	4,520	4,520	X	56	56	X
Malignant neoplasms of kidney and renal pelvis (C64-C65)	10,515	6,716	3,799	1,194	740	454	14	10	4
Malignant neoplasm of bladder (C67)	12,379	8,789	3,590	945	513	432	21	15	6
Malignant neoplasms of meninges, brain and other parts of central nervous system (C70-C72)	11,699	6,575	5,124	832	452	380	23	13	10
Malignant neoplasms of lymphoid, hematopoietic and related tissue (C81-C96)	45,058	25,102	19,956	5,206	2,770	2,436	90	49	41
Hodgkin's disease (C81)	907	495	412	118	63	55	2	2	-
Non-Hodgkin's lymphoma (C82-C85)	17,268	9,316	7,952	1,341	726	615	24	16	8
Leukemia (C91-C95)	18,532	10,606	7,926	1,870	1039	831	48	24	24
Multiple myeloma and immunoproliferative neoplasms (C88, C90)	8,302	4,655	3,647	1,872	938	934	16	7	9
Other and unspecified malignant neoplasms of lymphoid, hematopoietic and related tissue (C96)	49	30	19	5	4	1	-	-	-
All other and unspecified malignant neoplasms (C17, C23-C24, C26-C31, C37-C41, C44-C49, C51- C52, C57-C60, C62-C63, C66, C68-C69, C73-C80, C97)	51,150	26,771	24,379	6,818	3,505	3,313	119	66	53
In situ neoplasms, benign neoplasms and neoplasms of uncertain or unknown behavior (D00-D48)	12,255	6,393	5,862	1,148	550	598	9	3	6
Anemias (D50-D64)	3,645	1,434	2,211	1004	443	561	10	6	4
Diabetes mellitus (E10-E14)	49,388	25,303	24,085	11,934	5,378	6,556	161	94	67
Nutritional deficiencies (E40-E64)	2,381	868	1,513	370	173	197	2	1	1
Malnutrition (E40-E46)	2,195	802	1,393	352	164	188	2	1	1
Other nutritional deficiencies (E50-E64)	186	66	120	18	9	9	-	-	-
Meningitis (G00,G03)	397	214	183	118	62	56	2	2	-
Parkinson's disease (G20-G21)	18,474	10,845	7,629	739	394	345	24	14	10
Alzheimer's disease (G30)	73,219	21,780	51,439	5,024	1,394	3,630	107	31	76

Table B-15. Number of Deaths from Selected Causes by Hispanic Origin, Race for Non–Hispanic Population, and Sex, 2008—Continued

(Number.)

Cause of death (based on ICD–10, 2004)	All origins			Hispanic[1]			Non–Hispanic[2]		
	Both sexes	Male	Female	Both sexes	Male	Female	Both sexes	Male	Female
Major cardiovascular diseases (I00-I78)	804,483	388,514	415,969	38,724	20,119	18,605	764,061	367,406	396,655
Diseases of heart (I00-I09, I11, I13, I20-I51)	616,828	311,201	305,627	28,951	15,498	13,453	586,514	294,876	291,638
Acute rheumatic fever and chronic rheumatic heart diseases (I00-I09)	3,141	1,025	2,116	154	49	105	2,983	976	2,007
Hypertensive heart disease (I11)	32,391	15,201	17,190	1,779	1003	776	30,479	14,112	16,367
Hypertensive heart and renal disease (I13)	2,872	1,250	1,622	164	71	93	2,703	1,175	1,528
Ischemic heart diseases (I20-I25)	405,309	216,248	189,061	20,261	11,120	9,141	384,127	204,552	179,575
Acute myocardial infarction (I21-I22)	133,958	72,447	61,511	6,611	3,624	2,987	127,087	68,662	58,425
Other acute ischemic heart diseases (I24)	4,252	2,219	2,033	125	69	56	4,111	2,137	1,974
Other forms of chronic ischemic heart disease (I20, I25)	267,099	141,582	125,517	13,525	7,427	6,098	252,929	133,753	119,176
Atherosclerotic cardiovascular disease, so described (I25.0)	58,625	33,341	25,284	3,208	2,019	1,189	55,137	31,135	24,002
All other forms of chronic ischemic heart disease (I20,I25.1-I25.9)	208,474	108,241	100,233	10,317	5,408	4,909	197,792	102,618	95,174
Other heart diseases (I26-I51)	173,115	77,477	95,638	6,593	3,255	3,338	166,222	74,061	92,161
Acute and subacute endocarditis (I33)	1,180	662	518	77	57	20	1,101	603	498
Diseases of pericardium and acute myocarditis (I30-I31, I40)	827	406	421	71	34	37	754	372	382
Heart failure (I50)	56,830	23,017	33,813	1,966	843	1,123	54,769	22,130	32,639
All other forms of heart disease (I26-I28, I34-I38, I42-I49, I51)	114,278	53,392	60,886	4,479	2,321	2,158	109,598	50,956	58,642
Essential hypertension and hypertensive renal disease (I10, I12, I15)	25,742	10,325	15,417	1,522	666	856	24,180	9,641	14,539
Cerebrovascular diseases (I60-I69)	134,148	53,525	80,623	7,121	3,370	3,751	126,777	50,037	76,740
Atherosclerosis (I70)	7,836	3,012	4,824	282	112	170	7,546	2,896	4,650
Other diseases of circulatory system (I71-I78)	19,929	10,451	9,478	848	473	375	19,044	9,956	9,088
Aortic aneurysm and dissection (I71)	11,079	6,502	4,577	425	282	143	10,634	6,208	4,426
Other diseases of arteries, arterioles and capillaries (I72-I78)	8,850	3,949	4,901	423	191	232	8,410	3,748	4,662
Other disorders of circulatory system (I80-I99)	4,042	1,857	2,185	210	115	95	3,825	1,738	2,087
Influenza and pneumonia (J09-J18)[1]	56,284	25,571	30,713	3,176	1,544	1,632	53,024	23,983	29,041
Influenza (J09-J11)[1]	1722	690	1032	73	32	41	1645	656	989
Pneumonia (J12-J18)	54,562	24,881	29,681	3,103	1,512	1,591	51,379	23,327	28,052
Other acute lower respiratory infections (J20-J22, U04)[2]	284	126	158	22	9	13	261	116	145
Acute bronchitis and bronchiolitis (J20-J21)	235	106	129	21	9	12	213	96	117
Other and unspecified acute lower respiratory infections (J22, U04)[2,3]	49	20	29	1	-	1	48	20	28
Chronic lower respiratory diseases (J40-J47)	141,090	67,122	73,968	3,949	2,019	1,930	136,895	64,959	71,936
Bronchitis, chronic and unspecified (J40-J42)	731	311	420	47	29	18	682	281	401
Emphysema (J43)	12,448	6,467	5,981	284	174	110	12,143	6,280	5,863
Asthma (J45-J46)	3,397	1,186	2,211	271	116	155	3,115	1,067	2,048
Other chronic lower respiratory diseases (J44, J47)	124,514	59,158	65,356	3,347	1,700	1,647	120,955	57,331	63,624
Pneumoconioses and chemical effects (J60-J66, J68)	908	859	49	22	20	2	882	835	47
Pneumonitis due to solids and liquids (J69)	16,608	8,650	7,958	639	329	310	15,949	8,309	7,640
Other diseases of respiratory system (J00-J06, J30-J39, J67, J70-J98)	29,925	14,916	15,009	1,803	901	902	28,071	13,987	14,084
Peptic ulcer (K25-K28)	3,073	1,551	1,522	155	95	60	2,908	1,449	1,459
Diseases of appendix (K35-K38)	418	242	176	43	33	10	375	209	166
Hernia (K40-K46)	1,674	717	957	108	44	64	1,563	671	892
Chronic liver disease and cirrhosis (K70, K73-K74)	29,963	19,646	10,317	4,091	2,850	1,241	25,813	16,754	9,059
Alcoholic liver disease (K70)	14,864	10,817	4,047	2,152	1,757	395	12,675	9,029	3,646
Other chronic liver disease and cirrhosis (K73-K74)	15,099	8,829	6,270	1,939	1,093	846	13,138	7,725	5,413
Cholelithiasis and other disorders of gallbladder (K80-K82)	3,417	1,585	1,832	281	115	166	3,132	1,468	1,664
Nephritis, nephrotic syndrome and nephrosis (N00-N07, N17-N19, N25-N27)	48,237	23,533	24,704	2,903	1,456	1,447	45,245	22,035	23,210
Acute and rapidly progressive nephritic and nephrotic syndrome (N00-N01,N04)	160	73	87	7	4	3	153	69	84
Chronic glomerulonephritis, nephritis and nephropathy not specified as acute or chronic, and renal sclerosis unspecified (N02-N03, N05-N07, N26)	4,109	1,970	2,139	233	126	107	3,866	1,837	2,029
Renal failure (N17-N19)	43,935	21,477	22,458	2,661	1,325	1,336	41,195	20,117	21,078
Other disorders of kidney (N25, N27)	33	13	20	2	1	1	31	12	19
Infections of kidney (N10-N12,N13.6,N15.1)	627	179	448	59	18	41	566	161	405
Hyperplasia of prostate (N40)	502	502	X	21	21	X	477	477	X
Inflammatory diseases of female pelvic organs (N70-N76)	136	X	136	6	X	6	129	X	129
Pregnancy, childbirth and the puerperium (O00-O99)	795	X	795	154	X	154	636	X	636
Pregnancy with abortive outcome (O00-O07)	34	X	34	7	X	7	26	X	26
Other complications of pregnancy, childbirth and the puerperium (O10-O99)	761	X	761	147	X	147	610	X	610

Table B-15. Number of Deaths from Selected Causes by Hispanic Origin, Race for Non–Hispanic Population, and Sex, 2008—Continued

(Number.)

Cause of death (based on ICD–10, 2004)	Non–Hispanic White			Non–Hispanic Black			Orgin not stated[3]		
	Both sexes	Male	Female	Both sexes	Male	Female	Both sexes	Male	Female
Major cardiovascular diseases (I00-I78)	650,843	312,004	338,839	94,214	45,579	48,635	1,698	989	709
Diseases of heart (I00-I09, I11, I13, I20-I51)	503,096	252,572	250,524	69,918	34,965	34,953	1363	827	536
Acute rheumatic fever and chronic rheumatic heart diseases (I00-I09)	2,603	833	1,770	261	97	164	4	-	4
Hypertensive heart disease (I11)	22,331	9,977	12,354	7,361	3,722	3,639	133	86	47
Hypertensive heart and renal disease (I13)	1,783	763	1,020	830	372	458	5	4	1
Ischemic heart diseases (I20-I25)	333,378	178,052	155,326	41,373	21,131	20,242	921	576	345
Acute myocardial infarction (I21-I22)	110,461	60,166	50,295	13,645	6,811	6,834	260	161	99
Other acute ischemic heart diseases (I24)	3,447	1,781	1,666	558	299	259	16	13	3
Other forms of chronic ischemic heart disease (I20, I25)	219,470	116,105	103,365	27,170	14,021	13,149	645	402	243
Atherosclerotic cardiovascular disease, so described (I25.0)	45,179	25,335	19,844	8,469	4,864	3,605	280	187	93
All other forms of chronic ischemic heart disease (I20,I25.1-I25.9)	174,291	90,770	83,521	18,701	9,157	9,544	365	215	150
Other heart diseases (I26-I51)	143,001	62,947	80,054	20,093	9,643	10,450	300	161	139
Acute and subacute endocarditis (I33)	871	486	385	204	106	98	2	2	-
Diseases of pericardium and acute myocarditis (I30-I31, I40)	580	285	295	145	70	75	2	-	2
Heart failure (I50)	48,518	19,406	29,112	5,415	2,380	3,035	95	44	51
All other forms of heart disease (I26-I28, I34-I38, I42-I49, I51)	93,032	42,770	50,262	14,329	7,087	7,242	201	115	86
Essential hypertension and hypertensive renal disease (I10, I12, I15)	18,351	7,088	11,263	5,028	2,194	2,834	40	18	22
Cerebrovascular diseases (I60-I69)	106,134	41,092	65,042	16,527	7,135	9,392	250	118	132
Atherosclerosis (I70)	6,781	2,561	4,220	648	276	372	8	4	4
Other diseases of circulatory system (I71-I78)	16,481	8,691	7,790	2,093	1,009	1,084	37	22	15
Aortic aneurysm and dissection (I71)	9,409	5,515	3,894	910	503	407	20	12	8
Other diseases of arteries, arterioles and capillaries (I72-I78)	7,072	3,176	3,896	1,183	506	677	17	10	7
Other disorders of circulatory system (I80-I99)	3,007	1,343	1,664	756	363	393	7	4	3
Influenza and pneumonia (J09-J18)[1]	45,780	20,516	25,264	5,396	2,542	2,854	84	44	40
Influenza (J09-J11)[1]	1523	598	925	81	37	44	4	2	2
Pneumonia (J12-J18)	44,257	19,918	24,339	5,315	2,505	2,810	80	42	38
Other acute lower respiratory infections (J20-J22, U04)[2]	215	90	125	35	19	16	1	1	-
Acute bronchitis and bronchiolitis (J20-J21)	172	71	101	30	18	12	1	1	-
Other and unspecified acute lower respiratory infections (J22, U04)[2,3]	43	19	24	5	1	4	-	-	-
Chronic lower respiratory diseases (J40-J47)	126,146	59,284	66,862	8,679	4,497	4,182	246	144	102
Bronchitis, chronic and unspecified (J40-J42)	610	240	370	61	36	25	2	1	1
Emphysema (J43)	11,302	5,767	5,535	668	397	271	21	13	8
Asthma (J45-J46)	2,070	641	1,429	892	370	522	11	3	8
Other chronic lower respiratory diseases (J44, J47)	112,164	52,636	59,528	7,058	3,694	3,364	212	127	85
Pneumoconioses and chemical effects (J60-J66, J68)	839	796	43	37	34	3	4	4	-
Pneumonitis due to solids and liquids (J69)	14,135	7,369	6,766	1,466	751	715	20	12	8
Other diseases of respiratory system (J00-J06, J30-J39, J67, J70-J98)	24,564	12,301	12,263	2,753	1,292	1,461	51	28	23
Peptic ulcer (K25-K28)	2,491	1,210	1,281	300	181	119	10	7	3
Diseases of appendix (K35-K38)	305	164	141	56	37	19	-	-	-
Hernia (K40-K46)	1,391	588	803	146	73	73	3	2	1
Chronic liver disease and cirrhosis (K70, K73-K74)	22,210	14,452	7,758	2,464	1,653	811	59	42	17
Alcoholic liver disease (K70)	10,819	7,802	3,017	1,177	801	376	37	31	6
Other chronic liver disease and cirrhosis (K73-K74)	11,391	6,650	4,741	1,287	852	435	22	11	11
Cholelithiasis and other disorders of gallbladder (K80-K82)	2,713	1,266	1,447	303	142	161	4	2	2
Nephritis, nephrotic syndrome and nephrosis (N00-N07, N17-N19, N25-N27)	35,439	17,535	17,904	8,564	3,893	4,671	89	42	47
Acute and rapidly progressive nephritic and nephrotic syndrome (N00-N01,N04)	123	57	66	27	9	18	-	-	-
Chronic glomerulonephritis, nephritis and nephropathy not specified as acute or chronic, and renal sclerosis unspecified (N02-N03, N05-N07, N26)	3,077	1,479	1,598	680	306	374	10	7	3
Renal failure (N17-N19)	32,214	15,990	16,224	7,852	3,576	4,276	79	35	44
Other disorders of kidney (N25, N27)	25	9	16	5	2	3	-	-	-
Infections of kidney (N10-N12,N13.6,N15.1)	474	129	345	66	24	42	2	-	2
Hyperplasia of prostate (N40)	435	435	X	35	35	X	4	4	X
Inflammatory diseases of female pelvic organs (N70-N76)	105	X	105	19	X	19	1	X	1
Pregnancy, childbirth and the puerperium (O00-O99)	345	X	345	247	X	247	5	X	5
Pregnancy with abortive outcome (O00-O07)	10	X	10	15	X	15	1	X	1
Other complications of pregnancy, childbirth and the puerperium (O10-O99)	335	X	335	232	X	232	4	X	4

Table B-15. Number of Deaths from Selected Causes by Hispanic Origin, Race for Non–Hispanic Population, and Sex, 2008—Continued

(Number.)

Cause of death (based on ICD–10, 2004)	All origins			Hispanic[1]			Non–Hispanic[2]		
	Both sexes	Male	Female	Both sexes	Male	Female	Both sexes	Male	Female
Certain conditions originating in the perinatal period (P00-P96)	13,933	7,919	6,014	2,873	1,645	1,228	10,901	6,182	4,719
Congenital malformations, deformations and chromosomal abnormalities (Q00-Q99)	10,288	5,395	4,893	2,011	1,061	950	8,225	4,308	3,917
Symptoms, signs and abnormal clinical and laboratory findings, not elsewhere classified (R00-R99)	38,522	16,803	21,719	2,195	1,229	966	36,209	15,512	20,697
All other diseases (Residual)	252,490	101,521	150,969	12,561	5,866	6,695	239,433	95,428	144,005
Accidents (unintentional injuries) (V01-X59, Y85-Y86)	121,902	78,378	43,524	11,080	8,363	2,717	110,476	69,771	40,705
Transport accidents (V01-V99, Y85)	42,709	30,650	12,059	5,413	4,186	1,227	37,190	26,384	10,806
Motor vehicle accidents (V02-V04, V09.0, V09.2, V12-V14, V19.0-V19.2, V19.4-V19.6, V20-V79, V80.3-V80.5, V81.0-V81.1, V82.0-V82.1, V83- V86, V87.0-V87.8, V88.0-V88.8, V89.0, V89.2)	39,790	28,291	11,499	5,105	3,920	1,185	34,590	24,300	10,290
Other land transport accidents (V01,V05-V06, V09.1, V09.3-V09.9, V10-V11, V15-V18, V19.3, V19.8-V19.9, V80.0-V80.2, V80.6-V80.9, V81.2- V81.9, V82.2-V82.9, V87.9, V88.9, V89.1, V89.3, V89.9)	1,140	907	233	187	158	29	945	742	203
Water, air and space, and other and unspecified transport accidents and their sequelae (V90-V99, Y85)	1,779	1,452	327	121	108	13	1,655	1,342	313
Nontransport accidents (W00-X59, Y86)	79,193	47,728	31,465	5,667	4,177	1,490	73,286	43,387	29,899
Falls (W00-W19)	24,013	12,318	11,695	1,267	828	439	22,707	11,471	11,236
Accidental discharge of firearms (W32-W34)	592	510	82	39	33	6	551	475	76
Accidental drowning and submersion (W65-W74)	3,548	2,726	822	500	399	101	3,033	2,315	718
Accidental exposure to smoke, fire and flames (X00-X09)	2,912	1,705	1,207	189	118	71	2,707	1,576	1,131
Accidental poisoning and exposure to noxious substances (X40-X49)	31,116	20,533	10,583	2,564	2,007	557	28,432	18,439	9,993
Other and unspecified nontransport accidents and their sequelae (W20-W31, W35-W64, W75-W99, X10-X39, X50-X59, Y86)	17,012	9,936	7,076	1,108	792	316	15,856	9,111	6,745
Intentional self-harm (suicide) (*U03, X60-X84, Y87.0)	36,035	28,450	7,585	2,345	1,955	390	33,589	26,417	7,172
Intentional self-harm (suicide) by discharge of firearms (X72-X74)	18,223	15,931	2,292	863	786	77	17,318	15,109	2,209
Intentional self-harm (suicide) by other and unspecified means and their sequelae (*U03, X60-X71, X75-X84, Y87.0)	17,812	12,519	5,293	1,482	1,169	313	16,271	11,308	4,963
Assault (homicide) (*U01-*U02, X85-Y09, Y87.1)	17,826	14,135	3,691	3,331	2,777	554	14,427	11,305	3,122
Assault (homicide) by discharge of firearms (*U01.4, X93-X95)	12,179	10,361	1,818	2,260	2,003	257	9,882	8,327	1,555
Assault (homicide) by other and unspecified means and their sequelae (*U01.0-*U01.3, *U01.5-*U01.9, *U02, X85-X92, X96-Y09, Y87.1)	5,647	3,774	1,873	1,071	774	297	4,545	2,978	1,567
Legal intervention (Y35, Y89.0)	381	369	12	79	78	1	302	291	11
Events of undetermined intent (Y10-Y34, Y87.2,Y89.9)	5,051	3,144	1,907	326	251	75	4,707	2,879	1,828
Discharge of firearms, undetermined intent (Y22-Y24)	273	220	53	22	19	3	247	197	50
Other and unspecified events of undetermined intent and their sequelae (Y10-Y21, Y25-Y34, Y87.2, Y89.9)	4,778	2,924	1,854	304	232	72	4,460	2,682	1,778
Operations of war and their sequelae (Y36, Y89.1)	31	31	-	1	1	-	30	30	-
Complications of medical and surgical care (Y40-Y84, Y88)	2,590	1,183	1,407	151	64	87	2,435	1,117	1,318
Enterocolitis due to Clostridium difficile (A04.7)[4]	7,476	2,847	4,629	351	142	209	7,115	2,700	4,415
Drug-induced deaths[5]	38,649	23,928	14,721	2,761	2,033	728	35,735	21,791	13,944
Alcohol-induced deaths[5]	24,189	18,152	6,037	3,021	2,522	499	21,085	15,561	5,524
Injury by firearms[5]	31,593	27,336	4,257	3,256	2,912	344	28,252	24,351	3,901

Table B-15. Number of Deaths from Selected Causes by Hispanic Origin, Race for Non–Hispanic Population, and Sex, 2008—Continued

(Number.)

Cause of death (based on ICD–10, 2004)	Non–Hispanic White			Non–Hispanic Black			Orgin not stated[3]		
	Both sexes	Male	Female	Both sexes	Male	Female	Both sexes	Male	Female
Certain conditions originating in the perinatal period (P00-P96)	5,695	3,253	2,442	4,627	2,608	2,019	159	92	67
Congenital malformations, deformations and chromosomal abnormalities (Q00-Q99)	6,186	3,230	2,956	1,624	847	777	52	26	26
Symptoms, signs and abnormal clinical and laboratory findings, not elsewhere classified (R00-R99)	30,364	12,567	17,797	5,145	2,591	2,554	118	62	56
All other diseases (Residual)	207,369	81,906	125,463	26,781	11,171	15,610	496	227	269
Accidents (unintentional injuries) (V01-X59, Y85-Y86)	94,722	59,173	35,549	12,215	8,282	3,933	346	244	102
Transport accidents (V01-V99, Y85)	30,440	21,597	8,843	5,117	3,723	1,394	106	80	26
Motor vehicle accidents (V02-V04, V09.0, V09.2, V12-V14, V19.0-V19.2, V19.4-V19.6, V20-V79, V80.3-V80.5, V81.0-V81.1, V82.0-V82.1,V83- V86, V87.0-V87.8, V88.0-V88.8, V89.0, V89.2)	28,272	19,855	8,417	4,788	3,458	1,330	95	71	24
Other land transport accidents (V01,V05-V06, V09.1, V09.3-V09.9, V10-V11, V15-V18, V19.3, V19.8-V19.9, V80.0-V80.2, V80.6-V80.9, V81.2- V81.9, V82.2-V82.9, V87.9, V88.9, V89.1, V89.3, V89.9)	736	578	158	168	134	34	8	7	1
Water, air and space, and other and unspecified transport accidents and their sequelae (V90-V99, Y85)	1,432	1,164	268	161	131	30	3	2	1
Nontransport accidents (W00-X59, Y86)	64,282	37,576	26,706	7,098	4,559	2,539	240	164	76
Falls (W00-W19)	21,084	10,517	10,567	1,015	587	428	39	19	20
Accidental discharge of firearms (W32-W34)	441	378	63	93	84	9	2	2	-
Accidental drowning and submersion (W65-W74)	2,317	1,759	558	534	420	114	15	12	3
Accidental exposure to smoke, fire and flames (X00-X09)	2,037	1,181	856	603	356	247	16	11	5
Accidental poisoning and exposure to noxious substances (X40-X49)	24,855	16,047	8,808	2,938	1,948	990	120	87	33
Other and unspecified nontransport accidents and their sequelae (W20-W31, W35-W64, W75-W99, X10-X39, X50-X59, Y86)	13,548	7,694	5,854	1,915	1,164	751	48	33	15
Intentional self-harm (suicide) (*U03, X60-X84, Y87.0)	30,281	23,835	6,446	2,063	1,721	342	101	78	23
Intentional self-harm (suicide) by discharge of firearms (X72-X74)	15,968	13,891	2,077	1034	938	96	42	36	6
Intentional self-harm (suicide) by other and unspecified means and their sequelae (*U03, X60-X71, X75-X84, Y87.0)	14,313	9,944	4,369	1029	783	246	59	42	17
Assault (homicide) (*U01-*U02, X85-Y09, Y87.1)	5,656	3,855	1,801	8,206	7,047	1,159	68	53	15
Assault (homicide) by discharge of firearms (*U01.4, X93-X95)	3,117	2,256	861	6,481	5,851	630	37	31	6
Assault (homicide) by other and unspecified means and their sequelae (*U01.0-*U01.3, *U01.5-*U01.9, *U02, X85-X92, X96-Y09, Y87.1)	2,539	1,599	940	1,725	1,196	529	31	22	9
Legal intervention (Y35, Y89.0)	167	160	7	120	118	2	-	-	-
Events of undetermined intent (Y10-Y34, Y87.2,Y89.9)	3,909	2,343	1,566	664	449	215	18	14	4
Discharge of firearms, undetermined intent (Y22-Y24)	202	159	43	39	32	7	4	4	-
Other and unspecified events of undetermined intent and their sequelae (Y10-Y21, Y25-Y34, Y87.2, Y89.9)	3,707	2,184	1,523	625	417	208	14	10	4
Operations of war and their sequelae (Y36, Y89.1)	25	25	-	3	3	-	-	-	-
Complications of medical and surgical care (Y40-Y84, Y88)	1,997	904	1,093	396	191	205	4	2	2
Enterocolitis due to Clostridium difficile (A04.7)[4]	6,543	2,473	4,070	442	164	278	10	5	5
Drug-induced deaths[5]	31,448	19,044	12,404	3,589	2,326	1,263	153	104	49
Alcohol-induced deaths[5]	17,759	13,160	4,599	2,240	1,660	580	83	69	14
Injury by firearms[5]	19,873	16,822	3,051	7,741	6,997	744	85	73	12

X = Category not applicable.
- = Quantity zero
[1]Includes races other than White and Black.
[2]Persons of Hispanic origin may be of any race.
[3]Includes deaths for Hispanic origin was not reported on the death certificate.
[4]Included in certain other intestinal infections (A04, A07–A09).
[5]Included in selected categories above.

NOTE: Complete confirmation of deaths from selected causes of death, considered to be of public health concern, were not provided by the following states—Massachusetts, North Carolina, and West Virginia.

Table B-16. Death Rates from Selected Causes by Hispanic Origin, Race for Non-Hispanic Population, and Sex, 2008

(Rates per 100,000 population in specified group.)

Cause of death (based on ICD–10, 2004)	All origins[1]			Hispanic[2]			Non-Hispanic		
	Both sexes	Male	Female	Both sexes	Male	Female	Both sexes	Male	Female
ALL CAUSES	813.0	817.9	808.2	296.6	316.9	274.9	905.3	912.2	898.7
Salmonella infections (A01-A02)	0.0	0.0	0.0	*	*	*	0.0	0.0	0.0
Shigellosis and amebiasis (A03, A06)	*	*	*	*	*	*	*	*	*
Certain other intestinal infections (A04, A07-A09)	2.6	2.0	3.2	0.8	0.6	1.0	2.9	2.3	3.5
Tuberculosis (A16-A19)	0.2	0.3	0.1	0.2	0.3	0.1	0.2	0.2	0.1
Respiratory tuberculosis (A16)	0.1	0.2	0.1	0.2	0.2	0.1	0.1	0.2	0.1
Other tuberculosis (A17-A19)	0.0	0.1	0.0	0.1	0.1	*	0.0	0.0	0.0
Whooping cough (A37)	0.0	*	*	*	*	*	*	*	*
Scarlet fever and erysipelas (A38, A46)	*	*	*	*	*	*	*	*	*
Meningococcal infection (A39)	0.0	0.0	0.0	*	*	*	0.0	0.0	0.0
Septicemia (A40-A41)	11.8	10.9	12.7	4.3	4.0	4.5	13.2	12.2	14.1
Syphilis (A50-A53)	0.0	0.0	*	*	*	*	0.0	0.0	*
Acute poliomyelitis (A80)	*	*	*	*	*	*	*	*	*
Arthropod-borne viral encephalitis (A83-A84, A85.2)	*	*	*	*	*	*	*	*	*
Measles (B05)	*	*	*	*	*	*	*	*	*
Viral hepatitis (B15-B19)	2.5	3.3	1.7	2.5	3.2	1.8	2.5	3.4	1.7
Human immunodeficiency virus (HIV) disease (B20-B24)	3.4	4.9	1.9	2.9	4.3	1.4	3.4	5.0	1.9
Malaria (B50-B54)	*	*	*	*	*	*	*	*	*
Other and unspecified infectious and parasitic diseases and their sequelae (A00, A05, A20-A36, A42-A44, A48- A49, A54-A79, A81-A82, A85.0-A85.1, A85.8, A86-B04, B06-B09, B25-B49, B55-B99)	1.9	2.0	1.9	0.9	1.0	0.9	2.1	2.2	2.1
Malignant neoplasms (C00-C97)	186.0	196.9	175.3	61.5	63.0	59.8	208.3	222.4	194.9
Malignant neoplasms of lip, oral cavity and pharynx (C00-C14)	2.6	3.7	1.6	0.8	1.1	0.4	3.0	4.1	1.9
Malignant neoplasm of esophagus (C15)	4.5	7.2	1.9	1.2	1.9	0.5	5.1	8.2	2.1
Malignant neoplasm of stomach (C16)	3.7	4.5	3.0	3.0	3.3	2.6	3.9	4.7	3.1
Malignant neoplasms of colon, rectum and anus (C18-C21)	17.5	18.1	17.0	6.3	6.8	5.7	19.6	20.2	18.9
Malignant neoplasms of liver and intrahepatic bile ducts (C22)	6.0	8.2	3.8	4.4	5.7	3.0	6.3	8.7	4.0
Malignant neoplasm of pancreas (C25)	11.6	11.7	11.5	4.1	4.2	4.1	12.9	13.1	12.8
Malignant neoplasm of larynx (C32)	1.2	2.0	0.5	0.4	0.7	0.1	1.4	2.2	0.6
Malignant neoplasms of trachea, bronchus and lung (C33-C34)	52.2	59.1	45.5	10.2	12.4	7.9	59.7	68.0	51.9
Malignant melanoma of skin (C43)	2.8	3.8	1.9	0.4	0.5	0.3	3.3	4.4	2.2
Malignant neoplasm of breast (C50)	13.5	0.3	26.3	4.6	*	9.4	15.1	0.3	29.2
Malignant neoplasm of cervix uteri (C53)	1.3	X	2.6	1.0	X	2.1	1.4	X	2.7
Malignant neoplasms of corpus uteri and uterus, part unspecified (C54-C55)	2.5	X	5.0	1.0	X	2.1	2.8	X	5.5
Malignant neoplasm of ovary (C56)	4.7	X	9.3	1.7	X	3.5	5.3	X	10.3
Malignant neoplasm of prostate (C61)	9.4	19.0	X	3.1	5.9	X	10.5	21.5	X
Malignant neoplasms of kidney and renal pelvis (C64-C65)	4.2	5.5	3.0	1.8	2.2	1.4	4.7	6.1	3.3
Malignant neoplasm of bladder (C67)	4.6	6.5	2.8	1.0	1.3	0.7	5.3	7.5	3.1
Malignant neoplasms of meninges, brain and other parts of central nervous system (C70-C72)	4.5	5.1	3.9	1.8	1.9	1.7	5.0	5.7	4.3
Malignant neoplasms of lymphoid, hematopoietic and related tissue (C81-C96)	18.1	20.3	15.9	7.0	7.6	6.4	20.1	22.7	17.5
Hodgkin's disease (C81)	0.4	0.4	0.3	0.3	0.3	0.2	0.4	0.5	0.4
Non-Hodgkin's lymphoma (C82-C85)	6.7	7.3	6.1	2.6	2.8	2.4	7.4	8.2	6.7
Leukemia (C91-C95)	7.3	8.5	6.2	2.9	3.2	2.6	8.1	9.5	6.9
Multiple myeloma and immunoproliferative neoplasms (C88, C90)	3.6	4.0	3.2	1.3	1.4	1.2	4.0	4.6	3.6
Other and unspecified malignant neoplasms of lymphoid, hematopoietic and related tissue (C96)	0.0	0.0	0.0	*	*	*	0.0	0.0	0.0
All other and unspecified malignant neoplasms (C17, C23-C24, C26-C31, C37-C41, C44-C49, C51- C52, C57-C60, C62-C63, C66, C68-C69, C73-C80, C97)	20.9	22.0	19.7	7.7	7.5	7.9	23.2	24.8	21.7
In situ neoplasms, benign neoplasms and neoplasms of uncertain or unknown behavior (D00-D48)	4.8	5.0	4.5	1.5	1.4	1.6	5.4	5.7	5.1
Anemias (D50-D64)	1.7	1.4	1.9	0.5	0.5	0.5	1.9	1.5	2.2
Diabetes mellitus (E10-E14)	23.2	23.6	22.8	13.9	13.7	14.2	24.8	25.4	24.3
Nutritional deficiencies (E40-E64)	1.0	0.8	1.2	0.3	0.3	0.4	1.1	0.9	1.3
Malnutrition (E40-E46)	0.9	0.7	1.1	0.3	0.3	0.3	1.0	0.8	1.2
Other nutritional deficiencies (E50-E64)	0.1	0.1	0.1	*	*	*	0.1	0.1	0.1
Meningitis (G00,G03)	0.2	0.2	0.2	0.2	0.2	0.2	0.2	0.2	0.2
Parkinson's disease (G20-G21)	6.7	8.0	5.5	1.8	2.0	1.6	7.6	9.1	6.2
Alzheimer's disease (G30)	27.1	16.4	37.6	6.4	4.0	9.0	30.9	18.7	42.5

Table B-16. Death Rates from Selected Causes by Hispanic Origin, Race for Non-Hispanic Population, and Sex, 2008—Continued

(Rates per 100,000 population in specified group.)

Cause of death (based on ICD–10, 2004)	Non-Hispanic White			Non-Hispanic Black		
	Both sexes	Male	Female	Both sexes	Male	Female
ALL CAUSES	982.0	978.2	985.5	745.2	794.3	700.5
Salmonella infections (A01-A02)	0.0	*	*	*	*	*
Shigellosis and amebiasis (A03, A06)	*	*	*	*	*	*
Certain other intestinal infections (A04, A07-A09)	3.4	2.6	4.2	1.2	1.0	1.4
Tuberculosis (A16-A19)	0.1	0.1	0.1	0.3	0.5	0.2
Respiratory tuberculosis (A16)	0.1	0.1	0.1	0.3	0.4	0.2
Other tuberculosis (A17-A19)	0.0	0.0	0.0	0.1	*	*
Whooping cough (A37)	*	*	*	*	*	*
Scarlet fever and erysipelas (A38, A46)	*	*	*	*	*	*
Meningococcal infection (A39)	0.0	0.0	0.0	0.1	*	*
Septicemia (A40-A41)	13.2	12.2	14.2	16.6	15.5	17.6
Syphilis (A50-A53)	*	*	*	*	*	*
Acute poliomyelitis (A80)	*	*	*	*	*	*
Arthropod-borne viral encephalitis (A83-A84, A85.2)	*	*	*	*	*	*
Measles (B05)	*	*	*	*	*	*
Viral hepatitis (B15-B19)	2.4	3.3	1.6	2.9	3.9	1.9
Human immunodeficiency virus (HIV) disease (B20-B24)	1.5	2.5	0.5	14.8	20.4	9.8
Malaria (B50-B54)	*	*	*	*	*	*
Other and unspecified infectious and parasitic diseases and their sequelae (A00, A05, A20-A36, A42-A44, A48- A49, A54-A79, A81-A82, A85.0-A85.1, A85.8, A86-B04, B06-B09, B25-B49, B55-B99)	2.2	2.2	2.2	1.9	2.2	1.6
Malignant neoplasms (C00-C97)	226.6	241.1	212.6	165.2	178.7	152.8
Malignant neoplasms of lip, oral cavity and pharynx (C00-C14)	3.1	4.3	2.0	2.6	4.0	1.3
Malignant neoplasm of esophagus (C15)	5.7	9.3	2.2	3.7	5.5	2.1
Malignant neoplasm of stomach (C16)	3.5	4.3	2.7	5.3	6.5	4.2
Malignant neoplasms of colon, rectum and anus (C18-C21)	20.7	21.3	20.2	17.8	19.0	16.8
Malignant neoplasm of liver and intrahepatic bile ducts (C22)	6.1	8.3	4.0	6.4	9.5	3.5
Malignant neoplasm of pancreas (C25)	14.0	14.2	13.7	10.6	10.2	10.9
Malignant neoplasm of larynx (C32)	1.4	2.3	0.6	1.7	2.7	0.7
Malignant neoplasms of trachea, bronchus and lung (C33-C34)	66.4	74.4	58.6	42.0	52.2	32.7
Malignant melanoma of skin (C43)	4.1	5.5	2.7	0.3	0.3	0.3
Malignant neoplasm of breast (C50)	15.8	0.3	30.7	15.4	0.4	29.0
Malignant neoplasm of cervix uteri (C53)	1.3	X	2.5	2.1	X	4.0
Malignant neoplasms of corpus uteri and uterus, part unspecified (C54-C55)	2.8	X	5.6	3.3	X	6.4
Malignant neoplasm of ovary (C56)	5.9	X	11.6	3.1	X	5.9
Malignant neoplasm of prostate (C61)	10.9	22.2	X	11.8	24.7	X
Malignant neoplasms of kidney and renal pelvis (C64-C65)	5.2	6.8	3.7	3.1	4.0	2.3
Malignant neoplasm of bladder (C67)	6.1	8.9	3.5	2.5	2.8	2.2
Malignant neoplasms of meninges, brain and other parts of central nervous system (C70-C72)	5.8	6.6	5.0	2.2	2.5	1.9
Malignant neoplasms of lymphoid, hematopoietic and related tissue (C81-C96)	22.3	25.3	19.4	13.6	15.2	12.2
Hodgkin's disease (C81)	0.4	0.5	0.4	0.3	0.3	0.3
Non-Hodgkin's lymphoma (C82-C85)	8.6	9.4	7.7	3.5	4.0	3.1
Leukemia (C91-C95)	9.2	10.7	7.7	4.9	5.7	4.1
Multiple myeloma and immunoproliferative neoplasms (C88, C90)	4.1	4.7	3.6	4.9	5.1	4.7
Other and unspecified malignant neoplasms of lymphoid, hematopoietic and related tissue (C96)	0.0	0.0	*	*	*	*
All other and unspecified malignant neoplasms (C17, C23-C24, C26-C31, C37-C41, C44-C49, C51- C52, C57-C60, C62-C63, C66, C68-C69, C73-C80, C97)	25.4	27.0	23.7	17.8	19.2	16.5
In situ neoplasms, benign neoplasms and neoplasms of uncertain or unknown behavior (D00-D48)	6.1	6.5	5.7	3.0	3.0	3.0
Anemias (D50-D64)	1.8	1.4	2.2	2.6	2.4	2.8
Diabetes mellitus (E10-E14)	24.5	25.5	23.5	31.1	29.4	32.7
Nutritional deficiencies (E40-E64)	1.2	0.9	1.5	1.0	0.9	1.0
Malnutrition (E40-E46)	1.1	0.8	1.4	0.9	0.9	0.9
Other nutritional deficiencies (E50-E64)	0.1	0.1	0.1	*	*	*
Meningitis (G00,G03)	0.2	0.2	0.2	0.3	0.3	0.3
Parkinson's disease (G20-G21)	9.2	10.9	7.4	1.9	2.2	1.7
Alzheimer's disease (G30)	36.3	22.0	50.1	13.1	7.6	18.1

Table B-16. Death Rates from Selected Causes by Hispanic Origin, Race for Non-Hispanic Population, and Sex, 2008—Continued

(Rates per 100,000 population in specified group.)

Cause of death (based on ICD–10, 2004)	All origins[1]			Hispanic[2]			Non-Hispanic		
	Both sexes	Male	Female	Both sexes	Male	Female	Both sexes	Male	Female
Major cardiovascular diseases (I00-I78)	264.6	259.1	269.9	82.5	82.9	82.0	297.2	292.4	301.8
Diseases of heart (I00-I09, I11, I13, I20-I51)	202.9	207.6	198.3	61.7	63.9	59.3	228.1	234.6	221.9
Acute rheumatic fever and chronic rheumatic heart diseases (I00-I09)	1.0	0.7	1.4	0.3	0.2	0.5	1.2	0.8	1.5
Hypertensive heart disease (I11)	10.7	10.1	11.2	3.8	4.1	3.4	11.9	11.2	12.5
Hypertensive heart and renal disease (I13)	0.9	0.8	1.1	0.3	0.3	0.4	1.1	0.9	1.2
Ischemic heart diseases (I20-I25)	133.3	144.2	122.7	43.2	45.8	40.3	149.4	162.8	136.6
Acute myocardial infarction (I21-I22)	44.1	48.3	39.9	14.1	14.9	13.2	49.4	54.6	44.4
Other acute ischemic heart diseases (I24)	1.4	1.5	1.3	0.3	0.3	0.2	1.6	1.7	1.5
Other forms of chronic ischemic heart disease (I20, I25)	87.8	94.4	81.4	28.8	30.6	26.9	98.4	106.4	90.7
Atherosclerotic cardiovascular disease, so described (I25.0)	19.3	22.2	16.4	6.8	8.3	5.2	21.4	24.8	18.3
All other forms of chronic ischemic heart disease (I20,I25.1-I25.9)	68.6	72.2	65.0	22.0	22.3	21.6	76.9	81.7	72.4
Other heart diseases (I26-I51)	56.9	51.7	62.0	14.0	13.4	14.7	64.6	58.9	70.1
Acute and subacute endocarditis (I33)	0.4	0.4	0.3	0.2	0.2	0.1	0.4	0.5	0.4
Diseases of pericardium and acute myocarditis (I30-I31, I40)	0.3	0.3	0.3	0.2	0.1	0.2	0.3	0.3	0.3
Heart failure (I50)	18.7	15.4	21.9	4.2	3.5	4.9	21.3	17.6	24.8
All other forms of heart disease (I26-I28, I34-I38, I42-I49, I51)	37.6	35.6	39.5	9.5	9.6	9.5	42.6	40.5	44.6
Essential hypertension and hypertensive renal disease (I10, I12, I15)	8.5	6.9	10.0	3.2	2.7	3.8	9.4	7.7	11.1
Cerebrovascular diseases (I60-I69)	44.1	35.7	52.3	15.2	13.9	16.5	49.3	39.8	58.4
Atherosclerosis (I70)	2.6	2.0	3.1	0.6	0.5	0.7	2.9	2.3	3.5
Other diseases of circulatory system (I71-I78)	6.6	7.0	6.1	1.8	2.0	1.7	7.4	7.9	6.9
Aortic aneurysm and dissection (I71)	3.6	4.3	3.0	0.9	1.2	0.6	4.1	4.9	3.4
Other diseases of arteries, arterioles and capillaries (I72-I78)	2.9	2.6	3.2	0.9	0.8	1.0	3.3	3.0	3.5
Other disorders of circulatory system (I80-I99)	1.3	1.2	1.4	0.4	0.5	0.4	1.5	1.4	1.6
Influenza and pneumonia (J09-J18)[1]	18.5	17.1	19.9	6.8	6.4	7.2	20.6	19.1	22.1
Influenza (J09-J11)[1]	0.6	0.5	0.7	0.2	0.1	0.2	0.6	0.5	0.8
Pneumonia (J12-J18)	17.9	16.6	19.3	6.6	6.2	7.0	20.0	18.6	21.3
Other acute lower respiratory infections (J20-J22, U04)[2]	0.1	0.1	0.1	0.0	*	*	0.1	0.1	0.1
Acute bronchitis and bronchiolitis (J20-J21)	0.1	0.1	0.1	0.0	*	*	0.1	0.1	0.1
Other and unspecified acute lower respiratory infections (J22, U04)[2,3]	0.0	0.0	0.0	*	*	*	0.0	0.0	0.0
Chronic lower respiratory diseases (J40-J47)	46.4	44.8	48.0	8.4	8.3	8.5	53.2	51.7	54.7
Bronchitis, chronic and unspecified (J40-J42)	0.2	0.2	0.3	0.1	0.1	*	0.3	0.2	0.3
Emphysema (J43)	4.1	4.3	3.9	0.6	0.7	0.5	4.7	5.0	4.5
Asthma (J45-J46)	1.1	0.8	1.4	0.6	0.5	0.7	1.2	0.8	1.6
Other chronic lower respiratory diseases (J44, J47)	41.0	39.5	42.4	7.1	7.0	7.3	47.0	45.6	48.4
Pneumoconioses and chemical effects (J60-J66, J68)	0.3	0.6	0.0	0.0	0.1	*	0.3	0.7	0.0
Pneumonitis due to solids and liquids (J69)	5.5	5.8	5.2	1.4	1.4	1.4	6.2	6.6	5.8
Other diseases of respiratory system (J00-J06, J30-J39, J67, J70-J98)	9.8	9.9	9.7	3.8	3.7	4.0	10.9	11.1	10.7
Peptic ulcer (K25-K28)	1.0	1.0	1.0	0.3	0.4	0.3	1.1	1.2	1.1
Diseases of appendix (K35-K38)	0.1	0.2	0.1	0.1	0.1	*	0.1	0.2	0.1
Hernia (K40-K46)	0.6	0.5	0.6	0.2	0.2	0.3	0.6	0.5	0.7
Chronic liver disease and cirrhosis (K70, K73-K74)	9.9	13.1	6.7	8.7	11.8	5.5	10.0	13.3	6.9
Alcoholic liver disease (K70)	4.9	7.2	2.6	4.6	7.2	1.7	4.9	7.2	2.8
Other chronic liver disease and cirrhosis (K73-K74)	5.0	5.9	4.1	4.1	4.5	3.7	5.1	6.1	4.1
Cholelithiasis and other disorders of gallbladder (K80-K82)	1.1	1.1	1.2	0.6	0.5	0.7	1.2	1.2	1.3
Nephritis, nephrotic syndrome and nephrosis (N00-N07, N17-N19, N25-N27)	15.9	15.7	16.0	6.2	6.0	6.4	17.6	17.5	17.7
Acute and rapidly progressive nephritic and nephrotic syndrome (N00-N01,N04)	0.1	0.0	0.1	*	*	*	0.1	0.1	0.1
Chronic glomerulonephritis, nephritis and nephropathy not specified as acute or chronic, and renal sclerosis unspecified (N02-N03, N05-N07, N26)	1.4	1.3	1.4	0.5	0.5	0.5	1.5	1.5	1.5
Renal failure (N17-N19)	14.4	14.3	14.6	5.7	5.5	5.9	16.0	16.0	16.0
Other disorders of kidney (N25, N27)	0.0	*	0.0	*	*	*	0.0	0.0	*
Infections of kidney (N10-N12,N13.6,N15.1)	0.2	0.1	0.3	0.1	*	0.2	0.2	0.1	0.3
Hyperplasia of prostate (N40)	0.2	0.3	X	0.0	0.1	X	0.2	0.4	X
Inflammatory diseases of female pelvic organs (N70-N76)	0.0	X	0.1	*	X	*	0.1	X	0.1
Pregnancy, childbirth and the puerperium (O00-O99)	0.3	X	0.5	0.3	X	0.7	0.2	X	0.5
Pregnancy with abortive outcome (O00-O07)	0.0	X	0.0	*	X	*	0.0	X	0.0
Other complications of pregnancy, childbirth and the puerperium (O10-O99)	0.3	X	0.5	0.3	X	0.6	0.2	X	0.5

Table B-16. Death Rates from Selected Causes by Hispanic Origin, Race for Non-Hispanic Population, and Sex, 2008—Continued

(Rates per 100,000 population in specified group.)

Cause of death (based on ICD–10, 2004)	Non-Hispanic White			Non-Hispanic Black		
	Both sexes	Male	Female	Both sexes	Male	Female
Major cardiovascular diseases (I00-I78)	322.6	314.9	330.1	245.9	249.4	242.7
Diseases of heart (I00-I09, I11, I13, I20-I51)	249.4	254.9	244.0	182.5	191.3	174.4
Acute rheumatic fever and chronic rheumatic heart diseases (I00-I09)	1.3	0.8	1.7	0.7	0.5	0.8
Hypertensive heart disease (I11)	11.1	10.1	12.0	19.2	20.4	18.2
Hypertensive heart and renal disease (I13)	0.9	0.8	1.0	2.2	2.0	2.3
Ischemic heart diseases (I20-I25)	165.2	179.7	151.3	108.0	115.6	101.0
Acute myocardial infarction (I21-I22)	54.8	60.7	49.0	35.6	37.3	34.1
Other acute ischemic heart diseases (I24)	1.7	1.8	1.6	1.5	1.6	1.3
Other forms of chronic ischemic heart disease (I20, I25)	108.8	117.2	100.7	70.9	76.7	65.6
Atherosclerotic cardiovascular disease, so described (I25.0)	22.4	25.6	19.3	22.1	26.6	18.0
All other forms of chronic ischemic heart disease (I20,I25.1-I25.9)	86.4	91.6	81.4	48.8	50.1	47.6
Other heart diseases (I26-I51)	70.9	63.5	78.0	52.4	52.8	52.2
Acute and subacute endocarditis (I33)	0.4	0.5	0.4	0.5	0.6	0.5
Diseases of pericardium and acute myocarditis (I30-I31, I40)	0.3	0.3	0.3	0.4	0.4	0.4
Heart failure (I50)	24.0	19.6	28.4	14.1	13.0	15.1
All other forms of heart disease (I26-I28, I34-I38, I42-I49, I51)	46.1	43.2	49.0	37.4	38.8	36.1
Essential hypertension and hypertensive renal disease (I10, I12, I15)	9.1	7.2	11.0	13.1	12.0	14.1
Cerebrovascular diseases (I60-I69)	52.6	41.5	63.4	43.1	39.0	46.9
Atherosclerosis (I70)	3.4	2.6	4.1	1.7	1.5	1.9
Other diseases of circulatory system (I71-I78)	8.2	8.8	7.6	5.5	5.5	5.4
Aortic aneurysm and dissection (I71)	4.7	5.6	3.8	2.4	2.8	2.0
Other diseases of arteries, arterioles and capillaries (I72-I78)	3.5	3.2	3.8	3.1	2.8	3.4
Other disorders of circulatory system (I80-I99)	1.5	1.4	1.6	2.0	2.0	2.0
Influenza and pneumonia (J09-J18)[1]	22.7	20.7	24.6	14.1	13.9	14.2
Influenza (J09-J11)[1]	0.8	0.6	0.9	0.2	0.2	0.2
Pneumonia (J12-J18)	21.9	20.1	23.7	13.9	13.7	14.0
Other acute lower respiratory infections (J20-J22, U04)[2]	0.1	0.1	0.1	0.1	*	*
Acute bronchitis and bronchiolitis (J20-J21)	0.1	0.1	0.1	0.1	*	*
Other and unspecified acute lower respiratory infections (J22, U04)[2,3]	0.0	*	0.0	*	*	*
Chronic lower respiratory diseases (J40-J47)	62.5	59.8	65.1	22.7	24.6	20.9
Bronchitis, chronic and unspecified (J40-J42)	0.3	0.2	0.4	0.2	0.2	0.1
Emphysema (J43)	5.6	5.8	5.4	1.7	2.2	1.4
Asthma (J45-J46)	1.0	0.6	1.4	2.3	2.0	2.6
Other chronic lower respiratory diseases (J44, J47)	55.6	53.1	58.0	18.4	20.2	16.8
Pneumoconioses and chemical effects (J60-J66, J68)	0.4	0.8	0.0	0.1	0.2	*
Pneumonitis due to solids and liquids (J69)	7.0	7.4	6.6	3.8	4.1	3.6
Other diseases of respiratory system (J00-J06, J30-J39, J67, J70-J98)	12.2	12.4	11.9	7.2	7.1	7.3
Peptic ulcer (K25-K28)	1.2	1.2	1.2	0.8	1.0	0.6
Diseases of appendix (K35-K38)	0.2	0.2	0.1	0.1	0.2	*
Hernia (K40-K46)	0.7	0.6	0.8	0.4	0.4	0.4
Chronic liver disease and cirrhosis (K70, K73-K74)	11.0	14.6	7.6	6.4	9.0	4.0
Alcoholic liver disease (K70)	5.4	7.9	2.9	3.1	4.4	1.9
Other chronic liver disease and cirrhosis (K73-K74)	5.6	6.7	4.6	3.4	4.7	2.2
Cholelithiasis and other disorders of gallbladder (K80-K82)	1.3	1.3	1.4	0.8	0.8	0.8
Nephritis, nephrotic syndrome and nephrosis (N00-N07, N17-N19, N25-N27)	17.6	17.7	17.4	22.4	21.3	23.3
Acute and rapidly progressive nephritic and nephrotic syndrome (N00-N01,N04)	0.1	0.1	0.1	0.1	*	*
Chronic glomerulonephritis, nephritis and nephropathy not specified as acute or chronic, and renal sclerosis unspecified (N02-N03, N05-N07, N26)	1.5	1.5	1.6	1.8	1.7	1.9
Renal failure (N17-N19)	16.0	16.1	15.8	20.5	19.6	21.3
Other disorders of kidney (N25, N27)	0.0	*	*	*	*	*
Infections of kidney (N10-N12,N13.6,N15.1)	0.2	0.1	0.3	0.2	0.1	0.2
Hyperplasia of prostate (N40)	0.2	0.4	X	0.1	0.2	X
Inflammatory diseases of female pelvic organs (N70-N76)	0.1	X	0.1	*	X	*
Pregnancy, childbirth and the puerperium (O00-O99)	0.2	X	0.3	0.6	X	1.2
Pregnancy with abortive outcome (O00-O07)	*	X	*	*	X	*
Other complications of pregnancy, childbirth and the puerperium (O10-O99)	0.2	X	0.3	0.6	X	1.2

Table B-16. Death Rates from Selected Causes by Hispanic Origin, Race for Non-Hispanic Population, and Sex, 2008—Continued

(Rates per 100,000 population in specified group.)

Cause of death (based on ICD–10, 2004)	All origins[1]			Hispanic[2]			Non-Hispanic		
	Both sexes	Male	Female	Both sexes	Male	Female	Both sexes	Male	Female
Certain conditions originating in the perinatal period (P00-P96)	4.6	5.3	3.9	6.1	6.8	5.4	4.2	4.9	3.6
Congenital malformations, deformations and chromosomal abnormalities (Q00-Q99)	3.4	3.6	3.2	4.3	4.4	4.2	3.2	3.4	3.0
Symptoms, signs and abnormal clinical and laboratory findings, not elsewhere classified (R00-R99)	12.7	11.2	14.1	4.7	5.1	4.3	14.1	12.3	15.7
All other diseases (Residual)	83.0	67.7	97.9	26.8	24.2	29.5	93.1	75.9	109.6
Accidents (unintentional injuries) (V01-X59, Y85-Y86)	40.1	52.3	28.2	23.6	34.5	12.0	43.0	55.5	31.0
Transport accidents (V01-V99, Y85)	14.0	20.4	7.8	11.5	17.3	5.4	14.5	21.0	8.2
Motor vehicle accidents (V02-V04, V09.0, V09.2, V12-V14, V19.0-V19.2, V19.4-V19.6, V20-V79, V80.3-V80.5, V81.0-V81.1, V82.0-V82.1, V83-V86, V87.0-V87.8, V88.0-V88.8, V89.0, V89.2)	13.1	18.9	7.5	10.9	16.2	5.2	13.5	19.3	7.8
Other land transport accidents (V01,V05-V06, V09.1, V09.3-V09.9, V10-V11, V15-V18, V19.3, V19.8-V19.9, V80.0-V80.2, V80.6-V80.9, V81.2- V81.9, V82.2-V82.9, V87.9, V88.9, V89.1, V89.3, V89.9)	0.4	0.6	0.2	0.4	0.7	0.1	0.4	0.6	0.2
Water, air and space, and other and unspecified transport accidents and their sequelae (V90-V99, Y85)	0.6	1.0	0.2	0.3	0.4	*	0.6	1.1	0.2
Nontransport accidents (W00-X59, Y86)	26.0	31.8	20.4	12.1	17.2	6.6	28.5	34.5	22.7
Falls (W00-W19)	7.9	8.2	7.6	2.7	3.4	1.9	8.8	9.1	8.5
Accidental discharge of firearms (W32-W34)	0.2	0.3	0.1	0.1	0.1	*	0.2	0.4	0.1
Accidental drowning and submersion (W65-W74)	1.2	1.8	0.5	1.1	1.6	0.4	1.2	1.8	0.5
Accidental exposure to smoke, fire and flames (X00-X09)	1.0	1.1	0.8	0.4	0.5	0.3	1.1	1.3	0.9
Accidental poisoning and exposure to noxious substances (X40-X49)	10.2	13.7	6.9	5.5	8.3	2.5	11.1	14.7	7.6
Other and unspecified nontransport accidents and their sequelae (W20-W31, W35-W64, W75-W99, X10-X39, X50-X59, Y86)	5.6	6.6	4.6	2.4	3.3	1.4	6.2	7.2	5.1
Intentional self-harm (suicide) (*U03, X60-X84, Y87.0)	11.9	19.0	4.9	5.0	8.1	1.7	13.1	21.0	5.5
Intentional self-harm (suicide) by discharge of firearms (X72-X74)	6.0	10.6	1.5	1.8	3.2	0.3	6.7	12.0	1.7
Intentional self-harm (suicide) by other and unspecified means and their sequelae (*U03, X60-X71, X75-X84, Y87.0)	5.9	8.4	3.4	3.2	4.8	1.4	6.3	9.0	3.8
Assault (homicide) (*U01-*U02, X85-Y09, Y87.1)	5.9	9.4	2.4	7.1	11.4	2.4	5.6	9.0	2.4
Assault (homicide) by discharge of firearms (*U01.4, X93-X95)	4.0	6.9	1.2	4.8	8.3	1.1	3.8	6.6	1.2
Assault (homicide) by other and unspecified means and their sequelae (*U01.0-*U01.3, *U01.5-*U01.9, *U02, X85-X92, X96-Y09, Y87.1)	1.9	2.5	1.2	2.3	3.2	1.3	1.8	2.4	1.2
Legal intervention (Y35, Y89.0)	0.1	0.2	*	0.2	0.3	*	0.1	0.2	*
Events of undetermined intent (Y10-Y34, Y87.2,Y89.9)	1.7	2.1	1.2	0.7	1.0	0.3	1.8	2.3	1.4
Discharge of firearms, undetermined intent (Y22-Y24)	0.1	0.1	0.0	0.0	*	*	0.1	0.2	0.0
Other and unspecified events of undetermined intent and their sequelae (Y10-Y21, Y25-Y34, Y87.2, Y89.9)	1.6	2.0	1.2	0.6	1.0	0.3	1.7	2.1	1.4
Operations of war and their sequelae (Y36, Y89.1)	0.0	0.0	*	*	*	*	0.0	0.0	*
Complications of medical and surgical care (Y40-Y84, Y88)	0.9	0.8	0.9	0.3	0.3	0.4	0.9	0.9	1.0
Enterocolitis due to Clostridium difficile (A04.7)[3]	2.5	1.9	3.0	0.7	0.6	0.9	2.8	2.1	3.4
Drug-induced deaths[4,5]	12.7	16.0	9.6	5.9	8.4	3.2	13.9	17.3	10.6
Alcohol-induced deaths[4,6]	8.0	12.1	3.9	6.4	10.4	2.2	8.2	12.4	4.2
Injury by firearms[4,7]	10.4	18.2	2.8	6.9	12.0	1.5	11.0	19.4	3.0

Table B-16. Death Rates from Selected Causes by Hispanic Origin, Race for Non-Hispanic Population, and Sex, 2008—Continued

(Rates per 100,000 population in specified group.)

Cause of death (based on ICD–10, 2004)	Non-Hispanic White			Non-Hispanic Black		
	Both sexes	Male	Female	Both sexes	Male	Female
Certain conditions originating in the perinatal period (P00-P96)	2.8	3.3	2.4	12.1	14.3	10.1
Congenital malformations, deformations andchromosomal abnormalities (Q00-Q99)	3.1	3.3	2.9	4.2	4.6	3.9
Symptoms, signs and abnormal clinical and laboratory findings, not elsewhere classified (R00-R99)	15.1	12.7	17.3	13.4	14.2	12.7
All other diseases (Residual)	102.8	82.7	122.2	69.9	61.1	77.9
Accidents (unintentional injuries) (V01-X59, Y85-Y86)	47.0	59.7	34.6	31.9	45.3	19.6
Transport accidents (V01-V99, Y85)	15.1	21.8	8.6	13.4	20.4	7.0
Motor vehicle accidents (V02-V04, V09.0, V09.2, V12-V14, V19.0-V19.2, V19.4-V19.6, V20-V79, V80.3-V80.5, V81.0-V81.1, V82.0-V82.1,V83- V86, V87.0-V87.8, V88.0-V88.8, V89.0, V89.2)	14.0	20.0	8.2	12.5	18.9	6.6
Other land transport accidents (V01,V05-V06, V09.1, V09.3-V09.9, V10-V11, V15-V18, V19.3, V19.8-V19.9, V80.0-V80.2, V80.6-V80.9, V81.2- V81.9, V82.2-V82.9, V87.9, V88.9, V89.1, V89.3, V89.9)	0.4	0.6	0.2	0.4	0.7	0.2
Water, air and space, and other and unspecified transport accidents and their sequelae (V90-V99, Y85)	0.7	1.2	0.3	0.4	0.7	0.1
Nontransport accidents (W00-X59, Y86)	31.9	37.9	26.0	18.5	24.9	12.7
Falls (W00-W19)	10.5	10.6	10.3	2.6	3.2	2.1
Accidental discharge of firearms (W32-W34)	0.2	0.4	0.1	0.2	0.5	*
Accidental drowning and submersion (W65-W74)	1.1	1.8	0.5	1.4	2.3	0.6
Accidental exposure to smoke, fire and flames (X00-X09)	1.0	1.2	0.8	1.6	1.9	1.2
Accidental poisoning and exposure to noxious substances (X40-X49)	12.3	16.2	8.6	7.7	10.7	4.9
Other and unspecified nontransport accidents and their sequelae (W20-W31, W35-W64, W75-W99, X10-X39, X50-X59, Y86)	6.7	7.8	5.7	5.0	6.4	3.7
Intentional self-harm (suicide) (*U03, X60-X84, Y87.0)	15.0	24.1	6.3	5.4	9.4	1.7
Intentional self-harm (suicide) by discharge of firearms (X72-X74)	7.9	14.0	2.0	2.7	5.1	0.5
Intentional self-harm (suicide) by other and unspecified means and their sequelae (*U03, X60-X71, X75-X84, Y87.0)	7.1	10.0	4.3	2.7	4.3	1.2
Assault (homicide) (*U01-*U02, X85-Y09, Y87.1)	2.8	3.9	1.8	21.4	38.6	5.8
Assault (homicide) by discharge of firearms (*U01.4, X93-X95)	1.5	2.3	0.8	16.9	32.0	3.1
Assault (homicide) by other and unspecified means and their sequelae (*U01.0-*U01.3, *U01.5-*U01.9, *U02, X85-X92, X96-Y09, Y87.1)	1.3	1.6	0.9	4.5	6.5	2.6
Legal intervention (Y35, Y89.0)	0.1	0.2	*	0.3	0.6	*
Events of undetermined intent (Y10-Y34, Y87.2,Y89.9)	1.9	2.4	1.5	1.7	2.5	1.1
Discharge of firearms, undetermined intent (Y22-Y24)	0.1	0.2	0.0	0.1	0.2	*
Other and unspecified events of undetermined intent and their sequelae (Y10-Y21, Y25-Y34, Y87.2, Y89.9)	1.8	2.2	1.5	1.6	2.3	1.0
Operations of war and their sequelae (Y36, Y89.1)	0.0	0.0	*	*	*	*
Complications of medical and surgical care (Y40-Y84, Y88)	1.0	0.9	1.1	1.0	1.0	1.0
Enterocolitis due to Clostridium difficile (A04.7)[3]	3.2	2.5	4.0	1.2	0.9	1.4
Drug-induced deaths[4]	15.6	19.2	12.1	9.4	12.7	6.3
Alcohol-induced deaths[4]	8.8	13.3	4.5	5.8	9.1	2.9
Injury by firearms[4]	9.9	17.0	3.0	20.2	38.3	3.7

X = Category not applicable.
* = Figure does not meet standards of reliability or precision.
0.0 = Quantity more than zero but less than 0.05.
[1]Figures for origin not stated are included in "All origins" but not distributed among specified origins.
[2]Includes races other than white and black.
[3]Included in certain other intestinal infections (A04, A07–A09)
[4]Included in selected categories above.

PART B: MORTALITY 149

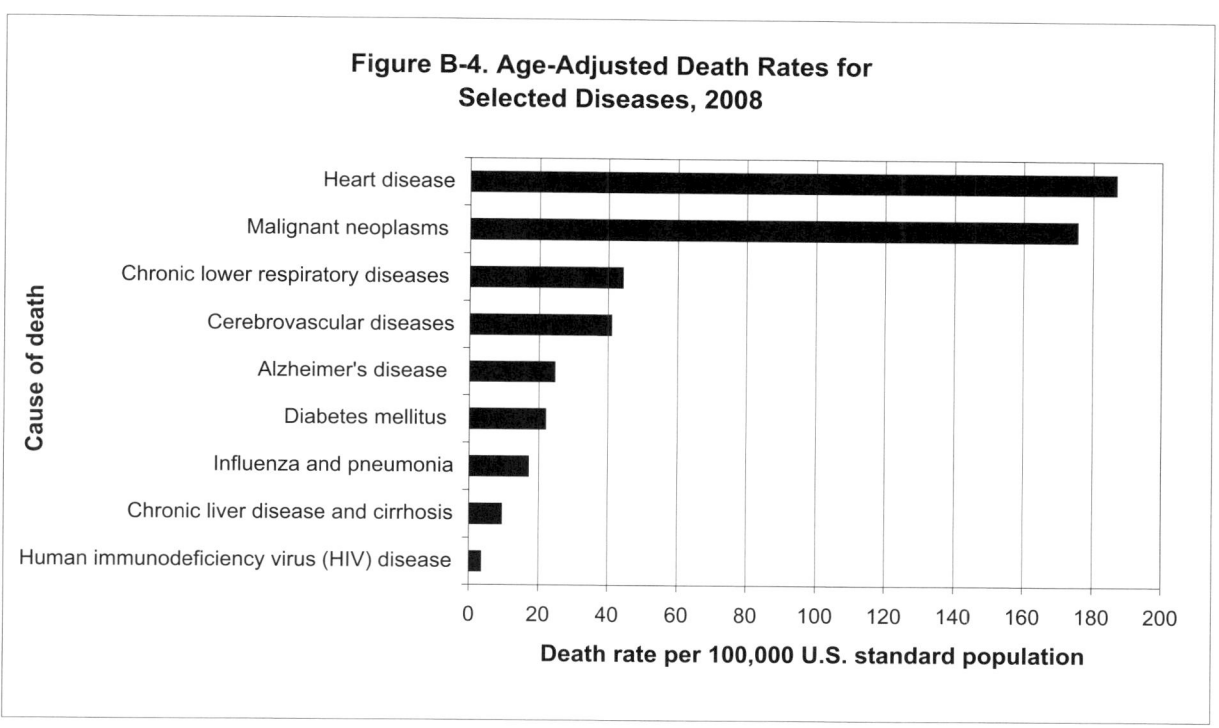

Figure B-4. Age-Adjusted Death Rates for Selected Diseases, 2008

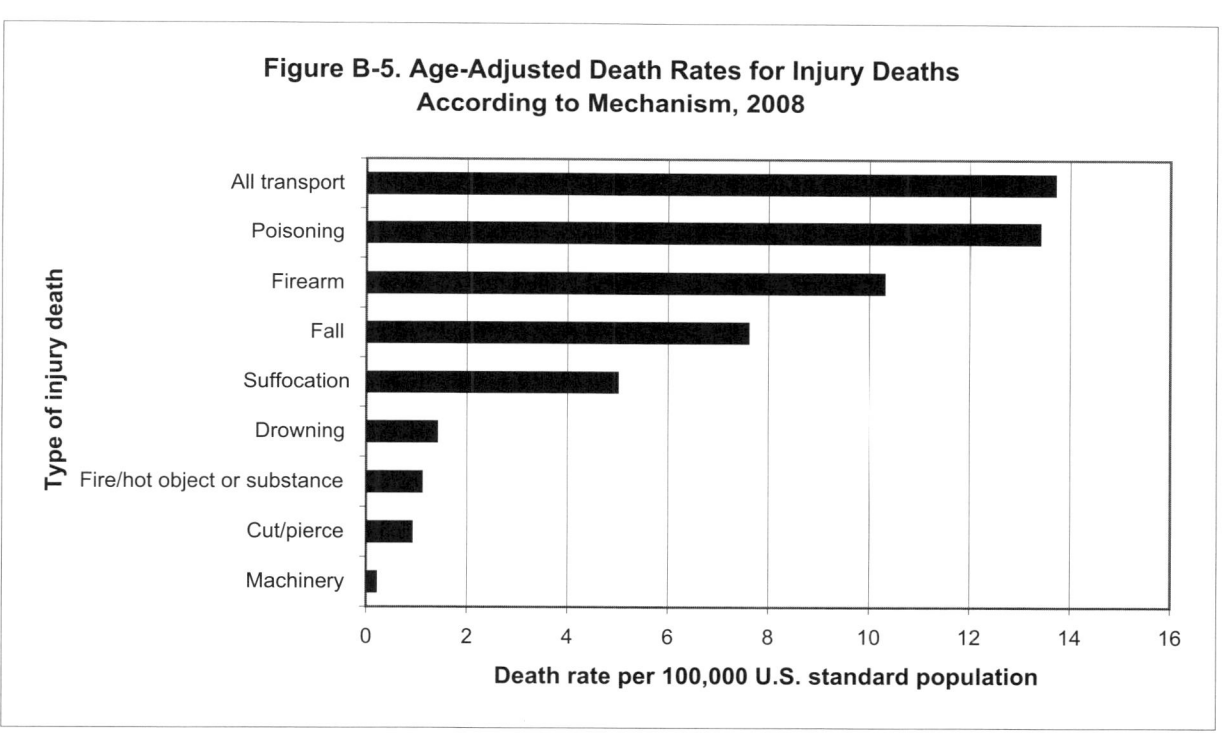

Figure B-5. Age-Adjusted Death Rates for Injury Deaths According to Mechanism, 2008

Table B-17. Age-Adjusted Death Rates from Selected Causes by Race and Sex, 2008

(Age-adjusted rates per 100,000 U.S. standard population.)

Cause of death (based on ICD–10, 2004)	All races Both sexes	All races Male	All races Female	White[1] Both sexes	White[1] Male	White[1] Female	Black[1] Both sexes	Black[1] Male	Black[1] Female
ALL CAUSES	758.3	900.6	643.4	750.3	889.2	636.9	934.9	1150.4	778.4
Salmonella infections (A01-A02)	0.0	0.0	0.0	0.0	0.0	*	*	*	*
Shigellosis and amebiasis (A03, A06)	*	*	*	*	*	*	*	*	*
Certain other intestinal infections (A04, A07-A09)	2.4	2.4	2.4	2.5	2.5	2.6	1.7	1.7	1.7
Tuberculosis (A16-A19)	0.2	0.3	0.1	0.1	0.2	0.1	0.4	0.7	0.3
Respiratory tuberculosis (A16)	0.1	0.2	0.1	0.1	0.1	0.0	0.3	0.6	0.2
Other tuberculosis (A17-A19)	0.0	0.1	0.0	0.0	0.0	0.0	0.1	*	*
Whooping cough (A37)	0.0	*	*	*	*	*	*	*	*
Scarlet fever and erysipelas (A38, A46)	*	*	*	*	*	*	*	*	*
Meningococcal infection (A39)	0.0	0.0	0.0	0.0	0.0	0.0	0.1	*	*
Septicemia (A40-A41)	11.1	12.1	10.3	10.2	11.2	9.5	21.6	24.4	19.8
Syphilis (A50-A53)	0.0	0.0	*	*	*	*	*	*	*
Acute poliomyelitis (A80)	*	*	*	*	*	*	*	*	*
Arthropod-borne viral encephalitis (A83-A84, A85.2)	*	*	*	*	*	*	*	*	*
Measles (B05)	*	*	*	*	*	*	*	*	*
Viral hepatitis (B15-B19)	2.3	3.1	1.5	2.2	3.0	1.4	3.1	4.4	2.0
Human immunodeficiency virus (HIV) disease (B20-B24)	3.3	4.8	1.9	1.7	2.8	0.7	15.3	21.9	9.8
Malaria (B50-B54)	*	*	*	*	*	*	*	*	*
Other and unspecified infectious and parasitic diseases and their sequelae (A00, A05, A20-A36, A42-A44, A48- A49, A54-A79, A81-A82, A85.0-A85.1, A85.8, A86-B04, B06-B09, B25-B49, B55-B99)	1.8	2.2	1.6	1.8	2.1	1.6	2.3	3.0	1.8
Malignant neoplasms (C00-C97)	175.3	213.6	148.5	174.7	211.7	148.5	209.1	272.4	170.0
Malignant neoplasms of lip, oral cavity and pharynx (C00-C14)	2.4	3.7	1.4	2.4	3.6	1.4	3.0	5.2	1.5
Malignant neoplasm of esophagus (C15)	4.2	7.5	1.6	4.3	7.7	1.5	4.5	7.7	2.3
Malignant neoplasms of stomach (C16)	3.5	4.8	2.5	3.0	4.2	2.1	6.8	9.9	4.8
Malignant neoplasms of colon, rectum and anus (C18-C21)	16.4	19.5	14.0	16.0	18.9	13.6	22.8	28.6	18.9
Malignant neoplasms of liver and intrahepatic bileducts (C22)	5.6	8.3	3.2	5.1	7.6	3.0	7.5	12.2	3.9
Malignant neoplasm of pancreas (C25)	10.9	12.5	9.6	10.8	12.4	9.4	13.6	15.1	12.5
Malignant neoplasm of larynx (C32)	1.1	2.1	0.5	1.1	1.9	0.4	2.0	3.9	0.8
Malignant neoplasms of trachea, bronchus and lung (C33-C34)	49.5	63.6	39.0	50.2	63.4	40.2	53.4	78.5	36.9
Malignant melanoma of skin (C43)	2.7	4.0	1.7	3.1	4.6	1.9	0.4	0.5	0.3
Malignant neoplasm of breast (C50)	12.6	0.3	22.5	12.2	0.3	21.9	18.4	0.6	31.1
Malignant neoplasm of cervix uteri (C53)	1.2	X	2.4	1.1	X	2.1	2.4	X	4.2
Malignant neoplasms of corpus uteri and uterus, part unspecified (C54-C55)	2.4	X	4.2	2.2	X	3.9	4.2	X	7.1
Malignant neoplasm of ovary (C56)	4.4	X	8.0	4.6	X	8.2	3.9	X	6.6
Malignant neoplasm of prostate (C61)	8.8	22.3	X	8.2	20.8	X	16.8	46.2	X
Malignant neoplasms of kidney and renal pelvis (C64-C65)	4.0	5.8	2.6	4.1	5.9	2.6	3.9	5.8	2.6
Malignant neoplasm of bladder (C67)	4.3	7.4	2.2	4.5	7.9	2.2	3.3	4.7	2.5
Malignant neoplasms of meninges, brain and other parts of central nervous system (C70-C72)	4.3	5.2	3.4	4.6	5.6	3.8	2.5	3.2	2.0
Malignant neoplasms of lymphoid, hematopoietic and related tissue (C81-C96)	17.2	22.4	13.3	17.5	22.8	13.5	17.2	22.3	13.8
Hodgkin's disease (C81)	0.4	0.4	0.3	0.4	0.5	0.3	0.3	0.4	0.3
Non-Hodgkin's lymphoma (C82-C85)	6.3	8.1	5.0	6.7	8.5	5.3	4.3	5.5	3.4
Leukemia (C91-C95)	7.0	9.4	5.3	7.2	9.7	5.4	6.2	8.4	4.7
Multiple myeloma and immunoproliferative neoplasms (C88, C90)	3.4	4.4	2.7	3.2	4.2	2.5	6.4	8.0	5.4
Other and unspecified malignant neoplasms of lymphoid, hematopoietic and related tissue (C96)	0.0	0.0	0.0	0.0	0.0	0.0	*	*	*
All other and unspecified malignant neoplasms (C17, C23-C24, C26-C31, C37-C41, C44-C49, C51-C52, C57-C60, C62-C63, C66, C68-C69, C73-C80, C97)	19.7	23.9	16.5	19.7	23.8	16.5	22.2	27.9	18.3
In situ neoplasms, benign neoplasms and neoplasms of uncertain or unknown behavior (D00-D48)	4.5	5.7	3.7	4.6	5.9	3.7	3.9	4.6	3.4
Anemias (D50-D64)	1.5	1.6	1.5	1.4	1.4	1.3	3.1	3.1	3.0
Diabetes mellitus (E10-E14)	21.8	25.6	18.8	19.9	23.9	16.7	40.5	44.8	37.2
Nutritional deficiencies (E40-E64)	0.9	0.9	0.9	0.9	0.8	0.9	1.3	1.7	1.1
Malnutrition (E40-E46)	0.8	0.8	0.8	0.8	0.8	0.8	1.3	1.6	1.1
Other nutritional deficiencies (E50-E64)	0.1	0.1	0.1	0.1	0.1	0.1	*	*	*
Meningitis (G00,G03)	0.2	0.2	0.2	0.2	0.2	0.2	0.3	0.4	0.3
Parkinson's disease (G20-G21)	6.4	9.7	4.3	6.8	10.3	4.5	2.9	4.3	2.1
Alzheimer's disease (G30)	24.4	20.1	26.7	25.4	21.0	27.9	19.7	16.3	21.1

Table B-17. Age-Adjusted Death Rates from Selected Causes by Race and Sex, 2008—Continued

(Age-adjusted rates per 100,000 U.S. standard population.)

Cause of death (based on ICD–10, 2004)	American Indian or Alaska Native[1,2]			Asian or Pacific Islander[1,3]		
	Both sexes	Male	Female	Both sexes	Male	Female
ALL CAUSES	610.1	717.3	515.1	413.7	492.8	353.1
Salmonella infections (A01-A02)	*	*	*	*	*	*
Shigellosis and amebiasis (A03, A06)	*	*	*	*	*	*
Certain other intestinal infections (A04, A07-A09)	1.4	*	*	1	1.2	0.9
Tuberculosis (A16-A19)	*	*	*	0.9	1.5	0.4
Respiratory tuberculosis (A16)	*	*	*	0.8	1.4	0.3
Other tuberculosis (A17-A19)	*	*	*	*	*	*
Whooping cough (A37)	*	*	*	*	*	*
Scarlet fever and erysipelas (A38, A46)	*	*	*	*	*	*
Meningococcal infection (A39)	*	*	*	*	*	*
Septicemia (A40-A41)	10.6	10.8	10.4	4.9	5.4	4.5
Syphilis (A50-A53)	*	*	*	*	*	*
Acute poliomyelitis (A80)	*	*	*	*	*	*
Arthropod-borne viral encephalitis (A83-A84, A85.2)	*	*	*	*	*	*
Measles (B05)	*	*	*	*	*	*
Viral hepatitis (B15-B19)	3.3	4.1	2.6	2.4	2.7	2
Human immunodeficiency virus (HIV) disease (B20-B24)	2.1	3.3	*	0.6	1	0.3
Malaria (B50-B54)	*	*	*	*	*	*
Other and unspecified infectious and parasitic diseases and their sequelae (A00, A05, A20-A36, A42-A44, A48- A49, A54-A79, A81-A82, A85.0-A85.1, A85.8, A86-B04, B06-B09, B25-B49, B55-B99)	2.3	2.4	2.2	1.4	1.6	1.2
Malignant neoplasms (C00-C97)	119.6	142.0	102.3	106.5	128.8	90.6
Malignant neoplasms of lip, oral cavity and pharynx (C00-C14)	2.0	3.3	*	2.0	2.9	1.2
Malignant neoplasm of esophagus (C15)	2.7	5.3	*	1.6	2.7	0.8
Malignant neoplasm of stomach (C16)	3.0	3.8	2.2	6.4	8.5	4.8
Malignant neoplasms of colon, rectum and anus (C18-C21)	13.8	15.0	12.6	11.3	13.4	9.7
Malignant neoplasms of liver and intrahepatic bile ducts (C22)	6.3	9.1	3.9	9.8	14.4	6.0
Malignant neoplasm of pancreas (C25)	5.6	6.5	4.9	7.4	8.3	6.7
Malignant neoplasm of larynx (C32)	*	*	*	0.3	0.6	*
Malignant neoplasms of trachea, bronchus and lung (C33-C34)	33.2	41.7	26.3	25.1	35.1	17.8
Malignant melanoma of skin (C43)	*	*	*	0.3	0.4	*
Malignant neoplasm of breast (C50)	6.9	*	12.6	6.5	*	11.7
Malignant neoplasm of cervix uteri (C53)	1.8	X	3.4	1.0	X	1.9
Malignant neoplasms of corpus uteri and uterus, part unspecified (C54-C55)	1.4	X	2.6	1.4	X	2.5
Malignant neoplasm of ovary (C56)	2.8	X	5.0	2.9	X	5.2
Malignant neoplasm of prostate (C61)	6.9	16.6	X	3.7	9.1	X
Malignant neoplasms of kidney and renal pelvis (C64-C65)	4.9	6.3	3.6	1.8	2.7	1.1
Malignant neoplasm of bladder (C67)	2.3	2.9	*	1.7	3.1	0.7
Malignant neoplasms of meninges, brain and other parts of central nervous system (C70-C72)	2.4	2.8	2.2	1.9	2.4	1.5
Malignant neoplasms of lymphoid, hematopoietic and related tissue (C81-C96)	8.6	11.1	6.7	9.5	11.6	7.8
Hodgkin's disease (C81)	*	*	*	0.2	*	*
Non-Hodgkin's lymphoma (C82-C85)	3.0	3.3	2.7	4.0	5.0	3.2
Leukemia (C91-C95)	3.5	4.5	2.7	3.6	4.2	3.1
Multiple myeloma and immunoproliferative neoplasms (C88, C90)	2.1	3.0	*	1.7	2.1	1.3
Other and unspecified malignant neoplasms of lymphoid, hematopoietic and related tissue (C96)	*	*	*	*	*	*
All other and unspecified malignant neoplasms (C17, C23-C24, C26-C31, C37-C41, C44-C49, C51- C52, C57-C60, C62-C63, C66, C68-C69, C73-C80, C97)	13.5	15.6	11.7	12.0	13.4	10.8
In situ neoplasms, benign neoplasms and neoplasms of uncertain or unknown behavior (D00-D48)	2.6	3.1	2.3	2.7	3.2	2.4
Anemias (D50-D64)	1.3	*	*	0.8	0.8	0.9
Diabetes mellitus (E10-E14)	34.5	36.4	32.6	16.0	18.2	14.2
Nutritional deficiencies (E40-E64)	1.1	*	*	0.5	0.5	0.5
Malnutrition (E40-E46)	1.1	*	*	0.5	*	0.5
Other nutritional deficiencies (E50-E64)	*	*	*	*	*	*
Meningitis (G00,G03)	*	*	*	0.2	*	*
Parkinson's disease (G20-G21)	4.0	5.6	2.9	3.3	4.7	2.3
Alzheimer's disease (G30)	11.4	9.2	12.9	8.9	7.4	9.9

Table B-17. Age-Adjusted Death Rates from Selected Causes by Race and Sex, 2008—Continued

(Age-adjusted rates per 100,000 U.S. standard population.)

Cause of death (based on ICD–10, 2004)	All races			White[1]			Black[1]		
	Both sexes	Male	Female	Both sexes	Male	Female	Both sexes	Male	Female
Major cardiovascular diseases (I00-I78)	243.5	291.3	204.9	238.3	286.0	199.4	323.0	387.7	275.3
Diseases of heart (I00-I09, I11, I13, I20-I51)	186.5	232.3	150.4	183.9	229.9	147.2	238.6	295.6	197.5
Acute rheumatic fever and chronic rheumatic heart diseases (I00-I09)	1.0	0.8	1.1	1.0	0.8	1.1	0.8	0.8	0.9
Hypertensive heart disease (I11)	9.8	10.7	8.5	8.3	9.1	7.3	23.9	28.7	20.1
Hypertensive heart and renal disease (I13)	0.9	0.9	0.8	0.7	0.7	0.6	2.8	3.0	2.5
Ischemic heart diseases (I20-I25)	122.7	161.2	93.0	122.5	161.7	91.9	143.7	183.7	115.6
Acute myocardial infarction (I21-I22)	40.7	53.2	30.9	40.9	53.7	30.5	47.0	58.3	38.9
Other acute ischemic heart diseases (I24)	1.3	1.6	1.0	1.2	1.5	1.0	1.9	2.4	1.4
Other forms of chronic ischemic heart disease (I20, I25)	80.7	106.4	61.1	80.3	106.4	60.3	94.8	122.9	75.1
Atherosclerotic cardiovascular disease, so described (I25.0)	17.7	23.7	12.6	16.9	22.5	12.0	28.4	39.9	20.3
All other forms of chronic ischemic heart disease (I20,I25.1-I25.9)	63.0	82.7	48.4	63.5	83.9	48.4	66.4	83.0	54.9
Other heart diseases (I26-I51)	52.3	58.7	46.9	51.5	57.7	46.2	67.5	79.5	58.5
Acute and subacute endocarditis (I33)	0.4	0.4	0.3	0.3	0.4	0.3	0.6	0.7	0.5
Diseases of pericardium and acute myocarditis (I30-I31, I40)	0.3	0.3	0.2	0.2	0.3	0.2	0.4	0.4	0.4
Heart failure (I50)	16.9	18.1	15.8	17.0	18.2	15.9	19.4	22.1	17.4
All other forms of heart disease (I26-I28, I34-I38, I42-I49, I51)	34.7	39.8	30.6	33.9	38.8	29.8	47.0	56.3	40.2
Essential hypertension and hypertensive renal disease (I10, I12, I15)	7.7	7.8	7.5	6.8	6.7	6.6	17.2	18.6	16.0
Cerebrovascular diseases (I60-I69)	40.7	40.9	39.9	39.1	39.0	38.6	57.4	62.1	53.4
Atherosclerosis (I70)	2.3	2.4	2.2	2.4	2.4	2.3	2.4	2.8	2.1
Other diseases of circulatory system (I71-I78)	6.1	7.8	4.8	6.1	7.9	4.8	7.2	8.7	6.2
Aortic aneurysm and dissection (I71)	3.4	4.9	2.4	3.5	5.0	2.4	3.0	4.0	2.3
Other diseases of arteries, arterioles and capillaries (I72-I78)	2.7	3.0	2.5	2.6	2.9	2.3	4.2	4.7	3.9
Other disorders of circulatory system (I80-I99)	1.2	1.3	1.2	1.1	1.2	1.1	2.3	2.6	2.1
Influenza and pneumonia (J09-J18)[1]	16.9	19.9	15.0	16.7	19.5	14.9	18.9	23.2	16.1
Influenza (J09-J11)[1]	0.5	0.5	0.5	0.6	0.5	0.5	0.2	0.3	0.2
Pneumonia (J12-J18)	16.4	19.3	14.4	16.2	19.0	14.3	18.6	22.9	15.9
Other acute lower respiratory infections (J20-J22, U04)[2]	0.1	0.1	0.1	0.1	0.1	0.1	0.1	*	*
Acute bronchitis and bronchiolitis (J20-J21)	0.1	0.1	0.1	0.1	0.1	0.1	0.1	*	*
Other and unspecified acute lower respiratory infections (J22, U04)[2,3]	0.0	0.0	0.0	0.0	*	0.0	*	*	*
Chronic lower respiratory diseases (J40-J47)	44.0	51.4	39.1	46.4	53.5	41.9	30.4	41.5	23.9
Bronchitis, chronic and unspecified (J40-J42)	0.2	0.2	0.2	0.2	0.2	0.2	0.2	0.3	0.1
Emphysema (J43)	3.9	4.9	3.2	4.2	5.1	3.5	2.3	3.5	1.6
Asthma (J45-J46)	1.0	0.8	1.2	0.9	0.6	1.0	2.5	2.1	2.7
Other chronic lower respiratory diseases (J44, J47)	38.8	45.5	34.5	41.2	47.5	37.1	25.4	35.6	19.5
Pneumoconioses and chemical effects (J60-J66, J68)	0.3	0.7	0.0	0.3	0.7	0.0	0.1	0.3	*
Pneumonitis due to solids and liquids (J69)	5.0	6.8	3.9	5.0	6.9	3.9	5.3	7.4	4.1
Other diseases of respiratory system (J00-J06, J30-J39, J67, J70-J98)	9.3	11.3	7.9	9.4	11.4	7.9	9.0	10.5	8.1
Peptic ulcer (K25-K28)	0.9	1.1	0.8	0.9	1.1	0.8	1.0	1.5	0.7
Diseases of appendix (K35-K38)	0.1	0.2	0.1	0.1	0.2	0.1	0.2	0.3	*
Hernia (K40-K46)	0.5	0.5	0.5	0.5	0.5	0.5	0.5	0.6	0.4
Chronic liver disease and cirrhosis (K70, K73-K74)	9.2	12.7	6.0	9.6	13.2	6.2	7.0	10.6	4.2
Alcoholic liver disease (K70)	4.5	6.9	2.4	4.8	7.2	2.5	3.3	5.1	1.9
Other chronic liver disease and cirrhosis (K73-K74)	4.6	5.9	3.5	4.8	6.0	3.7	3.7	5.6	2.3
Cholelithiasis and other disorders of gallbladder (K80-K82)	1.0	1.2	0.9	1.0	1.2	0.9	1.0	1.3	0.9
Nephritis, nephrotic syndrome and nephrosis (N00-N07, N17-N19, N25-N27)	14.8	18.0	12.6	13.4	16.7	11.2	29.4	33.8	26.4
Acute and rapidly progressive nephritic and nephrotic syndrome (N00-N01,N04)	0.0	0.0	0.0	0.0	0.0	0.0	0.1	*	*
Chronic glomerulonephritis, nephritis and nephropathy not specified as acute or chronic, and renal sclerosis unspecified (N02-N03, N05-N07, N26)	1.2	1.5	1.0	1.1	1.4	0.9	2.4	2.8	2.1
Renal failure (N17-N19)	13.5	16.4	11.5	12.2	15.2	10.2	26.9	31.0	24.2
Other disorders of kidney (N25, N27)	0.0	*	0.0	0.0	*	*	*	*	*
Infections of kidney (N10-N12,N13.6,N15.1)	0.2	0.1	0.2	0.2	0.1	0.2	0.2	0.2	0.2
Hyperplasia of prostate (N40)	0.1	0.4	X	0.1	0.4	X	0.1	0.4	X
Inflammatory diseases of female pelvic organs (N70-N76)	0.0	X	0.1	0.0	X	0.1	*	X	*
Pregnancy, childbirth and the puerperium (O00-O99)	0.3	X	0.6	0.2	X	0.4	0.6	X	1.2
Pregnancy with abortive outcome (O00-O07)	0.0	X	0.0	*	X	*	*	X	*
Other complications of pregnancy, childbirth and the puerperium (O10-O99)	0.3	X	0.5	0.2	X	0.4	0.6	X	1.1

Table B-17. Age-Adjusted Death Rates from Selected Causes by Race and Sex, 2008—Continued

(Age-adjusted rates per 100,000 U.S. standard population.)

Cause of death (based on ICD-10, 2004)	American Indian or Alaska Native[1,2]			Asian or Pacific Islander[1,3]		
	Both sexes	Male	Female	Both sexes	Male	Female
Major cardiovascular diseases (I00-I78)	155.0	185.6	128.0	144.5	171.4	123.5
Diseases of heart (I00-I09, I11, I13, I20-I51)	119.8	149.1	94.3	100.5	124.7	81.7
Acute rheumatic fever and chronic rheumatic heart diseases (I00-I09)	0.8	*	*	0.9	0.7	1.0
Hypertensive heart disease (I11)	5.8	6.9	4.6	5.9	6.7	5.2
Hypertensive heart and renal disease (I13)	*	*	*	0.7	0.7	0.7
Ischemic heart diseases (I20-I25)	79.5	105.1	57.8	70.9	92.7	54.2
Acute myocardial infarction (I21-I22)	26.8	36.1	19.0	22.1	28.0	17.5
Other acute ischemic heart diseases (I24)	2.6	3.1	2.0	0.4	0.4	0.4
Other forms of chronic ischemic heart disease (I20, I25)	50.1	65.9	36.9	48.4	64.2	36.3
Atherosclerotic cardiovascular disease, so described (I25.0)	14.6	20.3	9.6	10.2	14.2	7.0
All other forms of chronic ischemic heart disease (I20,I25.1-I25.9)	35.6	45.5	27.2	38.2	50.1	29.3
Other heart diseases (I26-I51)	33.1	35.4	30.8	22.1	24.0	20.6
Acute and subacute endocarditis (I33)	*	*	*	*	*	*
Diseases of pericardium and acute myocarditis (I30-I31, I40)	*	*	*	0.2	*	*
Heart failure (I50)	11.7	11.4	11.8	5.8	5.9	5.8
All other forms of heart disease (I26-I28, I34-I38, I42-I49, I51)	20.7	23.3	18.2	15.9	17.7	14.5
Essential hypertension and hypertensive renal disease (I10, I12, I15)	5.3	6.2	4.6	6.7	7.1	6.3
Cerebrovascular diseases (I60-I69)	24.5	24.5	24.0	33.0	34.0	32.1
Atherosclerosis (I70)	1.7	*	*	0.9	1.1	0.7
Other diseases of circulatory system (I71-I78)	3.8	4.3	3.4	3.5	4.6	2.8
Aortic aneurysm and dissection (I71)	2.0	2.3	*	2.5	3.5	1.7
Other diseases of arteries, arterioles and capillaries (I72-I78)	1.8	*	1.7	1.1	1.1	1.1
Other disorders of circulatory system (I80-I99)	0.9	*	*	0.3	0.4	0.3
Influenza and pneumonia (J09-J18)[1]	17.2	20.0	15.4	14.3	17.8	11.9
Influenza (J09-J11)[1]	*	*	*	0.2	*	*
Pneumonia (J12-J18)	16.5	19.0	14.9	14.1	17.5	11.7
Other acute lower respiratory infections (J20-J22, U04)[2]	*	*	*	*	*	*
Acute bronchitis and bronchiolitis (J20-J21)	*	*	*	*	*	*
Other and unspecified acute lower respiratory infections (J22, U04)[2,3]						
Chronic lower respiratory diseases (J40-J47)	*	*	*	*	*	*
Bronchitis, chronic and unspecified (J40-J42)	29.3	32.8	26.7	14.1	20.6	9.6
Emphysema (J43)	*	*	*	*	*	*
Asthma (J45-J46)	2.4	2.9	2.0	1.1	1.9	0.5
Other chronic lower respiratory diseases (J44, J47)	0.8	*	*	1.1	0.9	1.3
Pneumoconioses and chemical effects (J60-J66, J68)	26.0	29.1	23.7	11.8	17.8	7.7
Pneumonitis due to solids and liquids (J69)	*	*	*	*	*	*
Other diseases of respiratory system (J00-J06, J30-J39, J67, J70-J98)	3.9	4.9	3.1	2.7	3.8	2.0
Peptic ulcer (K25-K28)	9.2	11.3	7.7	5.1	6.2	4.2
Diseases of appendix (K35-K38)	1.1	*	*	0.9	1.0	0.8
Hernia (K40-K46)	*	*	*	*	*	*
Chronic liver disease and cirrhosis (K70, K73-K74)	*	*	*	*	*	*
Alcoholic liver disease (K70)	25.7	28.9	22.8	3.4	4.4	2.5
Other chronic liver disease and cirrhosis (K73-K74)	17.7	20.4	15.3	1.2	2.2	0.4
Cholelithiasis and other disorders of gallbladder (K80-K82)	8.0	8.5	7.5	2.2	2.1	2.1
Nephritis, nephrotic syndrome and nephrosis (N00-N07, N17-N19, N25-N27)	1.2	*	*	0.8	1.1	0.6
Acute and rapidly progressive nephritic and nephrotic syndrome (N00-N01,N04)	15.6	16.7	14.9	8.4	10.0	7.2
Chronic glomerulonephritis, nephritis and nephropathy not specified as acute or chronic, and renal sclerosis unspecified (N02-N03, N05-N07, N26)	*	*	*	*	*	*
Renal failure (N17-N19)	1.1	*	*	0.9	1.0	0.8
Other disorders of kidney (N25, N27)	14.4	15.2	13.9	7.5	9.0	6.4
Infections of kidney (N10-N12,N13.6,N15.1)	*	*	*	*	*	*
Hyperplasia of prostate (N40)	*	*	*	0.2	*	*
Inflammatory diseases of female pelvic organs (N70-N76)	*	*	X	*	*	X
Pregnancy, childbirth and the puerperium (O00-O99)	*	X	*	*	X	*
Pregnancy with abortive outcome (O00-O07)	*	X	*	0.2	X	0.4
Other complications of pregnancy, childbirth and the puerperium (O10-O99)	*	X	*	*	X	*

Table B-17. Age-Adjusted Death Rates from Selected Causes by Race and Sex, 2008—Continued

(Age-adjusted rates per 100,000 U.S. standard population.)

Cause of death (based on ICD–10, 2004)	All races			White[1]			Black[1]		
	Both sexes	Male	Female	Both sexes	Male	Female	Both sexes	Male	Female
Certain conditions originating in the perinatal period (P00-P96)	4.5	5.0	3.9	3.5	4.0	3.1	9.4	10.3	8.4
Congenital malformations, deformations and chromosomal abnormalities (Q00-Q99)	3.3	3.5	3.1	3.3	3.5	3.1	3.6	3.8	3.4
Symptoms, signs and abnormal clinical and laboratory findings, not elsewhere classified (R00-R99)	11.7	12.1	10.8	11.4	11.7	10.7	15.4	17.7	13.3
All other diseases (Residual)	76.3	75.8	75.1	76.2	75.4	74.9	90.6	94.5	86.7
Accidents (unintentional injuries) (V01-X59, Y85-Y86)	38.8	53.6	25.1	40.7	55.7	26.5	33.3	49.4	19.9
Transport accidents (V01-V99, Y85)	13.8	20.4	7.6	14.3	20.9	7.8	13.2	20.6	6.8
Motor vehicle accidents (V02-V04, V09.0, V09.2, V12-V14, V19.0-V19.2, V19.4-V19.6, V20-V79, V80.3-V80.5, V81.0-V81.1, V82.0-V82.1, V83- V86, V87.0-V87.8, V88.0-V88.8, V89.0, V89.2)	12.9	18.8	7.3	13.3	19.3	7.5	12.3	19.1	6.5
Other land transport accidents (V01,V05-V06, V09.1, V09.3-V09.9, V10-V11, V15-V18, V19.3, V19.8-V19.9, V80.0-V80.2, V80.6-V80.9, V81.2-V81.9, V82.2-V82.9, V87.9, V88.9, V89.1, V89.3, V89.9)	0.4	0.6	0.1	0.4	0.6	0.1	0.4	0.8	0.2
Water, air and space, and other and unspecified transport accidents and their sequelae (V90-V99, Y85)	0.6	0.9	0.2	0.6	1.0	0.2	0.4	0.7	0.1
Nontransport accidents (W00-X59, Y86)	25.0	33.2	17.5	26.4	34.8	18.6	20.1	28.9	13.1
Falls (W00-W19)	7.3	9.4	5.7	7.8	9.9	6.2	3.4	4.9	2.4
Accidental discharge of firearms (W32-W34)	0.2	0.4	0.1	0.2	0.3	0.1	0.2	0.4	*
Accidental drowning and submersion (W65-W74)	1.2	1.8	0.5	1.1	1.7	0.5	1.3	2.1	0.6
Accidental exposure to smoke, fire and flames (X00-X09)	0.9	1.2	0.7	0.8	1.1	0.7	1.7	2.4	1.3
Accidental poisoning and exposure to noxious substances (X40-X49)	10.2	13.5	6.8	11.1	14.6	7.5	7.8	11.3	4.9
Other and unspecified nontransport accidents and their sequelae (W20-W31, W35-W64, W75-W99, X10-X39, X50-X59, Y86)	5.3	7.0	3.7	5.3	7.1	3.7	5.6	7.7	3.9
Intentional self-harm (suicide) (*U03, X60-X84, Y87.0)	11.6	18.9	4.8	12.9	20.8	5.4	5.3	9.5	1.7
Intentional self-harm (suicide) by discharge of firearms (X72-X74)	5.8	10.7	1.4	6.5	11.8	1.7	2.7	5.2	0.5
Intentional self-harm (suicide) by other and unspecified means and their sequelae (*U03, X60-X71, X75-X84, Y87.0)	5.8	8.3	3.4	6.3	9.0	3.7	2.6	4.3	1.2
Assault (homicide) (*U01-*U02, X85-Y09, Y87.1)	5.9	9.3	2.4	3.7	5.4	1.9	19.5	34.4	5.5
Assault (homicide) by discharge of firearms (*U01.4, X93-X95)	4.0	6.8	1.2	2.2	3.4	0.9	15.2	28.1	2.9
Assault (homicide) by other and unspecified means and their sequelae (*U01.0-*U01.3, *U01.5-*U01.9, *U02, X85-X92, X96-Y09, Y87.1)	1.8	2.5	1.2	1.5	1.9	1.0	4.3	6.4	2.5
Legal intervention (Y35, Y89.0)	0.1	0.2	*	0.1	0.2	*	0.3	0.6	*
Events of undetermined intent (Y10-Y34, Y87.2,Y89.9)	1.6	2.1	1.2	1.7	2.1	1.3	1.7	2.5	1.0
Discharge of firearms, undetermined intent (Y22-Y24)	0.1	0.1	0.0	0.1	0.1	0.0	0.1	0.2	*
Other and unspecified events of undetermined intent and their sequelae (Y10-Y21, Y25-Y34, Y87.2, Y89.9)	1.5	1.9	1.2	1.6	1.9	1.3	1.6	2.3	1.0
Operations of war and their sequelae (Y36, Y89.1)	0.0	0.0	*	0.0	0.0	*	*	*	*
Complications of medical and surgical care (Y40-Y84, Y88)	0.8	0.9	0.8	0.8	0.8	0.8	1.3	1.5	1.1
Enterocolitis due to Clostridium difficile (A04.7)[4]	2.3	2.3	2.3	2.4	2.3	2.4	1.6	1.6	1.6
Drug-induced deaths[5]	12.6	15.7	9.4	13.8	17.1	10.5	9.5	13.4	6.2
Alcohol-induced deaths[5]	7.4	11.6	3.6	7.7	11.9	3.7	6.2	10.6	2.9
Injury by firearms[5]	10.3	18.2	2.7	9.1	15.9	2.7	18.4	34.4	3.5

Table B-17. Age-Adjusted Death Rates from Selected Causes by Race and Sex, 2008—Continued

(Age-adjusted rates per 100,000 U.S. standard population.)

Cause of death (based on ICD–10, 2004)	American Indian or Alaska Native[1,2]			Asian or Pacific Islander[1,3]		
	Both sexes	Male	Female	Both sexes	Male	Female
Certain conditions originating in the perinatal period (P00-P96)	*	X	*	0.2	X	0.4
Congenital malformations, deformations and chromosomal abnormalities (Q00-Q99)	2.8	3.1	2.4	3.0	3.3	2.7
Symptoms, signs and abnormal clinical and laboratory findings, not elsewhere classified (R00-R99)	2.7	3.1	2.3	2.1	2.2	1.9
All other diseases (Residual)	8.2	9.1	7.3	4.0	4.4	3.6
Accidents (unintentional injuries) (V01-X59, Y85-Y86)	64.7	67.5	61.0	34.8	35.0	34.4
Transport accidents (V01-V99, Y85)	22.4	29.9	15.0	6.7	8.9	4.7
Motor vehicle accidents (V02-V04, V09.0, V09.2, V12-V14, V19.0-V19.2, V19.4-V19.6, V20-V79, V80.3-V80.5, V81.0-V81.1, V82.0-V82.1,V83-V86, V87.0-V87.8, V88.0-V88.8, V89.0, V89.2)	21.1	27.6	14.6	6.3	8.3	4.4
Other land transport accidents (V01,V05-V06, V09.1, V09.3-V09.9, V10-V11, V15-V18, V19.3, V19.8-V19.9, V80.0-V80.2, V80.6-V80.9, V81.2-V81.9, V82.2-V82.9, V87.9, V88.9, V89.1, V89.3, V89.9)	0.7	*	*	0.1	*	*
Water, air and space, and other and unspecified transport accidents and their sequelae (V90-V99, Y85)	0.7	*	*	0.3	0.4	*
Nontransport accidents (W00-X59, Y86)	31.1	44.6	18.4	8.7	11.8	6.1
Falls (W00-W19)	6.4	9.0	4.3	4.4	6.1	3.2
Accidental discharge of firearms (W32-W34)	*	*	*	*	*	*
Accidental drowning and submersion (W65-W74)	1.8	3.0	*	0.9	1.2	0.5
Accidental exposure to smoke, fire and flames (X00-X09)	1.2	1.4	*	0.3	*	*
Accidental poisoning and exposure to noxious substances (X40-X49)	14.4	19.8	9.0	1.4	2.0	0.8
Other and unspecified nontransport accidents and their sequelae (W20-W31, W35-W64, W75-W99, X10-X39, X50-X59, Y86)	7.0	10.9	3.5	1.8	2.2	1.4
Intentional self-harm (suicide) (*U03, X60-X84, Y87.0)	11.7	17.7	5.8	5.8	8.2	3.7
Intentional self-harm (suicide) by discharge of firearms (X72-X74)	4.5	8.2	*	1.2	2.2	0.3
Intentional self-harm (suicide) by other and unspecified means and their sequelae (*U03, X60-X71, X75-X84, Y87.0)	7.2	9.5	4.8	4.6	5.9	3.5
Assault (homicide) (*U01-*U02, X85-Y09, Y87.1)	7.1	10.7	3.6	2.3	3.1	1.4
Assault (homicide) by discharge of firearms (*U01.4, X93-X95)	2.6	3.9	1.4	1.3	2.1	0.6
Assault (homicide) by other and unspecified means and their sequelae (*U01.0-*U01.3, *U01.5-*U01.9, *U02, X85-X92, X96-Y09, Y87.1)	4.5	6.8	2.2	0.9	1.0	0.8
Legal intervention (Y35, Y89.0)	*	*	*	*	*	*
Events of undetermined intent (Y10-Y34, Y87.2,Y89.9)	2.1	3.0	*	0.5	0.6	0.4
Discharge of firearms, undetermined intent (Y22-Y24)	*	*	*	*	*	*
Other and unspecified events of undetermined intent and their sequelae (Y10-Y21, Y25-Y34, Y87.2, Y89.9)	2.0	2.9	*	0.5	0.6	0.4
Operations of war and their sequelae (Y36, Y89.1)	*	*	*	*	*	*
Complications of medical and surgical care (Y40-Y84, Y88)	*	*	*	0.2	*	*
Enterocolitis due to Clostridium difficile (A04.7)[4]	1.3	*	*	1.0	1.1	0.9
Drug-induced deaths[5]	13.7	16.5	10.9	1.9	2.4	1.5
Alcohol-induced deaths[5]	28.5	37.2	20.4	1.8	3.3	0.6
Injury by firearms[5]	8.0	13.3	2.7	2.6	4.5	0.8

X = Category not applicable.
− = Quantity zero.
[1]Race categories are consistent with the 1977 Office of Management and Budget (OMB) standards.
[2]Includes Aleuts and Eskimos.
[3]Includes Chinese, Filipino, Hawaiian, Japanese, and Other Asian and Pacific Islander.
[4]Included in certain other intestinal infections (A04, A07–A09).
[5]Included in selected categories above.

NOTE: Complete confirmation of deaths from selected causes of death, considered to be of public health concern, were not provided by the following states—Massachusetts, North Carolina, and West Virginia.

Table B-18. Age-Adjusted Death Rates from Selected Causes by Hispanic Origin, Race for Non-Hispanic Population, and Sex, 2008

(Age-adjusted rates are per 100,000 U.S. standard population.)

Cause of death (based on ICD–10, 2004)	All origins[1]			Hispanic			Non-Hispanic[2]		
	Both sexes	Male	Female	Both sexes	Male	Female	Both sexes	Male	Female
ALL CAUSES	758.3	900.6	643.4	532.2	630.7	445.7	775.8	922.2	658.5
Salmonella infections (A01-A02)	0.0	0.0	0.0	-	-	-	0.0	0.0	0.0
Shigellosis and amebiasis (A03, A06)	-	-	-	-	-	-	-	-	-
Certain other intestinal infections (A04, A07-A09)	2.4	2.4	2.4	1.7	1.6	1.8	2.4	2.4	2.5
Tuberculosis (A16-A19)	0.2	0.3	0.1	0.3	0.6	0.2	0.1	0.2	0.1
Respiratory tuberculosis (A16)	0.1	0.2	0.1	0.3	0.4	0.1	0.1	0.2	0.1
Other tuberculosis (A17-A19)	0.0	0.1	0.0	0.1	0.1	-	0.0	0.0	0.0
Whooping cough (A37)	0.0	-	-	-	-	-	-	-	-
Scarlet fever and erysipelas (A38, A46)	-	-	-	-	-	-	-	-	-
Meningococcal infection (A39)	0.0	0.0	0.0	-	-	-	0.0	0.0	0.0
Septicemia (A40-A41)	11.1	12.1	10.3	8.2	8.9	7.6	11.3	12.4	10.6
Syphilis (A50-A53)	0.0	0.0	-	-	-	-	0.0	0.0	-
Acute poliomyelitis (A80)	-	-	-	-	-	-	-	-	-
Arthropod-borne viral encephalitis (A83-A84, A85.2)	-	-	-	-	-	-	-	-	-
Measles (B05)	-	-	-	-	-	-	-	-	-
Viral hepatitis (B15-B19)	2.3	3.1	1.5	3.8	4.8	2.7	2.1	2.9	1.4
Human immunodeficiency virus (HIV) disease (B20-B24)	3.3	4.8	1.9	3.6	5.4	1.7	3.3	4.7	1.9
Malaria (B50-B54)	-	-	-	-	-	-	-	-	-
Other and unspecified infectious and parasitic diseases and their sequelae (A00, A05, A20-A36, A42-A44, A48-A49, A54-A79, A81-A82, A85.0-A85.1, A85.8, A86-B04, B06-B09, B25-B49, B55-B99)	1.8	2.2	1.6	1.5	1.7	1.3	1.9	2.2	1.6
Malignant neoplasms (C00-C97)	175.3	213.6	148.5	114.6	139.6	96.6	180.1	219.3	152.5
Malignant neoplasms of lip, oral cavity and pharynx (C00-C14)	2.4	3.7	1.4	1.4	2.3	0.7	2.5	3.9	1.4
Malignant neoplasm of esophagus (C15)	4.2	7.5	1.6	2.3	4.1	0.8	4.4	7.8	1.6
Malignant neoplasm of stomach (C16)	3.5	4.8	2.5	5.3	6.9	4.1	3.3	4.6	2.3
Malignant neoplasms of colon, rectum and anus (C18-C21)	16.4	19.5	14.0	11.9	15.0	9.5	16.8	19.9	14.3
Malignant neoplasms of liver and intrahepatic bile ducts (C22)	5.6	8.3	3.2	8.1	11.5	5.1	5.4	8.1	3.1
Malignant neoplasm of pancreas (C25)	10.9	12.5	9.6	8.1	9.3	7.1	11.1	12.7	9.8
Malignant neoplasm of larynx (C32)	1.1	2.1	0.5	0.8	1.5	0.2	1.2	2.1	0.5
Malignant neoplasms of trachea, bronchus and lung (C33-C34)	49.5	63.6	39.0	20.5	29.7	13.7	51.8	66.3	41.0
Malignant melanoma of skin (C43)	2.7	4.0	1.7	0.7	0.9	0.5	2.8	4.3	1.8
Malignant neoplasm of breast (C50)	12.6	0.3	22.5	7.8	-	14.3	13.0	0.3	23.2
Malignant neoplasm of cervix uteri (C53)	1.2	X	2.4	1.5	X	2.8	1.2	X	2.3
Malignant neoplasms of corpus uteri and uterus, part unspecified (C54-C55)	2.4	X	4.2	1.8	X	3.3	2.4	X	4.2
Malignant neoplasm of ovary (C56)	4.4	X	8.0	3.0	X	5.5	4.6	X	8.1
Malignant neoplasm of prostate (C61)	8.8	22.3	X	6.7	16.5	X	9.0	22.7	X
Malignant neoplasms of kidney and renal pelvis (C64-C65)	4.0	5.8	2.6	3.3	4.6	2.3	4.0	5.9	2.6
Malignant neoplasm of bladder (C67)	4.3	7.4	2.2	2.0	3.2	1.2	4.5	7.7	2.3
Malignant neoplasms of meninges, brain and other parts of central nervous system (C70-C72)	4.3	5.2	3.4	2.8	3.2	2.4	4.4	5.5	3.5
Malignant neoplasms of lymphoid, hematopoietic and related tissue (C81-C96)	17.2	22.4	13.3	12.4	15.2	10.2	17.5	22.9	13.5
Hodgkin's disease (C81)	0.4	0.4	0.3	0.4	0.5	0.3	0.4	0.4	0.3
Non-Hodgkin's lymphoma (C82-C85)	6.3	8.1	5.0	4.8	5.9	4.0	6.5	8.3	5.1
Leukemia (C91-C95)	7.0	9.4	5.3	4.7	5.8	3.8	7.1	9.6	5.3
Multiple myeloma and immunoproliferative neoplasms (C88, C90)	3.4	4.4	2.7	2.5	3.0	2.0	3.5	4.5	2.7
Other and unspecified malignant neoplasms of lymphoid, hematopoietic and related tissue (C96)	0.0	0.0	0.0	-	-	-	0.0	0.0	0.0
All other and unspecified malignant neoplasms (C17, C23-C24, C26-C31, C37-C41, C44-C49, C51-C52, C57-C60, C62-C63, C66, C68-C69, C73-C80, C97)	19.7	23.9	16.5	14.0	15.5	12.9	20.1	24.5	16.8
In situ neoplasms, benign neoplasms and neoplasms of uncertain or unknown behavior (D00-D48)	4.5	5.7	3.7	2.8	3.1	2.5	4.6	5.9	3.7
Anemias (D50-D64)	1.5	1.6	1.5	1.0	1.0	0.9	1.6	1.6	1.6
Diabetes mellitus (E10-E14)	21.8	25.6	18.8	27.7	31.3	24.7	21.3	25.2	18.3
Nutritional deficiencies (E40-E64)	0.9	0.9	0.9	0.7	0.7	0.6	0.9	0.9	0.9
Malnutrition (E40-E46)	0.8	0.8	0.8	0.7	0.7	0.6	0.8	0.8	0.8
Other nutritional deficiencies (E50-E64)	0.1	0.1	0.1	-	-	-	0.1	0.1	0.1
Meningitis (G00,G03)	0.2	0.2	0.2	0.2	0.3	0.2	0.2	0.2	0.2
Parkinson's disease (G20-G21)	6.4	9.7	4.3	4.2	5.8	3.1	6.5	10.0	4.3
Alzheimer's disease (G30)	24.4	20.1	26.7	15.0	12.3	16.5	25.0	20.6	27.3

Table B-18. Age-Adjusted Death Rates from Selected Causes by Hispanic Origin, Race for Non-Hispanic Population, and Sex, 2008—*Continued*

(Age-adjusted rates are per 100,000 U.S. standard population.)

Cause of death (based on ICD–10, 2004)	Non-Hispanic White			Non-Hispanic Black		
	Both sexes	Male	Female	Both sexes	Male	Female
ALL CAUSES	766.2	908.5	650.8	955.2	1176.6	794.8
Salmonella infections (A01-A02)	0.0	-	-	-	-	-
Shigellosis and amebiasis (A03, A06)	-	-	-	-	-	-
Certain other intestinal infections (A04, A07-A09)	2.6	2.5	2.6	1.7	1.7	1.7
Tuberculosis (A16-A19)	0.1	0.1	0.1	0.4	0.7	0.3
Respiratory tuberculosis (A16)	0.1	0.1	0.0	0.3	0.6	0.2
Other tuberculosis (A17-A19)	0.0	0.0	0.0	0.1	-	-
Whooping cough (A37)	-	-	-	-	-	-
Scarlet fever and erysipelas (A38, A46)	-	-	-	-	-	-
Meningococcal infection (A39)	0.0	0.0	0.0	0.1	-	-
Septicemia (A40-A41)	10.3	11.3	9.6	22.1	24.9	20.2
Syphilis (A50-A53)	-	-	-	-	-	-
Acute poliomyelitis (A80)	-	-	-	-	-	-
Arthropod-borne viral encephalitis (A83-A84, A85.2)	-	-	-	-	-	-
Measles (B05)	-	-	-	-	-	-
Viral hepatitis (B15-B19)	2.0	2.7	1.3	3.1	4.5	2.0
Human immunodeficiency virus (HIV) disease (B20-B24)	1.4	2.3	0.5	15.7	22.4	10.1
Malaria (B50-B54)	-	-	-	-	-	-
Other and unspecified infectious and parasitic diseases and their sequelae (A00, A05, A20-A36, A42-A44, A48- A49, A54-A79, A81-A82, A85.0-A85.1, A85.8, A86-B04, B06-B09, B25-B49, B55-B99)	1.8	2.1	1.6	2.3	3.1	1.8
Malignant neoplasms (C00-C97)	179.4	217.3	152.6	213.5	278.3	173.6
Malignant neoplasms of lip, oral cavity and pharynx (C00-C14)	2.5	3.7	1.4	3.1	5.3	1.5
Malignant neoplasm of esophagus (C15)	4.5	8.1	1.6	4.6	7.9	2.3
Malignant neoplasm of stomach (C16)	2.8	3.9	1.9	7.0	10.1	4.9
Malignant neoplasms of colon, rectum and anus (C18-C21)	16.3	19.2	13.9	23.3	29.2	19.2
Malignant neoplasms of liver and intrahepatic bile ducts (C22)	4.8	7.2	2.8	7.6	12.6	4.0
Malignant neoplasm of pancreas (C25)	11.0	12.6	9.6	13.9	15.4	12.7
Malignant neoplasm of larynx (C32)	1.1	2.0	0.5	2.1	4.0	0.8
Malignant neoplasms of trachea, bronchus and lung (C33-C34)	52.8	66.3	42.6	54.6	80.3	37.7
Malignant melanoma of skin (C43)	3.3	4.9	2.1	0.4	0.4	0.4
Malignant neoplasm of breast (C50)	12.5	0.3	22.5	18.9	0.6	31.9
Malignant neoplasm of cervix uteri (C53)	1.1	X	2.1	2.5	X	4.3
Malignant neoplasms of corpus uteri and uterus, part unspecified (C54-C55)	2.2	X	4.0	4.3	X	7.2
Malignant neoplasm of ovary (C56)	4.7	X	8.5	4.0	X	6.8
Malignant neoplasm of prostate (C61)	8.3	21.0	X	17.1	47.0	X
Malignant neoplasms of kidney and renal pelvis (C64-C65)	4.1	6.0	2.6	4.0	5.9	2.6
Malignant neoplasm of bladder (C67)	4.7	8.2	2.3	3.4	4.8	2.5
Malignant neoplasms of meninges, brain and other parts of central nervous system (C70-C72)	4.8	5.9	3.9	2.6	3.3	2.1
Malignant neoplasms of lymphoid, hematopoietic and related tissue (C81-C96)	17.8	23.3	13.6	17.6	22.8	14.0
Hodgkin's disease (C81)	0.4	0.4	0.3	0.4	0.4	0.3
Non-Hodgkin's lymphoma (C82-C85)	6.8	8.6	5.3	4.4	5.6	3.5
Leukemia (C91-C95)	7.4	9.9	5.5	6.3	8.6	4.7
Multiple myeloma and immunoproliferative neoplasms (C88, C90)	3.2	4.3	2.5	6.6	8.2	5.5
Other and unspecified malignant neoplasms of lymphoid, hematopoietic and related tissue (C96)	0.0	0.0	-	-	-	-
All other and unspecified malignant neoplasms (C17, C23-C24, C26-C31, C37-C41, C44-C49, C51- C52, C57-C60, C62-C63, C66, C68-C69, C73-C80, C97)	20.1	24.5	16.8	22.6	28.6	18.7
In situ neoplasms, benign neoplasms and neoplasms of uncertain or unknown behavior (D00-D48)	4.7	6.1	3.8	4.0	4.8	3.4
Anemias (D50-D64)	1.4	1.4	1.3	3.1	3.2	3.1
Diabetes mellitus (E10-E14)	19.1	23.2	16.0	41.3	45.6	38.0
Nutritional deficiencies (E40-E64)	0.9	0.8	0.9	1.3	1.7	1.2
Malnutrition (E40-E46)	0.8	0.8	0.8	1.3	1.6	1.1
Other nutritional deficiencies (E50-E64)	0.1	0.1	0.1	-	-	-
Meningitis (G00,G03)	0.2	0.2	0.1	0.3	0.4	0.3
Parkinson's disease (G20-G21)	7.0	10.7	4.6	3.0	4.4	2.1
Alzheimer's disease (G30)	26.1	21.5	28.6	20.0	16.5	21.5

Table B-18. Age-Adjusted Death Rates from Selected Causes by Hispanic Origin, Race for Non-Hispanic Population, and Sex, 2008—Continued

(Age-adjusted rates are per 100,000 U.S. standard population.)

Cause of death (based on ICD–10, 2004)	All origins[1]			Hispanic			Non-Hispanic[2]		
	Both sexes	Male	Female	Both sexes	Male	Female	Both sexes	Male	Female
Major cardiovascular diseases (I00-I78)	243.5	291.3	204.9	169.0	197.6	144.4	248.7	298.2	209.0
Diseases of heart (I00-I09, I11, I13, I20-I51)	186.5	232.3	150.4	126.3	151.9	104.6	190.9	238.5	153.5
Acute rheumatic fever and chronic rheumatic heart diseases (I00-I09)	1.0	0.8	1.1	0.6	0.4	0.8	1.0	0.8	1.1
Hypertensive heart disease (I11)	9.8	10.7	8.5	7.1	8.6	5.8	9.9	10.9	8.8
Hypertensive heart and renal disease (I13)	0.9	0.9	0.8	0.7	0.7	0.7	0.9	1.0	0.8
Ischemic heart diseases (I20-I25)	122.7	161.2	93.0	90.0	111.5	72.0	125.0	164.9	94.4
Acute myocardial infarction (I21-I22)	40.7	53.2	30.9	29.1	35.8	23.5	41.7	54.6	31.5
Other acute ischemic heart diseases (I24)	1.3	1.6	1.0	0.5	0.6	0.4	1.4	1.7	1.1
Other forms of chronic ischemic heart disease (I20, I25)	80.7	106.4	61.1	60.4	75.1	48.1	82.0	108.7	61.9
Atherosclerotic cardiovascular disease, so described (I25.0)	17.7	23.7	12.6	13.3	17.9	9.2	18.0	24.1	12.8
All other forms of chronic ischemic heart disease (I20,I25.1-I25.9)	63.0	82.7	48.4	47.1	57.2	39.0	64.0	84.6	49.0
Other heart diseases (I26-I51)	52.3	58.7	46.9	27.9	30.7	25.3	54.1	60.9	48.4
Acute and subacute endocarditis (I33)	0.4	0.4	0.3	0.3	0.4	0.1	0.4	0.4	0.3
Diseases of pericardium and acute myocarditis (I30-I31, I40)	0.3	0.3	0.2	0.2	0.2	0.2	0.3	0.3	0.2
Heart failure (I50)	16.9	18.1	15.8	9.2	9.5	8.9	17.4	18.7	16.3
All other forms of heart disease (I26-I28, I34-I38, I42-I49, I51)	34.7	39.8	30.6	18.2	20.6	16.0	36.0	41.4	31.6
Essential hypertension and hypertensive renal disease (I10, I12, I15)	7.7	7.8	7.5	6.7	6.7	6.6	7.8	7.8	7.6
Cerebrovascular diseases (I60-I69)	40.7	40.9	39.9	30.9	33.1	28.9	41.3	41.4	40.6
Atherosclerosis (I70)	2.3	2.4	2.2	1.3	1.3	1.4	2.4	2.5	2.3
Other diseases of circulatory system (I71-I78)	6.1	7.8	4.8	3.6	4.6	2.9	6.3	8.1	5.0
Aortic aneurysm and dissection (I71)	3.4	4.9	2.4	1.8	2.7	1.1	3.6	5.0	2.5
Other diseases of arteries, arterioles and capillaries (I72-I78)	2.7	3.0	2.5	1.8	1.9	1.8	2.7	3.1	2.5
Other disorders of circulatory system (I80-I99)	1.2	1.3	1.2	0.8	0.9	0.6	1.3	1.3	1.2
Influenza and pneumonia (J09-J18)[1]	16.9	19.9	15.0	14.0	16.0	12.4	17.1	20.1	15.1
Influenza (J09-J11)[1]	0.5	0.5	0.5	0.2	0.2	0.2	0.6	0.6	0.5
Pneumonia (J12-J18)	16.4	19.3	14.4	13.8	15.8	12.2	16.6	19.6	14.6
Other acute lower respiratory infections (J20-J22, U04)[2]	0.1	0.1	0.1	0.0	-	-	0.1	0.1	0.1
Acute bronchitis and bronchiolitis (J20-J21)	0.1	0.1	0.1	0.0	-	-	0.1	0.1	0.1
Other and unspecified acute lower respiratory infections (J22, U04)[2,3]	0.0	0.0	0.0	-	-	-	0.0	0.0	0.0
Chronic lower respiratory diseases (J40-J47)	44.0	51.4	39.1	18.3	22.6	15.3	45.8	53.5	40.9
Bronchitis, chronic and unspecified (J40-J42)	0.2	0.2	0.2	0.2	0.2	-	0.2	0.2	0.2
Emphysema (J43)	3.9	4.9	3.2	1.3	2.0	0.9	4.1	5.1	3.4
Asthma (J45-J46)	1.0	0.8	1.2	0.9	0.8	1.0	1.1	0.8	1.3
Other chronic lower respiratory diseases (J44, J47)	38.8	45.5	34.5	15.8	19.6	13.2	40.4	47.4	36.0
Pneumoconioses and chemical effects (J60-J66, J68)	0.3	0.7	0.0	0.1	0.2	-	0.3	0.7	0.0
Pneumonitis due to solids and liquids (J69)	5.0	6.8	3.9	2.9	3.6	2.4	5.1	7.1	4.0
Other diseases of respiratory system (J00-J06, J30-J39, J67, J70-J98)	9.3	11.3	7.9	7.6	8.6	6.8	9.4	11.4	8.0
Peptic ulcer (K25-K28)	0.9	1.1	0.8	0.6	0.9	0.4	1.0	1.2	0.8
Diseases of appendix (K35-K38)	0.1	0.2	0.1	0.1	0.2	-	0.1	0.1	0.1
Hernia (K40-K46)	0.5	0.5	0.5	0.4	0.4	0.5	0.5	0.5	0.5
Chronic liver disease and cirrhosis (K70, K73-K74)	9.2	12.7	6.0	13.7	19.1	8.6	8.7	12.1	5.8
Alcoholic liver disease (K70)	4.5	6.9	2.4	6.5	11.0	2.3	4.3	6.4	2.5
Other chronic liver disease and cirrhosis (K73-K74)	4.6	5.9	3.5	7.2	8.1	6.3	4.4	5.6	3.3
Cholelithiasis and other disorders of gallbladder (K80-K82)	1.0	1.2	0.9	1.2	1.2	1.2	1.0	1.2	0.9
Nephritis, nephrotic syndrome and nephrosis (N00-N07, N17-N19, N25-N27)	14.8	18.0	12.6	12.5	14.6	11.0	14.9	18.2	12.7
Acute and rapidly progressive nephritic and nephrotic syndrome (N00-N01,N04)	0.0	0.0	0.0	-	-	-	0.0	0.0	0.0
Chronic glomerulonephritis, nephritis and nephropathy not specified as acute or chronic, and renal sclerosis unspecified (N02-N03, N05-N07, N26)	1.2	1.5	1.0	1.0	1.3	0.8	1.3	1.5	1.0
Renal failure (N17-N19)	13.5	16.4	11.5	11.4	13.2	10.1	13.6	16.6	11.6
Other disorders of kidney (N25, N27)	0.0	-	0.0	-	-	-	0.0	-	-
Infections of kidney (N10-N12,N13.6,N15.1)	0.2	0.1	0.2	0.2	-	0.3	0.2	0.1	0.2
Hyperplasia of prostate (N40)	0.1	0.4	X	0.1	0.3	X	0.1	0.4	X
Inflammatory diseases of female pelvic organs (N70-N76)	0.0	X	0.1	-	X	-	0.0	X	0.1
Pregnancy, childbirth and the puerperium (O00-O99)	0.3	X	0.6	0.3	X	0.6	0.3	X	0.5
Pregnancy with abortive outcome (O00-O07)	0.0	X	0.0	-	X	-	0.0	X	0.0
Other complications of pregnancy, childbirth and the puerperium (O10-O99)	0.3	X	0.5	0.3	X	0.6	0.2	X	0.5

Table B-18. Age-Adjusted Death Rates from Selected Causes by Hispanic Origin, Race for Non-Hispanic Population, and Sex, 2008—Continued

(Age-adjusted rates are per 100,000 U.S. standard population.)

Cause of death (based on ICD–10, 2004)	Non-Hispanic White			Non-Hispanic Black		
	Both sexes	Male	Female	Both sexes	Male	Female
Major cardiovascular diseases (I00-I78)	243.0	292.4	202.8	329.3	396.0	280.3
Diseases of heart (I00-I09, I11, I13, I20-I51)	188.0	235.9	150.0	243.2	301.8	201.1
Acute rheumatic fever and chronic rheumatic heart diseases (I00-I09)	1.0	0.8	1.1	0.8	0.8	0.9
Hypertensive heart disease (I11)	8.4	9.1	7.4	24.3	29.2	20.4
Hypertensive heart and renal disease (I13)	0.7	0.7	0.6	2.8	3.1	2.6
Ischemic heart diseases (I20-I25)	124.8	165.5	93.1	146.2	187.2	117.4
Acute myocardial infarction (I21-I22)	41.8	55.2	31.1	48.0	59.6	39.7
Other acute ischemic heart diseases (I24)	1.3	1.6	1.0	1.9	2.5	1.5
Other forms of chronic ischemic heart disease (I20, I25)	81.7	108.7	61.0	96.3	125.1	76.3
Atherosclerotic cardiovascular disease, so described (I25.0)	17.1	22.9	12.1	28.8	40.4	20.6
All other forms of chronic ischemic heart disease (I20,I25.1-I25.9)	64.6	85.8	48.9	67.5	84.6	55.7
Other heart diseases (I26-I51)	53.2	59.7	47.7	69.0	81.6	59.8
Acute and subacute endocarditis (I33)	0.4	0.4	0.3	0.6	0.7	0.5
Diseases of pericardium and acute myocarditis (I30-I31, I40)	0.2	0.3	0.2	0.4	0.4	0.4
Heart failure (I50)	17.4	18.7	16.3	19.8	22.7	17.7
All other forms of heart disease (I26-I28, I34-I38, I42-I49, I51)	35.1	40.3	30.9	48.2	57.8	41.1
Essential hypertension and hypertensive renal disease (I10, I12, I15)	6.7	6.7	6.6	17.6	19.1	16.3
Cerebrovascular diseases (I60-I69)	39.5	39.2	39.0	58.6	63.4	54.5
Atherosclerosis (I70)	2.4	2.5	2.4	2.4	2.8	2.2
Other diseases of circulatory system (I71-I78)	6.3	8.1	4.9	7.4	8.8	6.3
Aortic aneurysm and dissection (I71)	3.7	5.2	2.5	3.1	4.0	2.4
Other diseases of arteries, arterioles and capillaries (I72-I78)	2.6	3.0	2.4	4.3	4.8	4.0
Other disorders of circulatory system (I80-I99)	1.2	1.2	1.2	2.4	2.7	2.2
Influenza and pneumonia (J09-J18)[1]	16.9	19.7	15.0	19.3	23.7	16.4
Influenza (J09-J11)[1]	0.6	0.6	0.6	0.3	0.3	0.2
Pneumonia (J12-J18)	16.3	19.2	14.4	19.0	23.4	16.2
Other acute lower respiratory infections (J20-J22, U04)[2]	0.1	0.1	0.1	0.1	-	-
Acute bronchitis and bronchiolitis (J20-J21)	0.1	0.1	0.1	0.1	-	-
Other and unspecified acute lower respiratory infections(J22, U04)[2,3]	0.0	-	0.0	-	-	-
Chronic lower respiratory diseases (J40-J47)	48.7	55.8	44.1	31.1	42.3	24.4
Bronchitis, chronic and unspecified (J40-J42)	0.2	0.2	0.2	0.2	0.3	0.1
Emphysema (J43)	4.4	5.3	3.7	2.4	3.6	1.6
Asthma (J45-J46)	0.8	0.6	1.0	2.6	2.2	2.8
Other chronic lower respiratory diseases (J44, J47)	43.2	49.6	39.1	25.9	36.3	19.9
Pneumoconioses and chemical effects (J60-J66, J68)	0.3	0.8	0.0	0.1	0.4	-
Pneumonitis due to solids and liquids (J69)	5.2	7.2	4.0	5.4	7.6	4.2
Other diseases of respiratory system (J00-J06, J30-J39, J67, J70-J98)	9.5	11.6	8.0	9.2	10.7	8.3
Peptic ulcer (K25-K28)	0.9	1.1	0.8	1.0	1.4	0.7
Diseases of appendix (K35-K38)	0.1	0.1	0.1	0.2	0.3	-
Hernia (K40-K46)	0.5	0.5	0.5	0.5	0.6	0.4
Chronic liver disease and cirrhosis (K70, K73-K74)	9.1	12.4	6.0	7.1	10.9	4.2
Alcoholic liver disease (K70)	4.5	6.7	2.5	3.3	5.1	1.9
Other chronic liver disease and cirrhosis (K73-K74)	4.5	5.8	3.5	3.8	5.7	2.3
Cholelithiasis and other disorders of gallbladder (K80-K82)	1.0	1.2	0.9	1.1	1.3	0.9
Nephritis, nephrotic syndrome and nephrosis (N00-N07, N17-N19, N25-N27)	13.3	16.8	11.1	30.1	34.7	27.1
Acute and rapidly progressive nephritic and nephrotic syndrome (N00-N01,N04)	0.0	0.0	0.0	0.1	-	-
Chronic glomerulonephritis, nephritis and nephropathy not specified as acute or chronic, and renal sclerosis unspecified (N02-N03, N05-N07, N26)	1.1	1.4	0.9	2.4	2.9	2.2
Renal failure (N17-N19)	12.2	15.2	10.1	27.6	31.8	24.8
Other disorders of kidney (N25, N27)	0.0	-	-	-	-	-
Infections of kidney (N10-N12,N13.6,N15.1)	0.2	0.1	0.2	0.2	0.2	0.2
Hyperplasia of prostate (N40)	0.2	0.4	X	0.1	0.4	X
Inflammatory diseases of female pelvic organs (N70-N76)	0.0	X	0.1	-	X	-
Pregnancy, childbirth and the puerperium (O00-O99)	0.2	X	0.4	0.6	X	1.2
Pregnancy with abortive outcome (O00-O07)	-	X	-	-	X	-
Other complications of pregnancy, childbirth and the puerperium (O10-O99)	0.2	X	0.4	0.6	X	1.2

Table B-18. Age-Adjusted Death Rates from Selected Causes by Hispanic Origin, Race for Non-Hispanic Population, and Sex, 2008—Continued

(Age-adjusted rates are per 100,000 U.S. standard population.)

Cause of death (based on ICD–10, 2004)	All origins[1]			Hispanic			Non-Hispanic[2]		
	Both sexes	Male	Female	Both sexes	Male	Female	Both sexes	Male	Female
Certain conditions originating in the perinatal period (P00-P96)	4.5	5.0	3.9	3.6	4.0	3.1	4.7	5.2	4.2
Congenital malformations, deformations and chromosomal abnormalities (Q00-Q99)	3.3	3.5	3.1	3.0	3.1	2.8	3.3	3.5	3.1
Symptoms, signs and abnormal clinical and laboratory findings, not elsewhere classified (R00-R99)	11.7	12.1	10.8	6.4	6.9	5.6	12.1	12.6	11.3
All other diseases (Residual)	76.3	75.8	75.1	50.4	50.8	48.7	78.2	77.7	76.9
Accidents (unintentional injuries) (V01-X59, Y85-Y86)	38.8	53.6	25.1	27.9	40.4	14.9	40.2	55.2	26.4
Transport accidents (V01-V99, Y85)	13.8	20.4	7.6	12.1	18.0	5.9	14.1	20.6	7.9
Motor vehicle accidents (V02-V04, V09.0, V09.2, V12-V14, V19.0-V19.2, V19.4-V19.6, V20-V79, V80.3-V80.5, V81.0-V81.1, V82.0-V82.1, V83-V86, V87.0-V87.8, V88.0-V88.8, V89.0, V89.2)	12.9	18.8	7.3	11.4	16.7	5.7	13.1	19.0	7.5
Other land transport accidents (V01, V05-V06, V09.1, V09.3-V09.9, V10-V11, V15-V18, V19.3, V19.8-V19.9, V80.0-V80.2, V80.6-V80.9, V81.2- V81.9, V82.2-V82.9, V87.9, V88.9, V89.1, V89.3, V89.9)	0.4	0.6	0.1	0.4	0.7	0.1	0.3	0.6	0.2
Water, air and space, and other and unspecified transport accidents and their sequelae (V90-V99, Y85)	0.6	0.9	0.2	0.3	0.5	-	0.6	1.0	0.2
Nontransport accidents (W00-X59, Y86)	25.0	33.2	17.5	15.8	22.4	9.0	26.1	34.6	18.5
Falls (W00-W19)	7.3	9.4	5.7	5.0	6.8	3.4	7.4	9.5	5.9
Accidental discharge of firearms (W32-W34)	0.2	0.4	0.1	0.1	0.1	-	0.2	0.4	0.1
Accidental drowning and submersion (W65-W74)	1.2	1.8	0.5	1.0	1.5	0.4	1.2	1.8	0.5
Accidental exposure to smoke, fire and flames (X00-X09)	0.9	1.2	0.7	0.5	0.6	0.4	1.0	1.2	0.8
Accidental poisoning and exposure to noxious substances (X40-X49)	10.2	13.5	6.8	6.0	8.9	2.8	10.9	14.4	7.4
Other and unspecified nontransport accidents and their sequelae (W20-W31, W35-W64, W75-W99, X10-X39, X50-X59, Y86)	5.3	7.0	3.7	3.1	4.4	1.9	5.5	7.3	3.9
Intentional self-harm (suicide) (*U03, X60-X84, Y87.0)	11.6	18.9	4.8	5.6	9.3	1.9	12.5	20.5	5.2
Intentional self-harm (suicide) by discharge of firearms (X72-X74)	5.8	10.7	1.4	2.2	4.0	0.3	6.3	11.6	1.6
Intentional self-harm (suicide) by other and unspecified means and their sequelae (*U03, X60-X71, X75-X84, Y87.0)	5.8	8.3	3.4	3.5	5.4	1.5	6.2	8.8	3.6
Assault (homicide) (*U01-*U02, X85-Y09, Y87.1)	5.9	9.3	2.4	6.6	10.5	2.4	5.7	9.0	2.4
Assault (homicide) by discharge of firearms (*U01.4, X93-X95)	4.0	6.8	1.2	4.4	7.4	1.1	4.0	6.7	1.2
Assault (homicide) by other and unspecified means and their sequelae (*U01.0-*U01.3, *U01.5-*U01.9, *U02, X85-X92, X96-Y09, Y87.1)	1.8	2.5	1.2	2.2	3.2	1.3	1.8	2.4	1.2
Legal intervention (Y35, Y89.0)	0.1	0.2	-	0.2	0.3	-	0.1	0.2	-
Events of undetermined intent (Y10-Y34, Y87.2, Y89.9)	1.6	2.1	1.2	0.7	1.1	0.4	1.8	2.2	1.3
Discharge of firearms, undetermined intent (Y22-Y24)	0.1	0.1	0.0	0.0	-	-	0.1	0.1	0.0
Other and unspecified events of undetermined intent and their sequelae (Y10-Y21, Y25-Y34, Y87.2, Y89.9)	1.5	1.9	1.2	0.7	1.0	0.4	1.7	2.1	1.3
Operations of war and their sequelae (Y36, Y89.1)	0.0	0.0	-	-	-	-	0.0	0.0	-
Complications of medical and surgical care (Y40-Y84, Y88)	0.8	0.9	0.8	0.5	0.5	0.6	0.8	0.9	0.8
Enterocolitis due to Clostridium difficile (A04.7)[4]	2.3	2.3	2.3	1.6	1.6	1.7	2.3	2.3	2.3
Drug-induced deaths[5]	12.6	15.7	9.4	6.5	9.1	3.7	13.6	16.9	10.3
Alcohol-induced deaths[5]	7.4	11.6	3.6	8.8	15.1	2.9	7.2	11.1	3.7
Injury by firearms[5]	10.3	18.2	2.7	6.8	11.8	1.5	10.7	19.0	2.9

Table B-18. Age-Adjusted Death Rates from Selected Causes by Hispanic Origin, Race for Non-Hispanic Population, and Sex, 2008—Continued

(Age-adjusted rates are per 100,000 U.S. standard population.)

Cause of death (based on ICD-10, 2004)	Non-Hispanic White			Non-Hispanic Black		
	Both sexes	Male	Female	Both sexes	Male	Female
Certain conditions originating in the perinatal period (P00-P96)	3.4	3.8	3.0	9.9	10.9	8.9
Congenital malformations, deformations and chromosomal abnormalities (Q00-Q99)	3.2	3.4	3.1	3.8	4.0	3.6
Symptoms, signs and abnormal clinical and laboratory findings, not elsewhere classified (R00-R99)	11.9	12.2	11.2	15.9	18.3	13.7
All other diseases (Residual)	78.0	77.3	76.7	92.4	96.5	88.4
Accidents (unintentional injuries) (V01-X59, Y85-Y86)	42.6	57.9	28.2	34.2	50.7	20.4
Transport accidents (V01-V99, Y85)	14.6	21.2	8.2	13.6	21.2	7.0
Motor vehicle accidents (V02-V04, V09.0, V09.2, V12-V14, V19.0-V19.2, V19.4-V19.6, V20-V79, V80.3-V80.5, V81.0-V81.1, V82.0-V82.1,V83-V86, V87.0-V87.8, V88.0-V88.8, V89.0, V89.2)	13.6	19.6	7.8	12.7	19.7	6.7
Other land transport accidents (V01,V05-V06, V09.1, V09.3-V09.9, V10-V11, V15-V18, V19.3, V19.8-V19.9, V80.0-V80.2, V80.6-V80.9, V81.2- V81.9, V82.2-V82.9, V87.9, V88.9, V89.1, V89.3, V89.9)	0.3	0.6	0.1	0.5	0.8	0.2
Water, air and space, and other and unspecified transport accidents and their sequelae (V90-V99, Y85)	0.6	1.1	0.2	0.4	0.8	0.2
Nontransport accidents (W00-X59, Y86)	28.0	36.7	20.0	20.6	29.5	13.4
Falls (W00-W19)	7.9	10.1	6.3	3.5	4.9	2.5
Accidental discharge of firearms (W32-W34)	0.2	0.4	0.1	0.2	0.4	-
Accidental drowning and submersion (W65-W74)	1.1	1.7	0.5	1.4	2.2	0.6
Accidental exposure to smoke, fire and flames (X00-X09)	0.9	1.1	0.7	1.8	2.5	1.3
Accidental poisoning and exposure to noxious substances (X40-X49)	12.2	16.0	8.4	8.0	11.5	5.0
Other and unspecified nontransport accidents and their sequelae (W20-W31, W35-W64, W75-W99, X10-X39, X50-X59, Y86)	5.6	7.4	3.9	5.7	8.0	4.0
Intentional self-harm (suicide) (*U03, X60-X84, Y87.0)	14.1	22.9	6.0	5.4	9.8	1.7
Intentional self-harm (suicide) by discharge of firearms (X72-X74)	7.3	13.1	1.9	2.8	5.4	0.5
Intentional self-harm (suicide) by other and unspecified means and their sequelae (*U03, X60-X71, X75-X84, Y87.0)	6.9	9.7	4.0	2.7	4.3	1.2
Assault (homicide) (*U01-*U02, X85-Y09, Y87.1)	2.8	3.9	1.8	20.2	35.7	5.6
Assault (homicide) by discharge of firearms (*U01.4, X93-X95)	1.6	2.3	0.9	15.8	29.2	3.0
Assault (homicide) by other and unspecified means and their sequelae (*U01.0-*U01.3, *U01.5-*U01.9, *U02, X85-X92, X96-Y09, Y87.1)	1.3	1.6	0.9	4.4	6.6	2.6
Legal intervention (Y35, Y89.0)	0.1	0.2	-	0.3	0.6	-
Events of undetermined intent (Y10-Y34, Y87.2,Y89.9)	1.9	2.3	1.5	1.8	2.6	1.1
Discharge of firearms, undetermined intent (Y22-Y24)	0.1	0.2	0.0	0.1	0.2	-
Other and unspecified events of undetermined intent and their sequelae (Y10-Y21, Y25-Y34, Y87.2, Y89.9)	1.8	2.2	1.5	1.7	2.4	1.0
Operations of war and their sequelae (Y36, Y89.1)	0.0	0.0	-	-	-	-
Complications of medical and surgical care (Y40-Y84, Y88)	0.8	0.8	0.8	1.3	1.5	1.1
Enterocolitis due to Clostridium difficile (A04.7)[4]	2.4	2.4	2.5	1.6	1.7	1.6
Drug-induced deaths[5]	15.4	18.9	11.7	9.7	13.7	6.4
Alcohol-induced deaths[5]	7.5	11.4	3.8	6.4	10.8	3.0
Injury by firearms[5]	9.2	16.1	2.9	19.1	35.7	3.6

X = Category not applicable.
* = Figure does not meet standards of reliability or precision.
0.0 = Quantity more than zero but less than 0.05
[1]Figures for origin not stated are included in "All origins" but not distributed among specified origins.
[2]Includes races other than white and black.
[3]Race categories are consistent with the 1977 Office of Management and Budget (OMB) standards.
[4]Included in certain other intestinal infections (A04, A07-A09).
[5]Included in selected categories above.

NOTE: Complete confirmation of deaths from selected causes of death, considered to be of public health concern, were not provided by the following states—Massachusetts, North Carolina, and West Virginia.

Table B-19. Age-Adjusted Death Rates, by Race and Hispanic Origin, Average Annual Rates, 1979–1981, 1989–1991, and 2006–2008

(Age-adjusted death rate per 100,000 population.)

State	All persons			White	Black	American Indian or Alaska Native[1]	Asian or Pacific Islander	Hispanic or Latino[2,3]	White, not Hispanic or Latino
	1979–1981	1989–1991	2006–2008	2006–2008	2006–2008	2006–2008	2006–2008	2006–2008	2006–2008
United States	1,022.8	942.2	764.9	754.6	957.9	625.4	418.8	546.7	768.8
Alabama	1,091.2	1,037.9	937.7	904.7	1,076.8	307.6	373.4	299.6	910.0
Alaska	1,087.4	944.6	756.9	730.8	713.0	1,026.2	433.7	498.2	736.4
Arizona	951.5	873.5	685.6	682.3	771.0	789.2	341.2	610.2	689.9
Arkansas	1,017.0	996.3	890.5	868.3	1,089.4	374.0	467.5	305.7	879.0
California	975.5	911.0	678.0	699.3	941.3	410.3	435.1	541.6	732.4
Colorado	941.1	856.1	708.8	714.1	786.3	494.9	373.9	669.0	713.4
Connecticut	961.5	857.5	700.0	696.7	785.2	288.2	304.1	530.5	697.8
Delaware	1,069.7	1,001.9	779.4	763.6	891.9	*	316.8	451.1	763.0
District of Columbia	1,243.1	1,255.3	869.9	554.5	1,096.3	*	392.1	355.1	563.7
Florida	960.8	870.9	691.8	676.4	869.3	257.0	310.0	547.9	701.2
Georgia	1,094.3	1,037.4	843.3	813.0	965.5	248.8	382.1	248.2	829.8
Hawaii	801.2	752.2	608.7	648.7	441.2	*	601.1	896.6	667.7
Idaho	936.7	856.6	734.8	737.2	530.0	707.1	490.4	514.5	741.7
Illinois	1,063.7	973.8	770.6	745.6	1,020.8	255.1	347.7	441.1	760.3
Indiana	1,048.3	962.0	830.9	821.9	1,001.1	151.0	254.2	397.6	825.5
Iowa	919.9	848.2	731.1	729.0	975.5	686.8	328.9	375.0	732.4
Kansas	940.1	867.2	787.5	776.2	1,030.8	1,192.5	416.0	508.2	780.7
Kentucky	1,088.9	1,024.5	904.8	901.6	1,019.5	179.2	416.0	448.7	904.4
Louisiana	1,132.6	1,074.6	926.2	872.9	1,092.0	336.0	413.4	348.9	883.6
Maine	1,002.9	918.7	771.1	771.9	591.0	*	332.9	324.3	770.5
Maryland	1,063.3	985.2	782.4	747.1	932.9	305.0	362.8	320.4	759.6
Massachusetts	982.6	884.8	710.9	717.4	749.0	311.4	359.2	470.6	718.1
Michigan	1,050.2	966.0	810.6	781.3	1,050.6	890.9	345.0	672.4	781.1
Minnesota	892.9	825.2	669.9	661.5	864.6	985.2	502.1	400.8	662.6
Mississippi	1,108.7	1,071.4	951.5	893.6	1,091.5	749.7	403.5	260.9	898.2
Missouri	1,033.7	952.4	840.7	823.9	1,048.1	377.8	351.4	468.5	828.2
Montana	1,013.6	890.2	780.4	761.6	*	1,141.1	*	526.5	756.3
Nebraska	930.6	867.9	740.1	731.7	986.7	978.1	333.0	463.6	735.9
Nevada	1,077.4	1,017.4	818.3	840.2	883.6	630.4	434.0	425.2	892.4
New Hampshire	982.3	891.7	721.3	727.5	495.6	*	254.3	288.3	729.8
New Jersey	1,047.5	956.0	726.0	719.6	904.9	261.2	326.7	458.7	738.8
New Mexico	967.1	891.9	763.0	763.0	669.8	793.6	357.5	729.8	758.8
New York	1,051.8	973.7	687.7	694.3	741.7	253.9	358.5	534.7	696.3
North Carolina	1,050.4	986.0	834.4	801.4	997.4	806.2	343.0	280.1	810.4
North Dakota	922.4	818.4	706.4	685.7	*	1,282.9	*	422.2	673.0
Ohio	1,070.6	967.4	838.6	821.2	1,035.5	238.1	337.7	450.0	823.7
Oklahoma	1,025.6	961.4	923.9	915.8	1,068.8	921.1	455.6	499.0	927.4
Oregon	953.9	893.0	757.5	764.9	780.5	736.9	437.8	402.3	774.0
Pennsylvania	1,076.4	963.4	795.8	778.5	1,025.9	203.6	361.7	489.4	780.5
Rhode Island	990.8	889.6	748.9	752.8	731.0	*	366.0	401.7	758.5
South Carolina	1,104.6	1,030.0	851.1	802.2	1,021.1	415.7	347.5	401.4	805.9
South Dakota	941.9	846.4	713.8	678.4	645.3	1,294.1	*	341.0	680.1
Tennessee	1,045.5	1,011.8	894.0	872.3	1,070.3	272.2	380.2	277.8	878.2
Texas	1,014.9	947.6	779.1	771.5	976.9	207.3	372.4	626.7	812.1
Utah	924.9	823.2	685.8	688.4	688.5	709.2	510.9	513.0	695.6
Vermont	990.2	908.6	724.2	727.8	*	*	*	*	729.2
Virginia	1,054.0	963.1	771.3	748.0	955.4	279.6	387.6	367.4	755.5
Washington	947.7	869.4	722.8	731.0	853.5	885.8	451.7	468.7	738.0
West Virginia	1,100.3	1,031.5	950.6	952.3	1,059.1	*	225.3	232.5	956.6
Wisconsin	956.4	879.1	736.3	721.9	1,034.4	1,000.8	473.4	399.9	725.1
Wyoming	1,016.1	897.4	798.9	793.8	*	1,084.0	*	720.5	793.5

* = Prior to 2006–2008, data for states with populations under 10,000 in the middle year of a 3-year period, or fewer than 50 deaths for the 3-year period, are considered unreliable and are not shown.
[1] All data for the American Indian or Alaska Native (AIAN) category should be used with caution. Agreement between self-reported race and death certificate proxy reporting was found to be poor for the AIAN population.
[2] Persons of Hispanic origin may be of any race.
[3] Caution should also be used when comparing death rates by Hispanic origin and race among states. Estimates of death rates may be affected by several factors, including possible misreporting of race and Hispanic origin on the death certificate, migration patterns between United States and country of origin for persons who were born outside the United States, and possible biases in population estimates.

PART B: MORTALITY

Table B-20. Age-Adjusted Death Rates for Selected Causes of Death, by Sex, Race, and Hispanic Origin, Selected Years, 1950–2008

(Age-adjusted death rate per 100,000 population.)

Sex, race, Hispanic origin, and cause of death[1]	1950[2,3]	1960[2,3]	1970[3]	1980[3]	1985	1990	2000[4]	2005[4]	2006[4]	2007[4]	2008[4]
All Persons											
All causes	1,446.0	1,339.2	1,222.6	1,039.1	988.1	938.7	869.0	798.8	776.5	760.2	758.3
Diseases of heart	588.8	559.0	492.7	412.1	375.0	321.8	257.6	211.1	200.2	190.9	186.5
Ischemic heart disease	—	—	—	345.2	296.2	249.6	186.8	144.4	134.9	126.0	122.7
Cerebrovascular diseases	180.7	177.9	147.7	96.2	76.4	65.3	60.9	46.6	43.6	42.2	40.7
Malignant neoplasms	193.9	193.9	198.6	207.9	211.3	216.0	199.6	183.8	180.7	178.4	175.3
Trachea, bronchus, and lung	15.0	24.1	37.1	49.9	54.6	59.3	56.1	52.6	51.5	50.6	49.5
Colon, rectum, and anus	—	30.3	28.9	27.4	26.3	24.5	20.8	17.5	17.2	16.9	16.4
Chronic lower respiratory diseases	—	—	—	28.3	34.5	37.2	44.2	43.2	40.5	40.8	44.0
Influenza and pneumonia	48.1	53.7	41.7	31.4	34.5	36.8	23.7	20.3	17.8	16.2	16.9
Chronic liver disease and cirrhosis	11.3	13.3	17.8	15.1	12.3	11.1	9.5	9.0	8.8	9.1	9.2
Diabetes mellitus	23.1	22.5	24.3	18.1	17.4	20.7	25.0	24.6	23.3	22.5	21.8
Alzheimer's disease	—	—	—	*	*	*	18.1	22.9	22.6	22.7	24.4
Human immunodeficiency virus (HIV) disease	*	*	*	*	—	10.2	5.2	4.2	4.0	3.7	3.3
Unintentional injuries	78.0	62.3	60.1	46.4	38.5	36.3	34.9	39.1	39.8	40.0	38.8
Motor vehicle-related injuries	24.6	23.1	27.6	22.3	18.6	18.5	15.4	15.2	15.0	14.4	12.9
Poisoning	2.5	1.7	2.8	1.9	2.2	2.3	4.5	7.9	9.1	9.8	10.2
Suicide	13.2	12.5	13.1	12.2	12.5	12.5	10.4	10.9	10.9	11.3	11.6
Homicide	5.1	5.0	8.8	10.4	7.9	9.4	5.9	6.1	6.2	6.1	5.9
Male											
All causes	1,674.2	1,609.0	1,542.1	1,348.1	1,278.1	1,202.8	1,053.8	951.1	924.8	905.6	900.6
Diseases of heart	699.0	687.6	634.0	538.9	488.0	412.4	320.0	260.9	248.5	237.7	232.3
Ischemic heart disease	—	—	—	459.7	393.7	328.2	241.4	187.4	176.5	165.4	161.2
Cerebrovascular diseases	186.4	186.1	157.4	102.2	79.9	68.5	62.4	46.9	43.9	42.5	40.9
Malignant neoplasms	208.1	225.1	247.6	271.2	274.4	280.4	248.9	225.1	220.1	217.5	213.6
Trachea, bronchus, and lung	24.6	43.6	67.5	85.2	88.6	91.1	76.7	69.0	67.0	65.1	63.6
Colon, rectum, and anus	—	31.8	32.3	32.8	31.8	30.4	25.1	20.9	20.5	20.1	19.5
Prostate	28.6	28.7	28.8	32.8	33.4	38.4	30.4	24.5	23.5	23.5	22.3
Chronic lower respiratory diseases	—	—	—	49.9	56.2	55.4	55.3	51.2	47.6	48.0	51.4
Influenza and pneumonia	55.0	65.8	54.0	42.1	46.8	47.8	28.9	23.9	21.2	19.3	19.9
Chronic liver disease and cirrhosis	15.0	18.5	24.8	21.3	17.4	15.9	13.4	12.4	12.1	12.7	12.7
Diabetes mellitus	18.8	19.9	23.0	18.1	17.7	21.7	27.8	28.4	27.4	26.4	25.6
Alzheimer's disease	—	—	—	*	*	*	15.2	18.5	18.4	18.5	20.1
Human immunodeficiency virus (HIV) disease	*	*	*	*	—	18.5	7.9	6.2	5.9	5.4	4.8
Unintentional injuries	101.8	85.5	87.4	69.0	57.1	52.9	49.3	54.2	55.2	55.2	53.6
Motor vehicle-related injuries	38.5	35.4	41.5	33.6	27.2	26.5	21.7	21.7	21.4	20.9	18.8
Poisoning	3.3	2.3	3.9	2.7	3.2	3.5	6.6	10.7	12.4	13.0	13.5
Suicide	21.2	20.0	19.8	19.9	21.1	21.5	17.7	18.0	18.0	18.4	18.9
Homicide	7.9	7.5	14.3	16.6	12.2	14.8	9.0	9.6	9.7	9.6	9.3
Female											
All causes	1,236.0	1,105.3	971.4	817.9	784.5	750.9	731.4	677.6	657.8	643.4	643.4
Diseases of heart	486.6	447.0	381.6	320.8	294.5	257.0	210.9	172.3	162.2	154.0	150.4
Ischemic heart disease	—	—	—	263.1	227.0	193.9	146.5	111.7	103.1	95.7	93.0
Cerebrovascular diseases	175.8	170.7	140.0	91.7	73.3	62.6	59.1	45.6	42.6	41.3	39.9
Malignant neoplasms	182.3	168.7	163.2	166.7	171.2	175.7	167.6	155.6	153.6	151.3	148.5
Trachea, bronchus, and lung	5.8	7.5	13.1	24.4	30.6	37.1	41.3	40.5	40.0	40.0	39.0
Colon, rectum, and anus	—	29.1	26.5	23.8	22.7	20.6	17.7	14.8	14.7	14.4	14.0
Breast	31.9	31.7	32.1	31.9	33.0	33.3	26.8	24.1	23.5	22.9	22.5
Chronic lower respiratory diseases	—	—	—	14.9	21.7	26.6	37.4	38.1	35.9	36.0	39.1
Influenza and pneumonia	41.9	43.8	32.7	25.1	27.6	30.5	20.7	17.9	15.5	14.2	15.0
Chronic liver disease and cirrhosis	7.8	8.7	11.9	9.9	7.9	7.1	6.2	5.8	5.8	5.9	6.0
Diabetes mellitus	27.0	24.7	25.1	18.0	17.0	19.9	23.0	21.6	20.1	19.5	18.8
Alzheimer's disease	—	—	—	*	*	*	19.3	25.1	24.7	24.9	26.7
Human immunodeficiency virus (HIV) disease	*	*	*	*	—	2.2	2.5	2.3	2.2	2.1	1.9
Unintentional injuries	54.0	40.0	35.1	26.1	22.2	21.5	22.0	25.0	25.5	25.8	25.1
Motor vehicle-related injuries	11.5	11.7	14.9	11.8	10.7	11.0	9.5	8.9	8.8	8.2	7.3
Poisoning	1.7	1.1	1.8	1.3	1.2	1.2	2.5	5.1	5.9	6.6	6.8
Suicide	5.6	5.6	7.4	5.7	5.2	4.8	4.0	4.4	4.5	4.7	4.8
Homicide	2.4	2.6	3.7	4.4	3.8	4.0	2.8	2.5	2.5	2.5	2.4

Table B-20. Age-Adjusted Death Rates for Selected Causes of Death, by Sex, Race, and Hispanic Origin, Selected Years, 1950-2008—Continued

(Age-adjusted death rate per 100,000 population.)

Sex, race, Hispanic origin, and cause of death[1]	1950[2,3]	1960[2,3]	1970[3]	1980[3]	1985	1990	2000[4]	2005[4]	2006[4]	2007[4]	2008[4]
White[5]											
All causes	1,410.8	1,311.3	1,193.3	1,012.7	963.6	909.8	849.8	785.3	764.4	749.4	750.3
Diseases of heart	586.0	559.0	492.2	409.4	371.4	317.0	253.4	207.8	197.0	187.8	183.9
Ischemic heart disease	—	—	—	347.6	298.0	249.7	185.6	143.8	134.2	125.5	122.5
Cerebrovascular diseases	175.5	172.7	143.5	93.2	73.7	62.8	58.8	44.7	41.7	40.5	39.1
Malignant neoplasms	194.6	193.1	196.7	204.2	207.3	211.6	197.2	182.6	179.9	177.5	174.7
Trachea, bronchus, and lung	15.2	24.0	36.7	49.2	53.9	58.6	56.2	53.1	52.1	51.2	50.2
Colon, rectum, and anus	—	30.9	29.2	27.4	26.1	24.1	20.3	16.9	16.7	16.4	16.0
Chronic lower respiratory diseases	—	—	—	29.3	35.6	38.3	46.0	45.4	42.6	43.0	46.4
Influenza and pneumonia	44.8	50.4	39.8	30.9	34.3	36.4	23.5	20.2	17.7	16.0	16.7
Chronic liver disease and cirrhosis	11.5	13.2	16.6	13.9	11.4	10.5	9.6	9.2	9.1	9.4	9.6
Diabetes mellitus	22.9	21.7	22.9	16.7	15.9	18.8	22.8	22.5	21.2	20.5	19.9
Alzheimer's disease	—	—	—	*	*	*	18.8	23.7	23.4	23.5	25.4
Human immunodeficiency virus (HIV) disease	*	*	*	*	—	8.3	2.8	2.2	2.1	1.9	1.7
Unintentional injuries	77.0	60.4	57.8	45.3	37.7	35.5	35.1	40.1	41.0	41.5	40.7
Motor vehicle-related injuries	24.4	22.9	27.1	22.6	18.8	18.5	15.6	15.6	15.4	14.8	13.3
Poisoning	2.4	1.6	2.4	1.8	2.0	2.1	4.5	8.4	9.7	10.6	11.1
Suicide	13.9	13.1	13.8	13.0	13.4	13.4	11.3	12.0	12.1	12.5	12.9
Homicide	2.6	2.7	4.7	6.7	5.3	5.5	3.6	3.7	3.7	3.7	3.7
Black or African American[5]											
All causes	1,722.1	1,577.5	1,518.1	1,314.8	1,261.2	1,250.3	1,121.4	1,016.5	982.0	958.0	934.9
Diseases of heart	588.7	548.3	512.0	455.3	430.6	391.5	324.8	271.3	257.7	247.3	238.6
Ischemic heart disease	—	—	—	334.5	293.4	267.0	218.3	171.3	161.6	150.6	143.7
Cerebrovascular diseases	233.6	235.2	197.1	129.1	105.2	91.6	81.9	65.2	61.6	60.3	57.4
Malignant neoplasms	176.4	199.1	225.3	256.4	266.5	279.5	248.5	222.7	217.4	215.5	209.1
Trachea, bronchus, and lung	11.1	23.7	41.3	59.7	65.8	72.4	64.0	58.4	56.8	55.6	53.4
Colon, rectum, and anus	—	22.8	26.1	28.3	30.0	30.6	28.2	24.8	24.3	23.5	22.8
Chronic lower respiratory diseases	—	—	—	19.2	24.6	28.1	31.6	30.6	28.1	28.1	30.4
Influenza and pneumonia	76.7	81.1	57.2	34.4	35.8	39.4	25.6	21.7	19.6	18.4	18.9
Chronic liver disease and cirrhosis	9.0	13.6	28.1	25.0	19.3	16.5	9.4	7.7	7.0	7.4	7.0
Diabetes mellitus	23.5	30.9	38.8	32.7	33.0	40.5	49.5	46.9	45.1	42.8	40.5
Alzheimer's disease	—	—	—	*	*	*	13.0	19.4	18.3	19.0	19.7
Human immunodeficiency virus (HIV) disease	*	*	*	*	—	26.7	23.3	19.4	18.6	17.3	15.3
Unintentional injuries	79.9	74.0	78.3	57.6	47.1	43.8	37.7	38.7	38.3	36.6	33.3
Motor vehicle-related injuries	26.0	24.2	31.1	20.2	17.8	18.8	15.7	14.5	14.6	14.1	12.3
Poisoning	2.8	2.9	5.8	3.1	3.6	4.1	6.0	8.2	9.4	8.6	7.8
Suicide	4.5	5.0	6.2	6.5	6.6	7.1	5.5	5.2	5.1	5.0	5.3
Homicide	28.3	26.0	44.0	39.0	28.1	36.3	20.5	21.1	21.6	21.1	19.5
American Indian or Alaska Native[5]											
All causes	—	—	—	867.0	731.7	716.3	709.3	663.4	642.1	527.2	610.1
Diseases of heart	—	—	—	240.6	219.0	200.6	178.2	141.8	139.4	127.3	119.8
Ischemic heart disease	—	—	—	173.6	158.3	139.1	129.1	96.2	97.4	86.7	79.5
Cerebrovascular diseases	—	—	—	57.8	46.2	40.7	45.0	34.8	29.4	29.8	24.5
Malignant neoplasms	—	—	—	113.7	113.5	121.8	127.8	123.2	119.4	117.8	119.6
Trachea, bronchus, and lung	—	—	—	20.7	25.8	30.9	32.3	34.1	31.2	32.7	33.2
Colon, rectum, and anus	—	—	—	9.5	10.5	12.0	13.4	12.0	11.2	11.5	13.8
Chronic lower respiratory diseases	—	—	—	14.2	17.6	25.4	32.8	29.1	27.4	30.9	29.3
Influenza and pneumonia	—	—	—	44.4	33.6	36.1	22.3	20.4	14.2	13.8	17.2
Chronic liver disease and cirrhosis	—	—	—	45.3	27.9	24.1	24.3	22.6	22.1	24.8	25.7
Diabetes mellitus	—	—	—	29.6	29.0	34.1	41.5	41.5	39.6	37.2	34.5
Alzheimer's disease	—	—	—	*	*	*	9.1	12.0	11.0	11.3	11.4
Human immunodeficiency virus (HIV) disease	*	*	*	*	—	1.8	2.2	2.7	2.4	2.6	2.1
Unintentional injuries	—	—	—	99.0	67.4	62.6	51.3	54.7	56.7	55.7	53.5
Motor vehicle-related injuries	—	—	—	54.5	34.8	32.5	27.3	24.8	26.7	23.7	21.1
Poisoning	—	—	—	2.3	3.1	3.2	4.7	9.4	10.4	11.6	14.4
Suicide	—	—	—	11.9	10.9	11.7	9.8	11.7	11.6	11.5	11.7
Homicide	—	—	—	15.5	11.7	10.4	6.8	7.7	7.5	6.5	7.1

Table B-20. Age-Adjusted Death Rates for Selected Causes of Death, by Sex, Race, and Hispanic Origin, Selected Years, 1950–2008—Continued

(Age-adjusted death rate per 100,000 population.)

Sex, race, Hispanic origin, and cause of death[1]	1950[2,3]	1960[2,3]	1970[3]	1980[3]	1985	1990	2000[4]	2005[4]	2006[4]	2007[4]	2008[4]
Asian or Pacific Islander[5]											
All causes	—	—	—	589.9	586.5	582.0	506.4	440.2	428.6	415.0	413.7
Diseases of heart	—	—	—	202.1	196.7	181.7	146.0	113.3	108.5	101.2	100.5
Ischemic heart disease	—	—	—	168.2	153.3	139.6	109.6	81.0	77.1	71.0	70.9
Cerebrovascular diseases	—	—	—	66.1	58.7	56.9	52.9	38.6	37.0	34.3	33.0
Malignant neoplasms	—	—	—	126.1	132.3	134.2	121.9	110.5	106.5	106.7	106.5
Trachea, bronchus, and lung	—	—	—	28.4	27.2	30.2	28.1	25.7	25.2	25.3	25.1
Colon, rectum, and anus	—	—	—	16.4	16.6	14.4	12.7	11.2	10.9	10.9	11.3
Chronic lower respiratory diseases	—	—	—	12.9	17.6	19.4	18.6	14.9	14.4	13.4	14.1
Influenza and pneumonia	—	—	—	24.0	26.1	31.4	19.7	15.5	14.7	13.6	14.3
Chronic liver disease and cirrhosis	—	—	—	6.1	5.9	5.2	3.5	3.6	3.5	3.3	3.4
Diabetes mellitus	—	—	—	12.6	12.1	14.6	16.4	16.6	15.8	16.2	16.0
Alzheimer's disease	—	—	—	*	*	*	5.5	7.7	8.4	8.1	8.9
Human immunodeficiency virus (HIV) disease	*	*	*	*	—	2.2	0.6	0.6	0.6	0.5	0.6
Unintentional injuries	—	—	—	27.0	24.8	23.9	17.9	17.9	16.9	17.0	15.4
Motor vehicle-related injuries	—	—	—	13.9	12.9	14.0	8.6	7.6	7.5	7.2	6.3
Poisoning	—	—	—	0.5	0.6	0.7	0.7	1.3	1.4	1.5	1.4
Suicide	—	—	—	7.8	7.1	6.7	5.5	5.2	5.6	6.1	5.8
Homicide	—	—	—	5.9	4.1	5.0	3.0	2.9	2.8	2.3	2.3
Hispanic or Latino[5,6]											
All causes	—	—	—	—	698.8	692.0	665.7	590.7	564.0	546.1	532.2
Diseases of heart	—	—	—	—	239.8	217.1	196.0	157.3	144.1	136.0	126.3
Ischemic heart disease	—	—	—	—	187.9	173.3	153.2	118.0	106.4	97.8	90.0
Cerebrovascular diseases	—	—	—	—	51.9	45.2	46.4	35.7	34.2	32.7	30.9
Malignant neoplasms	—	—	—	—	125.9	136.8	134.9	122.8	118.0	116.2	114.6
Trachea, bronchus, and lung	—	—	—	—	22.9	26.5	24.8	22.4	20.7	20.9	20.5
Colon, rectum, and anus	—	—	—	—	13.0	14.7	14.1	12.4	12.6	12.0	11.9
Chronic lower respiratory diseases	—	—	—	—	17.4	19.3	21.1	19.3	17.3	17.5	18.3
Influenza and pneumonia	—	—	—	—	30.2	29.7	20.6	16.8	15.0	13.1	14.0
Chronic liver disease and cirrhosis	—	—	—	—	20.3	18.3	16.5	13.9	13.3	13.8	13.7
Diabetes mellitus	—	—	—	—	23.0	28.2	36.9	33.6	29.9	28.9	27.7
Alzheimer's disease	—	—	—	—	*	*	10.4	13.8	14.0	13.5	15.0
Human immunodeficiency virus (HIV) disease	*	*	*	*	—	16.3	6.7	4.7	4.5	4.1	3.6
Unintentional injuries	—	—	—	—	34.3	34.6	30.1	31.3	31.5	30.1	27.9
Motor vehicle-related injuries	—	—	—	—	17.1	19.5	14.7	14.7	14.6	13.3	11.4
Poisoning	—	—	—	—	3.2	3.2	4.1	5.2	5.7	5.8	6.0
Suicide	—	—	—	—	6.3	7.8	5.9	5.6	5.3	6.0	5.6
Homicide	—	—	—	—	14.6	16.2	7.5	7.5	7.3	6.9	6.6
White, Not Hispanic or Latino[6]											
All causes	—	—	—	—	942.1	914.5	855.5	796.6	777.0	763.3	766.2
Diseases of heart	—	—	—	—	366.7	319.7	255.5	210.7	200.3	191.4	188.0
Ischemic heart disease	—	—	—	—	296.0	251.9	186.6	145.2	136.0	127.4	124.8
Cerebrovascular diseases	—	—	—	—	72.2	63.5	59.0	45.0	41.9	40.7	39.5
Malignant neoplasms	—	—	—	—	202.1	215.4	200.6	187.0	184.6	182.3	179.4
Trachea, bronchus, and lung	—	—	—	—	53.2	60.3	58.2	55.5	54.7	53.9	52.8
Colon, rectum, and anus	—	—	—	—	25.7	24.6	20.5	17.2	17.0	16.7	16.3
Chronic lower respiratory diseases	—	—	—	—	36.3	39.2	47.2	47.2	44.4	44.9	48.7
Influenza and pneumonia	—	—	—	—	35.2	36.5	23.5	20.4	17.8	16.2	16.9
Chronic liver disease and cirrhosis	—	—	—	—	10.9	9.9	9.0	8.7	8.6	8.9	9.1
Diabetes mellitus	—	—	—	—	14.8	18.3	21.8	21.5	20.4	19.8	19.1
Alzheimer's disease	—	—	—	—	*	*	19.1	24.2	24.0	24.1	26.1
Human immunodeficiency virus (HIV) disease	*	*	*	*	—	7.4	2.2	1.8	1.7	1.5	1.4
Unintentional injuries	—	—	—	—	35.2	35.0	35.3	41.0	42.1	43.0	42.6
Motor vehicle-related injuries	—	—	—	—	17.4	18.2	15.6	15.5	15.3	14.9	13.6
Poisoning	—	—	—	—	2.2	2.0	4.6	9.0	10.5	11.6	12.2
Suicide	—	—	—	—	13.8	13.8	12.0	12.9	13.2	13.5	14.1
Homicide	—	—	—	—	4.4	4.0	2.8	2.7	2.7	2.8	2.8

— = Data not available.
* = Data for Alzheimer's disease are only presented for data years 1999 and beyond due to large differences in death rates caused by changes in the coding of the causes of death between ICD-9 and ICD-10.
X = Category not applicable.
[1] Underlying cause of death code numbers are based on the applicable revision of the International Classification of Diseases (ICD) for data years shown.
[2] Includes deaths of persons who were not residents of the 50 states and the District of Columbia (D.C.).
[3] Underlying cause of death was coded according to the 6th Revision of the ICD in 1950, 7th Revision in 1960, 8th Revision in 1970, and 9th Revision in 1980–1998.
[4] Starting with 1999 data, cause of death is coded according to ICD-10.
[5] The race groups, White, Black, Asian or Pacific Islander, and American Indian or Alaska Native, include persons of Hispanic and non-Hispanic origin. Persons of Hispanic origin may be of any race.
[6] Prior to 1997, excludes data from states lacking an Hispanic-origin item on the death certificate.

Table B-21. Number of Deaths, Death Rates, and Age–Adjusted Death Rates for Injury Deaths According to Mechanism and Intent of Death, 2008

(Number, rates are per 100,000 population, age–adjusted rates are per 100,000 U.S. standard population.)

Mechanism and intent of death (based on the International Classification of Diseases, Tenth Revision)	Number	Rate	Age-adjusted rate
All Injury (*U01–*U03, V01–Y36, Y85–Y87, Y89)	181,226	59.6	58.1
Unintentional (V01–X59, Y85–Y86)	121,902	40.1	38.8
Suicide (*U03,X60–X84, Y87.0)	36,035	11.9	11.6
Homicide (*U01–*U02, X85–Y09, Y87.1)	17,826	5.9	5.9
Undetermined (Y10–Y34, Y87.2, Y89.9)	5,051	1.7	1.6
Legal intervention/war (Y35–Y36, Y89[.0,.1])	412	0.1	0.1
Cut/Pierce (W25–W29, W45, X78, X99, Y28, Y35.4)	2,808	0.9	0.9
Unintentional (W25–W29, W45)	87	0.0	0.0
Suicide (X78)	666	0.2	0.2
Homicide (X99)	2,043	0.7	0.7
Undetermined (Y28)	12	*	*
Legal intervention/war (Y35.4)	-	*	*
Drowning (W65–W74, X71, X92, Y21)	4,251	1.4	1.4
Unintentional (W65–W74)	3,548	1.2	1.2
Suicide (X71)	407	0.1	0.1
Homicide (X92)	56	0.0	0.0
Undetermined (Y21)	240	0.1	0.1
Fall (W00–W19, X80, Y01, Y30)	24,820	8.2	7.6
Unintentional (W00–W19)	24,013	7.9	7.3
Suicide (X80)	709	0.2	0.2
Homicide (Y01)	20	0.0	0.0
Undetermined (Y30)	78	0.0	0.0
Fire/Hot Object or Substance (*U01.3, X00–X19, X76–X77, X97–X98, Y26–Y27, Y36.3)[1]	3,382	1.1	1.1
Unintentional (X00–X19)	2,992	1.0	1.0
Suicide (X76–X77)	170	0.1	0.1
Homicide (*U01.3, X97–X98)	97	0.0	0.0
Undetermined (Y26–Y27)	123	0.0	0.1
Legal intervention/war (Y36.3)	-	*	*
Fire/flame (X00–X09, X76, X97, Y26)	3,297	1.1	1.1
Unintentional (X00–X09)	2,912	1.0	0.9
Suicide (X76)	169	0.1	0.1
Homicide (X97)	94	0.0	0.0
Undetermined (Y26)	122	0.0	0.1
Hot object/substance (X10–X19, X77, X98,Y27)	85	0.0	0.0
Unintentional (X10–X19)	80	0.0	0.0
Suicide (X77)	1	*	*
Homicide (X98)	3	*	*
Undetermined (Y27)	1	*	*
Firearm (*U01.4, W32–W34, X72–X74, X93–X95, Y22–Y24, Y35.0)	31,593	10.4	10.3
Unintentional (W32–W34)	592	0.2	0.2
Suicide (X72–X74)	18,223	6.0	5.8
Homicide (*U01.4, X93–X95)	12,179	4.0	4.0
Undetermined (Y22–Y24)	273	0.1	0.1
Legal intervention/war (Y35.0)	326	0.1	0.1
Machinery (W24,W30–W31)[2]	693	0.2	0.2
All Transport (*U01.1, V01–V99, X82, Y03, Y32, Y36.1)	42,094	13.8	13.7
Unintentional (V01–V99)	41,911	13.8	13.6
Suicide (X82)	129	0.0	0.1
Homicide (*U01.1,Y03)	37	0.0	0.0
Undetermined (Y32)	17	*	*
Legal intervention/war (Y36.1)	-	*	*
Motor vehicle traffic (V02–V04[.1,.9], V09.2, V12–V14[.3–.9], V19[.4–.6], V20–V28[.3–.9], V29–V79[.4–.9], V80[.3–.5],V81.1, V82.1,V83–V86[.0–.3], V87[.0–.8],V89.2)[2]	37,985	12.5	12.3
Occupant (V30–V79[.4–.9], V83–V86[.0–3])[2]	13,677	4.5	4.5
Motorcyclist (V20–V28[.3–.9], V29[.4–.9])[2]	5,037	1.7	1.7
Pedal cyclist (V12–V14[.3–.9], V19[.4–.6])[2]	582	0.2	0.2
Pedestrian (V02–V04[.1,.9], V09.2)[2]	4,489	1.5	1.5
Other (V80[.3–.5], V81.1, V82.1)[2]	8	*	*
Unspecified (V87[.0–.8], V89.2)[2]	14,192	4.7	4.6
Pedal cyclist, other (V10–V11, V12–V14[.0–.2], V15–V18, V19[.0–.3,.8,.9])[2]	311	0.1	0.1
Pedestrian, other (V01, V02–V04[.0], V05, V06, V09[.0,.1,.3,.9])[2]	1,089	0.4	0.4
Other land transport (V20–V28[.0–.2], V29–V79[.0–.3],V80[.0–.2,.6–.9], V81–V82[.0,.2–.9], V83–V86[.4–.9],V87.9,V88[.0–.9], V89[.0,.1,.3,.9], X82, Y03, Y32)	1,728	0.6	0.5

Table B-21. Number of Deaths, Death Rates, and Age–Adjusted Death Rates for Injury Deaths According to Mechanism and Intent of Death, 2008—*Continued*

(Number, rates are per 100,000 population, age–adjusted rates are per 100,000 U.S. standard population.)

Mechanism and intent of death (based on the International Classification of Diseases, Tenth Revision)	Number	Rate	Age-adjusted rate
Unintentional (V20–V28[.0–.2], V29–V79[.0–.3], V80(.0–.2,.6–.9), V81–V82[.0,.2–.9], V83–V86[.4–.9], V87.9, V88[.0–.9], V89[.0,.1,.3,.9])	1,545	0.5	0.5
Suicide (X82)	129	0.0	0.1
Homicide (Y03)	37	0.0	0.0
Undetermined (Y32)	17	*	*
Other transport (*U01.1, V90–V99, Y36.1)	981	0.3	0.3
Unintentional (V90–V99)	981	0.3	0.3
Homicide (*U01.1)	-	*	*
Legal intervention/war (Y36.1)	-	*	*
Natural/Environmental (W42–W43, W53–W64, W92–W99, X20–X39, X51–X57)[2]	1,409	0.5	0.4
Overexertion (X50)[2]	7	*	*
Poisoning (*U01[.6–.7], X40–X49, X60–X69, X85–X90, Y10–Y19, Y35.2)	41,080	13.5	13.4
Unintentional (X40–X49)	31,116	10.2	10.2
Suicide (X60–X69)	6,442	2.1	2.1
Homicide (*U01[.6–.7], X85–X90)	101	0.0	0.0
Undetermined (Y10–Y19)	3,421	1.1	1.1
Legal intervention/war (Y35.2)	-	*	*
Struck by or Against (W20–W22, W50–W52, X79, Y00, Y04, Y29, Y35.3)	1,060	0.3	0.3
Unintentional (W20–W22, W50–W52)	891	0.3	0.3
Suicide (X79)	-	*	*
Homicide (Y00,Y04)	169	0.1	0.1
Undetermined (Y29)	-	*	*
Legal intervention/war (Y35.3)	-	*	*
Suffocation (W75–W84, X70, X91,Y20)	15,434	5.1	5.0
Unintentional (W75–W84)	6,125	2.0	1.9
Suicide (X70)	8,578	2.8	2.8
Homicide (X91)	562	0.2	0.2
Undetermined (Y20)	169	0.1	0.0
Other Specified, Classifiable (*U01[.0,.2,.5], *U03.0, W23, W35–W41, W44,W49, W85–W91, X75, X81, X96, Y02, Y05– Y07, Y25, Y31, Y35[.1,.5], Y36[.0,.2,.4–.8], Y85)	2,023	0.7	0.6
Unintentional (W23, W35–W41, W44, W49, W85–W91, Y85)	1,447	0.5	0.5
Suicide (*U03.0, X75, X81)	301	0.1	0.1
Homicide (*U01[.0,.2,.5], X96, Y02, Y05–Y07)	218	0.1	0.1
Undetermined (Y25, Y31)	16	*	*
Legal intervention/war (Y35[.1,.5], Y36[.0,.2,.4–.8])	41	0.0	0.0
Other Specified, Not Elsewhere Classified (*U01.8, *U02, X58, X83, Y08, Y33, Y35.6, Y86–Y87, Y89[.0–.1])	2,162	0.7	0.7
Unintentional (X58, Y86)	1,160	0.4	0.4
Suicide (X83, Y87.0)	222	0.1	0.1
Homicide (*U01.8, *U02, Y08, Y87.1)	549	0.2	0.2
Undetermined (Y33, Y87.2)	191	0.1	0.1
Legal intervention/war (Y35.6, Y89[.0,.1])	40	0.0	0.0
Unspecified (*U01.9, *U03.9, X59, X84, Y09, Y34, Y35.7, Y36.9, Y89.9)	8,410	2.8	2.6
Unintentional (X59)	5,911	1.9	1.8
Suicide (*U03.9, X84)	188	0.1	0.1
Homicide (*U01.9, Y09)	1,795	0.6	0.6
Undetermined (Y34, Y89.9)	511	0.2	0.2
Legal intervention/war (Y35.7, Y36.9)	5	*	*

– = Quantity zero.
* = Figure does not meet standard of reliability or precision.
0.0 = Quantity more than zero but less than 0.05.
[1]Codes *U01.3 and Y36.3 cannot be divided separately into the subcategories shown below; therefore, subcategories may not add to the total.
[2]Intent of death is unintentional.

Table B-22. Leading Causes of Death and Numbers of Death, by Sex, Race, and Hispanic Origin, 1980 and 2008

(Number.)

Sex, race, Hispanic origin, and rank order	1980		2008	
	Cause of death	Deaths	Cause of death	Deaths
All Persons				
Rank	All causes	1,989,841	All causes	2,471,984
1	Diseases of heart	761,085	Diseases of heart	616,828
2	Malignant neoplasms	416,509	Malignant neoplasms	565,469
3	Cerebrovascular diseases	170,225	Chronic lower respiratory diseases	141,090
4	Unintentional injuries	105,718	Cerebrovascular diseases	134,148
5	Chronic obstructive pulmonary diseases	56,050	Unintentional injuries	121,902
6	Pneumonia and influenza	54,619	Alzheimer's disease	82,435
7	Diabetes mellitus	34,851	Diabetes mellitus	70,553
8	Chronic liver disease and cirrhosis	30,583	Influenza and pneumonia	56,284
9	Atherosclerosis	29,449	Nephritis, nephrotic syndrome and nephrosis	48,237
10	Suicide	26,869	Suicide	36,035
Male				
Rank	All causes	1,075,078	All causes	1,226,197
1	Diseases of heart	405,661	Diseases of heart	311,201
2	Malignant neoplasms	225,948	Malignant neoplasms	295,259
3	Unintentional injuries	74,180	Unintentional injuries	78,378
4	Cerebrovascular diseases	69,973	Chronic lower respiratory diseases	67,122
5	Chronic obstructive pulmonary diseases	38,625	Cerebrovascular diseases	53,525
6	Pneumonia and influenza	27,574	Diabetes mellitus	35,346
7	Suicide	20,505	Suicide	28,450
8	Chronic liver disease and cirrhosis	19,768	Influenza and pneumonia	25,571
9	Homicide	18,779	Alzheimer's disease	24,516
10	Diabetes mellitus	14,325	Nephritis, nephrotic syndrome and nephrosis	23,533
Female				
Rank	All causes	914,763	All causes	1,245,787
1	Diseases of heart	355,424	Diseases of heart	305,627
2	Malignant neoplasms	190,561	Malignant neoplasms	270,210
3	Cerebrovascular diseases	100,252	Cerebrovascular diseases	80,623
4	Unintentional injuries	31,538	Chronic lower respiratory diseases	73,968
5	Pneumonia and influenza	27,045	Alzheimer's disease	57,919
6	Diabetes mellitus	20,526	Unintentional injuries	43,524
7	Atherosclerosis	17,848	Diabetes mellitus	35,207
8	Chronic obstructive pulmonary diseases	17,425	Influenza and pneumonia	30,713
9	Chronic liver disease and cirrhosis	10,815	Nephritis, nephrotic syndrome and nephrosis	24,704
10	Certain conditions originating in the perinatal period	9,815	Septicemia	19,599
White				
Rank	All causes	1,738,607	All causes	2,120,233
1	Diseases of heart	683,347	Diseases of heart	532,304
2	Malignant neoplasms	368,162	Malignant neoplasms	485,893
3	Cerebrovascular diseases	148,734	Chronic lower respiratory diseases	130,221
4	Unintentional injuries	90,122	Cerebrovascular diseases	113,244
5	Chronic obstructive pulmonary diseases	52,375	Unintentional injuries	105,715
6	Pneumonia and influenza	48,369	Alzheimer's disease	76,263
7	Diabetes mellitus	28,868	Diabetes mellitus	55,893
8	Atherosclerosis	27,069	Influenza and pneumonia	48,941
9	Chronic liver disease and cirrhosis	25,240	Nephritis, nephrotic syndrome and nephrosis	38,352
10	Suicide	24,829	Suicide	32,644
Black				
Rank	All causes	233,135	All causes	289,072
1	Diseases of heart	72,956	Diseases of heart	70,731
2	Malignant neoplasms	45,037	Malignant neoplasms	63,954
3	Cerebrovascular diseases	20,135	Cerebrovascular diseases	16,710
4	Unintentional injuries	13,480	Unintentional injuries	12,447
5	Homicide	10,172	Diabetes mellitus	12,064
6	Certain conditions originating in the perinatal period	6,961	Chronic lower respiratory diseases	8,766
7	Pneumonia and influenza	5,648	Nephritis, nephrotic syndrome and nephrosis	8,619
8	Diabetes mellitus	5,544	Homicide	8,335
9	Chronic liver disease and cirrhosis	4,790	Septicemia	6,426
10	Nephritis, nephrotic syndrome, and nephrosis	3,416	Human immunodeficiency virus (HIV) disease	5,780

Table B-22. Leading Causes of Death and Numbers of Death, by Sex, Race, and Hispanic Origin, 1980 and 2008—Continued

(Number.)

Sex, race, Hispanic origin, and rank order	1980 Cause of death	1980 Deaths	2008 Cause of death	2008 Deaths
American Indian or Alaska Native				
Rank	All causes	6,923	All causes	14,776
1	Diseases of heart	1,494	Malignant neoplasms	2,727
2	Unintentional injuries	1,290	Diseases of heart	2,657
3	Malignant neoplasms	770	Unintentional injuries	1,682
4	Chronic liver disease and cirrhosis	410	Diabetes mellitus	779
5	Cerebrovascular diseases	322	Chronic liver disease and cirrhosis	742
6	Pneumonia and influenza	257	Chronic lower respiratory diseases	619
7	Homicide	217	Cerebrovascular diseases	517
8	Diabetes mellitus	210	Suicide	409
9	Certain conditions originating in the perinatal period	199	Influenza and pneumonia	379
10	Suicide	181	Nephritis, nephrotic syndrome and nephrosis	338
Asian or Pacific Islander				
Rank	All causes	11,071	All causes	47,903
1	Diseases of heart	3,265	Malignant neoplasms	12,895
2	Malignant neoplasms	2,522	Diseases of heart	11,136
3	Cerebrovascular diseases	1,028	Cerebrovascular diseases	3,677
4	Unintentional injuries	810	Unintentional injuries	2,058
5	Pneumonia and influenza	342	Diabetes mellitus	1,817
6	Suicide	249	Influenza and pneumonia	1,508
7	Certain conditions originating in the perinatal period	246	Chronic lower respiratory diseases	1,484
8	Diabetes mellitus	227	Nephritis, nephrotic syndrome and nephrosis	928
9	Homicide	211	Alzheimer's disease	893
10	Chronic obstructive pulmonary diseases	207	Suicide	876
Hispanic or Latino				
Rank	—	—	All causes	139,241
1	—	—	Diseases of heart	28,951
2	—	—	Malignant neoplasms	28,851
3	—	—	Unintentional injuries	11,080
4	—	—	Cerebrovascular diseases	7,121
5	—	—	Diabetes mellitus	6,544
6	—	—	Chronic liver disease and cirrhosis	4,091
7	—	—	Chronic lower respiratory diseases	3,949
8	—	—	Homicide	3,331
9	—	—	Influenza and pneumonia	3,176
10	—	—	Alzheimer's disease	3,005
White Male				
Rank	All causes	933,878	All causes	1,046,183
1	Diseases of heart	364,679	Diseases of heart	268,317
2	Malignant neoplasms	198,188	Malignant neoplasms	254,124
3	Unintentional injuries	62,963	Unintentional injuries	67,471
4	Cerebrovascular diseases	60,095	Chronic lower respiratory diseases	61,383
5	Chronic obstructive pulmonary diseases	35,977	Cerebrovascular diseases	44,457
6	Pneumonia and influenza	23,810	Diabetes mellitus	28,598
7	Suicide	18,901	Suicide	25,801
8	Chronic liver disease and cirrhosis	16,407	Alzheimer's disease	22,752
9	Diabetes mellitus	12,125	Influenza and pneumonia	22,048
10	Atherosclerosis	10,543	Nephritis, nephrotic syndrome and nephrosis	18,992
Black or African American male				
Rank	All causes	130,138	All causes	147,143
1	Diseases of heart	37,877	Diseases of heart	35,387
2	Malignant neoplasms	25,861	Malignant neoplasms	33,019
3	Unintentional injuries	9,701	Unintentional injuries	8,453
4	Cerebrovascular diseases	9,194	Cerebrovascular diseases	7,222
5	Homicide	8,274	Homicide	7,148
6	Certain conditions originating in the perinatal period	3,869	Diabetes mellitus	5,457
7	Pneumonia and influenza	3,386	Chronic lower respiratory diseases	4,548
8	Chronic liver disease and cirrhosis	3,020	Nephritis, nephrotic syndrome and nephrosis	3,919
9	Chronic obstructive pulmonary diseases	2,429	Human immunodeficiency virus (HIV) disease	3,790
10	Diabetes mellitus	2,010	Septicemia	2,877

Table B-22. Leading Causes of Death and Numbers of Death, by Sex, Race, and Hispanic Origin, 1980 and 2008—Continued

(Number.)

Sex, race, Hispanic origin, and rank order	1980 Cause of death	1980 Deaths	2008 Cause of death	2008 Deaths
American Indian or Alaska Native Male				
Rank	All causes	4,193	All causes	8,163
1	Unintentional injuries	946	Diseases of heart	1,527
2	Diseases of heart	917	Malignant neoplasms	1,452
3	Malignant neoplasms	408	Unintentional injuries	1,158
4	Chronic liver disease and cirrhosis	239	Chronic liver disease and cirrhosis	406
5	Cerebrovascular diseases	163	Diabetes mellitus	388
6	Homicide	162	Chronic lower respiratory diseases	308
7[1]	Pneumonia and influenza	148	Suicide[1]	308
8	Suicide	147	Cerebrovascular diseases	234
9	Certain conditions originating in the perinatal period	107	Homicide	192
10	Diabetes mellitus	86	Influenza and pneumonia	186
Asian or Pacific Islander Male				
Rank	All causes	6,809	All causes	24,708
1	Diseases of heart	2,174	Malignant neoplasms	6,664
2	Malignant neoplasms	1,485	Diseases of heart	5,970
3	Unintentional injuries	556	Cerebrovascular diseases	1,612
4	Cerebrovascular diseases	521	Unintentional injuries	1,296
5	Pneumonia and influenza	227	Diabetes mellitus	903
6	Suicide	159	Chronic lower respiratory diseases	883
7	Chronic obstructive pulmonary diseases	158	Influenza and pneumonia	765
8	Homicide	151	Suicide	582
9	Certain conditions originating in the perinatal period	128	Nephritis, nephrotic syndrome and nephrosis	467
10	Diabetes mellitus	103	Essential hypertension and hypertensive renal disease	314
Hispanic or Latino Male				
Rank	—	—	All causes	76,861
1	—	—	Diseases of heart	15,498
2	—	—	Malignant neoplasms	15,283
3	—	—	Unintentional injuries	8,363
4	—	—	Cerebrovascular diseases	3,370
5	—	—	Diabetes mellitus	3,314
6	—	—	Chronic liver disease and cirrhosis	2,850
7	—	—	Homicide	2,777
8	—	—	Chronic lower respiratory diseases	2,019
9	—	—	Suicide	1,955
10	—	—	Certain conditions originating in the perinatal period	1,645
White Female				
Rank	All causes	804,729	All causes	1,074,050
1	Diseases of heart	318,668	Diseases of heart	263,987
2	Malignant neoplasms	169,974	Malignant neoplasms	231,769
3	Cerebrovascular diseases	88,639	Chronic lower respiratory diseases	68,838
4	Unintentional injuries	27,159	Cerebrovascular diseases	68,787
5	Pneumonia and influenza	24,559	Alzheimer's disease	53,511
6	Diabetes mellitus	16,743	Unintentional injuries	38,244
7	Atherosclerosis	16,526	Diabetes mellitus	27,295
8	Chronic obstructive pulmonary diseases	16,398	Influenza and pneumonia	26,893
9	Chronic liver disease and cirrhosis	8,833	Nephritis, nephrotic syndrome and nephrosis	19,360
10	Certain conditions originating in the perinatal period	6,512	Septicemia	15,631
Black or African American Female				
Rank	All causes	102,997	All causes	141,929
1	Diseases of heart	35,079	Diseases of heart	35,344
2	Malignant neoplasms	19,176	Malignant neoplasms	30,935
3	Cerebrovascular diseases	10,941	Cerebrovascular diseases	9,488
4	Unintentional injuries	3,779	Diabetes mellitus	6,607
5	Diabetes mellitus	3,534	Nephritis, nephrotic syndrome and nephrosis	4,700
6	Certain conditions originating in the perinatal period	3,092	Chronic lower respiratory diseases	4,218
7	Pneumonia and influenza	2,262	Unintentional injuries	3,994
8	Homicide	1,898	Alzheimer's disease	3,663
9	Chronic liver disease and cirrhosis	1,770	Septicemia	3,549
10	Nephritis, nephrotic syndrome, and nephrosis	1,722	Influenza and pneumonia	2,884

Table B-22. Leading Causes of Death and Numbers of Death, by Sex, Race, and Hispanic Origin, 1980 and 2008—*Continued*

(Number.)

Sex, race, Hispanic origin, and rank order	1980		2008	
	Cause of death	Deaths	Cause of death	Deaths
American Indian or Alaska Native Female				
Rank	All causes	2,730	All causes	6,613
1	Diseases of heart	577	Malignant neoplasms	1,275
2	Malignant neoplasms	362	Diseases of heart	1,130
3	Unintentional injuries	344	Unintentional injuries	524
4	Chronic liver disease and cirrhosis	171	Diabetes mellitus	391
5	Cerebrovascular diseases	159	Chronic liver disease and cirrhosis	336
6	Diabetes mellitus	124	Chronic lower respiratory diseases	311
7	Pneumonia and influenza	109	Cerebrovascular diseases	283
8	Certain conditions originating in the perinatal period	92	Influenza and pneumonia	193
9	Nephritis, nephrotic syndrome, and nephrosis	56	Nephritis, nephrotic syndrome and nephrosis	183
10	Homicide	55	Alzheimer's disease	142
Asian or Pacific Islander Female				
Rank	All causes	4,262	All causes	23,195
1	Diseases of heart	1,091	Malignant neoplasms	6,231
2	Malignant neoplasms	1,037	Diseases of heart	5,166
3	Cerebrovascular diseases	507	Cerebrovascular diseases	2,065
4	Unintentional injuries	254	Diabetes mellitus	914
5	Diabetes mellitus	124	Unintentional injuries	762
6	Certain conditions originating in the perinatal period	118	Influenza and pneumonia	743
7	Pneumonia and influenza	115	Alzheimer's disease	603
8	Congenital anomalies	104	Chronic lower respiratory diseases	601
9	Suicide	90	Nephritis, nephrotic syndrome and nephrosis	461
10	Homicide	60	Essential hypertension and hypertensive renal disease	393
Hispanic or Latina Female				
Rank	—	—	All causes	62,380
1	—	—	Malignant neoplasms	13,568
2	—	—	Diseases of heart	13,453
3	—	—	Cerebrovascular diseases	3,751
4	—	—	Diabetes mellitus	3,230
5	—	—	Unintentional injuries	2,717
6	—	—	Alzheimer's disease	2,039
7	—	—	Chronic lower respiratory diseases	1,930
8	—	—	Influenza and pneumonia	1,632
9	—	—	Nephritis, nephrotic syndrome and nephrosis	1,447
10	—	—	Chronic liver disease and cirrhosis	1,241

— = Data not available.
[1]Suicide is tied with chronic lower respiratory diseases for the 6th rank in 2008.

Table B-23. Leading Causes of Death and Numbers of Deaths, by Age, 1980 and 2008

(Number.)

Age and rank order	1980		2008	
	Cause of death	Deaths	Cause of death	Deaths
Under 1 Year Rank	All causes	45,526	All causes	28,059
1	Congenital anomalies	9,220	Congenital malformations, deformations and chromosomal abnormalities	5,638
2	Sudden infant death syndrome	5,510	Disorders related to short gestation and low birth weight, not elsewhere classified	4,754
3	Respiratory distress syndrome	4,989	Sudden infant death syndrome	2,353
4	Disorders relating to short gestation and unspecified low birthweight	3,648	Newborn affected by maternal complications of pregnancy	1,765
5	Newborn affected by maternal complications of pregnancy	1,572	Unintentional injuries	1,315
6	Intrauterine hypoxia and birth asphyxia	1,497	Newborn affected by complications of placenta, cord and membranes	1,080
7	Unintentional injuries	1,166	Bacterial sepsis of newborn	700
8	Birth trauma	1,058	Respiratory distress of newborn	630
9	Pneumonia and influenza	1,012	Diseases of circulatory system	594
10	Newborn affected by complications of placenta, cord, and membranes	985	Neonatal hemorrhage	556
1–4 Years Rank	All causes	8,187	All causes	4,730
1	Unintentional injuries	3,313	Unintentional injuries	1,469
2	Congenital anomalies	1,026	Congenital malformations, deformations and chromosomal abnormalities	521
3	Malignant neoplasms	573	Homicide	421
4	Diseases of heart	338	Malignant neoplasms	394
5	Homicide	319	Diseases of heart	186
6	Pneumonia and influenza	267	Influenza and pneumonia	142
7	Meningitis	223	Septicemia	93
8	Meningococcal infection	110	Cerebrovascular diseases	63
9	Certain conditions originating in the perinatal period	84	Chronic lower respiratory diseases	54
10	Septicemia	71	Certain conditions originating in the perinatal period	51
5–14 Years Rank	All causes	10,689	All causes	5,651
1	Unintentional injuries	5,224	Unintentional injuries	1,859
2	Malignant neoplasms	1,497	Malignant neoplasms	890
3	Congenital anomalies	561	Congenital malformations, deformations and chromosomal abnormalities	331
4	Homicide	415	Homicide	320
5	Diseases of heart	330	Diseases of heart	229
6	Pneumonia and influenza	194	Suicide	222
7	Suicide	142	Chronic lower respiratory diseases	119
8	Benign neoplasms	104	Cerebrovascular diseases	97
9	Cerebrovascular diseases	95	Influenza and pneumonia	89
10	Chronic obstructive pulmonary diseases	85	In situ neoplasms, benign neoplasms and neoplasms of uncertain or unknown behavior	88
15–24 Years Rank	All causes	49,027	All causes	32,198
1	Unintentional injuries	26,206	Unintentional injuries	14,089
2	Homicide	6,537	Homicide	5,275
3	Suicide	5,239	Suicide	4,298
4	Malignant neoplasms	2,683	Malignant neoplasms	1,663
5	Diseases of heart	1,223	Diseases of heart	1,065
6	Congenital anomalies	600	Congenital malformations, deformations and chromosomal abnormalities	467
7	Cerebrovascular diseases	418	Influenza and pneumonia	206
8	Pneumonia and influenza	348	Diabetes mellitus	204
9	Chronic obstructive pulmonary diseases	141	Cerebrovascular diseases	189
10	Anemias	133	Pregnancy, childbirth, and the puerperium	169

Table B-23. Leading Causes of Death and Numbers of Deaths, by Age, 1980 and 2008—Continued

(Number.)

Age and rank order	1980		2008	
	Cause of death	Deaths	Cause of death	Deaths
25–44 Years				
Rank	All causes	108,658	All causes	118,645
1	Unintentional injuries	26,722	Unintentional injuries	30,653
2	Malignant neoplasms	17,551	Malignant neoplasms	16,220
3	Diseases of heart	14,513	Diseases of heart	14,590
4	Homicide	10,983	Suicide	12,003
5	Suicide	9,855	Homicide	7,516
6	Chronic liver disease and cirrhosis	4,782	Human immunodeficiency virus (HIV) disease	3,813
7	Cerebrovascular diseases	3,154	Chronic liver disease and cirrhosis	2,985
8	Diabetes mellitus	1,472	Cerebrovascular diseases	2,574
9	Pneumonia and influenza	1,467	Diabetes mellitus	2,428
10	Congenital anomalies	817	Septicemia	1,251
			Influenza and pneumonia[1]	1,251
45–64 Years				
Rank	All causes	425,338	All causes	482,724
1	Diseases of heart	148,322	Malignant neoplasms	154,494
2	Malignant neoplasms	135,675	Diseases of heart	104,603
3	Cerebrovascular diseases	19,909	Unintentional injuries	33,136
4	Unintentional injuries	18,140	Chronic lower respiratory diseases	18,434
5	Chronic liver disease and cirrhosis	16,089	Diabetes mellitus	16,992
6	Chronic obstructive pulmonary diseases	11,514	Chronic liver disease and cirrhosis	16,746
7	Diabetes mellitus	7,977	Cerebrovascular diseases	16,571
8	Suicide	7,079	Suicide	13,752
9	Pneumonia and influenza	5,804	Septicemia	7,066
10	Homicide	4,019	Nephritis, nephrotic syndrome and nephrosis	7,023
65 Years and Over				
Rank	All causes	1,341,848	All causes	1,799,830
1	Diseases of heart	595,406	Diseases of heart	495,730
2	Malignant neoplasms	258,389	Malignant neoplasms	391,729
3	Cerebrovascular diseases	146,417	Chronic lower respiratory diseases	121,223
4	Pneumonia and influenza	45,512	Cerebrovascular diseases	114,508
5	Chronic obstructive pulmonary diseases	43,587	Alzheimer's disease	81,573
6	Atherosclerosis	28,081	Diabetes mellitus	50,883
7	Diabetes mellitus	25,216	Influenza and pneumonia	48,382
8	Unintentional injuries	24,844	Nephritis, nephrotic syndrome and nephrosis	39,921
9	Nephritis, nephrotic syndrome, and nephrosis	12,968	Unintentional injuries	39,359
10	Chronic liver disease and cirrhosis	9,519	Septicemia	27,028

X = Category not applicable.
[1] This cause is tied with Septicemia for the 10th rank in 2008.

Table B-24. Deaths from Selected Occupational Diseases Among Persons 15 Years of Age and Over, Selected Years, 1980–2008

(Number of deaths.)

Cause of death	1980[1]	1985[1]	1995[1]	2000[2]	2005[2]	2006[2]	2007[2]	2008[2]
Multiple Cause of Death								
Angiosarcoma of liver[3]	—	—	—	16	26	23	22	17
Malignant mesothelioma[4]	699	715	897	2,531	2,704	2,588	2,606	2,709
Pneumoconiosis[5]	4,151	3,783	3,151	2,859	2,425	2,308	2,189	2,155
Coal workers' pneumoconiosis	2,576	2,615	1,413	949	652	654	524	470
Asbestosis	339	534	1,169	1,486	1,416	1,340	1,393	1,341
Silicosis	448	334	242	151	160	126	122	146
Other (including unspecified)	814	321	343	290	222	206	163	215
Underlying Cause of Death								
Angiosarcoma of liver[3]	—	—	—	15	23	21	20	16
Malignant mesothelioma[4]	531	573	780	2,384	2,553	2,452	2,432	2,538
Pneumoconiosis	1,581	1,355	1,117	1,142	983	907	898	891
Coal workers' pneumoconiosis	982	958	533	389	270	266	209	183
Asbestosis	101	139	355	558	532	485	538	520
Silicosis	207	143	114	71	74	67	72	85
Other (including unspecified)	291	115	115	124	107	89	79	103

— =Data not available.

[1]For the period 1980–1998, underlying cause of death was coded according to the 9th Revision of the International Classification of Diseases (ICD).
[2]Starting with 1999 data, ICD-10 was introduced for coding cause of death. Discontinuities exist between 1998 and 1999 due to ICD-10 coding and classification changes.
[3]Prior to 1999, there was no discrete code for this condition.
[4]Prior to 1999, the combined ICD-9 categories of malignant neoplasm of peritoneum and malignant neoplasm of pleura served as a crude surrogate for malignant mesothelioma category under ICD-10.
[5]For multiple cause of death, counts for pneumoconiosis subgroups may sum to slightly more than total pneumoconiosis due to the reporting of more than one type of pneumoconiosis on some death certificates.

PART B: MORTALITY   175

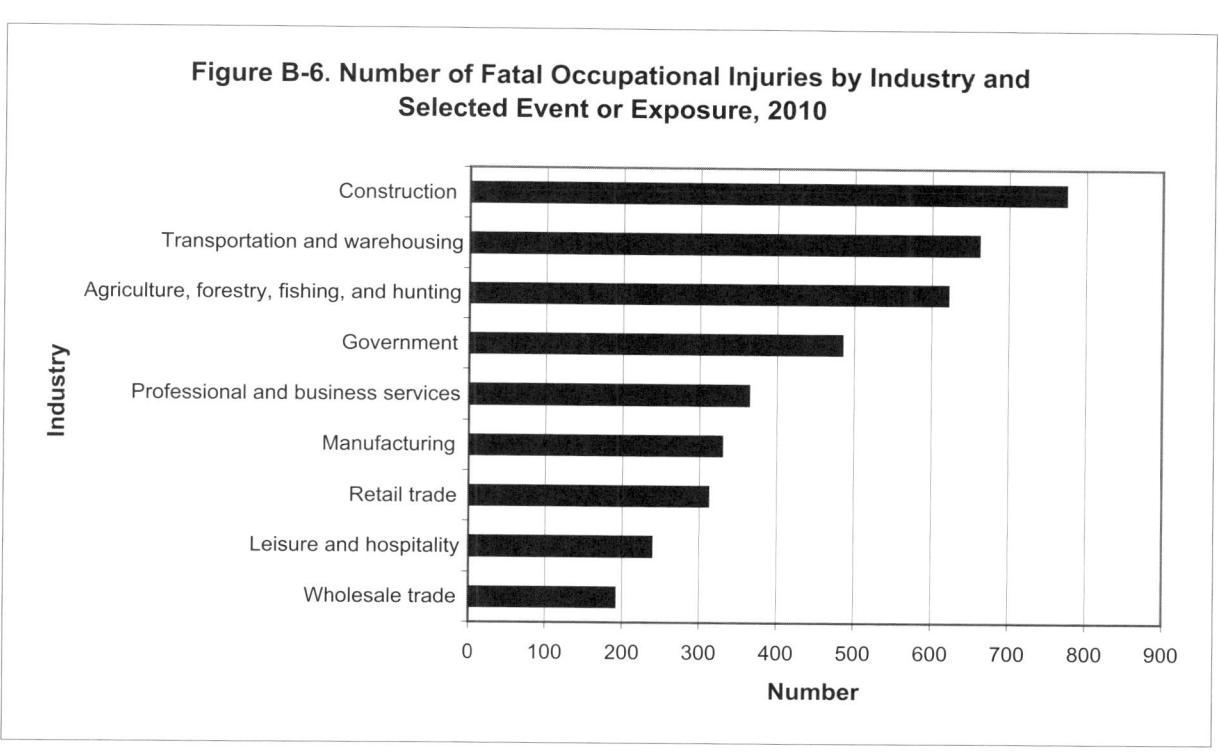

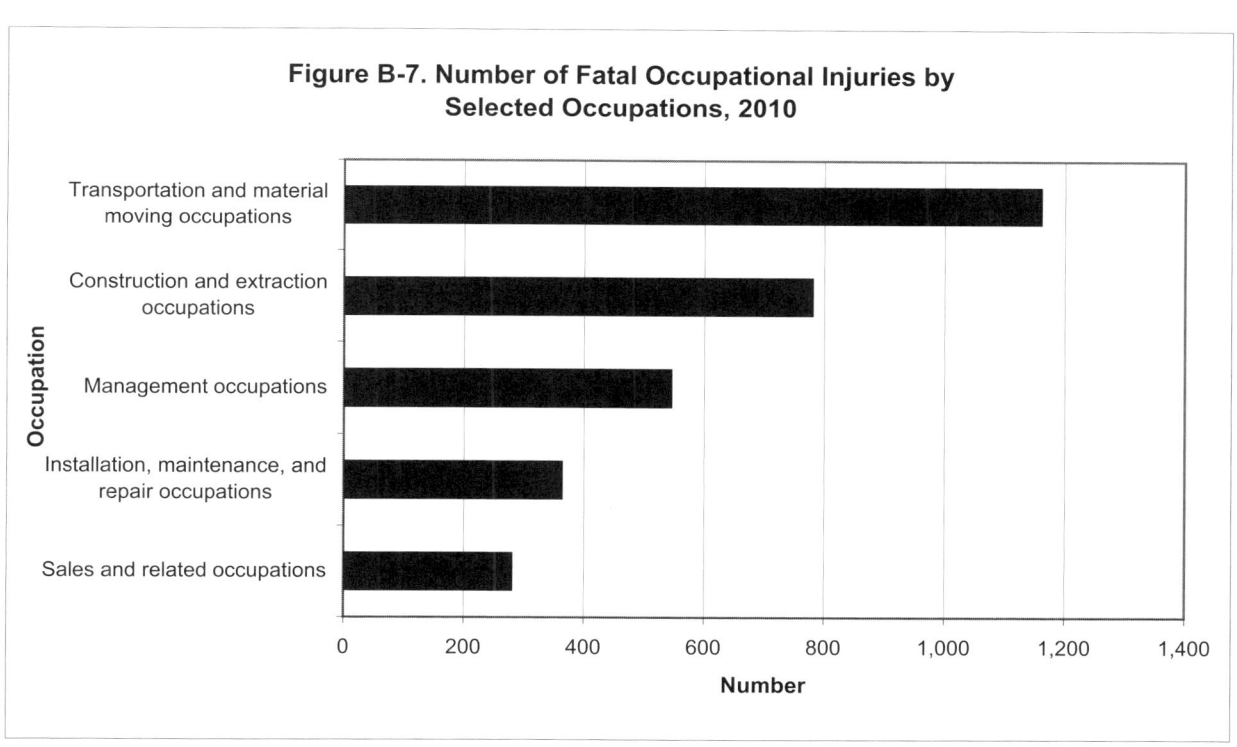

Table B-25. Fatal Occupational Injuries, Comparison of 2010 Preliminary and Final Figures, by Selected Characteristics

(Number, rate.)

Characteristic	Number			Rate[1]		
	Preliminary	Final	Difference	Preliminary	Final	Difference
Total	4,547	4,690	143	3.5	3.6	0.1
Employee status						
Wage and salary workers[2]	3,548	3,651	103	2.9	3	0.1
Self-employed[3]	999	1,039	40	12.1	12.6	0.5
Gender						
Men	4,192	4,322	130	5.7	5.8	0.1
Women	355	368	13	0.6	0.6	0.0
Age						
16 to 17 years	19	18	-1	3.1	3	-0.1
18 to 19 years	53	56	3	2.7	2.8	0.1
20 to 24 years	240	245	5	2.2	2.2	0.0
25 to 34 years	756	785	29	2.6	2.7	0.1
35 to 44 years	849	868	19	2.8	2.9	0.1
45 to 54 years	1,124	1,169	45	3.4	3.6	0.2
55 to 64 years	921	948	27	4.5	4.7	0.2
65 years and over	565	582	17	11.5	11.9	0.4
Race or Ethnic Origin[4]						
White, non-Hispanic	3,279	3,363	84	3.6	3.7	0.1
Black, non-Hispanic	384	412	28	2.8	3	0.2
Hispanic or Latino	682	707	25	3.7	3.9	0.2
Occupation[5]						
Management occupations	533	545	12	3.4	3.4	0.0
Protective service occupations	258	261	3	7.4	7.5	0.1
Sales and related occupations	274	280	6	1.9	2	0.1
Farming, fishing, and forestry occupations	260	276	16	25.3	27	1.7
Construction and extraction occupations	760	780	20	11.5	11.8	0.3
Installation, maintenance, and repair occupations	351	363	12	7	7.3	0.3
Transportation and material moving occupations	1,115	1,160	45	14.2	14.8	0.6
Military occupations	42	46	4	N/A	N/A	N/A
Industry[6]						
Private Industry	4,070	4,206	136	3.7	3.8	0.1
Goods-Producing	1,839	1,896	57	7.2	7.4	0.2
Agriculture, forestry, fishing, and hunting	596	621	25	26.8	27.9	1.1
Construction	751	774	23	9.5	9.8	0.3
Manufacturing	320	329	9	2.2	2.3	0.1
Service-Providing	2,231	2,310	79	2.6	2.7	0.1
Wholesale trade	185	191	6	4.8	4.9	0.1
Retail trade	301	311	10	2.2	2.2	0.0
Transportation and warehousing	631	661	30	13.1	13.7	0.6
Professional and business services	356	364	8	2.5	2.6	0.1
Leisure and hospitality	229	238	9	2.2	2.3	0.1
Government[7]	477	484	7	2.2	2.2	0.0
Event or exposure[8]						
Transportation accidents	1,766	1,857	91	—	—	—
Highway accidents[9]	968	1,044	76	—	—	—
Assaults and violent acts	808	832	24	—	—	—
Homicides	506	518	12	—	—	—
Contact with objects and equipment	732	738	6	—	—	—
Falls	635	646	11	—	—	—
Exposure to harmful substances or environments	409	414	5	—	—	—
Other events or exposures	197	203	6	—	—	—

— =Data not available.
[1]The rate represents the number of fatal occupational injuries per 100,000 full-time equivalent workers and was calculated as (N/EH) x 200,000,000 where N = the number of fatal work injuries EH = total hours worked by all employees during the calendar year. 200,000,000 = base for 100,000 equivalent full-time workers (working 40 hours per week, 50 weeks per year).
[2]May include volunteers and workers receiving other types of compensation.
[3]Includes self-employed workers, owners of unincorporated businesses and farms, paid and unpaid family workers, members of partnerships, and may include owners of incorporated businesses.
[4]Persons identified as Hispanic or Latino may be of any race. The race categories shown exclude Hispanic and Latino workers.
[5]Based on the 2000 Standard Occupational Classification system.
[6]Based on the North American Industry Classification System, 2007.
[7]Includes fatalities to workers employed by governmental organizations regardless of industry.
[8]Based on the Occupational Injury and Illness Classification System (OIICS).
[9]"Highway" includes deaths to vehicle occupants resulting from traffic incidents that occur on the public roadway.

Table B-26. Occupational Fatal Injuries and Rates, by Industry, Sex, Age, Race, and Hispanic Origin, Selected Years 1995–2009

(Rate.)

Characteristic	Deaths per 100,000 employed workers					Deaths per full-time equivalent workers	
	1995	2000	2005	2006	2007	2008	2009
Total workforce	4.9	4.3	4.0	4.0	3.8	3.7	3.5
Sex							
Male	8.3	7.4	6.9	6.9	6.6	6.1	5.7
Female	0.9	0.7	0.6	0.7	0.6	0.6	0.6
Age							
16–17 years	1.6	1.6	1.4	0.9	0.9	2.5	*
18–19 years	3.3	2.7	2.9	2.8	2.6	2.4	2.5
20–24 years	3.8	3.2	2.8	2.7	3.0	2.8	2.4
25–34 years	4.3	3.8	3.3	3.3	3.1	2.8	2.4
35–44 years	4.6	4.0	3.6	3.7	3.4	3.3	3.0
45–54 years	5.2	4.4	4.2	4.2	4.1	3.8	3.6
55–64 years	7.2	6.1	5.1	5.0	4.6	4.7	4.3
65 years and over	14.0	12.0	11.3	11.2	10.2	12.7	12.1
Race and Hispanic Origin							
Hispanic or Latino	5.5	5.6	4.9	5.0	4.6	4.2	4.0
Not Hispanic or Latino	—	—	—	—	—	—	—
White	—	4.2	3.9	4.0	3.8	3.8	3.5
Black or African American	—	3.8	3.9	3.7	3.9	3.7	3.1
Industry[1]							
Private sector	—	—	4.3	4.3	4.1	4.0	3.7
Agriculture, forestry, fishing, and hunting	—	—	32.5	30.0	27.9	30.4	27.2
Mining	—	—	25.6	28.1	25.1	18.1	12.4
Utilities	—	—	3.6	6.3	4.0	3.9	1.7
Construction	—	—	11.1	10.9	10.5	9.7	9.9
Manufacturing	—	—	2.4	2.8	2.5	2.5	2.3
Wholesale trade	—	—	4.6	4.9	4.7	4.4	5.0
Retail trade	—	—	2.4	2.2	2.1	2.0	2.2
Transportation and warehousing	—	—	17.7	16.8	16.9	14.9	13.3
Information	—	—	2.0	2.0	2.3	1.5	1.1
Finance and insurance	—	—	0.6	0.6	0.6	0.3	0.5
Real estate and rental and leasing	—	—	1.9	2.6	2.4	3.1	3.0
Professional, scientific, and technical services	—	—	1.0	0.9	0.9	0.8	1.0
Management of companies and enterprises	—	—	*	*	*	*	*
Administrative and support and waste management and remediation services	—	—	7.2	6.6	6.3	6.1	6.7
Educational services	—	—	1.3	1.3	0.9	0.9	0.7
Health care and social assistance	—	—	0.7	0.8	0.7	0.7	0.8
Arts, entertainment, and recreation	—	—	3.2	3.5	3.9	4.0	3.6
Accommodation and food services	—	—	1.5	2.0	1.7	1.8	1.9
Other services (except public administration)	—	—	3.0	2.6	2.5	2.6	2.8
Government[2]	—	—	2.4	2.4	2.5	2.4	1.9
Number of Deaths[3]							
Total workforce	6,275	5,920	5,734	5,840	5,657	5,214	4,551
Sex							
Male	5,736	5,471	5,328	5,396	5,228	4,827	4,216
Female	539	449	406	444	429	387	335
Age							
Under 16 years	26	29	23	11	18	11	13
16–17 years	42	44	31	21	20	23	14
18–19 years	130	127	111	106	97	66	57
20–24 years	486	446	403	390	424	353	275
25–34 years	1,409	1,163	1,017	1,041	991	850	704
35–44 years	1,571	1,473	1,243	1,288	1,168	1,113	908
45–54 years	1,256	1,313	1,389	1,417	1,425	1,292	1,173
55–64 years	827	831	933	963	934	920	853
65 years and over	515	488	578	599	574	580	551
Unspecified	13	6	6	4	6	6	3

Table B-26. Occupational Fatal Injuries and Rates, by Industry, Sex, Age, Race, and Hispanic Origin, Selected Years 1995–2009—Continued

(Rate.)

Characteristic	Deaths per 100,000 employed workers					Deaths per full-time equivalent workers	
	1995	2000	2005	2006	2007	2008	2009
Race and Hispanic Origin							
White	5,120	—	—	—	—	—	—
Black or African American	697	—	—	—	—	—	—
Hispanic or Latino	619	815	923	990	937	804	713
Not Hispanic or Latino	5,656	5,105	4,809	4,850	4,734	4,410	3,838
White	4,599	4,244	3,977	4,019	3,867	3,663	3,204
Black or African American	684	575	584	565	609	533	421
American Indian or Alaska Native	27	33	50	46	29	32	33
Asian[4]	188	171	154	148	166	145	141
Native Hawaiian or Other Pacific Islander	—	14	9	11	6	7	7
Multiple races	—	—	—	11	10	6	7
Other races or not reported	158	68	35	50	33	24	25
Industry							
Private sector	—	—	5,214	5,320	5,112	4,670	4,090
Agriculture, forestry, fishing, and hunting	—	—	715	655	585	672	575
Mining	—	—	159	192	183	176	99
Utilities	—	—	30	53	34	37	16
Construction	—	—	1,192	1,239	1,204	975	834
Manufacturing	—	—	393	456	400	411	319
Wholesale trade	—	—	209	222	207	180	190
Retail trade	—	—	400	359	348	301	307
Transportation and warehousing	—	—	885	860	890	796	633
Information	—	—	65	66	79	47	33
Finance and insurance	—	—	42	44	46	24	33
Real estate and rental and leasing	—	—	57	82	73	82	75
Professional, scientific, and technical services	—	—	83	78	77	69	85
Management of companies and enterprises	—	—	*	*	4	*	*
Administrative and support and waste management and remediation services	—	—	398	381	395	332	336
Educational services	—	—	46	49	34	28	27
Health care and social assistance	—	—	104	129	115	113	123
Arts, entertainment, and recreation	—	—	77	80	96	92	80
Accommodation and food services	—	—	136	185	164	146	151
Other services (except public administration)	—	—	210	183	175	178	173
Government[2]	—	—	520	520	545	544	461

— = Data not available.
* = Estimates are unreliable or data do not meet publication criteria.
[1]Starting with 2003 data, establishments were classified by industry according to the North American Industry Classification System (NAICS). Prior to 2003, the Standard Industrial Classification (SIC) system was used.
[2]Includes fatal work injuries to workers employed by governmental organizations, regardless of industry.
[3]Includes fatal work injuries to all workers, regardless of age.
[4]In 1999 and earlier years, category also included Native Hawaiian or Other Pacific Islander.

Table B-27. Number of Fatal Work Injuries by Most Frequent Type, 1992–2010

(Number.)

Year	Total	Highway incidents	Homicides	Falls	Struck by object
1992	6,217	1,158	1,044	600	557
1993	6,331	1,242	1,074	618	565
1994	6,632	1,343	1,080	665	591
1995	6,275	1,346	1,036	651	547
1996	6,202	1,346	927	691	582
1997	6,238	1,393	860	716	579
1998	6,055	1,442	714	706	520
1999	6,054	1,496	651	721	585
2000	5,920	1,365	677	734	571
2001	5,915	1,409	643	810	553
2002	5,534	1,373	609	719	505
2003	5,575	1,353	632	696	531
2004	5,764	1,398	559	822	602
2005	5,734	1,437	567	770	607
2006	5,840	1,356	540	827	589
2007	5,657	1,414	628	847	504
2008	5,214	1,215	526	700	520
2009	4,551	985	542	645	420
2010	4,690	1,044	518	646	404

Table B-28. Number and Rate of Fatal Occupational Injuries, by Industry Sector and Occupation, 2010

(Number, percent.)

Industry and Occupation	Number	Rate
Industry		
Construction	774	9.8
Transportation and warehousing	661	13.7
Agriculture, forestry, fishing and hunting	621	27.9
Government	484	2.2
Professional and business services	364	2.6
Manufacturing	329	2.3
Retail trade	311	2.2
Leisure and hospitality	238	2.3
Other services (exc. public administration)	192	3.0
Wholesale trade	191	4.9
Mining	172	19.8
Educational and health services	171	0.9
Financial activities	113	1.3
Information	43	1.5
Utilities	26	2.8
Occupation		
Fishers and related fishing workers	38	152.0
Logging workers	60	93.5
Aircraft pilots and flight engineers	78	70.6
Farmers and ranchers	308	42.5
Mining machine operators	22	37.0
Roofers	57	32.4
Refuse and recyclable material collectors	26	29.8
Driver/sales workers and truck drivers	718	23.0
Industrial machinery installation, repair, and maintenance workers	98	20.7
Police and sheriff's patrol officers	134	18.1

Table B-29. Number of Fatal Work Injuries, by State, 2010

(Number.)

State	2009	2010	Net change
Alabama	75	92	17
Alaska	17	39	22
Arizona	76	77	1
Arkansas	75	88	13
California	409	326	-83
Colorado	83	85	2
Connecticut	34	49	15
Delaware	7	8	1
District of Columbia	11	16	5
Florida	245	225	-20
Georgia	110	108	-2
Hawaii	13	19	6
Idaho	27	33	6
Illinois	158	206	48
Indiana	125	118	-7
Iowa	80	77	-3
Kansas	76	85	9
Kentucky	101	69	-32
Louisiana	140	111	-29
Maine	16	20	4
Maryland	65	71	6
Massachusetts	64	54	-10
Michigan	94	146	52
Minnesota	61	70	9
Mississippi	67	68	1
Missouri	142	106	-36
Montana	52	36	-16
Nebraska	57	54	-3
Nevada	24	38	14
New Hampshire	6	6	0
New Jersey	99	81	-18
New Mexico	42	38	-4
New York State	185	182	-3
North Carolina	129	139	10
North Dakota	25	30	5
Ohio	137	161	24
Oklahoma	82	94	12
Oregon	66	47	-19
Pennsylvania	168	221	53
Rhode Island	7	9	2
South Carolina	73	69	-4
South Dakota	24	36	12
Tennessee	111	138	27
Texas	482	461	-21
Utah	48	41	-7
Vermont	12	12	0
Virginia	119	107	-12
Washington	76	104	28
West Virginia	41	95	54
Wisconsin	94	91	-3
Wyoming	19	33	14

Table B-30. Years of Potential Life Lost Before Age 75 for Selected Causes of Death, by Sex, Race, and Hispanic Origin, Selected Years, 1980–2007

(Years lost before 75 per 100,000 population.)

Sex, race, Hispanic origin, and cause of death[2]	Crude	Age-adjusted[1]					
	2007[3]	1980	1990	2000[3]	2005[3]	2006[3]	2007[3]
ALL PERSONS							
All Causes	7,366.2	10,448.4	9,085.5	7,578.1	7,299.8	7,214.3	7,083.5
Diseases of heart	1,112.6	2,238.7	1,617.7	1,253.0	1,110.4	1,077.8	1,042.4
Ischemic heart disease	694.0	1,729.3	1,153.6	841.8	701.8	675.5	642.1
Cerebrovascular diseases	195.4	357.5	259.6	223.3	193.3	190.2	184.5
Malignant neoplasms	1,574.0	2,108.8	2,003.8	1,674.1	1,525.2	1,490.5	1,461.4
Trachea, bronchus, and lung	402.9	548.5	561.4	443.1	392.9	378.7	366.8
Colorectal	136.8	190.0	164.7	141.9	124.7	126.1	126.7
Prostate[4]	55.4	84.9	96.8	63.6	55.1	54.8	53.5
Breast[5]	300.0	463.2	451.6	332.6	296.2	286.7	275.4
Chronic lower respiratory diseases	185.5	169.1	187.4	188.1	181.2	171.0	172.1
Influenza and pneumonia	74.5	160.2	141.5	87.1	83.6	76.4	71.6
Chronic liver disease and cirrhosis	167.0	300.3	196.9	164.1	152.6	149.9	157.6
Diabetes mellitus	181.9	134.4	155.9	178.4	179.9	176.5	170.1
Human immunodeficiency virus (HIV) disease	113.7	—	383.8	174.6	133.6	126.0	115.2
Unintentional injuries	1,155.5	1,543.5	1,162.1	1,026.5	1,132.7	1,167.5	1,159.5
Motor vehicle-related injuries	536.4	912.9	716.4	574.3	564.4	561.2	538.4
Poisoning	351.2	68.0	81.2	163.6	287.3	332.5	354.3
Suicide[6]	357.2	392.0	393.1	334.5	347.3	348.7	357.5
Homicide[6]	276.0	425.5	417.4	266.5	276.8	281.8	278.3
MALE							
All Causes	9,171.1	13,777.2	11,973.5	9,572.2	9,206.1	9,092.6	8,919.9
Diseases of heart	1,528.7	3,352.1	2,356.0	1,766.0	1,561.6	1,517.5	1,468.2
Ischemic heart disease	1,008.8	2,715.1	1,766.3	1,255.4	1,044.3	1,009.2	962.1
Cerebrovascular diseases	213.1	396.7	286.6	244.6	213.7	212.0	206.2
Malignant neoplasms	1,642.2	2,360.8	2,214.6	1,810.8	1,639.7	1,595.2	1,565.1
Trachea, bronchus, and lung	459.1	821.1	764.8	554.9	476.3	454.5	434.0
Colorectal	155.7	214.9	194.3	167.3	146.2	145.4	148.5
Prostate	55.4	84.9	96.8	63.6	55.1	54.8	53.5
Chronic lower respiratory diseases	194.0	235.1	224.8	206.0	195.8	182.4	187.5
Influenza and pneumonia	85.6	202.5	180.0	102.8	97.8	88.9	83.5
Chronic liver disease and cirrhosis	231.9	415.0	283.9	236.9	216.1	210.9	222.4
Diabetes mellitus	215.3	140.4	170.4	203.8	216.5	213.2	207.1
Human immunodeficiency virus (HIV) disease	158.5	—	686.2	258.9	192	178	161
Unintentional injuries	1,648.6	2342.7	1,715.1	1,475.4	1,608.5	1,659.2	1,639.2
Motor vehicle-related injuries	774.0	1,359.7	1,018.4	796.4	795.9	790.9	766.5
Poisoning	479.2	96.4	123.6	242.1	395.6	461.6	480.7
Suicide[6]	564.1	605.6	634.8	539.1	548.0	549.0	561.5
Homicide[6]	444.2	675.0	658.0	410.5	439.0	447.1	439.4
FEMALE							
All Causes	5,560.6	7,350.3	6,333.1	5,644.6	5,425.7	5,364.7	5,274.2
Diseases of heart	696.4	1,246.0	948.5	774.6	682.6	660.6	637.9
Ischemic heart disease	379.2	852.1	600.3	457.6	379.0	360.6	339.7
Cerebrovascular diseases	177.7	324.0	235.9	203.9	174.4	169.8	164.3
Malignant neoplasms	1,505.7	1,896.8	1,826.6	1,555.3	1,424.3	1,398.6	1,370.3
Trachea, bronchus, and lung	346.8	310.4	382.2	342.1	316.9	309.7	305.6
Colorectal	117.9	168.7	138.7	118.7	104.9	108.4	106.6
Breast	300.0	463.2	451.6	332.6	296.2	286.7	275.4
Chronic lower respiratory diseases	177.0	114.0	155.9	172.3	168.2	160.5	158.0
Influenza and pneumonia	63.4	122.0	106.2	72.3	70.0	64.7	60.3
Chronic liver disease and cirrhosis	102.1	194.5	115.1	94.5	91.6	91.3	95.3
Diabetes mellitus	148.4	128.5	142.3	154.4	145.1	141.7	135.0
Human immunodeficiency virus (HIV) disease	68.8	—	87.8	92.0	76.2	74.5	70.1
Unintentional injuries	662.1	755.3	607.4	573.2	648.0	666.1	670.2
Motor vehicle-related injuries	298.8	470.4	411.6	348.5	327.1	325.4	304.5
Poisoning	223.1	40.2	39.1	85.0	177.2	201.0	225.3
Suicide[6]	150.4	184.2	153.3	129.1	144.1	145.7	150.8
Homicide[6]	107.7	181.3	174.3	118.9	108.7	110.4	111.2

Table B-30. Years of Potential Life Lost Before Age 75 for Selected Causes of Death, by Sex, Race, and Hispanic Origin, Selected Years, 1980–2007—Continued

(Years lost before 75 per 100,000 population.)

Sex, race, Hispanic origin, and cause of death[2]	Crude 2007[3]	Age-adjusted[1]					
		1980	1990	2000[3]	2005[3]	2006[3]	2007[3]
WHITE							
All Causes	6,985.7	9,554.1	8,159.5	6,949.5	6,775.6	6,713.1	6,614.2
Diseases of heart	1,052.9	2,100.8	1,490.3	1,149.4	1,011.7	985.9	952.2
Ischemic heart disease	693.0	1,682.7	1,113.4	805.3	672.0	648.2	617.1
Cerebrovascular diseases	168.4	300.7	213.1	187.1	160.4	158.1	154.0
Malignant neoplasms	1,593.8	2,035.9	1,929.3	1,627.8	1,485.9	1,456.6	1,428.3
Trachea, bronchus, and lung	419.1	529.9	544.2	436.3	389.4	374.8	364.8
Colorectal	133.9	186.8	157.8	134.1	117.3	118.9	119.6
Prostate[4]	50.6	74.8	86.6	54.3	47.0	47.3	46.2
Breast[5]	289.1	460.2	441.7	315.6	275.1	269.0	256.9
Chronic lower respiratory diseases	197.2	165.4	182.3	185.3	182.2	172.0	174.0
Influenza and pneumonia	69.2	130.8	116.9	77.7	76.3	70.4	65.2
Chronic liver disease and cirrhosis	177.9	257.3	175.8	162.7	156.7	155.3	163.6
Diabetes mellitus	163.7	115.7	133.7	155.6	156.3	152.8	147.7
Human immunodeficiency virus (HIV) disease	57.5	—	309.0	94.7	69.8	64.6	58.1
Unintentional injuries	1,193.3	1,520.4	1,139.7	1,031.8	1,170.9	1,209.8	1,208.5
Motor vehicle-related injuries	548.5	939.9	726.7	586.1	585.7	580.5	557.5
Poisoning	385.7	64.9	74.4	167.2	310.6	360.6	391.9
Suicide[6]	392.6	414.5	417.7	362.0	381.2	383.5	393.8
Homicide[6]	158.2	271.7	234.9	156.6	159.7	160.1	162.4
BLACK OR AFRICAN AMERICAN							
All Causes	11,005.6	17,873.4	16,593.0	12,897.1	11,890.7	11,646.3	11,259.8
Diseases of heart	1,728.1	3,619.9	2,891.8	2,275.2	2,046.0	1,969.3	1,906.3
Ischemic heart disease	864.8	2,305.1	1,676.1	1,300.1	1,080.2	1,034.5	972.4
Cerebrovascular diseases	375.0	883.2	656.4	507.0	441.7	431.8	416.5
Malignant neoplasms	1,768.4	2,946.1	2,894.8	2,294.7	2,069.7	2,003.1	1,966.9
Trachea, bronchus, and lung	415.8	776.0	811.3	593.0	511.8	496.4	470.9
Colorectal	178.4	232.3	241.8	222.4	199.6	198.9	199.5
Prostate[4]	103.3	200.3	223.5	171.0	144.8	140.0	138.8
Breast[5]	422.8	524.2	592.9	500.0	485.7	450.1	445.3
Chronic lower respiratory diseases	175.8	203.7	240.6	232.7	211.0	197.6	192.7
Influenza and pneumonia	117.4	384.9	330.8	161.2	145.3	127.6	123.7
Chronic liver disease and cirrhosis	119.9	644.0	371.8	185.6	138.4	127.0	130.4
Diabetes mellitus	321.7	305.3	361.5	383.4	379.9	375.4	358.6
Human immunodeficiency virus (HIV) disease	483.2	—	1,014.7	763.3	594.4	566.8	522.1
Unintentional injuries	1,139.3	1,751.5	1,392.7	1,152.8	1,134.6	1,170.7	1,116.5
Motor vehicle-related injuries	539.4	750.2	699.5	580.8	532.3	541.6	521.4
Poisoning	250.7	99.4	144.3	196.6	253.8	296.1	263.5
Suicide[6]	190.0	238.0	261.4	208.7	194.0	187.3	187.3
Homicide[6]	1,031.8	1,580.8	1,612.9	941.6	967.8	998.6	967.7
AMERICAN INDIAN OR ALASKAN NATIVE							
All Causes	8,164.2	13,390.9	9,506.2	7,758.2	8,624.4	8,517.6	8,463.6
Diseases of heart	885.5	1,819.9	1,391.0	1,030.1	1,010.2	1,008.6	985.4
Ischemic heart disease	514.5	1,208.2	901.8	709.3	625.2	614.2	587.1
Cerebrovascular diseases	148.7	269.3	223.3	198.1	209.4	178.2	170.0
Malignant neoplasms	881.4	1,101.3	1,141.1	995.7	1,084.3	983.9	991.1
Trachea, bronchus, and lung	190.1	181.1	268.1	227.8	268.2	225.3	226.3
Colorectal	89.2	78.8	82.4	93.8	109.7	88.1	100.5
Prostate[4]	26.6	66.7	42.0	44.5	37.6	38.8	33.5
Breast[5]	153.8	205.5	213.4	174.1	149.2	172.9	163.8
Chronic lower respiratory diseases	147.3	89.3	129.0	151.8	155.3	144.6	171.4
Influenza and pneumonia	103.3	307.9	206.3	124.0	113.6	101.6	110.9
Chronic liver disease and cirrhosis	529.3	1,190.3	535.1	519.4	498.9	479.2	576.3
Diabetes mellitus	253.0	305.5	292.3	305.6	347.3	324.8	292.6
Human immunodeficiency virus (HIV) disease	72.0	—	70.1	68.4	89.9	76.1	79.7
Unintentional injuries	1,955.0	3,541.0	2,183.9	1,700.1	1,875.6	1,885.1	1,870.6
Motor vehicle-related injuries	1,009.1	2,102.4	1,301.5	1,032.2	1,004.9	1,021.7	930.5
Poisoning	421.9	92.9	119.5	180.1	333.8	358.5	416.7
Suicide[6]	514.3	515.0	495.9	403.1	498.6	487.8	470.6
Homicide[6]	305.3	628.9	434.2	278.5	337.5	328.3	283.3

Table B-30. Years of Potential Life Lost Before Age 75 for Selected Causes of Death, by Sex, Race, and Hispanic Origin, Selected Years, 1980–2007—Continued

(Years lost before 75 per 100,000 population.)

Sex, race, Hispanic origin, and cause of death[2]	Crude 2007[3]	Age-adjusted[1]					
		1980	1990	2000[3]	2005[3]	2006[3]	2007[3]
ASIAN OR PACIFIC ISLANDER							
All Causes	3,388.3	5,378.4	4,705.2	3,811.1	3,533.2	3,450.6	3,404.9
Diseases of heart	445.5	952.8	702.2	567.9	513.8	471.8	454.5
Ischemic heart disease	286.7	697.7	486.6	381.1	326.5	305.7	295.4
Cerebrovascular diseases	149.5	266.9	233.5	199.4	162.8	163.9	153.5
Malignant neoplasms	882.2	1,218.6	1,166.4	1,033.8	945.3	912.7	895.8
Trachea, bronchus, and lung	156.5	238.2	204.7	185.8	169.2	171.3	162.5
Colorectal	81.1	115.9	105.1	91.6	78.7	81.2	82.1
Prostate[4]	13.4	17.0	32.4	18.8	20.4	18.3	16.6
Breast[5]	163.3	222.2	216.5	200.8	178.4	173.3	156.3
Chronic lower respiratory diseases	34.0	56.4	72.8	56.5	36.0	37.4	35.9
Influenza and pneumonia	35.4	79.3	74.0	48.6	40.3	36.8	37.1
Chronic liver disease and cirrhosis	41.8	85.6	72.4	44.8	43.6	44.3	41.3
Diabetes mellitus	77.0	83.1	74.0	77.0	78.1	80.8	79.5
Human immunodeficiency virus (HIV) disease	16.1	—	77.0	19.9	16.6	15.4	15.0
Unintentional injuries	418.2	742.7	636.6	425.7	413.7	411.0	417.4
Motor vehicle-related injuries	231.0	472.6	445.5	263.4	242.1	243.9	231.8
Poisoning	55.8	*	17.6	25.9	42.0	46.6	52.8
Suicide[6]	212.6	217.1	200.6	168.6	164.6	185.1	205.0
Homicide[6]	100.0	201.1	205.8	113.1	130.8	121.7	97.3
HISPANIC OR LATINO[7,8]							
All Causes	5,118.6	—	7,963.3	6,037.6	5,757.9	5,601.9	5,447.4
Diseases of heart	487.2	—	1,082.0	821.3	727.0	686.8	666.9
Ischemic heart disease	280.7	—	756.6	564.6	483.2	446.2	418.0
Cerebrovascular diseases	131.4	—	238.0	207.8	184.9	184.5	176.0
Malignant neoplasms	742.3	—	1,232.2	1,098.2	1,017.5	987.7	991.2
Trachea, bronchus, and lung	80.9	—	193.7	152.1	138.1	125.0	126.0
Colorectal	65.2	—	100.2	101.4	86.4	91.5	92.7
Prostate[4]	22.6	—	47.7	42.9	41.7	43.8	43.5
Breast[5]	150.7	—	299.3	230.7	197.3	203.2	194.7
Chronic lower respiratory diseases	40.9	—	78.8	68.5	62.2	56.9	56.5
Influenza and pneumonia	47.1	—	130.1	76.0	69.5	65.1	55.1
Chronic liver disease and cirrhosis	157.3	—	329.1	252.1	210.3	201.4	210.3
Diabetes mellitus	122.3	—	177.8	215.6	202.2	181.1	178.6
Human immunodeficiency virus (HIV) disease	100.6	—	600.1	209.4	139.3	129.0	115.6
Unintentional injuries	977.1	—	1,190.6	920.1	980.1	993.0	929.0
Motor vehicle-related injuries	551.1	—	740.8	540.2	569.2	564.7	509.1
Poisoning	196.7	—	121.9	145.9	179.5	195.6	202.1
Suicide[6]	205.4	—	256.2	188.5	193.2	185.1	200.3
Homicide[6]	362.2	—	720.8	335.1	343.0	335.3	322.6
WHITE, NOT HISPANIC OR LATINO[8]							
All Causes	7,341.4	—	8,022.5	6,960.5	6,853.3	6,813.8	6,736.5
Diseases of heart	1,171.7	—	1,504.0	1,175.1	1,046.4	1,024.0	989.1
Ischemic heart disease	780.2	—	1,127.2	824.7	694.4	673.5	643.5
Cerebrovascular diseases	174.9	—	210.1	183.0	155.5	152.5	149.3
Malignant neoplasms	1,774.1	—	1,974.1	1,668.4	1,534.3	1,505.9	1,474.4
Trachea, bronchus, and lung	493.3	—	566.8	460.3	416.3	402.4	392.3
Colorectal	148.5	—	162.1	136.2	120.8	121.8	122.9
Prostate[4]	56.8	—	89.2	54.9	47.3	47.6	46.3
Breast[5]	316.8	—	451.5	322.3	283.6	275.5	263.1
Chronic lower respiratory diseases	231.3	—	188.1	193.8	194.0	183.4	186.5
Influenza and pneumonia	73.6	—	112.3	76.4	76.8	70.4	66.6
Chronic liver disease and cirrhosis	180.1	—	162.4	150.9	147.8	147.4	155.5
Diabetes mellitus	171.4	—	131.2	150.2	151.5	150.1	144.5
Human immunodeficiency virus (HIV) disease	46.6	—	271.2	76.0	56.6	51.5	45.8
Unintentional injuries	1,228.8	—	1,114.7	1,041.4	1,199.6	1,246.6	1,263.4
Motor vehicle-related injuries	541.1	—	715.7	588.8	579.9	575.4	561.1
Poisoning	424.8	—	68.3	169.4	338.2	397.9	435.8
Suicide[6]	431.7	—	433.0	389.2	416.6	422.7	433.8
Homicide[6]	109.0	—	162.0	113.2	109.1	109.9	115.4

— = Data not available.
* = Figure does not meet standards of reliability or precision.
[1] Age-adjusted rates are calculated using the year 2000 standard population.
[2] Underlying cause of death code numbers are based on the applicable revision of the International Classification of Diseases (ICD) for data years shown. For the period 1980–1998, causes were coded using ICD-9 codes that are most nearly comparable with the 113 cause list for ICD-10.
[3] Starting with 1999 data, cause of death is coded according to ICD-10.
[4] Rate for male population only.
[5] Rate for female population only.
[6] Figures for 2001 include September 11th related deaths for which death certificates were filed as of October 24, 2002.
[7] Persons of Hispanic origin may be of any race.
[8] Prior to 1997, excludes data from states lacking an Hispanic origin item on the death certificate.

Table B-31. Number of Deaths, Death Rates, and Age–Adjusted Death Rates for Major Causes of Death, by State and Territory, 2008

(Number, rates per 100,000 population, age–adjusted rates per 100,000 U.S. standard population.)

Area	All causes			Human immunodeficiency virus (HIV) disease (B20–B24)			Malignant neoplasms (C00-C97)			Diabetes mellitus (E10-E14)		
	Number	Rate	Age-adjusted rate[1]	Number	Rate	Age-adjusted rate[1]	Number	Rate	Age-adjusted rate[1]	Number	Rate	Age-adjusted rate[1]
UNITED STATES[2]	2,471,984	813.0	758.3	10,285	3.4	3.3	565,469	186.0	175.3	70,553	23.2	21.8
Alabama	47,707	1,023.3	930.2	181	3.9	3.9	10,182	218.4	195.6	1,386	29.7	26.7
Alaska	3,494	509.1	742.0	14	*	*	867	126.3	180.0	93	13.6	21.8
Arizona	45,823	704.9	653.7	112	1.7	1.8	10,081	155.1	145.3	1,173	18.0	16.9
Arkansas	29,322	1,026.9	899.6	69	2.4	2.5	6,526	228.6	200.1	901	31.6	27.7
California	234,766	638.7	660.3	949	2.6	2.6	54,686	148.8	156.8	7,375	20.1	21.1
Colorado	31,274	633.1	709.0	57	1.2	1.1	6,719	136.0	150.8	767	15.5	17.6
Connecticut	28,794	822.4	691.4	115	3.3	3.0	6,830	195.1	169.7	624	17.8	15.2
Delaware	7,622	873.0	780.8	57	6.5	6.2	1,912	219.0	194.0	217	24.9	22.2
District of Columbia	5,140	868.5	850.0	164	27.7	27.0	1,143	193.1	192.1	156	26.4	26.0
Florida	170,703	931.4	679.1	1,417	7.7	7.6	40,814	222.7	166.2	5,161	28.2	20.8
Georgia	69,640	719.0	831.9	508	5.2	5.2	14,621	151.0	171.4	1,496	15.4	17.6
Hawaii	9,501	737.5	590.6	19	*	*	2,194	170.3	140.7	286	22.2	18.1
Idaho	10,962	719.4	723.0	6	*	*	2,511	164.8	166.0	356	23.4	23.6
Illinois	103,471	802.0	770.9	333	2.6	2.5	24,300	188.3	184.4	2,846	22.1	21.5
Indiana	56,752	890.0	835.3	121	1.9	1.9	13,137	206.0	194.8	1,683	26.4	24.8
Iowa	28,541	950.6	744.2	14	*	*	6,424	214.0	177.7	764	25.4	20.2
Kansas	24,975	891.3	784.9	30	1.1	1.1	5,294	188.9	173.2	706	25.2	22.7
Kentucky	41,329	968.1	902.4	84	2.0	1.9	9,589	224.6	205.9	1,214	28.4	26.2
Louisiana	41,220	934.5	922.1	326	7.4	7.6	9,197	208.5	204.3	1,332	30.2	29.7
Maine	12,541	952.6	764.8	12	*	*	3,093	234.9	187.8	344	26.1	21.1
Maryland	43,892	779.1	771.7	435	7.7	7.3	10,360	183.9	180.8	1,239	22.0	21.7
Massachusetts	53,518	823.6	705.9	144	2.2	2.0	13,031	200.5	178.3	1,079	16.6	14.5
Michigan	88,445	884.1	811.9	194	1.9	1.9	20,211	202.0	185.9	2,752	27.5	25.4
Minnesota	38,499	737.5	675.4	39	0.7	0.7	9,446	180.9	172.0	1,087	20.8	19.2
Mississippi	28,984	986.3	950.1	152	5.2	5.4	6,166	209.8	201.8	758	25.8	24.7
Missouri	56,578	957.1	847.1	116	2.0	2.0	12,523	211.8	190.0	1,348	22.8	20.3
Montana	8,913	921.3	786.9	9	*	*	1,862	192.5	163.2	254	26.3	22.5
Nebraska	15,461	866.9	741.4	18	*	*	3,376	189.3	170.0	470	26.4	23.1
Nevada	19,335	743.6	808.6	80	3.1	3.0	4,404	169.4	179.0	373	14.3	15.4
New Hampshire	10,268	780.4	712.5	5	*	*	2,576	195.8	177.9	297	22.6	20.6
New Jersey	70,026	806.5	717.2	448	5.2	4.7	16,876	194.4	176.0	2,242	25.8	23.2
New Mexico	16,005	806.6	758.6	49	2.5	2.6	3,355	169.1	158.6	582	29.3	27.5
New York	148,698	762.9	676.0	1,255	6.4	6.0	35,351	181.4	163.8	3,605	18.5	16.6
North Carolina	77,283	838.0	825.6	356	3.9	3.7	17,453	189.2	183.8	2,170	23.5	22.9
North Dakota	5,871	915.2	713.2	3	*	*	1,354	211.1	174.6	201	31.3	25.3
Ohio	109,767	955.7	844.1	192	1.7	1.7	24,998	217.6	193.7	3,565	31.0	27.4
Oklahoma	37,014	1,016.2	931.0	82	2.3	2.4	7,657	210.2	192.6	1,103	30.3	28.0
Oregon	31,967	843.4	748.6	39	1.0	1.0	7,479	197.3	177.2	1,025	27.0	23.9
Pennsylvania	127,462	1,023.9	796.5	315	2.5	2.3	28,964	232.7	186.3	3,313	26.6	20.9
Rhode Island	9,738	926.7	749.4	26	2.5	2.2	2,227	211.9	180.6	195	18.6	15.3
South Carolina	40,289	899.3	839.5	229	5.1	5.0	9,199	205.3	187.9	1,133	25.3	23.4
South Dakota	7,083	880.8	708.8	5	*	*	1,570	195.2	165.4	216	26.9	21.7
Tennessee	58,820	946.4	888.8	271	4.4	4.3	13,162	211.8	195.4	1,733	27.9	25.9
Texas	164,914	677.9	776.0	860	3.5	3.7	35,713	146.8	168.1	5,155	21.2	24.5
Utah	14,040	513.1	659.1	21	0.8	0.9	2,492	91.1	119.4	468	17.1	22.5
Vermont	5,211	838.8	721.9	4	*	*	1,279	205.9	176.8	151	24.3	21.1
Virginia	59,100	760.7	762.7	184	2.4	2.3	13,983	180.0	177.8	1,534	19.7	19.6
Washington	48,627	742.5	723.7	89	1.4	1.3	11,618	177.4	173.9	1,590	24.3	23.9
West Virginia	21,557	1,188.1	958.5	30	1.7	1.7	4,605	253.8	201.6	753	41.5	32.8
Wisconsin	46,815	831.8	729.9	45	0.8	0.8	11,185	198.7	178.8	1,152	20.5	18.2
Wyoming	4,227	793.6	773.4	2	*	*	874	164.1	158.3	130	24.4	24.2
Puerto Rico[3]	29,050	734.7	707.2	421	10.6	10.9	5,044	127.6	119.8	2,842	71.9	67.5
Virgin Islands[3]	749	681.9	729.0	11	*	*	124	112.9	112.5	47	42.8	45.4
Guam[3]	783	444.9	699.7	2	*	*	134	76.1	122.2	47	26.7	46.8
American Samoa[3]	241	371.8	958.9	-	*	*	40	61.7	158.2	33	50.9	134.8
Northern Marianas[3]	178	322.2	877.5	-	*	*	25	45.3	110.3	23	41.6	140.9

Table B-31. Number of Deaths, Death Rates, and Age–Adjusted Death Rates for Major Causes of Death, by State and Territory, 2008—Continued

(Number, rates per 100,000 population, age–adjusted rates per 100,000 U.S. standard population.)

Area	Parkinson's disease (G20–G21)			Alzheimer's disease (G30)			Disease of the heart (I00–I09, I11, I13, I20–I51)			Essential hypertension and hypertensive renal disease (I10, I12, I15)		
	Number	Rate	Age-adjusted rate[1]	Number	Rate	Age-adjusted rate[1]	Number	Rate	Age-adjusted rate[1]	Number	Rate	Age-adjusted rate[1]
UNITED STATES[2]	20,483	6.7	6.4	82,435	27.1	24.4	616,828	202.9	186.5	25,742	8.5	7.7
Alabama	348	7.5	6.8	1,518	32.6	29.3	12,074	259.0	233.1	501	10.7	9.7
Alaska	19	*	*	80	11.7	24.9	634	92.4	145.4	16	*	*
Arizona	488	7.5	6.9	2,099	32.3	28.3	10,385	159.8	145.6	475	7.3	6.6
Arkansas	167	5.8	5.2	893	31.3	26.1	7,516	263.2	226.2	256	9.0	7.6
California	2,026	5.5	5.9	10,098	27.5	27.9	60,709	165.2	170.2	3,423	9.3	9.6
Colorado	314	6.4	7.8	1,353	27.4	32.7	6,118	123.9	141.0	241	4.9	5.6
Connecticut	256	7.3	6.1	839	24.0	18.4	7,355	210.1	170.9	319	9.1	7.3
Delaware	50	5.7	5.2	204	23.4	20.5	1,777	203.5	179.4	51	5.8	5.1
District of Columbia	26	4.4	4.3	132	22.3	20.3	1,389	234.7	229.2	66	11.2	11.0
Florida	1,577	8.6	5.7	4,743	25.9	15.9	42,067	229.5	157.0	1,841	10.0	6.9
Georgia	427	4.4	5.7	1,929	19.9	25.6	15,721	162.3	190.5	945	9.8	11.3
Hawaii	79	6.1	4.8	218	16.9	11.8	2,313	179.6	141.0	101	7.8	5.9
Idaho	111	7.3	7.7	393	25.8	26.1	2,330	152.9	153.0	92	6.0	6.1
Illinois	886	6.9	6.7	3,192	24.7	22.8	26,078	202.1	191.9	930	7.2	6.7
Indiana	504	7.9	7.6	1,971	30.9	28.3	13,663	214.3	198.5	484	7.6	6.9
Iowa	305	10.2	7.6	1,332	44.4	30.4	7,284	242.6	182.2	268	8.9	6.4
Kansas	210	7.5	6.6	961	34.3	27.9	5,643	201.4	172.4	173	6.2	5.1
Kentucky	296	6.9	6.6	1,370	32.1	30.2	10,061	235.7	217.8	338	7.9	7.3
Louisiana	254	5.8	5.9	1,361	30.9	31.0	10,347	234.6	230.4	372	8.4	8.3
Maine	114	8.7	6.9	450	34.2	26.2	2,785	211.6	165.3	67	5.1	3.9
Maryland	351	6.2	6.5	1,016	18.0	18.2	11,157	198.0	195.5	441	7.8	7.7
Massachusetts	423	6.5	5.6	1,832	28.2	22.3	12,776	196.6	163.8	452	7.0	5.8
Michigan	766	7.7	7.2	2,739	27.4	24.7	24,344	243.4	220.3	899	9.0	8.1
Minnesota	466	8.9	8.4	1,344	25.7	22.2	7,367	141.1	126.6	509	9.8	8.6
Mississippi	152	5.2	5.1	916	31.2	29.8	7,997	272.1	260.2	459	15.6	15.0
Missouri	484	8.2	7.3	2,010	34.0	28.4	14,644	247.7	214.4	504	8.5	7.2
Montana	84	8.7	7.4	294	30.4	24.9	1,975	204.1	169.8	48	5.0	4.0
Nebraska	167	9.4	7.9	610	34.2	26.1	3,459	194.0	159.5	179	10.0	8.1
Nevada	119	4.6	5.5	279	10.7	13.2	4,646	178.7	195.7	129	5.0	5.8
New Hampshire	74	5.6	5.3	393	29.9	27.0	2,409	183.1	164.8	77	5.9	5.3
New Jersey	588	6.8	6.1	1,857	21.4	18.0	19,056	219.5	190.6	641	7.4	6.4
New Mexico	161	8.1	7.6	366	18.4	16.8	3,275	165.0	151.9	131	6.6	6.2
New York	929	4.8	4.2	2,303	11.8	9.9	49,324	253.1	218.9	1,850	9.5	8.2
North Carolina	534	5.8	6.0	2,624	28.5	28.8	17,335	188.0	184.9	760	8.2	8.1
North Dakota	48	7.5	5.7	312	48.6	31.6	1,391	216.8	158.8	65	10.1	6.8
Ohio	875	7.6	6.7	4,285	37.3	31.5	27,324	237.9	206.3	1,229	10.7	9.2
Oklahoma	241	6.6	6.1	1061	29.1	25.8	9,767	268.2	242.2	331	9.1	8.2
Oregon	352	9.3	8.4	1,302	34.4	29.4	6,519	172.0	149.5	408	10.8	9.2
Pennsylvania	1,204	9.7	7.2	3,863	31.0	21.5	33,308	267.6	200.0	1024	8.2	6.1
Rhode Island	95	9.0	7.4	359	34.2	24.5	2,657	252.9	195.2	71	6.8	5.3
South Carolina	292	6.5	6.3	1,492	33.3	31.6	8,996	200.8	186.0	446	10.0	9.2
South Dakota	69	8.6	6.8	402	50.0	35.3	1,681	209.0	160.8	68	8.5	6.4
Tennessee	395	6.4	6.2	2,423	39.0	37.3	14,661	235.9	220.1	555	8.9	8.4
Texas	1,272	5.2	6.5	5,280	21.7	26.3	38,384	157.8	183.3	1,589	6.5	7.6
Utah	178	6.5	9.0	409	14.9	20.5	2,844	103.9	138.0	108	3.9	5.2
Vermont	53	8.5	7.3	218	35.1	29.6	1,216	195.7	165.9	44	7.1	6.0
Virginia	490	6.3	6.7	1,763	22.7	23.5	13,675	176.0	176.6	570	7.3	7.3
Washington	518	7.9	8.0	3,105	47.4	45.7	10,916	166.7	161.0	525	8.0	7.8
West Virginia	165	9.1	7.2	662	36.5	28.3	5,264	290.1	228.1	235	13.0	10.1
Wisconsin	447	7.9	7.0	1,655	29.4	24.2	11,275	200.3	171.8	421	7.5	6.3
Wyoming	34	6.4	6.4	125	23.5	23.1	937	175.9	169.4	15	*	*
Puerto Rico[3]	118	3.0	2.9	1,589	40.2	39.8	5,351	135.3	129.2	518	13.1	12.7
Virgin Islands[3]	4	*	*	17	*	*	238	216.7	234.5	11	*	*
Guam[3]	4	*	*	11	*	*	194	110.2	193.1	9	*	*
American Samoa[3]	-	*	*	1	*	*	31	47.8	124.3	6	*	*
Northern Marianas[3]	-	*	*	-	*	*	26	47.1	147.4	1	*	*

Table B-31. Number of Deaths, Death Rates, and Age–Adjusted Death Rates for Major Causes of Death, by State and Territory, 2008—Continued

(Number, rates per 100,000 population, age–adjusted rates per 100,000 U.S. standard population.)

Area	Cerebrovascular disease (I60–I69)			Influenza and pneumonia (J09–J18)			Chronic lower respiratory disease (J40–J47)			Chronic liver disease and cirrhosis (K70,K73–K74)		
	Number	Rate	Age-adjusted rate[1]	Number	Rate	Age-adjusted rate[1]	Number	Rate	Age-adjusted rate[1]	Number	Rate	Age-adjusted rate[1]
UNITED STATES[2]	134,148	44.1	40.7	56,284	18.5	16.9	141,090	46.4	44.0	29,963	9.9	9.2
Alabama	2,863	61.4	55.4	912	19.6	17.6	2,733	58.6	52.9	489	10.5	9.3
Alaska	172	25.1	42.9	51	7.4	12.4	181	26.4	43.6	60	8.7	9.3
Arizona	2,147	33.0	30.1	1068	16.4	15.0	2,939	45.2	41.9	794	12.2	11.9
Arkansas	1,722	60.3	52.0	846	29.6	25.1	1,887	66.1	57.4	247	8.7	7.9
California	14,048	38.2	39.7	6,560	17.8	18.4	13,426	36.5	38.9	4,152	11.3	11.4
Colorado	1,565	31.7	36.9	678	13.7	15.7	2,188	44.3	52.3	540	10.9	10.6
Connecticut	1,433	40.9	33.1	694	19.8	15.6	1,505	43.0	36.6	298	8.5	7.4
Delaware	365	41.8	36.7	135	15.5	13.9	472	54.1	48.2	91	10.4	9.3
District of Columbia	222	37.5	36.0	78	13.2	12.9	139	23.5	23.7	52	8.8	8.4
Florida	8,589	46.9	32.0	2,300	12.5	8.5	10,198	55.6	38.9	2,335	12.7	10.6
Georgia	3,805	39.3	47.2	1,498	15.5	18.7	3,546	36.6	44.2	665	6.9	7.1
Hawaii	642	49.8	38.4	270	21.0	15.9	293	22.7	18.4	112	8.7	7.6
Idaho	609	40.0	40.4	206	13.5	13.5	703	46.1	47.5	155	10.2	10.1
Illinois	5,788	44.9	42.6	2,672	20.7	19.4	5,602	43.4	42.9	1,145	8.9	8.6
Indiana	3,114	48.8	45.2	1,318	20.7	19.0	3,878	60.8	57.8	523	8.2	7.7
Iowa	1,732	57.7	42.8	829	27.6	19.7	1,848	61.5	49.3	217	7.2	6.3
Kansas	1,574	56.2	47.6	743	26.5	21.8	1,626	58.0	52.7	242	8.6	8.2
Kentucky	2,098	49.1	45.9	943	22.1	20.6	2,926	68.5	64.0	367	8.6	7.7
Louisiana	2,084	47.2	46.6	894	20.3	20.0	1,896	43.0	43.1	389	8.8	8.4
Maine	671	51.0	40.6	263	20.0	15.5	794	60.3	48.4	138	10.5	8.3
Maryland	2,330	41.4	41.4	1,008	17.9	17.9	1,982	35.2	35.8	408	7.2	6.8
Massachusetts	2,747	42.3	35.0	1,598	24.6	20.0	2,587	39.8	34.7	598	9.2	8.2
Michigan	4,769	47.7	43.4	1,853	18.5	16.8	5,185	51.8	48.2	1,084	10.8	9.7
Minnesota	2,199	42.1	37.7	745	14.3	12.4	2,096	40.2	38.3	380	7.3	6.8
Mississippi	1,592	54.2	51.9	626	21.3	20.4	1,520	51.7	50.2	269	9.2	8.8
Missouri	3,261	55.2	47.7	1,414	23.9	20.5	3,765	63.7	57.1	514	8.7	7.9
Montana	466	48.2	39.8	168	17.4	14.3	691	71.4	61.2	136	14.1	12.4
Nebraska	863	48.4	40.1	366	20.5	16.5	1047	58.7	51.4	135	7.6	7.1
Nevada	906	34.8	39.2	496	19.1	21.2	1,257	48.3	54.8	323	12.4	11.9
New Hampshire	484	36.8	33.6	211	16.0	14.4	688	52.3	48.9	120	9.1	7.9
New Jersey	3,264	37.6	33.0	1,413	16.3	14.1	3,280	37.8	34.0	707	8.1	7.3
New Mexico	760	38.3	35.6	351	17.7	16.4	1,001	50.4	47.4	392	19.8	19.3
New York	6,123	31.4	27.4	4,609	23.6	20.4	6,919	35.5	31.8	1,369	7.0	6.3
North Carolina	4,637	50.3	50.2	1,737	18.8	18.8	4,572	49.6	49.6	961	10.4	9.7
North Dakota	325	50.7	36.6	148	23.1	16.7	355	55.3	43.8	58	9.0	8.5
Ohio	5,951	51.8	45.1	2,085	18.2	15.7	6,928	60.3	53.7	1,198	10.4	9.3
Oklahoma	2,079	57.1	51.5	938	25.8	23.0	2,694	74.0	67.9	463	12.7	11.8
Oregon	1,899	50.1	43.8	517	13.6	11.9	1,951	51.5	46.6	466	12.3	10.9
Pennsylvania	6,942	55.8	41.5	2,705	21.7	16.0	6,767	54.4	42.0	1,113	8.9	7.5
Rhode Island	462	44.0	34.4	257	24.5	18.3	478	45.5	37.8	113	10.8	9.5
South Carolina	2,394	53.4	50.0	727	16.2	15.3	2,266	50.6	47.2	470	10.5	9.5
South Dakota	396	49.2	37.6	177	22.0	16.0	491	61.1	49.3	101	12.6	11.7
Tennessee	3,356	54.0	51.0	1,424	22.9	21.7	3,545	57.0	53.7	665	10.7	9.6
Texas	9,629	39.6	46.7	3,554	14.6	17.2	8,874	36.5	43.8	2,646	10.9	11.6
Utah	748	27.3	36.8	343	12.5	16.6	638	23.3	31.5	127	4.6	5.8
Vermont	281	45.2	38.3	74	11.9	10.2	341	54.9	47.7	46	7.4	6.3
Virginia	3,301	42.5	43.3	1,324	17.0	17.3	3,023	38.9	39.9	640	8.2	7.6
Washington	2,773	42.3	41.4	771	11.8	11.3	2,930	44.7	44.9	678	10.4	9.6
West Virginia	1,096	60.4	47.2	448	24.7	19.5	1,590	87.6	69.1	221	12.2	10.1
Wisconsin	2,638	46.9	40.0	1,116	19.8	16.6	2,538	45.1	40.1	474	8.4	7.6
Wyoming	234	43.9	43.3	123	23.1	22.4	311	58.4	58.3	77	14.5	13.4
Puerto Rico[3]	1,529	38.7	37.4	946	23.9	23.2	1,199	30.3	29.4	263	6.7	6.0
Virgin Islands[3]	44	40.1	45.7	10	*	*	8	*	*	8	*	*
Guam[3]	66	37.5	67.1	20	11.4	17.8	29	16.5	26.4	19	*	*
American Samoa[3]	29	44.7	130.3	3	*	*	8	*	*	1	*	*
Northern Marianas[3]	15	*	*	4	*	*	5	*	*	2	*	*

Table B-31. Number of Deaths, Death Rates, and Age–Adjusted Death Rates for Major Causes of Death, by State and Territory, 2008—Continued

(Number, rates per 100,000 population, age–adjusted rates per 100,000 U.S. standard population.)

Area	Nephritis, nephrotic syndrome, and nephrosis (N00–N07, N–17–N19, N–25–N27)			Accidents (V01–X59, Y85–Y86)			Motor vehicle accidents[4]			Intentional self–harm (suicide) (*U03, X60–X84, Y87.0)		
	Number	Rate	Age-adjusted rate[1]	Number	Rate	Age-adjusted rate[1]	Number	Rate	Age-adjusted rate[1]	Number	Rate	Age-adjusted rate[1]
UNITED STATES[2]	48,237	15.9	14.8	121,902	40.1	38.8	39,790	13.1	12.9	36,035	11.9	11.6
Alabama	1,107	23.7	21.5	2,509	53.8	52.5	1,085	23.3	23.1	604	13.0	12.7
Alaska	50	7.3	13.0	332	48.4	53.5	73	10.6	11.3	169	24.6	24.2
Arizona	503	7.7	7.2	2,956	45.5	44.4	965	14.8	14.9	972	15.0	15.0
Arkansas	638	22.3	19.2	1,477	51.7	50.3	641	22.4	22.3	447	15.7	15.6
California	2,854	7.8	8.1	10,761	29.3	29.2	3,619	9.8	9.7	3,775	10.3	10.3
Colorado	483	9.8	11.4	2,172	44.0	45.7	588	11.9	12.1	803	16.3	16.0
Connecticut	589	16.8	13.9	1,386	39.6	36.4	330	9.4	9.3	315	9.0	8.6
Delaware	189	21.6	19.2	352	40.3	39.7	127	14.5	14.7	109	12.5	12.1
District of Columbia	78	13.2	13.0	160	27.0	26.2	48	8.1	7.8	43	7.3	7.1
Florida	2,946	16.1	11.3	8,939	48.8	45.0	3,040	16.6	16.3	2,740	14.9	14.0
Georgia	1,668	17.2	20.5	3,774	39.0	40.9	1,510	15.6	15.8	981	10.1	10.2
Hawaii	197	15.3	11.9	406	31.5	28.3	108	8.4	8.0	133	10.3	10.1
Idaho	173	11.4	11.4	649	42.6	42.9	250	16.4	16.8	252	16.5	16.7
Illinois	2,576	20.0	19.3	4,218	32.7	32.1	1,159	9.0	8.9	1,198	9.3	9.2
Indiana	1,363	21.4	19.9	2,558	40.1	39.3	870	13.6	13.6	809	12.7	12.6
Iowa	304	10.1	7.7	1,266	42.2	37.6	440	14.7	14.2	380	12.7	12.6
Kansas	620	22.1	19.4	1,174	41.9	39.7	421	15.0	14.9	337	12.0	12.0
Kentucky	993	23.3	21.8	2,379	55.7	54.7	871	20.4	20.3	612	14.3	14.0
Louisiana	1,195	27.1	26.9	2,409	54.6	54.7	926	21.0	20.9	532	12.1	12.1
Maine	263	20.0	15.7	628	47.7	43.5	175	13.3	12.7	181	13.7	12.8
Maryland	775	13.8	13.7	1,465	26.0	25.7	646	11.5	11.4	507	9.0	8.8
Massachusetts	1,377	21.2	17.9	2,040	31.4	28.8	383	5.9	5.6	509	7.8	7.5
Michigan	1,663	16.6	15.2	3,685	36.8	35.3	1,100	11.0	10.8	1,180	11.8	11.6
Minnesota	813	15.6	14.1	2,010	38.5	36.1	528	10.1	9.9	596	11.4	11.1
Mississippi	723	24.6	23.7	1,693	57.6	57.5	780	26.5	26.8	409	13.9	14.0
Missouri	1,274	21.6	18.6	2,997	50.7	48.5	992	16.8	16.6	779	13.2	13.0
Montana	151	15.6	12.9	592	61.2	59.0	220	22.7	22.9	203	21.0	20.6
Nebraska	270	15.1	12.5	714	40.0	36.9	244	13.7	13.3	191	10.7	10.7
Nevada	456	17.5	19.5	1,134	43.6	44.3	341	13.1	13.2	528	20.3	20.2
New Hampshire	174	13.2	12.3	488	37.1	35.2	149	11.3	11.1	179	13.6	13.1
New Jersey	1,715	19.8	17.5	2,436	28.1	26.7	585	6.7	6.7	615	7.1	6.8
New Mexico	287	14.5	13.4	1,366	68.8	68.1	373	18.8	18.9	419	21.1	21.2
New York	2,394	12.3	10.7	5,042	25.9	24.3	1,284	6.6	6.4	1,409	7.2	7.0
North Carolina	1,729	18.7	18.5	4,313	46.8	46.5	1,563	16.9	16.8	1,162	12.6	12.4
North Dakota	98	15.3	11.8	342	53.3	47.7	121	18.9	18.5	86	13.4	13.5
Ohio	1,865	16.2	14.3	5,093	44.3	42.1	1,301	11.3	11.1	1,412	12.3	12.1
Oklahoma	664	18.2	16.4	2,119	58.2	56.8	766	21.0	20.9	575	15.8	15.8
Oregon	397	10.5	9.3	1,674	44.2	41.3	443	11.7	11.4	572	15.1	14.4
Pennsylvania	3,138	25.2	19.0	5,787	46.5	42.3	1,584	12.7	12.3	1,539	12.4	11.9
Rhode Island	163	15.5	12.1	480	45.7	40.6	72	6.9	6.5	110	10.5	9.9
South Carolina	945	21.1	19.5	2,285	51.0	50.3	957	21.4	21.3	565	12.6	12.1
South Dakota	89	11.1	8.7	381	47.4	42.4	131	16.3	15.8	124	15.4	15.6
Tennessee	908	14.6	13.8	3,250	52.3	50.9	1,164	18.7	18.6	973	15.7	15.1
Texas	3,536	14.5	17.0	9,189	37.8	39.8	3,780	15.5	15.7	2,552	10.5	10.8
Utah	212	7.7	10.3	881	32.2	36.2	302	11.0	11.6	390	14.3	15.4
Vermont	39	6.3	5.4	306	49.3	44.4	76	12.2	11.7	94	15.1	14.0
Virginia	1,537	19.8	20.1	2,820	36.3	36.1	884	11.4	11.2	948	12.2	11.9
Washington	471	7.2	7.0	2,727	41.6	40.5	620	9.5	9.3	889	13.6	13.1
West Virginia	522	28.8	22.8	1,253	69.1	65.8	372	20.5	20.2	261	14.4	13.8
Wisconsin	1,007	17.9	15.5	2,484	44.1	40.7	642	11.4	11.2	743	13.2	12.8
Wyoming	56	10.5	10.5	351	65.9	65.1	141	26.5	25.8	124	23.3	23.1
Puerto Rico[3]	1,057	26.7	25.5	1,107	28.0	27.6	383	9.7	9.6	303	7.7	7.6
Virgin Islands[3]	10	*	*	37	33.7	33.9	18	*	*	7	*	*
Guam[3]	15	*	*	39	22.2	24.8	11	*	*	29	16.5	16.0
American Samoa[3]	9	*	*	9	*	*	-	*	*	-	*	*
Northern Marianas[3]	7	*	*	18	*	*	8	*	*	3	*	*

Table B-31. Number of Deaths, Death Rates, and Age–Adjusted Death Rates for Major Causes of Death, by State and Territory, 2008—Continued

(Number, rates per 100,000 population, age–adjusted rates per 100,000 U.S. standard population.)

Area	Assault (homicide) (*U01–*U02,X85–Y09, Y87.1)			Alcohol–induced causes[5]			Drug–induced causes[6]			Injury by firearms		
	Number	Rate	Age-adjusted rate[1]	Number	Rate	Age-adjusted rate[1]	Number	Rate	Age-adjusted rate[1]	Number	Rate	Age-adjusted rate[1]
UNITED STATES[2]	17,826	5.9	5.9	24,189	8.0	7.4	38,649	12.7	12.6	31,593	10.4	10.3
Alabama	454	9.7	10.0	250	5.4	4.9	646	13.9	13.9	820	17.6	17.6
Alaska	29	4.2	4.4	147	21.4	21.8	132	19.2	18.9	142	20.7	20.9
Arizona	474	7.3	7.4	784	12.1	12.0	853	13.1	13.5	907	14.0	14.0
Arkansas	214	7.5	7.7	200	7.0	6.6	390	13.7	14.1	444	15.5	15.6
California	2,280	6.2	6.0	4,167	11.3	11.3	4,147	11.3	11.1	3,171	8.6	8.5
Colorado	194	3.9	3.8	676	13.7	12.8	760	15.4	14.8	513	10.4	10.3
Connecticut	127	3.6	3.8	229	6.5	5.9	397	11.3	11.1	200	5.7	5.6
Delaware	65	7.4	7.8	75	8.6	7.7	125	14.3	14.6	95	10.9	10.9
District of Columbia	164	27.7	25.6	73	12.3	11.7	77	13.0	12.9	137	23.1	20.4
Florida	1,300	7.1	7.5	1,765	9.6	8.4	3,097	16.9	17.2	2,334	12.7	12.4
Georgia	712	7.4	7.3	481	5.0	4.8	977	10.1	9.9	1,177	12.2	12.3
Hawaii	28	2.2	2.2	75	5.8	5.3	129	10.0	9.9	41	3.2	3.1
Idaho	25	1.6	1.6	173	11.4	11.1	152	10.0	10.1	175	11.5	11.5
Illinois	872	6.8	6.7	707	5.5	5.3	1,412	10.9	10.9	1,105	8.6	8.4
Indiana	323	5.1	5.2	376	5.9	5.5	869	13.6	13.8	723	11.3	11.3
Iowa	81	2.7	2.8	205	6.8	6.2	214	7.1	7.3	224	7.5	7.3
Kansas	112	4.0	3.9	205	7.3	7.0	241	8.6	8.7	277	9.9	9.7
Kentucky	240	5.6	5.7	237	5.6	5.0	779	18.2	18.3	576	13.5	13.3
Louisiana	541	12.3	12.2	210	4.8	4.5	686	15.6	15.9	822	18.6	18.5
Maine	34	2.6	2.7	99	7.5	6.1	162	12.3	12.3	122	9.3	8.5
Maryland	523	9.3	9.3	269	4.8	4.5	731	13.0	12.5	665	11.8	11.8
Massachusetts	167	2.6	2.6	431	6.6	6.0	885	13.6	13.3	224	3.4	3.4
Michigan	644	6.4	6.5	780	7.8	7.0	1,575	15.7	15.5	1,081	10.8	10.8
Minnesota	128	2.5	2.5	408	7.8	7.3	398	7.6	7.4	371	7.1	7.0
Mississippi	330	11.2	11.3	172	5.9	5.7	321	10.9	11.3	568	19.3	19.4
Missouri	482	8.2	8.3	397	6.7	6.3	779	13.2	13.3	818	13.8	13.8
Montana	40	4.1	4.2	162	16.7	15.2	141	14.6	14.8	155	16.0	15.7
Nebraska	78	4.4	4.4	137	7.7	7.3	113	6.3	6.5	150	8.4	8.4
Nevada	161	6.2	6.2	281	10.8	10.2	529	20.3	20.0	404	15.5	15.6
New Hampshire	22	1.7	1.6	125	9.5	7.9	129	9.8	9.5	93	7.1	6.7
New Jersey	377	4.3	4.5	504	5.8	5.2	808	9.3	9.1	429	4.9	5.0
New Mexico	151	7.6	7.8	435	21.9	21.6	534	26.9	27.8	294	14.8	14.8
New York	882	4.5	4.5	1,249	6.4	5.8	1,856	9.5	9.2	963	4.9	4.9
North Carolina	668	7.2	7.3	723	7.8	7.3	1,217	13.2	13.1	1,160	12.6	12.5
North Dakota	3	*	*	80	12.5	12.1	48	7.5	7.9	59	9.2	8.8
Ohio	598	5.2	5.4	834	7.3	6.5	1,811	15.8	15.7	1,115	9.7	9.7
Oklahoma	230	6.3	6.5	421	11.6	10.8	585	16.1	16.3	513	14.1	14.1
Oregon	103	2.7	2.7	544	14.4	12.8	521	13.7	13.3	385	10.2	9.7
Pennsylvania	697	5.6	5.9	631	5.1	4.5	1,898	15.2	15.4	1,345	10.8	10.7
Rhode Island	29	2.8	2.7	86	8.2	7.5	193	18.4	18.0	44	4.2	3.9
South Carolina	354	7.9	8.0	325	7.3	6.6	588	13.1	13.1	615	13.7	13.4
South Dakota	20	2.5	2.5	103	12.8	12.3	57	7.1	7.7	83	10.3	10.5
Tennessee	479	7.7	7.8	458	7.4	6.7	977	15.7	15.4	985	15.8	15.6
Texas	1,487	6.1	6.1	1,344	5.5	5.7	2,199	9.0	9.2	2,598	10.7	10.9
Utah	46	1.7	1.7	170	6.2	7.3	483	17.7	19.1	238	8.7	9.4

Table B-31. Number of Deaths, Death Rates, and Age–Adjusted Death Rates for Major Causes of Death, by State and Territory, 2008—Continued

(Number, rates per 100,000 population, age–adjusted rates per 100,000 U.S. standard population.)

Area	Assault (homicide) (*U01–*U02,X85–Y09, Y87.1)			Alcohol–induced causes[6]			Drug–induced causes[7]			Injury by firearms		
	Number	Rate	Age-adjusted rate[1]	Number	Rate	Age-adjusted rate[1]	Number	Rate	Age-adjusted rate[1]	Number	Rate	Age-adjusted rate[1]
Vermont	17	*	*	62	10.0	8.8	76	12.2	11.2	54	8.7	8.1
Virginia	376	4.8	4.8	460	5.9	5.4	730	9.4	9.2	817	10.5	10.3
Washington	224	3.4	3.4	780	11.9	11.0	1,058	16.2	15.4	587	9.0	8.7
West Virginia	70	3.9	4.0	132	7.3	6.4	468	25.8	26.3	239	13.2	12.7
Wisconsin	153	2.7	2.8	463	8.2	7.4	622	11.1	10.8	443	7.9	7.7
Wyoming	18	*	*	89	16.7	15.7	74	13.9	14.4	93	17.5	17.1
Puerto Rico[3]	818	20.7	20.5	195	4.9	4.5	251	6.3	6.6	781	19.8	19.6
Virgin Islands[3]	47	42.8	47.4	11	*	*	1	*	*	45	41.0	45.1
Guam[3]	1	*	*	2	*	*	-	*	*	3	*	*
American Samoa[3]	-	*	*	2	*	*	2	*	*	-	*	*
Northern Marianas[3]	1	*	*	3	*	*	-	*	*	-	*	*

- = Quantity zero
* = Figure does not meet standards of reliability or precision.
[1]Death rates are affected by the population composition of the area. Age–adjusted death rates should be used for comparisons between areas.
[2]Excludes data for Puerto Rico, Virgin Islands, Guam, American Samoa and Northern Marianas.
[3]Age–adjusted death rates for Puerto Rico, Virgin Islands, Guam, American Samoa, and Northern Marianas are calculated using different age groups in the weighting procedure.
[4]ICD–10 codes for motor vehicle accidents are V02–V04, V09.0, V09.2, V12–V14, V19.0–V19.2, V19.4–V19.6, V20–V79, V80.3–V80.5, V81.0–V81.1, V82.0–V82.1, V83–V86, V87.0–V87.8, V88.0–V88.8, V89.0, and V89.2.
[5]Causes of death attributable to alcohol–induced mortality include ICD–10 codes E24.4, F10, G31.2, G62.1, G72.1, I42.6, K29.2, K70, K85.2, K86.0, R78.0, X45, X65, and Y15.
[6]Causes of death attributable to drug–induced mortality include ICD–10 codes D52.1, D59.0, D59.2, D61.1, D64.2, E06.4, E16.0, E23.1, E24.2, E27.3, E66.1, F11.0–F11.5, F11.7–F11.9, F12.0–F12.5, F12.7–F12.9, F13.0–F13.5, F13.7–F13.9, F14.0–F14.5, F14.7–F14.9, F15.0–F15.5, F15.7–F15.9, F16.0–F16.5, F16.7–F16.9, F17.0, F17.3–F17.5, F17.7–F17.9, F18.0–F18.5, F18.7–F18.9, F19.0–F19.5, F19.7–F19.9, G21.1, G24.0, G25.1, G25.4, G25.6, G44.4, G62.0, G72.0, I 95.2, J70.2–J70.4, K85.3, L10.5, L27.0–L27.1, M10.2, M32.0, M80.4, M81.4, M83.5, M87.1, R50.2, R78.1–R78.5, X40–X44, X60–X64, X85, and Y10–Y14.
[7]ICD–10 codes for Injury by firearms are *U01.4, W32–W34, X72–X74, X93–X95, Y22–Y24, and Y35.0.

Table B-32. Death Rates for All Causes, by Sex, Race, Hispanic Origin, and Age, Selected Years, 1950–2008

(Deaths per 100,000 resident population.)

Sex, race, Hispanic origin, and age	1950[1]	1960[1]	1970	1980	1985	1990	1995	2000	2005	2006	2007	2008
All Persons												
All ages, age-adjusted	1,446.0	1,339.2	1,222.6	1,039.1	988.1	938.7	909.8	869.0	798.8	776.5	760.2	758.3
All ages, crude	963.8	954.7	945.3	878.3	876.9	863.8	868.3	854.0	825.9	810.4	803.6	813.0
Under 1 year	3,299.2	2,696.4	2,142.4	1,288.3	1,088.1	971.9	780.3	736.7	692.5	690.7	684.5	650.5
1–4 years	139.4	109.1	84.5	63.9	51.8	46.8	40.4	32.4	29.4	28.4	28.6	28.3
5–14 years	60.1	46.6	41.3	30.6	26.5	24.0	22.2	18.0	16.3	15.2	15.3	14.1
15–24 years	128.1	106.3	127.7	115.4	94.9	99.2	93.4	79.9	81.4	82.2	79.9	75.6
25–34 years	178.7	146.4	157.4	135.5	124.4	139.2	137.3	101.4	104.4	106.3	104.9	103.3
35–44 years	358.7	299.4	314.5	227.9	207.7	223.2	239.4	198.9	193.3	190.2	184.4	179.7
45–54 years	853.9	756.0	730.0	584.0	519.3	473.4	454.3	425.6	432.0	427.5	420.9	420.4
55–64 years	1,901.0	1,735.1	1,658.8	1,346.3	1,294.2	1,196.9	1,104.7	992.2	906.9	890.9	877.7	879.2
65–74 years	4,104.3	3,822.1	3,582.7	2,994.9	2,862.8	2,648.6	2,549.0	2,399.1	2,137.1	2,062.1	2,011.3	1,995.6
75–84 years	9,331.1	8,745.2	8,004.4	6,692.6	6,398.7	6,007.2	5,811.3	5,666.5	5,260.0	5,115.0	5,011.6	5,017.7
85 years and over	20,196.9	19,857.5	16,344.9	15,980.3	15,712.4	15,327.4	15,248.6	15,524.4	13,798.6	13,253.1	12,946.5	13,015.1
Male												
All ages, age-adjusted	1,674.2	1,609.0	1,542.1	1,348.1	1,278.1	1,202.8	1,143.9	1,053.8	951.1	924.8	905.6	900.6
All ages, crude	1,106.1	1,104.5	1,090.3	976.9	948.6	918.4	900.8	853.0	827.2	814.8	809.9	817.9
Under 1 year	3,728.0	3,059.3	2,410.0	1,428.5	1,219.9	1,082.8	856.3	806.5	762.3	756.3	747.8	709.7
1–4 years	151.7	119.5	93.2	72.6	58.5	52.4	44.5	35.9	33.4	30.5	31.3	31.5
5–14 years	70.9	55.7	50.5	36.7	31.8	28.5	26.4	20.9	18.6	17.6	17.4	16.0
15–24 years	167.9	152.1	188.5	172.3	138.9	147.4	137.4	114.9	117.8	119.3	115.8	109.8
25–34 years	216.5	187.9	215.3	196.1	179.6	204.3	198.0	138.6	143.4	146.8	144.0	141.8
35–44 years	428.8	372.8	402.6	299.2	278.9	310.4	331.0	255.2	243.0	238.7	231.8	223.7
45–54 years	1,067.1	992.2	958.5	767.3	671.6	610.3	589.9	542.8	547.8	541.0	530.0	526.4
55–64 years	2,395.3	2,309.5	2,282.7	1,815.1	1,711.4	1,553.4	1,400.7	1,230.7	1,131.0	1,110.0	1,100.6	1,104.9
65–74 years	4,931.4	4,914.4	4,873.8	4,105.2	3,856.3	3,491.5	3,263.8	2,979.6	2,612.2	2,516.2	2,456.9	2,432.8
75–84 years	10,426.0	10,178.4	10,010.2	8,816.7	8,501.6	7,888.6	7,399.6	6,972.6	6,349.8	6,177.7	6,038.4	6,032.2
85 years and over	21,636.0	21,186.3	17,821.5	18,801.1	18,614.1	18,056.6	17,861.0	17,501.4	14,889.4	14,309.1	14,006.4	14,017.3
Female												
All ages, age-adjusted	1,236.0	1,105.3	971.4	817.9	784.5	750.9	739.4	731.4	677.6	657.8	643.4	643.4
All ages, crude	823.5	809.2	807.8	785.3	809.1	812.0	837.2	855.0	824.6	806.1	797.4	808.2
Under 1 year	2,854.6	2,321.3	1,863.7	1,141.7	950.6	855.7	700.5	663.4	619.4	622.0	618.1	588.5
1–4 years	126.7	98.4	75.4	54.7	44.8	41.0	36.0	28.7	25.1	26.3	25.7	25.0
5–14 years	48.9	37.3	31.8	24.2	21.0	19.3	17.9	15.0	13.9	12.8	13.1	12.1
15–24 years	89.1	61.3	68.1	57.5	49.6	49.0	47.3	43.1	42.7	42.8	42.0	39.5
25–34 years	142.7	106.6	101.6	75.9	69.4	74.2	76.1	63.5	64.1	64.3	64.2	63.1
35–44 years	290.3	229.4	231.1	159.3	138.7	137.9	149.3	143.2	143.6	141.6	136.9	135.4
45–54 years	641.5	526.7	517.2	412.9	375.2	342.7	324.1	312.5	319.9	317.7	315.2	317.5
55–64 years	1,404.8	1,196.4	1,098.9	934.3	925.6	878.8	835.2	772.2	698.5	687.0	670.1	668.9
65–74 years	3,333.2	2,871.8	2,579.7	2,144.7	2,096.9	1,991.2	1,975.8	1,921.2	1,736.3	1,677.9	1,633.0	1,622.6
75–84 years	8,399.6	7,633.1	6,677.6	5,440.1	5,162.1	4,883.1	4,818.6	4,814.7	4,520.0	4,388.3	4,304.1	4,313.7
85 years and over	19,194.7	19,008.4	15,518.0	14,746.9	14,553.9	14,274.3	14,242.3	14,719.2	13,297.7	12,759.0	12,442.3	12,531.0
White Male[2]												
All ages, age-adjusted	1,642.5	1,586.0	1,513.7	1,317.6	1,249.8	1,165.9	1,107.5	1,029.4	933.2	908.2	890.5	889.2
All ages, crude	1,089.5	1,098.5	1,086.7	983.3	963.6	930.9	921.0	887.8	864.5	852.3	848.1	860.3
Under 1 year	3,400.5	2,694.1	2,113.2	1,230.3	1,056.5	896.1	720.7	667.6	640.0	632.7	627.8	600.2
1–4 years	135.5	104.9	83.6	66.1	52.8	45.9	39.0	32.6	30.9	27.5	28.3	29.1
5–14 years	67.2	52.7	48.0	35.0	30.1	26.4	24.3	19.8	17.1	16.4	16.2	14.6
15–24 years	152.4	143.7	170.8	167.0	134.2	131.3	120.1	105.8	110.4	111.8	108.1	102.6
25–34 years	185.3	163.2	176.6	171.3	158.8	176.1	171.9	124.1	130.8	135.4	134.2	133.2
35–44 years	380.9	332.6	343.5	257.4	243.1	268.2	286.8	233.6	228.5	224.4	218.2	213.5
45–54 years	984.5	932.2	882.9	698.9	611.7	548.7	528.3	496.9	509.3	505.2	498.4	500.5
55–64 years	2,304.4	2,225.2	2,202.6	1,728.5	1,625.8	1,467.2	1,319.3	1,163.3	1,068.1	1,050.6	1,042.7	1,051.8
65–74 years	4,864.9	4,848.4	4,810.1	4,035.7	3,770.7	3,397.7	3,173.3	2,905.7	2,552.7	2,455.8	2,396.7	2,376.5
75–84 years	10,526.3	10,299.6	10,098.8	8,829.8	8,486.1	7,844.9	7,347.3	6,933.1	6,343.2	6,182.2	6,049.2	6,052.0
85 years and over	22,116.3	21,750.0	18,551.7	19,097.3	18,980.1	18,268.3	18,050.7	17,716.4	15,156.5	14,576.8	14,286.4	14,354.0
Black or African American Male[2]												
All ages, age-adjusted	1,909.1	1,811.1	1,873.9	1,697.8	1,634.5	1,644.5	1,585.7	1,403.5	1,252.9	1,215.6	1,184.4	1,150.4
All ages, crude	1,257.7	1,181.7	1,186.6	1,034.1	989.3	1,008.0	960.2	834.1	799.2	786.7	775.6	762.7
Under 1 year	—	5,306.8	4,298.9	2,586.7	2,219.9	2,112.4	1,664.7	1,567.6	1,437.2	1,407.1	1,363.2	1,298.7
1–4 years[3]	1,412.6	208.5	150.5	110.5	90.1	85.8	73.1	54.5	46.7	47.1	45.3	47.3
5–14 years	95.1	75.1	67.1	47.4	42.3	41.2	38.5	28.2	27.0	24.8	24.6	23.6
15–24 years	289.7	212.0	320.6	209.1	173.6	252.2	246.6	181.4	172.1	171.3	168.1	159.1
25–34 years	503.5	402.5	559.5	407.3	351.9	430.8	407.4	261.0	254.3	254.2	240.3	224.9
35–44 years	878.1	762.0	956.6	689.8	630.2	699.6	716.8	453.0	395.5	392.3	378.9	347.5
45–54 years	1,905.0	1,624.8	1,777.5	1,479.9	1,292.9	1,261.0	1,238.9	1,017.7	948.6	921.9	876.7	827.5
55–64 years	3,773.2	3,316.4	3,256.9	2,873.0	2,779.8	2,618.4	2,382.0	2,080.1	1,954.3	1,891.8	1,870.8	1,826.3
65–74 years	5,310.3	5,798.7	5,803.2	5,131.1	5,172.4	4,946.1	4,707.8	4,253.5	3,747.3	3,669.2	3,604.9	3,537.9
75–84 years[4]	10,101.9	8,605.1	9,454.9	9,231.6	9,262.3	9,129.5	8,862.0	8,486.0	7,667.1	7,393.2	7,169.0	7,102.0
85 years and over	—	14,844.8	12,222.3	16,098.8	15,774.2	16,954.9	17,016.0	16,791.0	13,809.8	13,206.0	12,964.7	12,528.3

Table B-32. Death Rates for All Causes, by Sex, Race, Hispanic Origin, and Age, Selected Years, 1950–2008—Continued

(Deaths per 100,000 resident population.)

Sex, race, Hispanic origin, and age	1950[1]	1960[1]	1970	1980	1985	1990	1995	2000	2005	2006	2007	2008
American Indian or Alaska Native Male[2]												
All ages, age-adjusted	—	—	—	1,111.5	926.1	916.2	932.0	841.5	775.3	739.9	736.7	717.3
All ages, crude	—	—	—	597.1	492.5	476.4	459.4	415.6	481.9	477.1	488.2	477.6
Under 1 year	—	—	—	1,598.1	1,080.0	1,056.6	696.0	700.2	882.4	1,057.8	1,009.9	659.7
1–4 years	—	—	—	82.7	105.3	77.4	73.3	44.9	72.4	58.1	63.6	38.4
5–14 years	—	—	—	43.7	39.2	33.4	27.0	20.2	22.7	17.2	23.2	18.5
15–24 years	—	—	—	311.1	214.4	219.8	182.1	136.2	145.1	156.1	143.7	150.7
25–34 years	—	—	—	360.6	275.0	256.1	263.6	179.1	206.3	194.0	198.3	198.2
35–44 years	—	—	—	556.8	363.5	365.4	377.4	295.2	336.6	338.5	332.5	315.9
45–54 years	—	—	—	871.3	687.9	619.9	601.0	520.0	588.9	591.9	573.0	617.8
55–64 years	—	—	—	1,547.5	1,319.1	1,211.3	1,276.0	1,090.4	1,124.1	1,029.5	1,037.0	1,037.8
65–74 years	—	—	—	2,968.4	2,692.3	2,461.7	2,660.8	2,478.3	2,254.1	2,146.7	2,131.7	2,169.8
75–84 years	—	—	—	5,607.0	5,572.7	5,389.2	5,787.7	5,351.2	4,373.3	4,198.0	4,193.4	4,150.2
85 years and over	—	—	—	12,635.2	8,900.0	11,243.9	10,604.7	10,725.8	8,419.0	7,540.2	7,638.6	6,513.8
Asian or Pacific Islander Male[2]												
All ages, age-adjusted	—	—	—	786.5	755.4	716.4	693.4	624.2	534.4	516.0	499.2	492.8
All ages, crude	—	—	—	375.3	344.6	334.3	341.4	332.9	333.9	330.6	331.4	337.7
Under 1 year	—	—	—	816.5	750.0	605.3	468.3	529.4	464.5	469.7	483.5	464.2
1–4 years	—	—	—	50.9	43.4	45.0	28.0	23.3	20.8	18.1	25.3	17.1
5–14 years	—	—	—	23.4	22.5	20.7	19.6	12.9	14.0	11.3	12.2	12.4
15–24 years	—	—	—	80.8	76.0	76.0	73.0	55.2	56.9	61.7	61.0	50.0
25–34 years	—	—	—	83.5	77.3	79.6	75.4	55.0	55.6	54.2	50.1	55.1
35–44 years	—	—	—	128.3	114.4	130.8	124.9	104.9	93.6	88.5	88.9	87.2
45–54 years	—	—	—	342.3	284.8	287.1	273.0	249.7	242.4	232.5	229.1	222.9
55–64 years	—	—	—	881.1	869.4	789.1	714.2	642.4	545.4	550.7	523.1	529.2
65–74 years	—	—	—	2,236.1	2,102.0	2,041.4	1,894.8	1,661.0	1,403.8	1,329.2	1,304.7	1,312.6
75–84 years	—	—	—	5,389.5	5,551.2	5,008.6	4,729.9	4,328.2	3,759.2	3,606.4	3,538.4	3,497.1
85 years and over	—	—	—	13,753.6	12,750.0	12,446.3	13,252.0	12,125.3	9,839.1	9,524.7	8,918.0	8,724.9
Hispanic or Latino Male[2,5]												
All ages, age-adjusted	—	—	—	—	889.2	886.4	897.6	818.1	717.0	675.6	654.5	630.7
All ages, crude	—	—	—	—	374.6	411.6	391.6	331.3	334.4	323.9	321.8	316.9
Under 1 year	—	—	—	—	1,044.6	921.8	684.6	637.1	670.2	640.7	632.7	578.5
1–4 years	—	—	—	—	53.8	53.8	39.3	31.5	33.2	28.8	28.0	27.5
5–14 years	—	—	—	—	23.0	26.0	24.6	17.9	15.3	16.4	15.8	12.7
15–24 years	—	—	—	—	147.5	159.3	147.3	107.7	120.4	120.7	115.3	103.9
25–34 years	—	—	—	—	202.1	234.0	196.7	120.2	115.5	112.7	110.1	107.2
35–44 years	—	—	—	—	290.1	341.8	333.6	211.0	182.0	176.5	166.3	158.9
45–54 years	—	—	—	—	495.7	533.9	528.5	439.0	417.4	403.8	399.2	372.5
55–64 years	—	—	—	—	1,129.4	1,123.7	1,076.9	965.7	875.8	843.6	831.4	831.3
65–74 years	—	—	—	—	2,484.9	2,368.2	2,429.3	2,287.9	2,029.4	1,910.7	1,862.7	1,826.9
75–84 years	—	—	—	—	5,696.1	5,369.1	5,557.4	5,395.3	4,856.8	4,492.6	4,364.8	4,264.0
85 years and over	—	—	—	—	12,156.2	12,272.1	13,295.9	13,086.2	10,140.5	9,435.5	8,953.7	8,379.0
White, not Hispanic or Latino Male[5]												
All ages, age-adjusted	—	—	—	—	1,215.6	1,170.9	1,105.6	1,035.4	945.4	922.8	906.8	908.5
All ages, crude	—	—	—	—	956.3	985.9	984.8	978.5	970.6	962.0	960.4	978.2
Under 1 year	—	—	—	—	1,002.0	865.4	703.8	658.7	625.7	621.9	616.8	594.4
1–4 years	—	—	—	—	48.8	43.8	37.8	32.4	29.9	26.7	28.1	29.3
5–14 years	—	—	—	—	28.9	25.7	23.5	20.0	17.4	16.2	16.1	15.0
15–24 years	—	—	—	—	125.0	123.4	111.5	103.5	105.8	107.6	104.6	100.8
25–34 years	—	—	—	—	151.2	165.3	163.5	123.0	134.1	141.1	140.8	140.4
35–44 years	—	—	—	—	231.8	257.1	276.5	233.9	236.1	233.1	228.4	225.3
45–54 years	—	—	—	—	587.7	544.5	520.7	497.7	517.2	515.1	508.7	515.8
55–64 years	—	—	—	—	1,550.7	1,479.7	1,322.7	1,170.9	1,079.6	1,064.0	1,057.5	1,067.2
65–74 years	—	—	—	—	3,648.1	3,434.5	3,188.5	2,930.5	2,584.5	2,490.3	2,432.7	2,413.0
75–84 years	—	—	—	—	8,361.0	7,920.4	7,367.4	6,977.8	6,420.4	6,278.3	6,152.7	6,166.5
85 years and over	—	—	—	—	18,635.3	18,505.4	18,132.6	17,853.2	15,401.3	14,841.1	14,588.3	14,721.8
White Female[2]												
All ages, age-adjusted	1,198.0	1,074.4	944.0	796.1	764.3	728.8	718.7	715.3	666.5	648.2	634.8	636.9
All ages, crude	803.3	800.9	812.6	806.1	840.1	846.9	883.2	912.3	882.8	863.9	854.9	868.7
Under 1 year	2,566.8	2,007.7	1,614.6	962.5	799.3	690.0	574.4	550.5	515.3	516.5	516.8	496.9
1–4 years	112.2	85.2	66.1	49.3	40.0	36.1	31.3	25.5	22.9	23.5	23.1	22.8
5–14 years	45.1	34.7	29.9	22.9	19.5	17.9	16.5	14.1	12.8	11.9	12.4	11.3
15–24 years	71.5	54.9	61.6	55.5	48.1	45.9	43.7	41.1	41.5	41.7	41.2	37.8
25–34 years	112.8	85.0	84.1	65.4	59.4	61.5	62.9	55.1	58.0	58.9	59.6	58.2
35–44 years	235.8	191.1	193.3	138.2	121.9	117.4	125.5	125.7	130.4	129.0	126.2	125.8
45–54 years	546.4	458.8	462.9	372.7	341.7	309.3	291.9	281.4	291.1	291.6	290.5	295.1
55–64 years	1,293.8	1,078.9	1,014.9	876.2	869.1	822.7	783.4	730.9	663.9	654.6	638.0	639.1
65–74 years	3,242.8	2,779.3	2,470.7	2,066.6	2,027.1	1,923.5	1,913.2	1,868.3	1,700.4	1,646.0	1,600.9	1,594.6
75–84 years	8,481.5	7,696.6	6,698.7	5,401.7	5,111.6	4,839.1	4,775.3	4,785.3	4,519.4	4,395.4	4,317.6	4,342.2
85 years and over	19,679.5	19,477.7	15,980.2	14,979.6	14,745.4	14,400.6	14,405.8	14,890.7	13,498.3	12,965.7	12,646.7	12,765.0

Table B-32. Death Rates for All Causes, by Sex, Race, Hispanic Origin, and Age, Selected Years, 1950–2008—Continued

(Deaths per 100,000 resident population.)

Sex, race, Hispanic origin, and age	1950[1]	1960[1]	1970	1980	1985	1990	1995	2000	2005	2006	2007	2008
Black or African American Female[2]												
All ages, age-adjusted	1,545.5	1,369.7	1,228.7	1,033.3	994.4	975.1	955.9	927.6	845.7	813.0	793.8	778.4
All ages, crude	1,002.0	905.0	829.2	733.3	734.2	747.9	743.2	733.0	703.9	684.0	675.7	673.5
Under 1 year	—	4,162.2	3,368.8	2,123.7	1,821.4	1,735.5	1,399.9	1,279.8	1,179.7	1,194.6	1,132.2	1,086.3
1–4 years[4]	1,139.3	173.3	129.4	84.4	71.1	67.6	59.5	45.3	36.7	39.4	39.0	35.7
5–14 years	72.8	53.8	43.8	30.5	28.6	27.5	25.4	20.0	19.4	17.4	17.0	16.4
15–24 years	213.1	107.5	111.9	70.5	59.6	68.7	68.9	58.3	51.2	51.3	48.9	50.5
25–34 years	393.3	273.2	231.0	150.0	137.6	159.5	162.8	121.8	109.8	106.6	102.1	97.4
35–44 years	758.1	568.5	533.0	323.9	276.5	298.6	324.9	271.9	250.0	245.0	229.1	221.5
45–54 years	1,576.4	1,177.0	1,043.9	768.2	667.6	639.4	612.1	588.3	568.4	548.1	537.2	525.0
55–64 years	3,089.4	2,510.9	1,986.2	1,561.0	1,532.5	1,452.6	1,354.3	1,227.2	1,103.6	1,076.3	1,047.6	1,028.8
65–74 years	4,000.2	4,064.2	3,860.9	3,057.4	2,967.8	2,865.7	2,837.5	2,689.6	2,341.5	2,239.7	2,209.5	2,155.1
75–84 years[4]	8,347.0	6,730.0	6,691.5	6,212.1	6,078.0	5,688.3	5,671.9	5,696.5	5,263.7	5,028.9	4,902.9	4,816.3
85 years and over	—	13,052.6	10,706.6	12,367.2	12,703.0	13,309.5	13,073.3	13,941.3	12,789.9	12,196.7	11,997.4	11,863.8
American Indian or Alaska Native Female[2]												
All ages, age-adjusted	—	—	—	662.4	577.2	561.8	643.9	604.5	567.7	555.7	533.2	515.1
All ages, crude	—	—	—	380.1	342.5	330.4	360.1	346.1	398.8	399.9	400.0	386.1
Under 1 year	—	—	—	1,352.6	910.5	688.7	780.6	492.2	752.9	689.9	830.3	495.3
1–4 years	—	—	—	87.5	54.8	37.8	54.4	39.8	45.6	50.5	46.0	39.5
5–14 years	—	—	—	33.5	23.0	25.5	20.0	17.7	16.8	16.6	13.0	16.5
15–24 years	—	—	—	90.3	72.8	69.0	60.4	58.9	67.9	63.5	61.3	58.4
25–34 years	—	—	—	178.5	121.5	102.3	106.3	84.8	90.6	92.1	90.6	99.1
35–44 years	—	—	—	286.0	185.6	156.4	171.9	171.9	194.1	204.6	196.0	217.6
45–54 years	—	—	—	491.4	415.5	380.9	349.1	284.9	366.2	342.4	346.4	342.3
55–64 years	—	—	—	837.1	851.9	805.9	876.2	772.1	699.4	686.6	693.5	667.6
65–74 years	—	—	—	1,765.5	1,630.3	1,679.4	1,935.6	1,899.8	1,780.5	1,657.3	1,611.9	1,561.8
75–84 years	—	—	—	3,612.9	3,200.0	3,073.2	4,067.6	3,850.0	3,602.6	3,746.4	3,436.8	3,261.2
85 years and over	—	—	—	8,567.4	7,740.0	8,201.1	9,201.8	9,118.2	7,065.0	6,633.7	6,248.2	5,997.1
Asian or Pacific Islander Female[2]												
All ages, age-adjusted	—	—	—	425.9	456.7	469.3	446.7	416.8	369.3	362.6	350.6	353.1
All ages, crude	—	—	—	222.5	224.9	234.3	250.4	262.3	282.8	285.6	287.2	300.7
Under 1 year	—	—	—	755.8	622.0	518.2	396.6	434.3	395.3	356.9	397.6	377.2
1–4 years	—	—	—	35.4	36.8	32.0	24.9	20.0	17.5	21.1	17.9	20.1
5–14 years	—	—	—	21.5	19.1	13.0	15.4	11.7	11.9	10.3	9.8	8.6
15–24 years	—	—	—	32.3	30.7	28.8	31.1	22.4	26.1	25.4	24.4	23.4
25–34 years	—	—	—	45.4	36.5	37.5	35.6	27.6	28.6	28.5	28.1	35.1
35–44 years	—	—	—	89.7	77.8	69.9	66.2	65.6	58.1	56.8	54.9	49.4
45–54 years	—	—	—	214.1	184.9	182.7	184.1	155.5	142.8	145.2	136.2	136.2
55–64 years	—	—	—	440.8	468.0	483.4	457.7	390.9	353.2	332.7	329.2	327.9
65–74 years	—	—	—	1,027.7	1,130.8	1,089.2	1,037.8	996.4	905.5	897.9	832.7	866.5
75–84 years	—	—	—	2,833.6	2,873.9	3,127.9	3,089.9	2,882.4	2,529.8	2,525.5	2,470.6	2,437.2
85 years and over	—	—	—	7,923.3	9,808.3	10,254.0	9,406.1	9,052.2	7,792.5	7,560.2	7,334.0	7,478.6
Hispanic or Latina Female[2,5]												
All ages, age-adjusted	—	—	—	—	546.1	537.1	546.1	546.0	485.3	468.6	452.7	445.7
All ages, crude	—	—	—	—	251.9	285.4	281.9	274.6	278.2	274.6	272.1	274.9
Under 1 year	—	—	—	—	791.4	746.6	572.0	553.6	555.4	538.3	539.9	482.2
1–4 years	—	—	—	—	42.3	42.1	33.1	27.5	24.5	24.0	23.8	21.6
5–14 years	—	—	—	—	16.0	17.3	15.0	13.4	12.0	11.8	12.3	11.4
15–24 years	—	—	—	—	36.2	40.6	37.5	31.7	36.6	35.2	33.5	31.3
25–34 years	—	—	—	—	56.3	62.9	58.6	43.4	41.1	43.1	43.4	42.4
35–44 years	—	—	—	—	100.0	109.3	118.9	100.5	90.6	87.1	82.7	82.2
45–54 years	—	—	—	—	251.3	253.3	238.8	223.8	216.4	215.3	204.0	200.8
55–64 years	—	—	—	—	619.7	607.5	602.3	548.4	493.9	486.5	476.9	477.2
65–74 years	—	—	—	—	1,449.5	1,453.8	1,457.2	1,423.2	1,291.6	1,222.7	1,162.1	1,153.1
75–84 years	—	—	—	—	3,551.8	3,351.3	3,506.4	3,624.5	3,365.8	3,222.9	3,196.2	3,118.7
85 years and over	—	—	—	—	10,228.6	10,098.7	10,540.5	11,202.8	9,068.4	8,803.5	8,318.9	8,254.9

Table B-32. Death Rates for All Causes, by Sex, Race, Hispanic Origin, and Age, Selected Years, 1950–2008—Continued

(Deaths per 100,000 resident population.)

Sex, race, Hispanic origin, and age	1950[1]	1960[1]	1970	1980	1985	1990	1995	2000	2005	2006	2007	2008
White, not Hispanic or Latina Female[5]												
All ages, age-adjusted	—	—	—	—	754.3	734.6	721.1	721.5	677.7	660.0	647.7	650.8
All ages, crude	—	—	—	—	861.7	903.6	951.7	1,007.3	992.6	974.7	967.6	985.5
Under 1 year	—	—	—	—	763.0	655.3	553.9	530.9	496.5	503.7	499.6	488.6
1–4 years	—	—	—	—	36.5	34.0	30.3	24.4	22.2	23.2	22.7	22.7
5–14 years	—	—	—	—	19.0	17.6	16.4	13.9	12.9	11.8	12.3	11.1
15–24 years	—	—	—	—	47.9	46.0	44.0	42.6	42.2	42.9	42.7	39.0
25–34 years	—	—	—	—	59.0	60.6	62.2	56.8	62.1	62.5	63.4	62.0
35–44 years	—	—	—	—	122.8	116.8	124.1	128.1	137.0	136.3	134.4	134.4
45–54 years	—	—	—	—	335.7	312.1	293.0	285.0	298.7	299.8	300.5	306.5
55–64 years	—	—	—	—	853.3	834.5	789.8	742.1	677.2	668.0	651.3	652.3
65–74 years	—	—	—	—	1,998.1	1,940.2	1,925.9	1,891.0	1,729.6	1,677.4	1,634.9	1,628.5
75–84 years	—	—	—	—	5,059.1	4,887.3	4,794.9	4,819.3	4,579.7	4,460.7	4,385.4	4,420.2
85 years and over	—	—	—	—	14,560.4	14,533.1	14,450.9	14,971.7	13,683.1	13,150.7	12,856.7	12,996.9

— = Data not available.

[1] Includes deaths of persons who were not residents of the 50 states and the District of Columbia (D.C.).
[2] The race groups, White, Black, Asian or Pacific Islander, and American Indian or Alaska Native, include persons of Hispanic and non-Hispanic origin. Persons of Hispanic origin may be of any race.
[3] In 1950, rate is for the age group under 5 years.
[4] In 1950, rate is for the age group 75 years and over.
[5] Prior to 1997, excludes data from states lacking an Hispanic-origin item on the death certificate.

Table B-33. Death Rates for Diseases of the Heart, by Sex, Race, Hispanic Origin, and Age, Selected Years, 1950–2008

(Deaths per 100,000 resident population.)

Sex, race, Hispanic origin, and age	1950[1,2]	1960[1,2]	1970[2]	1980[2]	1985	1990[2]	1995	2000[3]	2005[3]	2006[3]	2007[3]	2008[3]
All Persons												
All ages, age-adjusted	588.8	559.0	492.7	412.1	375.0	321.8	293.4	257.6	211.1	200.2	190.9	186.5
All ages, crude	356.8	369.0	362.0	336.0	324.1	289.5	277.0	252.6	220.0	211.0	204.3	202.9
Under 1 year	4.1	6.6	13.1	22.8	25.0	20.1	17.4	13.0	8.7	8.4	10.0	9.2
1–4 years	1.6	1.3	1.7	2.6	2.2	1.9	1.6	1.2	0.9	1.0	1.1	1.1
5–14 years	3.9	1.3	0.8	0.9	1.0	0.9	0.8	0.7	0.6	0.6	0.6	0.6
15–24 years	8.2	4.0	3.0	2.9	2.8	2.5	2.8	2.6	2.7	2.5	2.6	2.5
25–34 years	20.9	15.6	11.4	8.3	8.3	7.6	8.2	7.4	8.1	8.2	7.9	7.9
35–44 years	88.3	74.6	66.7	44.6	38.1	31.4	31.8	29.2	28.9	28.3	27.4	26.7
45–54 years	309.2	271.8	238.4	180.2	153.8	120.5	109.6	94.2	89.7	88.0	85.3	85.4
55–64 years	804.3	737.9	652.3	494.1	443.0	367.3	320.1	261.2	214.8	207.3	200.3	198.0
65–74 years	1,857.2	1,740.5	1,558.2	1,218.6	1,089.8	894.3	795.4	665.6	518.9	490.3	462.9	449.8
75–84 years	4,311.0	4,089.4	3,683.8	2,993.1	2,693.1	2,295.7	2,050.5	1,780.3	1,460.8	1,383.1	1,315.0	1,276.7
85 years and over	9,152.5	9,317.8	7,891.3	7,777.1	7,384.1	6,739.9	6,391.5	5,926.1	4,778.4	4,480.8	4,267.7	4,175.7
Male												
All ages, age-adjusted	699.0	687.6	634.0	538.9	488.0	412.4	371.0	320.0	260.9	248.5	237.7	232.3
All ages, crude	424.7	439.5	422.5	368.6	344.1	297.6	278.5	249.8	221.1	214.0	208.4	207.6
Under 1 year	4.7	7.8	15.1	25.5	27.8	21.9	17.7	13.3	9.4	8.8	10.9	9.8
1–4 years	1.7	1.4	1.9	2.8	2.2	1.9	1.7	1.4	1.0	1.1	1.0	1.1
5–14 years	3.5	1.4	0.9	1.0	0.9	0.9	0.8	0.8	0.6	0.7	0.6	0.6
15–24 years	8.3	4.2	3.7	3.7	3.5	3.1	3.5	3.2	3.6	3.3	3.2	3.4
25–34 years	24.4	20.1	15.2	11.4	11.6	10.3	11.0	9.6	10.8	11.2	10.5	10.4
35–44 years	120.4	112.7	103.2	68.7	58.6	48.1	46.9	41.4	40.7	39.5	38.6	36.8
45–54 years	441.2	420.4	376.4	282.6	237.8	183.0	166.1	140.2	131.5	128.9	124.6	123.0
55–64 years	1,100.5	1,066.9	987.2	746.8	659.1	537.3	460.1	371.7	306.9	296.8	288.8	284.7
65–74 years	2,310.2	2,291.3	2,170.3	1,728.0	1,535.8	1,250.0	1,095.3	898.3	692.3	660.5	624.9	609.2
75–84 years	4,825.8	4,742.4	4,534.8	3,834.3	3,496.9	2,968.2	2,622.9	2,248.1	1,829.4	1,743.5	1,656.5	1,609.1
85 years and over	9,661.4	9,788.9	8,426.2	8,752.7	8,251.8	7,418.4	6,993.5	6,430.0	5,143.4	4,819.9	4,621.8	4,535.9
Female												
All ages, age-adjusted	486.6	447.0	381.6	320.8	294.5	257.0	236.6	210.9	172.3	162.2	154.0	150.4
All ages, crude	289.7	300.6	304.5	305.1	305.2	281.8	275.5	255.3	218.9	208.0	200.2	198.3
Under 1 year	3.4	5.4	10.9	20.0	22.0	18.3	17.0	12.5	8.0	7.9	9.0	8.5
1–4 years	1.6	1.1	1.6	2.5	2.2	1.9	1.5	1.0	0.9	0.9	1.1	1.1
5–14 years	4.3	1.2	0.8	0.9	1.0	0.8	0.7	0.5	0.6	0.6	0.6	0.5
15–24 years	8.2	3.7	2.3	2.1	2.1	1.8	2.1	2.1	1.7	1.8	1.9	1.6
25–34 years	17.6	11.3	7.7	5.3	5.0	5.0	5.4	5.2	5.3	5.1	5.3	5.4
35–44 years	57.0	38.2	32.2	21.4	18.3	15.1	17.0	17.2	17.1	17.0	16.2	16.4
45–54 years	177.8	127.5	109.9	84.5	74.4	61.0	55.4	49.8	49.2	48.5	47.2	48.9
55–64 years	507.0	429.4	351.6	272.1	252.1	215.7	192.6	159.3	129.1	124.1	117.9	117.2
65–74 years	1,434.9	1,261.3	1,082.7	828.6	746.1	616.8	554.9	474.0	372.7	346.3	325.4	313.9
75–84 years	3,873.0	3,582.7	3,120.8	2,497.0	2,220.4	1,893.8	1,692.7	1,475.1	1,210.5	1,136.7	1,079.7	1,046.0
85 years and over	8,798.1	9,016.8	7,591.8	7,350.5	7,037.6	6,478.1	6,159.6	5,720.9	4,610.8	4,322.1	4,099.3	4,001.7
White Male[4]												
All ages, age-adjusted	701.4	694.5	640.2	539.6	487.3	409.2	367.0	316.7	258.0	245.2	234.8	229.9
All ages, crude	434.2	454.6	438.3	384.0	360.3	312.7	294.4	265.8	234.9	226.9	221.1	220.6
45–54 years	424.1	413.2	365.7	269.8	225.5	170.6	153.9	130.7	121.3	119.2	116.2	116.1
55–64 years	1,082.6	1,056.0	979.3	730.6	640.1	516.7	439.2	351.8	288.2	278.9	271.4	268.9
65–74 years	2,309.4	2,297.9	2,177.2	1,729.7	1,522.7	1,230.5	1,071.8	877.8	671.9	636.6	603.0	586.7
75–84 years	4,908.0	4,839.9	4,617.6	3,883.2	3,527.0	2,983.4	2,625.6	2,247.0	1,831.8	1,743.3	1,659.3	1,611.2
85 years and over	9,952.3	10,135.8	8,818.0	8,958.0	8,481.7	7,558.7	7,125.1	6,560.8	5,288.4	4,947.1	4,756.1	4,680.9
Black or African American Male[4]												
All ages, age-adjusted	641.5	615.2	607.3	561.4	533.9	485.4	451.3	392.5	329.8	320.6	305.9	295.6
All ages, crude	348.4	330.6	330.3	301.0	288.6	256.8	239.1	211.1	194.8	191.8	186.5	183.4
45–54 years	624.1	514.0	512.8	433.4	385.2	328.9	308.6	247.2	237.4	229.8	216.3	201.4
55–64 years	1,434.0	1,236.8	1,135.4	987.2	935.3	824.0	740.5	631.2	549.1	526.4	516.3	493.3
65–74 years	2,140.1	2,281.4	2,237.8	1,847.2	1,839.2	1,632.9	1,514.1	1,268.8	1,041.6	1,044.6	989.4	977.5
75–84 years[5]	4,107.9	3,533.6	3,783.4	3,578.8	3,436.6	3,107.1	2,908.7	2,597.6	2,204.1	2,129.9	1,999.2	1,963.5
85 years and over	—	6,037.9	5,367.6	6,819.5	6,393.5	6,479.6	6,088.5	5,633.5	4,230.5	4,073.1	3,879.6	3,681.1
American Indian or Alaska Native Male[4]												
All ages, age-adjusted	—	—	—	320.5	280.5	264.1	256.4	222.2	173.2	170.2	159.8	149.1
All ages, crude	—	—	—	130.6	117.9	108.0	101.0	90.1	93.2	95.8	94.1	89.3
45–54 years	—	—	—	238.1	209.1	173.8	136.2	108.5	112.2	119.5	112.4	122.4
55–64 years	—	—	—	496.3	438.3	411.0	375.7	285.0	275.0	256.2	235.8	236.7
65–74 years	—	—	—	1,009.4	984.6	839.1	938.2	748.2	554.4	573.6	521.5	530.6
75–84 years	—	—	—	2,062.2	2,118.2	1,788.8	1,858.5	1,655.7	1,123.9	1,176.6	1,129.5	928.8
85 years and over	—	—	—	4,413.7	2,766.7	3,860.3	3,306.5	3,318.3	2,509.3	2,066.9	1,901.1	1,769.8

Table B-33. Death Rates for Diseases of the Heart, by Sex, Race, Hispanic Origin, and Age, Selected Years, 1950–2008—Continued

(Deaths per 100,000 resident population.)

Sex, race, Hispanic origin, and age	1950[1,2]	1960[1,2]	1970[2]	1980[2]	1985	1990[2]	1995	2000[3]	2005[3]	2006[3]	2007[3]	2008[3]
Asian or Pacific Islander Male[4]												
All ages, age–adjusted	—	—	—	286.9	258.9	220.7	214.5	185.5	141.1	136.3	126.0	124.7
All ages, crude	—	—	—	119.8	103.5	88.7	93.2	90.6	83.5	82.4	79.6	81.6
45–54 years	—	—	—	112.0	81.1	70.4	69.8	61.1	58.1	55.7	51.5	51.6
55–64 years	—	—	—	306.7	291.2	226.1	205.4	182.6	145.3	145.4	131.5	134.6
65–74 years	—	—	—	852.4	753.5	623.5	581.0	482.5	374.9	344.3	321.3	317.5
75–84 years	—	—	—	2,010.9	2,025.6	1,642.2	1,533.8	1,354.7	984.3	963.3	906.3	898.9
85 years and over	—	—	—	5,923.0	4,937.5	4,617.8	4,888.9	4,154.2	3,052.0	2,985.9	2,665.8	2,636.6
Hispanic or Latino Male[4,6]												
All ages, age–adjusted	—	—	—	—	296.6	270.0	260.8	238.2	192.4	175.2	165.0	151.9
All ages, crude	—	—	—	—	92.1	91.0	83.1	74.7	72.1	67.7	66.6	63.9
45–54 years	—	—	—	—	128.1	116.4	102.0	84.3	77.9	75.6	73.3	67.6
55–64 years	—	—	—	—	398.8	363.0	311.2	264.8	219.3	202.3	201.9	195.3
65–74 years	—	—	—	—	971.1	829.9	784.6	684.8	561.5	505.6	477.0	452.1
75–84 years	—	—	—	—	2,150.0	1,971.3	1,854.0	1,733.2	1,469.2	1,308.4	1,233.4	1,139.8
85 years and over	—	—	—	—	4,912.5	4,711.9	5,104.0	4,897.5	3,534.2	3,257.9	2,960.8	2,611.7
White, Not Hispanic or Latino Male[6]												
All ages, age–adjusted	—	—	—	—	480.4	413.6	369.1	319.9	262.2	250.0	239.8	235.9
All ages, crude	—	—	—	—	362.8	336.5	320.6	297.5	267.8	260.3	254.3	254.9
45–54 years	—	—	—	—	219.9	172.8	155.9	134.3	126.2	124.5	121.6	122.4
55–64 years	—	—	—	—	610.6	521.3	443.2	356.3	293.0	284.5	276.6	274.4
65–74 years	—	—	—	—	1,471.3	1,243.4	1,077.0	885.1	677.6	644.3	610.9	595.1
75–84 years	—	—	—	—	3,512.8	3,007.7	2,635.3	2,261.9	1,849.3	1,767.4	1,685.0	1,641.1
85 years and over	—	—	—	—	8,538.4	7,663.4	7,156.4	6,606.6	5,374.1	5,032.8	4,858.5	4,808.9
White Female[4]												
All ages, age–adjusted	479.2	441.7	376.7	315.9	289.1	250.9	230.8	205.6	168.2	158.6	150.5	147.2
All ages, crude	290.5	306.5	313.8	319.2	321.8	298.4	294.7	274.5	235.5	224.2	215.5	213.5
45–54 years	142.4	103.4	91.4	71.2	62.5	50.2	45.5	40.9	40.8	40.7	40.0	41.2
55–64 years	460.7	383.0	317.7	248.1	227.1	192.4	172.0	141.3	114.5	111.4	105.3	104.4
65–74 years	1,401.6	1,229.8	1,044.0	796.7	713.3	583.6	523.5	445.2	351.8	325.8	304.4	295.8
75–84 years	3,926.2	3,629.7	3,143.5	2,493.6	2,207.5	1,874.3	1,670.3	1,452.4	1,193.3	1,123.9	1,068.9	1,035.9
85 years and over	9,086.9	9,280.8	7,839.9	7,501.6	7,170.0	6,563.4	6,251.3	5,801.4	4,691.0	4,402.6	4,169.6	4,084.5
Black or African American Female[4]												
All ages, age–adjusted	538.9	488.9	435.6	378.6	357.7	327.5	304.0	277.6	228.3	212.5	204.5	197.5
All ages, crude	289.9	268.5	261.0	249.7	250.3	237.0	226.3	212.6	185.2	174.3	170.0	167.7
45–54 years	526.8	360.7	290.9	202.4	176.2	155.3	141.5	125.0	115.4	111.0	107.0	111.8
55–64 years	1,210.7	952.3	710.5	530.1	510.7	442.0	386.0	332.8	272.0	251.3	242.5	240.8
65–74 years	1,659.4	1,680.5	1,553.2	1,210.3	1,149.9	1,017.5	938.2	815.2	614.9	578.3	563.5	527.0
75–84 years[5]	3,499.3	2,926.9	2,964.1	2,707.2	2,533.4	2,250.9	2,100.7	1,913.1	1,595.1	1,461.7	1,384.0	1,334.6
85 years and over	—	5,650.0	5,003.8	5,796.5	5,686.5	5,766.1	5,448.5	5,298.7	4,365.6	4,049.4	3,962.0	3,738.9
American Indian or Alaska Native Female[4]												
All ages, age–adjusted	—	—	—	175.4	170.0	153.1	164.8	143.6	115.9	113.2	99.8	94.3
All ages, crude	—	—	—	80.3	84.3	77.5	80.2	71.9	75.1	75.1	69.6	66.0
45–54 years	—	—	—	65.2	59.2	62.0	62.4	40.2	52.0	41.8	36.7	40.0
55–64 years	—	—	—	193.5	230.8	197.0	200.7	149.4	122.1	125.2	108.7	106.5
65–74 years	—	—	—	577.2	472.7	492.8	514.2	391.8	348.6	322.3	288.5	265.7
75–84 years	—	—	—	1,364.3	1,258.8	1,050.3	1,184.3	1,044.1	846.8	937.9	779.2	717.6
85 years and over	—	—	—	2,893.3	3,180.0	2,868.7	3,118.1	3,146.3	2,145.9	1,883.1	1,697.9	1,640.8
Asian or Pacific Islander Female[4]												
All ages, age–adjusted	—	—	—	132.3	149.4	149.2	137.6	115.7	91.9	87.3	82.0	81.7
All ages, crude	—	—	—	57.0	60.3	62.0	66.3	65.0	66.2	64.9	63.9	67.0
45–54 years	—	—	—	28.6	23.8	17.5	20.8	15.9	15.8	15.9	12.1	13.4
55–64 years	—	—	—	92.9	103.0	99.0	89.5	68.8	56.9	48.4	46.6	51.3
65–74 years	—	—	—	313.3	341.0	323.9	288.3	229.6	194.3	187.4	168.5	163.8
75–84 years	—	—	—	1,053.2	1,056.5	1,130.9	1,001.8	866.2	682.9	639.8	611.4	614.2
85 years and over	—	—	—	3,211.0	4,208.3	4,161.2	3,942.4	3,367.2	2,560.3	2,492.6	2,345.6	2,304.8

Table B-33. Death Rates for Diseases of the Heart, by Sex, Race, Hispanic Origin, and Age, Selected Years, 1950–2008—Continued

(Deaths per 100,000 resident population.)

Sex, race, Hispanic origin, and age	1950[1,2]	1960[1,2]	1970[2]	1980[2]	1985	1990[2]	1995	2000[3]	2005[3]	2006[3]	2007[3]	2008[3]
Hispanic or Latina Female[4,6]												
All ages, age–adjusted	—	—	—	—	195.9	177.2	173.8	163.7	129.1	118.9	111.8	104.6
All ages, crude	—	—	—	—	75.0	79.4	76.5	71.5	66.2	62.6	60.8	59.3
45–54 years	—	—	—	—	46.6	43.5	32.0	28.2	26.2	27.3	23.4	24.3
55–64 years	—	—	—	—	184.7	153.2	141.0	111.2	92.6	86.9	81.4	79.6
65–74 years	—	—	—	—	534.1	460.4	419.0	366.3	305.9	273.0	249.7	245.7
75–84 years	—	—	—	—	1,457.3	1,259.7	1,231.3	1,169.4	973.4	894.5	856.6	768.8
85 years and over	—	—	—	—	4,528.6	4,440.3	4,653.1	4,605.8	3,341.3	3,078.3	2,888.2	2,705.9
White, not Hispanic or Latina Female[6]												
All ages, age–adjusted	—	—	—	—	287.2	252.6	231.5	206.8	170.3	160.9	153.0	150.0
All ages, crude	—	—	—	—	334.2	320.0	319.7	304.9	266.4	254.7	245.5	244.0
45–54 years	—	—	—	—	61.3	50.2	46.1	41.9	42.4	42.2	42.1	43.3
55–64 years	—	—	—	—	219.6	193.6	172.0	142.9	116.1	113.2	107.1	106.3
65–74 years	—	—	—	—	700.5	584.7	525.2	448.5	354.6	329.1	308.1	299.1
75–84 years	—	—	—	—	2,201.7	1,890.2	1,674.9	1,458.9	1,203.6	1,135.8	1,081.0	1,052.9
85 years and over	—	—	—	—	7,164.2	6,615.2	6,265.8	5,822.7	4,745.1	4,460.8	4,230.8	4,154.9

— = Data not available.

[1] Includes deaths of persons who were not residents of the 50 states and the District of Columbia.
[2] Underlying cause of death was coded according to the 6th Revision of the International Classification of Diseases (ICD) in 1950, 7th Revision in 1960, 8th Revision in 1970, and 9th Revision in 1980–1998.
[3] Starting with 1999 data, cause of death is coded according to ICD-10.
[4] The race groups, White, Black, Asian or Pacific Islander, and American Indian or Alaska Native, include persons of Hispanic and non-Hispanic origin. Persons of Hispanic origin may be of any race.
[5] In 1950, rate is for the age group 75 years and over.
[6] Prior to 1997, excludes data from states lacking an Hispanic-origin item on the death certificate.

Table B–34. Death Rates for Cerebrovascular Diseases, by Sex, Race, Hispanic Origin, and Age, Selected Years, 1950–2008

(Deaths per 100,000 resident population.)

Sex, race, Hispanic origin, and age	1950[1,2]	1960[1,2]	1970[2]	1980[2]	1985	1990[2]	1995	2000[3]	2005[3]	2006[3]	2007[3]	2008[3]
All Persons												
All ages, age–adjusted	180.7	177.9	147.7	96.2	76.4	65.3	63.1	60.9	46.6	43.6	42.2	40.7
All ages, crude	104.0	108.0	101.9	75.0	64.2	57.8	59.2	59.6	48.4	45.8	45.1	44.1
Under 1 year	5.1	4.1	5.0	4.4	3.6	3.8	5.9	3.3	3.1	3.4	3.1	3.3
1–4 years	0.9	0.8	1.0	0.5	0.3	0.3	0.4	0.3	0.4	0.3	0.3	0.4
5–14 years	0.5	0.7	0.7	0.3	0.2	0.2	0.2	0.2	0.2	0.2	0.2	0.2
15–24 years	1.6	1.8	1.6	1.0	0.8	0.6	0.5	0.5	0.5	0.5	0.5	0.4
25–34 years	4.2	4.7	4.5	2.6	2.2	2.2	1.7	1.5	1.4	1.3	1.2	1.3
35–44 years	18.7	14.7	15.6	8.5	7.2	6.4	6.5	5.8	5.2	5.1	4.9	4.8
45–54 years	70.4	49.2	41.6	25.2	21.2	18.7	17.4	16.0	15.0	14.7	14.6	13.8
55–64 years	194.2	147.3	115.8	65.1	54.7	47.9	45.6	41.0	33.0	33.3	32.1	31.0
65–74 years	554.7	469.2	384.1	219.0	172.4	144.2	136.2	128.6	101.1	96.3	93.0	88.9
75–84 years	1,499.6	1,491.3	1,254.2	786.9	600.1	498.0	477.1	461.3	359.0	335.1	322.3	314.5
85 years and over	2,990.1	3,680.5	3,014.3	2,283.7	1,858.5	1,628.9	1,607.2	1,589.2	1,141.8	1,039.6	1,015.5	972.6
Male												
All ages, age–adjusted	186.4	186.1	157.4	102.2	79.9	68.5	65.9	62.4	46.9	43.9	42.5	40.9
All ages, crude	102.5	104.5	94.5	63.4	52.4	46.7	47.2	46.9	38.8	37.0	36.4	35.7
Under 1 year	6.4	5.0	5.8	5.0	4.6	4.4	6.4	3.8	3.5	3.9	3.5	3.1
1–4 years	1.1	0.9	1.2	0.4	0.4	0.3	0.4	*	0.5	0.3	0.2	0.3
5–14 years	0.5	0.7	0.8	0.3	0.2	0.2	0.2	0.2	0.3	0.3	0.2	0.2
15–24 years	1.8	1.9	1.8	1.1	0.7	0.7	0.5	0.5	0.4	0.5	0.5	0.5
25–34 years	4.2	4.5	4.4	2.6	2.2	2.1	1.8	1.5	1.5	1.4	1.2	1.4
35–44 years	17.5	14.6	15.7	8.7	7.4	6.8	7.0	5.8	5.2	5.3	5.3	5.1
45–54 years	67.9	52.2	44.4	27.2	23.1	20.5	19.5	17.5	16.5	16.4	16.2	15.3
55–64 years	205.2	163.8	138.7	74.6	63.4	54.3	52.7	47.2	38.5	38.7	38.0	36.0
65–74 years	589.6	530.7	449.5	258.6	201.0	166.6	154.7	145.0	113.6	108.0	105.2	100.1
75–84 years	1,543.6	1,555.9	1,361.6	866.3	659.4	551.1	517.7	490.8	372.9	345.5	333.2	325.4
85 years and over	3,048.6	3,643.1	2,895.2	2,193.6	1,723.8	1,528.5	1,522.1	1,484.3	1,023.3	932.4	895.7	861.3
Female												
All ages, age–adjusted	175.8	170.7	140.0	91.7	73.3	62.6	60.5	59.1	45.6	42.6	41.3	39.9
All ages, crude	105.6	111.4	109.0	85.9	75.3	68.4	70.7	71.8	57.8	54.4	53.5	52.3
Under 1 year	3.7	3.2	4.0	3.8	2.7	3.1	5.3	2.7	2.6	2.9	2.6	3.4
1–4 years	0.7	0.7	0.7	0.5	0.3	0.3	0.3	0.4	0.3	0.4	0.4	0.4
5–14 years	0.4	0.6	0.6	0.3	0.3	0.2	0.1	0.2	0.2	0.2	0.2	0.2
15–24 years	1.5	1.6	1.4	0.8	0.8	0.6	0.4	0.5	0.5	0.5	0.4	0.4
25–34 years	4.3	4.9	4.7	2.6	2.1	2.2	1.6	1.5	1.2	1.2	1.3	1.2
35–44 years	19.9	14.8	15.6	8.4	6.9	6.1	6.0	5.7	5.1	4.8	4.6	4.5
45–54 years	72.9	46.3	39.0	23.3	19.4	17.0	15.3	14.5	13.6	13.0	12.9	12.3
55–64 years	183.1	131.8	95.3	56.8	47.1	42.2	39.1	35.3	27.9	28.2	26.6	26.4
65–74 years	522.1	415.7	333.3	188.7	150.4	126.7	121.4	115.1	90.5	86.5	82.7	79.4
75–84 years	1,462.2	1,441.1	1,183.1	740.1	565.1	466.2	451.8	442.1	349.5	328.0	314.9	306.9
85 years and over	2,949.4	3,704.4	3,081.0	2,323.1	1,912.3	1,667.6	1,640.0	1,632.0	1,196.1	1,089.8	1,072.4	1,026.3
White Male[4]												
All ages, age–adjusted	182.1	181.6	153.7	98.7	77.1	65.5	62.9	59.8	44.7	41.7	40.2	39.0
All ages, crude	100.5	102.7	93.5	63.1	52.5	46.9	48.0	48.4	39.7	37.7	37.0	36.6
45–54 years	53.7	40.9	35.6	21.7	18.0	15.4	14.7	13.6	12.8	12.8	13.0	11.9
55–64 years	182.2	139.0	119.9	64.0	54.5	45.7	44.2	39.7	31.7	31.5	31.4	30.1
65–74 years	569.7	501.0	420.0	239.8	185.9	152.9	142.1	133.8	103.0	97.1	94.3	90.1
75–84 years	1,556.3	1,564.8	1,361.6	852.7	648.1	539.2	503.8	480.0	364.8	338.5	323.1	319.3
85 years and over	3,127.1	3,734.8	3,018.1	2,230.8	1,758.7	1,545.4	1,536.0	1,490.7	1,033.7	941.3	905.0	873.4
Black or African American Male[4]												
All ages, age–adjusted	228.8	238.5	206.4	142.0	112.5	102.2	97.0	89.6	70.5	67.1	67.1	62.1
All ages, crude	122.0	122.9	108.8	73.0	59.2	53.0	49.8	46.1	40.3	39.3	39.5	37.4
45–54 years	211.9	166.1	136.1	82.1	71.1	68.4	62.3	49.5	44.8	43.5	41.0	41.2
55–64 years	522.8	439.9	343.4	189.7	160.5	141.7	130.8	115.4	103.7	105.9	99.8	90.2
65–74 years	783.6	899.2	780.1	472.3	379.4	326.9	297.0	268.5	224.3	218.7	223.3	206.0
75–84 years[5]	1,504.9	1,475.2	1,445.7	1,066.3	813.2	721.5	705.9	659.2	503.7	471.1	491.9	444.6
85 years and over	—	2,700.0	1,963.1	1,873.2	1,427.4	1,421.5	1,410.1	1,458.8	983.5	882.0	866.9	816.9
American Indian or Alaska Native Male[4]												
All ages, age–adjusted	—	—	—	66.4	48.4	44.3	51.7	46.1	31.3	25.8	31.1	24.5
All ages, crude	—	—	—	23.1	18.4	16.0	18.4	16.8	15.8	14.4	16.5	13.7
45–54 years	—	—	—	*	*	*	25.5	13.3	13.7	16.3	13.9	15.0
55–64 years	—	—	—	72.0	0.0	39.8	42.6	48.6	36.0	35.0	37.0	30.3
65–74 years	—	—	—	170.5	196.2	120.3	156.4	144.7	113.0	82.9	83.3	96.3
75–84 years	—	—	—	523.9	372.7	325.9	351.2	373.3	229.6	174.3	266.0	170.1
85 years and over	—	—	—	1,384.7	733.3	949.8	1,072.4	834.9	466.2	344.5	481.0	324.6

Table B–34. Death Rates for Cerebrovascular Diseases, by Sex, Race, Hispanic Origin, and Age, Selected Years, 1950–2008—Continued

(Deaths per 100,000 resident population.)

Sex, race, Hispanic origin, and age	1950[1,2]	1960[1,2]	1970[2]	1980[2]	1985	1990[2]	1995	2000[3]	2005[3]	2006[3]	2007[3]	2008[3]
Asian or Pacific Islander Male[4]												
All ages, age-adjusted	—	—	—	71.4	65.2	59.1	64.0	58.0	41.5	39.8	35.5	34.0
All ages, crude	—	—	—	28.7	24.0	23.3	27.5	27.2	23.8	23.6	22.0	22.0
45–54 years	—	—	—	17.0	13.9	15.6	16.5	15.0	14.4	13.4	14.7	13.4
55–64 years	—	—	—	59.9	48.8	51.8	59.6	49.3	33.4	36.3	31.5	32.1
65–74 years	—	—	—	197.9	155.6	167.9	155.6	135.6	105.0	108.9	90.7	90.9
75–84 years	—	—	—	619.5	583.7	483.9	521.9	438.7	337.4	294.9	274.2	257.8
85 years and over	—	—	—	1,399.0	1,387.5	1,196.6	1,382.1	1,415.6	873.6	865.9	748.7	694.5
Hispanic or Latino Male[4,6]												
All ages, age-adjusted	—	—	—	—	57.5	46.5	51.2	50.5	38.0	35.9	34.4	33.1
All ages, crude	—	—	—	—	17.2	15.6	16.2	15.8	14.4	14.3	14.1	13.9
45–54 years	—	—	—	—	23.6	20.0	20.3	18.1	17.8	17.0	16.5	15.2
55–64 years	—	—	—	—	64.0	49.2	46.9	48.8	40.3	41.1	42.9	35.0
65–74 years	—	—	—	—	163.3	126.4	138.1	136.1	106.2	100.1	94.6	89.3
75–84 years	—	—	—	—	394.7	356.6	373.3	392.9	294.0	292.8	263.6	273.0
85 years and over	—	—	—	—	1,181.2	866.3	1,079.5	1,029.9	692.4	581.9	594.6	554.8
White, Not Hispanic or Latino Male[6]												
All ages, age-adjusted	—	—	—	—	74.8	66.3	62.8	59.9	44.8	41.7	40.3	39.2
All ages, crude	—	—	—	—	52.1	50.6	51.9	53.9	44.8	42.6	41.9	41.5
45–54 years	—	—	—	—	15.9	14.9	13.9	13.0	12.1	12.1	12.3	11.2
55–64 years	—	—	—	—	50.4	45.1	43.3	38.7	30.7	30.3	30.0	29.4
65–74 years	—	—	—	—	178.2	154.5	141.4	133.1	102.4	96.5	93.8	89.8
75–84 years	—	—	—	—	635.2	547.3	506.2	482.3	368.2	340.5	326.3	321.8
85 years and over	—	—	—	—	1,729.1	1,578.7	1,544.8	1,505.9	1,050.5	960.2	922.4	892.3
White Female[4]												
All ages, age-adjusted	169.7	165.0	135.5	89.0	70.7	60.3	58.6	57.3	44.0	41.1	39.9	38.6
All ages, crude	103.3	110.1	109.8	88.6	78.2	71.6	75.1	76.9	61.6	57.9	57.0	55.6
45–54 years	55.0	33.8	30.5	18.6	15.5	13.5	12.6	11.2	10.5	10.4	10.0	9.5
55–64 years	156.9	103.0	78.1	48.6	39.9	35.8	33.3	30.2	23.8	24.1	22.5	22.1
65–74 years	498.1	383.3	303.2	172.5	137.6	116.1	111.7	107.3	83.2	79.3	75.8	73.6
75–84 years	1,471.3	1,444.7	1,176.8	728.8	551.7	456.5	443.4	434.2	342.9	321.5	310.5	301.2
85 years and over	3,017.9	3,795.7	3,167.6	2,362.7	1,938.0	1,685.9	1,656.7	1,646.7	1,208.5	1,102.2	1,083.8	1,039.8
Black or African American Female[4]												
All ages, age-adjusted	238.4	232.5	189.3	119.6	99.2	84.0	79.4	76.2	60.7	57.0	55.0	53.4
All ages, crude	128.3	127.7	112.2	77.8	68.5	60.7	59.1	58.3	49.1	46.5	45.6	45.0
45–54 years	248.9	166.2	119.4	61.8	50.8	44.1	36.0	38.1	35.0	31.3	33.0	30.7
55–64 years	567.7	452.0	272.4	138.4	113.5	96.9	85.6	76.4	59.8	61.1	58.4	59.2
65–74 years	754.4	830.5	673.5	361.7	285.1	236.7	222.3	190.9	153.7	148.9	143.8	130.6
75–84 years[6]	1,496.7	1,413.1	1,338.3	917.5	752.4	595.0	565.1	549.2	450.2	415.6	387.9	397.1
85 years and over	—	2,578.9	2,210.5	1,891.6	1,653.4	1,495.2	1,518.4	1,556.5	1,156.5	1,060.5	1,050.6	996.1
American Indian or Alaska Native Female[4]												
All ages, age-adjusted	—	—	—	51.2	44.3	38.4	46.3	43.7	37.1	30.9	28.4	24.0
All ages, crude	—	—	—	22.0	21.5	19.3	22.0	21.5	23.9	19.8	19.7	16.5
45–54 years	—	—	—	*	*	*	*	14.4	17.7	*	10.0	10.7
55–64 years	—	—	—	*	40.4	40.7	41.5	37.9	35.8	16.2	23.7	26.0
65–74 years	—	—	—	128.3	118.2	100.5	114.8	79.5	115.2	78.8	83.4	55.7
75–84 years	—	—	—	404.2	317.6	282.0	364.4	391.1	287.9	267.6	198.7	207.8
85 years and over	—	—	—	1,095.5	980.0	776.2	983.9	931.5	627.3	648.1	599.9	408.9
Asian or Pacific Islander Female[4]												
All ages, age-adjusted	—	—	—	60.8	54.8	54.9	48.3	49.1	36.3	34.9	33.2	32.1
All ages, crude	—	—	—	26.4	23.3	24.3	24.2	28.7	26.6	26.7	26.4	26.8
45–54 years	—	—	—	20.3	15.1	19.7	15.6	13.3	9.9	10.4	9.9	10.7
55–64 years	—	—	—	43.7	49.0	42.1	37.6	33.3	27.2	28.8	25.2	26.0
65–74 years	—	—	—	136.1	129.9	124.0	101.0	102.8	81.0	80.8	72.6	77.7
75–84 years	—	—	—	446.6	387.0	396.6	381.8	386.0	269.2	284.2	259.7	238.1
85 years and over	—	—	—	1,545.2	1,383.3	1,395.0	1,197.0	1,246.6	928.3	777.0	802.4	758.2

Table B–34. Death Rates for Cerebrovascular Diseases, by Sex, Race, Hispanic Origin, and Age, Selected Years, 1950–2008—Continued

(Deaths per 100,000 resident population.)

Sex, race, Hispanic origin, and age	1950[1,2]	1960[1,2]	1970[2]	1980[2]	1985	1990[2]	1995	2000[3]	2005[3]	2006[3]	2007[3]	2008[3]
Hispanic or Latina Female[4,6]												
All ages, age-adjusted	—	—	—	—	47.5	43.7	42.7	43.0	33.5	32.3	30.8	28.9
All ages, crude	—	—	—	—	18.2	20.1	19.4	19.4	17.7	17.5	17.1	16.5
45–54 years	—	—	—	—	15.8	15.2	15.1	12.4	12.1	11.8	11.0	10.3
55–64 years	—	—	—	—	35.3	38.5	36.5	31.9	27.1	27.8	25.4	21.1
65–74 years	—	—	—	—	108.6	102.6	102.3	95.2	75.8	76.9	71.6	66.8
75–84 years	—	—	—	—	340.0	308.5	307.3	311.3	262.6	240.6	244.2	239.2
85 years and over	—	—	—	—	1,185.7	1,055.3	1,021.0	1,108.9	762.5	742.9	684.5	624.0
White, not Hispanic or Latina Female[6]												
All ages, age-adjusted	—	—	—	—	69.7	61.0	58.7	57.6	44.4	41.5	40.3	39.0
All ages, crude	—	—	—	—	80.8	77.2	81.5	85.5	69.6	65.5	64.7	63.4
45–54 years	—	—	—	—	14.3	13.2	12.3	10.9	10.2	10.1	9.8	9.2
55–64 years	—	—	—	—	37.8	35.7	32.6	29.9	23.3	23.5	22.1	22.1
65–74 years	—	—	—	—	133.2	116.9	111.4	107.6	83.6	79.0	75.9	73.9
75–84 years	—	—	—	—	550.8	461.9	445.9	438.3	347.2	325.9	314.4	304.9
85 years and over	—	—	—	—	1,920.7	1,714.7	1,666.8	1,661.6	1,227.3	1,118.7	1,103.7	1,061.5

* = Rates based on fewer than 20 deaths are considered unreliable and are not shown.
– = Data not available.
[1]Includes deaths of persons who were not residents of the 50 states and the District of Columbia.
[2]Underlying cause of death was coded according to the 6th Revision of the International Classification of Diseases (ICD) in 1950, 7th Revision in 1960, 8th Revision in 1970, and 9th Revision in 1980–1998.
[3]Starting with 1999 data, cause of death is coded according to ICD–10.
[4]The race groups, White, Black, Asian or Pacific Islander, and American Indian or Alaska Native, include persons of Hispanic and non–Hispanic origin. Persons of Hispanic origin may be of any race.
[5]In 1950, rate is for the age group 75 years and over.
[6]Prior to 1997, excludes data from states lacking an Hispanic-origin item on the death certificate.

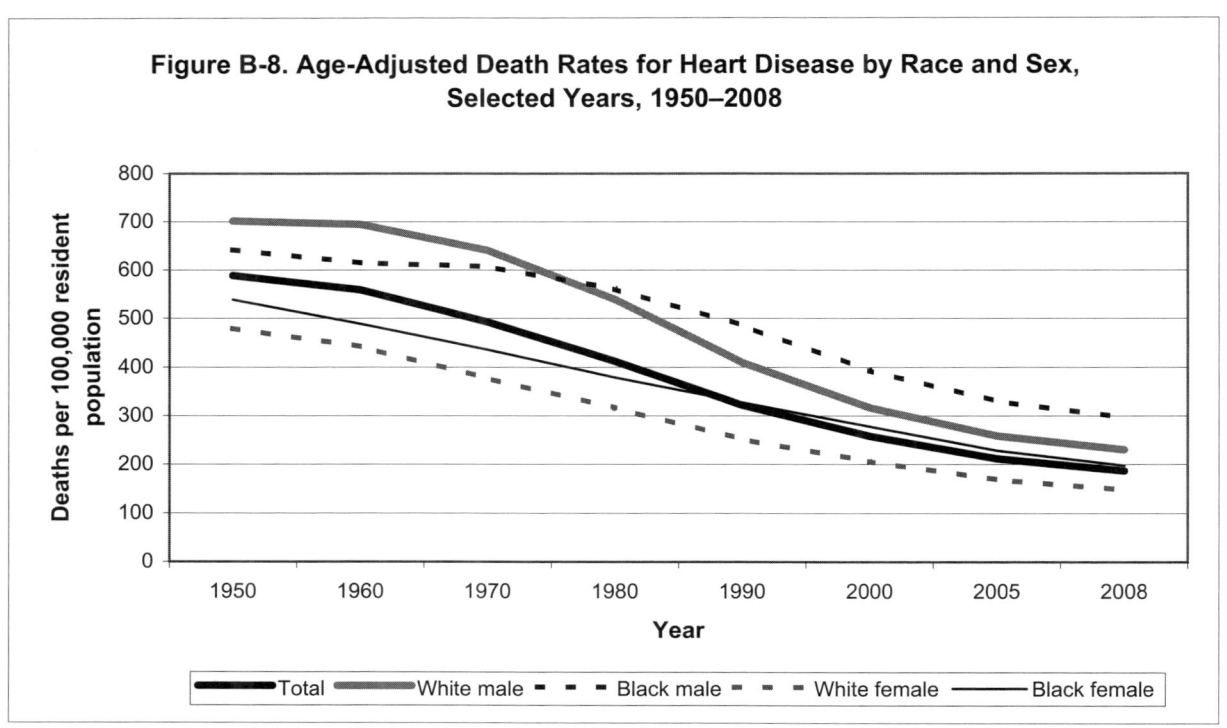

Figure B-8. Age-Adjusted Death Rates for Heart Disease by Race and Sex, Selected Years, 1950–2008

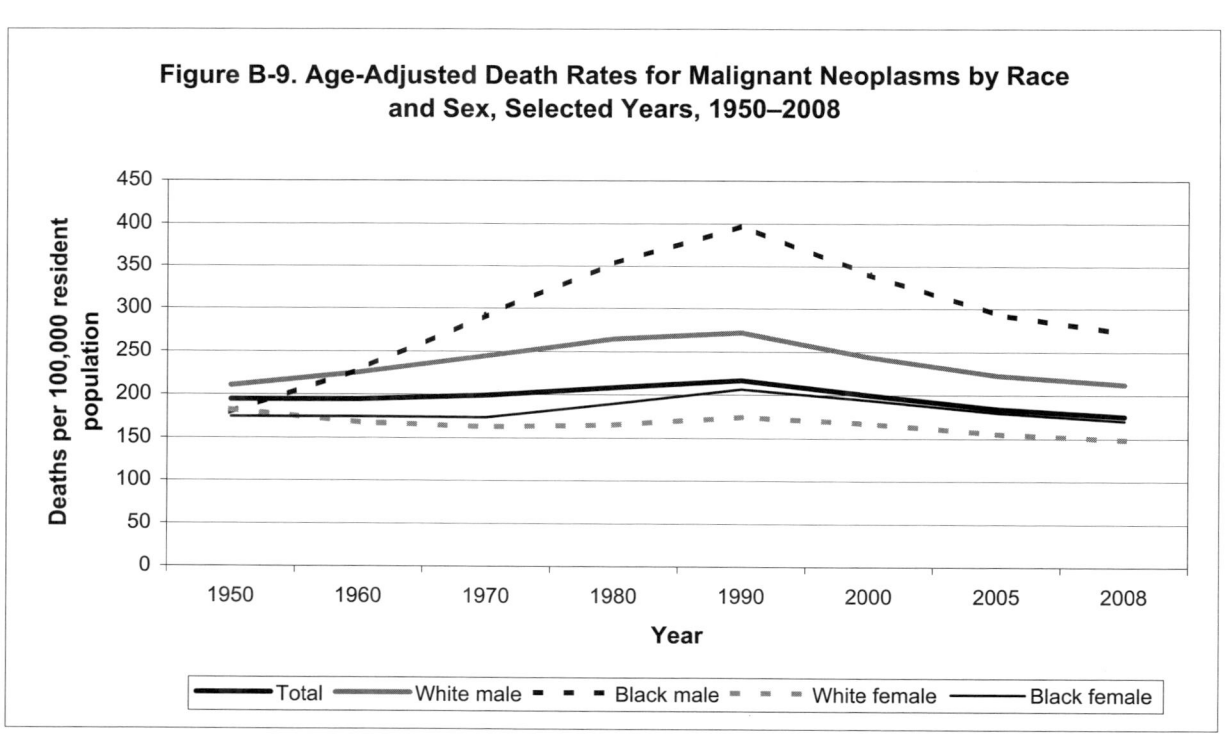

Figure B-9. Age-Adjusted Death Rates for Malignant Neoplasms by Race and Sex, Selected Years, 1950–2008

Table B–35. Death Rates for Malignant Neoplasms, by Sex, Race, Hispanic Origin, and Age, Selected Years, 1950–2008

(Deaths per 100,000 resident population.)

Sex, race, Hispanic origin, and age	1950[1,2]	1960[1,2]	1970[2]	1980[2]	1985	1990[2]	1995	2000[3]	2005[3]	2006[3]	2007[3]	2008[3]
All Persons												
All ages, age–adjusted	193.9	193.9	198.6	207.9	211.3	216.0	209.9	199.6	183.8	180.7	178.4	175.3
All ages, crude	139.8	149.2	162.8	183.9	194.0	203.2	202.2	196.5	188.7	187.0	186.6	186.0
Under 1 year	8.7	7.2	4.7	3.2	3.1	2.3	1.8	2.4	1.8	1.8	1.7	1.6
1–4 years	11.7	10.9	7.5	4.5	3.8	3.5	3.1	2.7	2.3	2.3	2.2	2.4
5–14 years	6.7	6.8	6.0	4.3	3.5	3.1	2.7	2.5	2.5	2.2	2.4	2.2
15–24 years	8.6	8.3	8.3	6.3	5.4	4.9	4.5	4.4	4.1	3.9	3.9	3.9
25–34 years	20.0	19.5	16.5	13.7	13.2	12.6	11.6	9.8	9.0	9.0	8.5	8.6
35–44 years	62.7	59.7	59.5	48.6	45.9	43.3	40.1	36.6	33.2	31.9	30.8	29.9
45–54 years	175.1	177.0	182.5	180.0	170.1	158.9	140.4	127.5	118.6	116.3	114.3	113.6
55–64 years	390.7	396.8	423.0	436.1	454.6	449.6	412.3	366.7	326.9	321.2	315.4	309.0
65–74 years	698.8	713.9	754.2	817.9	845.5	872.3	863.3	816.3	742.7	727.2	715.5	701.5
75–84 years	1,153.3	1,127.4	1,169.2	1,232.3	1,271.8	1,348.5	1,355.4	1,335.6	1,274.8	1,263.8	1,256.3	1,235.8
85 years and over	1,451.0	1,450.0	1,320.7	1,594.6	1,615.4	1,752.9	1,797.7	1,819.4	1,637.7	1,606.1	1,590.2	1,566.1
Male												
All ages, age–adjusted	208.1	225.1	247.6	271.2	274.4	280.4	267.5	248.9	225.1	220.1	217.5	213.6
All ages, crude	142.9	162.5	182.1	205.3	213.4	221.3	216.3	207.2	198.9	196.6	197.0	196.9
Under 1 year	9.7	7.7	4.4	3.7	3.0	2.4	1.9	2.6	2.1	1.8	1.8	2.2
1–4 years	12.5	12.4	8.3	5.2	4.3	3.7	3.6	3.0	2.6	2.5	2.3	2.6
5–14 years	7.4	7.6	6.7	4.9	3.9	3.5	3.0	2.7	2.7	2.5	2.4	2.2
15–24 years	9.7	10.2	10.4	7.8	6.4	5.7	5.4	5.1	4.8	4.6	4.5	4.7
25–34 years	17.7	18.8	16.3	13.4	13.2	12.6	11.3	9.2	8.8	8.6	8.2	8.5
35–44 years	45.6	48.9	53.0	44.0	42.4	38.5	36.3	32.7	28.9	27.4	26.4	25.8
45–54 years	156.2	170.8	183.5	188.7	175.2	162.5	141.5	130.9	121.6	119.0	117.5	117.7
55–64 years	413.1	459.9	511.8	520.8	536.9	532.9	475.1	415.8	369.5	363.6	358.5	354.1
65–74 years	791.5	890.5	1,006.8	1,093.2	1,105.2	1,122.2	1,083.0	1,001.9	899.1	870.4	854.3	837.8
75–84 years	1,332.6	1,389.4	1,588.3	1,790.5	1,839.7	1,914.4	1,847.9	1,760.6	1,649.7	1,631.3	1,617.4	1,587.5
85 years and over	1,668.3	1,741.2	1,720.8	2,369.5	2,451.8	2,739.9	2,818.7	2,710.7	2,319.3	2,248.7	2,249.2	2,181.0
Female												
All ages, age–adjusted	182.3	168.7	163.2	166.7	171.2	175.7	173.6	167.6	155.6	153.6	151.3	148.5
All ages, crude	136.8	136.4	144.4	163.6	175.7	186.0	188.8	186.2	178.8	177.6	176.5	175.3
Under 1 year	7.6	6.8	5.0	2.7	3.2	2.2	1.8	2.3	1.5	1.8	1.6	1.0
1–4 years	10.8	9.3	6.7	3.7	3.4	3.2	2.6	2.5	2.0	2.1	2.2	2.2
5–14 years	6.0	6.0	5.2	3.6	3.1	2.8	2.3	2.2	2.2	2.0	2.3	2.2
15–24 years	7.6	6.5	6.2	4.8	4.3	4.1	3.5	3.6	3.3	3.1	3.2	3.1
25–34 years	22.2	20.1	16.7	14.0	13.2	12.6	11.9	10.4	9.1	9.5	8.9	8.7
35–44 years	79.3	70.0	65.6	53.1	49.2	48.1	43.8	40.4	37.5	36.4	35.2	34.0
45–54 years	194.0	183.0	181.5	171.8	165.3	155.5	139.3	124.2	115.8	113.7	111.3	109.6
55–64 years	368.2	337.7	343.2	361.7	381.8	375.2	355.1	321.3	287.4	281.8	275.2	267.0
65–74 years	612.3	560.2	557.9	607.1	645.3	677.4	687.1	663.6	610.9	605.9	597.6	585.1
75–84 years	1,000.7	924.1	891.9	903.1	937.8	1,010.3	1,047.5	1,058.5	1,020.3	1,012.5	1,007.4	991.7
85 years and over	1,299.7	1,263.9	1,096.7	1,255.7	1,281.4	1,372.1	1,404.4	1,456.4	1,324.6	1,305.5	1,276.7	1,269.1
White Male[4]												
All ages, age–adjusted	210.0	224.7	244.8	265.1	267.1	272.2	260.6	243.9	222.3	217.9	215.1	211.7
All ages, crude	147.2	166.1	185.1	208.7	218.1	227.7	225.3	218.1	210.6	208.7	208.8	209.0
25–34 years	17.7	18.8	16.2	13.6	13.1	12.3	11.0	9.2	8.5	8.6	8.1	8.4
35–44 years	44.5	46.3	50.1	41.1	39.8	35.8	34.1	30.9	28.4	26.7	25.9	25.1
45–54 years	150.8	164.1	172.0	175.4	162.0	149.9	132.7	123.5	115.7	113.6	112.0	112.9
55–64 years	409.4	450.9	498.1	497.4	512.0	508.2	456.0	401.9	356.5	352.9	346.7	342.9
65–74 years	798.7	887.3	997.0	1,070.7	1,076.5	1,090.7	1,056.1	984.3	889.9	862.0	845.4	829.2
75–84 years	1,367.6	1,413.7	1,592.7	1,779.7	1,817.1	1,883.2	1,817.4	1,736.0	1,646.2	1,631.3	1,617.4	1,590.3
85 years and over	1,732.7	1,791.4	1,772.2	2,375.6	2,449.1	2,715.1	2,789.4	2,693.7	2,322.7	2,258.3	2,253.2	2,197.6
Black or African American Male[4]												
All ages, age–adjusted	178.9	227.6	291.9	353.4	373.9	397.9	374.3	340.3	293.7	284.9	282.3	272.4
All ages, crude	106.6	136.7	171.6	205.5	214.9	221.9	204.8	188.5	175.4	172.3	172.9	171.1
25–34 years	18.0	18.4	18.8	14.1	14.9	15.7	14.8	10.1	11.9	10.0	9.5	9.4
35–44 years	55.7	72.9	81.3	73.8	69.9	64.3	57.2	48.4	36.2	36.5	34.0	34.2
45–54 years	211.7	244.7	311.2	333.0	315.9	302.6	243.9	214.2	186.1	182.2	178.0	173.1
55–64 years	490.8	579.7	689.2	812.5	851.3	859.2	738.1	626.4	568.3	542.9	544.1	531.2
65–74 years	636.5	938.5	1,168.9	1,417.2	1,532.8	1,613.9	1,541.4	1,363.8	1,183.8	1,156.5	1,139.5	1,106.8
75–84 years[5]	853.5	1,053.3	1,624.8	2,029.6	2,229.6	2,478.3	2,449.8	2,351.8	2,017.5	1,979.1	1,936.9	1,880.4
85 years and over	—	1,155.2	1,387.0	2,393.9	2,629.0	3,238.3	3,395.5	3,264.8	2,683.7	2,543.3	2,637.1	2,408.5

Table B–35. Death Rates for Malignant Neoplasms, by Sex, Race, Hispanic Origin, and Age, Selected Years, 1950–2008—Continued

(Deaths per 100,000 resident population.)

Sex, race, Hispanic origin, and age	1950[1,2]	1960[1,2]	1970[2]	1980[2]	1985	1990[2]	1995	2000[3]	2005[3]	2006[3]	2007[3]	2008[3]
American Indian or Alaska Native Male[4]												
All ages, age–adjusted	—	—	—	140.5	142.1	145.8	169.0	155.8	147.6	135.5	139.4	142.0
All ages, crude	—	—	—	58.1	62.8	61.4	67.8	67.0	82.2	76.1	83.3	84.9
25–34 years	—	—	—	*	*	*	*	*	*	*	*	*
35–44 years	—	—	—	*	28.8	22.8	14.3	21.4	26.9	15.1	16.0	21.3
45–54 years	—	—	—	86.9	89.4	86.9	79.2	70.3	81.7	74.5	78.3	95.2
55–64 years	—	—	—	213.4	276.6	246.2	279.8	255.6	269.1	222.8	264.5	243.2
65–74 years	—	—	—	613.0	584.6	530.6	684.7	648.0	622.2	583.5	565.5	632.9
75–84 years	—	—	—	936.4	963.6	1,038.4	1,346.3	1,152.5	1,020.7	1,016.8	984.5	1,004.0
85 years and over	—	—	—	1,471.2	1,133.3	1,654.4	1,549.0	1,584.2	1,302.6	1,161.0	1,271.2	1,047.2
Asian or Pacific Islander Male[4]												
All ages, age–adjusted	—	—	—	165.2	173.4	172.5	164.3	150.8	133.0	126.7	130.2	128.8
All ages, crude	—	—	—	81.9	82.6	82.7	83.7	85.2	86.7	84.5	89.0	91.1
25–34 years	—	—	—	6.3	10.0	9.2	8.2	7.4	7.2	6.9	6.5	7.4
35–44 years	—	—	—	29.4	25.7	27.7	26.1	26.1	20.0	19.6	18.8	18.5
45–54 years	—	—	—	108.2	98.0	92.6	82.4	78.5	75.9	70.2	73.4	70.6
55–64 years	—	—	—	298.5	315.0	274.6	244.8	229.2	199.4	197.2	190.0	194.1
65–74 years	—	—	—	581.2	631.3	687.2	614.3	559.4	492.2	459.9	470.7	478.5
75–84 years	—	—	—	1,147.6	1,251.2	1,229.9	1,167.2	1,086.1	991.4	942.3	1,014.5	976.5
85 years and over	—	—	—	1,798.7	1,800.0	1,837.0	2,081.3	1,823.2	1,488.6	1,439.0	1,427.4	1,404.5
Hispanic or Latino Male[4,6]												
All ages, age–adjusted	—	—	—	—	161.3	174.7	180.9	171.7	152.7	143.4	141.4	139.6
All ages, crude	—	—	—	—	56.1	65.5	65.4	61.3	63.0	60.4	61.6	63.0
25–34 years	—	—	—	—	9.7	8.0	8.4	6.9	6.5	6.1	6.3	7.6
35–44 years	—	—	—	—	22.9	22.5	24.7	20.1	17.8	16.0	17.4	17.4
45–54 years	—	—	—	—	83.5	96.6	85.0	79.4	75.9	71.4	74.2	70.8
55–64 years	—	—	—	—	259.0	294.0	281.6	253.1	236.9	224.8	221.9	227.3
65–74 years	—	—	—	—	598.2	655.5	697.9	651.2	603.5	574.8	560.3	557.0
75–84 years	—	—	—	—	1,210.5	1,233.4	1,359.8	1,306.4	1,161.8	1,098.4	1,072.6	1,062.9
85 years and over	—	—	—	—	1,743.8	2,019.4	2,018.6	2,049.7	1,601.5	1,440.1	1,417.9	1,331.7
White, Not Hispanic or Latino Male[6]												
All ages, age–adjusted	—	—	—	—	259.0	276.7	263.5	247.7	227.3	223.4	220.8	217.3
All ages, crude	—	—	—	—	217.4	246.2	246.0	244.4	240.7	239.9	240.6	241.1
25–34 years	—	—	—	—	13.5	12.8	11.2	9.7	9.0	9.3	8.6	8.6
35–44 years	—	—	—	—	39.1	36.8	34.8	32.3	30.5	28.9	27.7	26.8
45–54 years	—	—	—	—	159.9	153.9	135.6	127.2	120.3	118.7	116.8	118.7
55–64 years	—	—	—	—	496.4	520.6	464.9	412.0	366.1	363.4	357.6	353.0
65–74 years	—	—	—	—	1,044.2	1,109.0	1,069.9	1,002.1	910.4	883.0	867.3	849.5
75–84 years	—	—	—	—	1,765.5	1,906.6	1,825.4	1,750.2	1,673.7	1,662.9	1,652.8	1,625.1
85 years and over	—	—	—	—	2,327.3	2,744.4	2,810.8	2,714.1	2,358.3	2,300.2	2,300.4	2,251.6
White Female[5]												
All ages, age–adjusted	182.0	167.7	162.5	165.2	169.9	174.0	172.1	166.9	155.2	153.6	151.2	148.5
All ages, crude	139.9	139.8	149.4	170.3	184.4	196.1	200.6	199.4	191.1	190.1	188.8	187.5
25–34 years	20.9	18.8	16.3	13.5	12.7	11.9	11.2	10.1	8.6	9.1	8.6	8.5
35–44 years	74.5	66.6	62.4	50.9	47.3	46.2	41.9	38.2	36.0	34.9	33.9	32.6
45–54 years	185.8	175.7	177.3	166.4	161.6	150.9	135.0	120.1	110.7	109.5	107.1	105.7
55–64 years	362.5	329.0	338.6	355.5	376.3	368.5	350.3	319.7	284.0	279.1	271.8	264.1
65–74 years	616.5	562.1	554.7	605.2	644.9	675.1	685.6	665.6	616.2	611.5	602.3	588.2
75–84 years	1,026.6	939.3	903.5	905.4	938.2	1,011.8	1,047.9	1,063.4	1,030.5	1,023.0	1,017.7	1,005.8
85 years and over	1,348.3	1,304.9	1,126.6	1,266.8	1,285.4	1,372.3	1,405.4	1,459.1	1,333.6	1,317.5	1,291.6	1,282.4
Black or African American Female[4]												
All ages, age–adjusted	174.1	174.3	173.4	189.5	195.5	205.9	203.8	193.8	179.6	176.1	174.9	170.0
All ages, crude	111.8	113.8	117.3	136.5	145.2	156.1	155.8	151.8	149.1	147.7	148.2	146.8
25–34 years	34.3	31.0	20.9	18.3	17.2	18.7	16.5	13.5	12.6	12.5	12.0	10.4
35–44 years	119.8	102.4	94.6	73.5	69.0	67.4	61.7	58.9	52.5	50.8	48.5	48.4
45–54 years	277.0	254.8	228.6	230.2	212.4	209.9	190.6	173.9	166.3	158.7	156.1	151.8
55–64 years	484.6	442.7	404.8	450.4	474.9	482.4	444.9	391.0	365.4	356.9	352.5	340.2
65–74 years	477.3	541.6	615.8	662.4	704.2	773.2	803.5	753.1	679.6	672.9	681.0	668.7
75–84 years[6]	605.3	696.3	763.3	923.9	986.3	1,059.9	1,120.8	1,124.0	1,071.9	1,065.3	1,071.7	1,015.6
85 years and over	—	728.9	791.5	1,159.8	1,284.2	1,431.3	1,446.2	1,527.7	1,365.8	1,324.4	1,265.2	1,285.4

Table B–35. Death Rates for Malignant Neoplasms, by Sex, Race, Hispanic Origin, and Age, Selected Years, 1950–2008—Continued

(Deaths per 100,000 resident population.)

Sex, race, Hispanic origin, and age	1950[1,2]	1960[1,2]	1970[2]	1980[2]	1985	1990[2]	1995	2000[3]	2005[3]	2006[3]	2007[3]	2008[3]
American Indian or Alaska Native Female[4]												
All ages, age–adjusted	—	—	—	94.0	93.0	106.9	117.7	108.3	105.9	108.3	102.1	102.3
All ages, crude	—	—	—	50.4	52.5	62.1	64.5	61.3	73.8	76.8	75.0	74.4
25–34 years	—	—	—	*	*	*	10.2	*	*	*	*	*
35–44 years	—	—	—	36.9	23.4	31.0	29.7	23.7	23.5	25.4	20.3	27.6
45–54 years	—	—	—	96.9	90.1	104.5	76.9	59.7	85.5	72.8	75.6	73.3
55–64 years	—	—	—	198.4	192.3	213.3	213.2	200.9	201.5	193.8	190.3	181.0
65–74 years	—	—	—	350.8	378.8	438.9	437.0	458.3	475.8	469.8	444.3	453.6
75–84 years	—	—	—	446.4	505.9	554.3	819.9	714.0	701.5	756.8	712.1	687.9
85 years and over	—	—	—	786.5	700.0	843.7	1,039.4	983.2	581.0	684.8	639.5	655.3
Asian or Pacific Islander Female[4]												
All ages, age–adjusted	—	—	—	93.0	99.6	103.0	107.4	100.7	94.5	92.2	90.0	90.6
All ages, crude	—	—	—	54.1	57.5	60.5	69.5	72.1	78.1	77.8	78.2	80.8
25–34 years	—	—	—	9.5	9.9	7.3	9.9	8.1	7.7	7.3	6.0	9.0
35–44 years	—	—	—	38.7	33.1	29.8	27.6	28.9	25.1	24.7	24.0	21.1
45–54 years	—	—	—	99.8	91.3	93.9	94.4	78.2	75.4	73.5	70.0	70.4
55–64 years	—	—	—	174.7	195.5	196.2	203.5	176.5	171.3	160.2	162.2	153.9
65–74 years	—	—	—	301.9	330.8	346.2	343.3	357.4	328.1	330.9	308.8	327.8
75–84 years	—	—	—	522.1	589.1	641.4	681.0	650.1	606.8	602.4	601.2	609.9
85 years and over	—	—	—	800.0	908.3	971.7	1,092.7	988.5	942.0	878.4	875.2	867.1
Hispanic or Latina Female[4,6]												
All ages, age–adjusted	—	—	—	—	101.5	111.9	110.8	110.8	101.9	100.4	98.6	96.6
All ages, crude	—	—	—	—	49.8	60.7	58.7	58.5	59.5	59.7	59.9	59.8
25–34 years	—	—	—	—	9.7	9.7	8.5	7.8	7.1	8.5	8.9	8.2
35–44 years	—	—	—	—	30.9	34.8	30.7	30.7	27.0	27.9	26.5	25.9
45–54 years	—	—	—	—	90.1	100.5	89.7	84.7	79.9	78.1	75.5	71.7
55–64 years	—	—	—	—	199.2	205.4	203.0	192.5	172.5	174.4	175.6	179.0
65–74 years	—	—	—	—	356.4	404.8	398.0	410.0	382.5	370.2	364.4	351.1
75–84 years	—	—	—	—	600.0	663.0	706.2	716.5	688.5	665.9	665.7	657.9
85 years and over	—	—	—	—	907.1	1,022.7	1,028.6	1,056.5	880.4	884.9	814.2	792.1
White, Not Hispanic or Latina Female[6]												
All ages, age–adjusted	—	—	—	—	167.1	177.5	174.7	170.0	159.1	157.6	155.3	152.6
All ages, crude	—	—	—	—	187.1	210.6	217.3	220.6	215.1	214.7	213.7	212.6
25–34 years	—	—	—	—	12.2	11.9	11.5	10.5	8.9	9.2	8.4	8.4
35–44 years	—	—	—	—	47.2	47.0	42.7	38.9	37.5	35.9	35.2	33.7
45–54 years	—	—	—	—	158.8	154.9	137.8	123.0	113.9	113.0	110.9	109.8
55–64 years	—	—	—	—	372.7	379.5	359.3	328.9	293.6	288.5	280.6	271.8
65–74 years	—	—	—	—	638.4	688.5	697.9	681.0	634.4	631.3	622.2	607.9
75–84 years	—	—	—	—	917.8	1,027.2	1,056.1	1,075.3	1,049.5	1,044.4	1,040.1	1,029.0
85 years and over	—	—	—	—	1,241.5	1,385.7	1,411.6	1,468.7	1,353.2	1,336.7	1,315.2	1,308.1

* = Rates based on fewer than 20 deaths are considered unreliable and are not shown.
– = Data not available.
[1]Includes deaths of persons who were not residents of the 50 states and the District of Columbia.
[2]Underlying cause of death was coded according to the 6th Revision of the International Classification of Diseases (ICD) in 1950, 7th Revision in 1960, 8th Revision in 1970.
[3]Starting with 1999 data, cause of death is coded according to ICD–10.
[4]The race groups, White, Black, Asian or Pacific Islander, and American Indian or Alaska Native, include persons of Hispanic and non–Hispanic origin. Persons of Hispanic origin may be of any race.
[5]In 1950, rate is for the age group 75 years and over.
[6]Prior to 1997, excludes data from states lacking an Hispanic–origin item on the death certificate.

Table B–36. Death Rates for Malignant Neoplasm of Breast Among Females, by Race, Hispanic Origin, and Age, Selected Years, 1950–2008

(Deaths per 100,000 resident population.)

Race, Hispanic origin, and age	1950[1,2]	1960[1,2]	1970[2]	1980[2]	1985	1990[2]	1995	2000[3]	2005[3]	2006[3]	2007[3]	2008[3]
All Females												
All ages, age–adjusted	31.9	31.7	32.1	31.9	33.0	33.3	30.5	26.8	24.1	23.5	22.9	22.5
All ages, crude	24.7	26.1	28.4	30.6	32.8	34.0	32.2	29.2	27.3	26.9	26.5	26.3
Under 25 years	*	*	*	*	0.0	*	*	*	*	*	*	*
25–34 years	3.8	3.8	3.9	3.3	3.0	2.9	2.6	2.3	1.8	1.8	1.7	1.6
35–44 years	20.8	20.2	20.4	17.9	17.5	17.8	14.9	12.4	11.3	10.8	10.1	10.1
45–54 years	46.9	51.4	52.6	48.1	47.1	45.4	41.0	33.0	28.7	27.6	26.7	26.3
55–64 years	69.9	70.8	77.6	80.5	84.2	78.6	69.4	59.3	54.5	53.7	51.3	49.9
65–74 years	95.0	90.0	93.8	101.1	107.8	111.7	102.8	88.3	79.2	76.9	77.3	76.6
75–84 years	139.8	129.9	127.4	126.4	136.2	146.3	140.1	128.9	119.2	119.2	116.3	113.3
85 years and over	195.5	191.9	157.1	169.3	178.5	196.8	200.2	205.7	177.9	169.9	170.4	167.3
White[4]												
All ages, age–adjusted	32.4	32.0	32.5	32.1	33.1	33.2	30.1	26.3	23.4	22.9	22.3	21.9
All ages, crude	25.7	27.2	29.9	32.3	34.7	35.9	33.8	30.7	28.3	27.9	27.6	27.3
35–44 years	20.8	19.7	20.2	17.3	16.8	17.1	14.0	11.3	10.2	9.8	9.1	9.0
45–54 years	47.1	51.2	53.0	48.1	46.8	44.3	38.9	31.2	26.2	25.6	24.7	24.4
55–64 years	70.9	71.8	79.3	81.3	84.7	78.5	68.3	57.9	52.4	52.0	49.4	48.2
65–74 years	96.3	91.6	95.9	103.7	109.9	113.3	103.3	89.3	79.3	77.1	77.3	75.7
75–84 years	143.6	132.8	129.6	128.4	138.8	148.2	141.4	130.2	120.7	120.4	117.3	114.1
85 years and over	204.2	199.7	161.9	171.7	180.9	198.0	202.6	205.5	179.1	170.3	172.1	168.3
Black or African American[4]												
All ages, age–adjusted	25.3	27.9	28.9	31.7	34.6	38.1	38.0	34.5	32.8	31.6	31.4	31.1
All ages, crude	16.4	18.7	19.7	22.9	25.9	29.0	29.6	27.9	28.4	27.5	27.7	27.8
35–44 years	21.0	24.8	24.4	24.1	26.1	25.8	22.9	20.9	20.2	19.0	18.2	18.0
45–54 years	46.5	54.4	52.0	52.7	55.5	60.5	61.9	51.5	50.0	44.5	44.3	43.0
55–64 years	64.3	63.2	64.7	79.9	90.4	93.1	89.1	80.9	81.1	76.3	75.7	71.2
65–74 years	67.0	72.3	77.3	84.3	100.7	112.2	117.9	98.6	96.2	91.2	96.0	100.3
75–84 years[5]	81.0	87.5	101.8	114.1	117.6	140.5	147.2	139.8	126.6	138.2	135.2	132.7
85 years and over	—	92.1	112.1	149.9	159.4	201.5	192.7	238.7	201.8	199.2	191.9	201.7
American Indian or Alaska Native[4]												
All ages, age–adjusted	—	—	—	10.8	12.1	13.7	15.0	13.6	15.2	12.8	12.7	12.6
All ages, crude	—	—	—	6.1	6.9	8.6	9.0	8.7	10.5	10.0	10.4	9.9
35–44 years	—	—	—	*	*	*	*	*	*	*	*	*
45–54 years	—	—	—	*	*	23.9	21.6	14.4	12.9	15.8	18.1	13.8
55–64 years	—	—	—	*	*	*	37.4	40.0	21.0	30.9	34.8	35.3
65–74 years	—	—	—	*	*	*	46.3	42.5	65.8	43.0	38.3	51.8
75–84 years	—	—	—	*	*	*	*	71.8	117.4	54.1	51.6	52.0
85 years and over	—	—	—	*	*	*	*	*	*	*	*	*
Asian or Pacific Islander[4]												
All ages, age–adjusted	—	—	—	11.9	13.2	13.7	13.9	12.3	12.2	12.1	11.1	11.7
All ages, crude	—	—	—	8.2	8.6	9.3	10.8	10.2	11.0	11.1	10.4	11.2
35–44 years	—	—	—	10.4	7.2	8.4	8.0	8.1	6.7	5.2	5.8	6.4
45–54 years	—	—	—	23.4	21.9	26.4	29.1	22.3	18.5	19.6	15.4	16.0
55–64 years	—	—	—	35.7	39.5	33.8	37.9	31.3	35.0	33.0	28.9	30.8
65–74 years	—	—	—	*	32.5	38.5	36.6	34.7	32.1	39.1	35.7	40.9
75–84 years	—	—	—	*	50.0	48.0	42.3	37.5	52.2	42.5	48.8	50.4
85 years and over	—	—	—	*	*	*	*	68.2	62.0	68.8	52.4	47.7
Hispanic or Latina[4,6]												
All ages, age–adjusted	—	—	—	—	16.3	19.5	18.7	16.9	15.0	15.0	14.5	14.3
All ages, crude	—	—	—	—	8.8	11.5	10.6	9.7	9.4	9.6	9.4	9.4
35–44 years	—	—	—	—	10.4	11.7	9.5	8.7	8.0	7.9	7.4	7.5
45–54 years	—	—	—	—	26.4	32.8	27.7	23.9	20.0	19.6	19.4	17.5
55–64 years	—	—	—	—	43.5	45.8	45.0	39.1	34.7	36.4	33.9	35.3
65–74 years	—	—	—	—	40.9	64.8	58.0	54.9	46.9	47.3	48.3	46.5
75–84 years	—	—	—	—	64.5	67.2	80.9	74.9	73.3	68.8	66.5	67.0
85 years and over	—	—	—	—	85.7	102.8	115.6	105.8	95.1	89.9	88.3	86.5

Table B–36. **Death Rates for Malignant Neoplasm of Breast Among Females, by Race, Hispanic Origin, and Age, Selected Years, 1950–2008**—Continued

(Deaths per 100,000 resident population.)

Race, Hispanic origin, and age	1950[1,2]	1960[1,2]	1970[2]	1980[2]	1985	1990[2]	1995	2000[3]	2005[3]	2006[3]	2007[3]	2008[3]
White, not Hispanic or Latina[6]												
All ages, age–adjusted	—	—	—	—	33.0	33.9	30.6	26.8	24.0	23.5	23.0	22.5
All ages, crude	—	—	—	—	35.6	38.5	36.6	33.8	31.8	31.4	31.1	30.7
35–44 years	—	—	—	—	16.9	17.5	14.4	11.6	10.6	10.0	9.3	9.3
45–54 years	—	—	—	—	46.8	45.2	39.5	31.7	26.8	26.3	25.3	25.2
55–64 years	—	—	—	—	85.1	80.6	69.5	59.2	53.9	53.4	50.8	49.3
65–74 years	—	—	—	—	108.6	115.7	105.4	91.4	81.9	79.6	79.8	78.1
75–84 years	—	—	—	—	139.4	151.4	143.2	132.2	123.4	123.6	120.7	117.3
85 years and over	—	—	—	—	175.6	201.5	204.4	208.3	182.9	174.1	176.3	172.7

* = Rates based on fewer than 20 deaths are considered unreliable and are not shown.
– = Data not available.
[1]Includes deaths of persons who were not residents of the 50 states and the District of Columbia.
[2]Underlying cause of death was coded according to the 6th Revision of the International Classification of Diseases (ICD) in 1950, 7th Revision in 1960, 8th Revision in 1970, and 9th Revision in 1980–1998.
[3]Starting with 1999 data, cause of death is coded according to ICD–10.
[4]The race groups, White, Black, Asian or Pacific Islander, and American Indian or Alaska Native, include persons of Hispanic and non–Hispanic origin. Persons of Hispanic origin may be of any race.
[5]In 1950, rate is for the age group 75 years and over.
[6]Prior to 1997, excludes data from states lacking an Hispanic-origin item on the death certificate.

Table B-37 Death Rates for Malignant Neoplasms of the Trachea, Bronchus, and Lung, by Sex, Race, Hispanic Origin, and Age, Selected Years, 1950–2008

(Deaths per 100,000 resident population.)

Sex, race, Hispanic origin, and age	1950[1,2]	1960[1,2]	1970[2]	1980[2]	1985	1990[2]	1995	2000[3]	2005[3]	2006[3]	2007[3]	2008[3]
All Persons												
All ages, age-adjusted	15.0	24.1	37.1	49.9	54.6	59.3	58.4	56.1	52.6	51.5	50.6	49.5
All ages, crude	12.2	20.3	32.1	45.8	51.5	56.8	56.8	55.3	53.7	53.0	52.6	52.2
Under 25 years	0.1	0.0	0.1	0.0	0.0	0.0	0.0	0.0	0.0	0.0	0.0	0.0
25–34 years	0.8	1.0	0.9	0.6	0.6	0.7	0.6	0.5	0.3	0.4	0.3	0.4
35–44 years	4.5	6.8	11.0	9.2	7.8	6.8	6.0	6.1	5.3	4.6	4.3	3.8
45–54 years	20.4	29.6	43.4	54.1	50.9	46.8	37.5	31.6	29.7	29.1	28.4	28.2
55–64 years	48.7	75.3	109.1	138.2	153.8	160.6	141.6	122.4	103.3	99.1	95.4	91.4
65–74 years	59.7	108.1	164.5	233.3	261.2	288.4	295.4	284.2	259.6	253.1	248.8	240.0
75–84 years	55.8	91.5	163.2	240.5	282.0	333.3	358.9	370.8	375.6	373.5	371.3	368.1
85 years and over	42.3	65.6	101.7	176.0	195.2	242.5	279.9	302.1	302.3	300.5	299.8	302.3
Male												
All ages, age-adjusted	24.6	43.6	67.5	85.2	88.6	91.1	84.2	76.7	69.0	67.0	65.1	63.6
All ages, crude	19.9	35.4	53.4	68.6	72.5	75.1	70.5	65.5	61.8	60.5	59.4	59.1
Under 25 years	0.0	0.0	0.1	0.1	*	0.0	0.1	*	*	*	0.0	0.1
25–34 years	1.1	1.4	1.3	0.8	0.7	0.9	0.7	0.5	0.4	0.4	0.4	0.4
35–44 years	7.1	10.5	16.1	11.9	10.0	8.5	7.0	6.9	5.5	4.7	4.2	3.9
45–54 years	35.0	50.6	67.5	76.0	67.5	59.7	46.3	38.5	35.1	33.8	32.1	32.3
55–64 years	83.8	139.3	189.7	213.6	223.5	222.9	185.3	154.0	127.6	121.6	116.2	112.6
65–74 years	98.7	204.3	320.8	403.9	416.2	430.4	414.3	377.9	330.7	319.4	310.2	298.7
75–84 years	82.6	167.1	330.8	488.8	537.6	572.9	553.8	532.2	515.1	509.9	498.3	489.5
85 years and over	62.5	107.7	194.0	368.1	433.2	513.2	540.3	521.2	468.0	457.7	453.0	456.0
Female												
All ages, age-adjusted	5.8	7.5	13.1	24.4	30.6	37.1	40.4	41.3	40.5	40.0	40.0	39.0
All ages, crude	4.5	6.4	11.9	24.3	31.7	39.4	43.6	45.4	45.9	45.7	46.0	45.5
Under 25 years	0.1	0.0	0.0	*	*	*	*	*	*	*	*	*
25–34 years	0.5	0.5	0.5	0.5	0.6	0.5	0.6	0.5	0.3	0.4	0.3	0.3
35–44 years	1.9	3.2	6.1	6.5	5.6	5.2	5.0	5.3	5.1	4.5	4.4	3.6
45–54 years	5.8	9.2	21.0	33.7	35.2	34.5	29.1	25.0	24.5	24.6	24.9	24.3
55–64 years	13.6	15.4	36.8	72.0	92.1	105.0	101.9	93.3	80.7	78.2	76.1	71.7
65–74 years	23.3	24.4	43.1	102.7	141.8	177.6	200.0	206.9	199.6	197.0	196.7	189.9
75–84 years	32.9	32.8	52.4	94.1	131.7	190.1	237.2	265.6	280.9	280.3	283.8	283.9
85 years and over	28.2	38.8	50.0	91.9	100.2	138.1	179.6	212.8	226.2	226.9	227.0	228.1
White Male[4]												
All ages, age-adjusted	25.1	43.6	67.1	83.8	86.8	89.0	82.6	75.7	68.7	66.8	64.8	63.4
All ages, crude	20.8	36.4	54.6	70.2	74.5	77.8	74.0	69.4	65.9	64.6	63.4	63.1
45–54 years	35.1	49.2	63.3	70.9	62.7	55.2	43.2	35.7	33.3	31.7	30.2	30.7
55–64 years	85.4	139.2	186.8	205.6	214.2	213.7	178.9	150.8	123.4	118.3	113.1	109.7
65–74 years	101.5	207.5	325.0	401.0	409.5	422.1	408.0	374.9	331.8	319.8	310.4	299.8
75–84 years	85.5	170.4	336.7	493.5	540.3	572.2	550.8	529.9	519.9	514.6	502.7	493.3
85 years and over	67.4	109.4	199.6	374.1	440.0	516.3	539.3	522.4	469.9	464.0	453.3	459.2
Black or African American Male[4]												
All ages, age-adjusted	17.8	42.6	75.4	107.6	117.2	125.4	115.1	101.1	86.4	83.7	82.2	78.5
All ages, crude	12.1	28.1	47.7	66.6	71.2	73.7	65.6	58.3	53.0	52.0	51.5	50.0
45–54 years	34.4	68.4	115.4	133.8	122.5	114.9	85.2	70.7	56.9	56.9	54.1	50.9
55–64 years	68.3	146.8	234.3	321.1	351.5	358.6	288.5	223.5	199.1	184.3	177.7	168.5
65–74 years	53.8	168.3	300.5	472.3	539.6	585.4	559.5	488.8	408.8	402.7	395.6	365.1
75–84 years[5]	36.2	107.3	271.6	472.9	556.4	645.4	667.1	642.5	565.2	563.9	546.2	545.6
85 years and over	—	82.8	137.0	311.3	382.3	499.5	583.0	562.8	495.5	442.3	504.8	481.5
American Indian or Alaska Native Male[4]												
All ages, age-adjusted	—	—	—	31.7	41.2	47.5	53.6	42.9	40.4	37.6	40.7	41.7
All ages, crude	—	—	—	14.2	18.4	20.0	21.8	18.1	22.6	21.2	23.8	24.3
45–54 years	—	—	—	*	*	26.6	23.8	14.5	19.8	18.3	14.4	19.2
55–64 years	—	—	—	72.0	85.1	97.8	98.9	86.0	83.0	64.4	82.4	71.4
65–74 years	—	—	—	202.8	223.1	194.3	261.5	184.8	191.2	202.2	202.6	225.3
75–84 years	—	—	—	*	263.6	356.2	409.7	367.9	305.8	294.1	300.5	317.2
85 years and over	—	—	—	*	*	*	*	*	*	*	286.3	219.9

Table B-37 Death Rates for Malignant Neoplasms of the Trachea, Bronchus, and Lung, by Sex, Race, Hispanic Origin, and Age, Selected Years, 1950–2008—Continued

(Deaths per 100,000 resident population.)

Sex, race, Hispanic origin, and age	1950[1,2]	1960[1,2]	1970[2]	1980[2]	1985	1990[2]	1995	2000[3]	2005[3]	2006[3]	2007[3]	2008[3]
Asian or Pacific Islander Male[4]												
All ages, age–adjusted	—	—	—	43.3	42.7	44.2	41.0	40.9	35.9	35.3	34.7	35.1
All ages, crude	—	—	—	22.1	20.4	20.7	20.7	22.7	22.9	23.2	22.9	24.2
45–54 years	—	—	—	33.3	21.7	18.8	18.6	17.2	15.6	18.0	17.1	16.6
55–64 years	—	—	—	94.4	98.1	74.4	64.4	61.4	57.3	56.2	44.1	50.7
65–74 years	—	—	—	174.3	180.8	215.8	184.0	183.2	144.1	141.2	135.2	140.7
75–84 years	—	—	—	301.3	295.3	307.5	296.6	323.2	286.1	285.6	301.5	294.9
85 years and over	—	—	—	*	350.0	421.3	439.0	378.0	381.2	342.6	357.3	346.4
Hispanic or Latino Male[4,6]												
All ages, age–adjusted	—	—	—	—	39.2	44.1	42.2	39.0	33.3	30.3	29.6	29.7
All ages, crude	—	—	—	—	12.9	16.2	14.8	13.3	13.0	12.0	12.0	12.4
45–54 years	—	—	—	—	16.7	21.5	17.5	14.8	11.9	10.5	10.3	9.6
55–64 years	—	—	—	—	68.6	80.7	69.9	58.6	52.3	44.8	42.1	43.2
65–74 years	—	—	—	—	169.9	195.5	192.0	167.3	151.4	140.1	140.7	135.2
75–84 years	—	—	—	—	292.1	313.4	324.4	327.5	281.6	254.2	246.1	259.8
85 years and over	—	—	—	—	393.8	420.7	382.8	368.8	269.0	263.9	256.1	247.1
White, not Hispanic or Latino Male[6]												
All ages, age–adjusted	—	—	—	—	84.2	91.1	84.1	77.9	71.4	69.7	67.7	66.3
All ages, crude	—	—	—	—	74.5	84.7	81.5	78.9	76.8	75.8	74.6	74.4
45–54 years	—	—	—	—	62.6	57.8	44.9	37.7	36.0	34.5	33.0	33.8
55–64 years	—	—	—	—	209.8	221.0	184.8	157.7	129.7	124.8	119.8	116.1
65–74 years	—	—	—	—	398.4	431.4	416.0	387.3	345.6	334.0	324.2	313.1
75–84 years	—	—	—	—	518.2	580.4	554.8	537.7	534.1	531.2	520.4	509.7
85 years and over	—	—	—	—	413.8	520.9	542.7	527.3	480.2	474.2	464.7	472.4
White Female[4]												
All ages, age–adjusted	5.9	6.8	13.1	24.5	31.0	37.6	41.1	42.3	41.5	41.1	41.2	40.2
All ages, crude	4.7	5.9	12.3	25.6	33.9	42.4	47.5	49.9	50.4	50.2	50.7	50.1
45–54 years	5.7	9.0	20.9	33.0	35.4	34.6	29.3	24.8	24.0	24.0	24.7	24.6
55–64 years	13.7	15.1	37.2	71.9	92.4	105.7	104.0	96.1	82.7	80.5	78.3	73.8
65–74 years	23.7	24.8	42.9	104.6	145.5	181.3	203.8	213.2	207.2	205.2	204.7	197.8
75–84 years	34.0	32.7	52.6	95.2	134.8	194.6	243.3	272.7	288.4	288.8	293.0	293.3
85 years and over	29.3	39.1	50.6	92.4	99.3	138.3	181.0	215.9	229.9	231.9	232.3	233.0
Black or African American Female[4]												
All ages, age–adjusted	4.5	6.8	13.7	24.8	29.7	36.8	38.8	39.8	40.0	39.0	38.1	36.9
All ages, crude	2.8	4.3	9.4	18.3	22.5	28.1	29.5	30.8	32.7	32.3	31.8	31.4
45–54 years	7.5	11.3	23.9	43.4	39.1	41.3	34.5	32.9	33.6	34.7	32.5	28.8
55–64 years	12.9	17.9	33.5	79.9	103.5	117.9	106.9	95.3	87.9	82.6	78.6	76.3
65–74 years	14.0	18.1	46.1	88.0	117.2	164.3	196.2	194.1	184.5	179.1	180.4	172.5
75–84 years[5]	*	31.3	49.1	79.4	101.2	148.1	183.2	224.3	253.5	251.3	249.3	247.6
85 years and over	—	34.2	44.8	85.8	114.3	134.9	158.9	185.9	205.9	191.9	190.9	203.7
American Indian or Alaska Native Female[4]												
All ages, age–adjusted	—	—	—	11.7	14.2	19.3	25.9	24.8	29.4	26.3	26.8	26.3
All ages, crude	—	—	—	6.0	8.2	11.2	13.8	14.0	20.0	18.5	19.2	18.4
45–54 years	—	—	—	*	*	22.9	*	12.1	18.6	12.1	10.9	12.4
55–64 years	—	—	—	*	38.5	53.7	45.7	52.6	56.8	59.7	52.3	43.9
65–74 years	—	—	—	*	93.9	78.5	134.6	151.5	166.1	144.7	160.0	129.6
75–84 years	—	—	—	*	*	111.8	209.5	136.3	192.8	173.0	180.6	205.4
85 years and over	—	—	—	*	*	*	*	*	*	*	*	157.3
Asian or Pacific Islander Female[4]												
All ages, age–adjusted	—	—	—	15.4	14.4	18.9	21.4	18.4	18.1	17.7	18.5	17.8
All ages, crude	—	—	—	8.4	7.9	10.5	13.0	12.6	14.5	14.5	15.7	15.4
45–54 years	—	—	—	13.5	12.5	11.3	11.6	9.9	10.9	10.2	10.6	10.0
55–64 years	—	—	—	24.6	26.0	38.3	37.6	30.4	28.1	27.5	33.2	27.2
65–74 years	—	—	—	62.4	60.7	71.6	84.2	77.0	74.7	75.0	74.7	76.5
75–84 years	—	—	—	117.7	97.8	137.9	153.5	135.0	140.0	130.0	139.8	143.1
85 years and over	—	—	—	*	*	172.9	235.5	175.3	163.9	166.4	166.2	142.1

Table B–37 Death Rates for Malignant Neoplasms of the Trachea, Bronchus, and Lung, by Sex, Race, Hispanic Origin, and Age, Selected Years, 1950–2008—Continued

(Deaths per 100,000 resident population.)

Sex, race, Hispanic origin, and age	1950[1,2]	1960[1,2]	1970[2]	1980[2]	1985	1990[2]	1995	2000[3]	2005[3]	2006[3]	2007[3]	2008[3]
Hispanic or Latina Female[4,6]												
All ages, age–adjusted	—	—	—	—	10.9	14.1	14.3	14.7	14.4	13.6	14.4	13.7
All ages, crude	—	—	—	—	4.9	7.2	7.1	7.2	7.8	7.5	8.2	7.9
45–54 years	—	—	—	—	6.8	8.7	7.1	7.1	7.1	6.3	6.7	7.3
55–64 years	—	—	—	—	17.4	25.1	25.5	22.2	20.4	19.0	22.2	21.3
65–74 years	—	—	—	—	49.1	66.8	59.2	66.0	63.1	65.2	56.7	62.9
75–84 years	—	—	—	—	73.6	94.3	111.0	112.3	114.9	107.6	111.7	106.9
85 years and over	—	—	—	—	110.7	118.2	128.3	137.5	129.0	106.0	123.0	106.9
White, not Hispanic or Latina Female[6]												
All ages, age–adjusted	—	—	—	—	31.7	39.0	42.5	44.1	43.7	43.5	43.5	42.6
All ages, crude	—	—	—	—	35.6	46.2	52.3	56.4	58.2	58.4	59.0	58.6
45–54 years	—	—	—	—	36.6	36.6	31.0	26.4	26.0	26.3	27.1	27.0
55–64 years	—	—	—	—	93.4	111.3	109.4	102.2	88.5	86.4	83.8	79.0
65–74 years	—	—	—	—	149.4	186.4	210.4	222.9	219.3	217.3	216.7	209.7
75–84 years	—	—	—	—	138.1	199.1	247.2	279.2	298.7	300.5	305.2	306.8
85 years and over	—	—	—	—	100.9	139.0	181.6	218.0	234.1	237.8	237.7	239.9

* = Rates based on fewer than 20 deaths are considered unreliable and are not shown.
– = Data not available.
0.0 = Quantity more than zero but less than 0.05.
[1]Includes deaths of persons who were not residents of the 50 states and the District of Columbia.
[2]Underlying cause of death was coded according to the 6th Revision of the International Classification of Diseases (ICD) in 1950, 7th Revision in 1960, 8th Revision in 1970, and 9th Revision in 1980–1998.
[3]Starting with 1999 data, cause of death is coded according to ICD–10.
[4]The race groups, White, Black, Asian or Pacific Islander, and American Indian or Alaska Native, include persons of Hispanic and non–Hispanic origin. Persons of Hispanic origin may be of any race.
[5]In 1950, rate is for the age group 75 years and over.
[6]Prior to 1997, excludes data from states lacking an Hispanic–origin item on the death certificate.

Table B–38. Death Rates for Human Immunodeficiency Virus (HIV) Disease, by Sex, Race, Hispanic Origin, and Age, Selected Years, 1987–2008

(Deaths per 100,000 resident population.)

Sex, race, Hispanic origin, and age[1]	1987[2]	1990[2]	1995[2]	2000[3]	2005[3]	2006[3]	2007[3]	2008[3]
All Persons								
All ages, age–adjusted[4]	5.6	10.2	16.2	5.2	4.2	4.0	3.7	3.3
All ages, crude	5.6	10.1	16.2	5.1	4.2	4.0	3.7	3.4
Under 1 year	2.3	2.7	1.5	*	*	*	*	*
1–4 years	0.7	0.8	1.3	*	*	*	*	*
5–14 years	0.1	0.2	0.5	0.1	*	*	*	*
15–24 years	1.3	1.5	1.7	0.5	0.4	0.5	0.4	0.4
25–34 years	11.7	19.7	28.3	6.1	3.3	2.9	2.7	2.4
35–44 years	14.0	27.4	44.2	13.1	9.9	9.2	8.3	6.7
45–54 years	8.0	15.2	26.0	11.0	10.6	10.1	9.5	8.4
55–64 years	3.5	6.2	10.9	5.1	5.3	5.5	5.3	5.7
65–74 years	1.3	2.0	3.6	2.2	2.3	2.5	2.3	2.6
75–84 years	0.8	0.7	0.7	0.7	0.8	0.8	0.8	0.9
85 years and over	*	*	*	*	*	*	*	0.5
Male								
All ages, age–adjusted	10.4	18.5	27.3	7.9	6.2	5.9	5.4	4.8
All ages, crude	10.2	18.5	27.6	7.9	6.3	5.9	5.4	4.9
Under 1 year	2.2	2.4	1.7	*	*	*	*	*
1–4 years	0.7	0.8	1.2	*	*	*	*	*
5–14 years	0.2	0.3	0.5	0.1	*	*	*	*
15–24 years	2.2	2.2	2.0	0.5	0.4	0.6	0.4	0.4
25–34 years	20.7	34.5	45.5	8.0	4.0	3.5	3.2	2.9
35–44 years	26.3	50.2	75.5	19.8	14.3	12.9	11.6	9.1
45–54 years	15.5	29.1	46.2	17.8	16.4	15.3	14.0	12.6
55–64 years	6.8	12.0	19.7	8.7	8.8	8.9	8.5	9.3
65–74 years	2.4	3.7	6.4	3.8	4.1	4.2	4.2	4.2
75–84 years	1.2	1.1	1.3	1.3	1.4	1.6	1.6	1.6
85 years and over	*	*	*	*	*	*	*	*
Female								
All ages, age–adjusted	1.1	2.2	5.3	2.5	2.3	2.2	2.1	1.9
All ages, crude	1.1	2.2	5.3	2.5	2.2	2.2	2.1	1.9
Under 1 year	2.5	3.0	1.2	*	*	*	*	*
1–4 years	0.7	0.8	1.5	*	*	*	*	*
5–14 years	*	0.2	0.5	0.1	*	*	*	*
15–24 years	0.3	0.7	1.4	0.4	0.3	0.4	0.3	0.4
25–34 years	2.8	4.9	10.9	4.2	2.6	2.3	2.2	1.8
35–44 years	2.1	5.2	13.3	6.5	5.6	5.4	4.9	4.2
45–54 years	0.8	1.9	6.6	4.4	5.1	5.1	5.1	4.3
55–64 years	0.5	1.1	2.8	1.8	2.0	2.3	2.2	2.3
65–74 years	0.5	0.8	1.4	0.8	0.9	1.1	0.8	1.2
75–84 years	0.5	0.4	0.3	0.3	0.4	0.3	0.3	0.4
85 years and over	*	*	*	*	*	*	*	*
All Ages, Age–Adjusted								
White male	8.7	15.7	20.4	4.6	3.6	3.4	3.1	2.8
Black or African American male	26.2	46.3	89.0	35.1	28.2	26.3	24.5	21.9
American Indian or Alaska Native male	*	3.3	10.5	3.5	4.0	3.3	3.6	3.3
Asian or Pacific Islander male	2.5	4.3	6.0	1.2	1.0	1.1	0.8	1.0
Hispanic or Latino male[4]	18.8	28.8	40.8	10.6	7.5	7.0	6.3	5.4
White, not Hispanic or Latino male[4]	10.7	14.1	17.9	3.8	3.0	2.8	2.5	2.3
White female	0.6	1.1	2.5	1.0	0.8	0.7	0.7	0.7
Black or African American female	4.6	10.1	24.4	13.2	12.0	12.2	11.3	9.8
American Indian or Alaska Native female	*	*	2.5	1.0	1.5	1.5	1.7	*
Asian or Pacific Islander female	*	*	0.6	0.2	*	*	*	0.3
Hispanic or Latina female[4]	2.1	3.8	8.8	2.9	1.9	1.9	1.8	1.7
White, not Hispanic or Latina female[4]	0.5	0.7	1.7	0.7	0.6	0.6	0.5	0.5
Age 25–44 Years								
All persons	12.7	23.2	36.3	9.8	6.8	6.2	5.6	4.6
White male	19.2	35.0	46.1	8.8	5.7	5.1	4.5	3.6
Black or African American male	60.2	102.0	179.4	55.4	36.2	32.9	29.4	23.5
American Indian or Alaska Native male	*	7.7	28.5	5.5	6.1	5.4	5.1	4.2
Asian or Pacific Islander male	4.1	8.1	12.1	1.9	1.4	1.0	0.9	1.6
Hispanic or Latino male[4]	36.8	59.3	73.9	14.3	8.3	7.6	6.5	5.3
White, not Hispanic or Latino male[4]	23.3	31.6	41.2	7.4	4.9	4.3	3.7	3.0

Table B-38. Death Rates for Human Immunodeficiency Virus (HIV) Disease, by Sex, Race, Hispanic Origin, and Age, Selected Years, 1987–2008—*Continued*

(Deaths per 100,000 resident population.)

Sex, race, Hispanic origin, and age	1987[2]	1990[2]	1995[2]	2000[3]	2005[3]	2006[3]	2007[3]	2008[3]
White female	1.2	2.3	5.9	2.1	1.5	1.3	1.2	1.1
Black or African American female	11.6	23.6	53.6	26.7	20.7	19.9	18.6	15.0
American Indian or Alaska Native female	*	*	*	*	*	*	*	*
Asian or Pacific Islander female	*	*	1.2	*	*	*	*	*
Hispanic or Latina female[4]	4.9	8.9	17.2	4.6	2.6	2.5	2.3	2.1
White, not Hispanic or Latina female[4]	1.0	1.5	4.2	1.6	1.2	1.0	0.9	0.8
Age 45–64 Years								
All persons	5.8	11.1	19.9	8.7	8.4	8.1	7.7	7.2
White male	9.9	18.6	26.0	8.1	7.3	7.2	6.4	6.2
Black or African American male	27.3	53.0	133.2	71.6	66.2	61.4	58.3	54.2
American Indian or Alaska Native male	*	*	*	*	8.9	6.4	7.6	7.4
Asian or Pacific Islander male	*	6.5	9.1	2.1	2.0	2.3	2.2	1.9
Hispanic or Latino male[4]	25.8	37.9	67.1	23.3	18.0	16.6	14.9	13.2
White, not Hispanic or Latino male[4]	12.6	16.9	22.4	6.5	6.0	5.9	5.2	5.3
White female	0.5	0.9	2.4	1.3	1.4	1.3	1.4	1.3
Black or African American female	2.6	7.5	27.0	19.6	22.0	23.4	22.1	19.2
American Indian or Alaska Native female	*	*	*	*	*	*	*	*
Asian or Pacific Islander female	*	*	*	*	*	*	*	*
Hispanic or Latina female[4]	*	3.1	12.6	5.8	4.1	3.9	4.1	3.8
White, not Hispanic or Latina female[4]	0.5	0.7	1.5	0.9	1.1	0.9	1.0	1.0

* = Rates based on fewer than 20 deaths are considered unreliable and are not shown.
[1]The race groups, White, Black, Asian or Pacific Islander, and American Indian or Alaska Native, include persons of Hispanic and non–Hispanic origin. Persons of Hispanic origin may be of any race.
[2]Categories for the coding and classification of human immunodeficiency virus (HIV) disease were introduced in the United States in 1987. For the period 1987–1998, underlying cause of death was coded according to the 9th Revision of the International Classification of Diseases (ICD).
[3]Starting with 1999 data, cause of death is coded according to ICD–10.
[4]Prior to 1997, excludes data from states lacking an Hispanic–origin item on the death certificate.

Table B–39. Death Rates for Drug Poisoning and Drug Poisoning Involving Opioid Analgesics, by Sex, Age, Race, and Hispanic Origin, Selected Years, 1999–2008

(Rate per 100,000 resident population.)

Sex, age, race, and Hispanic origin	Drug poisoning deaths per 100,000 resident population[1]									
	1999	2000	2001	2002	2003	2004	2005	2006	2007	2008
All Persons										
All ages, age-adjusted	6.1	6.2	6.8	8.1	8.9	9.3	10.0	11.4	11.8	11.9
All ages, crude	6.0	6.2	6.8	8.2	8.9	9.3	10.1	11.5	11.9	12.0
Under 15 years	0.1	0.1	0.2	0.2	0.2	0.2	0.2	0.2	0.2	0.2
15–24 years	3.2	3.7	4.3	5.2	6.0	6.6	6.9	8.2	8.4	8.2
25–34 years	8.1	7.9	8.6	10.3	11.3	11.7	13.3	15.7	16.4	16.5
35–44 years	14.0	14.3	15.5	18.0	18.8	19.1	19.4	21.5	21.2	20.9
45–54 years	11.1	11.6	13.1	16.1	18.0	19.3	21.1	24.1	25.1	25.3
55–64 years	4.2	4.2	4.7	6.0	7.0	7.9	9.1	10.6	12.4	13.0
65–74 years	2.4	2.0	2.4	2.8	2.9	3.0	3.3	3.6	4.1	4.7
75–84 years	2.8	2.4	2.5	2.8	2.7	2.9	3.1	3.3	3.2	3.3
85 years and over	3.8	4.4	3.6	4.2	3.9	3.8	3.8	4.0	4.1	3.7
Male										
All ages, age-adjusted	8.2	8.3	9.0	10.5	11.4	11.7	12.7	14.6	14.8	14.8
All ages, crude	8.2	8.4	9.1	10.6	11.5	11.8	12.8	14.8	15.0	15.0
Under 15 years	0.1	0.2	0.2	0.2	0.2	0.2	0.2	0.2	0.3	0.2
15–24 years	4.5	5.3	6.2	7.4	8.8	9.6	10.1	12.1	12.2	12.1
25–34 years	11.5	11.3	12.0	14.4	15.4	16.1	18.0	21.8	22.5	22.8
35–44 years	19.2	19.5	20.6	23.2	24.1	23.6	24.1	27.1	26.3	25.3
45–54 years	15.2	15.7	17.1	20.2	22.6	23.7	25.8	29.7	29.2	29.6
55–64 years	4.9	4.4	5.2	6.9	7.9	8.7	10.7	12.5	14.2	15.0
65–74 years	2.7	2.1	2.7	2.8	3.0	3.0	3.4	3.5	4.5	4.9
75–84 years	2.5	2.5	2.6	3.1	2.9	2.8	3.4	3.3	3.2	3.3
85 years and over	4.4	5.9	3.5	5.3	4.4	4.4	4.7	4.3	4.4	3.9
Female										
All ages, age-adjusted	3.9	4.1	4.7	5.8	6.4	6.9	7.3	8.2	8.9	9.0
All ages, crude	3.9	4.1	4.6	5.8	6.4	6.9	7.4	8.3	9.0	9.1
Under 15 years	0.1	0.1	0.1	0.2	0.1	0.2	0.2	0.2	0.2	0.2
15–24 years	1.8	1.9	2.3	2.8	3.2	3.4	3.6	4.0	4.3	4.1
25–34 years	4.6	4.6	5.2	6.1	7.0	7.2	8.4	9.4	10.1	9.9
35–44 years	8.7	9.2	10.4	12.7	13.6	14.7	14.7	15.9	16.1	16.5
45–54 years	7.2	7.7	9.2	12.2	13.5	15.0	16.5	18.6	21.1	21.1
55–64 years	3.5	3.9	4.2	5.2	6.1	7.1	7.6	8.9	10.7	11.2
65–74 years	2.1	2.0	2.2	2.8	2.9	3.0	3.2	3.6	3.8	4.5
75–84 years	3.0	2.3	2.4	2.7	2.6	2.9	2.9	3.3	3.2	3.3
85 years and over	3.5	3.9	3.7	3.7	3.6	3.5	3.4	3.9	4.0	3.7
All Ages, Age-Adjusted[2]										
Male:										
White	8.1	8.4	9.2	11.0	12.0	12.5	13.4	15.4	16.0	16.2
Black or African American	11.5	10.8	11.1	11.6	11.4	11.2	13.0	15.5	13.3	11.6
American Indian or Alaska Native	5.7	6.1	5.9	8.4	9.8	11.9	11.8	14.4	11.9	15.7
Asian or Pacific Islander	1.5	1.4	1.6	1.9	1.7	2.1	2.2	2.4	2.2	2.2
Hispanic or Latino	8.6	7.1	6.6	7.8	8.2	7.3	8.2	8.8	8.6	8.3
White, not Hispanic or Latino	8.0	8.6	9.6	11.6	12.8	13.6	14.5	17.0	17.7	18.0
Female:										
White	4.0	4.3	4.9	6.2	6.8	7.5	8.0	8.9	9.8	10.1
Black or African American	3.9	4.1	4.4	5.0	5.2	5.5	6.0	6.3	6.4	5.5
American Indian or Alaska Native	4.6	3.7	5.3	5.8	7.7	8.4	9.4	8.8	11.1	10.3
Asian or Pacific Islander	1.0	0.8	0.8	1.1	1.2	1.1	1.3	1.5	1.6	1.4
Hispanic or Latina	2.2	2.0	2.1	2.6	2.9	3.0	3.1	3.5	3.1	3.3
White, not Hispanic or Latina	4.3	4.5	5.3	6.7	7.5	8.3	8.8	9.9	10.9	11.3

Table B–39. Death Rates for Drug Poisoning and Drug Poisoning Involving Opioid Analgesics, by Sex, Age, Race, and Hispanic Origin, Selected Years, 1999–2008—Continued

(Rate per 100,000 resident population.)

Sex, age, race, and Hispanic origin	Drug poisoning deaths involving opioid analgesics per 100,000 resident population[3]									
	1999	2000	2001	2002	2003	2004	2005	2006	2007	2008
All Persons										
All ages, age-adjusted	1.4	1.5	1.9	2.6	2.9	3.4	3.7	4.5	4.7	4.8
All ages, crude	1.4	1.6	1.9	2.6	2.9	3.4	3.7	4.6	4.8	4.9
Under 15 years	*	0.0	0.0	0.1	0.1	0.1	0.1	0.1	0.1	0.1
15–24 years	0.7	0.8	1.3	1.7	2.2	2.7	2.7	3.8	3.9	3.7
25–34 years	1.9	1.9	2.3	3.3	3.7	4.4	5.2	6.7	7.1	7.1
35–44 years	3.5	3.7	4.4	5.7	6.2	6.8	6.9	8.2	8.3	8.3
45–54 years	2.9	3.2	4.0	5.4	6.2	7.1	7.9	9.6	9.8	10.4
55–64 years	1.0	1.1	1.4	1.8	2.2	2.6	3.1	3.9	4.7	5.0
65–74 years	0.4	0.4	0.4	0.7	0.7	0.8	1.0	1.1	1.2	1.5
75–84 years	0.3	0.2	0.3	0.4	0.4	0.5	0.6	0.6	0.6	0.6
85 years and over	*	*	*	0.6	0.6	0.5	0.8	0.6	0.8	0.6
Male										
All ages, age-adjusted	2.0	2.0	2.5	3.3	3.7	4.1	4.5	5.8	5.8	5.9
All ages, crude	2.0	2.1	2.5	3.3	3.7	4.2	4.6	5.9	5.9	6.0
Under 15 years	*	*	0.1	0.1	0.1	0.1	0.1	0.1	0.1	0.1
15–24 years	1.0	1.2	2.0	2.6	3.3	4.2	4.2	5.8	5.9	5.7
25–34 years	2.7	2.7	3.1	4.5	4.9	5.9	6.9	9.3	9.8	9.8
35–44 years	5.0	4.9	5.7	7.0	7.7	8.1	8.2	10.3	9.9	9.8
45–54 years	3.9	4.3	5.1	6.8	7.5	8.2	9.4	11.3	10.8	11.8
55–64 years	1.1	1.0	1.4	1.9	2.4	2.8	3.5	4.3	5.2	5.4
65–74 years	0.5	0.3	0.4	0.6	0.7	0.7	0.8	1.0	1.1	1.5
75–84 years	*	*	0.4	0.4	*	0.4	0.6	0.6	0.5	0.5
85 years and over	*	*	*	*	*	*	*	*	1.1	*
Female										
All ages, age-adjusted	0.9	1.1	1.4	1.9	2.1	2.5	2.8	3.3	3.6	3.7
All ages, crude	0.9	1.1	1.4	1.9	2.1	2.5	2.8	3.3	3.7	3.7
Under 15 years	*	*	*	*	*	0.1	*	0.1	0.1	0.1
15–24 years	0.3	0.4	0.6	0.8	1.0	1.1	1.2	1.7	1.9	1.6
25–34 years	1.1	1.2	1.5	2.0	2.4	2.8	3.3	4.0	4.3	4.2
35–44 years	2.1	2.5	3.2	4.4	4.7	5.4	5.6	6.2	6.6	6.8
45–54 years	1.9	2.2	3.0	4.2	4.9	5.9	6.6	8.0	8.9	9.0
55–64 years	0.8	1.1	1.3	1.6	2.0	2.4	2.8	3.6	4.3	4.6
65–74 years	0.3	0.4	0.4	0.8	0.7	0.9	1.2	1.1	1.3	1.4
75–84 years	0.4	*	0.3	0.4	0.5	0.6	0.6	0.6	0.7	0.7
85 years and over	*	*	*	*	*	0.6	*	0.8	0.7	0.6	0.7
All Ages, Age-Adjusted[2]										
Male:										
White	2.2	2.3	2.8	3.7	4.3	4.7	5.2	6.5	6.7	6.9
Black or African American	1.2	1.2	1.4	1.6	1.5	1.8	2.1	3.6	2.3	2.3
American Indian or Alaska Native	*	1.9	1.6	2.8	3.2	4.7	4.8	6.0	4.6	6.9
Asian or Pacific Islander	*	*	*	0.6	*	0.4	0.5	0.6	0.4	0.5
Hispanic or Latino	2.9	1.7	1.8	2.0	2.3	2.1	2.2	2.7	2.8	2.8
White, not Hispanic or Latino	2.1	2.3	3.0	4.0	4.6	5.3	5.8	7.4	7.7	7.8
Female:										
White	1.0	1.2	1.5	2.1	2.4	2.9	3.1	3.8	4.2	4.2
Black or African American	0.6	0.6	0.8	1.0	1.0	1.2	1.4	1.8	1.7	1.6
American Indian or Alaska Native	*	*	1.9	2.1	3.0	2.9	4.1	3.6	5.1	5.4
Asian or Pacific Islander	*	*	*	*	*	*	*	0.4	0.4	0.5
Hispanic or Latina	0.5	0.5	0.5	1.0	0.9	1.0	1.0	1.3	1.2	1.2
White, not Hispanic or Latina	1.1	1.3	1.7	2.3	2.7	3.2	3.5	4.2	4.7	4.8

* = Rates based on fewer than 20 deaths are considered unreliable and are not shown.
0.0 = Rate more than zero but less than 0.05.
[1]Drug poisoning was coded using underlying cause of death according to the 10th Revision of the International Classification of Diseases (ICD–10).
[2]The race groups, white, black, Asian or Pacific Islander, and American Indian or Alaska Native, include persons of Hispanic and non–Hispanic origin. Persons of Hispanic origin may be of any race.
[3]Opioid analgesics include pharmaceutical opioids such as hydrocodone, codeine, and methadone, and synthetic narcotics such as fentanyl and propoxyphene, an underlying cause of drug poisoning and with opioid analgesics mentioned in the (ICD–10) multiple causes of death.

Table B-40. Unintentional Motor Vehicle Deaths by States, Annual Averages, 2000–2007

(Deaths per 100,000 population.)

State	Deaths per 100,000 population
United States	14.7
Mississippi	30.6
Wyoming	25.7
Montana	24.9
Arkansas	24.7
Alabama	24.6
South Carolina	23.8
New Mexico	22.5
South Dakota	21.9
Louisiana	21.9
Tennessee	21.8
Kentucky	20.9
West Virginia	20.9
Oklahoma	20.6
North Carolina	19.3
Missouri	19.2
Idaho	19.0
Arizona	19.0
Florida	18.4
Georgia	17.8
Kansas	17.7
Texas	17.2
Nevada	16.7
North Dakota	16.5
Nebraska	15.6
Delaware	15.2
Alaska	14.9
Indiana	14.9
Colorado	14.7
Wisconsin	14.2
Iowa	14.1
Maine	13.8
Utah	13.2
Oregon	13.2
Virginia	12.9
Michigan	12.6
Pennsylvania	12.5
Vermont	12.3
Maryland	12.1
Ohio	12.0
Minnesota	12.0
California	11.7
Illinois	11.5
Washington	11.2
New Hampshire	10.4
Hawaii	10.3
Connecticut	9.1
New Jersey	8.7
District of Columbia	8.3
Rhode Island	8.1
New York	7.8
Massachusetts	7.4

NOTE: States listed are where deaths occurred, not state of residence.

Table B–41. Death Rates for Motor Vehicle–Related Injuries, by Sex, Race, Hispanic Origin, and Age, Selected Years, 1950–2008

(Deaths per 100,000 resident population.)

Sex, race, Hispanic origin, and age	1950[1,2]	1960[1,2]	1970[2]	1980[2]	1985	1990[2]	1995	2000[3]	2005[3]	2006[3]	2007[3]	2008[3]
All Persons												
All ages, age–adjusted	24.6	23.1	27.6	22.3	18.6	18.5	16.3	15.4	15.2	15.0	14.4	12.9
All ages, crude	23.1	21.3	26.9	23.5	19.3	18.8	16.3	15.4	15.3	15.1	14.6	13.1
Under 1 year	8.4	8.1	9.8	7.0	4.9	4.9	4.7	4.4	3.6	3.4	2.9	2.4
1–14 years	9.8	8.6	10.5	8.2	7.0	6.0	5.3	4.3	3.6	3.4	3.2	2.6
1–4 years	11.5	10.0	11.5	9.2	7.2	6.3	5.2	4.2	3.8	3.6	3.3	2.8
5–14 years	8.8	7.9	10.2	7.9	6.9	5.9	5.3	4.3	3.6	3.3	3.2	2.6
15–24 years	34.4	38.0	47.2	44.8	35.7	34.1	28.9	26.9	25.9	26.0	24.9	21.0
15–19 years	29.6	33.9	43.6	43.0	33.5	33.1	28.1	26.0	23.6	23.2	22.0	17.9
20–24 years	38.8	42.9	51.3	46.6	37.6	35.0	29.7	28.0	28.2	28.8	27.8	24.2
25–34 years	24.6	24.3	30.9	29.1	23.0	23.6	19.2	17.3	18.0	18.2	17.5	16.1
35–44 years	20.3	19.3	24.9	20.9	17.2	16.9	15.3	15.3	15.4	15.3	14.8	13.3
45–64 years	25.2	23.0	26.5	18.0	15.4	15.7	14.1	14.3	14.9	14.9	14.2	13.4
45–54 years	22.2	21.4	25.5	18.6	15.2	15.6	13.8	14.2	15.1	15.3	14.9	13.7
55–64 years	29.0	25.1	27.9	17.4	15.6	15.9	14.5	14.4	14.7	14.3	13.3	12.9
65 years and over	43.1	34.7	36.2	22.5	21.7	23.1	22.6	21.4	20.1	19.0	18.6	16.8
65–74 years	39.1	31.4	32.8	19.2	17.9	18.6	17.5	16.5	16.7	15.4	15.2	14.0
75–84 years	52.7	41.8	43.5	28.1	27.4	29.1	28.4	25.7	22.9	22.3	21.8	19.3
85 years and over	45.1	37.9	34.2	27.6	26.5	31.2	31.0	30.4	25.1	23.4	23.2	21.1
Male												
All ages, age–adjusted	38.5	35.4	41.5	33.6	27.2	26.5	22.8	21.7	21.7	21.4	20.9	18.8
All ages, crude	35.4	31.8	39.7	35.3	28.0	26.7	22.4	21.3	21.7	21.4	20.9	18.9
Under 1 year	9.1	8.6	9.3	7.3	5.0	5.0	4.9	4.6	3.5	3.3	2.6	2.8
1–14 years	12.3	10.7	13.0	10.0	8.5	7.0	6.1	4.9	4.1	3.7	3.7	3.1
1–4 years	13.0	11.5	12.9	10.2	8.3	6.9	5.6	4.7	4.2	3.8	3.7	3.1
5–14 years	11.9	10.4	13.1	9.9	8.6	7.0	6.3	5.0	4.1	3.7	3.7	3.1
15–24 years	56.7	61.2	73.2	68.4	52.7	49.5	40.5	37.4	36.5	36.6	35.1	29.8
15–19 years	46.3	51.7	64.1	62.6	46.5	45.5	36.1	33.9	30.7	30.2	28.5	23.4
20–24 years	66.7	73.2	84.4	74.3	58.2	53.3	45.0	41.2	42.3	42.9	41.7	36.3
25–34 years	40.8	40.1	49.4	46.3	35.9	35.7	28.1	25.5	26.9	27.4	26.2	24.3
35–44 years	32.5	29.9	37.7	31.7	25.2	24.7	21.7	22.0	22.2	21.8	21.7	19.6
45–64 years	37.7	33.3	38.9	26.5	22.0	21.9	19.5	20.2	21.6	21.7	21.0	19.8
45–54 years	33.6	31.6	37.2	27.6	21.9	22.0	19.3	20.4	22.2	22.6	22.2	20.2
55–64 years	43.1	35.6	40.9	25.4	22.1	21.7	19.6	19.8	20.9	20.5	19.4	19.3
65 years and over	66.6	52.1	54.4	33.9	30.4	32.1	30.7	29.5	28.5	26.5	27.1	24.3
65–74 years	59.1	45.8	47.3	27.3	23.0	24.2	22.2	21.7	23.2	21.1	21.6	19.9
75–84 years	85.0	66.0	68.2	44.3	41.3	41.2	39.9	35.6	32.4	30.8	31.9	27.8
85 years and over	78.1	62.7	63.1	56.1	55.3	64.5	61.5	57.5	44.1	41.0	39.8	35.8
Female												
All ages, age–adjusted	11.5	11.7	14.9	11.8	10.7	11.0	10.3	9.5	8.9	8.8	8.2	7.3
All ages, crude	10.9	11.0	14.7	12.3	11.0	11.3	10.4	9.7	9.1	9.0	8.4	7.5
Under 1 year	7.6	7.5	10.4	6.7	4.7	4.9	4.5	4.2	3.6	3.5	3.2	1.9
1–14 years	7.2	6.3	7.9	6.3	5.4	4.9	4.4	3.7	3.1	3.1	2.8	2.2
1–4 years	10.0	8.4	10.0	8.1	6.0	5.6	4.8	3.8	3.4	3.4	3.0	2.5
5–14 years	5.7	5.4	7.2	5.7	5.1	4.7	4.2	3.6	3.0	2.9	2.7	2.0
15–24 years	12.6	15.1	21.6	20.8	18.2	17.9	16.8	15.9	14.7	14.7	14.1	11.8
15–19 years	12.9	16.0	22.7	22.8	20.1	20.0	19.7	17.5	16.2	15.7	15.2	12.2
20–24 years	12.2	14.0	20.4	18.9	16.7	16.0	13.8	14.2	13.2	13.7	12.9	11.3
25–34 years	9.3	9.2	13.0	12.2	10.1	11.5	10.2	8.8	8.8	8.7	8.4	7.4
35–44 years	8.5	9.1	12.9	10.4	9.4	9.2	9.0	8.8	8.6	8.8	7.7	7.0
45–64 years	12.6	13.1	15.3	10.3	9.5	10.1	9.0	8.7	8.5	8.3	7.7	7.3
45–54 years	10.9	11.6	14.5	10.2	9.0	9.6	8.4	8.2	8.2	8.2	7.8	7.4
55–64 years	14.9	15.2	16.2	10.5	9.9	10.8	9.9	9.5	8.9	8.5	7.6	7.0
65 years and over	21.9	20.3	23.1	15.0	15.8	17.2	17.0	15.8	14.0	13.5	12.5	11.4
65–74 years	20.6	19.0	21.6	13.0	14.0	14.1	13.7	12.3	11.2	10.6	9.7	9.0
75–84 years	25.2	23.0	27.2	18.5	19.2	21.9	21.2	19.2	16.5	16.5	14.9	13.4
85 years and over	22.1	22.0	18.0	15.2	15.0	18.3	19.3	19.3	16.4	15.2	15.2	14.0
White Male[4]												
All ages, age–adjusted	37.9	34.8	40.4	33.8	27.2	26.3	22.6	21.8	22.2	21.8	21.3	19.3
All ages, crude	35.1	31.5	39.1	35.9	28.3	26.7	22.4	21.6	22.3	22.0	21.5	19.5
Under 1 year	9.1	8.8	9.1	7.0	4.6	4.8	4.3	4.2	3.3	3.2	2.7	2.7
1–14 years	12.4	10.6	12.5	9.8	8.3	6.6	5.9	4.8	4.1	3.5	3.7	3.1
15–24 years	58.3	62.7	75.2	73.8	56.5	52.5	42.4	39.6	39.1	39.2	37.4	31.8
25–34 years	39.1	38.6	47.0	46.6	35.8	35.4	27.9	25.1	27.3	27.6	26.5	25.1
35–44 years	30.9	28.4	35.2	30.7	24.3	23.7	21.1	21.8	22.4	22.2	21.8	19.8
45–64 years	36.2	31.7	36.5	25.2	20.8	20.6	18.7	19.7	21.7	21.6	21.1	20.0
65 years and over	67.1	52.1	54.2	32.7	29.9	31.4	30.1	29.4	28.7	26.8	27.2	24.7

Table B–41. Death Rates for Motor Vehicle–Related Injuries, by Sex, Race, Hispanic Origin, and Age, Selected Years, 1950–2008—Continued

(Deaths per 100,000 resident population.)

Sex, race, Hispanic origin, and age	1950[1,2]	1960[1,2]	1970[2]	1980[2]	1985	1990[2]	1995	2000[3]	2005[3]	2006[3]	2007[3]	2008[3]
Black or African American Male[4]												
All ages, age-adjusted	34.8	39.6	51.0	34.2	29.0	29.9	26.1	24.4	22.5	22.6	22.5	19.1
All ages, crude	37.2	33.1	44.3	31.1	27.1	28.1	24.1	22.5	21.2	21.5	21.2	18.3
Under 1 year	—	*	10.6	7.8	*	*	8.7	6.7	*	*	*	*
1–14 years[5]	10.4	11.2	16.3	11.4	9.7	8.9	7.5	5.5	4.4	4.8	4.1	3.2
15–24 years	42.5	46.4	58.1	34.9	32.0	36.1	33.9	30.2	28.0	27.2	27.3	22.8
25–34 years	54.4	51.0	70.4	44.9	37.7	39.5	32.2	32.6	30.8	33.0	30.6	25.7
35–44 years	46.7	43.6	59.5	41.2	34.7	33.5	28.7	27.2	25.9	25.3	27.6	23.4
45–64 years	54.6	47.8	61.7	39.5	32.9	33.3	26.2	27.1	24.8	26.2	25.1	22.7
65 years and over	52.6	48.2	53.4	42.4	35.2	36.3	36.9	32.1	29.3	26.4	27.8	23.3
American Indian or Alaska Native Male[4]												
All ages, age-adjusted	—	—	—	78.9	50.9	48.3	40.7	35.8	34.3	36.8	32.0	27.6
All ages, crude	—	—	—	74.6	51.7	47.6	40.1	33.6	35.2	37.1	32.4	27.5
1–14 years	—	—	—	15.1	16.2	11.6	7.6	7.8	11.7	5.8	6.0	5.6
15–24 years	—	—	—	126.1	77.3	75.2	69.0	56.8	50.6	56.2	48.2	46.3
25–34 years	—	—	—	107.0	84.0	78.2	67.8	49.8	52.8	49.7	48.2	35.3
35–44 years	—	—	—	82.8	55.8	57.0	45.2	36.3	40.7	38.9	37.2	35.2
45–64 years	—	—	—	77.4	52.2	45.9	38.8	32.0	34.1	45.1	30.8	29.0
65 years and over	—	—	—	97.0	*	43.0	*	48.5	26.4	35.5	36.5	23.2
Asian or Pacific Islander Male[4]												
All ages, age-adjusted	—	—	—	19.0	17.3	17.9	14.5	10.6	9.6	9.5	9.4	8.3
All ages, crude	—	—	—	17.1	16.0	15.8	12.6	9.8	8.9	8.8	8.6	7.9
1–14 years	—	—	—	8.2	5.2	6.3	4.5	2.5	1.8	2.7	1.9	1.7
15–24 years	—	—	—	27.2	28.1	25.7	18.5	17.0	16.1	16.8	18.4	14.0
25–34 years	—	—	—	18.8	18.4	17.0	12.4	10.4	9.0	8.5	7.3	9.2
35–44 years	—	—	—	13.1	12.0	12.2	9.9	6.9	6.4	5.8	5.9	6.2
45–64 years	—	—	—	13.7	13.4	15.1	14.3	10.1	9.1	8.6	7.7	7.6
65 years and over	—	—	—	37.3	37.3	33.6	32.1	21.1	20.5	19.3	20.7	16.0
Hispanic or Latino Male[4,6]												
All ages, age-adjusted	—	—	—	—	25.4	29.5	24.4	21.3	21.3	21.2	19.3	16.7
All ages, crude	—	—	—	—	25.6	29.2	22.4	20.1	20.7	20.7	18.7	16.2
1–14 years	—	—	—	—	7.7	7.2	5.7	4.4	4.7	4.4	4.1	2.9
15–24 years	—	—	—	—	44.9	48.2	37.1	34.7	40.3	41.1	36.3	30.5
25–34 years	—	—	—	—	31.2	41.0	28.8	24.9	26.3	25.6	24.3	23.6
35–44 years	—	—	—	—	26.3	28.0	23.2	21.6	20.2	20.6	17.8	15.7
45–64 years	—	—	—	—	25.9	28.9	23.0	21.7	20.1	21.4	18.6	16.7
65 years and over	—	—	—	—	22.9	35.3	37.0	28.9	26.6	23.7	24.4	18.6
White, not Hispanic or Latino Male[6]												
All ages, age-adjusted	—	—	—	—	24.9	25.7	22.1	21.7	22.0	21.6	21.4	19.6
All ages, crude	—	—	—	—	25.9	26.0	21.9	21.5	22.4	22.0	21.8	20.0
1–14 years	—	—	—	—	7.8	6.4	5.8	4.9	3.9	3.2	3.5	3.0
15–24 years	—	—	—	—	53.3	52.3	42.7	40.3	38.2	38.1	37.2	31.7
25–34 years	—	—	—	—	33.2	34.0	27.1	24.7	27.1	27.8	26.8	25.2
35–44 years	—	—	—	—	21.6	23.1	20.3	21.6	22.7	22.2	22.5	20.7
45–64 years	—	—	—	—	18.0	19.8	18.1	19.3	21.7	21.4	21.2	20.3
65 years and over	—	—	—	—	27.6	31.1	29.4	29.3	28.7	26.9	27.3	25.1
White Female[4]												
All ages, age-adjusted	11.4	11.7	14.9	12.2	10.9	11.2	10.4	9.8	9.2	9.1	8.5	7.5
All ages, crude	10.9	11.2	14.8	12.8	11.4	11.6	10.7	10.0	9.5	9.4	8.8	7.7
Under 1 year	7.8	7.5	10.2	7.1	3.9	4.7	4.5	3.5	2.9	3.0	2.8	1.7
1–14 years	7.2	6.2	7.5	6.2	5.4	4.8	4.3	3.7	3.1	3.0	2.7	2.1
15–24 years	12.6	15.6	22.7	23.0	20.0	19.5	18.1	17.1	15.8	15.9	15.1	12.6
25–34 years	9.0	9.0	12.7	12.2	10.1	11.6	10.2	8.9	9.3	8.9	8.8	7.5
35–44 years	8.1	8.9	12.3	10.6	9.4	9.2	8.9	8.9	8.9	9.1	8.0	7.3
45–64 years	12.7	13.1	15.1	10.4	9.5	9.9	8.9	8.7	8.6	8.3	7.8	7.4
65 years and over	22.2	20.8	23.7	15.3	16.2	17.4	17.5	16.2	14.4	13.9	12.9	11.7

Table B–41. Death Rates for Motor Vehicle–Related Injuries, by Sex, Race, Hispanic Origin, and Age, Selected Years, 1950–2008—Continued

(Deaths per 100,000 resident population.)

Sex, race, Hispanic origin, and age	1950[1,2]	1960[1,2]	1970[2]	1980[2]	1985	1990[2]	1995	2000[3]	2005[3]	2006[3]	2007[3]	2008[3]
Black or African American Female[4]												
All ages, age-adjusted	9.3	10.4	14.1	8.5	8.5	9.6	9.0	8.4	7.6	7.8	7.0	6.5
All ages, crude	10.2	9.7	13.4	8.3	8.3	9.4	8.8	8.2	7.5	7.7	7.0	6.4
Under 1 year	—	8.1	11.9	*	8.1	7.0	*	*	6.8	*	*	*
1–14 years[5]	7.2	6.9	10.2	6.3	5.1	5.3	4.9	3.9	3.4	3.4	3.3	2.5
15–24 years	11.6	9.9	13.4	8.0	9.1	9.9	10.5	11.7	10.7	10.0	9.8	8.7
25–34 years	10.8	9.8	13.3	10.6	9.3	11.1	10.3	9.4	7.5	8.7	7.5	7.1
35–44 years	11.1	11.0	16.1	8.3	9.1	9.4	9.7	8.2	7.7	8.1	7.1	6.8
45–64 years	11.8	12.7	16.7	9.2	9.0	10.7	9.3	9.0	8.3	8.9	7.6	7.2
65 years and over	14.3	13.2	15.7	9.5	11.2	13.5	11.4	10.4	9.8	9.4	8.7	8.3
American Indian or Alaska Native Female[4]												
All ages, age-adjusted	—	—	—	32.0	19.8	17.5	18.2	19.5	15.4	16.9	15.6	14.6
All ages, crude	—	—	—	32.0	20.6	17.3	18.8	18.6	15.5	17.1	15.9	14.4
1–14 years	—	—	—	15.0	9.2	8.1	8.1	6.5	*	*	*	*
15–24 years	—	—	—	42.3	29.5	31.4	30.4	30.3	24.3	27.7	24.7	20.6
25–34 years	—	—	—	52.5	30.2	18.8	33.7	22.3	24.8	21.8	22.5	22.7
35–44 years	—	—	—	38.1	27.0	18.2	17.2	22.0	17.8	20.6	22.5	18.7
45–64 years	—	—	—	32.6	19.5	17.6	15.7	17.8	11.2	14.5	11.8	11.5
65 years and over	—	—	—	*	*	*	*	24.0	*	16.2	*	16.8
Asian or Pacific Islander Female[4]												
All ages, age-adjusted	—	—	—	9.3	8.8	10.4	8.6	6.7	5.9	5.6	5.2	4.4
All ages, crude	—	—	—	8.2	7.9	9.0	7.7	5.9	5.5	5.3	4.9	4.3
1–14 years	—	—	—	7.4	5.0	3.6	3.2	2.3	1.5	1.8	*	1.5
15–24 years	—	—	—	7.4	7.4	11.4	11.5	6.0	7.9	7.3	8.0	5.5
25–34 years	—	—	—	7.3	8.4	7.3	4.8	4.5	3.6	3.4	3.2	3.5
35–44 years	—	—	—	8.6	7.0	7.5	5.9	4.9	4.3	4.1	2.7	2.2
45–64 years	—	—	—	8.5	8.6	11.8	10.4	6.4	6.6	6.2	5.6	4.7
65 years and over	—	—	—	18.6	20.5	24.3	18.9	18.5	13.6	13.3	13.2	12.0
Hispanic or Latina Female[5,6]												
All ages, age-adjusted	—	—	—	—	8.8	9.6	8.8	7.9	7.8	7.7	6.9	5.7
All ages, crude	—	—	—	—	7.9	8.9	8.0	7.2	7.4	7.2	6.5	5.2
1–14 years	—	—	—	—	4.8	4.8	4.3	3.9	3.3	3.2	2.8	2.1
15–24 years	—	—	—	—	10.1	11.6	11.8	10.6	13.4	11.6	10.9	8.6
25–34 years	—	—	—	—	7.5	9.4	7.2	6.5	7.2	6.8	6.8	5.7
35–44 years	—	—	—	—	8.8	8.0	7.9	7.3	7.4	7.2	6.8	5.0
45–64 years	—	—	—	—	9.4	11.4	9.3	8.3	7.5	8.0	6.8	5.2
65 years and over	—	—	—	—	14.8	14.9	14.6	13.4	11.1	11.7	10.2	10.3
White, not Hispanic or Latina Female[6]												
All ages, age-adjusted	—	—	—	—	10.4	11.3	10.5	10.0	9.4	9.3	8.7	7.8
All ages, crude	—	—	—	—	10.9	11.7	10.9	10.3	9.8	9.7	9.1	8.2
1–14 years	—	—	—	—	4.9	4.7	4.2	3.5	3.0	2.9	2.6	2.1
15–24 years	—	—	—	—	20.2	20.4	19.0	18.4	16.1	16.7	16.0	13.5
25–34 years	—	—	—	—	9.8	11.7	10.5	9.3	9.7	9.4	9.3	7.9
35–44 years	—	—	—	—	8.6	9.3	8.9	9.0	9.1	9.3	8.2	7.8
45–64 years	—	—	—	—	8.6	9.7	8.6	8.7	8.6	8.3	7.9	7.6
65 years and over	—	—	—	—	15.3	17.5	17.5	16.3	14.6	14.0	13.0	11.7

* = Rates based on fewer than 20 deaths are considered unreliable and are not shown.
– = Data not available.
[1]Includes deaths of persons who were not residents of the 50 states and the District of Columbia.
[2]Underlying cause of death was coded according to the 6th Revision of the International Classification of Diseases (ICD) in 1950, 7th Revision in 1960, 8th Revision in 1970.
[3]Starting with 1999 data, cause of death is coded according to ICD–10.
[4]The race groups, White, Black, Asian or Pacific Islander, and American Indian or Alaska Native, include persons of Hispanic and non–Hispanic origin. Persons of Hispanic origin may be of any race.
[5]In 1950, rate is for the age group under 15 years.
[6]Prior to 1997, excludes data from states lacking an Hispanic–origin item on the death certificate.

PART B: MORTALITY 217

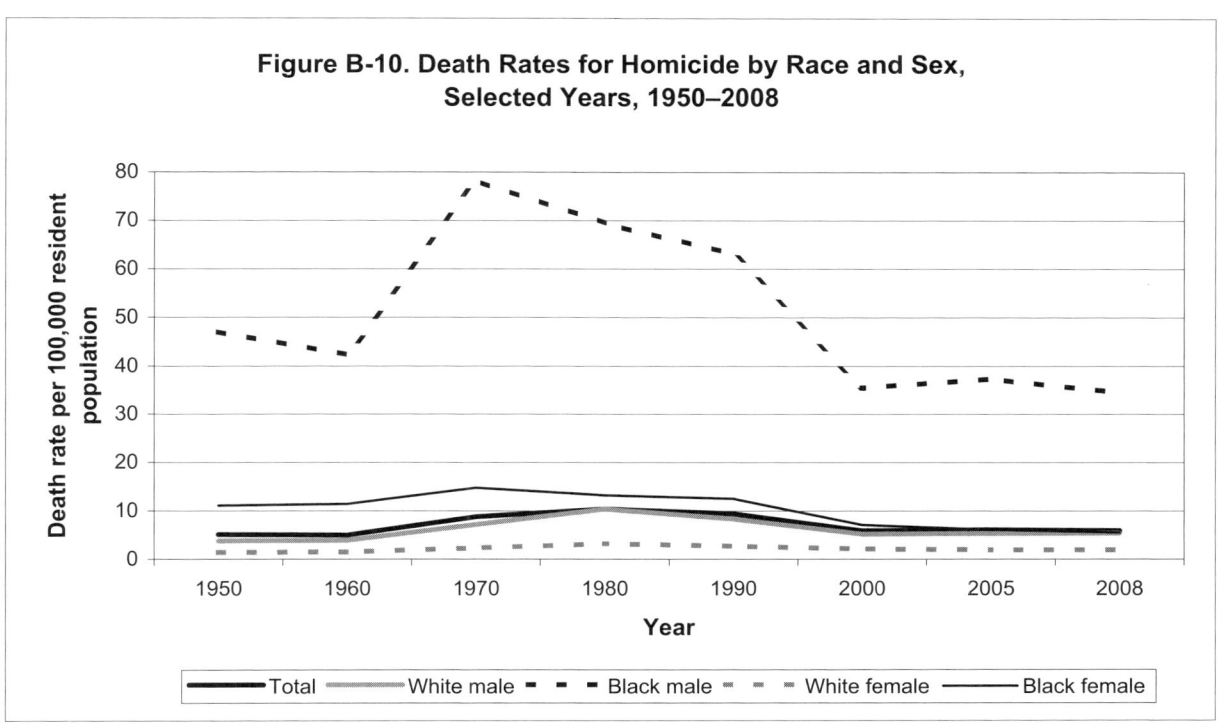

Figure B-10. Death Rates for Homicide by Race and Sex, Selected Years, 1950–2008

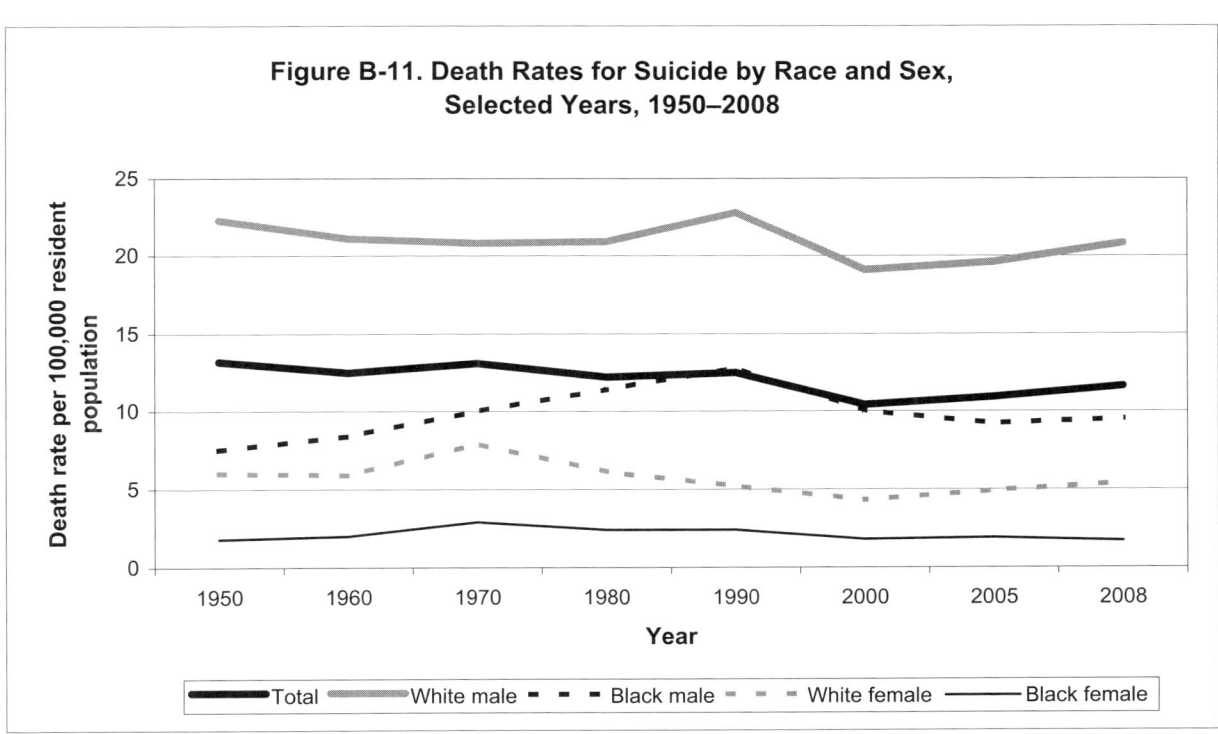

Figure B-11. Death Rates for Suicide by Race and Sex, Selected Years, 1950–2008

Table B-42. Death Rates for Homicide, by Sex, Race, Hispanic Origin, and Age, Selected Years, 1950–2008

(Deaths per 100,000 resident population.)

Sex, race, Hispanic origin, and age	1950[1,2]	1960[1,2]	1970[2]	1980[2]	1985	1990[2]	1995	2000[3]	2005[3]	2006[3]	2007[3]	2008[3]
All Persons												
All ages, age–adjusted	5.1	5.0	8.8	10.4	7.9	9.4	8.3	5.9	6.1	6.2	6.1	5.9
All ages, crude	5.0	4.6	8.1	10.6	8.2	9.9	8.5	6.0	6.1	6.2	6.1	5.9
Under 1 year	4.4	4.8	4.3	5.9	5.4	8.4	8.2	9.2	7.5	8.1	8.3	7.9
1–14 years	0.6	0.6	1.1	1.5	1.6	1.8	1.9	1.3	1.3	1.3	1.3	1.3
1–4 years	0.6	0.7	1.9	2.5	2.5	2.5	2.9	2.3	2.3	2.2	2.4	2.5
5–14 years	0.5	0.5	0.9	1.2	1.2	1.5	1.5	0.9	0.8	1.0	0.9	0.8
15–24 years	5.8	5.6	11.3	15.4	11.7	19.7	19.6	12.6	13.0	13.5	13.1	12.4
15–19 years	3.9	3.9	7.7	10.5	8.4	16.9	17.8	9.5	9.9	10.7	10.4	9.7
20–24 years	8.5	7.7	15.6	20.2	14.6	22.2	21.5	16.0	16.1	16.2	15.8	15.1
25–44 years	8.9	8.5	14.9	17.5	13.1	14.7	11.9	8.7	9.4	9.2	9.3	9.0
25–34 years	9.3	9.2	16.2	19.3	14.6	17.4	14.4	10.4	11.8	11.7	11.7	11.3
35–44 years	8.4	7.8	13.5	14.9	11.1	11.6	9.4	7.1	7.1	6.9	7.1	6.8
45–64 years	5.0	5.3	8.7	9.0	6.9	6.3	5.4	4.0	4.0	4.3	4.1	4.0
45–54 years	5.9	6.1	10.0	11.0	8.1	7.5	6.0	4.7	4.8	5.1	4.9	4.8
55–64 years	3.9	4.1	7.1	7.0	5.7	5.0	4.4	3.0	2.8	3.2	3.0	2.9
65 years and over	3.0	2.7	4.6	5.5	4.3	4.0	3.1	2.4	2.3	2.1	2.0	2.1
65–74 years	3.2	2.8	4.9	5.7	4.3	3.8	3.2	2.4	2.4	2.1	2.1	2.3
75–84 years	2.5	2.3	4.0	5.2	4.3	4.3	3.0	2.4	2.2	2.1	2.1	1.8
85 years and over	2.3	2.4	4.2	5.3	4.1	4.6	3.2	2.4	2.1	1.9	1.5	2.1
Male												
All ages, age–adjusted	7.9	7.5	14.3	16.6	12.2	14.8	12.8	9.0	9.6	9.7	9.6	9.3
All ages, crude	7.7	6.8	13.1	17.1	12.8	15.9	13.4	9.3	9.8	10.0	9.8	9.4
Under 1 year	4.5	4.7	4.5	6.3	5.6	8.8	9.0	10.4	8.2	9.4	9.5	8.9
1–14 years	0.6	0.6	1.2	1.6	1.8	2.0	2.2	1.5	1.4	1.6	1.5	1.5
1–4 years	0.5	0.7	1.9	2.7	2.5	2.7	3.1	2.5	2.6	2.5	2.5	2.7
5–14 years	0.6	0.5	1.0	1.2	1.4	1.7	1.9	1.1	1.0	1.2	1.0	1.0
15–24 years	8.6	8.4	18.2	24.0	18.2	32.5	32.8	20.9	22.0	22.8	22.1	20.9
15–19 years	5.5	5.7	12.1	15.9	12.8	27.8	29.1	15.5	16.8	18.2	17.6	16.4
20–24 years	13.5	11.8	25.6	32.2	23.0	36.9	36.5	26.7	27.2	27.5	26.7	25.5
25–44 years	13.8	12.8	24.4	28.9	20.6	23.5	18.2	13.3	14.9	14.7	14.9	14.6
25–34 years	14.4	13.9	26.8	31.9	22.8	27.7	22.5	16.7	19.6	19.4	19.4	18.6
35–44 years	13.2	11.7	21.7	24.5	17.6	18.6	14.0	10.3	10.6	10.4	10.6	10.5
45–64 years	8.1	8.1	14.8	15.2	11.0	10.2	8.3	6.0	6.2	6.5	6.2	6.1
45–54 years	9.5	9.4	16.8	18.4	12.7	11.9	9.2	6.9	7.6	7.6	7.3	7.3
55–64 years	6.3	6.4	12.1	11.8	9.1	8.0	7.0	4.6	4.3	4.8	4.6	4.4
65 years and over	4.8	4.3	7.7	8.8	6.2	5.8	4.2	3.3	3.0	2.8	2.8	2.8
65–74 years	5.2	4.6	8.5	9.2	6.5	5.8	4.5	3.4	3.3	3.0	3.1	3.1
75–84 years	3.9	3.7	5.9	8.1	5.7	5.7	3.7	3.2	2.6	2.7	2.8	2.5
85 years and over	2.5	3.6	7.4	7.5	5.0	6.7	4.1	3.3	2.7	2.3	1.5	2.2
Female												
All ages, age–adjusted	2.4	2.6	3.7	4.4	3.8	4.0	3.7	2.8	2.5	2.5	2.5	2.4
All ages, crude	2.4	2.4	3.4	4.5	3.9	4.2	3.8	2.8	2.5	2.5	2.5	2.4
Under 1 year	4.2	4.9	4.1	5.6	5.2	8.0	7.4	7.9	6.6	6.8	7.0	6.8
1–14 years	0.6	0.5	1.0	1.4	1.4	1.6	1.5	1.1	1.1	1.1	1.2	1.1
1–4 years	0.7	0.7	1.9	2.2	2.4	2.3	2.6	2.1	2.0	2.0	2.3	2.3
5–14 years	0.5	0.4	0.7	1.1	1.0	1.2	1.0	0.7	0.7	0.7	0.7	0.6
15–24 years	3.0	2.8	4.6	6.6	5.1	6.2	5.9	3.9	3.4	3.5	3.5	3.4
15–19 years	2.4	1.9	3.2	4.9	3.9	5.4	5.8	3.1	2.5	2.9	2.8	2.7
20–24 years	3.7	3.8	6.2	8.2	6.1	7.0	6.0	4.7	4.3	4.2	4.2	4.1
25–44 years	4.2	4.3	5.8	6.4	5.7	6.0	5.6	4.0	3.7	3.6	3.6	3.3
25–34 years	4.5	4.6	6.0	6.9	6.4	7.1	6.3	4.1	3.8	3.7	3.7	3.6
35–44 years	3.8	4.0	5.7	5.7	4.9	4.8	4.9	4.0	3.6	3.4	3.5	3.1
45–64 years	1.9	2.5	3.1	3.4	3.2	2.8	2.6	2.1	1.9	2.2	2.1	2.0
45–54 years	2.3	2.9	3.7	4.1	3.7	3.2	2.9	2.5	2.2	2.6	2.5	2.4
55–64 years	1.4	2.0	2.5	2.8	2.7	2.3	2.1	1.6	1.4	1.7	1.5	1.5
65 years and over	1.4	1.3	2.3	3.3	3.0	2.8	2.4	1.8	1.7	1.6	1.4	1.6
65–74 years	1.3	1.3	2.2	3.0	2.6	2.2	2.1	1.6	1.6	1.3	1.3	1.6
75–84 years	1.4	1.3	2.7	3.5	3.4	3.4	2.6	2.0	1.9	1.8	1.5	1.3
85 years and over	2.1	1.6	2.5	4.3	3.8	3.8	2.9	2.0	1.9	1.8	1.4	2.1
White Male[4]												
All ages, age–adjusted	3.8	3.9	7.2	10.4	7.7	8.3	7.3	5.2	5.3	5.4	5.4	5.4
All ages, crude	3.6	3.6	6.6	10.7	8.1	8.8	7.5	5.2	5.4	5.4	5.4	5.4
Under 1 year	4.3	3.8	2.9	4.3	3.8	6.4	7.1	8.2	6.7	7.4	7.7	7.3
1–14 years	0.4	0.5	0.7	1.2	1.3	1.3	1.5	1.2	1.0	1.1	1.0	1.0
15–24 years	3.2	5.0	7.6	15.1	10.7	15.2	15.9	9.9	10.6	10.6	10.5	10.2
25–44 years	5.4	5.5	11.6	17.2	12.7	13.0	10.4	7.4	8.0	7.8	8.1	8.1
25–34 years	4.9	5.7	12.5	18.5	13.7	14.7	12.1	8.4	9.8	9.3	9.9	9.5
35–44 years	6.1	5.2	10.8	15.2	11.3	11.1	8.7	6.5	6.3	6.4	6.4	6.7
45–64 years	4.8	4.6	8.3	9.8	7.4	6.9	5.5	4.1	4.3	4.4	4.2	4.4
65 years and over	3.8	3.1	5.4	6.7	4.4	4.1	2.9	2.5	2.2	2.2	2.2	2.3

Table B-42. Death Rates for Homicide, by Sex, Race, Hispanic Origin, and Age, Selected Years, 1950–2008—Continued

(Deaths per 100,000 resident population.)

Sex, race, Hispanic origin, and age	1950[1,2]	1960[1,2]	1970[2]	1980[2]	1985	1990[2]	1995	2000[3]	2005[3]	2006[3]	2007[3]	2008[3]
Black or African American Male[4]												
All ages, age-adjusted	47.0	42.3	78.2	69.4	48.4	63.1	51.1	35.4	37.3	37.8	37.1	34.4
All ages, crude	44.7	35.0	66.0	65.7	48.3	68.5	54.5	37.2	39.7	40.6	39.7	37.1
Under 1 year	—	10.3	14.3	18.6	16.7	21.4	20.3	23.3	15.9	20.7	19.2	17.0
1–14 years	1.8	1.5	4.4	4.1	4.2	5.8	5.8	3.1	3.9	4.0	3.9	3.8
15–24 years	53.8	43.2	98.3	82.6	64.8	137.1	129.4	85.3	84.1	88.2	85.3	78.1
25–44 years	92.8	80.5	140.2	130.0	86.1	105.4	75.8	55.8	63.4	63.2	62.3	59.2
25–34 years	104.3	86.4	154.5	142.9	94.0	123.7	95.1	73.9	86.2	86.2	82.5	78.4
35–44 years	80.0	74.4	124.0	109.3	74.0	81.2	54.9	38.5	40.6	39.8	41.2	38.6
45–64 years	46.0	44.6	82.3	70.6	46.0	41.4	33.4	21.9	22.3	23.3	22.5	21.0
65 years and over	16.5	17.3	33.3	30.9	26.1	25.7	20.3	12.8	11.9	10.0	10.8	8.6
American Indian or Alaska Native Male[4]												
All ages, age-adjusted	—	—	—	23.3	19.1	16.7	14.4	10.7	11.3	11.9	9.2	10.7
All ages, crude	—	—	—	23.1	18.4	16.6	15.7	10.7	12.2	12.9	10.1	11.2
15–24 years	—	—	—	35.4	27.1	25.1	28.0	17.0	22.1	22.5	14.7	16.3
25–44 years	—	—	—	39.2	28.2	25.7	24.6	17.0	16.1	17.9	17.1	18.9
45–64 years	—	—	—	22.1	21.2	14.8	12.0	*	10.8	9.1	6.5	8.8
Asian or Pacific Islander Male[5]												
All ages, age-adjusted	—	—	—	9.1	5.5	7.3	7.2	4.3	4.4	4.4	3.3	3.1
All ages, crude	—	—	—	8.3	5.7	7.9	7.5	4.4	4.6	4.5	3.5	3.3
15–24 years	—	—	—	9.3	8.0	14.9	17.2	7.8	10.8	11.5	7.4	7.1
25–44 years	—	—	—	11.3	8.6	9.6	7.4	4.6	4.9	4.0	3.9	3.6
45–64 years	—	—	—	10.4	5.2	7.0	7.7	6.1	4.2	4.7	3.3	2.9
Hispanic or Latino Male[4,6]												
All ages, age-adjusted	—	—	—	—	24.9	27.4	20.4	11.8	12.1	11.7	11.2	10.5
All ages, crude	—	—	—	—	27.2	31.0	23.5	13.4	13.6	13.1	12.4	11.4
Under 1 year	—	—	—	—	*	8.7	5.9	6.6	6.3	10.1	8.3	7.1
1–14 years	—	—	—	—	1.5	3.1	3.2	1.7	1.5	1.6	1.3	1.2
15–24 years	—	—	—	—	42.1	55.4	54.7	28.5	31.0	31.0	30.0	27.7
25–44 years	—	—	—	—	46.7	46.4	28.8	17.2	18.0	16.5	16.0	15.2
25–34 years	—	—	—	—	50.6	50.9	33.0	19.9	22.3	19.7	19.9	17.9
35–44 years	—	—	—	—	39.8	39.3	22.8	13.5	12.7	12.5	11.2	11.9
45–64 years	—	—	—	—	19.6	20.5	14.7	9.1	8.2	8.3	7.7	7.4
65 years and over	—	—	—	—	8.9	9.4	5.8	4.4	4.4	3.1	3.7	2.9
White, not Hispanic or Latino Male[6]												
All ages, age-adjusted	—	—	—	—	6.1	5.6	4.8	3.6	3.5	3.6	3.7	3.9
All ages, crude	—	—	—	—	6.2	5.8	4.9	3.6	3.6	3.6	3.7	3.9
Under 1 year	—	—	—	—	4.6	5.4	6.8	8.3	6.9	6.5	7.2	7.0
1–14 years	—	—	—	—	1.2	0.9	1.1	1.0	0.8	0.9	0.9	1.0
15–24 years	—	—	—	—	7.6	7.5	7.2	4.7	4.7	4.7	4.9	5.1
25–44 years	—	—	—	—	9.2	8.7	7.2	5.2	5.1	5.1	5.6	5.8
25–34 years	—	—	—	—	9.3	9.3	7.7	5.2	5.4	5.5	6.2	6.3
35–44 years	—	—	—	—	9.1	8.0	6.7	5.2	4.8	4.9	5.1	5.3
45–64 years	—	—	—	—	6.3	5.7	4.6	3.6	3.8	3.9	3.7	3.9
65 years and over	—	—	—	—	4.4	3.7	2.6	2.3	2.1	2.1	2.0	2.3
White Female[4]												
All ages, age-adjusted	1.4	1.5	2.3	3.2	2.9	2.7	2.7	2.1	1.9	1.9	2.0	1.9
All ages, crude	1.4	1.4	2.1	3.2	2.9	2.8	2.7	2.1	1.9	1.9	1.9	1.9
Under 1 year	3.9	3.5	2.9	4.3	4.3	5.1	5.1	5.0	5.5	6.3	6.1	5.3
1–14 years	0.4	0.4	0.7	1.1	1.1	1.0	1.1	0.8	0.8	0.8	0.9	0.8
15–24 years	1.3	1.5	2.7	4.7	3.6	4.0	4.0	2.7	2.3	2.4	2.5	2.2
25–44 years	2.0	2.1	3.3	4.2	4.1	3.8	3.7	2.9	2.8	2.5	2.7	2.7
45–64 years	1.5	1.7	2.1	2.6	2.6	2.3	2.2	1.8	1.5	1.8	1.7	1.8
65 years and over	1.2	1.2	1.9	2.9	2.6	2.2	2.0	1.6	1.6	1.5	1.3	1.5
Black or African American Female[4]												
All ages, age-adjusted	11.1	11.4	14.7	13.2	10.6	12.5	10.4	7.1	6.1	6.4	6.1	5.5
All ages, crude	11.5	10.4	13.2	13.5	11.0	13.4	10.9	7.2	6.2	6.6	6.2	5.6
Under 1 year	—	13.8	10.7	12.8	10.7	22.8	20.1	22.2	12.6	11.1	11.4	15.2
1–14 years[5]	1.8	1.2	3.1	3.3	3.3	4.7	3.4	2.7	2.3	2.5	2.7	2.6
15–24 years	16.5	11.9	17.7	18.4	14.2	18.9	16.4	10.7	8.8	9.5	8.9	9.7
25–44 years	22.5	22.7	25.3	22.6	17.8	21.0	17.1	11.0	9.3	10.1	9.1	7.7
45–64 years	6.8	10.3	13.4	10.8	7.9	6.5	5.9	4.5	4.9	5.2	4.9	3.8
65 years and over	3.6	3.0	7.4	8.0	7.8	9.4	6.8	3.5	2.9	2.5	2.6	2.3

Table B-42. Death Rates for Homicide, by Sex, Race, Hispanic Origin, and Age, Selected Years, 1950–2008—Continued

(Deaths per 100,000 resident population.)

Sex, race, Hispanic origin, and age	1950[1,2]	1960[1,2]	1970[2]	1980[2]	1985	1990[2]	1995	2000[3]	2005[3]	2006[3]	2007[3]	2008[3]
American Indian or Alaska Native Female[4]												
All ages, age–adjusted	—	—	—	8.1	4.8	4.6	5.3	3.0	4.0	2.9	3.6	3.6
All ages, crude	—	—	—	7.7	4.5	4.8	5.1	2.9	4.0	3.0	3.5	3.7
15–24 years	—	—	—	*	*	*	*	*	*	*	*	*
25–44 years	—	—	—	13.7	*	6.9	8.3	5.9	6.1	6.0	5.1	4.7
45–64 years	—	—	—	*	*	*	*	*	*	*	*	*
Asian or Pacific Islander Female[5]												
All ages, age–adjusted	—	—	—	3.1	2.6	2.8	2.4	1.7	1.6	1.4	1.3	1.4
All ages, crude	—	—	—	3.1	2.8	2.8	2.6	1.7	1.6	1.4	1.4	1.3
15–24 years	—	—	—	*	*	*	3.4	*	2.8	*	*	*
25–44 years	—	—	—	4.6	2.9	3.8	3.6	2.2	1.7	1.6	1.9	1.4
45–64 years	—	—	—	*	*	*	2.2	2.0	1.3	2.0	1.5	1.2
Hispanic or Latina Female[4,6]												
All ages, age–adjusted	—	—	—	—	4.1	4.3	4.0	2.8	2.4	2.3	2.3	2.4
All ages, crude	—	—	—	—	4.3	4.7	4.2	2.8	2.5	2.4	2.5	2.4
Under 1 year	—	—	—	—	*	*	*	7.4	6.6	6.5	7.3	5.2
1–14 years	—	—	—	—	1.5	1.9	1.8	1.0	1.0	1.0	1.3	1.1
15–24 years	—	—	—	—	5.7	8.1	6.4	3.7	3.6	3.8	3.5	3.6
25–44 years	—	—	—	—	6.8	6.1	5.6	3.7	3.4	3.1	3.3	3.3
45–64 years	—	—	—	—	3.2	3.3	3.4	2.9	1.9	1.9	1.7	2.1
65 years and over	—	—	—	—	*	*	2.4	2.4	*	*	*	1.5
White, not Hispanic or Latina Female[6]												
All ages, age–adjusted	—	—	—	—	2.9	2.5	2.3	1.9	1.8	1.8	1.8	1.8
All ages, crude	—	—	—	—	2.9	2.5	2.3	1.9	1.8	1.8	1.8	1.8
Under 1 year	—	—	—	—	4.1	4.4	4.4	4.1	5.0	6.2	5.7	5.4
1–14 years	—	—	—	—	1.0	0.8	0.9	0.8	0.7	0.8	0.8	0.7
15–24 years	—	—	—	—	3.5	3.3	3.4	2.3	2.0	2.0	2.2	1.8
25–44 years	—	—	—	—	3.9	3.5	3.3	2.7	2.6	2.3	2.5	2.5
45–64 years	—	—	—	—	3.6	2.2	1.9	1.6	1.5	1.8	1.7	1.7
65 years and over	—	—	—	—	2.6	2.2	1.9	1.6	1.6	1.5	1.3	1.5

* = Rates based on fewer than 20 deaths are considered unreliable and are not shown.
— = Data not available.
[1]Includes deaths of persons who were not residents of the 50 states and the District of Columbia.
[2]Underlying cause of death was coded according to the 6th Revision of the International Classification of Diseases (ICD) in 1950, 7th Revision in 1960, 8th Revision in 1970.
[3]Starting with 1999 data, cause of death is coded according to ICD–10.
[4]The race groups, White, Black, Asian or Pacific Islander, and American Indian or Alaska Native, include persons of Hispanic and non–Hispanic origin. Persons of Hispanic origin may be of any race.
[5]In 1950, rate is for the age group 75 years and over.
[6]Prior to 1997, excludes data from states lacking an Hispanic–origin item on the death certificate.

Table B–43. Death Rates for Suicide, by Sex, Race, Hispanic Origin, and Age, Selected Years, 1950–2008

(Deaths per 100,000 resident population.)

Sex, race, Hispanic origin, and age	1950[1,2]	1960[1,2]	1970[2]	1980[2]	1985	1990[2]	1995	2000[3]	2005[3]	2006[3]	2007[3]	2008[3]
All Persons												
All ages, age–adjusted	13.2	12.5	13.1	12.2	12.5	12.5	11.8	10.4	10.9	10.9	11.3	11.6
All ages, crude	11.4	10.6	11.6	11.9	12.4	12.4	11.7	10.4	11.0	11.1	11.5	11.9
Under 1 year	X	X	X	X	X	X	X	X	X	X	X	X
1–4 years	X	X	X	X	X	X	X	X	X	X	X	X
5–14 years	0.2	0.3	0.3	0.4	0.8	0.8	0.9	0.7	0.7	0.5	0.5	0.6
15–24 years	4.5	5.2	8.8	12.3	12.8	13.2	13.0	10.2	10.0	9.9	9.7	10.1
15–19 years	2.7	3.6	5.9	8.5	9.9	11.1	10.3	8.0	7.7	7.3	6.9	7.5
20–24 years	6.2	7.1	12.2	16.1	15.4	15.1	15.8	12.5	12.4	12.5	12.6	12.8
25–44 years	11.6	12.2	15.4	15.6	15.0	15.2	15.1	13.4	13.7	13.8	14.3	14.4
25–34 years	9.1	10.0	14.1	16.0	15.3	15.2	15.0	12.0	12.4	12.3	13.0	12.9
35–44 years	14.3	14.2	16.9	15.4	14.6	15.3	15.1	14.5	14.9	15.1	15.6	15.8
45–64 years	23.5	22.0	20.6	15.9	16.3	15.3	13.9	13.5	15.4	16.0	16.8	17.6
45–54 years	20.9	20.7	20.0	15.9	15.7	14.8	14.4	14.4	16.5	17.2	17.7	18.7
55–64 years	26.8	23.7	21.4	15.9	16.8	16.0	13.2	12.1	13.9	14.5	15.5	16.2
65 years and over	30.0	24.5	20.8	17.6	20.4	20.5	17.9	15.2	14.7	14.2	14.3	14.8
65–74 years	29.6	23.0	20.8	16.9	18.7	17.9	15.7	12.5	12.6	12.6	12.6	13.9
75–84 years	31.1	27.9	21.2	19.1	23.9	24.9	20.6	17.6	16.9	15.9	16.3	16.2
85 years and over	28.8	26.0	19.0	19.2	19.4	22.2	21.3	19.6	16.9	15.9	15.6	14.9
Male												
All ages, age–adjusted	21.2	20.0	19.8	19.9	21.1	21.5	20.3	17.7	18.0	18.0	18.4	18.9
All ages, crude	17.8	16.5	16.8	18.6	20.0	20.4	19.5	17.1	17.7	17.8	18.3	19.0
Under 1 year	X	X	X	X	X	X	X	X	X	X	X	X
1–4 years	X	X	X	X	X	X	X	X	X	X	X	X
5–14 years	0.3	0.4	0.5	0.6	1.2	1.1	1.3	1.2	1.0	0.7	0.6	0.8
15–24 years	6.5	8.2	13.5	20.2	21.0	22.0	22.0	17.1	16.2	16.2	15.9	16.3
15–19 years	3.5	5.6	8.8	13.8	15.8	18.1	17.1	13.0	12.1	11.5	11.1	11.6
20–24 years	9.3	11.5	19.3	26.8	25.7	25.7	27.0	21.4	20.2	20.8	20.8	21.0
25–44 years	17.2	17.9	20.9	24.0	23.7	24.4	24.4	21.3	21.6	21.5	22.3	22.3
25–34 years	13.4	14.7	19.8	25.0	24.7	24.8	24.8	19.6	19.9	19.7	20.7	20.4
35–44 years	21.3	21.0	22.1	22.5	22.3	23.9	24.0	22.8	23.1	23.2	23.8	24.0
45–64 years	37.1	34.4	30.0	23.7	25.3	24.3	22.2	21.3	24.0	24.8	25.8	27.5
45–54 years	32.0	31.6	27.9	22.9	23.6	23.2	22.5	22.4	25.2	26.2	27.0	28.6
55–64 years	43.6	38.1	32.7	24.5	27.1	25.7	21.8	19.4	22.2	22.7	24.3	26.1
65 years and over	52.8	44.0	38.4	35.0	40.9	41.6	36.2	31.1	29.5	28.5	28.6	29.4
65–74 years	50.5	39.6	36.0	30.4	33.9	32.2	28.5	22.7	22.7	22.7	22.5	25.0
75–84 years	58.3	52.5	42.8	42.3	53.1	56.1	44.9	38.6	35.8	33.3	34.3	34.0
85 years and over	58.3	57.4	42.4	50.6	56.2	65.9	62.7	57.5	45.0	43.2	41.8	38.4
Female												
All ages, age–adjusted	5.6	5.6	7.4	5.7	5.2	4.8	4.3	4.0	4.4	4.5	4.7	4.8
All ages, crude	5.1	4.9	6.6	5.5	5.2	4.8	4.3	4.0	4.5	4.6	4.8	4.9
Under 1 year	X	X	X	X	X	X	X	X	X	X	X	X
1–4 years	X	X	X	X	X	X	X	X	X	X	X	X
5–14 years	0.1	0.1	0.2	0.2	0.4	0.4	0.4	0.3	0.3	0.3	0.3	0.3
15–24 years	2.6	2.2	4.2	4.3	4.3	3.9	3.6	3.0	3.5	3.2	3.2	3.6
15–19 years	1.8	1.6	2.9	3.0	3.7	3.7	3.1	2.7	3.0	2.8	2.5	3.1
20–24 years	3.3	2.9	5.7	5.5	4.9	4.1	4.2	3.2	4.0	3.6	3.9	4.1
25–44 years	6.2	6.6	10.2	7.7	6.5	6.2	5.8	5.4	5.8	5.9	6.2	6.3
25–34 years	4.9	5.5	8.6	7.1	5.9	5.6	5.1	4.3	4.7	4.7	5.0	5.1
35–44 years	7.5	7.7	11.9	8.5	7.1	6.8	6.4	6.4	6.8	7.0	7.3	7.4
45–64 years	9.9	10.2	12.0	8.9	8.0	7.1	6.1	6.2	7.2	7.7	8.2	8.2
45–54 years	9.9	10.2	12.6	9.4	8.3	6.9	6.6	6.7	8.0	8.4	8.8	9.1
55–64 years	9.9	10.2	11.4	8.4	7.8	7.3	5.3	5.4	6.1	6.8	7.3	7.0
65 years and over	9.4	8.4	8.1	6.1	6.6	6.4	5.4	4.0	4.0	3.9	3.9	4.1
65–74 years	10.1	8.4	9.0	6.5	6.9	6.7	5.4	4.0	4.0	4.1	4.2	4.4
75–84 years	8.1	8.9	7.0	5.5	6.7	6.3	5.4	4.0	4.0	4.0	3.8	3.8
85 years and over	8.2	6.0	5.9	5.5	4.7	5.4	5.4	4.2	4.0	3.1	3.1	3.5
White Male[4]												
All ages, age–adjusted	22.3	21.1	20.8	20.9	22.4	22.8	21.6	19.1	19.6	19.6	20.2	20.8
All ages, crude	19.0	17.6	18.0	19.9	21.6	22.0	21.1	18.8	19.7	19.8	20.5	21.2
15–24 years	6.6	8.6	13.9	21.4	22.3	23.2	23.1	17.9	17.3	17.1	16.9	17.2
25–44 years	17.9	18.5	21.5	24.6	24.8	25.4	25.8	22.9	23.5	23.5	24.5	24.6
45–64 years	39.3	36.5	31.9	25.0	27.0	26.0	23.9	23.2	26.6	27.4	28.8	30.7
65 years and over	55.8	46.7	41.1	37.2	43.7	44.2	38.5	33.3	32.1	30.9	31.1	31.8
65–74 years	53.2	42.0	38.7	32.5	35.8	34.2	30.1	24.3	24.9	24.7	24.7	26.9
75–84 years	61.9	55.7	45.5	45.5	57.0	60.2	47.7	41.1	38.4	36.0	36.9	36.7
85 years and over	61.9	61.3	45.8	52.8	60.9	70.3	67.9	61.6	48.2	46.1	45.4	41.3

Table B–43. Death Rates for Suicide, by Sex, Race, Hispanic Origin, and Age, Selected Years, 1950–2008—Continued

(Deaths per 100,000 resident population.)

Sex, race, Hispanic origin, and age	1950[1,2]	1960[1,2]	1970[2]	1980[2]	1985	1990[2]	1995	2000[3]	2005[3]	2006[3]	2007[3]	2008[3]
Black or African American Male[4]												
All ages, age-adjusted	7.5	8.4	10.0	11.4	11.8	12.8	12.4	10.0	9.2	9.4	8.8	9.5
All ages, crude	6.3	6.4	8.0	10.3	11.0	12.0	11.7	9.4	8.7	8.8	8.4	9.1
15–24 years	4.9	4.1	10.5	12.3	13.3	15.1	17.8	14.2	11.5	10.6	10.3	12.3
25–44 years	9.8	12.6	16.1	19.2	17.8	19.6	18.3	14.3	13.7	14.3	13.7	13.7
45–64 years	12.7	13.0	12.4	11.8	12.9	13.1	11.5	9.9	9.4	9.9	9.4	10.3
65 years and over	9.0	9.9	8.7	11.4	15.8	14.9	14.6	11.5	10.2	10.4	8.7	11.0
65–74 years	10.0	11.3	8.7	11.1	16.7	14.7	13.8	11.1	8.4	8.8	8.3	11.0
75–84 years[5]	*	*	*	10.5	15.6	14.4	16.7	12.1	12.8	11.6	11.2	11.8
85 years and over	—	*	*	*	*	*	*	*	*	*	*	*
American Indian or Alaska Native Male[4]												
All ages, age-adjusted	—	—	—	19.3	17.9	20.1	17.4	16.0	18.9	18.3	18.1	17.7
All ages, crude	—	—	—	20.9	20.3	20.9	18.0	15.9	19.8	19.3	19.2	18.0
15–24 years	—	—	—	45.3	42.0	49.1	30.8	26.2	32.7	35.9	32.3	35.9
25–44 years	—	—	—	31.2	30.2	27.8	29.1	24.5	29.4	26.0	28.6	26.8
45–64 years	—	—	—	*	*	*	13.6	15.4	16.8	18.0	15.9	12.5
65 years and over	—	—	—	*	*	*	*	*	*	*	*	*
Asian or Pacific Islander Male[4]												
All ages, age-adjusted	—	—	—	10.7	9.3	9.6	9.6	8.6	7.3	7.9	9.0	8.2
All ages, crude	—	—	—	8.8	8.4	8.7	9.0	7.9	7.2	8.0	8.7	8.0
15–24 years	—	—	—	10.8	14.2	13.5	14.4	9.1	7.2	12.0	13.4	8.6
25–44 years	—	—	—	11.0	9.3	10.6	10.8	9.9	9.5	9.2	9.8	8.7
45–64 years	—	—	—	13.0	10.4	9.7	8.7	9.7	8.9	9.7	10.7	11.2
65 years and over	—	—	—	18.6	16.7	16.8	18.9	15.4	11.0	10.6	12.9	14.7
Hispanic or Latino Male[4,6]												
All ages, age-adjusted	—	—	—	—	11.0	13.7	12.7	10.3	9.4	8.8	10.1	9.3
All ages, crude	—	—	—	—	9.8	11.4	10.9	8.4	8.3	7.9	8.8	8.1
15–24 years	—	—	—	—	13.8	14.7	16.0	10.9	12.1	11.6	11.5	10.8
25–44 years	—	—	—	—	14.8	16.2	14.5	11.2	11.2	10.8	11.9	10.8
45–64 years	—	—	—	—	12.3	16.1	14.2	12.0	10.7	10.3	12.9	11.5
65 years and over	—	—	—	—	14.7	23.4	21.0	19.5	14.1	12.1	15.9	15.8
White, not Hispanic or Latino Male[6]												
All ages, age-adjusted	—	—	—	—	22.9	23.5	22.3	20.2	21.2	21.4	21.9	22.9
All ages, crude	—	—	—	—	22.3	23.1	22.2	20.4	22.0	22.3	22.9	24.1
15–24 years	—	—	—	—	22.6	24.4	24.0	19.5	18.4	18.5	18.2	18.8
25–44 years	—	—	—	—	25.1	26.4	27.1	25.1	26.6	26.9	28.0	28.5
45–64 years	—	—	—	—	27.3	26.8	24.5	24.0	28.2	29.3	30.6	33.1
65 years and over	—	—	—	—	46.4	45.4	39.0	33.9	33.2	32.3	32.2	32.9
White Female[4]												
All ages, age-adjusted	6.0	5.9	7.9	6.1	5.7	5.2	4.7	4.3	4.9	5.1	5.2	5.4
All ages, crude	5.5	5.3	7.1	5.9	5.6	5.3	4.8	4.4	5.0	5.2	5.4	5.5
15–24 years	2.7	2.3	4.2	4.6	4.7	4.2	3.8	3.1	3.7	3.4	3.4	3.6
25–44 years	6.6	7.0	11.0	8.1	7.0	6.6	6.3	6.0	6.5	6.8	7.0	7.1
45–64 years	10.6	10.9	13.0	9.6	8.7	7.7	6.7	6.9	8.1	8.8	9.3	9.4
65 years and over	9.9	8.8	8.5	6.4	6.9	6.8	5.7	4.3	4.2	4.1	4.2	4.3
Black or African American Female[4]												
All ages, age-adjusted	1.8	2.0	2.9	2.4	2.3	2.4	2.0	1.8	1.9	1.4	1.7	1.7
All ages, crude	1.5	1.6	2.6	2.2	2.1	2.3	2.0	1.7	1.8	1.4	1.7	1.6
15–24 years	1.8	*	3.8	2.3	2.0	2.3	2.2	2.2	1.7	1.8	1.6	2.5
25–44 years	2.3	3.0	4.8	4.3	3.2	3.8	3.3	2.6	2.8	2.0	2.7	2.5
45–64 years	2.7	3.1	2.9	2.5	2.8	2.9	2.0	2.1	2.5	1.9	2.3	1.6
65 years and over	*	*	2.6	*	2.7	1.9	2.1	1.3	1.4	*	*	1.2
American Indian or Alaska Native Female[4]												
All ages, age-adjusted	—	—	—	4.7	4.1	3.6	3.9	3.8	4.6	5.1	4.9	5.8
All ages, crude	—	—	—	4.7	4.4	3.7	3.8	4.0	5.0	5.4	5.1	5.9
15–24 years	—	—	—	*	*	*	*	*	10.1	8.9	7.8	10.1
25–44 years	—	—	—	10.7	*	*	6.4	7.2	7.4	8.0	6.9	7.4
45–64 years	—	—	—	*	*	*	*	*	*	*	*	7.2
65 years and over	—	—	—	*	*	*	*	*	*	*	*	*

Table B–43. Death Rates for Suicide, by Sex, Race, Hispanic Origin, and Age, Selected Years, 1950–2008—Continued

(Deaths per 100,000 resident population.)

Sex, race, Hispanic origin, and age	1950[1,2]	1960[1,2]	1970[2]	1980[2]	1985	1990[2]	1995	2000[3]	2005[3]	2006[3]	2007[3]	2008[3]
Asian or Pacific Islander Female[5]												
All ages, age–adjusted	—	—	—	5.5	5.0	4.1	4.1	2.8	3.3	3.4	3.5	3.7
All ages, crude	—	—	—	4.7	4.3	3.4	3.7	2.7	3.2	3.3	3.6	3.8
15–24 years	—	—	—	*	5.8	3.9	4.8	2.7	3.7	4.0	3.8	4.7
25–44 years	—	—	—	5.4	4.2	3.8	3.6	3.3	3.4	3.3	4.6	4.9
45–64 years	—	—	—	7.9	5.4	5.0	4.7	3.2	3.8	4.2	4.0	3.9
65 years and over	—	—	—	*	13.6	8.5	8.6	5.2	6.8	6.9	5.2	5.7
Hispanic or Latina Female[4,6]												
All ages, age–adjusted	—	—	—	—	1.9	2.3	2.0	1.7	1.8	1.8	1.9	1.9
All ages, crude	—	—	—	—	1.6	2.2	1.8	1.5	1.7	1.7	1.8	1.7
15–24 years	—	—	—	—	2.1	3.1	2.4	2.0	2.7	2.6	2.2	2.4
25–44 years	—	—	—	—	2.1	3.1	2.5	2.1	2.2	2.3	2.7	2.3
45–64 years	—	—	—	—	3.2	2.5	2.8	2.5	2.1	2.4	2.8	2.8
65 years and over	—	—	—	—	*	*	*	*	2.0	1.7	*	1.5
White, not Hispanic or Latina Female[6]												
All ages, age–adjusted	—	—	—	—	6.1	5.4	4.9	4.7	5.3	5.6	5.7	6.0
All ages, crude	—	—	—	—	6.2	5.6	5.1	4.9	5.6	5.9	6.1	6.3
15–24 years	—	—	—	—	4.7	4.3	4.0	3.3	3.9	3.5	3.7	3.9
25–44 years	—	—	—	—	7.7	7.0	6.6	6.7	7.4	7.8	8.0	8.3
45–64 years	—	—	—	—	9.2	8.0	6.9	7.3	8.7	9.5	10.0	10.2
65 years and over	—	—	—	—	7.5	7.0	5.8	4.4	4.3	4.3	4.4	4.5

X = Category not applicable.
* = Rates based on fewer than 20 deaths are considered unreliable and are not shown.
– = Data not available.
[1]Includes deaths of persons who were not residents of the 50 states and the District of Columbia.
[2]Underlying cause of death was coded according to the 6th Revision of the International Classification of Diseases (ICD) in 1950, 7th Revision in 1960, 8th Revision in 1970.
[3]Starting with 1999 data, cause of death is coded according to ICD–10.
[4]The race groups, White, Black, Asian or Pacific Islander, and American Indian or Alaska Native, include persons of Hispanic and non–Hispanic origin. Persons of Hispanic origin may be of any race.
[5]In 1950, rate is for the age group 75 years and over.
[6]Prior to 1997, excludes data from states lacking an Hispanic–origin item on the death certificate.

Table B–44. Death Rates for Firearm-Related Injuries, by Sex, Race, Hispanic Origin, and Age, Selected Years, 1970–2008

(Deaths per 100,000 resident population.)

Sex, race, Hispanic origin, and age	1970[1]	1980[1]	1985	1990[1]	1995[1]	2000[2]	2001[2]	2002[2]	2003[2]	2004[2]	2005[2]	2006[2]	2007[2]	2008[2]
All Persons														
All ages, age–adjusted	14.3	14.8	13.1	14.6	13.4	10.2	10.3	10.4	10.3	10.0	10.2	10.2	10.2	10.3
All ages, crude	13.1	14.9	13.3	14.9	13.5	10.2	10.4	10.5	10.4	10.1	10.4	10.3	10.4	10.4
Under 1 year	*	*	*	*	*	*	*	*	*	*	*	*	*	*
1–14 years	1.6	1.4	1.4	1.5	1.6	0.7	0.7	0.7	0.7	0.6	0.7	0.7	0.7	0.6
1–4 years	1.0	0.7	0.7	0.6	0.6	0.3	0.5	0.4	0.3	0.3	0.4	0.3	0.4	0.5
5–14 years	1.7	1.6	1.8	1.9	1.9	0.9	0.8	0.8	0.8	0.7	0.8	0.9	0.8	0.7
15–24 years	15.5	20.6	17.2	25.8	26.7	16.8	16.7	16.7	16.6	15.7	16.2	16.9	16.2	15.7
15–19 years	11.4	14.7	13.3	23.3	24.1	12.9	12.4	12.1	12.1	12.0	12.5	13.2	12.4	12.0
20–24 years	20.3	26.4	20.6	28.1	29.2	20.9	21.2	21.3	21.1	19.3	20.0	20.6	20.1	19.4
25–44 years	20.9	22.5	17.9	19.3	16.9	13.1	13.5	13.7	13.4	13.1	13.6	13.3	13.6	13.4
25–34 years	22.2	24.3	19.3	21.8	19.6	14.5	15.5	15.4	15.5	15.0	15.7	15.3	15.5	15.2
35–44 years	19.6	20.0	16.0	16.3	14.3	11.9	11.7	12.1	11.5	11.3	11.6	11.5	11.9	11.7
45–64 years	17.6	15.2	14.3	13.6	11.7	10.0	10.3	10.6	10.7	10.5	10.6	10.6	10.7	11.3
45–54 years	18.1	16.4	14.7	13.9	12.0	10.5	10.5	10.8	11.2	11.0	11.2	11.2	11.1	11.6
55–64 years	17.0	13.9	13.9	13.3	11.3	9.4	10.1	10.2	10.1	9.8	9.8	9.8	10.2	10.9
65 years and over	13.8	13.5	15.6	16.0	14.1	12.2	12.4	12.4	11.8	11.5	11.8	11.2	11.3	11.7
65–74 years	14.5	13.8	15.1	14.4	12.8	10.6	10.9	10.9	10.4	10.2	10.3	10.0	10.0	10.9
75–84 years	13.4	13.4	17.7	19.4	16.3	13.9	14.3	14.4	13.5	13.3	13.7	12.9	13.2	13.3
85 years and over	10.2	11.6	12.2	14.7	14.4	14.2	12.8	12.5	12.5	11.9	12.0	11.5	11.6	11.3
Male														
All ages, age–adjusted	24.8	25.9	23.1	26.1	23.8	18.1	18.5	18.6	18.4	17.7	18.3	18.1	18.2	18.2
All ages, crude	22.2	25.7	22.8	26.2	23.6	17.8	18.2	18.4	18.3	17.6	18.3	18.1	18.2	18.2
Under 1 year	*	*	*	*	*	*	*	*	*	*	*	*	*	*
1–14 years	2.3	2.0	2.1	2.2	2.3	1.1	1.0	1.0	1.0	0.9	1.0	1.0	1.0	0.9
1–4 years	1.2	0.9	0.8	0.7	0.8	0.4	0.5	0.5	0.3	0.4	0.5	0.5	0.5	0.6
5–14 years	2.7	2.5	2.7	2.9	2.9	1.4	1.2	1.2	1.2	1.1	1.2	1.2	1.2	1.0
15–24 years	26.4	34.8	29.1	44.7	46.5	29.4	29.6	29.3	29.2	27.5	28.7	29.8	28.5	27.5
15–19 years	19.2	24.5	22.4	40.1	41.6	22.4	21.8	21.1	21.2	20.7	22.0	23.3	21.8	21.1
20–24 years	35.1	45.2	35.0	49.1	51.5	37.0	37.7	37.6	37.1	34.2	35.3	36.2	35.3	34.0
25–44 years	34.1	38.1	29.7	32.6	28.4	22.0	22.8	23.1	22.9	22.3	23.1	22.6	23.2	22.7
25–34 years	36.5	41.4	32.1	37.0	33.2	24.9	26.7	26.5	27.1	26.1	27.2	26.6	27.0	26.2
35–44 years	31.6	33.2	26.6	27.4	23.6	19.4	19.2	20.1	19.1	18.7	19.2	18.9	19.5	19.3
45–64 years	31.0	25.9	24.5	23.4	20.0	17.1	17.6	18.1	18.3	17.8	18.3	17.9	18.3	19.3
45–54 years	30.7	27.3	24.4	23.2	20.1	17.6	17.8	18.2	18.8	18.3	18.9	18.5	18.6	19.4
55–64 years	31.3	24.5	24.6	23.7	19.8	16.3	17.4	18.0	17.7	17.1	17.4	17.0	17.9	19.3
65 years and over	29.7	29.7	34.2	35.3	30.7	26.4	26.8	26.9	25.4	24.8	25.1	24.1	24.2	24.9
65–74 years	29.5	27.8	30.0	28.2	25.1	20.3	21.1	21.3	20.3	19.7	19.7	19.2	19.1	20.8
75–84 years	31.0	33.0	42.7	46.9	37.8	32.2	32.8	32.9	30.2	29.8	30.8	29.1	29.5	29.5
85 years and over	26.2	34.9	38.2	49.3	47.1	44.7	40.2	38.9	37.8	35.9	35.4	33.6	33.5	31.7
Female														
All ages, age–adjusted	4.8	4.7	4.2	4.2	3.8	2.8	2.8	2.8	2.7	2.7	2.7	2.7	2.7	2.7
All ages, crude	4.4	4.7	4.2	4.3	3.8	2.8	2.8	2.8	2.7	2.7	2.7	2.8	2.7	2.8
Under 1 year	*	*	*	*	*	*	*	*	*	*	*	*	*	*
1–14 years	0.8	0.7	0.7	0.8	0.8	0.3	0.4	0.5	0.3	0.3	0.4	0.4	0.4	0.4
1–4 years	0.9	0.5	0.5	0.5	0.5	*	0.4	0.3	0.3	0.3	0.3	*	0.4	0.3
5–14 years	0.8	0.7	0.8	1.0	0.9	0.4	0.4	0.5	0.3	0.3	0.4	0.4	0.4	0.4
15–24 years	4.8	6.1	5.0	6.0	5.9	3.5	3.2	3.5	3.3	3.2	3.0	3.2	3.2	3.2
15–19 years	3.5	4.6	3.9	5.7	5.6	2.9	2.6	2.7	2.4	2.9	2.4	2.5	2.6	2.5
20–24 years	6.4	7.7	5.9	6.3	6.1	4.2	3.8	4.2	4.2	3.5	3.6	3.8	3.9	4.0
25–44 years	8.3	7.4	6.2	6.1	5.5	4.2	4.2	4.1	3.8	3.8	3.9	3.9	3.9	3.8
25–34 years	8.4	7.5	6.6	6.7	5.8	4.0	4.0	4.0	3.6	3.7	3.8	3.7	3.6	3.6
35–44 years	8.2	7.2	5.8	5.4	5.2	4.4	4.3	4.2	4.0	3.9	4.0	4.1	4.2	4.0
45–64 years	5.4	5.4	5.0	4.5	3.9	3.4	3.4	3.4	3.4	3.7	3.3	3.6	3.4	3.6
45–54 years	6.4	6.2	5.6	4.9	4.2	3.6	3.5	3.6	3.8	4.0	3.7	4.0	3.7	4.0
55–64 years	4.2	4.6	4.5	4.0	3.5	3.0	3.3	3.1	2.9	3.1	2.8	3.2	3.0	3.1
65 years and over	2.4	2.5	3.2	3.1	2.8	2.2	2.2	2.0	2.1	2.0	2.1	1.9	2.0	2.1
65–74 years	2.8	3.1	3.6	3.6	3.0	2.5	2.4	2.3	2.2	2.2	2.5	2.2	2.3	2.4
75–84 years	1.7	1.7	3.0	2.9	2.8	2.0	2.2	2.1	2.2	2.3	2.1	1.8	2.0	2.0
85 years and over	*	1.3	1.8	1.3	1.8	1.7	1.3	1.1	1.3	1.0	1.3	1.1	1.1	1.5
White Male[3]														
All ages, age–adjusted	19.7	22.1	21.0	22.0	20.1	15.9	16.3	16.2	16.0	15.4	15.7	15.3	15.6	15.9
All ages, crude	17.6	21.8	20.7	21.8	19.9	15.6	16.2	16.1	16.0	15.5	15.8	15.4	15.8	16.2
1–14 years	1.8	1.9	2.1	1.9	1.9	1.0	0.9	0.8	0.7	0.7	0.8	0.8	0.7	0.7
15–24 years	16.9	28.4	24.1	29.5	30.8	19.6	19.5	19.4	19.2	18.4	18.2	18.4	17.5	17.7
25–44 years	24.2	29.5	25.0	25.7	23.2	18.0	18.9	18.5	18.1	17.6	17.9	17.3	18.3	18.0
25–34 years	24.3	31.1	26.3	27.8	25.2	18.1	19.9	18.5	18.8	18.2	18.6	17.7	18.9	18.2
35–44 years	24.1	27.1	23.3	23.3	21.2	17.9	18.0	18.5	17.5	17.1	17.2	17.0	17.6	17.8
45–64 years	27.4	23.3	23.6	22.8	19.5	17.4	18.3	18.7	19.0	18.4	19.0	18.4	19.0	20.4
65 years and over	29.9	30.1	35.4	36.8	32.2	28.2	28.6	28.9	27.4	26.5	27.1	26.0	26.2	26.8

Table B–44. Death Rates for Firearm–Related Injuries, by Sex, Race, Hispanic Origin, and Age, Selected Years, 1970–2008—Continued

(Deaths per 100,000 resident population.)

Sex, race, Hispanic origin, and age	1970[1]	1980[1]	1985	1990[1]	1995[1]	2000[2]	2001[2]	2002[2]	2003[2]	2004[2]	2005[2]	2006[2]	2007[2]	2008[2]
Black or African American Male[3]														
All ages, age–adjusted	70.8	60.1	40.9	56.3	49.2	34.2	34.5	36.0	35.6	34.5	36.4	37.4	36.2	34.4
All ages, crude	60.8	57.7	41.3	61.9	52.9	36.1	36.4	37.8	37.8	36.4	38.7	40.0	38.9	36.7
1–14 years	5.3	3.0	2.7	4.4	4.4	1.8	1.6	1.8	2.1	2.0	2.1	2.2	2.2	2.1
15–24 years	97.3	77.9	61.3	138.0	138.7	89.3	90.3	87.1	87.6	80.7	86.8	91.8	89.1	81.3
25–44 years	126.2	114.1	71.8	90.3	70.2	54.1	54.8	60.6	60.5	59.2	63.6	63.8	62.3	59.9
25–34 years	145.6	128.4	79.8	108.6	92.3	74.8	77.7	85.6	87.2	83.6	88.4	89.0	84.8	81.4
35–44 years	104.2	92.3	59.2	66.1	46.3	34.3	33.2	36.9	34.8	35.1	38.7	38.1	38.9	36.8
45–64 years	71.1	55.6	36.9	34.5	28.3	18.4	17.2	18.6	18.1	18.3	17.8	19.3	19.0	17.7
65 years and over	30.6	29.7	26.3	23.9	21.8	13.8	14.9	14.2	12.1	14.6	13.6	13.4	11.1	13.4
American Indian or Alaska Native Male[3]														
All ages, age–adjusted	—	24.0	23.6	19.4	19.4	13.1	13.0	14.8	14.1	14.2	15.7	14.7	12.4	13.3
All ages, crude	—	27.5	24.4	20.5	20.9	13.2	12.9	15.3	14.7	15.0	16.7	15.8	13.2	13.6
15–24 years	—	55.3	39.8	49.1	40.9	26.9	24.3	30.0	27.6	25.7	32.7	32.7	25.1	27.4
25–44 years	—	43.9	40.3	25.4	31.2	16.6	18.8	21.7	21.8	23.5	23.2	21.2	16.3	20.3
45–64 years	—	*	21.2	*	14.2	12.2	9.6	12.4	10.5	9.5	13.0	11.0	11.7	8.0
65 years and over	—	*	*	*	*	*	*	*	*	*	*	*	*	*
Asian or Pacific Islander Male[3]														
All ages, age–adjusted	—	7.8	7.3	8.8	9.2	6.0	5.2	5.5	5.4	4.8	5.3	5.4	5.2	4.5
All ages, crude	—	8.2	7.3	9.4	10.0	6.2	5.4	5.7	5.7	5.0	5.5	5.7	5.3	4.6
15–24 years	—	10.8	12.6	21.0	24.3	9.3	9.6	11.7	10.5	8.8	12.1	14.5	11.4	9.0
25–44 years	—	12.8	9.8	10.9	10.6	8.1	6.6	6.3	6.9	5.7	6.4	5.7	5.9	5.4
45–64 years	—	10.4	6.7	8.1	8.2	7.4	5.7	5.8	5.7	6.1	5.7	5.6	5.7	4.8
65 years and over	—	*	*	*	*	5.3	*	*	*	4.2	*	*	4.4	4.4
Hispanic or Latino Male[4]														
All ages, age–adjusted	—	—	24.2	27.6	23.8	13.6	13.7	13.4	13.6	13.1	13.3	12.7	12.9	11.8
All ages, crude	—	—	26.0	29.9	26.2	14.2	14.6	14.2	14.6	13.9	14.2	13.7	13.4	12.0
1–14 years	—	—	1.4	2.6	2.8	1.0	0.7	0.9	0.8	0.7	0.7	1.1	0.8	0.5
15–24 years	—	—	42.0	55.5	61.7	30.8	31.4	32.1	32.8	32.4	33.0	33.6	31.4	28.2
25–44 years	—	—	43.2	42.7	31.4	17.3	19.1	17.6	18.6	17.6	18.8	17.4	17.2	15.9
25–34 years	—	—	47.3	47.3	36.4	20.3	22.7	21.2	22.8	21.3	22.9	20.9	21.1	18.5
35–44 years	—	—	35.9	35.4	24.2	13.2	14.4	12.9	13.3	12.9	13.4	12.9	12.4	12.7
45–64 years	—	—	19.2	21.4	17.2	12.0	10.0	9.9	10.3	9.9	9.1	8.5	9.6	8.9
65 years and over	—	—	12.4	19.1	16.5	12.2	12.0	12.3	10.6	10.0	9.8	7.6	10.7	9.7
White, not Hispanic or Latino Male[3]														
All ages, age–adjusted	—	—	20.2	20.6	18.6	15.5	16.0	16.0	15.6	15.1	15.3	15.0	15.4	16.1
All ages, crude	—	—	19.9	20.4	18.5	15.7	16.3	16.3	16.0	15.6	15.9	15.6	16.1	17.0
1–14 years	—	—	2.0	1.6	1.6	1.0	1.0	0.7	0.7	0.7	0.8	0.7	0.7	0.7
15–24 years	—	—	22.0	24.1	23.5	16.2	16.0	15.6	15.2	14.3	13.9	13.9	13.4	14.5
25–44 years	—	—	23.0	23.3	21.4	17.9	18.6	18.4	17.7	17.4	17.4	17.1	18.3	18.5
25–34 years	—	—	23.7	24.7	22.5	17.2	18.9	17.4	17.3	16.9	16.9	16.3	18.0	17.9
35–44 years	—	—	22.0	21.6	20.4	18.4	18.4	19.3	18.1	17.8	17.8	17.8	18.6	19.0
45–64 years	—	—	23.0	22.7	19.5	17.8	19.0	19.4	19.8	19.2	20.0	19.5	20.1	21.8
65 years and over	—	—	37.3	37.4	32.5	29.0	29.4	29.8	28.4	27.6	28.2	27.3	27.4	28.1
White Female[3]														
All ages, age–adjusted	4.0	4.2	3.9	3.8	3.5	2.7	2.7	2.7	2.6	2.7	2.6	2.6	2.6	2.7
All ages, crude	3.7	4.1	4.0	3.8	3.5	2.7	2.7	2.7	2.6	2.7	2.6	2.6	2.7	2.7
15–24 years	3.4	5.1	4.4	4.8	4.5	2.8	2.7	2.6	2.5	2.6	2.3	2.3	2.6	2.3
25–44 years	6.9	6.2	5.6	5.3	4.9	3.9	3.9	3.8	3.6	3.6	3.7	3.5	3.7	3.7
45–64 years	5.0	5.1	5.0	4.5	4.0	3.5	3.7	3.6	3.7	3.9	3.6	3.9	3.7	4.0
65 years and over	2.2	2.5	3.2	3.1	2.8	2.4	2.3	2.2	2.1	2.2	2.3	2.0	2.1	2.2

Table B–44. Death Rates for Firearm–Related Injuries, by Sex, Race, Hispanic Origin, and Age, Selected Years, 1970–2008—Continued

(Deaths per 100,000 resident population.)

Sex, race, Hispanic origin, and age	1970[1]	1980[1]	1985	1990[1]	1995[1]	2000[2]	2001[2]	2002[2]	2003[2]	2004[2]	2005[2]	2006[2]	2007[2]	2008[2]
Black or African American Female[3]														
All ages, age–adjusted	11.1	8.7	6.4	7.3	6.2	3.9	3.8	4.1	3.8	3.6	3.6	4.0	3.8	3.5
All ages, crude	10.0	8.8	6.5	7.8	6.5	4.0	3.8	4.2	3.9	3.7	3.7	4.1	3.9	3.6
15–24 years	15.2	12.3	8.3	13.3	13.2	7.6	6.1	8.1	7.4	6.9	6.7	7.7	7.1	8.2
25–44 years	19.4	16.1	11.4	12.4	9.8	6.5	6.9	6.7	6.1	5.7	6.0	7.0	6.4	5.4
45–64 years	10.2	8.2	5.8	4.8	4.1	3.1	2.6	3.0	2.7	3.0	2.7	2.6	2.8	2.1
65 years and over	4.3	3.1	3.7	3.1	2.6	1.3	1.4	1.2	1.8	*	1.3	1.0	1.2	1.3
American Indian or Alaska Native Female[3]														
All ages, age–adjusted	—	5.8	3.9	3.3	3.8	2.9	2.8	3.1	2.4	2.7	2.4	2.4	2.0	2.7
All ages, crude	—	5.8	4.1	3.4	4.1	2.9	2.9	3.4	2.6	2.9	2.6	2.4	2.0	2.7
15–24 years	—	*	*	*	*	*	*	*	*	*	*	*	*	*
25–44 years	—	10.2	*	*	7.0	5.5	5.0	*	*	*	*	*	*	4.2
45–64 years	—	*	*	*	*	*	*	*	*	*	*	*	*	*
65 years and over	—	*	*	*	*	*	*	*	*	*	*	*	*	*
Asian or Pacific Islander Female[3]														
All ages, age–adjusted	—	2.0	1.5	1.9	2.0	1.1	1.0	1.1	1.1	0.9	0.9	1.0	0.7	0.8
All ages, crude	—	2.1	1.7	2.1	2.1	1.2	1.1	1.2	1.2	1.0	0.9	1.0	0.7	0.9
15–24 years	—	*	*	*	3.9	*	*	*	2.1	*	2.3	*	*	*
25–44 years	—	3.2	2.2	2.7	2.7	1.5	1.5	1.7	1.3	1.4	1.0	1.2	1.0	1.2
45–64 years	—	*	*	*	*	*	*	*	1.5	1.3	*	1.3	*	*
65 years and over	—	*	*	*	*	*	*	*	*	*	*	*	*	*
Hispanic or Latina Female[3,4]														
All ages, age–adjusted	—	—	2.9	3.3	3.1	1.8	1.7	1.6	1.6	1.5	1.6	1.5	1.5	1.5
All ages, crude	—	—	3.2	3.6	3.3	1.8	1.7	1.6	1.7	1.5	1.6	1.5	1.5	1.5
15–24 years	—	—	5.1	6.9	6.1	2.9	3.3	2.8	3.5	2.6	2.6	2.7	2.9	2.9
25–44 years	—	—	5.5	5.1	4.7	2.5	2.5	2.4	2.2	2.2	2.7	2.3	2.3	2.0
45–64 years	—	—	2.2	2.4	2.4	2.2	1.6	1.6	1.5	1.5	1.2	1.4	1.5	1.7
65 years and over	—	—	*	*	*	*	*	*	*	*	*	*	*	*
White, not Hispanic or Latina Female[4]														
All ages, age–adjusted	—	—	4.0	3.7	3.4	2.8	2.8	2.8	2.7	2.8	2.7	2.7	2.8	2.9
All ages, crude	—	—	4.1	3.7	3.5	2.9	2.9	2.8	2.7	2.9	2.8	2.8	2.9	3.0
15–24 years	—	—	4.5	4.3	4.1	2.7	2.5	2.5	2.2	2.5	2.2	2.2	2.5	2.2
25–44 years	—	—	5.6	5.1	4.8	4.2	4.1	4.1	3.9	3.9	4.0	3.8	4.1	4.1
45–64 years	—	—	5.1	4.6	4.1	3.6	3.8	3.8	3.9	4.1	3.8	4.2	3.9	4.2
65 years and over	—	—	3.4	3.2	2.8	2.4	2.4	2.3	2.2	2.3	2.4	2.2	2.2	2.4

* = Rates based on fewer than 20 deaths are considered unreliable and are not shown.
– = Data not available.
[1]Underlying cause of death was coded according to the 8th Revision of the International Classification of Diseases (ICD) in 1970 and 9th Revision in 1980–1998.
[2]Starting with 1999 data, cause of death is coded according to ICD–10.
[3]The race groups, White, Black, Asian or Pacific Islander, and American Indian or Alaska Native, include persons of Hispanic and non–Hispanic origin. Persons of Hispanic origin may be of any race.
[4]Prior to 1997, excludes data from states lacking an Hispanic–origin item on the death certificate.

PART B: MORTALITY 227

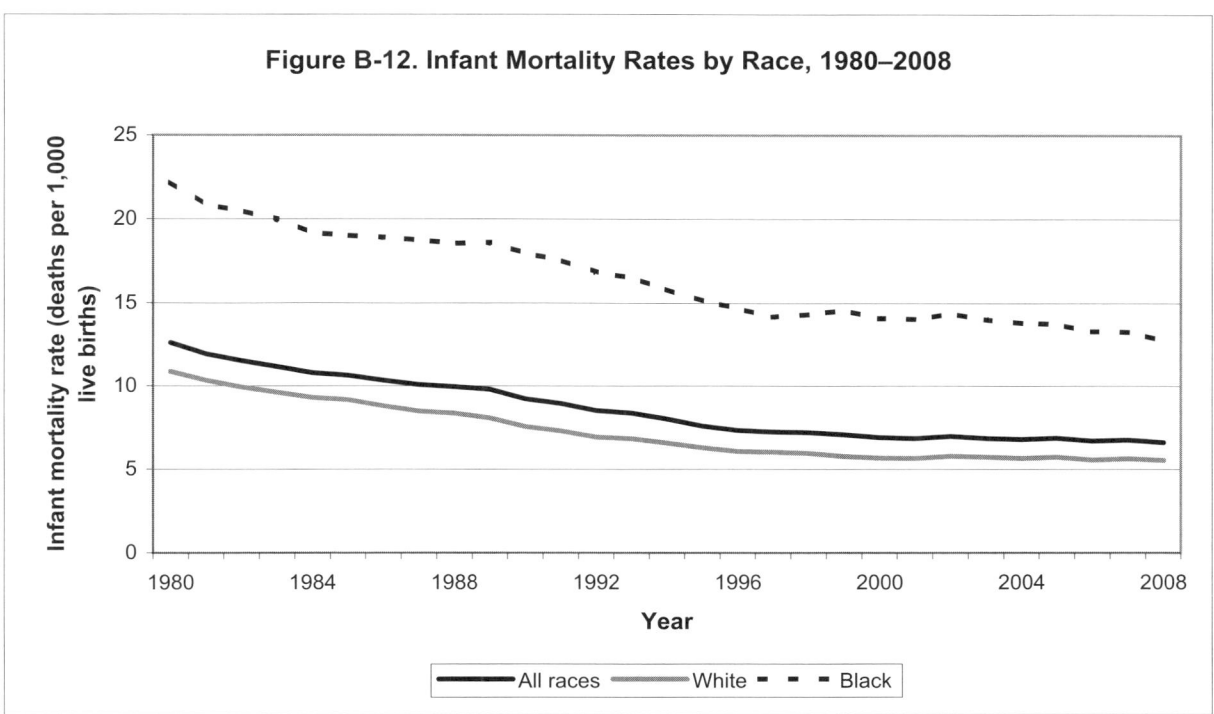

Figure B-12. Infant Mortality Rates by Race, 1980–2008

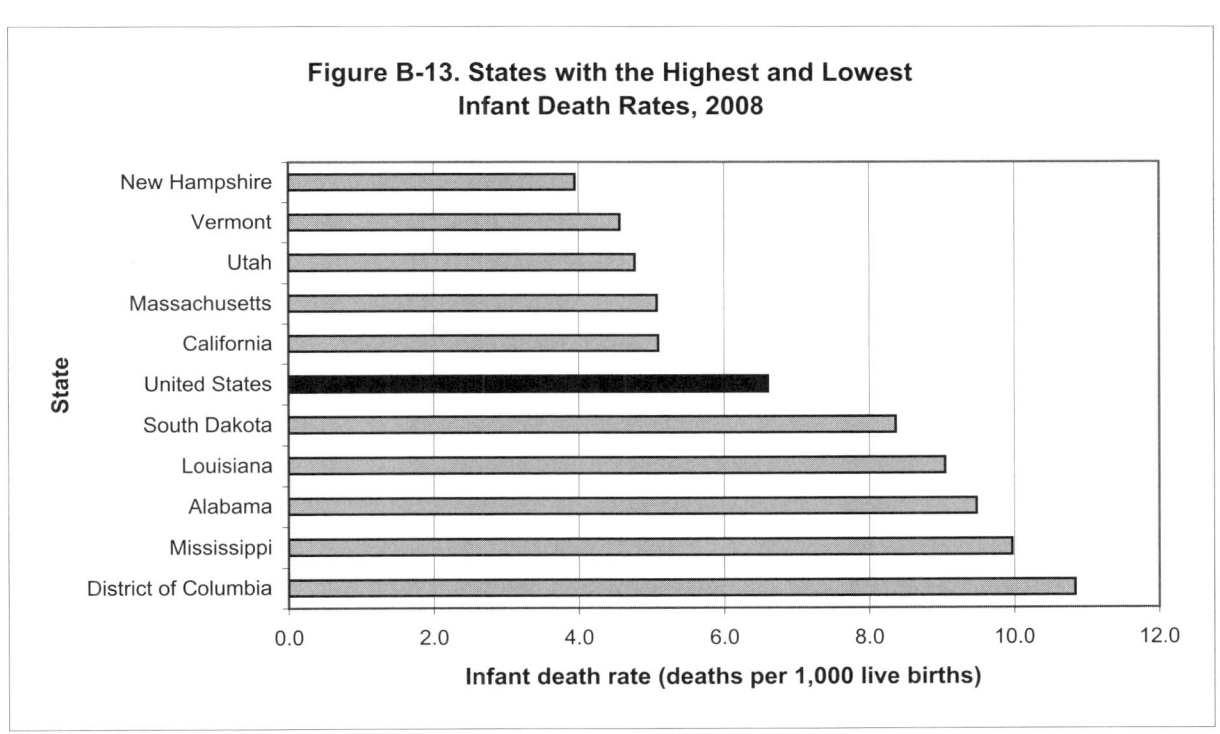

Figure B-13. States with the Highest and Lowest Infant Death Rates, 2008

Table B-45. Infant, Neonatal, and Postneonatal Mortality Rates, by Race and Sex, 1940–2008

(Rates are infant (under 1 year), neonatal (under 28 days), and postneonatal (28 days–11 months) deaths per 1,000 live births in specified group.)

Year	All races			White[1]			All other					
							Total[1]			Black[1]		
	Both sexes	Male	Female	Both sexes	Male	Female	Both sexes	Male	Female	Both sexes	Male	Female
INFANT MORTALITY RATE												
Race of Mother[2]												
1980	12.60	13.93	11.21	10.86	12.12	9.52	20.19	21.89	18.43	22.19	24.16	20.15
1981	11.93	13.14	10.66	10.34	11.50	9.12	18.82	20.36	17.24	20.81	22.54	19.03
1982	11.52	12.77	10.21	9.94	11.08	8.73	18.31	20.07	16.49	20.48	22.45	18.44
1983	11.16	12.31	9.96	9.61	10.66	8.49	17.80	19.44	16.11	19.98	21.95	17.96
1984	10.79	11.90	9.62	9.30	10.38	8.17	17.05	18.37	15.69	19.15	20.67	17.58
1985	10.64	11.91	9.32	9.17	10.39	7.88	16.84	18.33	15.28	19.01	20.76	17.22
1986	10.35	11.55	9.10	8.80	9.87	7.67	16.72	18.45	14.91	18.90	20.91	16.81
1987	10.08	11.17	8.94	8.48	9.45	7.45	16.46	18.06	14.80	18.75	20.63	16.83
1988	9.95	10.99	8.86	8.36	9.35	7.31	16.08	17.33	14.79	18.54	20.04	16.99
1989	9.81	10.81	8.77	8.08	9.01	7.10	16.33	17.60	15.02	18.61	20.02	17.15
1990	9.22	10.26	8.13	7.56	8.51	6.56	15.52	16.96	14.03	17.96	19.62	16.25
1991	8.94	10.00	7.84	7.30	8.26	6.30	15.07	16.53	13.57	17.57	19.38	15.71
1992	8.52	9.39	7.61	6.92	7.69	6.12	14.44	15.72	13.10	16.85	18.38	15.26
1993	8.37	9.25	7.43	6.82	7.56	6.05	14.07	15.58	12.52	16.52	18.33	14.67
1994	8.02	8.81	7.20	6.57	7.22	5.89	13.47	14.82	12.08	15.83	17.49	14.12
1995	7.59	8.33	6.81	6.29	6.99	5.55	12.61	13.53	11.65	15.12	16.34	13.86
1996	7.32	8.02	6.59	6.07	6.67	5.44	12.18	13.31	11.01	14.68	16.04	13.27
1997	7.23	7.95	6.47	6.03	6.67	5.36	11.76	12.83	10.65	14.16	15.47	12.82
1998	7.20	7.83	6.54	5.95	6.47	5.41	11.92	13.01	10.79	14.31	15.75	12.82
1999	7.06	7.72	6.36	5.77	6.35	5.15	11.94	12.94	10.90	14.56	15.92	13.16
2000	6.91	7.57	6.21	5.68	6.22	5.11	11.44	12.57	10.26	14.09	15.50	12.63
2001	6.85	7.52	6.14	5.65	6.21	5.06	11.33	12.44	10.18	14.02	15.48	12.52
2002	6.97	7.64	6.27	5.79	6.42	5.13	11.41	12.24	10.55	14.36	15.43	13.25
2003	6.85	7.60	6.07	5.72	6.36	5.05	11.09	12.24	9.90	14.01	15.53	12.43
2004	6.79	7.47	6.09	5.66	6.22	5.07	10.92	12.01	9.77	13.79	15.19	12.33
2005	6.87	7.56	6.15	5.73	6.32	5.11	10.92	11.98	9.82	13.73	15.15	12.27
2006	6.69	7.32	6.03	5.56	6.10	4.99	10.60	11.54	9.61	13.29	14.38	12.16
2007	6.75	7.38	6.09	5.64	6.17	5.08	10.55	11.51	9.54	13.24	14.49	11.94
2008	6.61	7.21	5.97	5.55	6.05	5.02	10.16	11.11	9.18	12.74	13.93	11.50
Race of Child[3]												
1940	47.02	52.45	41.29	43.23	48.32	37.84	73.78	82.21	65.19	72.94	81.07	64.61
1950	29.21	32.75	25.48	26.77	30.21	23.13	44.46	48.87	39.93	43.91	48.27	39.44
1960	26.04	29.33	22.59	22.91	26.01	19.64	43.21	47.88	38.46	44.32	49.12	39.43
1970	20.01	22.37	17.52	17.75	19.95	15.42	30.92	34.20	27.53	32.65	36.18	29.01
1975	16.07	17.86	14.18	14.17	15.94	12.30	24.23	26.24	22.17	26.21	28.32	24.03
1976	15.24	16.82	13.57	13.31	14.81	11.71	23.50	25.51	21.42	25.54	27.83	23.19
1977	14.12	15.75	12.40	12.34	13.90	10.68	21.68	23.71	19.58	23.64	25.91	21.30
1978	13.78	15.26	12.23	12.01	13.37	10.58	21.06	23.15	18.90	23.11	25.39	20.77
1979	13.07	14.50	11.56	11.42	12.82	9.94	19.81	21.47	18.09	21.78	23.66	19.85
1980	12.60	13.93	11.21	11.00	12.27	9.65	19.12	20.73	17.47	21.37	23.27	19.43
NEONATAL MORTALITY RATE												
Race of Mother[2]												
1980	8.48	9.31	7.60	7.39	8.19	6.54	13.21	14.27	12.13	14.62	15.91	13.29
1981	8.02	8.81	7.20	6.99	7.73	6.20	12.51	13.52	11.48	13.98	15.16	12.77
1982	7.70	8.48	6.88	6.69	7.39	5.94	12.04	13.15	10.88	13.62	14.86	12.34
1983	7.28	8.01	6.52	6.31	6.98	5.61	11.41	12.46	10.33	12.93	14.20	11.63
1984	7.00	7.66	6.31	6.09	6.72	5.41	10.87	11.66	10.06	12.32	13.22	11.40
1985	6.96	7.75	6.13	6.00	6.75	5.21	11.00	12.00	9.95	12.62	13.81	11.39
1986	6.71	7.42	5.97	5.72	6.34	5.05	10.79	11.83	9.70	12.31	13.59	10.98
1987	6.46	7.11	5.79	5.40	5.96	4.82	10.68	11.72	9.61	12.30	13.52	11.05
1988	6.32	6.95	5.65	5.27	5.84	4.67	10.33	11.22	9.42	12.05	13.14	10.93
1989	6.23	6.79	5.63	5.15	5.66	4.60	10.30	11.08	9.49	11.92	12.84	10.97

Table B-45. Infant, Neonatal, and Postneonatal Mortality Rates, by Race and Sex, 1940–2008—*Continued*

(Rates are infant (under 1 year), neonatal (under 28 days), and postneonatal (28 days–11 months) deaths per 1,000 live births in specified group.)

Year	All races			White[1]			All other					
							Total[1]			Black[1]		
	Both sexes	Male	Female	Both sexes	Male	Female	Both sexes	Male	Female	Both sexes	Male	Female
1990	5.85	6.50	5.16	4.79	5.38	4.17	9.86	10.79	8.89	11.55	12.69	10.38
1991	5.59	6.17	4.98	4.53	5.01	4.04	9.52	10.54	8.47	11.25	12.56	9.89
1992	5.37	5.84	4.89	4.35	4.72	3.96	9.19	10.02	8.32	10.83	11.83	9.79
1993	5.29	5.75	4.81	4.29	4.64	3.92	9.02	9.90	8.11	10.69	11.76	9.59
1994	5.12	5.58	4.64	4.20	4.55	3.83	8.60	9.51	7.65	10.21	11.32	9.07
1995	4.91	5.36	4.44	4.08	4.50	3.64	8.13	8.71	7.53	9.85	10.63	9.05
1996	4.77	5.18	4.34	3.97	4.31	3.62	7.86	8.59	7.12	9.56	10.45	8.65
1997	4.77	5.20	4.32	3.99	4.37	3.59	7.74	8.36	7.09	9.40	10.12	8.65
1998	4.80	5.21	4.37	3.98	4.31	3.63	7.91	8.63	7.17	9.55	10.51	8.56
1999	4.73	5.11	4.33	3.88	4.19	3.56	7.94	8.60	7.25	9.77	10.72	8.79
2000	4.63	5.06	4.17	3.82	4.16	3.46	7.60	8.39	6.79	9.38	10.39	8.35
2001	4.54	4.97	4.08	3.78	4.15	3.39	7.37	8.06	6.65	9.21	10.15	8.25
2002	4.66	5.06	4.25	3.89	4.27	3.50	7.55	8.03	7.05	9.51	10.13	8.87
2003	4.62	5.08	4.14	3.87	4.26	3.46	7.40	8.14	6.64	9.40	10.40	8.37
2004	4.52	4.94	4.09	3.78	4.14	3.41	7.19	7.82	6.54	9.13	9.95	8.27
2005	4.54	4.93	4.12	3.79	4.10	3.46	7.18	7.88	6.47	9.07	9.96	8.14
2006	4.45	4.84	4.05	3.72	4.05	3.37	7.00	7.58	6.40	8.82	9.49	8.12
2007	4.42	4.79	4.02	3.70	4.01	3.37	6.86	7.49	6.22	8.65	9.48	7.78
2008	4.29	4.67	3.89	3.62	3.94	3.28	6.54	7.14	5.92	8.23	8.99	7.45
Race of Child[3]												
1940	28.75	32.56	24.74	27.20	30.85	23.33	39.71	44.87	34.45	39.90	44.78	34.89
1950	20.50	23.34	17.50	19.37	22.18	16.40	27.54	30.76	24.23	27.80	31.09	24.44
1960	18.73	21.24	16.09	17.24	19.66	14.70	26.86	30.04	23.62	27.83	31.13	24.49
1970	15.08	16.96	13.10	13.77	15.55	11.88	21.43	23.87	18.91	22.76	25.37	20.07
1975	11.58	12.91	10.18	10.38	11.70	8.98	16.78	18.21	15.31	18.32	19.78	16.81
1976	10.92	12.03	9.75	9.66	10.73	8.52	16.31	17.68	14.90	17.92	19.47	16.32
1977	9.88	11.00	8.70	8.75	9.83	7.60	14.66	16.02	13.27	16.08	17.60	14.52
1978	9.49	10.54	8.38	8.39	9.34	7.38	14.01	15.54	12.43	15.47	17.17	13.72
1979	8.87	9.79	7.89	7.88	8.80	6.92	12.89	13.91	11.83	14.31	15.45	13.14
1980	8.48	9.31	7.60	7.48	8.29	6.62	12.52	13.51	11.49	14.08	15.32	12.81
POSTNEONATAL MORTALITY RATE												
Race of Mother[2]												
1980	4.13	4.62	3.61	3.47	3.93	2.98	6.97	7.62	6.30	7.57	8.25	6.87
1981	3.91	4.34	3.46	3.35	3.77	2.92	6.31	6.84	5.76	6.83	7.38	6.26
1982	3.82	4.29	3.33	3.25	3.68	2.79	6.28	6.92	5.61	6.86	7.59	6.10
1983	3.88	4.30	3.44	3.29	3.68	2.88	6.39	6.98	5.78	7.05	7.75	6.32
1984	3.79	4.23	3.31	3.22	3.65	2.76	6.18	6.71	5.63	6.83	7.46	6.18
1985	3.68	4.15	3.19	3.17	3.64	2.67	5.84	6.33	5.33	6.40	6.95	5.83
1986	3.64	4.13	3.13	3.08	3.53	2.62	5.93	6.62	5.21	6.59	7.33	5.83
1987	3.62	4.06	3.15	3.08	3.49	2.64	5.77	6.34	5.18	6.45	7.10	5.77
1988	3.64	4.04	3.21	3.09	3.51	2.65	5.75	6.11	5.37	6.49	6.90	6.07
1989	3.59	4.01	3.14	2.93	3.35	2.49	6.03	6.52	5.53	6.69	7.18	6.19
1990	3.38	3.76	2.97	2.78	3.14	2.39	5.66	6.16	5.13	6.41	6.93	5.87
1991	3.35	3.82	2.86	2.76	3.25	2.26	5.55	5.99	5.10	6.32	6.82	5.81
1992	3.14	3.55	2.72	2.58	2.97	2.16	5.25	5.69	4.78	6.02	6.54	5.47
1993	3.07	3.50	2.62	2.54	2.92	2.13	5.06	5.68	4.42	5.83	6.57	5.08
1994	2.90	3.22	2.56	2.37	2.67	2.06	4.88	5.32	4.42	5.61	6.17	5.04
1995	2.67	2.97	2.37	2.21	2.49	1.91	4.47	4.82	4.11	5.27	5.71	4.81
1996	2.55	2.84	2.24	2.09	2.36	1.81	4.32	4.72	3.90	5.11	5.60	4.62
1997	2.45	2.75	2.14	2.04	2.30	1.77	4.02	4.47	3.56	4.77	5.34	4.17
1998	2.40	2.62	2.16	1.97	2.16	1.78	4.01	4.38	3.62	4.76	5.24	4.26
1999	2.33	2.61	2.03	1.88	2.16	1.60	4.00	4.34	3.64	4.79	5.20	4.36

Table B-45. Infant, Neonatal, and Postneonatal Mortality Rates, by Race and Sex, 1940–2008—*Continued*

(Rates are infant (under 1 year), neonatal (under 28 days), and postneonatal (28 days–11 months) deaths per 1,000 live births in specified group.)

Year	All races			White[1]			All other					
							Total[1]			Black[1]		
	Both sexes	Male	Female	Both sexes	Male	Female	Both sexes	Male	Female	Both sexes	Male	Female
2000	2.28	2.51	2.04	1.86	2.06	1.66	3.83	4.18	3.47	4.70	5.11	4.28
2001	2.31	2.55	2.06	1.87	2.06	1.67	3.96	4.37	3.53	4.81	5.32	4.27
2002	2.31	2.58	2.03	1.89	2.15	1.63	3.86	4.21	3.50	4.85	5.30	4.38
2003	2.23	2.52	1.94	1.84	2.09	1.58	3.69	4.10	3.26	4.60	5.13	4.06
2004	2.27	2.53	2.00	1.87	2.07	1.66	3.72	4.19	3.23	4.66	5.24	4.06
2005	2.34	2.63	2.03	1.94	2.22	1.65	3.73	4.10	3.36	4.67	5.19	4.13
2006	2.24	2.48	1.98	1.84	2.05	1.62	3.60	3.96	3.22	4.47	4.89	4.04
2007	2.34	2.58	2.07	1.94	2.16	1.71	3.68	4.02	3.32	4.59	5.01	4.16
2008	2.32	2.54	2.08	1.93	2.12	1.73	3.62	3.97	3.26	4.50	4.93	4.06
Race of Child[3]												
1940	18.27	19.89	16.55	16.03	17.47	14.50	34.07	37.35	30.74	33.05	36.29	29.72
1950	8.71	9.41	7.98	7.40	8.04	6.73	16.92	18.11	15.70	16.10	17.18	15.00
1960	7.31	8.10	6.49	5.66	6.35	4.94	16.35	17.84	14.84	16.48	17.99	14.95
1970	4.93	5.41	4.42	3.98	4.40	3.54	9.49	10.33	8.62	9.89	10.81	8.94
1975	4.49	4.95	4.00	3.80	4.24	3.33	7.45	8.03	6.86	7.89	8.54	7.22
1976	4.32	4.79	3.83	3.65	4.08	3.19	7.19	7.83	6.52	7.63	8.36	6.88
1977	4.24	4.75	3.71	3.59	4.07	3.08	7.01	7.69	6.31	7.56	8.32	6.78
1978	4.30	4.72	3.85	3.63	4.03	3.20	7.05	7.60	6.48	7.64	8.22	7.05
1979	4.20	4.71	3.67	3.54	4.02	3.03	6.92	7.57	6.25	7.47	8.21	6.71
1980	4.13	4.62	3.61	3.52	3.98	3.02	6.61	7.22	5.97	7.29	7.95	6.62

[1]Multiple-race data were reported by 34 states and the District of Columbia in 2008, by 27 states and the District of Columbia in 2007, by 25 states and the District of Columbia in 2006, by 21 states and the District of Columbia in 2005, by 15 states in 2004, and by 7 states in 2003.
[2]Infant deaths are based on race of child as stated on the death certificate; live births are based on race of mother as stated on the birth certificate.
[3]Infant deaths are based on race of child as stated on the death certificate; live births are based on race of parents as stated on the birth certificate.

PART B: MORTALITY

Table B-46. Number of Infant Deaths and Infant Mortality Rates for 130 Selected Causes by Race, 2008

(Rates are infant deaths (under 1 year) per 100,000 live births in specified group. Infant deaths are based on race of decedent; live births are based on race of mother.)

Cause of death (based on ICD-10, 2004)	Number			Rate		
	All races[1]	White	Black	All races[1]	White	Black
ALL CAUSES	28,059	18,164	8,543	660.6	554.8	1,273.50
Certain infectious and parasitic diseases (A00–B99)	478	306	151	11.3	9.3	22.5
Certain intestinal infectious diseases (A00–A08)	12	8	3	*	*	*
Diarrhea and gastroenteritis of infectious origin (A09)	-	-	-	*	*	*
Tuberculosis (A16–A19)	-	-	-	*	*	*
Tetanus (A33, A35)	-	-	-	*	*	*
Diphtheria (A36)	-	-	-	*	*	*
Whooping cough (A37)	18	16	-	*	*	*
Meningococcal infection (A39)	9	9	-	*	*	*
Septicemia (A40–A41)	289	170	108	6.8	5.2	16.1
Congenital syphilis (A50)	-	-	-	*	*	*
Gonococcal infection (A54)	-	-	-	*	*	*
Viral diseases (A80–B34)	102	77	20	2.4	2.4	3
Acute poliomyelitis (A80)	-	-	-	*	*	*
Varicella (chickenpox) (B01)	-	-	-	*	*	*
Measles (B05)	-	-	-	*	*	*
Human immunodeficiency virus (HIV) disease (B20–B24)	-	-	-	*	*	*
Mumps (B26)	-	-	-	*	*	*
Other and unspecified viral diseases (A81–B00, B02–B04, B06–B19, B25,B27–B34)	102	77	20	2.4	2.4	3
Candidiasis (B37)	7	4	2	*	*	*
Malaria (B50–B54)	-	-	-	*	*	*
Pneumocystosis (B59)	3	3	-	*	*	*
All other and unspecified infectious and parasitic diseases (A20–A32, A38, A42–A49, A51–A53, A55–A79, B35–B36, B38–B49, B55–B58, B60–B99)	38	19	18	0.9	*	*
Neoplasms (C00–D48)	131	99	23	3.1	3	3.4
Malignant neoplasms (C00–C97)	70	51	15	1.6	1.6	*
Hodgkin's disease and non-Hodgkin's lymphomas (C81–C85)	1	-	1	*	*	*
Leukemia (C91–C95)	27	21	4	0.6	0.6	*
Other and unspecified malignant neoplasms (C00–C80, C88, C90, C96–C97)	42	30	10	1	0.9	*
In situ neoplasms, benign neoplasms and neoplasms of uncertain or unknown behavior (D00–D48)	61	48	8	1.4	1.5	*
Diseases of the blood and blood–forming organs and certain disorders involving the immune mechanism (D50–D89)	80	52	22	1.9	1.6	3.3
Anemias (D50–D64)	15	7	5	*	*	*
Hemorrhagic conditions and other diseases of blood and blood–forming organs (D65–D76)	56	41	13	1.3	1.3	*
Certain disorders involving the immune mechanism (D80–D89)	9	4	4	*	*	*
Endocrine, nutritional and metabolic diseases (E00–E88)	248	165	62	5.8	5	9.2
Short stature, not elsewhere classified (E34.3)	9	7	1	*	*	*
Nutritional deficiencies (E40–E64)	10	4	5	*	*	*
Cystic fibrosis (E84)	4	3	1	*	*	*
Volume depletion, disorders of fluid, electrolyte and acid–base balance (E86–E87)	78	50	28	1.8	1.5	4.2
All other endocrine, nutritional and metabolic diseases (E00–E32, E34.0–E34.2, E34.4–E34.9, E65–E83, E85, E88)	147	101	27	3.5	3.1	4
Diseases of the nervous system (G00–G98)	415	296	89	9.8	9	13.3
Meningitis (G00,G03)	68	49	13	1.6	1.5	*
Infantile spinal muscular atrophy, type I (Werdnig–Hoffman) (G12.0)	5	5	-	*	*	*
Infantile cerebral palsy (G80)	8	3	4	*	*	*
Anoxic brain damage, not elsewhere classified (G93.1)	56	28	24	1.3	0.9	3.6
Other diseases of nervous system (G04, G06–G11, G12.1–G12.9, G20–G72, G81–G92, G93.0, G93.2–G93.9, G95–G98)	278	211	48	6.5	6.4	7.2
Diseases of the ear and mastoid process (H60–H93)	6	4	2	*	*	*
Diseases of the circulatory system (I00–I99)	594	385	169	14	11.8	25.2
Pulmonary heart disease and diseases of pulmonary circulation (I26–I28)	88	48	36	2.1	1.5	5.4
Pericarditis, endocarditis and myocarditis (I30, I33, I40)	18	11	5	*	*	*
Cardiomyopathy (I42)	115	80	24	2.7	2.4	3.6
Cardiac arrest (I46)	25	14	11	0.6	*	*
Cerebrovascular diseases (I60–I69)	141	95	38	3.3	2.9	5.7
All other diseases of circulatory system (I00–I25, I31, I34–I38, I44–I45, I47–I51, I70–I99)	207	137	55	4.9	4.2	8.2
Diseases of the respiratory system (J00–J98,U04)	578	342	196	13.6	10.4	29.2
Acute upper respiratory infections (J00–J06)	12	7	4	*	*	*
Influenza and pneumonia (J09–J18)	226	147	64	5.3	4.5	9.5
Influenza (J09–J11)	16	13	2	*	*	*
Pneumonia (J12–J18)	210	134	62	4.9	4.1	9.2
Acute bronchitis and acute bronchiolitis (J20–J21)	43	27	10	1	0.8	*
Bronchitis, chronic and unspecified (J40–J42)	23	13	8	0.5	*	*
Asthma (J45–J46)	6	4	2	*	*	*
Pneumonitis due to solids and liquids (J69)	11	8	3	*	*	*
Other and unspecified diseases of respiratory system (J22, J30–J39, J43–J44, J47–J68, J70–J98, U04)4	257	136	105	6.1	4.2	15.7
Diseases of the digestive system (K00–K92)	579	331	207	13.6	10.1	30.9
Gastritis, duodenitis, and noninfective enteritis and colitis (K29, K50–K55)	354	192	141	8.3	5.9	21
Hernia of abdominal cavity and intestinal obstruction without hernia (K40–K46, K56)	46	28	16	1.1	0.9	*

Table B-46. Number of Infant Deaths and Infant Mortality Rates for 130 Selected Causes by Race, 2008—Continued

(Rates are infant deaths (under 1 year) per 100,000 live births in specified group. Infant deaths are based on race of decedent; live births are based on race of mother.)

Cause of death (based on ICD-10, 2004)	Number			Rate		
	All races	White	Black	All races	White	Black
All other and unspecified diseases of digestive system (K00–K28, K30–K38, K57–K92)	179	111	50	4.2	3.4	7.5
Diseases of the genitourinary system (N00–N95)	169	100	61	4	3.1	9.1
Renal failure and other disorders of kidney (N17–N19, N25, N27)	139	84	51	3.3	2.6	7.6
Other and unspecified diseases of genitourinary system (N00–N15, N20–N23, N26, N28–N95)	30	16	10	0.7	*	*
Certain conditions originating in the perinatal period (P00–P96)	13,800	8,359	4,811	324.9	255.3	717.2
Newborn affected by maternal factors and by complications of pregnancy, labor and delivery (P00–P04)	3,168	2,027	1,002	74.6	61.9	149.4
Newborn affected by maternal hypertensive disorders (P00.0)	85	51	29	2	1.6	4.3
Newborn affected by other maternal conditions which may be unrelated to present pregnancy (P00.1–P00.9)	88	58	24	2.1	1.8	3.6
Newborn affected by maternal complications of pregnancy (P01)	1,765	1,124	574	41.6	34.3	85.6
Newborn affected by incompetent cervix (P01.0)	446	287	140	10.5	8.8	20.9
Newborn affected by premature rupture of membranes (P01.1)	841	512	292	19.8	15.6	43.5
Newborn affected by multiple pregnancy (P01.5)	257	170	79	6.1	5.2	11.8
Newborn affected by other maternal complications of pregnancy (P01.2–P01.4, P01.6–P01.9)	221	155	63	5.2	4.7	9.4
Newborn affected by complications of placenta, cord and membranes (P02)	1,080	697	330	25.4	21.3	49.2
Newborn affected by complications involving placenta (P02.0–P02.3)	539	364	145	12.7	11.1	21.6
Newborn affected by complications involving cord (P02.4–P02.6)	55	41	12	1.3	1.3	*
Newborn affected by chorioamnionitis (P02.7)	485	291	173	11.4	8.9	25.8
Newborn affected by other and unspecified abnormalities of membranes (P02.8–P02.9)	1	1	-	*	*	*
Newborn affected by other complications of labor and delivery (P03)	99	69	25	2.3	2.1	3.7
Newborn affected by noxious influences transmitted via placenta or breast milk (P04)	51	28	20	1.2	0.9	3
Disorders related to length of gestation and fetal malnutrition (P05–P08)	4,836	2,703	1,910	113.9	82.6	284.7
Slow fetal growth and fetal malnutrition (P05)	82	47	29	1.9	1.4	4.3
Disorders related to short gestation and low birth weight, not elsewhere classified (P07)	4,754	2,656	1,881	111.9	81.1	280.4
Extremely low birth weight or extreme immaturity (P07.0, P07.2)	3,645	2,034	1,444	85.8	62.1	215.3
Other low birth weight or preterm (P07.1, P07.3)	1,109	622	437	26.1	19	65.1
Disorders related to long gestation and high birth weight (P08)	-	-	-	*	*	*
Birth trauma (P10–P15)	18	11	6	*	*	*
Intrauterine hypoxia and birth asphyxia (P20–P21)	385	258	106	9.1	7.9	15.8
Intrauterine hypoxia (P20)	143	99	38	3.4	3	5.7
Birth asphyxia (P21)	242	159	68	5.7	4.9	10.1
Respiratory distress of newborn (P22)	630	391	221	14.8	11.9	32.9
Other respiratory conditions originating in the perinatal period (P23–P28)	1,099	672	376	25.9	20.5	56.1
Congenital pneumonia (P23)	73	49	21	1.7	1.5	3.1
Neonatal aspiration syndromes (P24)	58	42	12	1.4	1.3	*
Interstitial emphysema and related conditions originating in the perinatal period (P25)	122	81	32	2.9	2.5	4.8
Pulmonary hemorrhage originating in the perinatal period (P26)	196	110	79	4.6	3.4	11.8
Chronic respiratory disease originating in the perinatal period (P27)	237	122	105	5.6	3.7	15.7
Atelectasis (P28.0–P28.1)	334	222	102	7.9	6.8	15.2
All other respiratory conditions originating in the perinatal period (P28.2–P28.9)	79	46	25	1.9	1.4	3.7
Infections specific to the perinatal period (P35–P39)	903	567	287	21.3	17.3	42.8
Bacterial sepsis of newborn (P36)	700	433	226	16.5	13.2	33.7
Omphalitis of newborn with or without mild hemorrhage (P38)	2	1	1	*	*	*
All other infections specific to the perinatal period (P35, P37, P39)	201	133	60	4.7	4.1	8.9
Hemorrhagic and hematological disorders of newborn (P50–P61)	648	432	188	15.3	13.2	28
Neonatal hemorrhage (P50–P52,P54)	556	365	166	13.1	11.1	24.7
Hemorrhagic disease of newborn (P53)	2	1	1	*	*	*
Hemolytic disease of newborn due to isoimmunization and other perinatal jaundice (P55–P59)	10	8	2	*	*	*
Hematological disorders (P60–P61)	80	58	19	1.9	1.8	*
Syndrome of infant of a diabetic mother and neonatal diabetes mellitus (P70.0–P70.2)	11	9	2	*	*	*
Necrotizing enterocolitis of newborn (P77)	549	307	221	12.9	9.4	32.9
Hydrops fetalis not due to hemolytic disease (P83.2)	169	131	26	4	4	3.9
Other perinatal conditions (P29, P70.3–P70.9, P71–P76, P78–P81, P83.0–P83.1, P83.3–P83.9, P90–P96)	1,384	851	466	32.6	26	69.5
Congenital malformations, deformations and chromosomal abnormalities (Q00–Q99)	5,638	4,291	1,069	132.7	131.1	159.4
Anencephaly and similar malformations (Q00)	338	286	41	8	8.7	6.1
Congenital hydrocephalus (Q03)	106	70	28	2.5	2.1	4.2
Spina bifida (Q05)	23	19	4	0.5	*	*
Other congenital malformations of nervous system (Q01–Q02, Q04, Q06–Q07)	355	273	64	8.4	8.3	9.5
Congenital malformations of heart (Q20–Q24)	1,305	982	260	30.7	30	38.8
Other congenital malformations of circulatory system (Q25–Q28)	222	161	52	5.2	4.9	7.8
Congenital malformations of respiratory system (Q30–Q34)	371	284	64	8.7	8.7	9.5

Table B-46. Number of Infant Deaths and Infant Mortality Rates for 130 Selected Causes by Race, 2008—Continued

(Rates are infant deaths (under 1 year) per 100,000 live births in specified group. Infant deaths are based on race of decedent; live births are based on race of mother.)

Cause of death (based on ICD–10, 2004)	Number			Rate		
	All races	White	Black	All races	White	Black
Congenital malformations of digestive system (Q35–Q45)	83	57	20	2	1.7	3
Congenital malformations of genitourinary system (Q50–Q64)	515	401	93	12.1	12.2	13.9
Congenital malformations and deformations of musculoskeletal system, limbs and integument (Q65–Q85)	664	499	128	15.6	15.2	19.1
Down's syndrome (Q90)	88	66	17	2.1	2	*
Edward's syndrome (Q91.0–Q91.3)	554	430	91	13	13.1	13.6
Patau's syndrome (Q91.4–Q91.7)	275	210	55	6.5	6.4	8.2
Other congenital malformations and deformations (Q10–Q18, Q86–Q89)	538	393	117	12.7	12	17.4
Other chromosomal abnormalities, not elsewhere classified (Q92–Q99)	201	160	35	4.7	4.9	5.2
Symptoms, signs and abnormal clinical and laboratory findings, not elsewhere classified (R00–R99)	3,546	2,280	1,117	83.5	69.6	166.5
Sudden infant death syndrome (R95)	2,353	1,497	758	55.4	45.7	113
Other symptoms, signs and abnormal clinical and laboratory findings, not elsewhere classified (R00–R53, R55–R94, R96–R99)	1,193	783	359	28.1	23.9	53.5
All other diseases (Residual)	24	21	3	0.6	0.6	*
External causes of mortality (*U01, V01–Y84)	1,773	1,133	561	41.7	34.6	83.6
Accidents (unintentional injuries) (V01–X59)	1,315	846	409	31	25.8	61
Transport accidents (V01–V99)	104	73	18	2.4	2.2	*
Motor vehicle accidents (V02–V04, V09.0, V09.2, V12–V14, V19.0–V19.2, V19.4–V19.6, V20–V79, V80.3–V80.5, V81.0–V81.1, V82.0–V82.1, V83–V86, V87.0–V87.8, V88.0–V88.8, V89.0, V89.2)	103	73	18	2.4	2.2	*
Other and unspecified transport accidents (V01, V05–V06,V09.1, V09.3–V09.9, V10– V11, V15–V18, V19.3, V19.8–V19.9, V80.0–V80.2, V80.6–V80.9, V81.2–V81.9, V82.2–V82.9, V87.9, V88.9, V89.1, V89.3, V89.9, V90–V99)	1	-	-	*	*	*
Falls (W00–W19)	13	10	3	*	*	*
Accidental discharge of firearms (W32–W34)	-	-	-	*	*	*
Accidental drowning and submersion (W65–W74)	41	29	8	1	0.9	*
Accidental suffocation and strangulation in bed (W75)	736	455	252	17.3	13.9	37.6
Other accidental suffocation and strangulation (W76–W77, W81–W84)	260	175	79	6.1	5.3	11.8
Accidental inhalation and ingestion of food or other objects causing obstruction of respiratory tract (W78–W80)	62	38	19	1.5	1.2	*
Accidents caused by exposure to smoke, fire and flames (X00–X09)	20	13	7	0.5	*	*
Accidental poisoning and exposure to noxious substances (X40–X49)	11	8	3	*	*	*
Other and unspecified accidents (W20–W31, W35–W64, W85–W99, X10–X39, X50–X59)	68	45	20	1.6	1.4	3
Assault (homicide) (*U01, X85–Y09)	340	208	115	8	6.4	17.1
Assault (homicide) by hanging, strangulation and suffocation (X91)	32	22	10	0.8	0.7	*
Assault (homicide) by discharge of firearms (*U01.4, X93–X95)	9	2	7	*	*	*
Neglect, abandonment and other maltreatment syndromes (Y06–Y07)	98	56	36	2.3	1.7	5.4
Assault (homicide) by other and unspecified means (*U01.0–*U01.3, *U01.5–*U01.9, X85–X90, X92, X96–X99, Y00–Y05, Y08–Y09)	201	128	62	4.7	3.9	9.2
Complications of medical and surgical care (Y40–Y84)	24	17	7	0.6	*	*
Other external causes (Y10–Y36)	94	62	30	2.2	1.9	4.5

– = Quantity zero.

* = Figure does not meet standards of reliability or precision.

NOTE: Complete confirmation of deaths from selected causes of death, considered to be of public health concern, were not provided by the following states—Massachusetts, North Carolina, and West Virginia.

Table B-47. Number of Infant and Neonatal Deaths and Mortality Rates, by Race, State, and Territory, 2008

(Rates are infant [under 1 year] and neonatal [under 28 days] deaths per 1,000 live births in specified group. Infant and neonatal deaths are based on race of decedent; live births are based on race of mother.)

Sex and area	Infant deaths						Neonatal deaths					
	All races		White		Black		All races		White		Black	
	Number	Rate	Number	Rate	Number	Rate	Number	Rate	Number	Rate	Number	Rate
UNITED STATES[1]	28,059	6.61	18,164	5.55	8,543	12.74	18,211	4.29	11,843	3.62	5,523	8.23
Male	15,669	7.21	10,151	6.05	4,748	13.93	10,144	4.67	6,598	3.94	3,066	8.99
Female	12,390	5.97	8,013	5.02	3,795	11.50	8,067	3.89	5,245	3.28	2,457	7.45
Alabama	612	9.48	328	7.55	279	13.98	377	5.84	202	4.65	171	8.57
Alaska	67	5.86	24	3.35	3	*	26	2.27	12	*	1	*
Arizona	635	6.39	478	5.63	77	17.14	426	4.28	323	3.80	52	11.58
Arkansas	300	7.38	190	6.01	107	13.22	178	4.38	112	3.54	65	8.03
California	2,814	5.10	2,112	4.80	417	12.06	1,909	3.46	1,450	3.29	269	7.78
Colorado	437	6.24	365	5.76	52	14.93	314	4.48	263	4.15	38	10.91
Connecticut	242	5.99	154	4.78	70	12.40	180	4.46	115	3.57	51	9.04
Delaware	101	8.35	50	6.06	51	15.50	68	5.62	33	4.00	35	10.64
District of Columbia	99	10.84	14	*	83	15.60	75	8.21	13	*	60	11.28
Florida	1,669	7.21	953	5.76	686	11.94	1,061	4.58	615	3.72	425	7.40
Georgia	1,182	8.06	485	5.57	674	12.64	767	5.23	304	3.49	449	8.42
Hawaii	108	5.54	25	4.26	5	*	71	3.64	20	3.40	4	*
Idaho	149	5.92	143	5.95	5	*	102	4.06	98	4.08	4	*
Illinois	1,256	7.10	773	5.71	439	14.08	820	4.64	514	3.79	271	8.69
Indiana	614	6.92	451	5.93	157	14.70	380	4.28	280	3.68	97	9.08
Iowa	228	5.67	197	5.32	27	14.16	141	3.51	125	3.37	12	*
Kansas	304	7.27	243	6.62	46	13.73	195	4.66	150	4.09	32	9.55
Kentucky	402	6.89	334	6.48	62	10.91	246	4.21	208	4.03	33	5.80
Louisiana	591	9.05	252	6.66	331	12.85	317	4.86	125	3.30	189	7.34
Maine	75	5.51	70	5.44	3	*	51	3.75	47	3.65	3	*
Maryland	619	8.01	246	5.42	352	13.17	453	5.86	174	3.84	260	9.73
Massachusetts	391	5.08	283	4.62	89	9.43	298	3.87	222	3.62	65	6.89
Michigan	894	7.38	537	5.76	333	14.51	609	5.03	373	4.00	220	9.59
Minnesota	434	5.99	296	5.09	82	11.59	275	3.80	193	3.32	52	7.35
Mississippi	448	9.97	182	7.48	261	13.15	257	5.72	97	3.99	158	7.96
Missouri	585	7.23	392	5.95	189	15.01	358	4.42	234	3.55	121	9.61
Montana	86	6.83	71	6.59	-	*	48	3.81	40	3.71	-	*
Nebraska	146	5.41	113	4.77	29	14.55	90	3.33	75	3.17	13	*
Nevada	211	5.34	155	4.86	48	12.65	128	3.24	99	3.11	26	6.85
New Hampshire	54	3.95	53	4.13	-	*	39	2.85	38	2.96	-	*
New Jersey	626	5.55	357	4.48	248	11.98	401	3.56	237	2.97	151	7.30
New Mexico	169	5.60	146	5.84	5	*	99	3.28	88	3.52	3	*
New York	1,374	5.49	787	4.45	521	10.50	929	3.71	545	3.08	339	6.83
North Carolina	1,073	8.20	567	6.06	462	14.71	685	5.24	365	3.90	295	9.39
North Dakota	52	5.82	38	5.01	1	*	41	4.59	33	4.35	1	*
Ohio	1,144	7.69	716	6.03	422	16.29	754	5.07	463	3.90	287	11.08
Oklahoma	397	7.25	270	6.43	75	14.95	249	4.55	166	3.95	49	9.77
Oregon	253	5.15	212	4.82	19	*	155	3.16	137	3.12	10	*
Pennsylvania	1,100	7.37	749	6.45	325	12.25	783	5.25	530	4.57	233	8.78
Rhode Island	71	5.89	53	5.28	15	*	53	4.40	38	3.79	12	*
South Carolina	507	8.04	254	6.36	245	11.39	310	4.92	154	3.85	150	6.97
South Dakota	101	8.37	63	6.56	3	*	61	5.05	41	4.27	3	*
Tennessee	693	8.10	410	6.38	279	14.71	425	4.97	239	3.72	184	9.70
Texas	2,504	6.17	1,962	5.80	483	9.77	1,563	3.85	1,211	3.58	317	6.41
Utah	266	4.78	243	4.63	7	*	177	3.18	163	3.11	5	*
Vermont	29	4.57	27	4.42	1	*	21	3.31	19	*	1	*
Virginia	732	6.86	411	5.46	288	12.17	485	4.55	265	3.52	197	8.32
Washington	491	5.44	377	5.12	50	10.29	301	3.33	244	3.31	22	4.53
West Virginia	165	7.67	148	7.23	17	*	95	4.42	83	4.05	12	*
Wisconsin	503	6.96	358	5.90	116	15.77	330	4.57	239	3.94	73	9.92
Wyoming	56	6.97	47	6.24	4	*	35	4.35	29	3.85	3	*
Puerto Rico	388	8.51	377	9.20	11	*	278	6.09	274	6.69	4	*
Virgin Islands	9	*	1	*	8	*	8	*	1	*	7	*
Guam	30	8.68	1	*	-	*	14	*	-	*	-	*
American Samoa	13	*	-	*	-	*	6	*	-	*	-	*
Northern Marianas	5	*	-	*	-	*	4	*	-	*	-	*

- = Quantity zero.
* = Figure does not meet standards of reliability or precision.
[1]Excludes data for Puerto Rico, Virgin Islands, Guam, American Samoa, and Northern Marianas.

Table B-48. Selected Charactersistics of Discharged Hospice Care Patients, 2007

(Percent.)

Characteristic	Percent
Age	
Under 65 years	16.9
65 years and over	83.1
65–74 years	15.4
75–84 years	29.5
85 years and over	38.2
Sex	
Male	44.9
Female	55.1
Race and Hispanic Origin	
Hispanic or Latino	4.1
Not Hispanic or Latino:	
White	86.6
Black or African American	7.6
Marital Status	
Married or living with partner	45.4
Single, divorced, or separated	14.2
Widowed	40.4
Vital Status at Discharge	
Deceased	84.4
Alive	15.6
Medicare Beneficiary	
Yes	84.3
No	15.7
Place of Care on First Day	
Private home	55.3
Nursing home/skilled nursing facility	21.1
Other place	23.6

Table B-49. Primary Admission Diagnosis of Discharged Hospice Care Patients, 1998 and 2007

(Percent.)

Admission diagnosis	1998	2007
Cancer (malignant neoplasms)	64.8	42.9
Noncancer	35.2	57.1
Alzheimer's, mental disorders, and other dementia	*3.1	11.2
Heart disease	8.6	11.1
CLRD (chronic lower respiratory diseases)	*3.5	4.8
Stroke (cerebrovascular diseases)	*2.6	4.5
All other	17.4	25.6

* = Figures do not meet standards of reliability and precision. Data preceded by an asterisk have a relative standard error of 20%–30%.

Table B-50. Services Offered or Provided to Hospice Care Patients' Family Members or Friends, 2007

(Percent.)

Type of service	Percent
Bereavement	85.1
Spiritual	66.8
Medication management or administration	66.7
Patient activities of daily living	58.1
Safety training	53.3
Equipment use	47.8
Caregiver health or wellness	25.7
Dietary	19.6
Referral or resource information	19.1
Dealing with difficult behaviors	17.8

Table B-51. Hospice Care Patients Symptoms at the Last Hospice Care Visit Before Death, 2007

(Percent.)

Symptom	Percent
Difficulty breathing	50.7
Pain	33.3
Restlessness	25.0
Anorexia	23.9
Constipation	10.0

NOTE: Data were collected through in-person interviews with agency directors and their designated staffs who were familiar with the patients and the care they received. Information was also abstracted from patients' medical records. No information was obtained from family members or friends.

Table B-52. Selected Drugs Prescribed to Hospice Care Patients in the Last Week of Life, 2007

(Percent.)

Multum Lexicon Plus Therapeutic Class	Percent
Narcotic analgesic (severe pain)	90.9
Antiemetic (vomiting or dizziness)	78.6
Laxative (constipation)	52.6
Antipsychotic (restlessness, agitation)	36.1
Diuretic (fluid retention, high blood pressure, cardiac, kidney conditions)	25.5
Proton pump inhibitor (antiulcer, antiitch)	25.3
Bronchodilator (breathing difficulties)	24.0
Antidepressant (depression, pain)	23.4
Antacid (stomach acid, antiulcer)	17.6
Antiarrythmic (heart rhythm disturbances)	15.9
Corticosteroid (anti-inflammatory, pain)	14.2
Antidiabetic (elevated blood sugar)	10.4
Antianginal (chest pain)	7.4
Antihyperlipidemia (elevated cholesterol)	7.1
Nonsteroidal anti-inflammatory drug (inflammation, mild pain)	6.7
Baby aspirin or Plavix (clopidogrel) (clot prevention)	3.4

NOTE: Information is collected from the patient's medical record based on the question: "What are the names of all the medications and drugs he/she was taking the 7 days prior to and on the day of his/her death? Please include any standing routine, or PRN (as needed) medications." Up to 25 medication names could be recorded.

NOTES AND DEFINITIONS

SOURCES OF DATA

Four different publications were used to obtain the mortality data in Part B. The majority of the tables came from Miniño AM, Murphy SL, Xu JQ, Kochanek KD. *Deaths: Final Data for 2008*. National Vital Statistics Reports; vol 59 no 10. Hyattsville, MD: National Center for Health Statistics.

Tables B-25, B-27, B-28, and B-29 come from *Fatal Occupational Injuries and Workers Memorial Day*, U.S. Department of Labor, Bureau of Labor Statistics.

Tables B-9, B-19, B-20, B-22 through B-24, B-26, B-32 through B-39, and B-41 through B-44 are from National Center for Health Statistics. *Health, United States, 2011: With Special Feature on Socioeconomic Status and Health*. Hyattsville, MD. 2012

In addition, Tables B-30 and B-40 through B-44 and B-48 through B-52 come from National Center for Health Statistics. *Health, United States, 2010: With Special Feature on Death and Dying*. Hyattsville, MD. 2011

NOTES ON THE DATA

Final data in Part B are based on information from all resident death certificates filed in the 50 states and the District of Columbia. It is believed that more than 99 percent of all deaths that occur in the United States are registered. Data for 2008 are based on records of deaths that occurred during 2008 and were received as of February 28, 2011.

Data shown for geographic areas are by place of residence. Beginning with 1970, mortality statistics for the United States exclude deaths of nonresidents of the United States. All data exclude fetal deaths. Mortality statistics for Puerto Rico, Virgin Islands, American Samoa, and Northern Marianas exclude deaths of nonresidents for each area. For Guam, however, mortality statistics exclude deaths that occurred to a resident of any place other than Guam or the United States.

Race and Hispanic origin are reported separately on the death certificate. Therefore, data shown by race include persons of Hispanic and non-Hispanic origin, and data for Hispanic origin include persons of any race. Unless otherwise specified, deaths of Hispanic origin are included in the totals for each race group—White, Black, American Indian or Alaska Native (AIAN), and Asian or Pacific Islander (API)—according to the decedent's race as reported on the death certificate. Data shown for Hispanic persons include all persons of Hispanic origin of any race.

Cause of death statistics are in accordance with the *International Classification of Diseases, Tenth Revision (ICD-10)*.

CONCEPTS AND DEFINITIONS

Age-adjusted death rate—the death rate used to make comparisons of relative mortality risks across groups and over time. This rate should be viewed as a construct or an index rather than as a direct or actual measure of mortality risk. Statistically, it is a weighted average of the age-specific death rates, where the weights represent the fixed population proportions by age.

Age-specific death rate—deaths per 100,000 population in a specified age group, such as 1–4 years or 5–9 years for a specified period.

Cause of death—for the purpose of national mortality statistics, every death is attributed to one underlying condition, based on information reported on the death certificate and using the international rules for selecting the underlying cause of death from the conditions stated on the death certificate. The underlying cause is defined by the World Health Organization as the disease or injury that initiated the train of events leading directly to death, or the circumstances of the accident or violence that produced the fatal injury. Generally more medical information is reported on death certificates than is directly reflected in the underlying cause of death. The conditions that are not selected as underlying cause of death constitute the nonunderlying causes of death, also known as multiple cause of death.

Cause-of-death ranking—selected causes of death of public health and medical importance comprise tabulation lists and are ranked according to the number of deaths assigned to these causes. The top-ranking causes determine the leading causes of death. Certain causes on the tabulation lists are not ranked if, for example, the category title represents a group title (such as major cardiovascular diseases and symptoms, signs, and abnormal clinical and laboratory findings, not elsewhere classified); or the category title begins with the words "other" and "all other". In addition, when one of the titles that represents a subtotal (such as malignant neoplasms) is ranked, its component parts are not ranked.

Crude death rate—total deaths per 100,000 population for a specified period. The crude death rate represents the average chance of dying during a specified period for persons in the entire population.

Fetal death rate—the number of fetal deaths with stated or presumed gestation of 20 weeks or more, divided by the sum of live births plus fetal deaths, per 1,000 live births plus fetal deaths.

Infant deaths—deaths of infants under 1 year of age.

International Classification of Diseases (ICD)—used to code and classify cause-of-death data. It is developed collaboratively by the World Health Organization and 10 international centers, one of which is housed at NCHS. The purpose of it is to promote international comparability in the collection, classification, processing, and presentation of health statistics. Since 1900, it has been modified about once every 10 years, except for the 20-year interval between the ninth and tenth editions. The purpose of the revisions is to stay abreast with advances in medical science. New revisions usually introduce major disruptions in time series of mortality statistics.

Hispanic origin—includes persons of Mexican, Puerto Rican, Cuban, Central and South American, and other or unknown Latin American or Spanish origins. Persons of Hispanic origin may be of any race.

Late fetal death rate—the number of fetal deaths with stated or presumed gestation of 28 weeks or more, divided by the sum of live births plus late fetal deaths per 1,000 live births plus late fetal deaths.

Life expectancy—the average number of years of life remaining to a person at a particular age and is based on a given set of age-specific death rates, generally the mortality conditions existing in the period mentioned.

Maternal mortality rate—the number of maternal deaths per 100,000 live births. The maternal mortality rate is the measure of the likelihood that a pregnant woman will die from maternal causes.

Neonatal deaths—deaths of infants aged 0–27 days.

Perinatal mortality rate—the sum of late fetal deaths plus infant deaths within 7 days of birth divided by the sum of live births plus late fetal deaths, per 1,000 live births plus late fetal deaths.

Perinatal mortality ratio—the sum of late fetal deaths plus infant deaths within 7 days of birth divided by the number of live births, per 1,000 live births.

Postneonatal deaths—deaths of infants aged 28 days–1 year old.

Years of potential life lost (YPLL)—a measure of premature mortality. YPLL is presented for persons under 75 years of age because the average life expectancy in the United States is over 75 years. YPLL-75 is calculated using the following eight age groups: under 1 year, 1–14 years, 15–24 years, 25–34 years, 35–44 years, 45–54 years, 55–64 years, and 65–74 years. The number of deaths for each age group is multiplied by years of life lost, calculated as the difference between age 75 years and the midpoint of the age group. For the eight age groups, the midpoints are 0.5, 7.5, 19.5, 29.5, 39.5, 49.5, 59.5, and 69.5. For example, the death of a person 15–24 years of age counts as 55.5 years of life lost. Years of potential life lost is derived by summing years of life lost over all age groups.

PART C:
HEALTH

HEALTH

DETERMINANTS AND MEASURES OF HEALTH

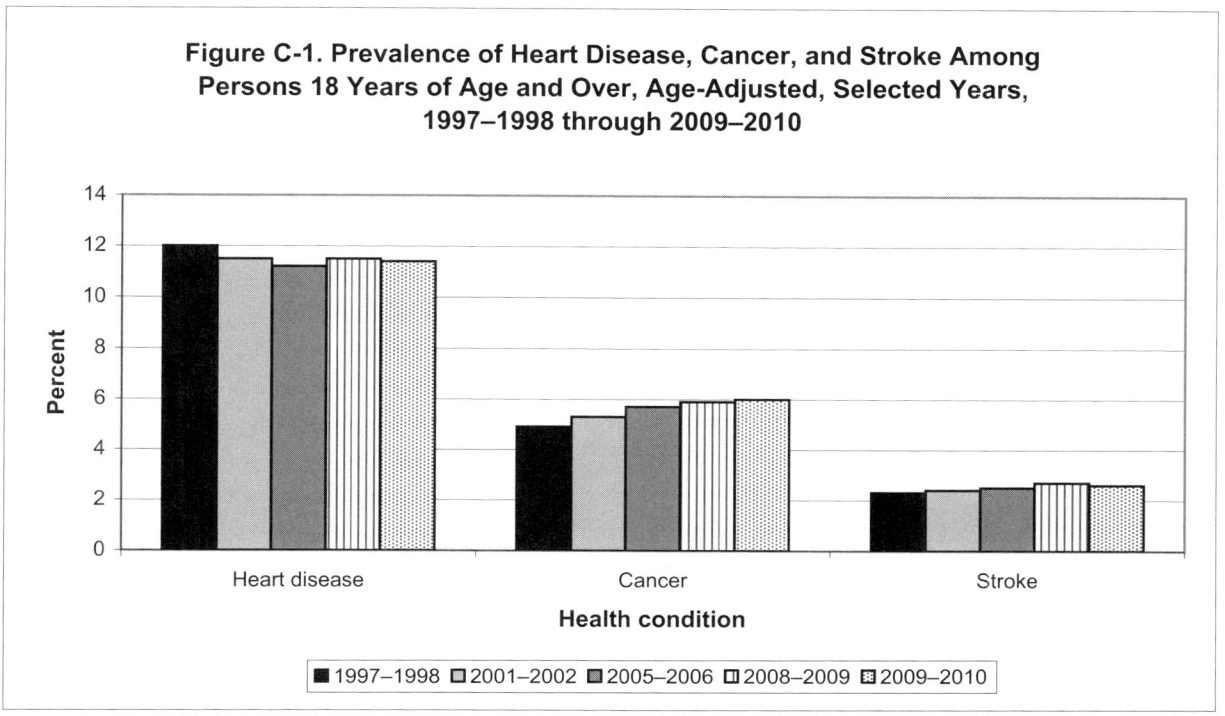

Figure C-1. Prevalence of Heart Disease, Cancer, and Stroke Among Persons 18 Years of Age and Over, Age-Adjusted, Selected Years, 1997–1998 through 2009–2010

HIGHLIGHTS

- In 2009–2010, 11.4 percent of people suffered from heart disease, a decline from 12.0 percent in 1997–1998. Although the percent of people with heart disease declined, the percent of people suffering from cancer increased from 4.9 percent to 6.0 percent and the percent of people suffering from a stroke increased from 2.3 percent to 2.6 percent in the same time period. (Determinants and Measures of Health, Table C-6)

- In 2010, 41.2 percent of high school seniors reported drinking alcohol, 21.4 percent of high school students reported using marijuana, 1.4 percent reported using inhalants, and 1.3 percent reported using cocaine. The percent of students using most drugs declined significantly from 1980 to 2010. (Use of Addictive Substances, Table C-32)

- Nearly 27 percent of American Indian or Alaska Natives had no usual source of health care compared to 19.7 percent of Whites and 22.4 percent of Blacks. (Ambulatory Care, Table C-34)

- The average length of stay in the hospital gradually declined from 7.5 days in 1980 to 4.8 days in 2008–2009. (Inpatient Care, Table C-57)

- The mean annual wage for healthcare practitioners and technical occupations in May 2011 was $72,730. Anesthesiologists earned the most at $234,950 while dietetic technicians earned the least at $29,200. (Health Personnel, Table C-64)

- National health care expenditures continued to climb in 2009 increasing to $2.48 billion dollars, an 80.4 percent increase from 2000. (Health Expenditures, Table C-70)

- The number of people with private health insurance declined for the second consecutive year in 2010, dropping to 163.9 million people. (Health Insurance, Tables C-84)

Table C-1. Nonfatal Occupational Injuries and Illnesses with Days Away from Work, Job Transfer, or Restriction, by Industry, Selected Years, 2005–2009

(Cases per 100 full-time workers, number.)

Industry	Injuries and illnesses with days away from work, job transfer, or restriction									
	Cases per 100 full-time workers[1]					Number of cases in thousands[2]				
	2005	2006	2007	2008	2009	2005	2006	2007	2008	2009
Total Private Sector[3]	2.4	2.3	2.1	2.0	1.8	2,184.8	2,114.6	2,036.0	1,900.8	1,667.4
Agriculture, forestry, fishing, and hunting[4]	3.3	3.2	2.8	2.9	2.9	29.5	27.6	26.6	26.0	24.2
Mining	2.2	2.1	2.0	2.0	1.5	13.7	14.0	14.1	16.4	10.7
Utilities	2.4	2.2	2.1	1.9	1.8	12.9	11.8	11.4	10.6	10.0
Construction	3.4	3.2	2.8	2.5	2.3	222.5	223.7	197.5	171.6	136.5
Manufacturing	3.5	3.3	3.0	2.7	2.3	490.8	473.4	427.1	372.9	285.6
Wholesale trade	2.7	2.5	2.4	2.2	2.0	146.8	140.6	139.3	130.9	112.2
Retail trade	2.6	2.6	2.5	2.3	2.2	314.2	308.6	309.1	283.4	254.3
Transportation and warehousing	4.6	4.3	4.3	3.9	3.5	185.6	176.3	179.4	164.3	141.0
Information	1.1	1.0	1.1	1.1	1.0	30.9	28.3	29.1	28.0	25.1
Finance and insurance	0.4	0.3	0.4	0.3	0.2	19.1	17.7	20.7	18.7	12.3
Real estate and rental and leasing	2.1	1.8	1.6	1.8	1.9	37.1	33.0	29.0	32.1	33.3
Professional, scientific, and technical services	0.6	0.5	0.5	0.5	0.5	38.4	34.5	31.8	33.5	34.0
Management of companies and enterprises	1.3	1.1	0.9	0.7	0.8	20.8	17.9	15.1	12.7	14.0
Administrative and support and waste management and remediation services	2.0	1.9	1.8	1.8	1.6	89.5	87.0	89.2	87.0	74.7
Educational services	1.0	0.9	1.0	1.0	0.8	14.8	14.5	15.8	16.0	14.5
Health care and social assistance	2.8	2.7	2.5	2.5	2.4	318.4	310.0	303.7	302.6	304.0
Arts, entertainment, and recreation	2.9	2.5	2.5	2.4	2.3	34.1	28.7	31.9	31.9	29.5
Accommodation and food services	1.7	1.7	1.6	1.5	1.5	120.8	124.6	119.6	116.0	108.5
Other services, except public administration	1.5	1.4	1.5	1.5	1.4	44.8	42.4	45.7	46.2	43.0

[1]Incidence rate calculated as (N/EH) x 200,000, where N = total number of injuries and illnesses, EH = total hours worked by all employees during the calendar year, and 200,000 = base for 100 full-time equivalent employees working 40 hours per week, 50 weeks per year.
[2]Because of rounding, components may not add to total number of cases in private sector.
[3]Totals include data for industries not shown separately. Excludes self-employed, private households, and employees in federal, state, and local government agencies.
[4]Excludes farms with fewer than 11 employees.

Table C-2. Selected Notifiable Disease Rates and Number of New Cases, Selected Years, 1950–2009

(Cases per 100,000 population.)

Disease	1950	1960	1970	1980	1985	1988	1989	1990	1991	1992	1993	1994	1995
Rate													
Diphtheria	3.83	0.51	0.21	0.00	0.00	0.00	0.00	0.00	0.00	0.00	-	0.00	-
Haemophilus influenzae, invasive	—	—	—	—	—	—	—	—	1.10	0.55	0.55	0.45	0.45
Hepatitis A	—	—	27.87	12.84	10.03	11.60	14.43	12.64	9.67	9.06	9.40	10.29	12.13
Hepatitis B	—	—	4.08	8.39	11.50	9.43	9.43	8.48	7.14	6.32	5.18	4.81	4.19
Lyme disease[1]	—	—	—	—	—	—	—	—	3.80	3.93	3.20	5.01	4.49
Meningococcal disease	—	—	1.23	1.25	1.04	1.21	1.10	0.99	0.84	0.84	1.02	1.11	1.25
Mumps	—	—	55.55	3.86	1.30	2.05	2.34	2.17	1.72	1.03	0.66	0.60	0.35
Pertussis (whooping cough)	79.82	8.23	2.08	0.76	1.50	1.40	1.67	1.84	1.08	1.60	2.55	1.77	1.97
Poliomyelitis, paralytic[2]	—	1.40	0.02	0.00	0.00	0.00	0.00	0.00	0.00	0.00	0.00	0.00	0.00
Rocky Mountain spotted fever[3]	—	—	0.19	0.52	0.30	0.25	0.25	0.26	0.25	0.20	0.18	0.18	0.23
Rubella (German measles)	—	—	27.75	1.72	0.26	0.09	0.16	0.45	0.56	0.06	0.07	0.09	0.05
Rubeola (measles)	211.01	245.42	23.23	5.96	1.18	1.38	7.33	11.17	3.82	0.88	0.12	0.37	0.12
Salmonellosis, excluding typhoid fever	—	3.85	10.84	14.88	27.37	19.91	19.26	19.54	19.10	16.04	16.15	16.64	17.66
Shigellosis	15.45	6.94	6.79	8.41	7.14	12.46	10.07	10.89	9.34	9.38	12.48	11.44	12.32
Tuberculosis[4]	—	30.83	18.28	12.25	9.30	9.13	9.46	10.33	10.42	10.46	9.82	9.36	8.70
Sexually transmitted diseases[5]													
Syphilis[6]	146.02	68.78	44.80	30.30	28.39	42.75	46.63	54.32	50.88	44.73	39.48	31.43	26.05
Primary and secondary	16.73	9.06	10.80	12.00	11.40	16.55	18.57	20.26	16.98	13.26	10.21	7.84	6.21
Early latent	39.71	10.11	8.00	8.90	9.11	14.71	18.39	22.19	21.29	19.46	16.13	12.17	10.01
Late and late latent[7]	70.22	45.91	24.70	9.20	7.74	11.19	8.93	10.32	10.87	10.42	11.83	10.49	9.12
Congenital[8]	368.30	103.70	52.30	7.70	8.75	18.95	45.46	92.95	107.62	100.05	85.49	62.03	47.77
Chlamydia[9]	—	—	—	—	17.42	87.13	102.45	160.19	179.66	182.35	178.05	192.49	187.84
Gonorrhea[10]	192.50	145.40	294.20	442.10	382.98	301.86	297.09	276.43	245.84	196.04	171.07	163.93	147.46
Chancroid	3.34	0.94	0.70	0.30	0.87	2.00	1.90	1.69	1.37	0.74	0.50	0.30	0.23
Number													
Diphtheria	5,796	918	435	3	3	2	3	4	5	4	-	2	-
Haemophilus influenzae, invasive	—	—	—	—	—	—	—	—	2,764	1,412	1,419	1,174	1,180
Hepatitis A	—	—	56,797	29,087	23,210	28,507	35,821	31,441	24,378	23,112	24,238	26,796	31,582
Hepatitis B	—	—	8,310	19,015	26,611	23,177	23,419	21,102	18,003	16,126	13,361	12,517	10,805
Lyme disease[1]	—	—	—	—	—	—	—	—	9,465	9,895	8,257	13,043	11,700
Meningococcal disease	—	—	2,505	2,840	2,479	2,964	2,727	2,451	2,130	2,134	2,637	2,886	3,243
Mumps	—	—	104,953	8,576	2,982	4,866	5,712	5,292	4,264	2,572	1,692	1,537	906
Pertussis (whooping cough)	120,718	14,809	4,249	1,730	3,589	3,450	4,157	4,570	2,719	4,083	6,586	4,617	5,137
Poliomyelitis, paralytic[2]	—	2,525	31	9	8	9	11	6	10	6	4	8	7
Rocky Mountain spotted fever[3]	—	—	380	1,163	714	609	623	651	628	502	456	465	590
Rubella (German measles)	—	—	56,552	3,904	630	225	396	1,125	1,401	160	192	227	128
Rubeola (measles)	319,124	441,703	47,351	13,506	2,822	3,396	18,193	27,786	9,643	2,237	312	963	309
Salmonellosis, excluding typhoid fever	—	6,929	22,096	33,715	65,347	48,948	47,812	48,603	48,154	40,912	41,641	43,323	45,970
Shigellosis	23,367	12,487	13,845	19,041	17,057	30,617	25,010	27,077	23,548	23,931	32,198	29,769	32,080
Tuberculosis[4]	—	55,494	37,137	27,749	22,201	22,436	23,495	25,701	26,283	26,673	25,313	24,361	22,860
Sexually transmitted diseases[5]													
Syphilis[6]	217,558	122,538	91,382	68,832	67,563	104,546	115,089	135,590	128,719	114,730	102,612	82,713	69,359
Primary and secondary	23,939	16,145	21,982	27,204	27,131	40,474	45,826	50,578	42,950	34,009	26,527	20,641	16,543
Early latent	59,256	18,017	16,311	20,297	21,689	35,968	45,394	55,397	53,855	49,929	41,919	32,017	26,657
Late and late latent[7]	113,569	81,798	50,348	20,979	18,414	27,363	22,032	25,750	27,490	26,725	30,746	27,603	24,296
Congenital[8]	13,377	4,416	1,953	277	329	741	1,837	3,865	4,424	4,067	3,420	2,452	1,863
Chlamydia[9]	—	—	—	—	25,848	157,854	200,904	323,663	381,228	409,694	405,332	451,785	478,577
Gonorrhea[10]	286,746	258,933	600,072	1,004,029	911,419	738,160	733,294	690,042	621,918	502,858	444,649	419,602	392,651
Chancroid	4,977	1,680	1,416	788	2,067	4,891	4,697	4,212	3,476	1,906	1,292	782	607

Table C-2. Selected Notifiable Disease Rates and Number of New Cases, Selected Years, 1950–2009—Continued

(Cases per 100,000 population.)

Disease	1996	1997	1998	1999	2000	2001	2002	2003	2004	2005	2006	2007	2008	2009
Rate														
Diphtheria	0.01	0.01	0.00	0.00	0.00	0.00	0.00	0.00	-	-	-	-	-	-
Haemophilus influenzae, invasive	0.45	0.44	0.44	0.48	0.51	0.57	0.62	0.70	0.72	0.78	0.82	0.85	0.96	0.99
Hepatitis A	11.70	11.22	8.59	6.25	4.91	3.77	3.13	2.66	1.95	1.53	1.21	1.00	0.86	0.65
Hepatitis B	4.01	3.90	3.80	2.82	2.95	2.79	2.84	2.61	2.14	1.78	1.62	1.51	1.34	1.12
Lyme disease[1]	6.21	4.79	6.39	5.99	6.53	6.05	8.44	7.39	6.84	7.94	6.75	9.21	11.67	12.71
Meningococcal disease	1.30	1.24	1.01	0.92	0.83	0.83	0.64	0.61	0.47	0.42	0.40	0.36	0.39	0.32
Mumps	0.29	0.27	0.25	0.14	0.13	0.10	0.10	0.08	0.09	0.11	2.22	0.27	0.15	0.65
Pertussis (whooping cough)	2.94	2.46	2.74	2.67	2.88	2.69	3.47	4.04	8.88	8.72	5.27	3.49	4.40	5.54
Poliomyelitis, paralytic[2]	0.03	0.02	0.01	0.00	-	-	-	-	-	-	-	-	-	0.00
Rocky Mountain spotted fever[3]	0.32	0.16	0.14	0.21	0.18	0.25	0.39	0.38	0.60	0.66	0.80	0.77	0.85	0.60
Rubella (German measles)	0.10	0.07	0.13	0.10	0.06	0.01	0.01	0.00	0.00	0.00	0.00	0.00	0.01	0.00
Rubeola (measles)	0.20	0.06	0.04	0.04	0.03	0.04	0.02	0.02	0.01	0.02	0.02	0.01	0.05	0.02
Salmonellosis, excluding typhoid fever	17.15	15.66	16.17	14.89	14.51	14.39	15.73	15.16	14.47	15.43	15.45	16.03	16.92	16.18
Shigellosis	9.80	8.64	8.74	6.43	8.41	7.19	8.37	8.19	4.99	5.51	5.23	6.60	7.50	5.24
Tuberculosis[4]	8.04	7.42	6.79	6.43	6.01	5.68	5.36	5.17	5.09	4.80	4.65	4.44	4.28	3.80
Sexually transmitted diseases[5]														
Syphilis[6]	19.76	17.13	13.88	12.68	11.20	11.32	11.42	11.79	11.38	11.23	12.34	13.57	15.22	14.74
Primary and secondary	4.23	3.14	2.54	2.37	2.12	2.14	2.38	2.47	2.72	2.94	3.26	3.80	4.44	4.60
Early latent	7.49	6.10	4.60	4.13	3.35	3.05	2.92	2.88	2.65	2.76	3.07	3.57	4.08	4.30
Late and late latent[7]	7.56	7.50	6.43	5.97	5.53	5.95	5.95	6.30	5.89	5.41	5.89	6.05	6.56	5.70
Congenital[8]	32.94	27.88	21.39	14.62	14.29	12.52	11.44	10.56	9.12	8.19	8.72	10.20	10.43	10.01
Chlamydia[9]	190.57	205.49	231.83	247.16	251.38	274.52	289.41	301.74	316.51	329.42	344.33	367.47	398.12	409.19
Gonorrhea[10]	121.82	120.18	129.23	129.31	128.67	126.77	122.01	115.23	112.42	114.57	119.70	118.03	110.75	99.05
Chancroid	0.14	0.09	0.07	0.04	0.03	0.01	0.02	0.02	0.01	0.01	0.01	0.01	0.01	0.01
Number														
Diphtheria	2	4	1	1	1	2	1	1	-	-	-	0	0	0
Haemophilus influenzae, invasive	1,170	1,162	1,194	1,309	1,398	1,597	1,743	2,013	2,085	2,304	2,496	2,541	2,886	3,022
Hepatitis A	31,032	30,021	23,229	17,047	13,397	10,609	8,795	7,653	5,683	4,488	3,579	2,979	2,585	1,987
Hepatitis B	10,637	10,416	10,258	7,694	8,036	7,843	7,996	7,526	6,212	5,119	4,713	4,519	4,033	3,405
Lyme disease[1]	16,455	12,801	16,801	16,273	17,730	17,029	23,763	21,273	19,804	23,305	19,931	27,444	35,198	38,468
Meningococcal disease	3,437	3,308	2,725	2,501	2,256	2,333	1,814	1,756	1,361	1,245	1,194	1,077	1,172	980
Mumps	751	683	666	387	338	266	270	231	258	314	6,584	800	454	1,991
Pertussis (whooping cough)	7,796	6,564	7,405	7,288	7,867	7,580	9,771	11,647	25,827	25,616	15,632	10,454	13,278	16,858
Poliomyelitis, paralytic[2]	7	6	3	2	0	0	0	0	0	0	0	0	0	1
Rocky Mountain spotted fever[3]	831	409	365	579	495	695	1,104	1,091	1,713	1,936	2,288	2,221	2,563	1,815
Rubella (German measles)	238	181	364	267	176	23	18	7	10	11	11	12	16	3
Rubeola (measles)	508	138	100	100	86	116	44	56	37	66	55	43	140	71
Salmonellosis, excluding typhoid fever	45,471	41,901	43,694	40,596	39,574	40,495	44,264	43,657	42,197	45,322	45,808	47,995	51,040	49,192
Shigellosis	25,978	23,117	23,626	17,521	22,922	20,221	23,541	23,581	14,627	16,168	15,503	19,758	22,625	15,931
Tuberculosis[4]	21,337	19,851	18,361	17,531	16,377	15,989	15,075	14,874	14,517	14,097	13,779	13,299	12,904	11,545
Sexually transmitted diseases[5]														
Syphilis[6]	53,240	46,716	38,289	35,385	31,618	32,284	32,919	34,289	33,423	33,288	36,958	40,925	46,291	44,828
Primary and secondary	11,405	8,556	7,007	6,617	5,979	6,103	6,862	7,177	7,980	8,724	9,756	11,466	13,500	13,997
Early latent	20,187	16,631	12,696	11,534	9,465	8,701	8,429	8,361	7,768	8,176	9,186	10,768	12,401	13,066
Late and late latent[7]	20,366	20,447	17,743	16,655	15,594	16,976	17,168	18,319	17,300	16,049	17,644	18,256	19,945	17,338
Congenital[8]	1,282	1,082	843	579	580	504	460	432	375	339	372	435	445	427
Chlamydia[9]	492,631	537,904	614,250	662,647	709,452	783,242	834,555	877,478	929,462	976,445	1,030,911	1,108,374	1,210,523	1,244,180
Gonorrhea[10]	328,169	327,665	356,492	360,813	363,136	361,705	351,852	335,104	330,132	339,593	358,366	355,991	336,742	301,174
Chancroid	386	246	189	110	78	38	48	54	30	17	19	23	25	28

0.00 = Rate more than zero but less than 0.005.
- = Quantity zero.
— = Data not available.
[1]National surveillance case definition revised in 2008; probable cases not previously reported.
[2]Cases of vaccine-associated paralytic poliomyelitis caused by polio vaccine virus.
[3]Revision of national surveillance case definition distinguishing between confirmed and probable cases; total case count includes two case reports with unknown case status.
[4]Case reporting for tuberculosis began in 1953. Data prior to 1975 are not comparable with subsequent years because of changes in reporting criteria effective in 1975.
[5]Starting with 1991, data include both civilian and military cases.
[6]Includes stage of syphilis not stated.
[7]Includes cases of unknown duration.
[8]Rates include all cases of congenitally acquired syphilis per 100,000 live births.
[9]Prior to 1994, chlamydia was not notifiable. In 1994–1999, cases for New York were exclusively reported by New York City. Starting with 2000 data, includes cases for the entire state.
[10]Data for 1994 do not include cases from Georgia.

NOTES: The total resident population was used to calculate all rates except sexually transmitted diseases (STDs), which used the civilian resident population prior to 1991.

Table C-3. Acquired Immunodeficiency Syndrome (AIDS) Cases, by Year of Diagnosis and Selected Characteristics, 2006–2009

(Number, percent distribution.)

Characteristic	All years[1]	2006	2007	2008	2009
Estimated number of AIDS diagnoses[2]					
All persons[3]	1,108,611	36,151	35,434	34,755	34,247
Sex and Age					
Male, 13 years and over	878,366	26,473	25,871	25,612	25,587
Female, 13 years and over	220,795	9,639	9,531	9,102	8,647
Children, under 13 years	9,448	39	31	40	13
Male, 13 Years and Over					
Hispanic origin and race					
Not Hispanic or Latino					
White	381,898	8,923	8,511	8,239	8,121
Black or African American	323,872	11,093	10,968	11,042	11,093
Asian[4]	7,068	348	370	399	349
Native Hawaiian or Other Pacific Islander	695	35	42	35	43
American Indian or Alaska Native	2,879	115	100	137	127
Hispanic or Latino[5]	152,310	5,483	5,418	5,313	5,359
Multiple race	9,382	477	462	448	495
Age at Diagnosis					
13–14 years	712	27	31	27	25
15–24 years	34,949	1,454	1,728	1,795	2,031
25–34 years	272,485	5,404	5,386	5,452	5,648
35–44 years	346,798	10,043	9,168	8,550	7,864
45–54 years	161,665	6,712	6,870	6,837	7,060
55–64 years	48,138	2,209	2,124	2,343	2,358
65 years and over	13,618	625	564	610	603
Female, 13 Years and Over					
Hispanic origin and race					
Not Hispanic or Latina					
White	42,602	1,558	1,534	1,421	1,344
Black or African American	136,690	6,177	6,179	6,000	5,639
Asian[4]	1,208	73	84	88	80
Native Hawaiian or Other Pacific Islander	136	15	10	5	7
American Indian or Alaska Native	789	30	41	39	28
Hispanic or Latina[5]	36,091	1,578	1,490	1,385	1,357
Multiple race	3,234	208	194	164	192
Age at Diagnosis					
13–14 years	609	51	50	31	33
15–24 years	15,185	580	601	554	548
25–34 years	71,302	2,227	2,088	2,124	1,871
35–44 years	81,013	3,371	3,253	3,038	2,718
45–54 years	37,042	2,439	2,460	2,342	2,389
55–64 years	11,518	759	852	823	844
65 years and over	4,125	211	228	190	243
Children, Under 13 Years					
Hispanic origin and race:					
Not Hispanic or Latino:					
White	1,602	3	4	7	1
Black or African American	5,787	30	22	23	8
Asian[4]	48	1	0	2	0
Native Hawaiian or Other Pacific Islander	7	0	0	0	0
American Indian or Alaska Native	31	0	0	0	0
Hispanic or Latino[5]	1,862	4	4	3	3
Multiple race	109	1	0	4	0
Region of Residence					
Northeast	340,357	9,369	9,082	8,064	8,171
Midwest	116,029	4,154	4,006	4,218	4,394
South	430,141	16,453	16,383	16,506	15,806
West	222,083	6,174	5,964	5,967	5,875
Percent Distribution					
All Persons[3]	100.0	100.0	100.0	100.0	100.0
Sex and Age					
Male, 13 years and over	79.2	73.2	73.0	73.7	74.7
Female, 13 years and over	19.9	26.7	26.9	26.2	25.2
Children, under 13 years	0.9	0.1	0.1	0.1	0.0

Table C-3. Acquired Immunodeficiency Syndrome (AIDS) Cases, by Year of Diagnosis and Selected Characteristics, 2006–2009—*Continued*

(Number, percent distribution.)

Characteristic	All years[1]	2006	2007	2008	2009
Male, 13 Years and Over					
Hispanic origin and race					
Not Hispanic or Latino					
White	43.5	33.7	32.9	32.2	31.7
Black or African American	36.9	41.9	42.4	43.1	43.4
Asian[4]	0.8	1.3	1.4	1.6	1.4
Native Hawaiian or Other Pacific Islander	0.1	0.1	0.2	0.1	0.2
American Indian or Alaska Native	0.3	0.4	0.4	0.5	0.5
Hispanic or Latino[5]	17.3	20.7	20.9	20.7	20.9
Multiple race	1.1	1.8	1.8	1.7	1.9
Age at Diagnosis					
13–14 years	0.1	0.1	0.1	0.1	0.1
15–24 years	4.0	5.5	6.7	7.0	7.9
25–34 years	31.0	20.4	20.8	21.3	22.1
35–44 years	39.5	37.9	35.4	33.4	30.7
45–54 years	18.4	25.4	26.6	26.7	27.6
55–64 years	5.5	8.3	8.2	9.1	9.2
65 years and over	1.6	2.4	2.2	2.4	2.4
Female, 13 Years and Over					
Hispanic origin and race					
Not Hispanic or Latina					
White	19.3	16.2	16.1	15.6	15.5
Black or African American	61.9	64.1	64.8	65.9	65.2
Asian[4]	0.5	0.8	0.9	1.0	0.9
Native Hawaiian or Other Pacific Islander	0.1	0.2	0.1	0.1	0.1
American Indian or Alaska Native	0.4	0.3	0.4	0.4	0.3
Hispanic or Latina[5]	16.3	16.4	15.6	15.2	15.7
Multiple race	1.5	2.2	2.0	1.8	2.2
Age at Diagnosis					
13–14 years	0.3	0.5	0.5	0.3	0.4
15–24 years	6.9	6.0	6.3	6.1	6.3
25–34 years	32.3	23.1	21.9	23.3	21.6
35–44 years	36.7	35.0	34.1	33.4	31.4
45–54 years	16.8	25.3	25.8	25.7	27.6
55–64 years	5.2	7.9	8.9	9.0	9.8
65 years and over	1.9	2.2	2.4	2.1	2.8
Children, Under 13 Years					
Hispanic origin and race					
Not Hispanic or Latino					
White	17.0	8.0	13.8	18.6	8.5
Black or African American	61.3	75.9	72.5	57.0	64.8
Asian[4]	0.5	2.6	-	5.5	-
Native Hawaiian or Other Pacific Islander	0.1	-	-	-	-
American Indian or Alaska Native	0.3	-	-	-	-
Hispanic or Latino[5]	19.7	10.8	13.8	8.2	26.7
Multiple race	1.2	2.6	-	10.8	-
Region of Residence					
Northeast	30.7	25.9	25.6	23.2	23.9
Midwest	10.5	11.5	11.3	12.1	12.8
South	38.8	45.5	46.2	47.5	46.2
West	20.0	17.1	16.8	17.2	17.2

0.0 = Quantity more than zero but less than 0.05.
- = Quantity zero.
[1]Based on diagnoses reported to CDC from the beginning of the epidemic (1981) through June 30, 2010.
[2]Numbers are point estimates that result from statistical adjustments for reporting delays and missing risk factor information. The estimates do not include adjustments for incomplete reporting.
[3]Total for all years includes 306 persons of unknown races and 2 persons of unknown sex. All persons totals were calculated independent of values for sub-populations.
[4]Includes Asian and Pacific Islander legacy cases.
[5]Persons of Hispanic origin may be of any race.

Table C-4. Age-Adjusted[1] Cancer Incidence Rates for Selected Cancer Sites, by Sex, Race, and Hispanic Origin, Selected Geographic Areas, Selected Years, 1990–2008 and Annual Percent Change (APC)[2], 1990–2008

(Number of new cases per 100,000 population.)

Site, sex, race, and Hispanic origin	1990	1991	1992	1993	1994	1995	1996	1997	1998	1999
All Sites										
All persons	475.5	495.0	503.0	486.7	474.9	470.7	472.5	478.0	479.4	480.5
White	483.1	504.2	510.9	491.3	480.5	477.4	479.8	485.8	488.9	490.2
Black or African American	512.7	536.3	551.8	557.2	541.4	534.6	532.8	536.8	528.3	532.3
American Indian or Alaska Native[3]	346.8	356.7	358.1	382.1	358.6	367.6	367.0	388.6	367.1	405.3
Asian or Pacific Islander	334.1	338.9	356.9	351.2	345.3	336.3	333.6	345.2	336.8	340.5
Hispanic or Latino[4]	356.9	365.4	377.9	369.0	358.8	359.2	363.7	358.6	373.6	371.4
White, not Hispanic or Latino[4]	494.9	517.4	524.1	503.9	493.6	491.1	494.0	502.0	504.4	506.7
Male	583.7	625.6	648.5	610.9	579.2	563.7	563.0	565.0	562.2	567.5
White	590.8	635.0	654.5	609.2	578.8	563.3	565.3	565.9	565.3	570.2
Black or African American	685.8	750.6	788.0	792.2	746.8	735.0	714.9	723.8	710.7	710.4
American Indian or Alaska Native[3]	394.5	412.7	403.3	487.8	412.6	420.6	396.8	447.9	391.2	467.4
Asian or Pacific Islander	385.2	399.6	429.3	423.4	410.6	394.2	384.3	395.7	380.9	393.0
Hispanic or Latino[4]	415.8	438.5	469.8	457.7	439.8	438.4	436.9	428.1	441.0	441.2
White, not Hispanic or Latino[4]	606.5	653.0	672.2	623.8	593.3	577.3	580.5	582.6	581.1	587.2
Female	411.2	413.3	409.3	405.4	406.9	410.2	413.7	421.3	425.8	423.0
White	421.3	424.6	420.1	415.9	417.9	423.3	425.7	435.0	441.1	438.4
Black or African American	404.1	403.4	399.7	404.0	407.3	400.7	413.3	413.8	410.3	414.7
American Indian or Alaska Native[3]	314.7	317.2	326.6	303.4	319.1	334.0	347.6	347.2	351.5	364.0
Asian or Pacific Islander	294.0	290.5	300.6	295.3	296.2	293.9	297.3	309.8	307.0	304.9
Hispanic or Latina[4]	325.5	324.1	323.0	313.7	309.8	311.0	319.7	316.6	332.6	329.7
White, not Hispanic or Latina[4]	430.2	434.2	429.8	426.8	429.6	436.6	438.9	450.7	456.0	454.1
Lung and Bronchus										
Male	95.0	94.2	93.0	89.7	87.2	86.9	84.4	82.6	83.3	80.3
White	94.2	92.8	90.8	88.2	86.6	85.1	82.9	81.0	82.2	78.9
Black or African American	133.9	141.8	142.6	130.9	123.1	136.7	129.6	125.0	123.3	120.0
Asian or Pacific Islander	64.2	63.0	69.4	64.4	60.6	60.0	60.6	62.0	61.2	62.2
Hispanic or Latino[4]	59.3	54.1	53.9	51.2	49.0	52.3	48.6	48.1	50.5	44.4
White, not Hispanic or Latino[4]	97.4	96.5	94.5	91.8	90.4	88.4	86.7	84.6	85.7	83.0
Female	47.2	48.3	48.7	48.8	48.9	49.3	50.1	50.3	50.9	50.4
White	48.4	49.8	50.5	50.7	50.4	51.8	52.3	52.9	53.1	52.5
Black or African American	52.9	54.6	51.7	53.0	55.1	49.7	54.0	50.6	56.9	58.2
Asian or Pacific Islander	28.3	26.3	29.4	26.4	29.1	27.1	28.0	29.8	28.5	28.8
Hispanic or Latina[4]	26.4	28.1	26.4	28.3	22.8	25.1	26.2	25.0	26.5	26.0
White, not Hispanic or Latina[4]	50.8	52.2	53.2	53.2	53.6	54.9	55.4	56.4	56.7	56.0
Colon and Rectum										
Male	72.2	71.4	69.0	66.5	65.3	63.2	64.5	66.4	65.9	64.2
White	73.0	71.6	69.4	66.1	65.2	62.6	65.0	66.2	65.7	64.2
Black or African American	72.7	78.5	75.5	76.4	73.0	74.3	67.7	74.4	77.4	73.1
Asian or Pacific Islander	60.9	60.0	57.8	58.3	57.7	58.1	56.2	59.3	57.6	54.1
Hispanic or Latino[4]	47.3	51.4	48.9	46.1	45.6	45.7	49.5	50.4	52.4	49.0
White, not Hispanic or Latino[4]	75.1	73.2	71.1	67.8	67.0	64.0	66.3	67.4	67.0	65.8
Female	50.2	49.3	48.0	47.6	46.5	45.9	46.0	47.2	48.6	47.0
White	49.7	48.9	47.5	47.2	45.8	45.5	45.7	47.0	48.3	46.2
Black or African American	61.1	56.7	56.6	55.4	57.7	54.7	54.2	57.9	56.0	58.4
Asian or Pacific Islander	37.7	41.9	41.0	40.9	38.8	38.4	39.1	35.7	40.5	40.1
Hispanic or Latina[4]	34.9	34.1	33.7	33.0	33.4	32.1	33.7	32.6	34.6	35.2
White, not Hispanic or Latina[4]	50.8	50.0	48.6	48.4	46.8	46.7	46.8	48.4	49.8	47.4
Prostate										
Male	166.7	210.2	234.0	206.9	177.3	166.1	166.4	171.6	169.3	179.9
White	168.4	212.5	234.8	201.0	170.9	161.1	162.2	167.4	164.5	175.4
Black or African American	218.4	279.3	321.4	336.8	302.1	275.4	273.8	277.3	282.4	285.0
American Indian or Alaska Native[3]	99.6	113.9	117.7	144.8	84.3	92.6	110.9	100.7	79.6	100.6
Asian or Pacific Islander	88.4	107.6	125.0	123.3	112.6	102.9	94.2	96.2	92.2	105.2
Hispanic or Latino[4]	118.4	137.5	161.8	162.4	148.9	139.7	140.4	141.8	148.8	150.6
White, not Hispanic or Latino[4]	172.1	218.7	241.2	204.6	173.1	163.6	165.2	170.9	167.0	179.0
Breast										
Female	129.3	130.6	129.9	127.2	128.7	130.8	132.0	135.9	138.8	138.3
White	134.2	136.4	134.5	132.1	134.3	136.4	137.2	141.6	145.0	145.1
Black or African American	116.6	115.7	121.3	117.2	121.8	122.2	122.8	124.8	124.2	124.0
American Indian or Alaska Native[3]	68.0	72.3	96.2	97.6	86.3	94.5	116.9	82.5	87.2	83.6
Asian or Pacific Islander	87.3	81.8	89.3	85.4	81.6	86.6	90.1	99.6	99.0	98.1
Hispanic or Latina[4]	91.6	94.6	91.9	83.5	86.1	89.8	93.4	91.3	95.2	95.7
White, not Hispanic or Latina[4]	138.5	140.6	138.9	137.5	139.7	141.9	142.8	148.2	151.8	152.1
Cervix Uteri										
Female	11.9	10.8	11.0	10.7	10.5	9.9	10.7	9.8	9.8	9.4
White	11.3	10.2	10.5	10.1	9.9	9.2	9.9	9.2	9.3	9.1
Black or African American	16.4	16.1	14.3	14.8	13.6	14.7	14.2	13.2	12.7	12.9
Asian or Pacific Islander	12.0	10.8	12.2	11.8	14.1	11.0	13.1	11.2	10.7	8.2
Hispanic or Latina[4]	21.4	19.8	21.0	20.0	20.2	17.4	18.8	16.6	15.5	17.1
White, not Hispanic or Latina[4]	9.7	8.6	8.9	8.5	8.1	7.8	8.5	7.9	8.1	7.6

Table C-4. Age-Adjusted[1] Cancer Incidence Rates for Selected Cancer Sites, by Sex, Race, and Hispanic Origin, Selected Geographic Areas, Selected Years, 1990–2008 and Annual Percent Change (APC)[2], 1990–2008—Continued

(Number of new cases per 100,000 population.)

Site, sex, race, and Hispanic origin	2000	2001	2002	2003	2004	2005	2006	2007	2008	1990–2008 APC[2]
All Sites										
All persons	473.8	477.2	472.5	461.1	461.9	455.5	454.5	459.9	449.9	*-0.4
White	485.1	489.2	482.8	471.3	471.4	466.4	465.0	468.7	458.1	*-0.4
Black or African American	518.8	511.0	519.1	506.4	510.5	489.9	485.2	493.2	482.0	*-0.7
American Indian or Alaska Native[3]	358.7	387.8	350.6	371.5	396.6	394.9	376.3	349.7	363.6	0.1
Asian or Pacific Islander	336.0	342.3	343.4	332.6	336.2	330.1	325.8	335.1	327.7	*-0.3
Hispanic or Latino[4]	360.1	362.7	367.5	353.9	362.0	356.9	345.3	349.9	343.1	*-0.3
White, not Hispanic or Latino[4]	503.0	508.0	500.6	489.8	489.2	485.0	485.8	490.0	479.2	*-0.3
Male	563.5	564.5	556.3	543.0	542.4	527.3	527.5	537.0	513.7	*-0.9
White	568.5	571.1	561.4	547.3	547.5	534.6	533.4	541.2	516.6	*-0.9
Black or African American	697.8	683.2	684.3	661.7	660.8	615.8	607.1	627.2	611.1	*-1.3
American Indian or Alaska Native[3]	367.9	442.5	376.3	431.5	397.0	415.5	377.4	380.8	390.7	-0.5
Asian or Pacific Islander	393.1	388.2	385.4	383.2	380.0	367.3	367.2	371.3	352.9	*-0.7
Hispanic or Latino[4]	431.4	429.2	433.0	412.2	422.8	407.0	393.1	398.8	382.3	*-0.8
White, not Hispanic or Latino[4]	587.9	590.7	580.1	567.1	566.6	554.7	556.2	565.8	540.4	*-0.8
Female	413.1	417.6	415.8	405.6	406.9	406.7	404.2	405.9	406.3	-0.1
White	429.9	434.3	430.4	420.5	419.8	420.8	418.3	418.3	418.9	0.0
Black or African American	398.3	394.5	409.5	402.7	411.1	406.3	402.7	403.1	394.8	0.0
American Indian or Alaska Native[3]	358.6	353.7	330.5	331.7	402.0	380.7	380.5	332.3	350.1	*0.8
Asian or Pacific Islander	296.6	311.8	317.4	299.6	308.6	307.2	300.3	313.0	314.3	*0.3
Hispanic or Latina[4]	318.2	321.5	327.3	318.6	325.0	326.5	316.6	320.8	321.2	0.0
White, not Hispanic or Latina[4]	445.8	451.8	446.8	437.4	435.9	437.6	436.9	436.1	437.2	0.1
Lung and Bronchus										
Male	77.7	77.2	75.6	75.3	71.5	71.0	69.2	67.9	65.5	*-2.0
White	76.3	76.2	74.9	74.2	70.2	70.3	67.9	67.3	64.2	*-2.0
Black or African American	110.6	112.3	108.9	111.4	102.0	97.0	97.6	93.1	92.9	*-2.4
Asian or Pacific Islander	63.2	57.1	57.7	58.4	59.3	57.7	57.2	54.6	55.1	*-0.9
Hispanic or Latino[4]	45.1	42.4	48.1	45.3	39.7	41.9	37.7	40.9	36.9	*-2.1
White, not Hispanic or Latino[4]	80.3	80.8	78.5	78.0	74.6	74.4	72.5	71.4	68.4	*-1.8
Female	48.6	48.8	49.3	49.7	48.9	49.7	48.8	48.7	46.7	0.0
White	50.8	50.8	51.5	52.3	50.4	51.6	50.7	51.3	49.1	0.0
Black or African American	54.6	54.7	55.0	54.4	57.0	57.4	56.6	53.5	51.3	0.2
Asian or Pacific Islander	27.2	30.0	29.3	29.1	31.1	31.0	30.1	28.3	27.4	0.3
Hispanic or Latina[4]	24.0	25.2	24.9	25.0	26.2	23.6	23.5	24.5	23.6	*-0.6
White, not Hispanic or Latina[4]	54.4	54.4	55.4	56.4	54.2	56.0	55.2	55.7	53.4	*0.3
Colon and Rectum										
Male	62.6	61.6	60.0	58.2	56.5	54.1	52.7	52.2	50.5	*-1.8
White	62.2	61.0	58.8	56.9	55.5	53.6	51.5	50.9	49.3	*-2.0
Black or African American	72.7	71.5	72.5	75.4	73.6	65.6	64.3	65.4	63.3	*-0.8
Asian or Pacific Islander	57.3	56.5	58.1	52.8	50.0	47.3	51.2	48.5	46.7	*-1.3
Hispanic or Latino[4]	50.1	49.0	45.1	46.3	46.9	45.1	44.3	43.3	44.1	*-0.6
White, not Hispanic or Latino[4]	63.6	62.5	60.3	58.2	56.5	54.6	52.5	51.8	50.0	*-2.0
Female	46.0	45.3	45.1	43.4	41.9	41.1	40.9	39.8	39.1	*-1.2
White	45.6	44.4	44.0	42.8	40.7	39.9	39.9	38.7	38.2	*-1.3
Black or African American	57.8	56.2	55.9	54.7	53.5	52.9	52.9	51.5	47.6	*-0.7
Asian or Pacific Islander	37.2	40.9	41.5	36.5	37.5	37.1	35.5	35.4	35.2	*-0.7
Hispanic or Latina[4]	34.2	32.9	31.8	34.3	32.8	33.0	32.3	33.7	31.3	-0.2
White, not Hispanic or Latina[4]	46.8	45.8	45.5	43.7	41.7	41.0	41.0	39.2	39.3	*-1.3
Prostate										
Male	178.2	179.4	177.3	164.8	164.6	151.7	161.3	164.0	148.4	*-1.4
White	174.3	176.9	173.7	160.6	161.0	147.1	157.1	157.4	142.5	*-1.6
Black or African American	287.0	269.7	278.2	250.6	248.1	231.4	231.3	244.3	227.7	*-1.4
American Indian or Alaska Native[3]	66.8	92.2	91.5	107.6	88.2	86.2	85.3	84.9	71.4	*-2.0
Asian or Pacific Islander	105.5	107.0	102.2	103.4	100.8	94.5	95.4	97.5	84.2	*-1.0
Hispanic or Latino[4]	147.9	145.0	148.2	135.0	145.0	126.7	126.1	123.8	117.5	*-1.0
White, not Hispanic or Latino[4]	178.3	181.2	177.3	164.5	163.6	150.3	162.2	163.7	147.6	*-1.6
Breast										
Female	134.0	135.6	132.5	123.9	124.5	123.9	122.3	125.2	125.4	-0.3
White	140.8	142.6	138.6	128.8	128.7	129.0	126.4	128.4	128.2	-0.4
Black or African American	120.4	116.3	121.9	121.4	121.4	116.7	121.6	123.5	122.4	0.1
American Indian or Alaska Native[3]	98.1	94.3	79.3	91.6	100.8	104.0	83.8	89.3	88.9	0.3
Asian or Pacific Islander	93.1	100.3	100.3	91.8	97.3	95.1	94.0	100.8	104.1	*0.9
Hispanic or Latina[4]	96.8	91.7	92.9	87.7	91.2	93.1	91.1	91.3	93.3	0.1
White, not Hispanic or Latina[4]	147.2	150.4	145.7	135.4	135.2	135.5	132.6	135.1	134.8	-0.2
Cervix Uteri										
Female	8.9	8.8	8.4	8.2	7.8	7.9	7.6	7.4	7.5	*-2.6
White	8.9	8.4	8.3	7.9	7.8	7.7	7.5	7.3	7.4	*-2.3
Black or African American	10.6	10.8	10.0	10.6	9.7	9.0	8.1	8.2	8.9	*-3.8
Asian or Pacific Islander	7.9	9.6	8.2	8.1	7.2	8.0	7.1	7.0	6.4	*-3.9
Hispanic or Latina[4]	17.1	15.0	14.7	14.2	13.2	13.8	11.8	10.9	11.9	*-3.4
White, not Hispanic or Latina[4]	7.1	7.0	6.9	6.4	6.5	6.3	6.6	6.4	6.2	*-2.3

PART C: HEALTH

Table C-4. Age-Adjusted[1] Cancer Incidence Rates for Selected Cancer Sites, by Sex, Race, and Hispanic Origin, Selected Geographic Areas, Selected Years, 1990–2008 and Annual Percent Change (APC)[2], 1990–2008—Continued

(Number of new cases per 100,000 population.)

Site, sex, race, and Hispanic origin	1990	1991	1992	1993	1994	1995	1996	1997	1998	1999
Corpus Uteri[5]										
Female	24.2	23.8	24.1	23.4	23.9	24.4	24.1	24.8	24.4	24.2
White	26.0	25.5	26.0	24.9	25.4	26.0	25.6	26.5	26.1	25.8
Black or African American	16.2	15.8	15.2	16.9	17.1	17.0	18.4	17.3	17.8	17.6
Asian or Pacific Islander	13.0	15.2	15.1	14.6	15.5	17.1	16.2	17.0	17.1	17.3
Hispanic or Latina[4]	17.8	18.0	16.9	16.2	15.2	16.2	16.5	17.1	17.6	16.3
White, not Hispanic or Latina[4]	26.6	26.3	26.8	25.9	26.5	27.1	26.5	27.6	27.1	27.1
Ovary										
Female	15.5	15.3	14.9	15.1	14.4	14.5	14.0	14.2	14.1	14.3
White	16.4	16.2	15.8	15.9	15.1	15.4	15.1	15.0	15.1	15.1
Black or African American	11.3	10.4	10.5	11.8	11.6	10.8	9.2	10.3	10.7	10.4
Asian or Pacific Islander	11.2	10.5	10.1	11.1	9.9	10.4	9.3	11.5	10.2	11.0
Hispanic or Latina[4]	12.3	11.9	13.0	11.6	12.1	11.7	12.2	11.2	12.3	11.0
White, not Hispanic or Latina[4]	16.7	16.6	16.0	16.4	15.4	15.9	15.4	15.5	15.4	15.7
Oral Cavity and Pharynx										
Male	18.5	17.7	18.0	17.7	17.2	16.5	17.2	16.8	16.4	15.4
White	18.0	17.6	17.7	17.4	16.7	16.4	16.8	16.7	16.2	15.3
Black or African American	25.4	21.3	23.5	22.9	23.5	22.3	22.7	19.3	21.5	19.2
Asian or Pacific Islander	14.8	13.0	13.5	12.6	13.7	11.7	14.1	14.5	13.0	11.2
Hispanic or Latino[4]	10.8	11.0	11.2	10.5	11.4	12.3	11.4	11.0	9.9	10.1
White, not Hispanic or Latino[4]	18.8	18.3	18.4	18.2	17.3	16.9	17.5	17.4	16.9	16.1
Female	7.3	7.3	6.8	7.2	6.8	7.0	6.9	6.9	6.7	6.3
White	7.4	7.3	6.8	7.3	6.8	7.1	6.9	6.9	6.8	6.2
Black or African American	6.4	6.9	6.5	7.3	6.9	6.7	7.3	7.0	6.7	6.0
Asian or Pacific Islander	6.1	6.7	6.3	6.0	5.7	5.2	5.9	6.6	4.6	6.4
Hispanic or Latina[4]	4.1	4.0	4.2	5.5	4.6	3.7	3.9	4.3	3.8	4.7
White, not Hispanic or Latina[4]	7.8	7.7	7.1	7.5	7.1	7.5	7.2	7.2	7.2	6.5
Stomach										
Male	14.6	14.7	14.3	14.3	14.2	13.5	13.7	13.4	12.8	12.8
White	12.8	12.7	12.4	12.3	12.2	11.9	11.9	11.3	11.0	11.2
Black or African American	21.4	24.2	20.8	20.6	23.0	18.6	22.2	22.1	20.4	17.0
Asian or Pacific Islander	26.8	25.8	27.9	28.3	24.6	24.3	23.3	24.8	21.3	22.6
Hispanic or Latino[4]	20.2	19.8	19.3	20.2	21.6	19.4	17.3	19.0	19.2	20.4
White, not Hispanic or Latino[4]	12.1	12.0	11.6	11.4	11.2	11.1	11.2	10.4	10.1	10.1
Female	6.7	7.0	6.6	6.4	6.2	6.2	6.1	6.1	6.4	6.6
White	5.7	5.9	5.6	5.4	5.0	5.1	5.1	4.9	5.2	5.5
Black or African American	9.9	11.3	9.2	8.9	9.9	9.8	9.1	10.8	10.9	10.4
Asian or Pacific Islander	15.4	15.4	14.6	15.3	15.1	13.0	13.8	12.0	12.9	12.1
Hispanic or Latina[4]	10.8	11.2	11.0	10.9	9.2	11.3	10.4	10.2	11.0	9.6
White, not Hispanic or Latina[4]	5.1	5.4	5.0	4.7	4.5	4.4	4.4	4.3	4.6	4.9
Pancreas										
Male	13.0	12.7	12.8	12.6	13.0	12.7	12.5	12.9	12.9	12.5
White	12.7	12.6	12.6	12.2	12.4	12.4	12.2	12.6	12.8	12.4
Black or African American	19.3	17.9	18.8	18.4	19.0	19.1	18.9	18.1	17.3	18.1
Asian or Pacific Islander	11.0	10.3	10.7	11.9	14.2	10.3	10.5	12.0	10.5	9.2
Hispanic or Latino[4]	10.7	9.9	11.3	10.4	9.7	12.0	11.4	11.8	9.9	9.2
White, not Hispanic or Latino[4]	12.8	12.8	12.7	12.3	12.7	12.4	12.3	12.7	13.2	12.7
Female	10.0	10.3	10.0	9.9	9.9	9.9	10.1	10.2	10.1	9.6
White	9.8	10.0	9.7	9.6	9.7	9.6	9.7	9.7	9.9	9.3
Black or African American	12.9	15.8	16.0	15.8	15.0	15.5	15.2	16.7	13.7	13.4
Asian or Pacific Islander	9.9	8.5	7.2	8.1	6.7	8.1	7.9	8.4	8.5	8.5
Hispanic or Latina[4]	9.9	10.8	9.3	10.0	9.8	8.9	9.1	10.0	10.1	9.8
White, not Hispanic or Latina[4]	9.7	9.8	9.7	9.5	9.7	9.7	9.8	9.6	9.8	9.3
Urinary Bladder										
Male	37.2	37.4	36.9	36.8	36.1	35.4	35.8	35.9	36.8	36.5
White	40.7	41.2	40.5	40.0	39.6	38.9	39.5	39.7	40.7	40.1
Black or African American	19.5	21.3	18.4	23.5	19.7	19.3	19.1	21.5	20.7	22.1
Asian or Pacific Islander	15.4	12.4	16.5	16.7	15.6	16.4	15.7	15.3	15.7	17.3
Hispanic or Latino[4]	22.1	19.9	20.2	20.6	21.4	17.6	18.2	18.8	18.2	19.5
White, not Hispanic or Latino[4]	42.4	43.2	42.4	41.8	41.5	41.0	41.6	41.9	43.2	42.4
Female	9.5	9.2	9.4	9.4	9.1	9.3	9.0	9.3	9.0	9.3
White	10.0	9.8	10.1	10.1	9.8	10.1	9.8	10.0	9.8	10.0
Black or African American	8.6	8.5	7.2	7.7	7.0	7.2	7.0	8.4	6.5	8.7
Asian or Pacific Islander	5.3	4.0	4.9	3.9	3.9	4.4	3.7	5.1	4.7	4.1
Hispanic or Latina[4]	5.8	5.5	6.1	5.6	5.8	5.3	5.9	5.4	4.9	4.8
White, not Hispanic or Latina[4]	10.3	10.3	10.5	10.6	10.3	10.6	10.3	10.6	10.4	10.6

Table C-4. Age-Adjusted[1] Cancer Incidence Rates for Selected Cancer Sites, by Sex, Race, and Hispanic Origin, Selected Geographic Areas, Selected Years, 1990–2008 and Annual Percent Change (APC)[2], 1990–2008—Continued

(Number of new cases per 100,000 population.)

Site, sex, race, and Hispanic origin	2000	2001	2002	2003	2004	2005	2006	2007	2008	2008
Corpus Uteri[5]										
Female	23.4	24.2	23.5	23.0	23.5	23.7	23.5	23.9	24.7	-0.1
White	25.2	25.6	24.4	24.4	24.7	24.9	24.9	24.8	25.6	*-0.2
Black or African American	16.3	19.2	21.3	18.8	19.2	20.2	17.8	21.5	22.3	*1.6
Asian or Pacific Islander	16.2	17.4	18.7	16.6	19.1	18.8	18.1	19.3	20.1	*1.7
Hispanic or Latina[4]	15.5	16.5	17.4	17.7	19.1	19.0	17.5	18.7	18.8	*0.7
White, not Hispanic or Latina[4]	26.4	26.9	25.3	25.3	25.3	25.7	26.0	25.7	26.6	-0.2
Ovary										
Female	14.2	14.2	13.8	13.5	13.1	13.1	12.7	12.9	12.5	*-1.0
White	15.1	15.3	14.6	14.2	13.7	13.7	13.5	13.6	13.3	*-1.1
Black or African American	10.7	9.4	9.8	11.4	11.0	10.4	8.8	11.2	9.7	-0.5
Asian or Pacific Islander	10.1	9.7	12.1	10.2	10.0	10.9	10.5	10.5	10.1	-0.1
Hispanic or Latina[4]	10.8	13.5	14.0	11.9	11.9	11.7	10.9	11.1	11.9	-0.2
White, not Hispanic or Latina[4]	15.6	15.7	14.6	14.6	14.0	14.0	14.0	13.9	13.5	*-1.1
Oral Cavity and Pharynx										
Male	15.8	15.1	15.7	15.1	15.3	14.9	14.6	15.0	15.5	*-1.2
White	15.6	15.3	15.8	15.2	15.6	15.2	14.7	15.4	15.8	*-0.9
Black or African American	19.3	18.1	18.0	17.3	16.2	15.6	15.5	15.4	14.2	*-2.9
Asian or Pacific Islander	13.3	9.9	12.8	11.7	11.4	11.4	11.5	11.0	12.8	*-1.1
Hispanic or Latino[4]	8.9	9.2	9.3	8.8	10.0	9.4	7.5	8.7	9.4	*-1.7
White, not Hispanic or Latino[4]	16.7	16.2	16.8	16.3	16.6	16.2	16.0	16.7	17.1	*-0.7
Female	6.2	6.7	6.5	5.9	6.1	6.1	6.2	6.0	6.2	*-1.1
White	6.2	6.6	6.6	5.8	6.1	5.9	6.2	6.0	6.2	*-1.1
Black or African American	5.3	6.5	6.3	6.7	5.8	6.8	5.4	5.5	5.0	*-1.3
Asian or Pacific Islander	6.1	5.8	5.9	5.2	5.8	5.9	5.3	5.2	5.8	-0.6
Hispanic or Latina[4]	3.7	4.1	3.8	3.9	3.6	3.4	4.0	4.0	4.3	-0.7
White, not Hispanic or Latina[4]	6.6	7.0	7.1	6.2	6.5	6.4	6.6	6.5	6.6	*-1.0
Stomach										
Male	12.6	11.8	12.0	11.7	11.9	11.3	11.2	11.3	10.4	*-1.8
White	10.7	10.3	10.4	10.1	10.3	9.5	9.6	9.6	9.1	*-1.9
Black or African American	18.4	17.5	15.8	18.5	16.4	17.2	16.0	17.4	16.3	*-2.0
Asian or Pacific Islander	22.5	19.1	20.4	19.1	20.1	20.0	18.0	18.0	15.5	*-2.7
Hispanic or Latino[4]	16.0	15.7	16.1	15.8	16.5	14.7	14.6	16.5	14.8	*-1.9
White, not Hispanic or Latino[4]	10.0	9.4	9.6	9.2	9.3	8.7	8.7	8.5	8.1	*-2.1
Female	6.1	5.8	6.2	6.0	5.9	5.7	5.9	5.5	5.5	*-1.0
White	5.0	4.7	5.1	4.9	5.0	4.7	4.9	4.5	4.4	*-1.1
Black or African American	8.6	9.0	9.9	9.5	7.5	8.0	9.4	7.7	7.9	*-1.3
Asian or Pacific Islander	13.0	12.2	11.3	11.2	11.2	10.5	9.2	10.4	9.9	*-2.6
Hispanic or Latina[4]	10.8	10.3	10.7	10.2	10.3	10.3	9.8	9.4	8.2	*-0.9
White, not Hispanic or Latina[4]	4.2	3.8	4.2	4.1	4.1	3.7	4.0	3.5	3.6	*-1.9
Pancreas										
Male	12.8	12.8	12.8	12.5	13.4	13.5	13.6	13.8	13.6	*0.4
White	12.6	12.9	13.0	12.3	13.2	13.3	13.7	13.7	13.4	*0.5
Black or African American	18.1	15.5	13.7	17.2	18.0	18.0	17.1	16.5	15.2	-0.6
Asian or Pacific Islander	10.7	9.8	9.8	10.2	11.9	11.7	10.3	11.8	11.5	0.0
Hispanic or Latino[4]	12.2	9.6	10.7	9.7	11.2	11.7	12.2	11.2	10.9	0.4
White, not Hispanic or Latino[4]	12.7	13.3	13.3	12.7	13.4	13.5	13.9	14.1	13.8	*0.6
Female	9.9	9.8	10.4	10.3	10.3	10.8	10.8	10.6	10.6	*0.4
White	9.6	9.5	10.1	10.1	10.1	10.5	10.5	10.3	10.3	*0.4
Black or African American	12.6	13.5	15.8	14.3	14.4	16.1	15.1	14.4	14.9	-0.1
Asian or Pacific Islander	9.2	9.1	8.9	8.2	9.0	8.0	9.7	8.8	8.9	0.6
Hispanic or Latina[4]	9.2	9.9	10.8	8.8	9.2	11.3	9.5	10.6	9.2	0.1
White, not Hispanic or Latina[4]	9.6	9.5	10.0	10.4	10.3	10.4	10.6	10.3	10.5	*0.5
Urinary Bladder										
Male	36.8	36.8	35.7	36.8	36.8	36.6	35.6	36.6	34.6	-0.1
White	40.8	41.0	39.2	40.6	40.8	40.4	39.1	40.4	37.8	-0.1
Black or African American	20.1	19.3	20.6	22.6	22.5	22.5	19.2	21.4	21.9	0.4
Asian or Pacific Islander	16.5	17.1	19.3	17.5	17.0	17.0	18.5	17.5	18.0	*1.1
Hispanic or Latino[4]	20.4	21.3	20.5	19.6	18.9	18.9	19.5	19.4	15.7	-0.6
White, not Hispanic or Latino[4]	43.2	43.4	41.6	43.3	43.8	43.3	41.9	43.6	41.1	0.1
Female	9.1	9.1	9.1	9.2	9.2	8.9	8.8	8.5	8.6	*-0.4
White	9.9	9.9	10.1	9.9	10.0	9.6	9.4	9.3	9.4	*-0.3
Black or African American	7.7	7.2	8.4	7.7	8.2	7.7	8.6	7.5	6.2	-0.2
Asian or Pacific Islander	4.2	4.6	3.2	4.9	3.9	5.1	3.7	3.7	4.9	-0.2
Hispanic or Latina[4]	5.7	5.3	6.4	4.4	5.7	6.2	5.3	5.3	5.3	-0.3
White, not Hispanic or Latina[4]	10.5	10.6	10.6	10.8	10.6	10.1	10.1	9.9	10.1	-0.1

Table C-4. **Age-Adjusted[1] Cancer Incidence Rates for Selected Cancer Sites, by Sex, Race, and Hispanic Origin, Selected Geographic Areas, Selected Years, 1990–2008 and Annual Percent Change (APC)[2], 1990–2008**—Continued

(Number of new cases per 100,000 population.)

Site, sex, race, and Hispanic origin	1990	1991	1992	1993	1994	1995	1996	1997	1998	1999
Non-Hodgkin's Lymphoma										
Male	22.6	23.2	23.3	23.4	24.8	25.0	24.6	23.9	23.0	24.3
White	23.6	24.5	24.4	24.5	25.8	26.2	25.9	24.8	24.2	25.3
Black or African American	17.4	17.1	18.9	17.7	20.3	21.4	18.7	22.9	17.3	18.5
Asian or Pacific Islander	16.7	16.0	16.3	15.7	18.2	16.5	16.7	16.3	15.4	19.1
Hispanic or Latino[4]	17.3	17.9	21.9	17.9	19.0	21.0	21.3	18.5	20.0	18.1
White, not Hispanic or Latino[4]	24.3	25.2	24.6	25.1	26.5	26.7	26.2	25.5	24.7	26.3
Female	14.5	14.4	14.6	14.5	15.2	15.2	15.2	15.9	16.3	16.1
White	15.4	15.1	15.6	15.3	16.2	15.9	16.0	16.8	17.2	17.2
Black or African American	10.3	10.3	9.2	9.9	8.5	10.1	11.6	11.8	12.9	11.1
Asian or Pacific Islander	9.1	10.1	9.0	11.0	12.2	11.9	9.5	10.9	11.0	11.3
Hispanic or Latina[4]	13.8	11.6	12.4	13.7	13.9	13.1	13.8	15.0	14.5	14.6
White, not Hispanic or Latina[4]	15.6	15.5	16.0	15.4	16.3	16.2	16.3	17.1	17.6	17.6
Leukemia										
Male	17.1	16.8	17.5	16.7	16.7	17.5	16.8	17.1	17.2	16.7
White	18.0	17.8	18.7	17.7	17.8	18.9	17.6	18.3	18.3	17.6
Black or African American	16.1	12.5	14.4	13.9	11.6	13.1	14.2	14.0	13.3	13.7
Asian or Pacific Islander	8.5	11.1	9.0	9.7	10.1	10.0	11.1	9.1	10.3	10.6
Hispanic or Latino[4]	12.1	12.0	11.8	10.7	10.9	14.6	12.7	12.4	12.3	11.8
White, not Hispanic or Latino[4]	18.2	18.1	19.1	18.1	18.2	19.2	17.9	18.7	18.8	18.1
Female	9.9	10.3	9.6	10.1	9.9	10.2	10.1	10.0	10.0	9.4
White	10.3	10.8	10.0	10.4	10.4	10.8	10.6	10.7	10.7	9.9
Black or African American	8.4	9.3	8.0	9.8	7.7	8.2	8.6	8.1	7.5	7.8
Asian or Pacific Islander	5.8	5.6	6.9	7.3	6.9	6.3	6.4	5.8	6.6	6.4
Hispanic or Latina[4]	8.6	8.2	8.2	7.4	8.4	8.1	7.3	8.8	9.1	8.1
White, not Hispanic or Latina[4]	10.2	10.8	10.0	10.4	10.5	11.0	10.8	10.8	10.6	10.1

Table C-4. **Age-Adjusted[1] Cancer Incidence Rates for Selected Cancer Sites, by Sex, Race, and Hispanic Origin, Selected Geographic Areas, Selected Years, 1990–2008 and Annual Percent Change (APC)[2], 1990–2008**—Continued

(Number of new cases per 100,000 population.)

Site, sex, race, and Hispanic origin	2000	2001	2002	2003	2004	2005	2006	2007	2008	1990–2008 APC
Non-Hodgkin's Lymphoma										
Male	23.4	24.0	23.7	24.0	25.0	24.3	23.6	24.5	24.0	0.2
White	24.8	25.1	25.0	25.4	26.2	25.4	24.9	26.1	25.1	0.2
Black or African American	17.5	18.2	18.0	18.9	21.9	19.1	19.3	17.0	17.7	-0.1
Asian or Pacific Islander	15.9	17.6	16.2	16.3	16.3	17.9	15.1	16.6	17.7	0.1
Hispanic or Latino[4]	20.2	18.4	20.1	19.0	21.0	18.6	18.2	20.0	19.6	0.1
White, not Hispanic or Latino[4]	25.4	26.0	25.6	26.3	26.9	26.6	26.0	27.2	26.0	*0.3
Female	15.9	16.1	16.4	17.1	17.2	16.3	16.7	16.5	16.2	*0.9
White	16.9	16.9	17.4	17.9	18.2	17.5	17.8	17.4	16.9	*0.9
Black or African American	11.8	12.4	11.8	13.2	13.3	12.9	12.2	12.9	12.6	*1.7
Asian or Pacific Islander	11.4	12.8	12.3	12.7	12.3	9.6	10.9	11.5	12.1	0.8
Hispanic or Latina[4]	13.6	14.4	13.8	15.2	15.7	15.0	15.2	14.5	14.5	*0.8
White, not Hispanic or Latina[4]	17.3	17.4	17.9	18.3	18.6	17.8	18.3	18.0	17.2	*0.9
Leukemia										
Male	16.8	17.6	16.8	16.9	16.8	16.6	15.5	16.3	15.9	*-0.3
White	17.9	18.9	18.2	18.0	17.6	17.9	16.6	17.6	16.8	*-0.3
Black or African American	13.7	13.0	12.5	14.1	16.0	12.2	13.5	12.8	12.8	-0.3
Asian or Pacific Islander	10.4	10.4	9.3	10.2	10.1	9.0	8.6	9.1	9.3	-0.5
Hispanic or Latino[4]	12.8	10.9	12.1	11.8	12.3	12.7	12.3	11.1	11.3	-0.2
White, not Hispanic or Latino[4]	18.4	19.6	18.8	18.6	18.1	18.3	16.8	18.4	17.3	-0.2
Female	10.2	10.4	9.8	9.8	10.2	9.6	10.3	9.5	10.0	-0.1
White	10.8	11.2	10.6	10.4	10.7	10.0	11.0	10.1	10.4	0.0
Black or African American	9.5	9.0	7.4	8.8	9.2	8.9	8.1	7.3	7.2	-0.5
Asian or Pacific Islander	6.3	5.1	6.3	6.4	6.4	6.4	6.5	6.0	6.9	0.0
Hispanic or Latina[4]	7.6	7.5	8.5	7.0	9.1	8.2	8.8	7.6	9.1	0.2
White, not Hispanic or Latina[4]	10.9	11.5	10.6	10.8	10.8	10.1	11.3	10.4	10.4	0.1

^ =Annual percent change (APC) is significantly different from 0 (p<0.05).
0.0 = APC is greater than -0.05 but less than 0.05
[1]Age-adjusted by 5-year age groups to the year 2000 U.S. standard population.
[2]APC has been calculated by fitting a linear regression model to the natural logarithm of the yearly rates from 1990–2006.
[3]Starting with Health, United States, 2007, estimates for American Indian or Alaska Native population are based on the Contract Health Service Delivery Area (CHSDA) counties within SEER areas. Estimates for American Indian or Alaska Native are not shown for some sites because of the small number of annual cases.
[4]Hispanic data exclude cases from Alaska. Persons of Hispanic origin may be of any race.

Table C-5. Five-Year Relative Cancer Survival Rates for Selected Cancer Sites, by Race and Sex, Selected Geographic Areas, Selected Years, 1975–1977 through 2001–2007

(Percent.)

Sex and site	White								
	1975–1977	1978–1980	1981–1983	1984–1986	1987–1989	1990–1992	1993–1995	1996–2000	2001–2007
BOTH SEXES									
All Sites	50.0	50.1	51.5	53.8	56.8	61.5	62.5	65.4	68.6
Oral cavity and pharynx	54.4	55.5	54.2	56.4	56.3	58.1	60.3	60.9	65.1
Esophagus	5.5	5.3	7.3	10.4	10.7	13.1	13.5	16.3	19.6
Stomach	14.2	15.5	16.2	17.0	18.5	18.8	19.9	21.0	26.1
Colon	51.1	52.6	55.7	59.2	60.9	63.0	60.8	64.4	66.5
Rectum	48.4	49.9	52.4	57.3	58.8	60.2	60.8	65.0	68.7
Pancreas	2.5	2.5	2.6	2.6	3.2	4.4	3.9	4.3	5.9
Lung and bronchus	12.3	12.9	13.4	13.1	13.4	14.0	14.6	15.2	16.7
Urinary bladder	73.5	74.9	77.7	77.5	80.0	80.6	81.4	80.3	81.1
Non-Hodgkin's lymphoma	47.0	48.1	51.1	52.1	51.6	51.7	53.4	61.4	70.7
Leukemia	34.8	36.9	38.4	41.8	44.0	46.4	48.3	49.0	57.1
MALE									
All Sites	42.9	44.5	46.8	48.8	53.0	61.0	62.1	65.4	69.3
Oral cavity and pharynx	54.0	54.6	53.1	54.9	54.2	56.5	59.7	60.4	65.2
Esophagus	4.8	5.3	6.5	9.2	11.1	12.5	13.7	15.9	19.7
Stomach	13.2	13.7	15.4	14.6	15.6	16.1	18.9	19.5	24.2
Colon	50.7	51.6	56.4	59.8	61.7	63.3	61.0	64.9	67.2
Rectum	47.5	49.5	51.3	56.7	59.1	59.3	59.7	64.3	69.5
Pancreas	2.6	2.6	2.2	2.1	3.1	4.2	3.6	4.8	5.8
Lung and bronchus	11.1	11.5	11.8	11.4	12.1	12.5	12.7	13.2	14.5
Prostate gland	69.0	71.7	73.5	76.8	84.8	94.4	96.1	98.9	99.9
Urinary bladder	74.6	75.7	78.9	78.7	82.2	83.0	82.8	81.3	82.4
Non-Hodgkin's lymphoma	46.4	46.4	50.7	50.8	48.4	47.7	50.0	59.5	69.6
Leukemia	33.8	35.9	38.2	41.5	45.7	46.3	49.2	49.4	57.2
Female									
All Sites	56.7	55.7	56.1	58.7	60.8	62.2	63.0	65.5	67.8
Colon	51.4	53.5	55.0	58.6	60.1	62.7	60.6	63.9	65.8
Rectum	49.5	50.3	53.6	57.9	58.5	61.4	62.2	65.7	67.8
Pancreas	2.3	2.5	3.0	3.1	3.3	4.6	4.3	3.8	6.1
Lung and bronchus	15.6	16.3	16.7	16.3	15.4	16.2	17.2	17.5	19.2
Melanoma of skin	86.2	87.8	87.2	91.0	91.3	91.8	92.6	93.4	95.3
Breast	75.9	75.3	77.3	80.2	85.3	86.6	87.8	90.2	91.4
Cervix uteri	69.8	68.2	67.9	69.0	72.5	70.9	74.2	73.8	70.3
Corpus uteri[1]	88.7	84.5	83.0	84.7	84.9	86.4	85.9	86.6	86.3
Ovary	35.3	36.9	38.8	37.6	38.2	40.5	40.7	42.9	43.3
Non-Hodgkin's lymphoma	47.6	49.9	51.4	53.7	55.5	56.7	57.8	63.7	72.0

Table C-5. **Five-Year Relative Cancer Survival Rates for Selected Cancer Sites, by Race and Sex, Selected Geographic Areas, Selected Years, 1975–1977 through 2001–2007**—*Continued*

(Percent.)

Sex and site	Black or African American								
	1975–1977	1978–1980	1981–1983	1984–1986	1987–1989	1990–1992	1993–1995	1996–2000	2001–2007
BOTH SEXES									
All Sites	39.2	39.0	39.0	40.2	43.1	47.9	52.7	56.0	59.4
Oral cavity and pharynx	36.1	34.9	31.4	35.1	33.9	32.5	38.0	39.8	44.7
Esophagus	3.2	4.3	4.3	8.7	6.6	9.2	7.5	11.1	12.8
Stomach	16.1	16.5	16.6	19.1	18.8	22.9	19.5	22.1	27.2
Colon	45.3	49.0	48.7	49.2	52.5	53.5	51.5	53.5	54.8
Rectum	44.6	34.9	39.8	45.8	52.3	51.3	54.0	54.8	60.9
Pancreas	2.3	5.6	3.6	4.6	5.5	3.7	3.4	4.6	3.8
Lung and bronchus	11.4	11.8	11.4	11.2	11.0	10.4	12.8	12.6	13.3
Urinary bladder	50.3	54.6	59.7	59.6	62.5	63.4	60.0	62.6	64.1
Non-Hodgkin's lymphoma	48.4	51.1	49.9	46.9	46.4	42.1	41.9	53.6	62.1
Leukemia	33.1	28.7	33.9	32.9	35.5	36.0	41.1	38.3	50.3
MALE									
All Sites	32.8	33.4	34.3	35.6	39.0	47.7	54.4	58.7	63.2
Oral cavity and pharynx	29.8	30.0	26.0	29.5	29.8	27.8	33.1	34.5	40.5
Esophagus	1.6	3.4	3.7	8.2	5.3	9.4	7.8	9.6	10.6
Stomach	16.1	15.6	16.5	17.0	16.6	22.1	17.5	21.2	23.2
Colon	43.9	47.5	44.9	48.8	50.8	55.0	51.0	54.8	53.0
Rectum	41.8	34.0	37.3	43.5	47.7	53.5	51.8	54.2	59.0
Pancreas	2.6	4.1	3.7	3.9	5.1	3.2	3.3	3.6	3.3
Lung and bronchus	10.7	9.8	10.2	10.5	10.8	9.3	11.3	11.1	12.1
Prostate gland	61.0	62.1	63.2	65.8	71.5	84.6	91.7	95.6	97.9
Urinary bladder	56.5	62.7	64.9	62.6	67.6	66.1	67.0	66.0	67.9
Non-Hodgkin's lymphoma	42.6	47.1	49.4	44.5	41.7	38.2	35.8	50.1	57.9
Leukemia	30.0	28.2	33.4	31.9	33.7	31.0	41.0	38.9	52.0
Female									
All Sites	46.3	45.7	44.6	45.5	47.8	48.3	50.6	52.9	55.1
Colon	46.1	50.0	51.7	49.5	53.8	52.3	51.8	52.4	56.1
Rectum	46.9	35.6	42.4	48.0	57.1	48.7	56.5	55.3	62.7
Pancreas	1.9	7.0	3.2	5.1	5.8	4.1	3.4	5.4	4.3
Lung and bronchus	13.8	17.9	14.9	12.8	11.2	12.5	15.5	14.8	15.0
Melanoma of skin	*	*	*	*	90.3	*	*	76.0	73.7
Breast	62.2	63.4	63.8	65.2	71.3	71.7	72.7	77.5	77.4
Cervix uteri	64.5	60.9	59.6	57.6	57.3	57.9	63.0	66.6	60.9
Corpus uteri[1]	61.3	55.4	52.7	56.9	57.9	56.0	60.5	63.4	62.0
Ovary	41.9	38.9	37.6	39.6	33.8	36.2	41.7	37.6	36.0
Non-Hodgkin's lymphoma	54.9	56.7	50.4	50.1	52.1	47.6	53.5	58.4	67.0

* = Figure does not meet standards of reliability or precision.
[1]Includes corpus uteri only cases and not uterus, not elsewhere specified cases.

NOTE: Rates are based on followup of patients through 2008. The rate is the ratio of the observed survival rate for the patient group to the expected survival rate for persons in the general population similar to the patient group with respect to age, sex, race, and calendar year of observation. It estimates the chance of surviving the effects of cancer. The site variable distinguishes Kaposi Sarcoma and Mesothelioma as individual cancer sites. As a result, Kaposi Sarcoma and Mesothelioma cases are excluded from each of the sites shown except all sites combined.

Table C-6 Respondent-Reported Prevalence of Heart Disease, Cancer, and Stroke Among Adults 18 Years of Age and Over, by Selected Characteristics, Selected Years 1997–1998 through 2009–2010

(Percent.)

Characteristic	Heart disease[1]							
	1997–1998	1999–2000	2001–2002	2003–2004	2005–2006	2007–2008	2008–2009	2009–2010
18 years and over, age-adjusted[2,3]	12.0	11.1	11.5	11.3	11.2	11.3	11.5	11.4
18 years and over, crude[3]	11.6	10.9	11.3	11.3	11.4	11.6	11.8	11.8
Age								
18–44 years	4.6	4.3	4.3	4.1	4.0	4.4	4.5	4.4
18–24 years	3.2	3.3	3.3	3.0	3.2	3.1	3.3	3.4
25–44 years	5.0	4.6	4.6	4.5	4.2	4.8	4.9	4.8
45–64 years	13.5	12.6	12.9	12.5	12.9	12.2	12.7	13.1
45–54 years	10.9	10.0	10.0	9.4	9.4	8.8	9.5	10.1
55–64 years	17.4	16.6	17.4	17.0	17.8	16.8	16.8	17.0
65 years and over	31.8	29.6	31.3	31.8	31.2	31.8	31.7	30.4
65–74 years	27.8	25.8	26.6	27.3	26.5	26.9	26.2	25.1
75 years and over	37.0	34.3	36.8	36.8	36.6	37.5	38.0	37.0
Sex[2]								
Male	12.3	11.9	12.4	12.3	12.2	12.5	12.8	12.8
Female	11.8	10.5	10.8	10.7	10.5	10.5	10.5	10.3
Sex and Age								
Male								
18–44 years	3.7	3.6	3.6	3.6	3.3	3.8	4.4	4.3
45–54 years	11.0	10.0	10.1	8.7	9.8	9.2	10.0	10.4
55–64 years	18.7	19.7	19.9	20.4	20.5	18.3	18.8	19.0
65–74 years	32.0	30.4	31.9	33.1	31.6	32.0	30.5	30.8
75 years and over	40.8	39.2	43.6	42.6	43.1	46.5	46.6	45.3
Female								
18–44 years	5.5	4.9	4.9	4.7	4.7	4.9	4.7	4.5
45–54 years	10.8	9.9	9.9	10.1	9.1	8.4	9.0	9.8
55–64 years	16.2	13.8	15.2	13.9	15.4	15.4	14.9	15.1
65–74 years	24.5	22.0	22.2	22.5	22.2	22.5	22.6	20.2
75 years and over	34.6	31.2	32.6	33.1	32.4	31.7	32.3	31.3
Race[2,4]								
White only	12.2	11.3	11.7	11.6	11.5	11.7	11.9	11.6
Black or African American only	11.4	10.6	10.6	9.8	10.1	10.2	10.7	11.0
American Indian or Alaska Native only	18.6	14.7	11.4	12.8	15.9	11.1	10.2	10.3
Asian only	6.9	6.3	8.8	6.3	6.8	6.0	5.7	6.7
Native Hawaiian or Other Pacific Islander only	—	*	*	*	*	*	*	*
2 or more races	—	17.0	16.5	12.5	14.7	16.9	15.2	15.5
Hispanic Origin and Race[2,4]								
Hispanic or Latino	8.7	8.0	8.0	8.5	8.0	8.5	8.4	8.3
Mexican	7.5	7.4	7.8	8.9	7.5	8.3	8.4	8.4
Not Hispanic or Latino	12.2	11.4	11.8	11.6	11.6	11.7	11.9	11.8
White only	12.5	11.6	12.1	12.0	12.0	12.1	12.4	12.1
Black or African American only	11.4	10.5	10.5	9.8	10.2	10.2	10.8	11.1
Education[5,6]								
No high school diploma or GED	15.1	13.8	14.3	14.3	14.2	14.9	14.5	14.5
High school diploma or GED	12.8	11.9	12.4	12.3	12.6	11.9	12.7	12.7
Some college or more	12.7	12.0	12.4	12.2	11.9	12.4	12.4	12.2
Percent of Poverty Level[2,7]								
Below 100%	15.3	13.6	14.4	14.3	14.6	14.0	14.1	14.5
100%–199%	13.2	12.0	12.4	12.8	12.5	13.0	13.2	12.8
200%–399%	11.5	11.0	11.3	11.4	11.0	11.7	11.6	11.3
400% or more	11.0	10.2	10.9	10.0	10.1	10.0	10.1	10.0

Table C-6 Respondent-Reported Prevalence of Heart Disease, Cancer, and Stroke Among Adults 18 Years of Age and Over, by Selected Characteristics, Selected Years 1997–1998 through 2009–2010—*Continued*

(Percent.)

Characteristic	Heart disease[1]							
	1997–1998	1999–2000	2001–2002	2003–2004	2005–2006	2007–2008	2008–2009	2009–2010
Hispanic Origin and Race and Percent of Poverty Level[2,4,7]								
Hispanic or Latino								
Below 100%	9.7	9.7	8.7	11.3	11.0	11.0	10.3	10.3
100%–199%	8.7	8.4	9.0	8.0	8.1	9.6	8.8	7.9
200%–399%	8.4	8.2	6.5	8.2	6.9	7.1	7.7	8.4
400% or more	8.4	5.6	6.9	5.4	5.1	8.0	7.1	7.2
Not Hispanic or Latino								
White only:								
Below 100%	17.8	15.2	16.5	15.9	16.9	16.0	15.9	16.3
100%–199%	14.1	12.8	13.5	14.8	14.3	14.7	15.6	15.1
200%–399%	12.2	11.6	12.1	12.3	11.9	12.9	12.8	12.1
400% or more	11.3	10.6	11.3	10.3	10.6	10.5	10.6	10.5
Black or African American only:								
Below 100%	14.6	13.0	14.1	14.1	13.2	13.2	15.2	15.7
100%–199%	12.9	11.2	12.3	10.5	10.7	11.3	10.9	10.5
200%–399%	9.2	10.2	9.0	8.0	9.1	9.3	9.3	10.2
400% or more	9.5	8.9	8.0	7.7	8.5	7.7	8.9	8.7
Geographic Region[2]								
Northeast	11.6	10.6	10.9	10.8	11.0	10.9	11.1	10.8
Midwest	12.1	11.4	12.1	11.8	12.3	12.4	12.4	12.1
South	12.5	11.5	11.7	11.7	11.5	11.7	12.3	12.3
West	11.1	10.4	10.9	10.5	9.8	9.9	9.7	9.8
Location of Residence[2]								
Within MSA[8]	11.7	10.7	11.2	10.9	10.9	10.8	11.2	11.2
Outside MSA[8]	12.8	12.5	12.7	13.0	13.0	14.1	13.1	12.5

Table C-6 Respondent-Reported Prevalence of Heart Disease, Cancer, and Stroke Among Adults 18 Years of Age and Over, by Selected Characteristics, Selected Years 1997–1998 through 2009–2010—*Continued*

(Percent.)

Characteristic	Cancer[9]							
	1997–1998	1999–2000	2001–2002	2003–2004	2005–2006	2007–2008	2008–2009	2009–2010
18 years and over, age-adjusted[2,3]	4.9	5.1	5.3	5.2	5.7	5.6	5.9	6.0
18 years and over, crude[3]	4.8	4.9	5.2	5.2	5.7	5.8	6.1	6.3
Age								
18–44 years	1.7	1.7	1.7	1.5	1.8	1.7	1.6	1.6
18–24 years	0.8	1.0	0.8	0.7	0.9	0.8	0.8	0.7
25–44 years	2.0	1.9	2.1	1.7	2.2	2.0	1.9	2.0
45–64 years	5.4	5.2	5.7	5.8	6.0	6.3	6.7	7.1
45–54 years	4.0	4.0	4.2	4.2	4.4	4.6	4.9	5.3
55–64 years	7.4	7.2	7.9	8.1	8.2	8.6	9.2	9.3
65 years and over	14.1	15.2	15.6	15.9	17.1	17.0	17.7	18.1
65–74 years	12.4	13.1	13.9	13.8	14.3	14.6	15.8	16.1
75 years and over	16.2	17.7	17.6	18.3	20.2	19.8	20.0	20.5
Sex[2]								
Male	4.1	4.4	4.7	4.7	5.1	4.8	5.0	5.5
Female	5.8	5.8	6.0	5.9	6.4	6.5	6.8	6.6
Sex and Age								
Male								
18–44 years	0.8	0.8	0.7	0.7	0.8	0.8	0.7	0.8
45–54 years	2.0	2.0	2.2	2.7	2.6	2.6	2.9	3.3
55–64 years	5.8	5.9	6.5	6.7	6.8	7.2	7.0	7.8
65–74 years	12.8	13.9	16.1	14.3	15.5	14.3	16.2	17.6
75 years and over	18.3	20.3	20.8	22.1	24.3	21.9	22.2	24.8
Female								
18–44 years	2.6	2.5	2.7	2.3	2.9	2.5	2.5	2.4
45–54 years	6.0	5.9	6.1	5.7	6.2	6.4	6.8	7.3
55–64 years	8.8	8.4	9.1	9.5	9.5	10.0	11.2	10.7
65–74 years	12.1	12.5	12.1	13.4	13.3	14.8	15.6	14.9
75 years and over	14.9	16.1	15.5	15.9	17.6	18.5	18.5	17.6
Race[2,4]								
White only	5.2	5.4	5.6	5.5	6.0	6.0	6.2	6.3
Black or African American only	3.5	3.5	3.3	4.0	3.9	4.4	4.3	4.7
American Indian or Alaska Native only	*6.5	*5.7	*	7.0	*7.4	*4.3	*5.4	7.0
Asian only	2.4	*2.3	*1.6	3.0	2.9	3.1	3.0	2.9
Native Hawaiian or Other Pacific Islander only	—	*	*	*	*	*	*	*
2 or more races	—	*4.7	7.1	*3.4	7.8	5.8	9.1	9.8
Hispanic Origin and Race[2,4]								
Hispanic or Latino	2.9	3.0	2.9	3.0	3.5	3.7	3.6	3.4
Mexican	3.0	2.8	2.9	2.6	3.1	3.6	3.3	3.2
Not Hispanic or Latino	5.1	5.2	5.5	5.5	5.9	5.9	6.1	6.3
White only	5.4	5.5	5.9	5.8	6.3	6.3	6.5	6.7
Black or African American only	3.6	3.6	3.3	3.9	3.9	4.3	4.2	4.7
Education[5,6]								
No high school diploma or GED	5.3	5.5	5.4	5.6	5.7	5.8	6.1	5.9
High school diploma or GED	5.5	5.8	6.3	5.7	6.4	6.1	6.4	6.7
Some college or more	6.0	5.9	6.2	6.4	6.9	6.9	7.1	7.4
Percent of Poverty Level[2,7]								
Below 100%	4.9	4.9	5.4	5.6	5.3	6.2	6.2	5.4
100%–199%	4.8	5.3	5.0	5.6	5.7	5.8	6.0	6.1
200%–399%	4.9	5.1	5.6	5.2	5.5	5.4	5.5	5.9
400% or more	5.2	5.1	5.2	5.0	6.1	5.8	6.0	6.3

Table C-6 Respondent-Reported Prevalence of Heart Disease, Cancer, and Stroke Among Adults 18 Years of Age and Over, by Selected Characteristics, Selected Years 1997–1998 through 2009–2010—*Continued*

(Percent.)

Characteristic	Cancer[9]							
	1997–1998	1999–2000	2001–2002	2003–2004	2005–2006	2007–2008	2008–2009	2009–2010
Hispanic Origin and Race and Percent of Poverty Level[2,4,7]								
Hispanic or Latino								
Below 100%	2.2	2.3	2.9	2.9	3.5	5.0	3.8	2.8
100%–199%	2.8	3.2	2.3	3.7	3.3	3.2	3.2	2.5
200%–399%	2.7	2.7	3.5	2.8	3.6	3.2	3.3	4.3
400% or more	*5.5	*4.5	*3.1	*1.9	*3.4	3.6	4.2	4.2
Not Hispanic or Latino								
White only:								
Below 100%	6.3	6.2	7.2	6.9	6.9	8.0	8.1	6.9
100%–199%	5.6	6.2	5.9	6.6	6.7	7.4	7.4	7.3
200%–399%	5.2	5.5	6.1	5.7	6.0	6.0	6.1	6.5
400% or more	5.4	5.3	5.5	5.3	6.5	6.0	6.2	6.6
Black or African American only:								
Below 100%	4.4	4.0	3.2	4.6	3.6	4.6	4.9	4.9
100%–199%	3.3	3.2	3.2	4.1	4.3	3.5	3.6	4.9
200%–399%	3.2	3.7	3.6	3.5	4.2	4.4	4.0	4.3
400% or more	4.0	4.3	*3.3	4.5	3.6	5.4	5.0	5.2
Geographic Region[2]								
Northeast	4.5	5.0	5.0	5.3	5.6	6.1	6.2	5.9
Midwest	5.1	5.2	5.7	5.3	5.7	5.5	5.8	6.4
South	5.0	5.0	5.3	5.2	5.6	5.8	5.9	6.1
West	5.1	5.0	5.1	5.2	5.7	5.3	5.6	5.6
Location of Residence[2]								
Within MSA[8]	4.9	5.0	5.1	5.1	5.6	5.6	5.7	5.9
Outside MSA[8]	5.1	5.5	6.0	5.7	6.0	6.2	7.0	6.8

Table C-6 Respondent-Reported Prevalence of Heart Disease, Cancer, and Stroke Among Adults 18 Years of Age and Over, by Selected Characteristics, Selected Years 1997–1998 through 2009–2010—*Continued*

(Percent.)

Characteristic	Stroke[10]							
	1997–1998	1999–2000	2001–2002	2003–2004	2005–2006	2007–2008	2008–2009	2009–2010
18 years and over, age-adjusted[2,3]	2.3	2.2	2.4	2.5	2.5	2.6	2.7	2.6
18 years and over, crude[3]	2.2	2.1	2.4	2.5	2.5	2.7	2.8	2.7
Age								
18–44 years	0.4	0.4	0.4	0.4	0.4	0.5	0.6	0.6
18–24 years	*	*	*	*	*	*	*	*
25–44 years	0.4	0.5	0.5	0.5	0.5	0.6	0.7	0.7
45–64 years	2.3	2.0	2.4	2.4	2.3	2.9	2.7	2.8
45–54 years	1.4	1.3	1.8	1.5	1.5	2.0	1.8	1.9
55–64 years	3.8	3.1	3.3	3.7	3.5	4.0	3.8	3.8
65 years and over	8.1	8.1	8.8	9.2	9.2	8.8	9.2	8.6
65–74 years	6.7	6.2	6.6	7.1	6.9	6.3	6.3	6.3
75 years and over	9.8	10.3	11.2	11.6	11.8	11.8	12.5	11.4
Sex[2]								
Male	2.6	2.4	2.6	2.7	2.6	2.5	2.7	2.7
Female	2.1	2.1	2.3	2.4	2.4	2.6	2.7	2.6
Sex and Age								
Male								
18–44 years	0.3	0.3	0.4	0.4	0.4	*0.3	0.5	0.5
45–54 years	1.2	1.3	1.9	1.5	1.5	2.0	1.6	1.6
55–64 years	4.6	3.7	3.5	4.2	3.9	4.2	4.4	4.1
65–74 years	8.1	6.7	7.2	8.3	7.7	7.0	6.7	6.9
75 years and over	11.2	11.3	12.6	12.5	12.5	11.1	12.8	12.1
Female								
18–44 years	0.4	0.4	0.5	0.5	0.5	0.6	0.8	0.6
45–54 years	1.5	1.4	1.6	1.5	1.4	2.1	2.1	2.3
55–64 years	3.2	2.6	3.2	3.3	3.1	3.8	3.3	3.5
65–74 years	5.5	5.8	6.1	6.1	6.3	5.7	6.0	5.7
75 years and over	9.0	9.6	10.4	11.0	11.5	12.2	12.3	10.9
Race[2,4]								
White only	2.2	2.1	2.3	2.4	2.3	2.5	2.6	2.5
Black or African American only	3.3	3.5	3.3	3.4	4.0	3.6	3.7	3.9
American Indian or Alaska Native only	*5.0	*5.4	*	*	*	*	*	*
Asian only	*1.2	*1.2	*3.1	*2.2	1.9	2.1	1.5	1.6
Native Hawaiian or Other Pacific Islander only	—	*	*	*	*	*	*	*
2 or more races	—	*4.0	*4.9	4.0	*4.6	*4.1	*3.5	*3.3
Hispanic Origin and Race[2,4]								
Hispanic or Latino	2.1	1.9	2.5	2.6	2.1	2.6	2.3	2.3
Mexican	2.5	2.0	2.7	2.9	2.5	2.5	2.5	2.4
Not Hispanic or Latino	2.3	2.2	2.4	2.5	2.5	2.6	2.7	2.6
White only	2.2	2.1	2.3	2.4	2.3	2.4	2.7	2.5
Black or African American only	3.3	3.5	3.3	3.4	4.1	3.6	3.7	3.9
Education[5,6]								
No high school diploma or GED	3.9	3.8	3.8	4.4	4.1	4.4	4.5	4.2
High school diploma or GED	2.5	2.5	2.9	2.8	2.9	3.2	3.3	3.2
Some college or more	2.1	1.9	2.3	2.3	2.3	2.3	2.5	2.5
Percent of Poverty Level[2,7]								
Below 100%	4.3	3.7	3.7	4.4	4.1	4.4	4.4	4.4
100%–199%	3.1	3.2	3.3	3.5	3.2	3.9	3.6	3.5
200%–399%	2.1	2.1	2.4	2.3	2.4	2.5	2.7	2.6
400% or more	1.6	1.5	1.9	1.8	1.8	1.6	1.8	1.7

Table C-6 Respondent-Reported Prevalence of Heart Disease, Cancer, and Stroke Among Adults 18 Years of Age and Over, by Selected Characteristics, Selected Years 1997–1998 through 2009–2010—*Continued*

(Percent.)

Characteristic	Stroke[10]							
	1997–1998	1999–2000	2001–2002	2003–2004	2005–2006	2007–2008	2008–2009	2009–2010
Hispanic Origin and Race and Percent of Poverty Level[2,4,7]								
Hispanic or Latino								
Below 100%	3.0	2.0	2.7	3.9	3.1	3.8	2.5	2.9
100%–199%	2.2	2.2	3.2	2.8	1.8	2.6	2.5	2.3
200%–399%	*1.8	*2.3	2.0	*2.0	*2.0	*2.2	2.4	2.0
400% or more	*	*	*	*	*	*2.7	*	*2.6
Not Hispanic or Latino								
White only:								
Below 100%	4.4	3.8	3.6	4.3	4.1	4.3	4.4	4.4
100%–199%	3.2	3.0	3.2	3.5	3.2	4.1	4.0	3.9
200%–399%	2.1	2.1	2.3	2.3	2.3	2.6	2.8	2.5
400% or more	1.6	1.5	1.8	1.8	1.8	1.5	1.8	1.7
Black or African American only:								
Below 100%	5.0	4.5	4.8	5.6	5.3	5.5	6.4	6.2
100%–199%	4.2	5.1	3.9	3.8	4.6	4.7	4.0	3.9
200%–399%	2.5	2.7	2.8	2.4	4.1	2.7	2.8	3.7
400% or more	*	*	*	*2.0	*2.6	*2.6	*2.5	*2.6
Geographic Region[2]								
Northeast	1.8	1.8	2.1	2.2	1.9	2.4	2.3	2.1
Midwest	2.3	2.2	2.4	2.5	2.5	2.5	2.6	2.6
South	2.6	2.5	2.5	2.8	2.9	3.0	3.2	3.0
West	2.1	2.0	2.7	2.4	2.1	2.2	2.2	2.3
Location of Residence[2]								
Within MSA[8]	2.2	2.1	2.4	2.4	2.4	2.5	2.6	2.4
Outside MSA[8]	2.7	2.5	2.5	2.8	2.9	2.9	3.0	3.3

* = Figure does not meet standards of reliability or precision.
—- = Data not available.
[1]Heart disease is based on self-reported responses to questions about whether respondents had ever been told by a doctor or other health professional that they had coronary heart disease, angina (angina pectoris), a heart attack (myocardial infarction), or any other kind or heart disease or heart condition.
[2]Estimates are age-adjusted to the year 2000 standard population using five age groups: 18–44 years, 45–54 years, 55–64 years, 65–74 years, and 75 years and over.
[3]Includes all other races not shown separately and unknown education level.
[4]The race groups, White, Black, American Indian or Alaska Native, Asian, Native Hawaiian or Other Pacific Islander, and 2 or more races, include persons of Hispanic and non-Hispanic origin. Persons of Hispanic origin may be of any race.
[5]Estimates are for persons 25 years of age and over and are age-adjusted to the year 2000 standard population using five age groups: 25–44 years, 45–54 years, 55–64 years, 65–74 years, and 75 years and over.
[6]GED is General Educational Development high school equivalency diploma.
[7]Percent of poverty level is based on family income and family size and composition sing U.S. Census Bureau poverty thresholds.
[8]MSA = metropolitan statistical area.
[9]Cancer is based on self-reported responses to a question about whether respondents had ever been told by a doctor or other health professional that they had cancer or a malignancy of any kind. Excludes squamous cell and basal cell carcinomas.
[10]Stroke is based on self-reported responses to a question about whether respondents had ever been told by a doctor or other health professional that they had a stroke.

Table C-7. Diabetes Prevalence and Glycemic Control Among Adults 20 Years of Age and Over, by Sex, Age, Race, and Hispanic Origin, Selected Years, 1988–1994 through 2003–2006

(Percent.)

Characteristic	Physician-diagnosed and undiagnosed diabetes[1,2]				Physician-diagnosed diabetes[1]				Undiagnosed diabetes[2]			
	1988–1994	1999–2002	2001–2004	2003–2006	1988–1994	1999–2002	2001–2004	2003–2006	1988–1994	1999–2002	2001–2004	2003–2006
20 Years and Over, Age-Adjusted[3]												
All persons[4]	9.1	9.8	10.7	10.6	5.5	6.6	7.3	7.6	3.6	3.2	3.3	2.9
Sex												
Male	9.6	10.8	12.0	11.5	5.5	7.0	7.5	7.5	4.1	3.8	4.5	4.0
Female	8.7	8.8	9.5	9.8	5.6	6.2	7.2	7.8	3.1	2.6	2.3	2.0
Hispanic Origin												
Not Hispanic or Latino												
White only	8.0	8.3	9.1	9.0	5.1	5.3	6.2	6.3	2.9	3.0	2.9	2.7
Black or African American only	16.0	16.3	15.4	16.4	8.8	11.9	11.3	12.6	7.2	4.4	4.1	3.8
Mexican[5]	14.9	13.2	15.2	16.3	9.8	10.1	11.7	12.1	5.0	*3.1	3.5	4.2
Percent of Poverty Level[6]												
Below 100%	14.2	14.5	14.8	15.1	8.8	9.1	10.2	12.8	5.4	5.4	4.6	*
100% or more	8.4	8.9	9.8	9.9	5.1	6.0	6.7	6.9	3.3	2.9	3.1	3.0
100%–199%	10.9	12.6	12.9	13.3	6.6	9.0	9.2	8.9	4.3	*3.6	3.7	4.4
200% or more	7.7	7.7	8.8	8.8	4.6	5.1	5.8	6.2	3.1	2.7	2.9	2.6
200%–399%	8.4	10.0	10.5	10.1	4.8	6.8	6.9	7.1	3.6	3.2	3.6	*3.0
400% or more	6.8	5.9	7.5	7.4	4.3	3.6	5.2	5.6	2.6	2.3	*2.3	*
20 Years and Over, Crude												
All persons[4]	8.4	9.7	10.4	10.7	5.1	6.5	7.2	7.7	3.3	3.2	3.2	3.0
Sex												
Male	8.6	10.4	11.5	11.4	4.8	6.7	7.2	7.4	3.7	3.7	4.3	4.0
Female	8.3	9.0	9.5	10.1	5.4	6.3	7.1	8.1	3.0	2.7	2.3	2.0
Hispanic Origin												
Not Hispanic or Latino:												
White only	7.8	8.7	9.5	9.8	5.0	5.5	6.4	6.9	2.8	3.2	3.1	2.9
Black or African American only	12.9	14.1	13.7	15.2	6.9	10.1	10.1	11.8	6.0	4.0	3.6	3.4
Mexican	9.7	8.5	9.8	11.6	5.6	6.5	7.0	7.9	4.1	1.9	*2.8	*3.6
Percent of Poverty Level[5]												
Below 100%	11.3	13.0	11.9	12.8	7.0	8.1	8.2	10.7	4.3	4.9	3.7	*
100% or more	7.8	8.8	9.7	10.2	4.7	5.9	6.7	7.1	3.0	2.8	3.0	3.1
100%–199%	10.1	12.6	12.8	14.3	6.4	9.1	9.2	9.7	3.8	*3.5	3.6	4.6
200% or more	7.0	7.5	8.7	9.0	4.2	4.9	5.8	6.3	2.8	2.6	2.9	2.6
200%–399%	7.3	9.6	10.3	10.5	4.3	6.5	6.7	7.3	3.1	*3.1	3.6	*3.2
400% or more	6.5	6.0	7.3	7.6	4.1	3.7	5.1	5.5	*2.4	2.2	*2.3	*2.1
Age												
20–44 years	2.6	3.4	3.6	3.6	1.6	2.3	2.5	2.6	*1.0	*	*1.1	*1.1
45–64 years	13.9	13.0	13.4	13.5	7.9	8.5	9.2	9.9	6.0	4.5	4.2	3.5
65 years and over	19.6	22.4	26.4	25.7	12.9	15.8	18.1	18.3	6.7	6.6	8.3	7.3

Table C-7. Diabetes Prevalence and Glycemic Control Among Adults 20 Years of Age and Over, by Sex, Age, Race and Hispanic Origin, Selected Years, 1988–1994 through 2003–2006—*Continued*

(Percent.)

Characteristic	Poor glycemic control (A1c greater than 9%) among persons with diagnosed diabetes			
	Percent of population with diagnosed diabetes			
	1988–1994	1999–2002	2001–2004	2003–2006
20 Years and Over, Crude[7]				
All persons[4]	23.3	18.4	14.4	13.0
Sex				
Male	20.2	20.2	17.5	14.8
Female	25.8	16.6	11.6	11.4
Hispanic Origin				
Not Hispanic or Latino:				
White only	20.6	13.6	11.5	8.6
Black or African American only	34.2	25.4	20.0	21.0
Mexican	29.2	26.5	22.9	24.0
Percent of Poverty Level[6]				
Below 100%	30.2	25.6	16.3	17.6
100% or more	21.4	15.9	13.8	12.2
100%–199%	24.2	*14.9	*10.5	*11.5
200% or more	20.0	16.4	15.5	12.5
200%–399%	*21.2	*17.3	15.5	*10.6
400% or more	*18.3	*	15.5	14.8
Age				
20–44 years	29.5	*32.1	*19.7	24.7
45–64 years	26.0	19.9	19.5	16.6
65 years and over	18.0	*10.2	*6.3	*4.1

* = Figure does not meet standards of reliability or precision.
[1]Physician-diagnosed diabetes was obtained by self-report and excludes women who reported having diabetes only during pregnancy.
[2]Undiagnosed diabetes is defined as a fasting plasma glucose (FPG) of at least 126 mg/dL or a hemoglobin A1c of at least 6.5% and no reported physician diagnosis.
[3]Estimates are age-adjusted to the year 2000 standard population using three age groups: 20–44 years, 45–64 years, and 65 years and over. Age-adjusted estimates in this table may differ from other
[4]Includes all other races and Hispanic origins not shown separately.
[5]Persons of Mexican origin may be of any race.
[6]Percent of poverty level is based on family income and family size.
[7]Age-adjusted estimates are not provided because the 2000 standard population used for age adjustment.

Table C-8. End-Stage Renal Disease Patients, by Selected Characteristics, Selected Years, 1980–2008

(Number, rate per million.)

| Characteristic | Incidence |||||||
| | Number of new patients |||||||
	1980	1985	1990	1995	2000	2005	2008
TOTAL	17,337	29,858	49,759	68,701	92,050	104,725	110,175
Age							
Under 20 years	738	870	1,050	1,122	1,172	1,235	1,277
20–44 years	4,701	6,945	10,346	12,227	12,800	13,301	13,410
45–64 years	6,949	11,123	17,156	24,093	32,126	38,529	42,081
65–74 years	3,644	7,289	13,338	18,303	23,341	24,243	25,369
75 years and over	1,305	3,631	7,869	12,956	22,611	27,417	28,038
Sex							
Male	9,661	16,177	26,671	36,169	49,150	58,082	62,117
Female	7,676	13,681	23,088	32,532	42,900	46,643	48,058
Race[1]							
White	12,295	20,369	33,133	44,101	61,043	69,150	72,391
Black or African American	4,814	8,614	14,831	21,502	26,659	30,325	31,620
American Indian or Alaska Native	124	304	599	884	1,201	1,220	1,261
Asian or Pacific Islander	104	571	1,196	2,214	3,147	4,030	4,903
Hispanic Origin[1,2]							
Hispanic	—	—	—	—	10,723	12,138	14,158
Not Hispanic[3]	—	—	—	—	81,327	92,587	96,017
Primary Diagnosis							
Diabetes	2,590	8,511	17,708	28,459	41,108	46,141	48,303
Hypertension	3,092	8,140	15,195	18,533	24,686	28,646	31,085
Glomerulonephritis	2,725	4,992	6,913	8,116	8,433	8,016	7,350
Cystic kidney	756	1,205	1,550	1,899	2,137	2,476	2,648
Other urologic	460	1,150	1,261	1,981	2,669	2,121	1,533
Other cause	1,787	3,502	4,800	7,025	8,911	12,165	14,128
Unknown cause	1,512	1,488	1,857	2,412	3,662	4,606	4,355
Missing disease	4,415	870	475	276	444	554	773

| Characteristic | New patients per million population |||||||
	1980	1985	1990	1995	2000	2005	2008
TOTAL	76.3	125.5	199.3	258.0	326.2	354.3	362.4
Age							
Under 20 years	10.2	12.4	14.6	14.6	14.6	15.1	15.5
20–44 years	55.6	73.4	103.3	118.6	122.9	127.4	128.3
45–64 years	156.2	249.4	370.5	456.3	514.8	529.5	539.1
65–74 years	232.8	432.4	736.7	970.2	1,270.7	1,300.6	1,260.7
75 years and over	129.8	314.2	598.7	869.3	1,353.3	1,513.7	1,495.6
Sex							
Male	87.5	139.8	219.1	277.8	355.0	399.3	414.3
Female	65.7	112.0	180.5	239.1	298.5	310.8	311.8
Race[1]							
White	63.0	100.8	158.3	200.1	264.7	288.7	295.2
Black or African American	179.8	301.5	483.9	635.3	726.0	780.0	783.3
American Indian or Alaska Native	86.7	177.0	291.0	362.0	404.3	376.7	368.5
Asian or Pacific Islander	27.1	101.9	158.4	230.5	265.1	290.4	326.2
Hispanic Origin[1,2]							
Hispanic	—	—	—	—	300.8	285.4	301.6
Not Hispanic[3]	—	—	—	—	329.9	365.9	373.4
Primary Diagnosis							
Diabetes	11.4	35.8	70.9	106.9	145.7	156.1	158.9
Hypertension	13.6	34.2	60.9	69.6	87.5	96.9	102.2
Glomerulonephritis	12.0	21.0	27.7	30.5	29.9	27.1	24.2
Cystic kidney	3.3	5.1	6.2	7.1	7.6	8.4	8.7
Other urologic	2.0	4.8	5.1	7.4	9.5	7.2	5.0
Other cause	7.9	14.7	19.2	26.4	31.6	41.2	46.5
Unknown cause	6.7	6.3	7.4	9.1	13.0	15.6	14.3
Missing disease	19.4	3.7	1.9	1.0	1.6	1.9	2.5

— =Data not available.
[1]The race groups, White, Black, American Indian or Alaska Native, and Asian or Pacific Islander, include persons of Hispanic and non-Hispanic origin. Persons of Hispanic origin may be of any race.
[2]Centers for Medicare & Medicaid Services began collecting Hispanic ethnicity data in April 1995.
[3]Not Hispanic includes unknown ethnicity.

Table C-8. End-Stage Renal Disease Patients, by Selected Characteristics, Selected Years 1980–2008—Continued

(Number, rate per million.)

Characteristic	Prevalence — Number of patients alive on December 31						
	1980	1985	1990	1995	2000	2005	2008
TOTAL	58,258	110,531	182,609	281,914	383,824	474,744	535,166
Age							
Under 20 years	2,368	3,475	4,485	5,467	6,287	6,995	7,216
20–44 years	20,212	37,113	57,142	76,188	87,827	92,464	95,870
45–64 years	23,683	42,430	67,095	107,546	156,691	207,054	239,158
65–74 years	9,205	19,221	35,577	57,920	76,241	92,509	108,212
75 years and over	2,790	8,292	18,310	34,793	56,778	75,722	84,710
Sex							
Male	32,181	60,462	98,438	151,624	209,491	264,255	301,436
Female	26,077	50,069	84,171	130,290	174,333	210,489	233,730
Race[1]							
White	41,051	74,423	118,535	175,868	237,068	293,187	328,250
Black or African American	16,432	33,203	57,368	92,640	126,137	153,593	172,719
American Indian or Alaska Native	374	1,085	2,175	3,787	5,393	6,519	7,220
Asian or Pacific Islander	401	1,820	4,531	9,619	15,226	21,445	26,977
Hispanic Origin[1,2]							
Hispanic	—	—	—	—	42,417	60,035	74,583
Not Hispanic[3]	—	—	—	—	341,407	414,709	460,583
Primary Diagnosis							
Diabetes	5,580	20,530	46,943	88,528	135,995	175,464	201,003
Hypertension	9,425	25,258	47,246	73,927	94,728	116,707	131,585
Glomerulonephritis	13,359	26,354	39,704	54,615	67,650	76,795	81,253
Cystic kidney	3,625	6,816	9,969	13,854	17,856	22,172	25,713
Other urologic	1,586	4,111	6,087	8,288	11,652	13,287	12,776
Other cause	6,576	14,212	21,429	30,376	39,375	49,172	58,411
Unknown cause	5,852	7,143	8,212	10,120	13,868	17,793	20,556
Missing disease	12,255	6,107	3,019	2,206	2,700	3,354	3,869

Characteristic	Patients alive on December 31 per million population						
	1980	1985	1990	1995	2000	2005	2008
TOTAL	255.0	462.4	726.7	1,052.6	1,353.4	1,598.7	1,752.1
Age							
Under 20 years	32.7	49.4	62.1	70.9	78.0	85.6	87.1
20–44 years	236.6	389.1	565.9	738.6	841.7	885.5	917.3
45–64 years	530.9	950.8	1,440.2	2,006.6	2,471.1	2,806.9	3,035.4
65–74 years	583.3	1,130.8	1,954.9	3,073.5	4,155.7	4,926.6	5,278.8
75 years and over	273.4	707.9	1,373.5	2,302.5	3,367.9	4,153.6	4,497.8
Sex							
Male	289.9	519.9	803.2	1,157.3	1,504.8	1,807.4	2,000.9
Female	222.1	408.0	653.8	952.2	1,207.4	1,396.2	1,510.0
Race[1]							
White	209.5	367.1	563.2	794.3	1,023.8	1,219.1	1,333.5
Black or African American	609.0	1,154.7	1,852.4	2,714.2	3,413.6	3,926.4	4,252.9
American Indian or Alaska Native	255.7	619.6	1,039.3	1,521.9	1,799.3	1,994.8	2,091.1
Asian or Pacific Islander	99.9	314.2	584.4	980.1	1,259.5	1,523.9	1,772.4
Hispanic Origin[1,2]							
Hispanic	—	—	—	—	1,167.0	1,387.9	1,564.3
Not Hispanic[3]	—	—	—	—	1,380.8	1,634.6	1,786.8
Primary Diagnosis							
Diabetes	24.4	85.9	186.8	330.5	479.5	590.9	658.1
Hypertension	41.3	105.7	188.0	276.0	334.0	393.0	430.8
Glomerulonephritis	58.5	110.3	158.0	203.9	238.5	258.6	266.0
Cystic kidney	15.9	28.5	39.7	51.7	63.0	74.7	84.2
Other urologic	6.9	17.2	24.2	30.9	41.1	44.7	41.8
Other cause	28.8	59.5	85.3	113.4	138.8	165.6	191.1
Unknown cause	25.6	29.9	32.7	37.8	48.9	59.9	67.3
Missing disease	53.7	25.6	12.0	8.2	9.5	11.3	12.7

— =Data not available.
[1]The race groups, White, Black, American Indian or Alaska Native, and Asian or Pacific Islander, include persons of Hispanic and non-Hispanic origin. Persons of Hispanic origin may be of any race
[2]Centers for Medicare & Medicaid Services began collecting Hispanic ethnicity data in April 1995.
[3]Not Hispanic includes unknown ethnicity.

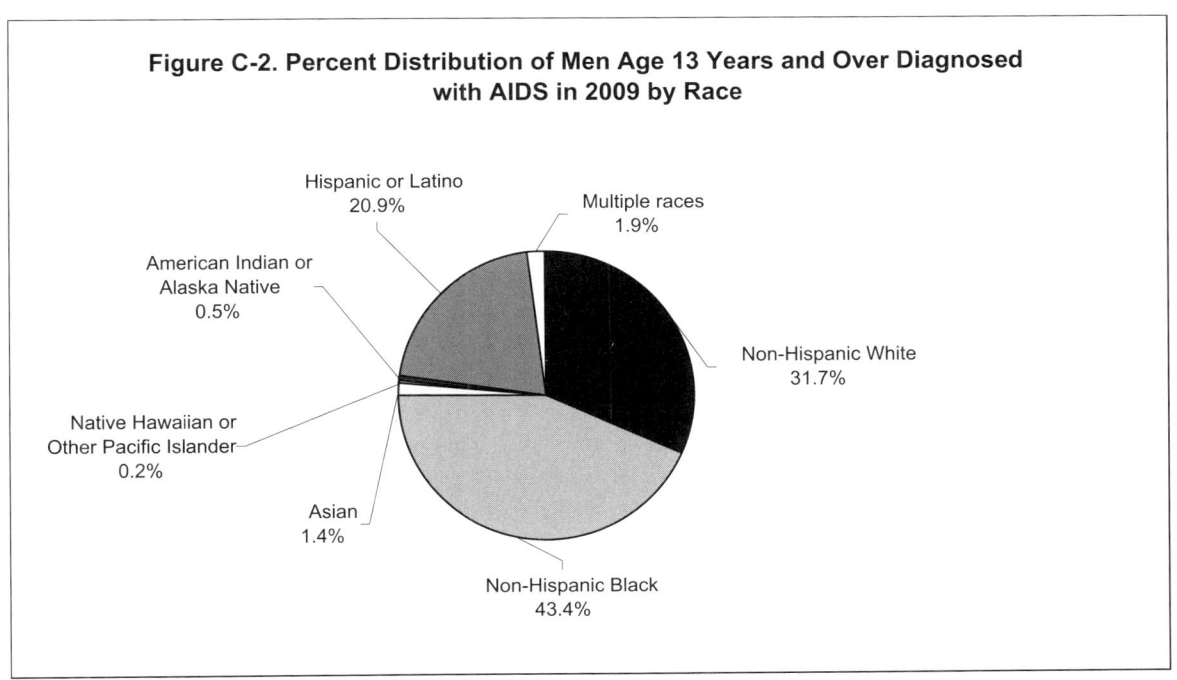

Figure C-2. Percent Distribution of Men Age 13 Years and Over Diagnosed with AIDS in 2009 by Race

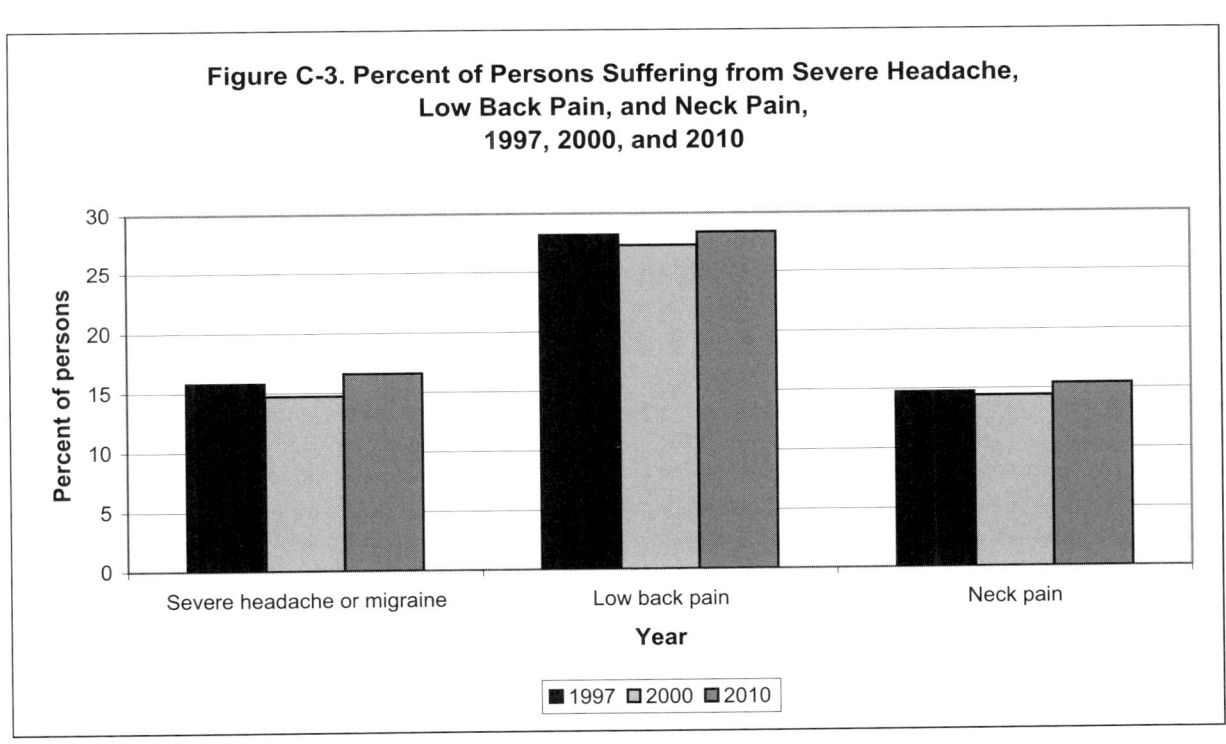

Figure C-3. Percent of Persons Suffering from Severe Headache, Low Back Pain, and Neck Pain, 1997, 2000, and 2010

Table C-9. Severe Headache or Migraine, Low Back Pain, and Neck Pain Among Adults 18 Years of Age and Over, by Selected Characteristics, 1997, 2000, and 2010

(Percent.)

Characteristic	Severe headache or migraine[1]			Low back pain[1]			Neck pain[1]		
	1997	2000	2010	1997	2000	2010	1997	2000	2010
18 years and over, age–adjusted[2,3]	15.8	14.7	16.6	28.2	27.3	28.4	14.7	14.4	15.4
18 years and over, crude[3]	16.0	14.8	16.4	28.1	27.2	28.8	14.6	14.4	15.8
Age									
18–44 years	18.7	17.2	20.4	26.1	24.6	25.2	13.3	12.6	13.1
18–24 years	18.7	16.1	19.6	21.9	20.9	19.4	9.8	8.7	8.3
25–44 years	18.7	17.6	20.7	27.3	25.8	27.2	14.3	13.9	14.8
45–64 years	15.8	14.8	15.6	31.3	30.4	32.4	17.0	17.7	20.0
45–54 years	17.8	16.3	16.7	31.3	29.4	31.3	17.3	17.8	19.1
55–64 years	12.7	12.3	14.1	31.2	32.0	33.8	16.6	17.6	21.0
65 years and over	7.0	7.0	6.4	29.5	30.0	31.8	15.0	14.0	14.8
65–74 years	8.2	7.9	7.4	30.2	29.6	32.5	15.0	13.9	15.5
75 years and over	5.4	6.0	5.1	28.6	30.6	30.9	15.0	14.2	14.0
Sex[2]									
Male	9.9	8.9	11.0	26.5	25.5	26.3	12.6	12.1	13.1
Female	21.4	20.3	22.1	29.6	28.8	30.3	16.6	16.5	17.6
Sex and Age									
Male									
18–44 years	11.9	10.4	13.5	24.8	23.4	23.2	11.6	10.6	11.0
45–54 years	10.3	9.1	10.4	29.4	27.4	29.6	13.9	14.8	16.3
55–64 years	8.8	7.6	9.6	30.7	29.6	32.8	14.6	15.1	17.6
65–74 years	5.0	5.1	5.5	29.0	27.5	28.4	13.6	12.0	12.8
75 years and over	*2.4	4.5	4.0	22.5	26.3	27.4	12.6	12.4	13.0
Female									
18–44 years	25.4	23.9	27.3	27.3	25.7	27.1	14.9	14.6	15.2
45–54 years	24.9	23.2	22.9	33.1	31.3	33.0	20.6	20.7	21.8
55–64 years	16.3	16.7	18.2	31.7	34.2	34.7	18.4	19.8	24.1
65–74 years	10.7	10.1	9.1	31.1	31.2	36.1	16.1	15.5	17.8
75 years and over	7.4	6.9	5.8	32.4	33.2	33.2	16.5	15.2	14.6
Race[2,4]									
White only	15.9	15.0	16.7	28.7	28.0	29.1	15.1	15.0	16.0
Black or African American only	16.7	13.9	18.2	26.9	24.3	27.2	13.3	10.7	13.3
American Indian or Alaska Native only	18.9	21.1	18.8	33.3	31.4	33.6	16.2	19.6	16.9
Asian only	11.7	12.0	10.1	21.0	19.0	19.1	9.2	11.0	9.6
Native Hawaiian or Other Pacific Islander only	—	*	*	—	*	*	—	*	*
2 or more races	—	19.9	21.5	—	41.8	35.6	—	22.1	22.0
Hispanic Origin and Race[2,4]									
Hispanic or Latino	15.5	13.5	16.2	26.4	25.0	27.4	13.9	13.4	15.1
Mexican	14.6	12.3	15.7	25.2	21.5	26.5	12.9	11.6	14.7
Not Hispanic or Latino	15.9	15.0	16.8	28.4	27.7	28.7	14.9	14.7	15.5
White only	16.1	15.4	17.0	29.1	28.4	29.7	15.4	15.4	16.3
Black or African American only	16.8	13.8	18.4	26.9	24.2	27.1	13.3	10.6	13.3
Education[5,6]									
25 years and over									
No high school diploma or GED	19.2	17.9	18.2	33.6	32.4	34.5	16.5	15.9	18.9
High school diploma or GED	16.0	14.8	17.4	30.2	29.4	31.9	15.5	15.4	16.8
Some college or more	13.8	13.4	15.1	26.9	26.3	28.0	14.6	15.0	15.8
Percent of Poverty Level[2,7]									
Below 100%	23.3	19.9	22.7	35.4	32.4	34.9	18.6	16.5	20.2
100%–199%	18.9	17.7	19.5	30.8	30.6	32.5	16.1	15.3	17.7
200%–399%	15.5	15.4	16.6	27.9	27.4	28.5	14.8	14.7	15.2
400% or more	12.4	11.8	13.3	24.8	24.5	24.7	12.8	13.4	13.1

Table C-9. Severe Headache or Migraine, Low Back Pain, and Neck Pain Among Adults 18 Years of Age and Over, by Selected Characteristics, 1997, 2000, and 2010—Continued

(Percent.)

Characteristic	Severe headache or migraine[1]			Low back pain[1]			Neck pain[1]		
	1997	2000	2010	1997	2000	2010	1997	2000	2010
Hispanic Origin and Race and Percent of Poverty Level[2,4,7]									
Hispanic or Latino									
Below 100%	18.9	18.1	19.6	29.5	28.4	29.0	16.4	15.6	17.4
100%–199%	15.7	12.9	15.1	26.8	24.8	27.2	12.9	13.3	15.7
200%–399%	14.0	13.6	16.5	25.0	23.5	27.5	13.8	13.6	12.9
400% or more	13.0	9.6	14.0	21.6	24.1	25.6	12.1	11.6	15.3
Not Hispanic or Latino									
White only									
Below 100%	26.1	21.3	24.8	38.9	36.6	40.5	20.5	18.7	23.7
100%–199%	20.4	20.3	22.0	33.3	34.6	35.9	18.0	17.6	19.9
200%–399%	16.3	16.5	16.9	29.1	28.5	30.5	15.9	16.0	16.8
400% or more	12.5	12.3	13.8	25.4	25.2	25.2	13.1	14.0	13.6
Black or African American only									
Below 100%	22.7	21.1	24.0	34.5	27.5	32.5	17.9	13.7	18.6
100%–199%	17.6	16.3	19.6	27.7	26.2	31.2	14.0	11.1	14.4
200%–399%	14.0	11.4	17.6	24.3	23.8	23.7	10.2	9.8	11.7
400% or more	12.9	8.2	12.2	21.5	20.3	21.0	11.9	8.1	8.5
Disability Measure[2,8]									
Any basic actions difficulty or complex activity limitation	29.3	28.3	30.1	48.0	49.0	49.5	27.2	29.0	28.1
Any basic actions difficulty	30.0	29.3	30.9	49.3	50.0	51.1	27.9	29.9	29.0
Any complex activity limitation	34.6	32.7	36.0	55.1	54.3	54.5	33.1	33.9	34.3
No disability	11.0	10.4	11.7	19.4	18.7	19.0	9.1	9.1	9.7
Geographic Region[2]									
Northeast	14.5	12.7	15.4	27.1	26.0	28.0	14.0	13.5	14.9
Midwest	15.6	15.1	16.8	28.7	28.2	28.1	15.3	14.5	16.0
South	17.1	14.9	18.2	27.5	26.5	28.3	13.9	13.7	14.6
West	15.3	15.9	15.1	30.0	28.6	29.3	16.1	16.5	16.5
Location of Residence[2]									
Within MSA[9]	15.2	14.4	16.3	27.0	26.6	27.5	14.2	14.3	14.9
Outside MSA[9]	18.1	16.1	18.6	32.5	29.6	33.8	16.4	14.9	18.1

* = Figure does not meet standards of reliability or precision.
— = Data not available.
[1] In three separate questions, respondents were asked, "During the past 3 months, did you have a severe headache or migraine? low back pain? neck pain?" Respondents were instructed to report pain that had lasted a whole day or more, and not to report fleeting or minor aches or pains.
[2] Estimates are age-adjusted to the year 2000 standard population using five age groups: 18–44 years, 45–54 years, 55–64 years, 65–74 years, and 75 years and over.
[3] Includes all other races not shown separately, unknown education level, and unknown disability status.
[4] The race groups, White, Black, American Indian or Alaska Native, Asian, Native Hawaiian or Other Pacific Islander, and 2 or more races, include persons of Hispanic and non-Hispanic origin. Persons of Hispanic origin may be of any race.
[5] Estimates are for persons 25 years of age and over and are age-adjusted to the year 2000 standard population using five age groups: 25–44 years, 45–54 years, 55–64 years, 65–74 years, and 75 years and over.
[6] GED is General Educational Development high school equivalency diploma.
[7] Percent of poverty level is based on family income and family size and composition using U.S. Census Bureau poverty thresholds.
[8] Any basic actions difficulty or complex activity limitation is defined as having one or more of the following limitations or difficulties: movement difficulty, emotional difficulty, sensory (seeing or hearing) difficulty, cognitive difficulty, self-care (activities of daily living or instrumental activities of daily living) limitation, social limitation, or work limitation.
[9] MSA = metropolitan statistical area.

Table C-10. Joint Pain Among Adults 18 Years of Age and Over, by Selected Characteristics, Selected Years, 2002–2010

(Percent.)

Characteristic	Any joint pain[1]			Knee pain[1]			Shoulder pain[1]		
	2002	2005	2010	2002	2005	2010	2002	2005	2010
18 years and over, age-adjusted[2,3]	29.5	30.7	32.1	16.5	18.2	19.6	8.6	9.2	9.0
18 years and over, crude[3]	29.5	31.1	33.3	16.5	18.5	20.3	8.7	9.3	9.4
Age									
18–44 years	19.3	19.1	20.6	10.5	11.6	12.6	4.9	4.9	5.2
18–24 years	14.2	14.0	15.2	8.3	8.8	9.8	3.4	2.4	3.5
25–44 years	21.0	20.9	22.6	11.2	12.6	13.6	5.4	5.8	5.8
45–64 years	37.5	39.9	42.9	20.4	23.2	26.1	12.3	12.9	13.2
45–54 years	34.3	35.8	39.3	18.4	20.6	23.5	10.5	11.5	12.0
55–64 years	42.3	45.7	47.3	23.4	26.9	29.3	15.1	14.9	14.8
65 years and over	47.2	50.9	49.6	28.6	30.2	30.5	14.1	16.0	13.6
65–74 years	46.0	49.3	49.5	27.6	29.7	30.2	14.0	15.7	13.5
75 years and over	48.7	52.6	49.8	29.7	30.8	30.9	14.1	16.2	13.7
Sex[2]									
Male	28.0	28.9	30.8	15.2	16.8	18.7	8.4	9.3	9.3
Female	30.7	32.2	33.2	17.6	19.4	20.3	8.8	9.0	8.6
Sex and Age									
Male									
18–44 years	20.1	19.3	21.6	10.7	12.0	12.9	5.5	5.4	6.1
45–54 years	31.1	33.4	37.3	16.2	18.9	22.3	9.5	11.4	12.2
55–64 years	37.3	40.7	42.5	20.1	23.1	27.4	13.7	14.7	15.3
65–74 years	41.7	45.1	42.9	24.1	25.1	25.3	13.3	15.7	11.8
75 years and over	43.9	47.0	46.6	25.7	25.7	28.7	11.4	15.1	13.1
Female									
18–44 years	18.4	18.9	19.7	10.2	11.2	12.2	4.2	4.5	4.3
45–54 years	37.3	38.2	41.3	20.5	22.3	24.8	11.4	11.5	11.8
55–64 years	46.8	50.4	51.8	26.4	30.5	31.0	16.3	15.1	14.3
65–74 years	49.6	52.9	55.2	30.5	33.6	34.4	14.7	15.7	15.0
75 years and over	51.6	56.2	51.9	32.1	34.0	32.4	15.7	16.9	14.1
Race[2,4]									
White only	29.8	31.3	32.6	16.3	18.5	19.7	8.8	9.5	9.1
Black or African American only	30.8	28.5	32.0	20.2	18.2	21.0	8.3	7.6	8.9
American Indian or Alaska Native only	36.7	34.8	38.1	24.5	15.0	26.9	*11.3	*8.1	10.1
Asian only	18.1	18.5	20.4	8.5	10.2	12.8	3.9	5.3	6.9
Native Hawaiian or Other Pacific Islander only	*	*	*	*	*	*	*	*	*
2 or more races	42.7	46.2	43.5	28.1	28.6	27.1	15.4	18.9	13.9
Hispanic Origin and Race[2,4]									
Hispanic or Latino	23.4	24.2	25.4	13.6	14.9	15.5	7.6	8.2	7.4
Mexican	24.6	23.8	25.0	14.1	14.9	15.4	8.3	8.5	7.3
Not Hispanic or Latino	30.4	31.7	33.3	17.0	18.9	20.3	8.9	9.4	9.3
White only	30.8	32.8	34.3	16.9	19.4	20.7	9.1	9.8	9.5
Black or African American only	30.8	28.5	32.1	20.1	18.1	21.0	8.3	7.6	8.9
Education[5,6]									
25 years of age and over:									
No high school diploma or GED	33.0	33.3	33.8	19.5	20.7	22.0	10.8	11.7	10.9
High school diploma or GED	32.9	33.1	36.8	18.6	19.7	22.7	10.2	10.5	10.9
Some college or more	31.1	33.2	34.0	16.9	19.2	20.1	8.8	9.7	9.1
Percent of Poverty Level[2,7]									
Below 100%	31.7	33.7	35.6	19.9	21.4	22.9	11.2	11.2	11.1
100%–199%	31.7	31.9	34.0	19.0	19.8	21.9	10.4	10.5	10.9
200%–399%	30.1	31.0	32.2	16.4	18.4	19.3	8.8	9.2	9.0
400% or more	27.6	29.3	30.5	14.9	16.6	18.1	7.3	8.1	7.7

Table C-10. Joint Pain Among Adults 18 Years of Age and Over, by Selected Characteristics, Selected Years, 2002–2010—Continued

(Percent.)

Characteristic	Finger pain[1]			Hip pain[1]		
	2002	2005	2010	2002	2005	2010
18 years and over, age-adjusted[2,3]	7.5	7.4	7.1	6.6	7.1	7.0
18 years and over, crude[3]	7.5	7.6	7.5	6.6	7.2	7.3
Age						
18–44 years	3.4	2.8	3.1	3.2	3.2	3.2
18–24 years	2.0	*1.0	1.7	1.6	2.1	*1.5
25–44 years	3.9	3.5	3.6	3.8	3.6	3.8
45–64 years	11.0	11.2	10.5	9.1	9.7	10.0
45–54 years	9.1	9.2	8.4	7.8	7.6	9.0
55–64 years	13.9	14.0	13.2	11.0	12.6	11.3
65 years and over	13.9	15.2	14.2	12.9	14.6	13.5
65–74 years	14.4	14.9	15.3	12.6	13.7	13.3
75 years and over	13.3	15.4	12.8	13.3	15.7	13.7
Sex[2]						
Male	5.8	6.0	5.8	5.1	5.4	5.3
Female	8.9	8.7	8.2	8.0	8.6	8.6
Sex and Age						
Male						
18–44 years	3.0	2.6	3.0	2.5	2.4	2.0
45–54 years	6.6	7.5	7.3	5.6	5.7	6.8
55–64 years	10.5	10.4	9.9	8.0	9.5	8.7
65–74 years	11.2	11.4	10.9	10.5	10.8	10.3
75 years and over	10.0	12.1	9.5	10.1	12.7	12.9
Female						
18–44 years	3.8	3.0	3.1	3.9	4.0	4.5
45–54 years	11.5	10.9	9.4	9.9	9.5	11.1
55–64 years	17.0	17.4	16.2	13.7	15.4	13.7
65–74 years	17.1	17.9	19.0	14.2	16.2	15.8
75 years and over	15.3	17.5	15.1	15.2	17.5	14.3
Race[2,4]						
White only	7.6	7.8	7.4	6.9	7.4	7.2
Black or African American only	6.5	4.6	5.6	5.6	6.1	6.0
American Indian or Alaska Native only	*12.9	*13.0	*7.2	*10.4	*	*9.9
Asian only	*3.2	4.1	3.3	*2.3	*2.1	*2.4
Native Hawaiian or Other Pacific Islander only	*	*	*	*	*	*
2 or more races	12.8	10.5	12.2	10.0	13.7	11.7
Hispanic Origin and Race[2,4]						
Hispanic or Latino	6.8	6.0	6.0	3.8	4.1	4.3
Mexican	7.8	7.0	6.3	4.0	4.1	3.9
Not Hispanic or Latino	7.6	7.6	7.3	6.9	7.4	7.3
White only	7.8	8.2	7.7	7.3	7.8	7.7
Black or African American only	6.5	4.7	5.6	5.7	6.2	6.1
Education[5,6]						
25 years of age and over:						
No high school diploma or GED	9.5	8.8	8.5	7.3	8.5	7.9
High school diploma or GED	8.3	8.8	9.1	7.3	7.5	9.0
Some college or more	8.2	8.1	7.4	7.5	7.8	7.3
Percent of Poverty Level[2,7]						
Below 100%	9.8	8.0	9.1	8.5	8.9	9.7
100%–199%	8.9	8.2	8.3	7.5	8.1	8.5
200%–399%	7.9	7.9	7.2	6.8	6.9	6.8
400% or more	6.2	6.6	6.0	5.8	6.3	5.7

Table C-10. Joint Pain Among Adults 18 Years of Age and Over, by Selected Characteristics, Selected Years, 2002–2010

(Percent.)

Characteristic	Any joint pain[1]			Knee pain[1]			Shoulder pain[1]		
	2002	2005	2010	2002	2005	2010	2002	2005	2010
Hispanic Origin and Race and Percent of Poverty Level[2,4,7]									
Hispanic or Latino									
Below 100%	26.8	24.5	25.3	16.1	15.7	15.9	11.5	10.5	7.6
100%–199%	24.5	24.1	25.4	14.4	15.2	16.1	8.2	8.3	8.0
200%–399%	21.6	23.6	24.8	11.7	13.1	14.5	5.7	8.2	6.8
400% or more	21.9	24.7	27.4	12.3	15.6	16.3	4.9	*6.4	7.4
Not Hispanic or Latino									
White only									
Below 100%	34.2	39.3	40.1	21.3	24.7	25.2	12.4	13.4	12.6
100%–199%	34.9	36.2	38.7	20.3	22.8	24.8	11.6	12.0	12.2
200%–399%	32.0	33.6	34.8	17.0	20.1	20.9	9.6	10.1	10.0
400% or more	28.2	30.1	31.8	15.1	17.0	18.8	7.6	8.4	8.0
Black or African American only									
Below 100%	31.6	33.0	37.6	20.8	22.5	25.1	9.1	9.0	11.9
100%–199%	34.0	28.6	33.0	23.2	18.3	22.6	10.9	8.3	10.0
200%–399%	29.1	27.2	30.8	19.1	16.6	19.8	7.4	7.2	7.8
400% or more	29.8	25.8	26.8	18.2	15.8	15.7	*8.0	*5.7	6.5
Disability Measure[2,8]									
Any basic actions difficulty or complex activity limitation	52.5	54.8	54.6	32.1	35.7	35.9	17.8	18.8	16.8
Any basic actions difficulty	54.0	56.7	56.2	33.4	37.3	37.3	18.3	19.5	17.2
Any complex activity limitation	56.4	57.8	56.5	35.2	38.2	37.5	22.0	23.5	20.6
No disability	19.6	20.3	21.5	9.4	10.4	11.6	4.6	4.8	4.9
Geographic Region[2]									
Northeast	27.5	28.6	28.9	15.8	16.7	17.9	7.9	8.1	8.3
Midwest	32.1	34.8	35.7	18.4	21.6	22.3	8.6	10.1	10.0
South	29.3	29.8	32.4	16.7	17.9	19.8	9.1	8.9	9.0
West	28.4	29.2	30.6	14.6	16.3	17.9	8.6	9.6	8.5
Location of Residence[2]									
Within MSA[9]	28.3	29.2	31.1	16.0	17.2	19.0	8.1	8.4	8.3
Outside MSA[9]	33.9	36.3	37.4	18.7	22.3	23.0	10.8	12.2	12.3

Table C-10. Joint Pain Among Adults 18 Years of Age and Over, by Selected Characteristics, Selected Years, 2002–2010—Continued

(Percent.)

Characteristic	Finger pain[1]			Hip pain[1]		
	2002	2005	2010	2002	2005	2010
Hispanic Origin and Race and Percent of Poverty Level[2,4,7]						
Hispanic or Latino						
Below 100%	8.6	6.4	6.4	5.9	4.4	5.6
100%–199%	8.2	5.7	5.2	3.9	3.9	4.5
200%–399%	6.2	6.5	6.8	3.2	4.2	3.1
400% or more	*5.3	*5.1	5.8	*1.8	*4.3	*5.2
Not Hispanic or Latino						
White only						
Below 100%	10.9	9.9	11.1	9.9	11.6	12.0
100%–199%	9.9	9.6	9.8	9.1	9.8	10.6
200%–399%	8.5	8.9	7.8	7.5	7.8	7.8
400% or more	6.5	7.0	6.3	6.2	6.8	6.0
Black or African American only						
Below 100%	7.9	5.7	7.8	8.1	7.7	9.0
100%–199%	7.4	6.0	6.2	6.4	6.3	5.9
200%–399%	6.0	3.9	4.3	4.7	6.0	5.2
400% or more	*4.8	*2.8	*4.2	*4.5	*5.5	4.7
Disability Measure[2,8]						
Any basic actions difficulty or complex activity limitation	14.5	14.2	12.8	13.8	14.6	14.2
Any basic actions difficulty	14.9	14.8	13.3	14.4	15.2	14.6
Any complex activity limitation	17.8	16.9	15.0	17.8	19.7	18.7
No disability	4.0	4.1	4.2	3.1	3.3	3.1
Geographic Region[2]						
Northeast	6.6	6.2	5.5	5.7	6.4	5.5
Midwest	7.5	8.5	7.9	6.9	7.9	8.5
South	7.6	7.3	7.4	7.0	7.1	7.2
West	8.0	7.5	7.1	6.4	6.6	6.3
Location of Residence[2]						
Within MSA[9]	7.2	7.0	7.0	6.2	6.5	6.5
Outside MSA[9]	8.4	9.1	7.9	8.0	9.3	9.4

* = Figure does not meet standards of reliability or precision.
[1]Starting with 2002 data, respondents were asked, "During the past 30 days, have you had any symptoms of pain, aching, or stiffness in or around a joint?" Respondents were instructed not to include the back or neck.
[2]Estimates are age-adjusted to the year 2000 standard population using five age groups: 18–44 years, 45–54 years, 55–64 years, 65–74 years, and 75 years and over.
[3]Includes all other races not shown separately, unknown education level, and unknown disability status.
[4]The race groups, White, Black, American Indian or Alaska Native, Asian, Native Hawaiian or Other Pacific Islander, and 2 or more races, include persons of Hispanic and non-Hispanic origin. Persons of Hispanic origin may be of any race.
[5]Estimates are for persons 25 years of age and over and are age-adjusted to the year 2000 standard population using five age groups: 25–44 years, 45–54 years, 55–64 years, 65–74 years, and 75 years and over.
[6]GED is General Educational Development high school equivalency diploma.
[7]Percent of poverty level is based on family income and family size and composition using U.S. Census Bureau poverty thresholds.
[8]Any basic actions difficulty or complex activity limitation is defined as having one or more of the following limitations or difficulties: movement difficulty, emotional difficulty, sensory (seeing or hearing) difficulty, cognitive difficulty, self-care (activities of daily living or instrumental activities of daily living) limitation, social limitation, or work limitation.
[9]MSA = metropolitan statistical area.

Table C-11. Basic Actions Difficulty and Complex Activity Limitation Among Adults 18 Years of Age and Over, by Selected Characteristics, Selected Years, 1997–2010

(Number, percent.)

Characteristic	18 years and over			18–64 years			65 years and over		
	1997	2005	2010[1]	1997	2005	2010[1]	1997	2005	2010[1]
Number in Millions									
At least one basic actions difficulty or complex activity limitation[2,3]	60.9	66.5	73.7	41.3	45.4	50.7	19.6	21.1	23.0
At least one basic actions difficulty[2]	56.7	62.4	69.2	38.1	42.1	47.2	18.6	20.3	22.0
At least one complex activity limitation[3]	29.0	31.3	35.0	18.1	19.9	22.9	11.0	11.5	12.1
Percent with At Least One Basic Actions Difficulty or Complex Activity Limitation[2,3]									
Total, age-adjusted[4,5]	32.5	31.0	31.9						
Total, crude[4]	31.8	31.2	32.8	25.8	25.3	27.1	62.2	62.4	61.7
Percent with At Least One Basic Actions Difficulty[2]									
Total, age-adjusted[4,5]	30.1	29.1	29.9						
Total, crude[4]	29.4	29.3	30.8	23.6	23.5	25.1	58.8	60.1	59.3
Sex									
Male	25.6	25.2	26.3	20.7	20.3	21.4	54.5	55.2	53.8
Female	32.9	33.1	35.1	26.4	26.6	28.8	61.9	63.7	63.6
Race[6]									
White only	29.6	29.7	31.2	23.5	23.5	25.1	58.5	60.0	59.2
Black or African American only	31.4	30.4	32.3	26.9	26.1	28.4	64.4	63.2	62.9
American Indian or Alaska Native only	43.8	25.6	41.6	41.9	25.2	38.5	66.0	*	74.0
Asian only	15.5	15.7	17.5	13.0	11.8	12.8	46.4	46.2	50.1
Native Hawaiian or Other Pacific Islander only	—	*	*	—	*	*	—	*	*
2 or more races	—	40.0	36.3	—	34.9	33.9	—	90.4	65.4
Hispanic Origin and Race[6]									
Hispanic or Latino	23.8	21.6	24.7	21.0	18.7	21.2	54.6	56.2	61.5
Not Hispanic or Latino	30.0	30.4	31.8	23.9	24.3	25.9	59.0	60.3	59.1
White only	30.3	31.1	32.4	23.8	24.5	26.0	58.7	60.3	59.0
Black or African American only	31.5	30.7	32.6	27.0	26.3	28.6	64.4	63.5	63.2
Percent of Poverty Level[7]									
Below 100%	41.9	40.2	40.6	36.2	34.9	36.3	74.1	73.1	72.7
100%–199%	38.2	38.4	38.7	29.2	29.6	30.5	66.6	68.5	69.5
200%–399%	28.4	29.7	31.1	22.0	22.8	24.1	56.1	59.0	58.9
400% or more	21.0	21.4	23.0	18.2	18.1	19.3	45.5	48.2	47.0
Location of Residence									
Within MSA[8]	27.7	27.5	29.2	22.3	22.1	23.6	56.6	58.3	59.2
Outside MSA[8]	35.6	36.3	39.3	28.6	29.5	33.8	65.8	65.5	59.9
Percent with At Least One Complex Activity Limitation[3]									
Total, age-adjusted[4,5]	15.6	14.5	14.9						
Total, crude[4]	15.1	14.6	15.5	11.2	11.0	12.1	35.1	33.6	32.3
Sex									
Male	13.7	12.9	14.0	10.6	10.1	11.3	31.9	29.4	30.1
Female	16.5	16.1	16.8	11.9	11.8	12.9	37.4	36.7	34.0
Race[6]									
White only	15.0	14.4	15.2	10.9	10.7	11.7	34.3	33.1	31.7
Black or African American only	19.0	17.1	19.7	15.2	14.0	17.0	47.1	40.9	39.9
American Indian or Alaska Native only	23.7	14.2	15.4	22.1	13.0	14.5	*42.6	*	*
Asian only	5.7	6.6	7.7	4.9	4.7	5.0	*14.8	*20.8	26.7
Native Hawaiian or Other Pacific Islander only	—	*	*	—	*	*	—	*	*
2 or more races	—	26.2	19.6	—	21.8	17.0	—	69.7	53.6
Hispanic Origin and Race[6]									
Hispanic or Latino	11.9	9.8	10.4	9.8	7.6	7.9	33.9	35.0	37.6
Not Hispanic or Latino	15.5	15.3	16.3	11.4	11.5	12.9	35.1	33.5	31.9
White only	15.4	15.2	16.1	11.1	11.3	12.5	34.4	32.9	31.1
Black or African American only	18.8	17.3	20.0	15.0	14.1	17.3	46.8	40.9	40.0

Table C-11. Basic Actions Difficulty and Complex Activity Limitation Among Adults 18 Years of Age and Over, by Selected Characteristics, Selected Years, 1997–2010—Continued

(Number, percent.)

Characteristic	18 years and over			18–64 years			65 years and over		
	1997	2005	2010[1]	1997	2005	2010[1]	1997	2005	2010[1]
Percent of Poverty Level[7]									
Below 100%	30.0	27.3	27.5	25.2	23.4	24.0	56.9	51.5	54.5
100%–199%	23.3	22.7	23.7	16.7	17.2	18.4	43.9	41.3	43.7
200%–399%	13.3	14.0	14.5	9.3	9.9	10.8	30.6	31.8	29.3
400% or more	7.3	7.3	7.7	5.8	5.5	5.8	20.2	21.5	19.8
Location of Residence									
Within MSA[8]	14.1	13.2	14.2	10.6	9.9	10.9	32.7	31.7	31.6
Outside MSA[8]	19.0	20.0	22.2	13.6	15.4	18.8	42.8	39.7	35.2

X = Category not applicable.
* = Figure does not meet standards of reliability or precision.
— = Data not available.
[1] Starting with 2007 data, the hearing question, a component of the basic actions difficulty measure, was revised. Consequently, data for basic actions difficulty prior to 2007 are not comparable with 2007 data and beyond.
[2] A basic actions difficulty is defined as having one or more of the following difficulties: movement, emotional, sensory (seeing or hearing), or cognitive.
[3] A complex activity limitation is defined as having one or more of the following limitations: self-care (activities of daily living or instrumental activities of daily living), social, or work.
[4] Includes all other races not shown separately.
[5] Estimates are age-adjusted to the year 2000 standard population using five age groups: 18–44 years, 45–54 years, 55–64 years, 65–74 years, and 75 years and over.
[6] The race groups, White, Black, American Indian or Alaska Native, Asian, Native Hawaiian or Other Pacific Islander, and 2 or more races, include persons of Hispanic and non-Hispanic origin. Persons of Hispanic origin may be of any race.
[7] Percent of poverty level is based on family income and family size and composition using U.S. Census Bureau poverty thresholds.
[8] MSA = metropolitan statistical area.

Table C-12. Vision and Hearing Limitations Among Adults 18 Years of Age and Over, by Selected Characteristics, Selected Years, 1997–2010

(Percent.)

Characteristic	Any trouble seeing, even with glasses or contacts[1]				A lot of trouble hearing or deaf[2]			
	1997	2000	2005	2010	1997	2000	2005	2010
Percent of Adults								
18 years and over, age-adjusted[3,4]	10.0	9.0	9.2	9.1	3.2	3.2	3.5	2.1
18 years and over, crude[4]	9.8	8.9	9.3	9.4	3.1	3.1	3.5	2.2
Age								
18–44 years	6.2	5.3	5.5	6.2	1.0	0.9	0.9	0.5
18–24 years	5.4	4.2	5.0	5.8	*0.5	*0.7	*1.0	*
25–44 years	6.5	5.7	5.7	6.3	1.2	1.0	0.9	0.5
45–64 years	12.0	10.7	11.2	11.6	3.1	3.0	3.4	1.9
45–54 years	12.2	10.9	11.0	10.7	2.6	2.3	2.3	1.2
55–64 years	11.6	10.5	11.5	12.7	3.9	4.0	4.8	2.7
65 years and over	18.1	17.4	17.4	13.9	9.8	10.5	11.9	7.6
65–74 years	14.2	13.6	13.2	12.2	6.6	7.4	6.4	4.6
75 years and over	23.1	21.9	22.0	16.1	14.1	14.3	18.1	11.1
Sex[3]								
Male	8.8	7.9	7.9	7.9	4.2	4.3	4.8	2.8
Female	11.1	10.1	10.5	10.3	2.4	2.3	2.5	1.6
Sex and Age								
Male								
18–44 years	5.3	4.4	4.5	5.2	1.2	1.1	1.2	*0.7
45–54 years	10.1	8.8	8.8	9.1	3.6	2.9	3.3	*1.1
55–64 years	10.5	9.5	10.5	10.7	5.4	6.2	7.3	3.9
65–74 years	13.2	12.8	11.4	10.5	9.4	10.8	9.5	6.7
75 years and over	21.4	20.7	20.4	15.7	17.7	18.0	23.3	14.5
Female								
18–44 years	7.1	6.2	6.5	7.1	0.9	0.8	0.7	*0.3
45–54 years	14.2	12.8	13.2	12.3	1.7	1.8	1.5	*1.3
55–64 years	12.6	11.5	12.4	14.6	2.6	1.9	2.6	1.6
65–74 years	15.0	14.4	14.8	13.6	4.4	4.5	3.8	2.9
75 years and over	24.2	22.7	23.0	16.4	11.7	12.1	14.7	8.9
Race[3,5]								
White only	9.7	8.8	9.1	8.8	3.4	3.4	3.8	2.3
Black or African American only	12.8	10.6	10.9	12.1	2.0	1.6	1.4	1.1
American Indian or Alaska Native only	19.2	16.6	*14.9	15.0	14.1	*	*	*
Asian only	6.2	6.3	5.5	5.3	*	*2.4	*2.2	*1.0
Native Hawaiian or Other Pacific Islander only	—	*	*	*	—	*	*	*
2 or more races	—	16.2	16.4	13.1	—	*5.7	*5.8	*
Hispanic Origin and Race[3,5]								
Hispanic or Latino	10.0	9.7	9.6	9.2	1.5	2.3	2.8	1.4
Mexican	10.2	8.3	9.9	9.0	1.8	3.0	3.3	*1.5
Not Hispanic or Latino	10.0	9.1	9.2	9.2	3.3	3.3	3.6	2.2
White only	9.8	8.9	9.1	8.9	3.5	3.5	3.9	2.4
Black or African American only	12.8	10.6	10.9	12.2	2.0	1.6	1.4	1.1
Education[6,7]								
25 years of age and over								
No high school diploma or GED	15.0	12.2	13.5	14.1	4.8	4.6	4.6	3.2
High school diploma or GED	10.6	9.5	10.3	10.5	3.7	3.9	4.1	2.5
Some college or more	8.9	8.9	8.6	8.0	2.9	2.8	3.5	2.0
Percent of Poverty Level[3,8]								
Below 100%	17.0	12.9	15.3	14.8	4.5	3.7	4.5	2.7
100%–199%	12.9	11.6	11.5	12.2	3.6	4.2	4.2	2.5
200%–399%	9.1	8.8	8.9	9.0	3.3	3.3	3.6	2.1
400% or more	7.3	7.1	6.9	6.4	2.7	2.5	3.0	1.8

Table C-12. Vision and Hearing Limitations Among Adults 18 Years of Age and Over, by Selected Characteristics, Selected Years, 1997–2010—Continued

(Percent.)

Characteristic	Any trouble seeing, even with glasses or contacts[1]				A lot of trouble hearing or deaf[2]			
	1997	2000	2005	2010	1997	2000	2005	2010
Hispanic Origin and Race and Percent of Poverty Level[3,5,8]								
Hispanic or Latino								
Below 100%	12.8	11.0	13.6	10.8	*1.9	3.3	3.7	*
100%–199%	11.2	9.4	8.8	10.8	*1.5	*2.3	*2.7	*2.3
200%–399%	8.1	9.2	8.2	8.9	*	*	*	*
400% or more	*8.1	10.5	8.0	5.3	*	*	*	*
Not Hispanic or Latino								
White only:								
Below 100%	17.9	13.1	16.2	16.8	5.8	4.5	5.7	3.7
100%–199%	13.1	12.0	12.7	12.6	4.3	5.0	5.1	3.0
200%–399%	9.2	9.2	9.0	8.8	3.7	3.7	4.0	2.3
400% or more	7.3	7.0	6.9	6.7	2.7	2.6	3.2	2.0
Black or African American only								
Below 100%	17.9	13.6	16.0	15.8	3.3	*1.6	*1.9	*1.5
100%–199%	16.0	12.9	11.3	14.9	*2.0	*2.0	*	*0.7
200%–399%	9.3	7.7	9.7	12.0	*	*	*	*
400% or more	7.7	8.3	6.4	6.6	*	*	*	*
Geographic Region[3]								
Northeast	8.6	7.4	8.1	7.8	2.2	2.4	2.9	1.4
Midwest	9.5	9.6	9.7	9.1	3.5	3.5	3.7	2.3
South	11.4	9.2	9.8	10.6	3.5	3.3	3.7	2.6
West	9.7	9.9	8.6	8.0	3.4	3.5	3.8	1.9
Location of Residence[3]								
Within MSA[9]	9.5	8.5	8.6	8.6	2.9	3.0	3.1	1.9
Outside MSA[9]	12.0	11.1	11.7	11.6	4.5	3.9	4.9	3.0

* = Figure does not meet standards of reliability or precision.
—— = Data not available.
[1] Respondents were asked, "Do you have any trouble seeing, even when wearing glasses or contact lenses?" Respondents were also asked, "Are you blind or unable to see at all?"
[2] Prior to 2007, respondents were asked, "Which statement best describes your hearing without a hearing aid: good, a little trouble, a lot of trouble, or deaf?" In this analysis, a lot of trouble and deaf are combined into one category. Starting with 2007, the question was revised to expand the response categories. Respondents were asked, "Which statement best describes your hearing without a hearing aid: excellent, good, a little trouble, moderate trouble, a lot of trouble, or deaf?"
[3] Estimates are age-adjusted to the year 2000 standard population using five age groups: 18–44 years, 45–54 years, 55–64 years, 65–74 years, and 75 years and over.
[4] Includes all other races not shown separately and unknown education level.
[5] The race groups, White, Black, American Indian or Alaska Native, Asian, Native Hawaiian or Other Pacific Islander, and 2 or more races, include persons of Hispanic and non-Hispanic origin. Persons of Hispanic origin may be of any race.
[6] Estimates are for persons 25 years of age and over and are age-adjusted to the year 2000 standard population using five age groups: 25–44 years, 45–54 years, 55–64 years, 65–74 years, and 75 years and over.
[7] GED is General Educational Development high school equivalency diploma.
[8] Percent of poverty level is based on family income and family size and composition using U.S. Census Bureau poverty thresholds.
[9] MSA = metropolitan statistical area.

Table C-13. Respondent-Assessed Health Status, by Selected Characteristics, Selected Years, 1991–2010

(Percent.)

Characteristic	1991[1]	1995[1]	2000	2005	2006	2007	2008	2009	2010
Percent of Persons with Fair or Poor Health									
All ages, age-adjusted[2,3]	10.4	10.6	9.0	9.2	9.2	9.5	9.5	9.4	9.6
All ages, crude[3]	10.0	10.1	8.9	9.3	9.5	9.8	9.9	9.9	10.1
Age									
Under 18 years	2.6	2.6	1.7	1.8	1.9	1.7	1.8	1.8	2.0
Under 6 years	2.7	2.7	1.5	1.6	1.9	1.5	1.2	1.3	1.8
6–17 years	2.6	2.5	1.8	1.9	1.9	1.7	2.1	2.0	2.2
18–44 years	6.1	6.6	5.1	5.5	5.7	5.9	6.3	6.3	6.3
18–24 years	4.8	4.5	3.3	3.3	3.7	3.3	4.0	3.6	3.9
25–44 years	6.4	7.2	5.7	6.3	6.3	6.8	7.2	7.2	7.2
45–54 years	13.4	13.4	11.9	11.6	12.9	13.3	12.9	13.1	13.3
55–64 years	20.7	21.4	17.9	18.3	18.8	17.9	18.8	19.1	19.4
65 years and over	29.0	28.3	26.9	26.6	24.8	26.8	24.9	24.0	24.4
65–74 years	26.0	25.6	22.5	23.4	21.9	23.4	21.8	19.9	21.2
75 years and over	33.6	32.2	32.1	30.2	28.1	30.7	28.4	28.9	28.3
Sex[2]									
Male	10.0	10.1	8.8	8.8	9.0	9.1	9.1	9.1	9.2
Female	10.8	11.1	9.3	9.5	9.5	9.9	9.8	9.7	10.0
Race[2,4]									
White only	9.6	9.7	8.2	8.6	8.6	8.8	8.9	8.7	8.8
Black or African American only	16.8	17.2	14.6	14.3	14.4	14.2	14.6	14.2	14.9
American Indian or Alaska Native only	18.3	18.7	17.2	13.2	12.1	17.1	14.5	16.3	17.8
Asian only	7.8	9.3	7.4	6.8	6.9	7.1	6.7	8.4	8.1
Native Hawaiian or Other Pacific Islander only	—	—	*	*	*	*	*	*	*
2 or more races	—	—	16.2	14.5	13.1	16.8	12.9	15.3	15.6
Black or African American; White	—	—	*14.5	8.3	*15.0	*16.6	20.2	18.0	*16.7
American Indian or Alaska Native; White	—	—	18.7	17.2	13.9	19.2	14.6	15.2	19.0
Hispanic Origin and Race[2,4]									
Hispanic or Latino	15.6	15.1	12.8	13.3	13.0	13.0	12.8	13.3	13.1
Mexican	17.0	16.7	12.8	14.3	14.1	13.2	13.4	13.7	13.7
Not Hispanic or Latino	10.0	10.1	8.7	8.7	8.8	9.1	9.1	8.9	9.2
White only	9.1	9.1	7.9	8.0	8.0	8.3	8.4	8.0	8.2
Black or African American only	16.8	17.3	14.6	14.4	14.4	14.1	14.6	14.2	14.9
Percent of Poverty Level[2,5]									
Below 100%	22.8	23.7	19.6	20.4	20.3	21.0	21.8	21.8	20.9
100%–199%	14.7	15.5	14.1	14.4	14.4	15.3	15.4	14.9	15.2
200%–399%	7.9	7.9	8.4	8.3	8.1	9.0	8.7	8.6	8.3
400% or more	4.9	4.7	4.5	4.7	4.5	4.7	4.4	4.3	4.3
Hispanic Origin and Race and Percent of Poverty Level[2,4,5]									
Hispanic or Latino									
Below 100%	23.6	22.7	18.7	20.2	20.6	21.0	21.0	22.1	19.2
100%–199%	18.0	16.9	15.3	15.3	14.4	15.1	14.6	16.2	15.6
200%–399%	10.3	10.1	10.3	10.3	10.5	10.5	10.7	9.7	10.3
400% or more	6.6	4.0	5.5	7.6	5.7	7.2	5.6	5.6	6.4
Not Hispanic or Latino									
White only									
Below 100%	21.9	22.8	18.8	20.1	19.5	20.9	22.1	20.5	20.9
100%–199%	14.0	14.8	13.4	13.8	14.2	15.2	15.7	14.6	14.8
200%–399%	7.5	7.3	7.9	7.9	7.5	8.4	8.3	8.1	7.7
400% or more	4.7	4.6	4.2	4.3	4.2	4.3	4.1	4.0	4.0
Black or African American only									
Below 100%	25.8	27.7	23.8	23.3	23.0	22.6	25.1	25.2	23.9
100%–199%	17.0	19.3	18.2	17.6	16.9	17.7	18.1	16.6	18.3
200%–399%	12.0	11.4	11.7	11.2	11.0	11.3	11.2	11.0	11.2
400% or more	5.9	6.5	7.3	7.1	7.0	7.2	6.9	5.9	6.8

Table C-13. Respondent-Assessed Health Status, by Selected Characteristics, Selected Years, 1991–2010—*Continued*

(Percent.)

Characteristic	1991[1]	1995[1]	2000	2005	2006	2007	2008	2009	2010
Disability Measure Among Adults 18 Years and Over[2,6]									
Any basic actions difficulty or complex activity limitation.....	—	—	27.6	28.5	27.2	31.2	28.5	30.3	28.7
Any basic actions difficulty.................	—	—	27.7	29.1	27.6	31.6	28.7	30.9	28.9
Any complex activity limitation	—	—	45.6	46.3	45.4	50.8	47.9	48.8	46.0
No disability........................	—	—	3.8	3.6	4.0	4.0	4.2	3.6	3.5
Geographic Region[2]									
Northeast................	8.3	9.1	7.6	7.5	8.2	8.4	8.0	8.4	7.9
Midwest.................	9.1	9.7	8.0	8.3	8.8	8.6	8.8	8.6	9.0
South...................	13.1	12.3	10.7	11.0	10.4	11.0	11.0	10.9	11.1
West....................	9.7	10.1	8.8	8.6	8.5	9.0	9.0	8.8	9.2
Location of Residence[2]									
Within MSA[7]................	9.9	10.1	8.5	8.7	8.7	9.0	9.1	9.1	9.2
Outside MSA[7]................	11.9	12.6	11.1	11.2	11.7	12.0	11.7	11.2	11.9

— = Data not available.
* = Figure does not meet standards of reliability or precision.
[1]Data prior to 1997 are not strictly comparable with data for later years due to the 1997 questionnaire redesign.
[2]Estimates are age-adjusted to the year 2000 standard population using six age groups: under 18 years, 18–44 years, 45–54 years, 55–64 years, 65–74 years, and 75 years and over. The disability measure is age-adjusted using the five adult age groups.
[3]Includes all other races not shown separately and unknown disability status.
[4]The race groups, White, Black, American Indian or Alaska Native, Asian, Native Hawaiian or Other Pacific Islander, and 2 or more races, include persons of Hispanic and non-Hispanic origin. Persons of Hispanic origin may be of any race.
[5]Percent of poverty level is based on family income and family size and composition using U.S. Census Bureau poverty thresholds.
[6]Any basic actions difficulty or complex activity limitation is defined as having one or more of the following limitations or difficulties: movement difficulty, emotional difficulty, sensory (seeing or hearing) difficulty, cognitive difficulty, self-care (activities of daily living or instrumental activities of daily living) limitation, social limitation, or work limitation.
[7]MSA = metropolitan statistical area.

Table C-14. Selected Measures of Disability and Health Status Among Adults 18–64 Years of Age, by Urbanization Level and Selected Characteristics, Average Annual, 2002–2004 through 2008–2010

(Percent.)

Urbanization level and selected characteristic	Any basic actions difficulty or complex activity limitation[1]			Fair or poor respondent-assessed health status[2]		
	2002–2004	2005–2007	2008–2010	2002–2004	2005–2007	2008–2010
PERCENT OF POPULATION, CRUDE						
Geographic Region						
All regions						
Metropolitan counties						
Large central	21.5	21.8	22.8	8.7	9.0	9.5
Large fringe	22.4	23.1	24.6	6.9	7.1	7.9
Medium and small	27.4	27.3	28.3	9.6	9.8	10.9
Nonmetropolitan counties						
Micropolitan	30.4	31.2	33.0	11.4	12.4	13.3
Nonmicropolitan	30.9	33.7	36.0	14.0	14.6	15.7
Northeast						
Metropolitan counties						
Large central	20.1	21.0	21.5	9.0	10.1	9.5
Large fringe	22.3	22.8	23.5	6.9	6.1	6.8
Medium and small	25.9	24.6	29.7	7.6	7.5	9.3
Nonmetropolitan counties						
Micropolitan	31.0	31.0	37.4	9.7	9.8	11.4
Nonmicropolitan	27.4	34.1	33.5	8.9	10.6	11.5
Midwest						
Metropolitan counties						
Large central	26.1	25.7	26.6	8.9	8.8	10.7
Large fringe	24.4	26.2	26.4	6.3	8.0	8.3
Medium and small	28.1	27.1	26.6	8.1	8.1	9.5
Nonmetropolitan counties						
Micropolitan	27.0	28.3	29.6	8.0	9.8	11.2
Nonmicropolitan	28.6	29.1	30.4	9.1	10.9	10.1
South						
Metropolitan counties						
Large central	21.5	21.9	24.3	8.9	9.9	10.0
Large fringe	20.9	21.4	23.0	7.1	7.2	8.3
Medium and small	27.8	28.0	29.6	11.9	11.9	12.6
Nonmetropolitan counties						
Micropolitan	32.3	31.4	32.5	14.3	14.6	14.7
Nonmicropolitan	34.7	36.5	42.4	20.2	18.2	21.8
West						
Metropolitan counties						
Large central	20.0	19.9	20.4	8.3	7.9	8.5
Large fringe	23.1	23.0	27.3	7.3	7.7	8.3
Medium and small	26.8	28.3	27.1	8.7	9.4	10.3
Nonmetropolitan counties						
Micropolitan	30.8	37.1	38.5	10.9	13.1	14.8
Nonmicropolitan	*24.2	36.1	33.7	*7.6	14.1	13.6
Age						
18–44 years						
Metropolitan counties						
Large central	15.4	15.1	16.2	5.3	5.6	6.0
Large fringe	16.1	16.2	17.3	4.3	4.3	5.1
Medium and small	20.0	19.0	20.2	6.0	6.0	6.6
Nonmetropolitan counties						
Micropolitan	22.5	21.6	23.0	6.6	7.3	7.8
Nonmicropolitan	21.5	23.4	23.8	9.3	8.5	9.1
45–64 years						
Metropolitan counties						
Large central	33.2	33.7	33.8	15.1	15.1	15.2
Large fringe	32.2	33.0	34.0	10.9	11.2	11.4
Medium and small	39.0	39.8	40.1	15.3	15.3	16.9
Nonmetropolitan counties						
Micropolitan	42.0	42.8	45.1	18.4	19.0	19.9
Nonmicropolitan	42.6	45.2	48.5	20.0	21.3	22.6

Table C-14. Selected Measures of Disability and Health Status Among Adults 18–64 Years of Age, by Urbanization Level and Selected Characteristics, Average Annual, 2002–2004 through 2008–2010—Continued

(Percent.)

Urbanization level and selected characteristic	Any basic actions difficulty or complex activity limitation[1]			Fair or poor respondent-assessed health status[2]		
	2002–2004	2005–2007	2008–2010	2002–2004	2005–2007	2008–2010
Sex						
Men						
Metropolitan counties						
Large central	18.2	18.9	19.2	7.6	8.3	8.5
Large fringe	19.7	20.3	22.1	6.3	6.6	7.2
Medium and small	23.8	24.9	25.1	8.9	8.9	10.4
Nonmetropolitan counties						
Micropolitan	28.3	28.2	29.9	11.2	11.8	12.6
Nonmicropolitan	28.5	31.0	35.0	13.5	14.7	14.7
Women						
Metropolitan counties						
Large central	24.8	24.6	26.4	9.8	9.7	10.5
Large fringe	25.0	25.8	27.0	7.5	7.7	8.5
Medium and small	30.8	29.7	31.5	10.3	10.5	11.4
Nonmetropolitan counties						
Micropolitan	32.3	34.1	35.9	11.6	13.0	13.9
Nonmicropolitan	33.2	36.4	36.8	14.5	14.5	16.6
Hispanic Origin and Race[3]						
Hispanic or Latino						
Metropolitan counties						
Large central	17.7	17.9	20.5	10.4	11.3	11.5
Large fringe	18.3	17.5	21.8	9.0	8.1	10.2
Medium and small	21.5	23.6	23.6	11.6	11.2	11.6
Nonmetropolitan counties						
Micropolitan	23.1	22.8	22.7	13.1	10.6	9.9
Nonmicropolitan	21.8	29.4	30.0	10.3	13.8	13.8
Not Hispanic or Latino						
White only						
Metropolitan counties						
Large central	22.4	23.1	23.2	6.4	6.5	7.3
Large fringe	23.5	24.3	25.9	6.5	6.8	7.2
Medium and small	27.8	27.8	28.5	8.7	8.9	9.7
Nonmetropolitan counties						
Micropolitan	30.6	31.8	33.3	10.5	11.8	13.0
Nonmicropolitan	30.9	33.4	35.9	13.1	13.7	15.3
Black or African American only						
Metropolitan counties						
Large central	26.9	27.5	29.1	13.6	14.3	14.5
Large fringe	21.0	23.1	24.5	8.8	9.1	10.6
Medium and small	30.5	29.1	33.5	14.5	15.5	17.2
Nonmetropolitan counties						
Micropolitan	33.8	31.4	36.1	18.7	17.4	16.3
Nonmicropolitan	31.6	37.6	43.7	23.3	26.4	24.8
Percent of Poverty Level[4]						
Below 100%						
Metropolitan counties						
Large central	31.8	31.4	32.6	19.7	18.6	19.4
Large fringe	33.2	38.9	39.4	17.4	19.1	21.8
Medium and small	38.8	37.8	41.4	21.1	20.1	22.6
Nonmetropolitan counties						
Micropolitan	42.0	46.8	46.5	23.1	23.8	26.4
Nonmicropolitan	47.6	51.8	56.5	27.8	31.3	32.8
100%–199%						
Metropolitan counties						
Large central	24.7	25.2	28.3	12.7	13.3	14.3
Large fringe	30.8	31.1	34.5	13.6	14.1	15.3
Medium and small	32.9	33.8	34.1	15.1	15.5	16.8
Nonmetropolitan counties						
Micropolitan	38.2	39.0	39.6	17.2	19.3	19.7
Nonmicropolitan	39.5	40.8	45.4	19.8	19.6	22.3
200%–399%						
Metropolitan counties						
Large central	20.3	20.4	20.9	7.9	8.3	8.6
Large fringe	23.8	23.2	25.7	7.5	7.3	8.3
Medium and small	27.3	26.3	27.7	8.5	8.7	9.8
Nonmetropolitan counties						
Micropolitan	27.1	28.0	31.2	8.7	10.1	10.2
Nonmicropolitan	26.6	29.0	30.5	10.9	10.8	11.1

Table C-14. Selected Measures of Disability and Health Status Among Adults 18–64 Years of Age, by Urbanization Level and Selected Characteristics, Average Annual, 2002–2004 through 2008–2010—*Continued*

(Percent.)

Urbanization level and selected characteristic	Any basic actions difficulty or complex activity limitation[1]			Fair or poor respondent-assessed health status[2]		
	2002–2004	2005–2007	2008–2010	2002–2004	2005–2007	2008–2010
Percent of Poverty Level[4]						
400% or more						
Metropolitan counties						
Large central	17.6	17.7	18.0	4.0	4.4	4.4
Large fringe	18.4	19.0	19.1	3.7	3.9	3.7
Medium and small	21.2	21.1	21.3	4.5	4.5	4.9
Nonmetropolitan counties						
Micropolitan	22.8	22.4	22.7	4.8	5.3	5.0
Nonmicropolitan	20.0	23.4	22.2	5.2	5.9	6.0
PERCENT OF POPULATION, AGE-ADJUSTED[5]						
Geographic Region						
All regions						
Metropolitan counties						
Large central	22.0	22.1	22.8	8.9	9.1	9.5
Large fringe	21.9	22.2	23.4	6.7	6.8	7.4
Medium and small	27.0	26.7	27.7	9.4	9.5	10.5
Nonmetropolitan counties						
Micropolitan	29.8	29.4	31.2	10.9	11.6	12.3
Nonmicropolitan	29.1	31.2	32.8	13.2	13.1	14.0
Northeast						
Metropolitan counties						
Large central	20.0	20.9	20.9	8.9	10.1	9.4
Large fringe	21.3	21.7	21.9	6.6	5.8	6.3
Medium and small	24.6	23.1	27.9	7.1	7.2	8.6
Nonmetropolitan counties						
Micropolitan	31.0	29.4	34.9	9.4	9.1	10.4
Nonmicropolitan	24.8	32.9	28.3	8.2	9.6	10.7
Midwest						
Metropolitan counties						
Large central	26.3	26.4	26.9	9.1	9.0	10.7
Large fringe	24.0	25.4	25.1	6.2	7.6	7.8
Medium and small	28.2	26.9	26.1	8.1	8.0	9.4
Nonmetropolitan counties						
Micropolitan	26.5	26.8	28.3	7.7	9.1	10.5
Nonmicropolitan	26.9	26.8	27.7	8.5	9.5	8.8
South						
Metropolitan counties						
Large central	22.0	22.4	24.5	9.1	10.3	10.2
Large fringe	20.7	20.9	21.9	7.0	6.8	7.8
Medium and small	27.4	27.4	29.1	11.6	11.6	12.2
Nonmetropolitan counties						
Micropolitan	31.4	29.8	31.0	13.7	13.8	13.6
Nonmicropolitan	33.1	34.2	39.3	19.4	16.6	19.7
West						
Metropolitan counties						
Large central	20.8	19.9	20.3	8.7	7.9	8.5
Large fringe	22.6	21.7	26.5	7.1	7.3	7.9
Medium and small	26.6	27.8	26.7	8.6	9.2	10.1
Nonmetropolitan counties						
Micropolitan	30.1	34.5	35.7	10.3	12.1	13.6
Nonmicropolitan	*22.7	32.4	29.8	*7.3	13.0	12.3
Sex						
Men						
Metropolitan counties						
Large central	18.7	19.3	19.3	7.9	8.5	8.6
Large fringe	19.4	19.7	21.2	6.1	6.2	6.9
Medium and small	23.5	24.4	24.6	8.7	8.7	10.0
Nonmetropolitan counties						
Micropolitan	27.6	26.6	28.2	10.7	10.9	11.6
Nonmicropolitan	27.1	28.5	31.3	12.8	13.1	13.0
Women						
Metropolitan counties						
Large central	25.1	24.8	26.2	9.9	9.8	10.4
Large fringe	24.2	24.6	25.4	7.2	7.3	8.0
Medium and small	30.3	28.9	30.6	10.1	10.2	11.0
Nonmetropolitan counties						
Micropolitan	31.7	32.1	34.0	11.2	12.2	13.0
Nonmicropolitan	31.1	33.8	34.0	13.6	13.1	15.1

Table C-14. Selected Measures of Disability and Health Status Among Adults 18–64 Years of Age, by Urbanization Level and Selected Characteristics, Average Annual, 2002–2004 through 2008–2010—Continued

(Percent.)

Urbanization level and selected characteristic	Any basic actions difficulty or complex activity limitation[1]			Fair or poor respondent-assessed health status[2]		
	2002–2004	2005–2007	2008–2010	2002–2004	2005–2007	2008–2010
Hispanic Origin and Race[3]						
Hispanic or Latino						
Metropolitan counties						
Large central	19.9	19.9	22.0	12.4	12.8	12.6
Large fringe	20.9	19.2	22.9	10.7	9.3	11.3
Medium and small	24.3	26.1	26.0	13.7	13.0	13.1
Nonmetropolitan counties						
Micropolitan	26.0	24.7	26.7	15.5	12.7	11.5
Nonmicropolitan	27.5	30.0	32.1	12.3	14.5	14.9
Not Hispanic or Latino						
White only						
Metropolitan counties						
Large central	21.8	22.3	22.5	6.1	6.2	7.0
Large fringe	22.3	22.7	24.0	6.0	6.2	6.6
Medium and small	26.9	26.6	27.4	8.3	8.3	9.1
Nonmetropolitan counties						
Micropolitan	29.6	29.4	31.0	9.9	10.8	11.8
Nonmicropolitan	28.7	30.7	32.3	12.1	12.1	13.4
Black or African American only						
Metropolitan counties						
Large central	27.4	27.8	28.9	13.8	14.5	14.6
Large fringe	22.0	23.3	25.0	9.4	9.2	10.6
Medium and small	30.9	29.7	33.2	15.0	16.0	17.2
Nonmetropolitan counties						
Micropolitan	34.0	31.6	35.5	18.6	17.3	16.1
Nonmicropolitan	33.3	32.5	42.3	24.1	24.6	23.0
Percent of Poverty Level[4]						
Below 100%						
Metropolitan counties						
Large central	36.3	37.2	38.0	23.5	22.6	22.8
Large fringe	39.4	43.5	43.1	20.9	22.0	24.1
Medium and small	45.3	45.1	47.6	25.6	25.0	27.6
Nonmetropolitan counties						
Micropolitan	48.7	51.1	50.6	27.3	26.3	29.2
Nonmicropolitan	49.9	51.3	56.7	29.5	31.5	33.1
100%–199%						
Metropolitan counties						
Large central	27.9	28.2	30.1	14.6	15.0	15.8
Large fringe	33.0	31.8	35.8	14.8	14.7	16.0
Medium and small	36.0	36.6	36.8	16.9	17.2	18.4
Nonmetropolitan counties						
Micropolitan	39.4	39.3	40.3	18.0	19.9	19.5
Nonmicropolitan	39.4	39.9	41.6	19.8	18.6	21.0
200%–399%						
Metropolitan counties						
Large central	21.4	20.9	21.4	8.4	8.6	8.7
Large fringe	24.0	23.5	25.3	7.6	7.3	8.1
Medium and small	27.6	26.2	27.6	8.6	8.6	9.6
Nonmetropolitan counties						
Micropolitan	26.9	26.6	29.5	8.5	9.5	9.5
Nonmicropolitan	25.0	26.3	26.8	10.2	9.5	9.6
400% or more						
Metropolitan counties						
Large central	16.7	16.7	16.7	3.8	4.0	3.9
Large fringe	17.0	17.5	16.8	3.4	3.5	3.2
Medium and small	19.3	18.3	18.7	3.9	3.7	4.1
Nonmetropolitan counties						
Micropolitan	19.9	17.8	18.8	3.9	4.2	4.0
Nonmicropolitan	16.1	19.1	18.7	4.3	4.8	4.5

* = Figure does not meet standards of reliability or precision.
[1]Any basic actions difficulty or complex activity limitation is defined as having one or more of the following limitations or difficulties: movement difficulty, emotional difficulty, sensory (seeing or hearing) difficulty, cognitive difficulty, self-care (activities of daily living or instrumental activities of daily living) limitation, social limitation, or work limitation.
[2]Based on responses to the question, "Would you say person's health in general is excellent, very good, good, fair, or poor?"
[3]Persons of Hispanic origin may be of any race.
[4]Percent of poverty level is based on family income and family size and composition using U.S. Census Bureau poverty thresholds.
[5]Estimates are age-adjusted to the year 2000 standard population using four age groups: 18–24 years, 25–34 years, 35–44 years, and 45–64 years.

Table C-15. Serious Psychological Distress[1] in the Past 30 Days Among Adults 18 Years of Age and Over, by Selected Characteristics, Average Annual, Selected Years, 1997–1998 through 2009–2010

(Percent.)

Characteristic	1997–1998	1999–2000	2000–2001	2001–2002	2002–2003	2003–2004	2004–2005	2006–2007	2007–2008	2008–2009	2009–2010
18 years and over, age-adjusted[2,3]	3.2	2.6	3.0	3.1	3.1	3.1	3.0	2.8	2.9	3.2	3.2
18 years and over, crude[3]	3.2	2.6	3.0	3.1	3.1	3.1	3.0	2.9	2.9	3.2	3.3
Age											
18–44 years	2.9	2.3	2.7	2.9	2.9	2.9	2.8	2.5	2.7	3.1	3.1
18–24 years	2.7	2.2	2.6	2.8	2.8	2.8	2.5	2.0	2.3	2.5	2.4
25–44 years	3.0	2.4	2.8	3.0	2.9	2.9	2.9	2.7	2.8	3.3	3.4
45–64 years	3.7	3.2	3.6	3.9	4.0	3.9	3.7	3.7	3.6	3.7	4.1
45–54 years	3.9	3.5	3.7	4.2	4.2	3.9	3.9	3.7	3.6	3.9	4.1
55–64 years	3.4	2.6	3.4	3.4	3.6	3.9	3.4	3.8	3.6	3.6	4.0
65 years and over	3.1	2.4	2.7	2.4	2.3	2.4	2.5	2.1	2.4	2.4	2.1
65–74 years	2.5	2.3	2.8	2.4	2.3	2.3	2.2	2.1	2.4	2.2	2.0
75 years and over	3.8	2.5	2.5	2.4	2.3	2.5	2.9	2.0	2.4	2.6	2.3
Sex[2]											
Male	2.5	2.0	2.4	2.4	2.3	2.3	2.3	2.1	2.2	2.7	2.8
Female	3.8	3.1	3.5	3.8	3.9	3.9	3.7	3.4	3.5	3.6	3.7
Race[2,4]											
White only	3.1	2.5	2.9	3.0	3.0	3.1	2.9	2.7	2.9	3.2	3.2
Black or African American only	4.0	2.9	3.1	3.5	3.4	3.4	3.6	3.2	3.2	3.7	3.8
American Indian or Alaska Native only	7.8	*7.2	*7.4	8.1	*7.1	*5.5	*3.5	*3.9	*	*3.8	*5.2
Asian only	2.0	*1.4	*2.0	*1.8	*1.9	*1.8	1.7	2.0	*1.0	*1.1	1.6
Native Hawaiian or Other Pacific Islander only	—	*	*	*	*	*	*	*	*	*	*
2 or more races	—	4.8	5.5	5.0	7.3	9.1	7.9	6.5	5.9	*4.9	5.2
Hispanic Origin and Race[2,4]											
Hispanic or Latino	5.0	3.5	4.0	4.0	3.9	3.9	3.7	3.4	3.6	3.4	3.6
Mexican	5.2	2.9	3.4	3.8	3.7	3.6	3.6	3.2	3.3	2.9	2.8
Not Hispanic or Latino	3.0	2.5	2.9	3.1	3.1	3.1	3.0	2.8	2.8	3.1	3.2
White only	2.9	2.4	2.9	3.0	3.0	3.0	2.9	2.7	2.9	3.2	3.1
Black or African American only	3.9	2.9	3.1	3.5	3.4	3.3	3.6	3.2	3.1	3.7	3.8
Percent of Poverty Level[2,5]											
Below 100%	9.1	6.8	7.7	8.4	8.6	8.8	8.6	7.2	8.3	9.0	8.4
100%–199%	5.0	4.4	5.0	5.2	5.2	5.2	5.0	5.0	4.7	4.9	4.8
200%–399%	2.5	2.3	2.7	2.8	2.6	2.5	2.5	2.1	2.4	2.7	2.8
400% or more	1.3	1.2	1.2	1.3	1.3	1.2	1.1	1.2	1.1	1.1	1.2
Hispanic Origin and Race and Percent of Poverty Level[2,4,5]											
Hispanic or Latino											
Below 100%	8.6	6.1	6.9	7.5	7.6	7.4	6.6	6.0	7.0	6.7	6.4
100%–199%	5.4	3.8	4.4	4.1	3.8	3.7	3.9	2.9	4.5	4.5	4.1
200%–399%	3.4	2.1	3.0	3.5	3.0	2.5	2.6	2.8	2.2	1.8	2.6
400% or more	*	2.3	*1.6	*	*	*1.8	*1.9	*2.2	*1.6	*1.0	*1.5
Not Hispanic or Latino											
White only											
Below 100%	9.6	7.8	8.9	9.2	9.6	10.4	10.2	8.8	10.7	11.2	10.1
100%–199%	5.2	4.9	5.5	5.9	6.1	6.1	5.6	6.0	5.4	5.7	5.5
200%–399%	2.5	2.3	2.9	2.9	2.7	2.6	2.6	2.1	2.6	3.1	3.2
400% or more	1.3	1.1	1.2	1.3	1.3	1.2	1.1	1.1	1.0	1.0	1.1
Black or African American only											
Below 100%	8.7	6.0	6.3	7.2	7.1	7.4	7.6	6.2	6.2	8.0	8.3
100%–199%	4.3	3.6	4.3	4.9	4.5	4.1	4.8	4.3	3.6	3.1	3.5
200%–399%	2.2	*1.7	1.9	2.3	2.0	1.9	2.1	2.0	2.4	2.9	2.5
400% or more	*	*1.0	*	*	*1.2	*	*	*	*	*	*1.6
Geographic Region[2]											
Northeast	2.7	1.9	2.5	2.8	3.0	2.9	2.5	2.6	2.6	2.9	3.1
Midwest	2.6	2.5	2.8	2.9	2.7	2.7	2.7	2.9	2.7	3.2	3.3
South	3.8	2.9	3.2	3.5	3.5	3.5	3.7	3.1	3.3	3.5	3.5
West	3.3	2.8	3.2	3.0	3.0	3.0	2.8	2.5	2.7	2.8	2.9
Location of Residence[2]											
Within MSA[6]	3.0	2.3	2.8	3.0	2.9	2.9	2.8	2.6	2.7	3.0	3.1
Outside MSA[6]	3.9	3.5	3.6	3.8	3.9	3.8	4.0	3.7	3.7	4.0	4.1

* = Figure does not meet standards of reliability or precision.
— = Data not available.
[1]Serious psychological distress is measured by a six-question scale that asks respondents how often they experienced each of six symptoms of psychological distress in the past 30 days.
[2]Estimates are age-adjusted to the year 2000 standard population using five age groups: 18–44 years, 45–54 years, 55–64 years, 65–74 years, and 75 years and over.
[3]Includes all other races not shown separately.
[4]The race groups, White, Black, American Indian or Alaska Native, Asian, Native Hawaiian or Other Pacific Islander, and 2 or more races, include persons of Hispanic and non-Hispanic origin. Persons of Hispanic origin may be of any race.
[5]Percent of poverty level is based on family income and family size and composition using U.S. Census Bureau poverty thresholds.
[6]MSA = metropolitan statistical area.

Table C-16. Children Under 18 Years of Age Who Suffer From Asthma, by Selected Characteristics, Average Annual, Selected Years, 1997–1999 through 2008–2010

(Rate.)

Characteristic	Current asthma[1]				Asthma attack in the past 12 months[2]			
	1997–1999	2000–2002	2003–2005	2008–2010	1997–1999	2000–2002	2003–2005	2008–2010
Under 18 Years[3]	—	—	8.7	9.5	5.4	5.7	5.4	5.6
Age								
0–4 years	—	—	6.1	6.2	4.3	4.7	4.2	4.4
5–17 years	—	—	9.6	10.8	5.7	6.1	5.8	6.1
5–9 years	—	—	9.1	10.7	5.6	6.3	6.1	6.5
10–17 years	—	—	9.9	10.9	5.8	5.9	5.7	5.8
Sex								
Male	—	—	9.9	11.1	6.2	6.6	6.3	6.5
Female	—	—	7.3	7.8	4.5	4.7	4.4	4.6
Race[4]								
White only	—	—	7.7	8.2	5.0	5.2	4.9	4.9
Black or African American only	—	—	13.0	16.0	7.0	8.0	7.6	8.7
American Indian or Alaska Native only	—	—	12.2	*10.3	6.4	*8.7	*6.1	*
Asian only	—	—	4.8	6.7	4.3	4.7	3.3	4.8
Native Hawaiian or Other Pacific Islander only	—	—	*	*	—	*	*	*
2 or more races	—	—	13.5	12.8	—	7.3	8.8	9.0
Hispanic Origin and Race[4]								
Hispanic or Latino	—	—	7.6	7.5	4.8	4.2	4.6	4.4
Not Hispanic or Latino	—	—	8.9	10.0	5.5	6.0	5.6	5.9
White only	—	—	7.9	8.5	5.1	5.5	5.0	5.1
Black or African American only	—	—	13.0	16.2	7.0	7.9	7.5	8.8
Percent of Poverty Level[5]								
Below 100%	—	—	10.4	12.4	6.1	7.1	6.5	7.4
100%–199%	—	—	8.6	9.9	5.3	5.4	5.2	6.0
200%–399%	—	—	8.3	8.2	5.0	5.3	5.2	4.6
400% or more	—	—	7.9	8.2	5.2	5.5	4.9	5.0
Health Insurance Status at the Time of Interview[6]								
Insured	—	—	9.0	9.8	5.6	5.9	5.6	5.8
Private	—	—	8.0	8.4	5.0	5.3	5.0	5.1
Medicaid	—	—	11.4	12.0	7.7	7.7	7.1	7.0
Uninsured	—	—	5.6	6.6	3.9	4.3	3.3	3.6

— = Data not available.
* = Figure does not meet standard of reliability or precision.
[1]Based on parent or knowledgeable adult responding to both questions, "Has a doctor or other health professional ever told you that your child had asthma?" and "Does your child still have asthma?"
[2]Based on parent or knowledgeable adult responding to both questions, "Has a doctor or other health professional ever told you that your child had asthma?" and "During the past 12 months, did your child have an episode of asthma or an asthma attack?"
[3]Includes all other races not shown separately, unknown poverty level, and unknown health insurance status.
[4]The race groups, White, Black, American Indian or Alaska Native, Asian, Native Hawaiian or Other Pacific Islander, and 2 or more races, include persons of Hispanic and non-Hispanic origin. Persons of Hispanic origin may be of any race.
[5]Percent of poverty level is based on family income and family size and composition using U.S. Census Bureau poverty thresholds. Missing family income data were imputed for 1997 and beyond.
[6]Health insurance categories are mutually exclusive. Persons who reported both Medicaid and private coverage are classified as having private coverage.

Table C-17. Hypertension Among Persons 20 Years of Age and Over, by Selected Characteristics, Selected Years, 1988–1994 through 2007–2010

(Percent.)

Characteristic	Hypertension[1,2]			Uncontrolled high blood pressure among persons with hypertension[3]		
	1988–1994	2001–2004	2007–2010	1988–1994	2001–2004	2005–2008
20 Years and Over, Age-Adjusted[4]						
Both sexes[5]	25.5	30.9	30.6	77.2	66.0	59.4
Male	26.4	30.3	31.3	83.2	68.3	63.8
Female	24.4	31.0	29.6	68.5	57.6	48.5
Not Hispanic or Latino:						
White only, male	25.6	29.3	31.1	82.6	67.8	60.8
White only, female	23.0	29.0	28.1	67.0	52.7	47.4
Black or African American only, male	37.5	41.5	40.5	84.0	70.8	70.6
Black or African American only, female	38.3	44.3	44.3	71.1	65.4	51.5
Mexican male[6]	26.9	26.1	28.6	87.9	76.4	68.8
Mexican female[6]	25.0	29.7	27.8	77.6	63.8	65.3
Percent of Poverty Level[7]						
Below 100%	31.7	35.5	33.8	75.0	66.1	57.7
100%–199%	26.6	34.0	33.4	76.0	70.1	65.7
200%–399%	24.7	31.4	31.7	76.2	67.8	58.8
400% or more	22.6	27.9	28.5	81.5	60.8	56.7
20 Years and Over, Crude						
Both sexes[6]	24.1	30.8	32.2	73.9	63.0	54.1
Male	23.8	29.0	31.7	79.3	62.1	56.3
Female	24.4	32.5	32.8	68.8	63.7	52.1
Not Hispanic or Latino:						
White only, male	24.3	29.9	33.7	78.0	59.4	53.6
White only, female	24.6	32.9	33.4	67.8	63.8	51.1
Black or African American only, male	31.1	36.7	37.6	83.3	68.7	64.2
Black or African American only, female	32.5	41.6	44.4	70.0	61.9	51.8
Mexican male	16.4	15.8	19.9	86.5	73.6	64.0
Mexican female	15.9	19.0	21.4	80.6	69.8	62.8
Percent of Poverty Level[7]						
Below 100%	25.7	28.3	27.5	74.0	67.3	58.8
100%–199%	26.7	34.6	36.2	75.1	64.5	61.9
200%–399%	22.4	31.5	34.2	73.4	63.4	52.0
400% or more	22.0	28.4	30.6	74.3	59.2	49.5
Male						
20–44 years	10.9	12.3	12.5	90.5	71.0	72.5
20–34 years	7.1	7.0	6.8	92.6	87.1	81.4
35–44 years	17.1	19.2	20.7	89.0	63.2	66.9
45–64 years	34.2	39.9	41.2	73.1	61.1	52.8
45–54 years	29.2	35.9	35.5	76.2	64.9	55.4
55–64 years	40.6	47.5	49.5	70.3	55.5	50.0
65–74 years	54.4	61.7	64.1	74.3	49.5	47.7
75 years and over	60.4	67.1	71.7	82.5	68.3	53.5
Female						
20–44 years	6.5	7.7	8.3	63.4	51.0	42.6
20–34 years	2.9	*2.7	3.8	82.2	*50.2	49.1
35–44 years	11.2	14.0	14.2	56.8	51.2	40.9
45–64 years	32.8	42.6	39.7	62.1	60.9	49.5
45–54 years	23.9	35.2	31.2	58.5	66.1	46.3
55–64 years	42.6	54.4	50.4	64.3	55.6	52.4
65–74 years	56.2	72.9	69.3	68.7	67.2	51.2
75 years and over	73.6	82.0	81.3	81.9	72.4	62.9

* = Figure does not meet standards of reliability or precision.
[1]Hypertension is defined as having measured high blood pressure and/or taking antihypertensive medication.
[2]Respondents were asked, "Are you now taking prescribed medicine for your high blood pressure?"
[3]Uncontrolled high blood pressure among persons with hypertension is defined as measured systolic pressure of at least 140 mmHg or diastolic pressure of at least 90 mmHg, among those with measured high blood pressure or reporting taking antihypertensive medication.
[4]Age-adjusted to the 2000 standard population using five age groups: 20–34 years, 35–44 years, 45–54 years, 55–64 years, and 65 years and over.
[5]Includes persons of all races and Hispanic origins, not just those shown separately.
[6]Persons of Mexican origin may be of any race.
[7]Percent of poverty level is based on family income and family size.

Table C-18. Cholesterol Among Persons 20 Years of Age and Over, by Selected Characteristics, Selected Years, 1988–1994 through 2007–2010

(Percent.)

Characteristic	1988–1994	1999–2002	2001–2004	2003–2006	2005–2008	2007–2010
PERCENT OF POPULATION WITH HIGH CHOLESTEROL (GREATER THAN OR EQUAL TO 240 MG/DL OR TAKING CHOLESTEROL-LOWERING MEDICATIONS)[1]						
20 Years and Over, Age-Adjusted[2]						
Both sexes	22.8	25.0	26.3	27.7	27.5	27.4
Male	21.1	25.3	27.1	27.7	27.3	28.0
Female	24.0	24.3	25.2	27.4	27.5	26.7
Not Hispanic or Latino						
White only, male	21.1	26.0	27.7	28.7	27.9	28.1
White only, female	24.2	25.1	25.8	28.2	28.1	27.4
Black or African American only, male	18.6	20.1	22.5	22.8	24.1	25.4
Black or African American only, female	23.1	22.0	22.3	23.3	25.3	25.6
Mexican male[3]	19.9	21.6	23.3	24.2	26.2	28.6
Mexican female[3]	19.8	19.3	21.7	24.1	25.0	25.5
Percent of Poverty Level[4]						
Below 100%	23.0	25.0	27.2	27.9	27.1	26.5
100%–199%	22.1	25.9	26.9	27.6	26.3	27.6
200%–399%	23.1	26.5	26.8	27.5	28.7	28.9
400% or more	21.7	23.1	25.7	27.9	27.5	26.6
20 Years and Over, Crude						
Both sexes	21.5	25.0	26.1	28.0	28.4	28.7
Male	19.6	25.1	26.7	27.5	27.7	28.7
Female	23.2	24.8	25.5	28.5	29.1	28.7
Not Hispanic or Latino						
White only, male	20.0	26.8	28.5	29.7	29.7	30.4
White only, female	24.5	27.0	27.6	30.8	31.2	31.4
Black or African American only, male	16.0	18.5	20.9	21.3	22.7	24.1
Black or African American only, female	19.7	19.9	20.0	21.9	24.5	24.7
Mexican male[3]	16.2	17.0	18.4	19.3	21.1	23.7
Mexican female[3]	14.9	13.8	15.2	18.7	20.6	21.0
Percent of Poverty Level[4]						
Below 100%	19.4	21.6	22.8	24.1	23.1	22.3
100%–199%	21.3	25.4	26.2	28.3	27.8	28.7
200%–399%	21.3	26.2	26.8	28.1	29.8	30.6
400% or more	21.9	24.2	26.8	28.7	28.9	29.6
Male						
20–44 years	13.1	16.1	16.4	16.5	14.9	14.3
20–34 years	8.2	10.4	9.6	10.2	10.1	8.5
35–44 years	21.0	23.1	25.3	25.2	21.5	22.5
45–64 years	30.1	36.0	36.9	35.7	37.0	39.0
45–54 years	29.6	34.1	33.3	32.4	33.2	34.0
55–64 years	30.8	39.1	43.8	41.6	43.4	46.2
65–74 years	27.4	36.3	42.9	49.4	49.5	48.9
75 years and over	24.4	29.0	34.4	37.1	39.4	45.2
Female						
20–44 years	9.9	11.4	11.4	12.9	12.7	10.6
20–34 years	7.3	9.1	9.4	10.8	9.5	6.8
35–44 years	13.5	14.4	14.3	15.8	17.0	15.7
45–64 years	36.4	31.7	33.5	37.3	38.2	39.1
45–54 years	28.2	27.2	26.8	29.6	29.9	29.1
55–64 years	45.8	39.2	43.9	49.2	50.0	51.4
65–74 years	46.9	51.9	54.4	55.3	51.8	53.3
75 years and over	41.2	44.0	45.3	47.3	51.7	52.5
MEAN SERUM TOTAL CHOLESTEROL LEVEL, MG/DL						
20 Years and Over, Age-Adjusted[2]						
Both sexes	206	203	202	200	198	196
Male	204	202	201	198	195	194
Female	207	204	202	202	200	198
Not Hispanic or Latino:						
White only, male	205	202	201	198	194	193
White only, female	208	205	203	203	201	199
Black or African American only, male	202	195	198	193	190	191
Black or African American only, female	207	202	199	195	193	192
Mexican male[3]	206	204	201	203	202	200
Mexican female[3]	206	199	200	200	198	196

Table C-18. Cholesterol Among Persons 20 Years of Age and Over, by Selected Characteristics, Selected Years, 1988–1994 through 2007–2010—Continued

(Percent.)

Characteristic	1988–1994	1999–2002	2001–2004	2003–2006	2005–2008	2007–2010
Percent of Poverty Level[4]						
Below 100%	205	201	203	203	198	196
100%–199%	205	204	202	201	199	198
200%–399%	207	205	202	199	197	196
400% or more	205	202	201	201	197	195
20 Years and Over, Crude						
Both sexes	204	203	202	200	198	197
Male	202	202	201	198	195	194
Female	206	204	203	202	201	199
Not Hispanic or Latino:						
White only, male	203	203	201	198	195	193
White only, female	208	206	205	205	203	201
Black or African American only, male	198	194	197	192	190	191
Black or African American only, female	201	199	196	194	193	191
Mexican male[3]	199	200	198	200	201	200
Mexican female[3]	198	194	194	196	196	195
Percent of Poverty Level[4]						
Below 100%	200	198	199	200	196	194
100%–199%	202	202	200	199	198	197
200%–399%	205	204	202	199	197	197
400% or more	206	204	203	203	200	198
Male						
20–44 years	194	196	197	196	194	194
20–34 years	186	188	186	186	186	186
35–44 years	206	207	210	209	205	205
45–64 years	216	213	211	206	203	202
45–54 years	216	215	213	208	205	204
55–64 years	216	212	208	202	199	199
65–74 years	212	202	194	191	184	182
75 years and over	205	195	194	187	179	176
Female						
20–44 years	189	191	191	192	190	187
20–34 years	184	185	186	188	186	181
35–44 years	195	198	198	197	196	195
45–64 years	225	215	213	213	212	211
45–54 years	217	211	209	208	209	208
55–64 years	235	221	219	219	216	214
65–74 years	233	224	219	214	209	207
75 years and over	229	217	213	206	203	203

[1]High cholesterol is defined as measured serum total cholesterol as greater than or equal to 240 mg/dL or reporting taking cholesterol-lowering medications. Respondents were asked, "Are you now following this advice [from a doctor of health professional] to take prescribed medicine [to lower your cholesterol]?"
[2]Age-adjusted to the 2000 standard population using five age groups: 20–34 years, 35–44 years, 45–54 years, 55–64 years, and 65 years and over.
[3]Persons of Mexican origin may be of any race.
[4]Percent of poverty level is based on family income and family size. Persons with unknown percent of poverty level are excluded.

PART C: HEALTH

Table C-19. Mean Energy and Macronutrient Intake Among Persons 20 Years of Age and Over, by Sex and Age, Selected Years, 1971–1974 through 2005–2008

(Number, percent.)

Sex and age	1971–1974	1976–1980	1988–1994	1999–2002	2003–2006	2005–2008
Mean Energy Intake in Kilocalories (kcal)						
Male, age-adjusted[1]	2,450	2,439	2,592	2,570	2,654	2,656
Male, crude	2,461	2,459	2,648	2,593	2,671	2,672
20–39 years	2,784	2,753	2,964	2,854	2,978	2,946
40–59 years	2,303	2,315	2,567	2,601	2,693	2,702
60–74 years	1,918	1,906	2,104	2,124	2,137	2,170
75 years and over	—	—	1,814	1,876	1,865	1,941
Female, age-adjusted[1]	1,542	1,522	1,762	1,837	1,836	1,811
Female, crude	1,540	1,525	1,772	1,832	1,828	1,803
20–39 years	1,652	1,643	1,956	2,031	2,001	1,973
40–59 years	1,510	1,473	1,734	1,823	1,823	1,798
60–74 years	1,325	1,322	1,520	1,582	1,633	1,605
75 years and over	—	—	1,401	1,435	1,472	1,466
Percent Kcal from Carbohydrates						
Male, age-adjusted[1]	42.4	42.6	48.5	49.1	47.7	47.4
Male, crude	42.4	42.7	48.4	49.0	47.6	47.4
20–39 years	42.2	43.1	48.1	50.1	48.5	48.0
40–59 years	41.6	41.5	47.8	47.7	46.4	46.5
60–74 years	44.8	44.1	49.7	48.9	47.0	47.3
75 years and over	—	—	50.9	50.8	50.4	49.0
Female, age-adjusted[1]	45.4	46.0	51.0	51.7	49.7	49.5
Female, crude	45.5	46.1	51.0	51.7	49.7	49.4
20–39 years	45.8	46.0	50.6	52.6	50.0	50.0
40–59 years	44.4	45.0	50.0	50.4	48.5	48.0
60–74 years	46.8	48.6	52.6	51.4	50.2	49.9
75 years and over	—	—	54.2	53.5	52.6	52.6
Percent Kcal from Protein						
Male, age-adjusted[1]	16.5	16.1	15.5	15.3	15.5	15.6
Male, crude	16.4	16.0	15.4	15.3	15.5	15.6
20–39 years	16.1	15.8	15.0	14.8	15.4	15.5
40–59 years	16.9	16.3	15.7	15.5	15.4	15.5
60–74 years	16.5	16.3	15.9	16.2	16.0	16.2
75 years and over	—	—	16.3	15.7	15.8	15.7
Female, age-adjusted[1]	16.9	16.0	15.4	15.1	15.6	15.8
Female, crude	16.8	16.0	15.4	15.1	15.6	15.9
20–39 years	16.4	15.8	14.8	14.6	15.3	15.4
40–59 years	17.3	16.3	15.6	15.3	15.7	16.4
60–74 years	17.0	16.1	16.4	16.0	15.9	15.9
75 years and over	—	—	15.9	15.3	15.6	15.6
Percent Kcal from Total Fat						
Male, age-adjusted[1]	36.9	36.7	33.8	33.0	33.5	33.6
Male, crude	36.9	36.7	33.9	33.0	33.5	33.6
20–39 years	37.0	36.2	34.0	32.1	32.5	32.7
40–59 years	36.9	37.2	34.2	33.7	34.2	34.1
60–74 years	36.4	36.8	32.9	33.8	34.7	34.2
75 years and over	—	—	32.9	33.5	33.1	34.1
Female, age-adjusted[1]	36.1	36.0	33.2	33.2	33.9	33.8
Female, crude	36.0	35.9	33.2	33.2	33.9	33.8
20–39 years	36.3	36.0	33.6	32.5	33.6	33.6
40–59 years	36.3	36.4	34.0	33.9	34.4	34.2
60–74 years	34.9	34.7	31.6	33.4	34.2	34.2
75 years and over	—	—	31.5	32.8	32.7	32.5
Percent Kcal from Saturated Fat						
Male, age-adjusted[1]	13.5	13.2	11.3	10.8	11.1	11.1
Male, crude	13.5	13.2	11.4	10.8	11.1	11.1
20–39 years	13.6	13.1	11.5	10.7	10.9	11.0
40–59 years	13.5	13.4	11.3	10.8	11.2	11.2
60–74 years	13.3	13.1	10.9	10.7	11.3	11.2
75 years and over	—	—	11.2	10.8	11.1	11.5
Female, age-adjusted[1]	13.0	12.5	11.1	10.7	11.2	11.3
Female, crude	12.9	12.5	11.1	10.7	11.2	11.3
20–39 years	13.0	12.6	11.4	10.8	11.1	11.2
40–59 years	13.1	12.6	11.3	10.9	11.5	11.5
60–74 years	12.4	11.8	10.4	10.5	11.1	11.3
75 years and over	—	—	10.5	10.2	10.8	10.9

— = Data not available.

[1] Age-adjusted to the 2000 standard population using four age groups: 20–39 years, 40–59 years, 60–74 years, and 75 years and over. Age-adjusted estimates in this table may differ from other age-adjusted estimates based on the same data and presented elsewhere if different age groups are used in the adjustment procedure.

Table C-20. Participation in Leisure-Time Aerobic and Muscle-Strengthening Activities that Meet the 2008 Federal Physical Activity Guidelines for Adults 18 Years of Age and Over, by Selected Characteristics, Selected Years, 1998–2010

(Percent.)

Characteristic	Met both aerobic activity and muscle-strengthening guidelines		Met neither aerobic activity nor muscle-strengthening guideline		Met aerobic activity guideline		Met muscle-strengthening guideline	
	2000	2010	2000	2010	2000	2010	2000	2010
18 years and over, age-adjusted[1,2]	15.0	20.7	54.7	49.1	42.2	47.3	18.0	24.4
18 years and over, crude[2]	15.1	20.4	54.6	49.5	42.4	46.9	18.1	24.0
Age								
18–44 years	18.9	25.7	49.1	43.1	47.7	53.8	22.1	28.8
18–24 years	23.8	29.6	44.5	39.4	52.2	57.2	27.2	32.8
25–44 years	17.3	24.3	50.6	44.4	46.3	52.5	20.5	27.4
45–64 years	12.8	17.7	57.6	51.0	39.7	45.2	15.5	21.5
45–54 years	14.5	19.2	55.4	48.9	42.1	47.6	17.0	22.6
55–64 years	10.1	15.9	61.0	53.7	36.1	42.1	13.1	20.1
65 years and over	6.8	10.4	67.0	64.6	30.1	30.5	9.8	15.4
65–74 years	8.4	13.6	60.3	59.9	36.8	35.9	11.3	17.9
75 years and over	4.9	6.4	75.0	70.3	22.1	23.9	8.0	12.3
Sex[1]								
Male	17.9	25.1	49.6	43.8	47.4	52.1	20.8	29.1
Female	12.3	16.5	59.4	54.0	37.6	42.7	15.4	19.8
Sex and Age								
Male								
18–44 years	23.0	31.8	43.0	37.1	53.6	59.0	26.3	35.6
45–54 years	16.0	20.9	52.7	45.2	45.2	50.7	18.0	24.8
55–64 years	11.3	19.1	58.7	50.1	38.9	46.0	13.8	22.9
65–74 years	9.4	16.6	55.3	55.6	41.8	40.7	12.2	20.6
75 years and over	7.1	9.1	66.7	62.8	30.7	32.3	10.1	14.5
Female								
18–44 years	15.0	19.6	55.0	49.0	42.0	48.5	17.9	22.1
45–54 years	13.1	17.5	57.9	52.4	39.1	44.7	16.1	20.4
55–64 years	9.0	13.1	63.1	57.0	33.5	38.6	12.4	17.5
65–74 years	7.7	11.0	64.3	63.6	32.6	31.8	10.5	15.6
75 years and over	3.6	4.6	80.0	75.3	16.8	18.3	6.7	10.8
Race[1,3]								
White only	15.7	21.4	53.1	47.6	44.1	48.9	18.5	24.8
Black or African American only	12.2	17.2	64.6	58.5	31.7	37.3	16.0	21.4
American Indian or Alaska Native only	*10.6	*12.7	67.1	54.0	29.7	42.0	13.9	16.7
Asian only	14.1	17.8	55.0	51.7	41.7	44.2	17.2	21.9
Native Hawaiian or Other Pacific Islander only	*	*	*	*	*	*	*	*
2 or more races	19.0	25.9	52.8	45.0	43.9	50.2	22.2	30.4
Hispanic Origin and Race[1,3]								
Hispanic or Latino	9.2	14.4	66.5	60.2	30.8	36.2	11.9	18.1
Mexican	8.1	13.2	67.0	60.7	30.0	35.9	11.3	16.7
Not Hispanic or Latino	15.8	21.9	53.2	47.2	43.7	49.1	18.8	25.5
White only	16.5	22.9	51.4	45.0	45.7	51.5	19.3	26.3
Black or African American only	12.2	17.4	64.6	58.4	31.7	37.3	16.0	21.6
Education[4]								
No high school diploma or GED	4.3	7.7	74.0	69.8	23.9	27.1	6.6	10.9
High school diploma or GED	9.5	12.7	61.7	59.0	35.7	37.3	12.1	16.2
Some college or more	18.9	25.0	47.1	42.1	49.4	53.9	22.4	28.9
Percent of Poverty Level[1,5]								
Below 100%	9.3	12.0	68.0	63.9	29.3	32.2	12.3	15.8
100%–199%	9.0	12.7	65.5	60.6	32.0	36.0	11.5	16.1
200%–399%	13.2	19.2	56.8	50.6	39.9	45.5	16.5	23.1
400% or more	20.5	29.1	45.0	36.9	52.0	59.3	23.4	32.8

Table C-20. Participation in Leisure-Time Aerobic and Muscle-Strengthening Activities that Meet the 2008 Federal Physical Activity Guidelines for Adults 18 Years of Age and Over, by Selected Characteristics, Selected Years, 1998–2010—*Continued*

(Percent.)

Characteristic	Met both aerobic activity and muscle-strengthening guidelines		Met neither aerobic activity nor muscle-strengthening guideline		Met aerobic activity guideline		Met muscle-strengthening guideline	
	2000	2010	2000	2010	2000	2010	2000	2010
Hispanic Origin and Race and Percent of Poverty Level[1,3,5]								
Hispanic or Latino								
Below 100%	4.4	8.9	75.2	68.6	22.1	27.8	7.2	12.4
100%–199%	5.0	9.3	72.2	66.7	25.8	30.1	7.1	12.6
200%–399%	10.2	15.7	63.1	57.6	33.0	38.8	14.0	19.5
400% or more	19.6	28.1	52.8	42.5	45.1	53.4	21.7	32.1
Not Hispanic or Latino								
White only								
Below 100%	11.7	13.7	63.5	60.5	34.0	35.5	14.7	17.5
100%–199%	10.3	14.1	62.6	56.4	34.8	40.6	12.9	17.0
200%–399%	13.9	20.0	54.7	48.6	42.3	47.8	16.9	23.6
400% or more	21.0	29.9	43.7	35.2	53.4	61.0	23.8	33.5
Black or African American only								
Below 100%	9.5	11.3	72.1	66.9	25.4	29.3	12.1	15.3
100%–199%	9.5	11.7	69.2	67.0	28.0	28.5	12.3	16.0
200%–399%	11.8	20.8	64.3	53.3	31.4	41.9	16.2	25.7
400% or more	17.6	26.1	54.9	47.7	40.3	48.5	22.4	29.8
Disability Measure[1,6]								
Any basic actions difficulty or complex activity limitation	10.3	13.6	62.2	59.1	34.2	36.4	14.0	18.0
Any basic actions difficulty	10.3	13.8	62.1	59.2	34.0	36.6	14.2	18.1
Any complex activity limitation	7.2	8.9	71.2	67.2	24.9	27.9	11.3	13.9
No disability	17.0	24.2	50.6	43.3	46.6	53.4	19.8	27.4
Geographic Region[1]								
Northeast	17.0	20.2	51.8	49.1	45.3	46.9	20.0	24.3
Midwest	16.4	20.7	53.4	49.7	43.5	46.1	19.3	24.7
South	12.1	18.8	59.7	51.8	37.3	45.0	15.1	22.0
West	16.7	24.0	50.1	44.5	46.9	52.0	19.7	27.5
Location of residence[1]								
Within MSA[7]	15.7	21.8	54.1	47.8	42.9	48.7	18.6	25.4
Outside MSA[7]	12.3	14.5	56.9	56.9	39.9	39.1	15.5	18.5

* = Figure does not meet standards of reliability or precision.
— = Data not available.
[1]Estimates are age-adjusted to the year 2000 standard population using five age groups: 18–44 years, 45–54 years, 55–64 years, 65–74 years, and 75 years and over.
[2]Includes all other races not shown separately, unknown education level, and unknown disability status.
[3]The race groups, White, Black, American Indian or Alaska Native, Asian, Native Hawaiian or Other Pacific Islander, and 2 or more races, include persons of Hispanic and non-Hispanic origin. Persons of Hispanic origin may be of any race.
[4]Estimates are for persons 25 years of age and over and are age-adjusted to the year 2000 standard population using five age groups: 25–44 years, 45–54 years, 55–64 years, 65–74 years, and 75 years and over.
[5]Percent of poverty level is based on family income and family size and composition using U.S. Census Bureau poverty thresholds.
[6]Any basic actions difficulty or complex activity limitation is defined as having one or more of the following limitations or difficulties: movement difficulty, emotional difficulty, sensory (seeing or hearing) difficulty, cognitive difficulty, self-care (activities of daily living or instrumental activities of daily living) limitation, social limitation, or work limitation.
[7]MSA = metropolitan statistical area.

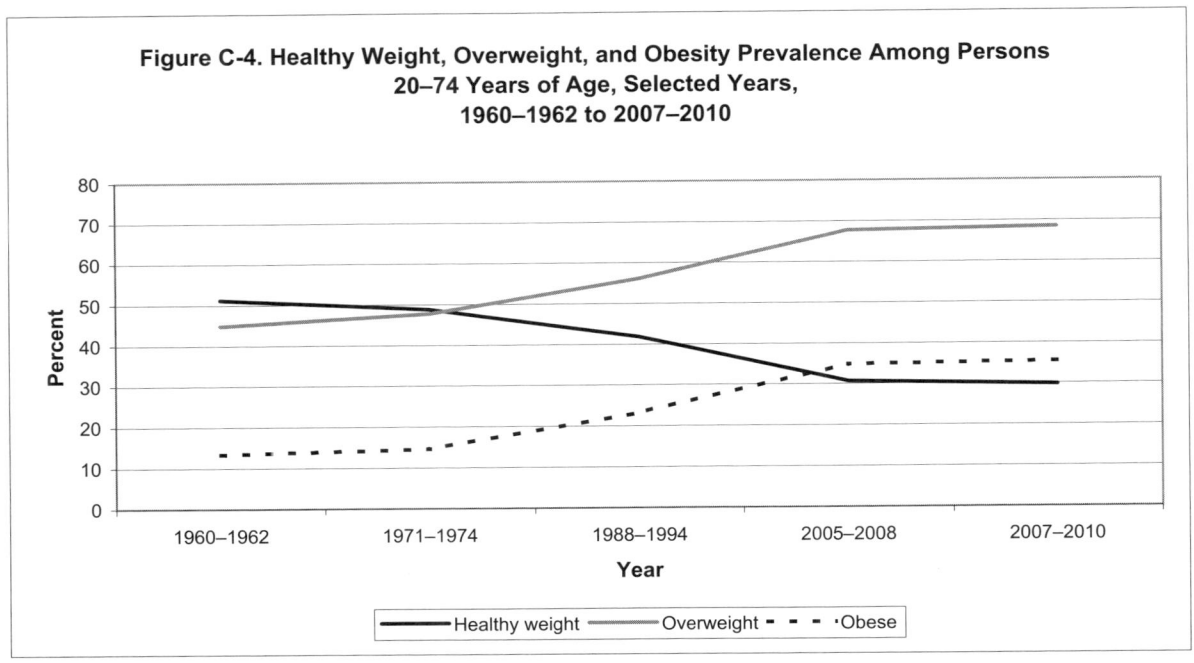

Figure C-4. Healthy Weight, Overweight, and Obesity Prevalence Among Persons 20–74 Years of Age, Selected Years, 1960–1962 to 2007–2010

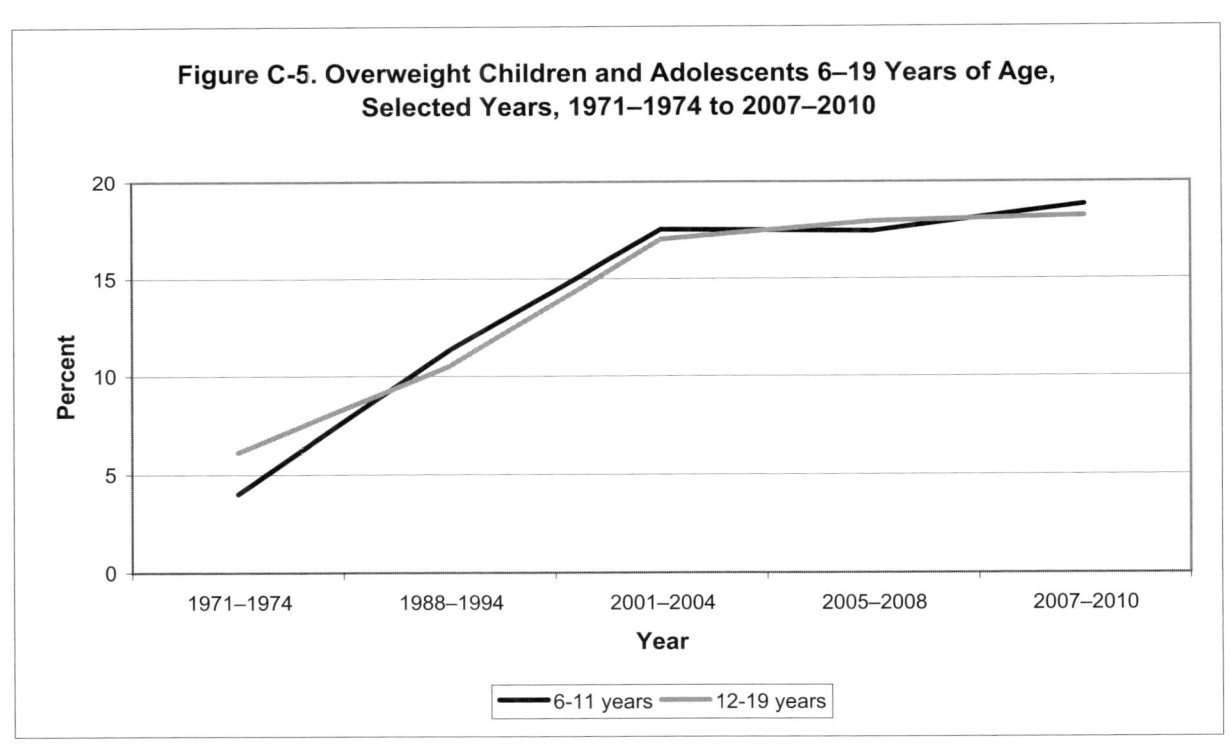

Figure C-5. Overweight Children and Adolescents 6–19 Years of Age, Selected Years, 1971–1974 to 2007–2010

Table C-21. Healthy Weight, Overweight, and Obesity Among Persons 20 Years of Age and Over, by Selected Characteristics, Selected Years, 1960–1962 through 2007–2010

(Percent.)

Characteristic	1960–1962	1971–1974	1976–1980	1988–1994	1999–2002	2001–2004	2003–2006	2005–2008	2007–2010
PERCENT OF POPULATION WITH A HEALTHY WEIGHT (BMI FROM 18.5 TO 24.9)[1]									
20–74 Years, Age-Adjusted[2]									
Both sexes	51.2	48.8	49.6	41.7	32.9	32.2	31.4	30.6	29.8
Male	48.3	43.0	45.4	37.9	30.2	28.1	26.1	26.0	25.8
Female	54.1	54.3	53.7	45.3	35.6	36.2	36.6	35.1	33.6
Not Hispanic or Latino									
White only, male	—	—	45.3	37.4	29.5	27.8	26.5	26.0	25.6
White only, female	—	—	56.7	49.2	39.7	40.2	40.0	38.0	36.9
Black or African American only, male	—	—	46.6	40.0	35.5	31.3	26.8	26.6	28.3
Black or African American only, female	—	—	35.0	28.9	21.2	18.9	18.4	19.3	17.7
Mexican male[3]	—	—	36.6	29.8	25.6	24.2	22.4	20.3	18.0
Mexican female[3]	—	—	35.9	29.0	27.6	26.3	24.5	23.1	20.2
Percent of Poverty Level[4]									
Below 100%	—	45.8	45.1	37.3	32.4	33.7	31.7	29.3	27.5
100%–199%	—	45.1	47.6	39.2	29.7	31.8	31.1	27.7	27.2
200%–399%	—	48.3	50.1	41.9	29.5	29.3	29.4	29.7	29.4
400% or more	—	53.9	53.0	46.0	36.9	35.2	33.8	33.9	32.3
20 Years and Over, Age-Adjusted[2]									
Both sexes	—	—	—	41.6	33.0	32.3	31.6	30.8	29.8
Male	—	—	—	37.9	30.2	28.3	26.6	26.1	25.7
Female	—	—	—	45.0	35.7	36.1	36.5	35.2	33.7
Not Hispanic or Latino									
White only, male	—	—	—	37.3	29.6	28.0	26.8	26.0	25.5
White only, female	—	—	—	48.7	39.5	39.8	39.6	37.8	36.9
Black or African American only, male	—	—	—	40.1	34.7	30.8	27.0	26.7	28.5
Black or African American only, female	—	—	—	29.2	21.6	18.9	19.2	20.4	17.9
Mexican male[3]	—	—	—	30.2	26.5	25.3	23.8	21.8	18.5
Mexican female[3]	—	—	—	29.7	27.5	26.5	25.1	24.1	21.3
Percent of Poverty Level[4]									
Below 100%	—	—	—	37.5	32.7	34.3	32.1	29.1	27.3
100%–199%	—	—	—	39.3	30.5	31.9	31.3	28.3	27.6
200%–399%	—	—	—	41.8	29.6	29.4	29.7	30.0	29.7
400% or more	—	—	—	45.5	36.5	35.1	33.7	33.5	32.1
20 Years and Over, Crude									
Both sexes	—	—	—	42.6	32.9	32.2	31.4	30.5	29.6
Male	—	—	—	39.4	30.4	28.4	26.6	26.1	25.8
Female	—	—	—	45.7	35.4	35.8	35.9	34.8	33.2
Not Hispanic or Latino:									
White only, male	—	—	—	38.2	29.2	27.4	26.2	25.4	24.8
White only, female	—	—	—	48.8	38.7	38.8	38.2	36.9	35.7
Black or African American only, male	—	—	—	41.5	35.9	31.5	27.1	27.4	29.4
Black or African American only, female	—	—	—	31.2	21.8	19.3	19.2	20.3	17.6
Mexican male[3]	—	—	—	35.2	29.4	28.1	25.2	22.8	19.5
Mexican female[3]	—	—	—	32.4	29.5	28.0	25.8	24.7	22.3
Percent of Poverty Level[4]									
Below 100%	—	—	—	39.8	34.5	36.2	33.2	30.9	29.2
100%–199%	—	—	—	41.5	31.5	32.6	31.7	28.8	28.0
200%–399%	—	—	—	42.9	29.7	29.3	29.6	30.0	29.5
400% or more	—	—	—	44.6	35.3	33.5	32.1	31.8	30.5
Male									
20–34 years	55.3	54.7	57.1	51.1	40.3	38.3	35.9	38.0	37.5
35–44 years	45.2	35.2	41.3	33.4	29.0	26.5	24.1	20.9	19.8
45–54 years	44.8	38.5	38.7	33.6	24.0	21.2	20.8	21.7	21.8
55–64 years	44.9	38.3	38.7	28.6	23.8	22.2	19.3	18.5	19.4
65–74 years	46.2	42.1	42.3	30.1	22.8	23.1	21.2	20.2	21.6
75 years and over	—	—	—	40.9	32.0	32.1	33.1	28.1	25.4
Female									
20–34 years	67.6	65.8	65.0	57.9	42.5	44.2	45.1	40.5	41.1
35–44 years	58.4	56.7	55.6	47.1	37.1	38.3	37.6	36.2	34.4
45–54 years	47.6	49.3	48.7	37.2	33.1	31.0	31.1	32.1	30.7
55–64 years	38.1	41.1	43.5	31.5	27.6	29.2	29.5	29.9	26.7
65–74 years	36.4	40.6	37.8	37.0	26.4	27.0	28.5	28.8	23.9
75 years and over	—	—	—	43.0	36.9	34.6	35.4	36.3	35.4

Table C-21. Healthy Weight, Overweight, and Obesity Among Persons 20 Years of Age and Over, by Selected Characteristics, Selected Years, 1960–1962 through 2007–2010—Continued

(Percent.)

Characteristic	1960–1962	1971–1974	1976–1980[3]	1988–1994	1999–2002	2001–2004	2003–2006	2005–2008	2007–2010
PERCENT OF POPULATION OVERWEIGHT (INCLUDES OBESITY; BMI GREATER THAN OR EQUAL TO 25.0)[1]									
20–74 Years, Age-Adjusted[2]									
Both sexes	44.8	47.7	47.4	56.0	65.2	66.0	66.9	67.7	68.5
Male	49.5	54.7	52.9	61.0	68.8	70.7	72.6	73.0	73.3
Female	40.2	41.1	42.0	51.2	61.7	61.4	61.2	62.6	63.9
Not Hispanic or Latino:									
White only, male	—	—	53.4	61.6	69.5	71.1	72.1	72.9	73.5
White only, female	—	—	38.7	47.2	57.0	57.1	57.4	59.4	60.2
Black or African American only, male	—	—	51.3	58.2	62.0	66.8	72.0	71.8	70.2
Black or African American only, female	—	—	62.6	68.5	77.6	79.5	80.5	79.1	80.3
Mexican male[3]	—	—	62.2	69.4	74.1	75.8	77.3	79.2	81.8
Mexican female[3]	—	—	62.2	69.6	71.4	73.2	74.4	75.6	79.2
Percent of Poverty Level[4]									
Below 100%	—	49.3	50.0	59.8	65.2	63.9	66.0	67.6	69.5
100%–199%	—	50.9	49.0	58.2	68.0	66.2	66.6	70.3	70.9
200%–399%	—	48.4	47.3	56.0	68.7	68.9	69.3	69.0	68.8
400% or more	—	43.4	45.0	51.8	61.8	63.5	64.7	65.1	66.7
20 Years and Over, Age–Adjusted[2]									
Both sexes	—	—	—	56.0	65.1	66.0	66.7	67.5	68.5
Male	—	—	—	60.9	68.8	70.5	72.1	72.9	73.3
Female	—	—	—	51.4	61.6	61.6	61.3	62.5	63.9
Not Hispanic or Latino									
White only, male	—	—	—	61.6	69.4	71.0	71.8	72.9	73.6
White only, female	—	—	—	47.5	57.2	57.6	57.9	59.6	60.3
Black or African American only, male	—	—	—	57.8	62.6	67.0	71.6	71.7	70.0
Black or African American only, female	—	—	—	68.2	77.2	79.6	79.8	78.0	80.0
Mexican male[3]	—	—	—	68.9	73.2	74.6	75.8	77.7	81.3
Mexican female[3]	—	—	—	68.9	71.2	73.0	73.9	74.8	78.0
Percent of Poverty Level[4]									
Below 100%	—	—	—	59.6	64.7	63.4	65.7	67.7	69.7
100%–199%	—	—	—	58.0	67.3	66.2	66.5	69.6	70.5
200%–399%	—	—	—	56.0	68.6	68.8	69.0	68.7	68.6
400% or more	—	—	—	52.4	62.2	63.7	64.7	65.3	66.9
20 Years and Over, Crude									
Both sexes	—	—	—	54.9	65.2	66.1	66.9	67.8	68.7
Male	—	—	—	59.4	68.6	70.4	72.1	72.8	73.2
Female	—	—	—	50.7	62.0	61.9	61.9	63.0	64.5
Not Hispanic or Latino:									
White only, male	—	—	—	60.6	69.9	71.6	72.5	73.4	74.2
White only, female	—	—	—	47.4	58.2	58.7	59.4	60.7	61.7
Black or African American only, male	—	—	—	56.7	61.7	66.3	71.6	71.1	69.1
Black or African American only, female	—	—	—	66.0	76.9	79.1	79.7	78.1	80.2
Mexican male[3]	—	—	—	63.9	70.1	71.8	74.6	76.8	80.2
Mexican female[3]	—	—	—	65.9	69.3	71.4	73.0	73.9	77.1
Percent of Poverty Level[4]									
Below 100%	—	—	—	56.8	62.5	61.4	64.4	65.9	67.8
100%–199%	—	—	—	55.7	66.2	65.3	66.0	69.1	70.1
200%–399%	—	—	—	54.9	68.5	69.0	69.0	68.7	68.8
400% or more	—	—	—	53.3	63.7	65.5	66.5	67.2	68.5
Male									
20–34 years	42.7	42.8	41.2	47.5	57.4	59.0	61.6	60.5	61.1
35–44 years	53.5	63.2	57.2	65.5	70.5	72.9	75.2	78.8	80.2
45–54 years	53.9	59.7	60.2	66.1	75.7	78.5	78.5	76.8	76.8
55–64 years	52.2	58.5	60.2	70.5	75.4	77.3	79.7	80.5	79.8
65–74 years	47.8	54.6	54.2	68.5	76.2	76.1	78.0	79.1	77.5
75 years and over	—	—	—	56.5	67.4	66.8	65.8	70.8	73.2
Female									
20–34 years	21.2	25.8	27.9	37.0	52.9	51.6	50.9	55.6	55.4
35–44 years	37.2	40.5	40.7	49.6	60.6	60.1	60.7	62.1	63.9
45–54 years	49.3	49.0	48.7	60.3	65.1	67.4	67.3	65.8	66.2
55–64 years	59.9	54.5	53.7	66.3	72.2	69.9	69.6	69.4	72.2
65–74 years	60.9	55.9	59.5	60.3	70.9	71.5	70.5	69.6	74.2
75 years and over	—	—	—	52.3	59.9	63.7	62.6	61.3	63.2

Table C-21. Healthy Weight, Overweight, and Obesity Among Persons 20 Years of Age and Over, by Selected Characteristics, Selected Years, 1960–1962 through 2007–2010—Continued

(Percent.)

Characteristic	1960–1962	1971–1974	1976–1980[3]	1988–1994	1999–2002	2001–2004	2003–2006	2005–2008	2007–2010
PERCENT OF POPULATION SUFFERING FROM OBESITY (BMI GREATER THAN OR EQUAL TO 30.0)[1]									
20–74 Years, Age-Adjusted[2]									
Both sexes	13.3	14.6	15.1	23.3	31.1	32.1	34.1	34.7	35.3
Male	10.7	12.2	12.8	20.6	28.1	30.2	33.1	33.3	34.4
Female	15.7	16.8	17.1	26.0	34.0	34.0	35.2	36.2	36.1
Not Hispanic or Latino									
White only, male	—	—	12.4	20.7	28.7	31.0	33.0	33.2	34.7
White only, female	—	—	15.4	23.3	31.3	31.5	32.5	33.8	32.9
Black or African American only, male	—	—	16.5	21.3	27.9	31.2	36.3	37.6	38.7
Black or African American only, female	—	—	31.0	39.1	49.4	51.6	54.3	51.8	54.4
Mexican male[3]	—	—	16.0	24.4	29.0	30.5	30.4	32.2	36.5
Mexican female[3]	—	—	26.6	36.1	38.9	40.3	42.6	44.0	45.8
Percent of Poverty Level[4]									
Below 100%	—	20.7	21.9	29.2	36.0	34.9	35.9	36.3	37.9
100%–199%	—	18.4	18.7	26.6	35.4	34.6	36.7	39.2	38.2
200%–399%	—	13.7	14.1	23.2	33.0	34.4	36.9	36.7	37.6
400% or more	—	10.1	10.0	18.9	25.8	27.4	29.4	29.9	31.4
20 Years and Over, Age–Adjusted[2]									
Both sexes[5]	—	—	—	22.9	30.4	31.4	33.4	34.0	34.7
Male	—	—	—	20.2	27.5	29.5	32.4	32.7	33.9
Female	—	—	—	25.5	33.2	33.2	34.3	35.4	35.5
Not Hispanic or Latino:									
White only, male	—	—	—	20.3	28.0	30.2	32.4	32.6	34.1
White only, female	—	—	—	22.9	30.7	30.7	31.6	33.1	32.5
Black or African American only, male	—	—	—	20.9	27.8	30.8	35.7	37.5	38.3
Black or African American only, female	—	—	—	38.3	48.6	51.1	53.4	51.0	54.0
Mexican male[3]	—	—	—	23.8	27.8	29.1	29.5	32.0	36.3
Mexican female[3]	—	—	—	35.2	38.0	39.4	41.8	43.3	44.6
Percent of Poverty Level[4]									
Below 100%	—	—	—	28.1	34.7	33.7	35.0	35.9	37.2
100%–199%	—	—	—	26.1	34.1	33.6	35.9	38.0	37.3
200%–399%	—	—	—	22.7	32.1	33.3	35.7	35.7	36.8
400% or more	—	—	—	18.7	25.5	27.3	28.9	29.4	31.3
20 Years and Over, Crude									
Both sexes	—	—	—	22.3	30.5	31.5	33.5	34.3	34.9
Male	—	—	—	19.5	27.5	29.5	32.4	32.8	33.9
Female	—	—	—	25.0	33.4	33.3	34.6	35.6	35.9
Not Hispanic or Latino									
White only, male	—	—	—	19.9	28.4	30.5	32.6	33.1	34.4
White only, female	—	—	—	22.7	31.3	31.2	32.2	33.3	33.2
Black or African American only, male	—	—	—	20.7	27.5	30.7	35.8	37.2	38.1
Black or African American only, female	—	—	—	36.7	48.7	51.1	53.2	51.0	54.2
Mexican male[3]	—	—	—	20.6	26.0	27.8	29.0	30.9	35.6
Mexican female[3]	—	—	—	33.3	37.0	38.5	41.2	42.9	44.2
Percent of Poverty Level[4]									
Below 100%	—	—	—	25.9	33.0	33.0	34.6	35.4	36.5
100%–199%	—	—	—	24.3	32.8	32.6	35.0	37.0	36.8
200%–399%	—	—	—	22.1	31.8	33.2	35.5	35.6	36.8
400% or more	—	—	—	19.3	27.2	28.6	30.7	31.7	32.4
Male									
20–34 years	9.2	9.7	8.9	14.1	21.7	23.2	26.2	25.4	27.1
35–44 years	12.1	13.5	13.5	21.5	28.5	33.8	37.0	35.9	37.2
45–54 years	12.5	13.7	16.7	23.2	30.6	31.8	34.6	35.9	36.6
55–64 years	9.2	14.1	14.1	27.2	35.5	36.0	39.3	40.4	37.3
65–74 years	10.4	10.9	13.2	24.1	31.9	32.1	33.0	36.2	41.5
75 years and over	—	—	—	13.2	18.0	19.9	24.0	25.6	26.6
Female									
20–34 years	7.2	9.7	11.0	18.5	28.3	28.6	28.4	31.4	30.4
35–44 years	14.7	17.7	17.8	25.5	32.1	33.3	36.1	36.7	37.1
45–54 years	20.3	18.9	19.6	32.4	36.9	38.0	40.0	39.1	36.9
55–64 years	24.4	24.1	22.9	33.7	42.1	39.0	41.0	42.3	43.4
65–74 years	23.2	22.0	21.5	26.9	39.3	37.9	36.4	35.6	40.3
75 years and over	—	—	—	19.2	23.6	23.2	24.2	25.9	28.7

— =Data not available.
* = Figure does not meet standards of reliability or precision.
[1] Body mass index (BMI) equals weight in kilograms divided by height in meters squared.
[2] Age-adjusted to the year 2000 standard population using five age groups: 20–34 years, 35–44 years, 45–54 years, 55–64 years, and 65 years and over (65-74 years for estimates for 20-74 years).
[3] Persons of Mexican origin may be of any race.
[4] Percent of poverty level is based on family income and family size using U.S. Census Bureau poverty thresholds.

Table C-22. Obesity Among Children and Adolescents 2–19 Years of Age, by Selected Characteristics, Selected Years, 1963–1965 through 2007–2010

(Percent.)

Characteristic	1963–1965, 1966–1970[1]	1971–1974	1976–1980[2]	1988–1994	1999–2002	2001–2004	2003–2006	2005–2008	2007–2010
AGE									
2–5 years									
Both sexes	—	—	—	7.2	10.3	12.4	12.5	10.5	11.1
Not Hispanic or Latino									
White only	—	—	—	5.2	8.7	10.2	10.8	9.3	9.0
Black or African American only	—	—	—	7.7	8.8	11.0	14.9	14.0	15.0
Mexican[3]	—	—	—	12.3	13.1	17.7	16.7	14.1	14.6
Boys	—	—	—	6.1	10.0	13.1	12.8	9.8	11.9
Not Hispanic or Latino									
White only	—	—	—	*4.5	*8.2	*11.5	11.1	*7.4	8.8
Black or African American only	—	—	—	7.7	*8.0	9.7	13.3	13.7	15.7
Mexican[3]	—	—	—	12.4	14.1	19.8	18.8	17.1	19.1
Girls	—	—	—	8.2	10.6	11.7	12.2	11.2	10.2
Not Hispanic or Latina									
White only	—	—	—	5.9	*9.0	*9.1	10.4	11.3	*9.2
Black or African American only	—	—	—	7.6	9.6	12.2	16.6	14.3	*14.2
Mexican[3]	—	—	—	12.3	*12.2	*15.7	14.5	10.8	*9.9
Percent of Poverty Level[4]									
Below 100%	—	—	—	9.7	10.9	14.4	14.3	12.3	13.2
100%–199%	—	—	—	7.2	*13.8	13.3	12.7	10.0	11.8
200%–399%	—	—	—	5.6	*7.6	13.6	11.9	11.6	13.9
400% or more	—	—	—	*	*	*	*10.0	*	*5.8
6–11 Years									
Both sexes	4.2	4.0	6.5	11.3	15.9	17.5	17.0	17.4	18.8
Boys	4.0	*4.3	6.6	11.6	16.9	18.7	18.0	18.7	20.7
Not Hispanic or Latino									
White only	—	—	6.1	10.7	14.0	16.9	15.5	16.5	18.6
Black or African American only	—	—	6.8	12.3	17.0	17.2	18.6	18.7	23.3
Mexican[3]	—	—	13.3	17.5	26.5	25.6	27.5	28.4	24.3
Girls	4.5	*3.6	6.4	11.0	14.7	16.3	15.8	16.0	16.9
Not Hispanic or Latina									
White only	—	—	5.2	*9.8	13.1	15.6	14.4	14.5	14.0
Black or African American only	—	—	11.2	17.0	22.8	24.8	24.0	21.3	24.5
Mexican[3]	—	—	9.8	15.3	17.1	16.6	19.7	21.2	22.4
Percent of Poverty Level[4]									
Below 100%	—	—	—	11.4	19.1	20.0	22.0	21.5	22.2
100%–199%	—	—	—	11.1	16.4	18.4	19.2	22.2	20.7
200%–399%	—	—	—	11.7	15.3	18.2	16.7	16.8	18.9
400% or more	—	—	—	*	12.9	11.4	9.2	*9.5	*12.5
12–19 Years									
Both sexes	4.6	6.1	5.0	10.5	16.0	17.0	17.6	17.9	18.2
Boys	4.5	6.1	4.8	11.3	16.7	17.9	18.2	18.7	19.4
Not Hispanic or Latino									
White only	—	—	3.8	11.6	14.6	17.9	17.3	16.1	17.1
Black or African American only	—	—	6.1	10.7	18.8	17.6	18.4	19.1	21.2
Mexican[3]	—	—	7.7	14.1	24.7	20.0	22.1	26.2	27.9
Girls	4.7	6.2	5.3	9.7	15.3	16.0	16.8	17.0	16.9
Not Hispanic or Latina									
White only	—	—	4.6	8.9	12.6	14.6	14.5	14.0	14.6
Black or African American only	—	—	10.7	16.3	23.5	23.8	27.7	29.5	27.1
Mexican[3]	—	—	8.8	*13.4	19.6	17.1	19.9	21.3	18.0
Percent of Poverty Level[4]									
Below 100%	—	—	—	15.8	19.8	18.2	19.3	23.1	24.3
100%–199%	—	—	—	11.2	15.1	17.0	18.4	19.8	20.1
200%–399%	—	—	—	9.4	15.7	19.0	19.3	17.2	16.3
400% or more	—	—	—	*	13.9	13.2	12.6	14.0	14.0

— = Data not available.
* = Figure does not meet standards of reliability or precision.
[1] Data for 1963–1965 are for children 6–11 years of age; data for 1966–1970 are for adolescents 12–17 years of age, not 12–19 years.
[2] Data for Mexican-origin persons are for 1982–1984.
[3] Persons of Mexican origin may be of any race.
[4] Percent of poverty level is based on family income and family size.

Table C-23. Untreated Dental Caries, by Selected Characteristics, Selected Years, 1971–1974 through 2005–2008

(Percent.)

Sex, race and Hispanic origin, and percent of poverty level	Age 2–5 years		Age 6–19 years		Age 20-64 years		Age 65-74 years		Age 75 years and over	
	1971–1974	2005–2008	1971–1974	2005–2008	1971–1974	2005–2008	1971–1974	2005–2008	1971–1974	2005–2008
TOTAL	25.0	X	54.7	16.2	48.0	23.7	29.7	19.6	—	20.2
Sex										
Male	26.4	X	54.9	17.0	50.5	27.2	32.6	24.8	—	25.7
Female	23.6	X	54.5	15.3	45.6	20.2	27.4	15.3	—	16.1
Race and Hispanic Origin[1]										
Not Hispanic or Latino										
White only	23.7	X	51.6	12.9	45.3	19.3	28.3	17.8	—	17.7
Black or African American only	29.0	X	71.0	22.1	67.3	39.7	41.5	32.4	—	42.6
Mexican	—	X	—	22.2	—	35.2	—	33.2	—	43.4
Percent of Poverty Level[2]										
Below 100%	32.0	X	68.0	25.4	63.5	41.9	34.3	42.5	—	39.3
100%-199%	29.9	X	60.3	18.4	56.2	37.7	35.6	22.9	—	22.1
200% or more	17.8	X	46.2	11.9	42.7	16.6	26.2	15.7	—	14.5
200%-399%	—	X	—	14.2	—	24.3	—	*17.9	—	14.8
400% or more	—	X	—	9.3	—	11.1	—	12.8	—	*13.8
Race and Hispanic Origin, and Percent of Poverty Level[2]										
Not Hispanic or Latino										
White only										
Below 100% of poverty level	32.1	X	65.9	25.4	60.2	39.8	33.3	*39.4	—	*29.6
100% or more of poverty level	22.0	X	49.9	11.0	44.2	17.1	28.3	16.4	—	15.6
Black or African American only										
Below 100% of poverty level	29.1	X	73.9	27.1	71.9	52.7	39.8	56.2	—	*
100% or more of poverty level	27.9	X	67.3	19.1	65.3	36.8	41.1	28.1	—	36.4

X = Category not applicable.
— =Data not available.
* = Figure does not meet standards of reliability or precision.
[1]Persons of Hispanic origin may be of any race.
[2]Percent of poverty level is based on family income and family size.

Table C-24. Health-Related Behaviors of Children 6–11 Years of Age, by Selected Characteristics, 2003 and 2007

(Percent.)

Characteristic	Did not get daily vigorous physical activity[1]		Greater than 2 hours of screen time per day[2]		Did not get enough sleep nightly[3]	
	2003	2007	2003	2007	2003	2007
Age						
6–11 years	68.7	62.3	36.2	39.5	24.5	27.6
6–8 years	67.0	59.2	33.8	35.1	22.8	26.1
9–11 years	70.3	65.4	38.5	44.0	26.1	29.1
Sex						
Male	63.7	57.8	37.0	39.4	24.6	27.6
Female	74.0	67.0	35.4	39.7	24.4	27.6
Sex and Age						
Male						
6–8 years	62.3	55.4	34.9	34.9	22.4	25.2
9–11 years	65.0	60.4	39.0	44.1	26.7	30.1
Female						
6–8 years	72.0	63.3	32.8	35.3	23.2	27.0
9–11 years	75.8	70.5	37.9	44.0	25.5	28.1
Hispanic Origin and Race[4]						
Hispanic or Latino	70.1	69.3	35.5	41.7	21.7	24.4
Not Hispanic or Latino	68.5	60.4	36.3	38.9	25.2	28.4
White only	68.3	59.7	33.0	34.7	25.8	29.1
Black or African American only	66.2	62.1	48.8	58.2	25.4	27.1
Sex and Hispanic Origin and Race[4]						
Male						
Hispanic or Latino	66.2	61.7	34.4	39.9	21.1	24.6
Not Hispanic or Latino	63.4	56.8	37.6	39.2	25.4	28.4
White only	62.7	54.9	34.7	35.0	25.8	29.3
Black or African American only	60.3	61.4	49.1	58.3	25.4	27.4
Female						
Hispanic or Latina	73.9	76.5	36.6	43.4	22.2	24.3
Not Hispanic or Latina	74.0	64.4	35.0	38.6	25.1	28.3
White only	74.4	64.9	31.2	34.4	25.8	29.0
Black or African American only	71.9	62.8	48.6	58.1	25.5	26.8
Percent of Poverty Level[5]						
Below 100%	63.3	62.6	38.2	43.9	22.4	25.9
100%–199%	66.7	63.1	41.8	44.4	22.8	25.6
200%–399%	70.7	60.8	36.8	40.1	25.0	28.9
400% or more	71.6	63.1	29.3	32.6	26.8	28.7
Sex and Percent of Poverty Level[5]						
Male						
Below 100%	57.9	59.3	39.0	43.1	21.7	26.7
100%–199%	61.2	58.0	42.8	44.6	23.7	26.2
200%–399%	65.4	57.6	38.1	40.1	24.6	29.0
400% or more	67.6	57.1	29.3	32.6	27.3	27.6
Female						
Below 100%	68.9	66.2	37.5	44.7	23.2	25.1
100%–199%	72.4	68.4	40.9	44.2	22.0	24.9
200%–399%	76.3	64.4	35.5	40.3	25.4	28.7
400% or more	75.8	69.3	29.3	32.8	26.2	29.7

[1]Based on respondent's answer to question, "During the past week, on how many days did CHILD exercise, play a sport, or participate in physical activity for at least 20 minutes that made him/her sweat and breathe hard?" Children whose parent/guardian responded that the child did not exercise, play a sport, or participate in physical activity every day were classified as not getting daily vigorous physical activity.
[2]Based on respondent's answer to question, "On an average weekday, about how much time does CHILD use a computer for purposes other than schoolwork?" and "On an average weekday, about how much time does CHILD usually watch TV, watch videos, or play video games?" Children whose parent's/guardian's combined responses to both questions equaled more than 2 hours were classified as watching more than 2 hours of screen time daily.
[3]Based on respondent's answer to question, "In the past week, on how many nights did CHILD get enough sleep for a child of his/her age?" Children whose parent/guardian responded that the child did not get enough sleep on at least one night were classified as not getting enough sleep nightly.
[4]Persons of Hispanic origin may be of any race.
[5]Percent of poverty level is based on total household income and family composition using U.S. Census Bureau poverty thresholds.

Table C-25. Selected Health Conditions and Risk Factors, Selected Years, 1988–1994 through 2009–2010

(Percent.)

Health condition	1988–1994	1999–2000	2001–2002	2003–2004	2005–2006	2007–2008	2009–2010
Diabetes[1]							
Total, age-adjusted[2]	9.1	9.0	10.5	10.8	10.4	—	—
Total, crude	8.4	8.5	10.1	10.8	10.7	—	—
High Cholesterol[3]							
Total, age-adjusted[4]	22.8	25.0	24.4	27.5	27.0	27.2	26.7
Total, crude	21.5	24.0	23.9	27.5	27.6	28.3	27.9
High Serum Total Cholesterol[5]							
Total, age-adjusted[4]	20.8	18.3	16.5	16.9	15.6	14.2	13.2
Total, crude	19.6	17.7	16.4	17.0	15.9	14.6	13.6
Hypertension[6]							
Total, age-adjusted[4]	25.5	30.0	29.7	32.1	30.5	31.2	30.0
Total, crude	24.1	28.9	28.9	32.5	31.7	32.6	31.9
Uncontrolled High Blood Pressure Among Persons with Hypertension[7]							
Total, age-adjusted[4]	77.2	71.9	68.3	63.8	63.0	56.2	55.7
Total, crude	73.9	69.1	65.4	60.8	56.6	51.8	46.7
Overweight (Includes Obesity)[8]							
Total, age-adjusted[4]	56.0	64.5	65.6	66.4	66.9	68.1	68.8
Total, crude	54.9	64.1	65.6	66.5	67.3	68.3	69.2
Obesity[9]							
Total, age-adjusted[4]	22.9	30.5	30.5	32.3	34.4	33.7	35.7
Total, crude	22.3	30.3	30.6	32.3	34.7	33.9	35.9
Untreated Dental Caries[10]							
Total, age-adjusted[4]	27.7	24.3	21.3	30.0	24.4	21.7	—
Total, crude	28.2	25.0	21.6	30.3	24.5	21.8	—
PERCENT OF PERSONS UNDER 20 YEARS OLD							
Obesity[11]							
2–5 years	7.2	10.3	10.6	14.0	11.0	10.1	12.1
6–11 years	11.3	15.1	16.3	18.8	15.1	19.6	18.0
12–19 years	10.5	14.8	16.7	17.4	17.8	18.1	18.4
Untreated Dental Caries[10,12]							
6–19 years	23.6	22.7	20.6	25.2	—	16.2	—

— = Data not available.

[1] Undiagnosed diabetes is defined as a fasting plasma glucose (FPG) of at least 126 mg/dL or a hemoglobin A1c of at least 6.5% and no reported physician diagnosis.
[2] Age-adjusted to the 2000 standard population using three age groups: 20–44 years, 45–64 years, and 65 years and over.
[3] High cholesterol is defined as measured serum total cholesterol greater than or equal to 240 mg/dL or reporting taking cholesterol-lowering medication. Respondents were asked, "Are you now following this advice [from a doctor of health professional] to take prescribed medicine [to lower your cholesterol]?"
[4] Age-adjusted to the 2000 standard population using five age groups: 20–34 years, 35–44 years, 45–54 years, 55–64 years, and 65 years and over.
[5] High serum total cholesterol is defined as greater than or equal to 240 mg/dL (6.20 mmol/L).
[6] Hypertension is defined as having measured high blood pressure and/or taking antihypertensive medication.
[7] Uncontrolled high blood pressure among persons with hypertension is defined as measured systolic pressure of at least 140 mmHg or diastolic pressure of at least 90 mmHg, among those with measured high blood pressure or reporting taking antihypertensive medication.
[8] Excludes pregnant women. Overweight is defined as body mass index (BMI) greater than or equal to 25.
[9] Excludes pregnant women. Obesity is defined as body mass index (BMI) greater than or equal to 30.
[10] Untreated dental caries refers to untreated coronal caries.
[11] Obesity is defined as body mass index (BMI) at or above the sex- and age-specific 5th percentile BMI cutoff points from the 2000 CDC growth charts for the United States.
[12] The estimate in the 2007–2008 column is for 2005–2008. The 4-year estimate is shown for children because it is more reliable than the 2-year estimates.

Table C-26. Health Risk Behaviors Among Students in Grades 9–12, by Sex, Grade Level, Race, and Hispanic Origin, Selected Years, 1991–2009

(Percent.)

Sex, grade level, race, and Hispanic origin	Seriously considered suicide			In a physical fight[1]			Carried a weapon[2,3]		
	1991	1999	2009	1991	1999	2009	1991	1999	2009
TOTAL	29.0	19.3	13.8	42.5	35.7	31.5	26.1	17.3	17.5
Male									
Total	20.8	13.7	10.5	50.2	44.0	39.3	40.6	28.6	27.1
9th grade	17.6	11.9	10.0	57.8	49.5	45.1	44.4	28.7	27.3
10th grade	19.5	13.7	10.0	50.2	46.0	41.2	41.5	30.7	28.5
11th grade	25.3	13.7	11.4	51.0	38.9	36.2	44.0	26.9	25.6
12th grade	20.7	15.6	10.5	42.3	39.0	32.5	33.1	27.3	26.5
Not Hispanic or Latino									
White	21.7	12.5	10.5	49.1	43.2	36.0	41.2	28.6	29.3
Black or African American	13.3	11.7	7.8	58.4	44.4	48.3	43.4	23.1	21.0
Hispanic or Latino	18.0	13.6	10.7	48.5	50.5	43.8	40.0	29.5	26.5
Female									
Total	37.2	24.9	17.4	34.4	27.3	22.9	10.9	6.0	7.1
9th grade	40.3	24.4	20.3	42.9	32.5	27.8	10.4	6.5	7.6
10th grade	39.7	30.1	17.2	35.4	29.4	24.8	11.2	7.1	7.2
11th grade	38.4	23.0	17.8	34.5	23.4	20.5	12.9	5.2	6.3
12th grade	30.7	21.2	13.6	25.4	21.9	17.0	9.5	4.8	6.4
Not Hispanic or Latina									
White	38.6	23.2	16.1	32.2	22.3	18.2	7.5	3.6	6.5
Black or African American	29.4	18.8	18.1	43.8	38.6	33.9	23.6	11.7	7.8
Hispanic or Latina	34.6	26.1	20.2	34.8	29.7	28.5	12.9	8.4	7.9

Sex, grade level, race, and Hispanic origin	Rarely or never wore a seatbelt[4]			Rode with a driver who had been drinking alcohol[2,5]			Drove while drinking alcohol[2,5]		
	1991	1999	2009	1991	1999	2009	1991	1999	2009
TOTAL	25.9	16.4	9.7	39.9	33.1	28.3	16.7	13.1	9.7
Male									
Total	30.0	20.8	11.5	40.0	34.4	27.8	21.5	17.4	11.6
9th grade	30.0	19.8	11.2	40.0	29.9	25.3	8.6	6.1	5.1
10th grade	25.5	17.7	11.7	33.9	34.8	28.3	16.1	15.0	11.0
11th grade	29.5	17.7	11.2	36.6	33.4	29.2	26.4	20.5	13.0
12th grade	34.7	28.1	12.0	45.0	39.7	28.6	34.5	31.2	19.3
Not Hispanic or Latino									
White	28.6	19.6	11.2	40.2	33.0	25.5	23.3	18.7	12.7
Black or African American	37.5	27.9	14.8	37.4	34.0	31.2	14.0	10.6	8.7
Hispanic or Latino	37.1	19.6	9.8	47.2	41.8	33.5	25.1	17.2	11.0
Female									
Total	21.6	11.9	7.7	39.8	31.7	28.8	11.7	8.7	7.6
9th grade	25.0	14.4	9.8	36.0	32.0	30.0	3.3	4.5	4.8
10th grade	20.4	12.3	6.8	38.8	32.0	27.6	7.3	5.3	5.3
11th grade	20.8	9.8	6.0	39.7	28.1	29.6	14.2	12.3	9.6
12th grade	20.2	10.3	8.0	44.8	34.8	27.9	21.7	14.4	11.4
Not Hispanic or Latina									
White	18.7	11.2	7.6	40.9	31.7	26.9	13.6	10.3	8.7
Black or African American	31.9	17.4	8.3	33.8	34.8	28.7	6.2	5.4	4.1
Hispanic or Latina	25.9	9.5	7.8	46.7	37.3	34.9	9.5	8.3	7.9

Table C-26. Health Risk Behaviors Among Students in Grades 9–12, by Sex, Grade Level, Race, and Hispanic Origin, Selected Years, 1991–2009—*Continued*

(Percent.)

Sex, grade level, race, and Hispanic origin	Ever had sexual intercourse			Did not use a condom at last sex[6]			Physically forced to have sex		
	1991	1999	2009	1991	1999	2009	1991	1999	2009
TOTAL	54.1	49.9	46.0	53.8	42.0	38.9	—	8.8	7.4
Male									
Total	57.4	52.2	46.1	45.5	34.5	31.4	—	5.2	4.5
9th grade	45.6	44.5	33.6	44.1	30.5	30.1	—	5.6	4.1
10th grade	50.9	51.1	41.9	43.1	30.0	28.1	—	4.6	4.0
11th grade	64.5	51.4	53.4	43.2	30.7	31.1	—	5.0	5.4
12th grade	68.3	63.9	59.6	49.3	44.1	35.0	—	5.6	4.9
Not Hispanic or Latino									
White	52.7	45.4	39.6	44.8	37.0	29.0	—	3.5	3.2
Black or African American	88.1	75.7	72.1	43.0	24.7	27.5	—	9.7	7.9
Hispanic or Latino	64.1	62.9	52.8	53.0	33.9	38.2	—	5.9	5.7
Female									
Total	50.8	47.7	45.7	62.0	49.3	46.1	—	12.5	10.5
9th grade	32.2	32.5	29.3	49.7	36.9	42.3	—	10.4	9.4
10th grade	45.3	42.6	39.6	63.6	44.7	36.5	—	12.4	10.6
11th grade	60.2	53.8	52.5	59.3	50.0	46.0	—	14.5	11.2
12th grade	65.2	65.8	65.0	67.4	58.9	53.7	—	12.8	10.8
Not Hispanic or Latina									
White	47.1	44.8	44.7	62.0	52.4	43.9	—	10.1	10.0
Black or African American	75.9	66.9	58.3	60.6	35.5	48.2	—	13.5	12.0
Hispanic or Latina	43.3	45.5	45.4	73.1	57.0	52.0	—	15.1	11.2

— = Data not available.
[1] During the last 12 months.
[2] During the last 30 days.
[3] Weapon refers to gun, knife, or club.
[4] When riding in a car driven by someone else.
[5] In car or other vehicle.
[6] Among students who had sexual intercourse in the last 3 months.

USE OF ADDICTIVE SUBSTANCES

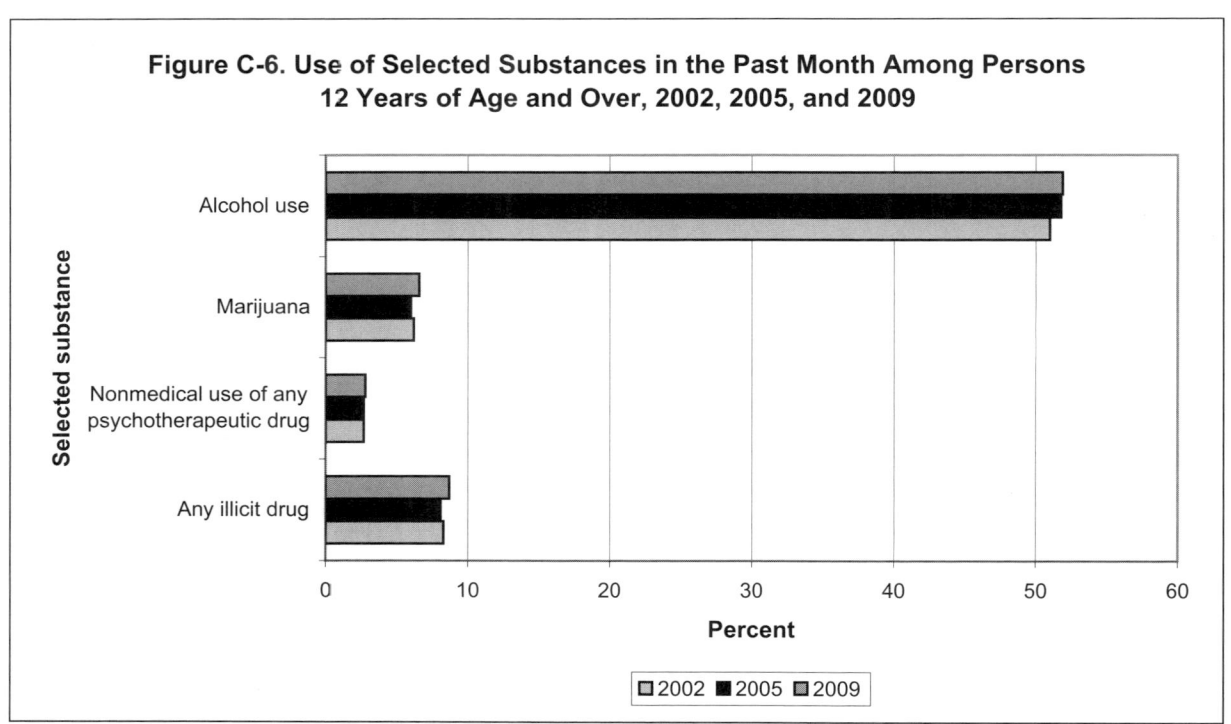

Figure C-6. Use of Selected Substances in the Past Month Among Persons 12 Years of Age and Over, 2002, 2005, and 2009

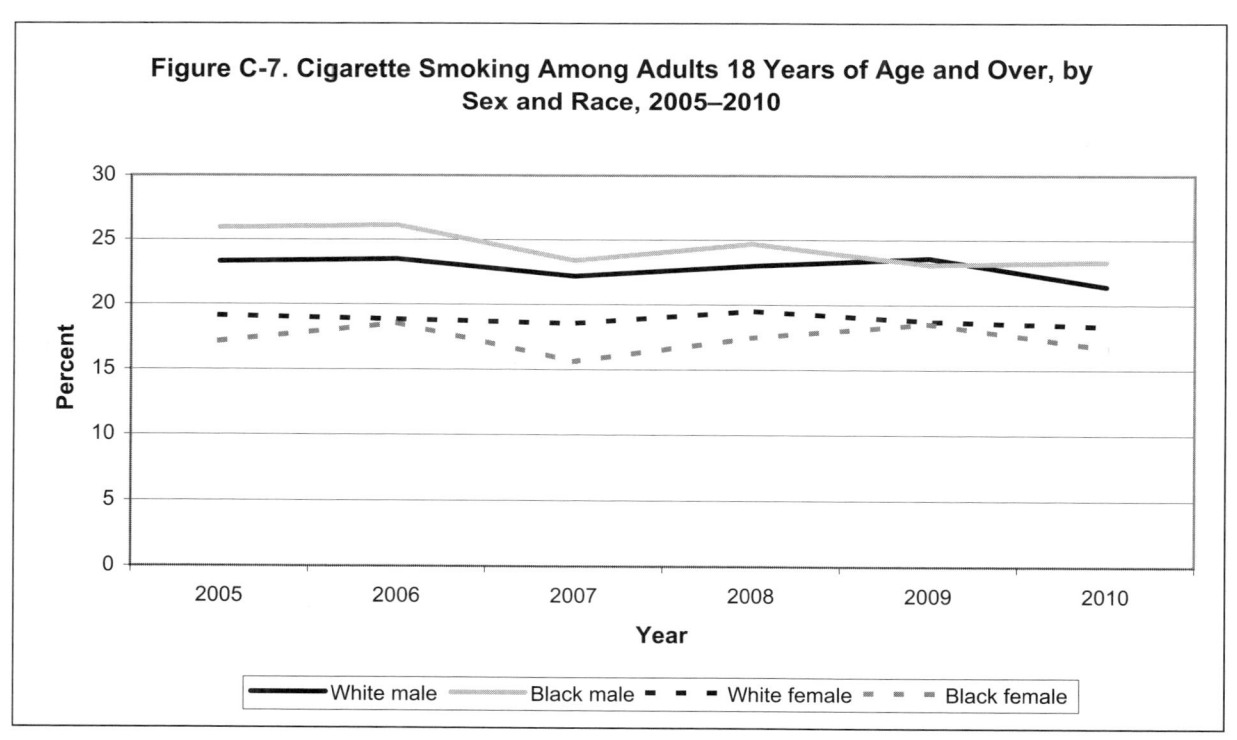

Figure C-7. Cigarette Smoking Among Adults 18 Years of Age and Over, by Sex and Race, 2005–2010

Table C-27. Use of Selected Substances in the Past Month Among Persons 12 Years of Age and Over, by Age, Sex, Race, and Hispanic Origin, Selected Years, 2002–2009

(Percent.)

Age, sex, race, and Hispanic origin	Any illicit drug[1]			Marijuana			Nonmedical use of any psychotherapeutic drug[2]		
	2002	2005	2009	2002	2005	2009	2002	2005	2009
12 years and over	8.3	8.1	8.7	6.2	6.0	6.6	2.7	2.7	2.8
Age									
12–13 years	4.2	3.8	3.6	1.4	0.9	0.8	1.7	1.7	1.6
14–15 years	11.2	8.9	9.0	7.6	5.9	6.3	4.0	2.8	3.3
16–17 years	19.8	17.0	16.7	15.7	13.6	14.0	6.3	5.4	4.3
18–25 years	20.2	20.1	21.2	17.3	16.6	18.1	5.5	6.3	6.3
26–34 years	10.5	11.0	12.3	7.7	8.6	9.6	3.7	3.5	3.8
35 years and over	4.6	4.5	4.9	3.1	3.0	3.4	1.6	1.6	1.7
Sex									
Male	10.3	10.2	10.8	8.1	8.2	8.6	2.8	2.8	3.1
Female	6.4	6.1	6.6	4.4	4.0	4.8	2.6	2.5	2.4
Age and Sex									
12–17 years	11.6	9.9	10.0	8.2	6.8	7.3	4.0	3.3	3.1
Male	12.3	10.1	10.6	9.1	7.5	8.3	3.6	3.1	2.8
Female	10.9	9.7	9.4	7.2	6.2	6.3	4.4	3.6	3.5
Hispanic Origin and Race[3]									
Not Hispanic or Latino									
White only	8.5	8.1	8.8	6.5	6.1	6.8	2.8	2.9	3.0
Black or African American only	9.7	9.7	9.6	7.4	7.6	7.8	2.0	1.8	2.0
American Indian or Alaska Native only	10.1	12.8	18.3	6.7	9.8	10.6	3.2	5.0	6.2
Native Hawaiian or Other Pacific Islander only	7.9	8.7	*	4.4	5.7	4.3	3.8	4.0	*
Asian only	3.5	3.1	3.7	1.8	1.6	2.4	0.7	1.5	1.4
2 or more races	11.4	12.2	14.3	9.0	10.6	12.2	3.5	2.9	3.4
Hispanic or Latino	7.2	7.6	7.9	4.3	5.1	5.8	2.9	2.5	2.4

Age, sex, race, and Hispanic origin	Alcohol use			Binge alcohol use[4]			Heavy alcohol use[5]		
	2002	2005	2009	2002	2005	2009	2002	2005	2009
12 years and over	51.0	51.8	51.9	22.9	22.7	23.7	6.7	6.6	6.8
Age									
12–13 years	4.3	4.2	3.5	1.8	2.0	1.6	0.3	0.2	0.2
14–15 years	16.6	15.1	13.0	9.2	8.0	7.0	1.9	1.7	1.4
16–17 years	32.6	30.1	26.3	21.4	19.7	17.0	5.6	5.3	4.5
18–25 years	60.5	60.9	61.8	40.9	41.9	41.7	14.9	15.3	13.7
26–34 years	61.4	62.5	64.3	33.1	32.9	36.3	9.0	9.6	10.1
35 years and over	52.1	53.3	52.7	18.6	18.3	19.2	5.2	4.7	5.3
Sex									
Male	57.4	58.1	57.6	31.2	30.5	31.6	10.8	10.3	10.3
Female	44.9	45.9	46.5	15.1	15.2	16.1	3.0	3.1	3.5
Age and Sex									
12–17 years	17.6	16.5	14.7	10.7	9.9	8.8	2.5	2.4	2.1
Male	17.4	15.9	15.1	11.4	10.4	9.6	3.1	3.0	2.3
Female	17.9	17.2	14.3	9.9	9.4	8.0	1.9	1.8	1.9
Hispanic Origin and Race[3]									
Not Hispanic or Latino									
White only	55.0	56.5	56.7	23.4	23.4	24.8	7.5	7.4	7.9
Black or African American only	39.9	40.8	42.8	21.0	20.3	19.8	4.4	4.2	4.5
American Indian or Alaska Native only	44.7	42.4	37.1	27.9	32.8	22.2	8.7	11.5	8.3
Native Hawaiian or Other Pacific Islander only	*	37.3	*	25.2	25.7	*	8.3	5.3	3.6
Asian only	37.1	38.1	37.6	12.4	12.7	11.1	2.6	2.0	1.5
2 or more races	49.9	47.3	47.6	19.8	20.8	24.1	7.5	5.6	6.4
Hispanic or Latino	42.8	42.6	41.7	24.8	23.7	25.0	5.9	5.6	5.2

Table C-27. **Use of Selected Substances in the Past Month Among Persons 12 Years of Age and Over, by Age, Sex, Race, and Hispanic Origin, Selected Years, 2002–2009**—*Continued*

(Percent.)

Age, sex, race, and Hispanic origin	Any tobacco[6]			Cigarettes			Cigars		
	2002	2005	2009	2002	2005	2009	2002	2005	2009
12 years and over	30.4	29.4	27.7	26.0	24.9	23.3	5.4	5.6	5.3
Age									
12–13 years	3.8	3.0	2.3	3.2	2.4	1.4	0.7	0.7	0.7
14–15 years	13.4	11.3	9.8	11.2	9.2	7.5	3.8	3.3	3.1
16–17 years	29.0	24.8	21.6	24.9	20.6	16.9	9.3	8.6	7.7
18–25 years	45.3	44.3	41.6	40.8	39.0	35.8	11.0	12.0	11.4
26–34 years	38.2	37.7	39.6	32.7	33.0	34.0	6.6	6.8	7.4
35 years and over	27.9	27.0	24.5	23.4	22.3	20.4	4.1	4.2	3.7
Sex									
Male	37.0	35.8	33.5	28.7	27.4	25.3	9.4	9.6	8.7
Female	24.3	23.4	22.2	23.4	22.5	21.4	1.7	1.8	2.0
Age and Sex									
12–17 years	15.2	13.1	11.6	13.0	10.8	8.9	4.5	4.2	4.0
Male	16.0	14.2	13.6	12.3	10.7	9.2	6.2	5.8	5.2
Female	14.4	11.9	9.5	13.6	10.8	8.6	2.7	2.5	2.7
Hispanic Origin and Race[3]									
Not Hispanic or Latino									
White only	32.0	31.2	29.6	26.9	26.0	24.5	5.5	5.9	5.2
Black or African American only	28.8	28.4	26.5	25.3	24.5	22.8	6.8	6.4	7.2
American Indian or Alaska Native only	44.3	41.7	41.8	37.1	36.0	33.0	5.2	10.6	6.9
Native Hawaiian or Other Pacific Islander only	28.8	30.3	*	*	28.8	15.4	4.1	3.7	*
Asian only	18.6	14.6	11.9	17.7	13.4	10.9	1.1	1.6	1.5
2 or more races	38.1	33.9	36.6	35.0	30.9	30.7	5.5	7.8	7.7
Hispanic or Latino	25.2	24.5	23.2	23.0	22.1	21.2	5.0	4.3	4.7

* = Figure does not meet standards of reliability or precision.
[1]Any illicit drug includes marijuana/hashish, cocaine (including crack), heroin, hallucinogens (including LSD and PCP), inhalants, or any prescription-type psychotherapeutic drug used nonmedically.
[2]Nonmedical use of prescription-type psychotherapeutic drugs includes the nonmedical use of pain relievers, tranquilizers, stimulants, or sedatives and does not include over-the-counter drugs.
[3]Persons of Hispanic origin may be of any race.
[4]Binge alcohol use is defined as drinking five or more drinks on the same occasion on at least 1 day in the past 30 days. Occasion is defined as at the same time or within a couple of hours of each other.
[5]Heavy alcohol use is defined as drinking five or more drinks on the same occasion on each of 5 or more days in the past 30 days. By definition, all heavy alcohol users are also binge alcohol users.
[6]Any tobacco product includes cigarettes, smokeless tobacco (i.e., chewing tobacco or snuff), cigars, or pipe tobacco.

Table C-28. Heavier Drinking and Drinking Five or More Drinks in a Day Among Adults 18 Years of Age and Over, by Selected Characteristics, Selected Years, 1997–2010

(Percent.)

Characteristic	Heavier drinker[1]				Five or more drinks in a day on at least 1 day in the past year[1]				Five or more drinks in a day on at least 12 days in the past year[1]			
	1997	2000	2005	2010	1997	2000	2005	2010	1997	2000	2005	2010
BOTH SEXES												
18 years and over, age–adjusted[2]	4.9	4.3	4.8	5.2	21.1	19.2	20.1	23.8	9.7	8.7	8.9	10.1
18 years and over, crude	5.0	4.3	4.9	5.2	21.5	19.3	19.9	23.2	9.8	8.7	8.8	9.9
Age												
All persons:												
18–44 years	5.2	4.7	5.2	5.7	29.2	26.9	28.5	32.5	13.2	12.2	12.7	13.7
18–24 years	5.3	5.8	6.6	6.2	31.8	30.3	31.4	34.0	15.2	15.5	15.7	16.2
25–44 years	5.2	4.3	4.8	5.5	28.5	25.8	27.5	31.9	12.6	11.1	11.6	12.7
45–64 years	5.5	4.6	5.2	5.4	15.9	14.4	14.7	19.0	7.6	6.4	6.3	8.1
45–54 years	5.5	4.4	5.4	5.9	19.0	16.4	17.5	22.9	8.7	7.0	7.7	9.3
55–64 years	5.4	5.0	4.9	4.7	11.1	11.3	10.8	14.1	5.8	5.4	4.4	6.7
65 years and over	3.1	2.6	3.0	3.7	4.9	3.8	3.6	5.5	2.2	1.8	1.7	2.6
65–74 years	3.9	3.1	4.0	4.4	6.7	5.2	5.4	7.9	3.0	2.5	2.7	3.5
75 years and over	2.1	2.0	2.0	2.8	2.4	2.1	1.6	2.7	1.1	*0.9	*0.7	*1.4
Race[2,3]												
White only	5.2	4.5	5.2	5.6	22.9	20.8	21.9	26.3	10.3	9.2	9.6	11.1
Black or African American only	4.0	3.5	3.0	4.1	11.7	11.6	12.0	14.0	6.5	6.5	5.6	6.1
American Indian or Alaska Native only	*	*	*	*	29.2	23.7	22.8	15.3	17.4	*12.1	*11.9	*9.5
Asian only	*1.9	*2.3	*2.1	*1.3	11.4	8.8	9.8	12.1	*4.8	3.6	3.8	4.3
Native Hawaiian or Other Pacific Islander only	—	*	*	*	—	*	*	*	—	*	*	*
2 or more races	—	*7.5	*5.0	*5.9	—	28.0	18.8	25.7	—	15.9	*9.0	12.5
Hispanic Origin and Race[2,3]												
Hispanic or Latino	3.9	3.2	2.4	2.8	20.4	17.3	17.4	19.7	11.2	9.0	8.4	9.2
Mexican	4.4	3.8	2.5	3.1	21.2	19.9	18.5	21.4	12.6	10.8	9.9	10.1
Not Hispanic or Latino	5.1	4.5	5.2	5.6	21.3	19.7	20.7	24.7	9.5	8.8	9.0	10.3
White only	5.4	4.7	5.8	6.2	23.5	21.5	23.0	27.9	10.3	9.3	9.9	11.5
Black or African American only	3.9	3.4	3.0	4.2	11.6	11.5	11.7	13.9	6.5	6.5	5.6	6.1
Percent of Poverty Level[2,4]												
Below 100%	4.8	4.3	4.2	4.7	17.3	15.0	15.3	17.6	9.7	8.6	8.1	8.5
100%–199%	4.9	4.2	4.5	4.9	18.4	15.7	15.9	20.9	9.8	8.0	8.4	9.8
200%–399%	4.9	4.2	4.8	4.8	21.0	18.7	19.4	23.3	9.8	8.9	8.7	10.1
400% or more	5.1	4.4	5.3	6.0	24.3	22.1	23.8	28.1	9.7	8.9	9.5	10.9
Disability Measure[2,5]												
Any basic actions difficulty or complex activity limitation	5.7	5.2	5.8	5.5	20.2	18.8	19.7	21.9	10.2	9.3	9.3	9.5
Any basic actions difficulty	5.8	5.3	5.9	5.5	20.6	19.1	20.0	22.3	10.5	9.4	9.5	9.7
Any complex activity limitation	4.5	4.3	4.4	5.5	16.4	14.3	14.6	16.2	8.8	7.3	6.9	7.8
No disability	4.9	4.1	4.6	5.3	21.8	19.7	20.5	25.0	9.6	8.7	8.8	10.4
MALE												
18 years and over, age–adjusted[2]	6.1	5.1	5.6	5.7	30.7	28.3	28.5	32.4	15.8	14.4	14.2	15.6
18 years and over, crude	6.1	5.2	5.6	5.7	31.7	29.0	28.8	32.2	16.3	14.7	14.4	15.6
Age												
All persons												
18–44 years	6.5	5.6	6.2	6.1	40.6	37.8	39.0	42.5	21.1	19.6	19.8	20.6
18–24 years	6.0	6.3	8.1	6.0	40.6	38.0	41.4	39.9	22.9	22.9	22.8	21.5
25–44 years	6.6	5.3	5.6	6.2	40.6	37.7	38.1	43.5	20.6	18.5	18.8	20.2
45–64 years	6.6	5.5	5.8	5.8	25.3	23.5	22.3	27.3	12.7	11.3	10.6	13.2
45–54 years	6.6	5.7	5.9	5.9	29.4	26.3	25.9	32.0	14.5	12.3	12.7	14.5
55–64 years	6.6	5.4	5.6	5.7	18.9	19.0	17.1	21.4	10.0	9.8	7.5	11.6
65 years and over	3.7	3.1	3.1	4.0	9.3	7.4	6.9	9.8	4.7	3.7	3.5	4.7
65–74 years	4.8	3.9	4.0	4.4	12.2	9.5	9.6	13.5	6.1	4.9	5.0	6.3
75 years and over	*2.1	*2.0	*2.1	*3.5	5.1	4.4	3.4	4.6	*2.5	*2.0	*1.4	*2.5
Race[2,3]												
White only	6.3	5.1	5.8	6.1	32.8	29.9	30.4	35.3	16.7	14.9	15.2	17.1
Black or African American only	5.3	5.4	4.4	4.6	18.4	19.8	20.0	20.2	11.0	12.4	10.5	9.8
American Indian or Alaska Native only	*	*	*	*	45.7	29.2	30.1	*20.5	30.4	*14.0	*19.0	*15.7
Asian only	*2.3	*3.5	*	*1.4	17.8	14.1	13.6	17.2	*7.5	*5.9	*5.7	6.8
Native Hawaiian or Other Pacific Islander only	—	*	*	*	—	*	*	*	—	*	*	*
2 or more races	—	*12.1	*	*8.4	—	39.2	28.2	37.6	—	23.7	*13.2	20.3

Table C-28. Heavier Drinking and Drinking Five or More Drinks in a Day Among Adults 18 Years of Age and Over, by Selected Characteristics, Selected Years, 1997–2010—Continued

(Percent.)

Characteristic	Heavier drinker[1]				Five or more drinks in a day on at least 1 day in the past year[1]				Five or more drinks in a day on at least 12 days in the past year[1]			
	1997	2000	2005	2010	1997	2000	2005	2010	1997	2000	2005	2010
Hispanic Origin and Race[2,3]												
Hispanic or Latino	5.7	5.2	3.8	3.9	30.9	27.9	27.4	28.8	18.8	15.9	14.4	14.6
Mexican	6.9	6.6	4.2	4.4	34.2	32.2	29.7	32.2	21.9	19.1	17.3	16.3
Not Hispanic or Latino	6.1	5.2	5.9	6.0	30.7	28.6	28.8	33.3	15.5	14.3	14.3	15.9
White only	6.4	5.2	6.3	6.5	33.3	30.6	31.4	36.9	16.6	15.0	15.5	17.6
Black or African American only	5.3	5.4	4.4	4.7	18.4	19.7	19.6	20.3	11.1	12.3	10.4	9.9
Percent of Poverty Level[2,4]												
Below 100%	6.8	6.4	6.2	6.5	26.9	24.8	24.4	26.0	16.5	15.7	14.4	14.1
100%–199%	7.1	5.8	6.0	5.8	27.3	23.6	23.7	29.1	16.4	13.3	14.0	14.8
200%–399%	6.6	5.3	5.7	5.8	30.4	27.4	27.1	31.8	16.0	14.7	13.9	16.4
400% or more	5.0	4.4	5.2	5.4	33.6	31.3	32.2	36.4	15.4	14.4	14.6	15.8
Disability Measure[2,5]												
Any basic actions difficulty or complex activity limitation	7.2	6.8	7.8	6.6	29.4	28.9	29.2	30.6	17.0	16.5	15.9	14.8
Any basic actions difficulty	7.5	6.8	8.1	6.7	30.4	29.8	30.1	31.8	17.7	16.8	16.5	15.5
Any complex activity limitation	5.4	5.8	6.0	6.6	23.1	20.5	20.6	21.1	14.2	11.9	11.4	11.3
No disability	5.8	4.8	4.9	5.4	31.5	28.5	28.7	33.5	15.6	14.1	13.9	15.9
FEMALE												
18 years and over, age-adjusted[2]	3.9	3.5	4.1	4.8	12.2	10.8	12.2	15.6	3.9	3.4	3.8	4.8
18 years and over, crude	3.9	3.5	4.1	4.8	12.1	10.6	11.8	14.9	3.9	3.3	3.7	4.6
Age												
All persons												
18–44 years	4.0	3.8	4.3	5.2	18.3	16.5	18.3	22.6	5.5	5.2	5.7	6.9
18–24 years	4.5	5.2	5.0	6.4	23.0	22.8	21.6	28.1	7.6	8.3	8.8	10.9
25–44 years	3.9	3.4	4.0	4.8	16.9	14.5	17.2	20.6	4.9	4.2	4.7	5.4
45–64 years	4.4	3.8	4.6	4.9	7.2	6.0	7.7	11.1	2.9	1.9	2.4	3.4
45–54 years	4.5	3.2	5.0	5.9	9.2	7.1	9.6	14.3	3.3	2.1	3.0	4.3
55–64 years	4.4	4.6	4.2	3.8	4.1	4.4	5.2	7.3	2.1	1.5	1.6	2.3
65 years and over	2.6	2.2	3.0	3.4	1.6	1.2	1.1	2.3	*0.4	*0.4	*	*
65–74 years	3.1	2.5	4.0	4.5	2.3	1.7	1.8	*3.1	*	*	*	*
75 years and over	2.0	1.9	1.9	2.3	*0.7	*	*	*1.4	*	*	*	*
Race[2,3]												
White only	4.2	4.0	4.6	5.2	13.5	12.1	13.6	17.4	4.2	3.7	4.2	5.2
Black or African American only	2.9	2.0	1.9	3.8	6.5	5.2	5.5	9.0	2.9	1.9	1.7	3.1
American Indian or Alaska Native only	*	*	*	*	18.1	*19.0	*16.6	*11.7	*	*	*	*
Asian only	*	*	*	*	*5.2	*3.7	*5.9	7.3	*	*	*	*
Native Hawaiian or Other Pacific Islander only	—	*	*	*	—	*	*	*	—	*	*	*
2 or more races	—	*	*	*	—	17.0	*10.7	16.4	—	*8.2	*	*6.3
Hispanic Origin and Race[2,3]												
Hispanic or Latina	2.2	1.2	1.0	1.7	9.7	6.8	7.2	10.3	3.5	2.1	2.2	3.6
Mexican	*1.9	*1.1	*0.9	*1.7	8.2	7.1	7.1	10.4	3.2	*2.2	2.3	3.7
Not Hispanic or Latina	4.1	3.8	4.6	5.3	12.6	11.5	13.1	16.6	4.0	3.6	4.1	5.0
White only	4.4	4.3	5.2	5.9	14.2	13.0	15.1	19.1	4.3	4.0	4.7	5.6
Black or African American only	2.9	2.0	1.9	3.8	6.2	5.2	5.4	8.9	2.9	1.9	1.7	3.0
Percent of Poverty Level[2,4]												
Below 100%	3.6	2.8	2.8	3.4	10.8	8.2	9.0	11.3	5.1	3.6	3.7	4.2
100%–199%	3.1	2.9	3.2	4.1	10.5	9.0	9.3	13.5	4.0	3.5	3.7	5.1
200%–399%	3.3	3.2	3.8	3.9	12.1	10.7	12.1	15.3	4.0	3.5	3.8	4.2
400% or more	5.2	4.5	5.4	6.7	14.2	12.6	14.8	19.2	3.4	3.3	4.0	5.6
Disability Measure[2,5]												
Any basic actions difficulty or complex activity limitation	4.5	4.1	4.3	4.7	13.1	11.3	12.7	15.2	5.0	4.1	4.4	5.4
Any basic actions difficulty	4.5	4.2	4.4	4.7	13.2	11.6	12.7	15.4	5.1	4.1	4.5	5.4
Any complex activity limitation	3.7	*3.2	3.0	4.6	10.8	9.1	9.7	12.3	4.2	*3.1	3.1	5.0
No disability	3.9	3.5	4.3	5.1	12.0	10.9	12.2	16.1	3.6	3.3	3.7	4.7

* = Figure does not meet standards of reliability or precision.
— = Data not available.
[1]Heavier drinking is based on self-reported responses to questions about average alcohol consumption and is defined as more than 14 drinks per week for men and more than seven drinks per week for women on average.
[2]Estimates are age-adjusted to the year 2000 standard population using four age groups: 18–24 years, 25–44 years, 45–64 years, and 65 years and over. Age-adjusted estimates in this table may differ from other age-adjusted estimates based on the same data and presented elsewhere if different age groups are used in the adjustment procedure.
[3]The race groups, White, Black, American Indian or Alaska Native, Asian, Native Hawaiian or Other Pacific Islander, and 2 or more races, include persons of Hispanic and non-Hispanic origin. Persons of Hispanic origin may be of any race.
[4]Percent of poverty level is based on family income and family size and composition using U.S. Census Bureau poverty thresholds.
[5]Any basic actions difficulty or complex activity limitation is defined as having one or more of the following limitations or difficulties: movement difficulty, emotional difficulty, sensory (seeing or hearing) difficulty, cognitive difficulty, self-care (activities of daily living or instrumental activities of daily living) limitation, social limitation, or work limitation.

Table C-29. Age-Adjusted Prevalence of Current Cigarette Smoking[1] Among Adults 25 Years of Age and Over, by Sex, Race, and Education Level, Selected Years, 1974–2010

(Percent.)

Sex, race, and education level	1974[2]	1979[2]	1985[2]	1990[2]	1995[2]	2000	2005	2006	2007	2008	2009	2010
25 YEARS AND OVER, AGE ADJUSTED[3]												
All Persons[4]	36.9	33.1	30.0	25.4	24.5	22.6	20.3	20.3	19.3	20.5	20.4	19.2
No high school diploma or GED	43.7	40.7	40.8	36.7	35.6	31.6	28.2	28.8	26.9	29.8	28.9	26.9
High school diploma or GED	36.2	33.6	32.0	29.1	29.1	29.2	27.0	26.5	26.6	28.1	28.7	27.0
Some college, no bachelor's degree	35.9	33.2	29.5	23.4	22.6	21.7	21.8	22.1	20.1	22.1	21.4	21.3
Bachelor's degree or higher	27.2	22.6	18.5	13.9	13.6	10.9	9.1	8.2	9.0	8.5	9.0	8.3
All Males[4]	42.9	37.3	32.8	28.2	26.4	24.7	22.7	22.9	21.4	22.6	22.4	21.0
No high school diploma or GED	52.3	47.6	45.7	42.0	39.7	36.0	31.7	31.6	30.8	32.5	32.3	29.7
High school diploma or GED	42.4	38.9	35.5	33.1	32.7	32.1	29.9	29.7	29.4	31.4	31.4	29.3
Some college, no bachelor's degree	41.8	36.5	32.9	25.9	23.7	23.3	24.9	25.2	21.6	24.3	23.0	23.2
Bachelor's degree or higher	28.3	22.7	19.6	14.5	13.8	11.6	9.7	9.2	10.4	9.1	9.6	8.7
White Males[4,5]	41.9	36.7	31.7	27.6	25.9	24.7	22.4	22.7	21.6	22.6	22.7	21.0
No high school diploma or GED	51.5	47.6	45.0	41.8	38.7	38.2	31.6	31.4	30.8	33.1	32.2	29.4
High school diploma or GED	42.0	38.5	34.8	32.9	32.9	32.4	30.0	29.2	29.9	31.9	32.4	29.6
Some college, no bachelor's degree	41.6	36.4	32.2	25.4	23.3	23.5	24.5	25.8	21.8	23.7	22.4	23.4
Bachelor's degree or higher	27.8	22.5	19.1	14.4	13.4	11.3	9.3	8.9	10.5	9.1	9.6	8.8
Black or African American Males[4,5]	53.4	44.4	42.1	34.5	31.6	26.4	26.5	25.4	23.7	25.9	23.7	23.9
No high school diploma or GED	58.1	49.7	50.5	41.6	41.9	38.2	35.9	35.2	30.4	35.0	39.1	34.4
High school diploma or GED	*50.7	48.6	41.8	37.4	36.6	29.0	30.1	31.3	29.6	28.3	26.0	28.8
Some college, no bachelor's degree	*45.3	39.2	41.8	28.1	26.4	19.9	27.4	21.0	23.6	29.5	26.5	24.2
Bachelor's degree or higher	*41.4	*36.8	*32.0	*20.8	*17.3	14.6	10.0	12.9	*13.5	*10.0	9.9	8.1
All Females[4]	32.0	29.5	27.5	22.9	22.9	20.5	18.0	17.9	17.2	18.4	18.5	17.5
No high school diploma or GED	36.6	34.8	36.5	31.8	31.7	27.1	24.6	26.0	22.7	27.0	24.8	23.7
High school diploma or GED	32.2	29.8	29.5	26.1	26.4	26.6	24.1	23.4	23.8	25.0	26.1	24.9
Some college, no bachelor's degree	30.1	30.0	26.3	21.0	21.6	20.4	19.1	19.6	18.9	20.1	20.0	19.6
Bachelor's degree or higher	25.9	22.5	17.1	13.3	13.3	10.1	8.5	7.2	7.7	8.1	8.4	7.9
White Females[4,5]	31.7	29.7	27.3	23.3	23.1	21.0	18.6	18.5	18.0	19.4	19.0	18.3
No high school diploma or GED	36.8	35.8	36.7	33.4	32.4	28.4	24.6	25.9	23.8	28.4	24.4	24.0
High school diploma or GED	31.9	29.9	29.4	26.5	26.8	27.8	25.9	24.6	25.2	27.1	26.5	25.8
Some college, no bachelor's degree	30.4	30.7	26.7	21.2	22.2	21.1	19.5	20.5	19.6	21.6	21.2	21.0
Bachelor's degree or higher	25.5	21.9	16.5	13.4	13.5	10.2	9.1	7.7	8.2	8.5	9.1	8.7
Black or African American Females[4,5]	35.6	30.3	32.0	22.4	25.7	21.6	17.5	19.1	16.6	17.5	19.3	17.0
No high school diploma or GED	36.1	31.6	39.4	26.3	32.3	31.1	27.8	31.2	23.1	28.9	31.0	25.8
High school diploma or GED	40.9	32.6	32.1	24.1	27.8	25.4	18.2	18.6	19.8	20.0	27.3	22.9
Some college, no bachelor's degree	32.3	*28.9	23.9	22.7	20.8	20.4	17.5	18.9	17.2	15.9	16.2	15.0
Bachelor's degree or higher	*36.3	*43.3	26.6	17.0	17.3	10.8	*6.6	*8.5	*6.0	*9.3	*7.3	*6.6

* = Figure does not meet standards of reliability or precision.
[1] Starting with 1993 data current cigarette smokers were defined as ever smoking 100 cigarettes in their lifetime and smoking now every day or some days.
[2] Data prior to 1997 are not strictly comparable with data for later years due to the 1997 questionnaire redesign.
[3] Estimates are age-adjusted to the year 2000 standard population using four age groups: 25–34 years, 35–44 years, 45–64 years, and 65 years and over.
[4] Includes unknown education level. Education categories shown are for 1997 and subsequent years.
[5] The race groups, White and Black, include persons of Hispanic and non-Hispanic origin.

Table C-30. Current Cigarette Smoking[1] Among Adults, by Sex, Race, Hispanic Origin, Age, and Education Level, Average Annual, Selected Years, 1990–1992 through 2008–2010

(Percent.)

Characteristic	Male				Female			
	1990–1992[2]	1999–2001	2006–2008	2008–2010	1990–1992[2]	1999–2001	2006–2008	2008–2010
18 Years and Over, Age–Adjusted[3]								
All persons[4]	27.9	25.0	22.8	22.4	23.7	21.1	18.0	18.0
Race[5]								
White only	27.4	25.1	22.9	22.6	24.3	22.2	18.9	18.8
Black or African American only	33.9	27.2	24.8	23.7	23.1	19.7	17.2	17.5
American Indian or Alaska Native only	34.2	30.3	31.5	25.1	36.7	34.7	22.2	21.0
Asian only	24.8	20.3	15.6	15.3	6.3	6.7	4.4	5.5
Native Hawaiian or Other Pacific Islander only	—	*	*	*	—	*	*	*
2 or more races	—	34.4	25.1	27.7	—	30.7	24.6	20.9
American Indian or Alaska Native; White	—	38.7	34.6	34.6	—	38.9	28.6	26.5
Hispanic Origin and Race[5]								
Hispanic or Latino	25.7	22.2	18.6	17.3	15.8	12.1	9.5	9.6
Mexican	26.2	21.9	18.7	17.5	14.8	10.6	8.8	8.4
Not Hispanic or Latino	28.1	25.5	23.7	23.4	24.4	22.3	19.4	19.5
White only	27.7	25.5	24.0	23.9	25.2	23.5	20.9	20.9
Black or African American only	33.9	27.2	25.1	24.0	23.2	19.7	17.2	17.7
18 Years and Over, Crude								
All persons[4]	28.4	25.5	23.1	22.7	23.6	21.0	17.9	17.8
Race[5]								
White only	27.8	25.4	23.0	22.7	24.1	21.7	18.5	18.4
Black or African American only	33.2	27.5	25.6	24.4	23.3	19.8	17.5	17.9
American Indian or Alaska Native only	35.5	31.8	30.7	25.6	37.3	36.9	23.0	21.6
Asian only	24.9	21.4	16.5	15.7	6.3	6.9	4.6	5.6
Native Hawaiian or Other Pacific Islander only	—	*	*	*	—	*	*	*
2 or more races	—	35.9	27.0	29.2	—	31.5	25.3	21.9
American Indian or Alaska Native; White	—	41.1	33.5	33.9	—	40.1	30.0	27.5
Hispanic Origin and Race[5]								
Hispanic or Latino	26.5	23.2	19.6	18.4	16.6	12.6	9.7	9.8
Mexican	27.1	22.8	19.4	18.6	15.0	11.0	8.8	8.5
Not Hispanic or Latino	28.5	25.8	23.7	23.4	24.2	21.9	19.1	19.0
White only	28.0	25.5	23.7	23.6	24.8	22.7	20.1	20.0
Black or African American only	33.3	27.5	26.0	24.7	23.3	19.8	17.6	18.0
Age and Hispanic Origin and Race[5]								
18–24 Years								
Hispanic or Latino	19.3	22.6	18.4	19.3	12.8	12.9	8.0	8.0
Not Hispanic or Latino								
White only	28.9	32.7	29.1	28.2	28.7	30.8	24.1	21.2
Black or African American only	17.7	21.9	23.6	18.4	10.8	13.0	13.5	14.9
25–34 Years								
Hispanic or Latino	29.9	23.2	20.4	20.1	19.2	12.5	9.5	9.6
Not Hispanic or Latino								
White only	32.7	30.8	31.6	30.8	30.9	27.4	26.7	26.5
Black or African American only	34.6	23.3	28.5	25.7	29.2	16.9	16.2	19.1
35–44 Years								
Hispanic or Latino	32.1	25.3	20.5	18.2	19.9	14.1	10.2	10.4
Not Hispanic or Latino								
White only	32.3	29.6	25.9	26.5	27.3	28.3	24.1	24.7
Black or African American only	44.1	32.0	20.9	23.2	31.3	27.5	19.4	19.0
45–64 Years								
Hispanic or Latino	26.6	24.7	21.4	19.2	17.1	13.5	12.5	12.2
Not Hispanic or Latino								
White only	28.4	25.1	23.5	24.1	26.1	22.1	20.7	21.0
Black or African American only	38.0	34.0	31.8	31.7	26.1	23.6	23.2	21.6
65 Years and Over								
Hispanic or Latino	16.1	12.6	9.4	8.2	6.6	5.9	4.7	5.5
Not Hispanic or Latino								
White only	14.2	10.0	10.5	9.8	12.3	9.8	8.6	9.5
Black or African American only	25.2	17.6	16.3	13.7	10.7	11.0	7.8	9.8
Percent of Poverty Level[2,6]								
Below 100%	40.5	36.5	32.1	32.5	30.7	29.1	28.1	28.6
100%–199%	35.0	32.8	29.4	29.3	26.9	25.6	22.4	22.8
200%–399%	26.5	27.3	24.8	24.3	22.6	22.3	18.5	18.5
400% or more	22.5	18.8	17.0	16.0	19.0	15.9	12.5	11.8

Table C-30. Current Cigarette Smoking[1] Among Adults, by Sex, Race, Hispanic Origin, Age, and Education Level, Average Annual, Selected Years, 1990–1992 through 2008–2010—Continued

(Percent.)

Characteristic	Male				Female			
	1990–1992[2]	1999–2001	2006–2008	2008–2010	1990–1992[2]	1999–2001	2006–2008	2008–2010
Hispanic Origin and Race and Percent of Poverty Level[2,4,6]								
Hispanic or Latino								
Below 100%	29.2	25.3	20.8	20.2	16.3	14.4	11.9	11.4
100%–199%	29.5	22.0	18.4	17.8	16.0	11.8	8.3	8.7
200%–399%	23.7	23.6	19.7	16.6	15.9	12.0	8.6	10.2
400% or more	19.7	18.1	15.7	15.1	13.6	9.4	9.9	7.9
Not Hispanic or Latino								
White only								
Below 100%	44.2	40.7	38.6	40.6	37.8	38.3	38.0	39.4
100%–199%	36.3	37.5	35.0	35.3	31.1	32.0	30.7	30.7
200%–399%	26.4	28.5	27.0	27.4	23.7	24.8	22.1	21.9
400% or more	22.5	19.1	17.4	16.3	19.5	17.1	13.6	13.1
Black or African American only								
Below 100%	43.5	40.6	38.2	36.5	28.9	27.7	27.0	29.1
100%–199%	36.0	33.9	30.9	30.4	20.3	21.3	18.6	19.6
200%–399%	31.4	24.9	21.8	20.7	21.4	17.3	13.5	13.2
400% or more	24.3	17.9	18.4	15.6	19.2	12.6	10.3	8.2
Disability Measure[7]								
Any basic actions difficulty or complex activity limitation	—	33.1	32.1	30.3	—	28.1	26.8	26.8
Any basic actions difficulty	—	33.2	32.5	30.5	—	28.2	27.0	27.0
Any complex activity limitation	—	37.6	34.2	33.2	—	30.6	31.8	31.5
No disability	—	22.8	20.1	19.8	—	18.8	14.9	14.6
Education, Hispanic Origin, and Race[5,8]								
25 years and over, age–adjusted[9]								
No high school diploma or GED								
Hispanic or Latino	30.2	24.3	19.5	18.5	15.8	12.1	8.6	8.6
Not Hispanic or Latino								
White only	46.1	43.5	42.0	45.1	40.4	39.3	42.9	44.0
Black or African American only	45.4	40.0	35.9	37.2	31.3	29.4	28.7	29.9
High school diploma or GED								
Hispanic or Latino	29.6	24.1	21.7	20.3	18.4	12.5	10.7	11.4
Not Hispanic or Latino								
White only	32.9	31.8	32.7	34.4	28.4	29.2	28.8	30.3
Black or African American only	38.2	31.4	29.5	27.8	25.4	23.0	19.8	23.7
Some college or more								
Hispanic or Latino	20.4	17.1	15.8	12.9	14.3	11.1	10.3	9.9
Not Hispanic or Latino								
White only	19.3	17.6	16.2	15.9	18.1	16.7	14.7	15.5
Black or African American only	25.6	19.2	19.3	19.8	22.8	16.9	13.7	12.7

— = Data not available.
* = Figure does not meet standards of reliability or precision.
[2] Estimates are age–adjusted to the year 2000 standard population using five age groups: 18–24 years, 25–34 years, 35–44 years, 45–64 years, and 65 years and over.
[3] Starting with 1993 data, current cigarette smokers were defined as ever smoking 100 cigarettes in their lifetime and smoking now every day or some days.
[4] Includes all other races not shown separately, unknown education level, and unknown disability measure.
[5] The race groups, White, Black, American Indian or Alaska Native, Asian, Native Hawaiian or Other Pacific Islander, and 2 or more races, include persons of Hispanic and non–Hispanic origin. Persons of Hispanic origin may be of any race.
[6] Percent of poverty level is based on family income and family size and composition using U.S. Census Bureau poverty thresholds.
[7] Any basic actions difficulty or complex activity limitation is defined as having one or more of the following limitations or difficulties: movement difficulty, emotional difficulty, sensory (seeing or hearing) difficulty, cognitive difficulty, self–care (activities of daily living or instrumental activities of daily living) limitation, social limitation, or work limitation.
[8] Education categories shown are for 1997 and subsequent years.
[9] Estimates are age–adjusted to the year 2000 standard using four age groups: 25–34 years, 35–44 years, 45–64 years, and 65 years and over.

Table C-31. Current Cigarette Smoking[1] Among Adults 18 Years of Age and Over, by Sex, Race, and Age, Selected Years, 1965–2010

(Percent.)

Sex, race, and age	1965[2]	1974[2]	1983[2]	1985[2]	1990[2]	1995[2]	2000	2005	2006	2007	2008	2009	2010
18 Years and Over, Age-Adjusted[3]													
All persons	41.9	37.0	31.9	29.9	25.3	24.6	23.1	20.8	20.8	19.7	20.6	20.6	19.3
Male	51.2	42.8	34.8	32.2	28.0	26.5	25.2	23.4	23.6	22.0	22.8	23.2	21.2
Female	33.7	32.2	29.4	27.9	22.9	22.7	21.1	18.3	18.1	17.5	18.5	18.1	17.5
White male[4]	50.4	41.7	34.2	31.3	27.6	26.2	25.4	23.3	23.5	22.2	23.0	23.6	21.4
Black or African American male[4]	58.8	53.6	41.7	40.2	32.8	29.4	25.7	25.9	26.1	23.4	24.7	23.1	23.3
White female[4]	33.9	32.0	29.6	27.9	23.5	23.4	22.0	19.1	18.8	18.5	19.5	18.7	18.3
Black or African American female[4]	31.8	35.6	31.3	30.9	20.8	23.5	20.7	17.1	18.5	15.6	17.4	18.5	16.6
18 Years and Over, Crude													
All persons	42.4	37.1	32.1	30.1	25.5	24.7	23.2	20.9	20.8	19.8	20.6	20.6	19.3
Male	51.9	43.1	35.1	32.6	28.4	27.0	25.6	23.9	23.9	22.3	23.1	23.5	21.5
Female	33.9	32.1	29.5	27.9	22.8	22.6	20.9	18.1	18.0	17.4	18.3	17.9	17.3
White male[4]	51.1	41.9	34.5	31.7	28.0	26.6	25.7	23.6	23.6	22.3	23.1	23.6	21.4
Black or African American male[4]	60.4	54.3	40.6	39.9	32.5	28.5	26.2	26.5	27.0	24.6	25.3	23.7	24.3
White female[4]	34.0	31.7	29.4	27.7	23.4	23.1	21.4	18.7	18.4	18.1	19.1	18.3	17.9
Black or African American female[4]	33.7	36.4	32.2	31.0	21.2	23.5	20.8	17.3	18.8	15.9	17.8	18.8	17.0
All Males													
18–44 years	57.3	47.9	37.7	35.2	31.4	29.9	29.2	27.1	26.7	25.8	25.6	26.9	23.9
18–24 years	54.1	42.1	32.9	28.0	26.6	27.8	28.1	28.0	28.5	25.4	23.6	28.0	22.8
25–34 years	60.7	50.5	38.8	38.2	31.6	29.5	28.9	27.7	27.4	28.8	28.5	27.6	26.1
35–44 years	58.2	51.0	41.0	37.6	34.5	31.5	30.2	26.0	26.8	23.2	24.3	25.4	22.5
45–64 years	51.9	42.6	35.9	33.4	29.3	27.1	26.4	25.2	24.5	22.6	24.8	24.5	23.2
45–54 years	55.9	46.8	39.0	34.9	32.1	27.2	28.8	28.1	26.6	24.8	26.4	27.3	25.2
55–64 years	46.6	37.7	32.6	31.9	25.9	26.9	22.6	21.1	21.5	19.6	22.6	20.8	20.7
65 years and over	28.5	24.8	22.0	19.6	14.6	14.9	10.2	8.9	12.6	9.3	10.5	9.5	9.7
White Male[4]													
18–44 years	57.1	46.8	37.5	34.6	31.3	30.1	30.2	27.7	27.1	26.6	26.7	28.1	24.6
18–24 years	53.0	40.8	32.5	28.4	27.4	28.4	30.4	29.7	28.9	26.5	25.2	30.0	23.8
25–34 years	60.1	49.5	38.6	37.3	31.6	29.9	29.7	27.7	27.9	29.0	29.5	28.4	26.6
35–44 years	57.3	50.1	40.8	36.6	33.5	31.2	30.6	26.3	25.3	24.4	24.9	26.3	23.1
45–64 years	51.3	41.2	35.0	32.1	28.7	26.3	25.8	24.5	23.4	22.1	24.0	24.0	22.5
45–54 years	55.3	45.0	38.0	33.7	31.3	25.9	28.0	27.4	25.7	24.4	26.1	27.1	24.5
55–64 years	46.1	36.6	31.9	30.5	25.6	27.0	22.5	20.4	20.4	19.1	21.2	20.1	20.1
65 years and over	27.7	24.3	20.6	18.9	13.7	14.1	9.8	7.9	12.6	8.9	9.9	9.3	9.6
Black or African American Male[4]													
18–44 years	66.3	58.1	39.4	39.6	32.9	26.4	25.5	25.1	26.2	24.2	22.0	22.5	22.6
18–24 years	62.8	54.9	34.2	27.2	21.3	*	20.9	21.6	31.2	21.4	*17.0	18.9	18.8
25–34 years	68.4	58.5	39.9	45.6	33.8	25.1	23.2	29.8	26.3	32.3	25.9	24.1	25.7
35–44 years	67.3	61.5	45.5	45.0	42.0	36.3	30.7	23.3	22.2	17.4	21.8	24.0	22.6
45–64 years	57.9	57.8	44.8	46.1	36.7	33.9	32.2	32.4	32.6	28.3	33.6	28.9	31.8
45–54 years	62.4	63.6	47.8	47.7	42.0	36.9	35.6	33.9	32.0	29.3	31.7	28.1	33.2
55–64 years	51.8	50.1	41.1	44.4	30.2	29.1	26.3	29.8	33.5	26.8	36.6	30.1	29.6
65 years and over	36.4	29.7	38.9	27.7	21.5	28.5	14.2	16.8	16.0	14.3	17.5	14.0	10.0
All Females													
18–44 years	42.1	37.5	33.8	31.4	25.6	25.6	24.5	21.2	20.6	19.5	20.6	20.0	19.1
18–24 years	38.1	34.1	35.5	30.4	22.5	21.8	24.9	20.7	19.3	19.1	19.0	15.6	17.4
25–34 years	43.7	38.8	32.6	32.0	28.2	26.4	22.3	21.5	21.5	19.6	21.4	21.8	20.6
35–44 years	43.7	39.8	33.8	31.5	24.8	27.1	26.2	21.3	20.6	19.6	20.9	21.2	19.0
45–64 years	32.0	33.4	31.0	29.9	24.8	24.0	21.7	18.8	19.3	19.5	20.5	19.5	19.1
45–54 years	37.5	36.0	34.1	32.4	28.5	24.3	22.2	20.9	22.5	22.1	23.7	22.3	21.3
55–64 years	25.0	30.4	28.0	27.4	20.5	23.7	20.9	16.1	14.9	16.2	16.3	16.1	16.5
65 years and over	9.6	12.0	13.1	13.5	11.5	11.5	9.3	8.3	8.3	7.6	8.3	9.5	9.3

Table C-31. Current Cigarette Smoking[1] Among Adults 18 Years of Age and Over, by Sex, Race, and Age, Selected Years, 1965–2010—Continued

(Percent.)

Sex, race, and age	1965[2]	1974[2]	1983[2]	1985[2]	1990[2]	1995[2]	2000	2005	2006	2007	2008	2009	2010
White Female[4]													
18–44 years	42.2	37.3	34.2	31.6	26.5	26.6	26.5	22.6	22.2	21.2	22.1	21.2	20.5
18–24 years	38.4	34.0	36.5	31.8	25.4	24.9	28.5	22.6	20.7	21.6	20.1	16.7	18.4
25–34 years	43.4	38.6	32.2	32.0	28.5	27.3	24.9	23.1	23.7	21.4	23.1	22.7	22.0
35–44 years	43.9	39.3	34.8	31.0	25.0	27.0	26.6	22.2	21.7	20.7	22.6	22.9	20.5
45–64 years	32.7	33.0	30.6	29.7	25.4	24.3	21.4	18.9	18.8	19.6	20.9	19.4	19.5
45–54 years	38.2	34.9	33.3	32.4	29.1	24.6	21.9	21.0	22.1	22.2	24.2	22.4	22.4
55–64 years	25.7	30.6	28.1	27.2	21.2	23.8	20.6	16.2	14.4	16.2	16.8	15.8	15.9
65 years and over	9.8	12.3	13.2	13.3	11.5	11.7	9.1	8.4	8.4	8.0	8.6	9.6	9.4
Black or African American Female[4]													
18–44 years	42.9	41.1	34.6	33.5	22.8	24.0	20.8	16.9	17.3	14.2	18.0	18.3	17.1
18–24 years	37.1	35.6	32.0	23.7	10.0	*8.8	14.2	14.2	14.8	*8.7	16.6	13.3	14.2
25–34 years	47.8	42.2	38.0	36.2	29.1	26.7	15.5	16.9	15.4	14.9	17.6	20.1	19.3
35–44 years	42.8	46.4	32.7	40.2	25.5	31.9	30.2	19.0	21.0	17.7	19.6	20.0	17.2
45–64 years	25.7	38.9	36.3	33.4	22.6	27.5	25.6	21.0	25.5	22.6	21.3	22.7	19.8
45–54 years	32.3	46.2	43.6	36.4	26.5	28.3	26.5	22.2	29.3	26.3	24.9	23.5	20.4
55–64 years	16.5	29.3	28.0	29.8	17.6	26.3	24.2	19.1	19.5	17.0	15.9	21.4	18.9
65 years and over	7.1	*8.9	*13.1	14.5	11.1	13.3	10.2	10.0	9.3	6.4	8.1	11.5	9.4

* = Figure does not meet standards of reliability or precision.
[1] Starting with 1993 data, current cigarette smokers were defined as ever smoking 100 cigarettes in their lifetime and smoking now every day or some days.
[2] Data prior to 1997 are not strictly comparable with data for later years due to the 1997 questionnaire redesign.
[3] Estimates are age-adjusted to the year 2000 standard population using five age groups: 18–24 years, 25–34 years, 35–44 years, 45–64 years, 65 years and over.
[4] The race groups, White and Black, include persons of Hispanic and non–Hispanic origin.

Table C-32. Use of Selected Substances Among High School Seniors, 10th Graders, and 8th Graders, by Sex and Race, Selected Years, 1980–2010

(Percent.)

Substance, grade in school, sex, and race	1980	1985	1990	1995	2000	2005	2006	2007	2008	2009	2010
Cigarettes											
All high school seniors	30.5	30.1	29.4	33.5	31.4	23.2	21.6	21.6	20.4	20.1	19.2
Male	26.8	28.2	29.1	34.5	32.8	24.8	22.4	23.1	21.5	22.1	21.9
Female	33.4	31.4	29.2	32.0	29.7	20.7	20.1	19.6	19.1	17.6	15.7
White	31.0	31.7	32.5	37.3	36.6	27.0	24.7	25.2	24.1	23.7	22.2
Black or African American	25.2	18.7	12.0	15.0	13.6	10.0	11.0	10.6	10.1	9.3	10.7
All 10th graders	—	—	—	27.9	23.9	14.9	14.5	14.0	12.3	13.1	13.6
Male	—	—	—	27.7	23.8	14.5	13.4	14.6	12.7	13.7	15.0
Female	—	—	—	27.9	23.6	15.1	15.5	13.3	11.9	12.5	12.1
White	—	—	—	31.2	27.3	17.0	16.3	16.1	14.1	14.6	14.8
Black or African American	—	—	—	12.2	11.3	7.7	8.5	5.8	7.1	6.4	7.0
All 8th graders	—	—	—	19.1	14.6	9.3	8.7	7.1	6.8	6.5	7.1
Male	—	—	—	18.8	14.3	8.7	8.1	7.5	6.7	6.7	7.4
Female	—	—	—	19.0	14.7	9.7	8.9	6.4	6.7	6.0	6.8
White	—	—	—	21.7	16.4	9.5	9.1	7.1	7.3	7.3	7.9
Black or African American	—	—	—	8.2	8.4	6.7	5.4	4.8	4.4	4.5	4.0
Marijuana											
All high school seniors	33.7	25.7	14.0	21.2	21.6	19.8	18.3	18.8	19.4	20.6	21.4
Male	37.8	28.7	16.1	24.6	24.7	23.6	19.7	22.3	22.2	24.3	25.2
Female	29.1	22.4	11.5	17.2	18.3	15.8	16.4	15.0	16.2	16.8	16.9
White	34.2	26.4	15.6	21.5	22.0	21.7	19.2	19.9	20.4	21.2	21.6
Black or African American	26.5	21.7	5.2	17.8	17.5	15.1	16.7	15.4	17.1	20.6	19.7
All 10th graders	—	—	—	17.2	19.7	15.2	14.2	14.2	13.8	15.9	16.7
Male	—	—	—	19.2	23.3	16.7	15.7	15.8	15.2	18.7	20.1
Female	—	—	—	15.0	16.2	13.4	12.6	12.5	12.3	13.2	13.3
White	—	—	—	17.7	20.1	15.7	14.7	14.8	13.5	15.6	15.9
Black or African American	—	—	—	15.1	17.0	13.5	14.2	11.0	12.3	15.1	15.9
All 8th graders	—	—	—	9.1	9.1	6.6	6.5	5.7	5.8	6.5	8.0
Male	—	—	—	9.8	10.2	7.6	6.7	6.2	6.6	7.5	9.2
Female	—	—	—	8.2	7.8	5.7	6.0	4.9	4.8	5.3	6.8
White	—	—	—	9.0	8.3	6.0	5.7	5.1	4.9	5.9	7.1
Black or African American	—	—	—	7.0	8.5	8.2	6.7	6.0	6.2	7.2	8.2
Cocaine											
All high school seniors	5.2	6.7	1.9	1.8	2.1	2.3	2.5	2.0	1.9	1.3	1.3
Male	6.0	7.7	2.3	2.2	2.7	2.6	3.0	2.4	2.3	1.5	1.9
Female	4.3	5.6	1.3	1.3	1.6	1.8	2.1	1.5	1.3	0.9	0.7
White	5.4	7.0	1.8	1.7	2.2	2.3	2.6	2.3	2.0	1.2	1.2
Black or African American	2.0	2.7	0.5	0.4	1.0	0.5	1.0	0.5	0.5	0.2	0.9
All 10th graders	—	—	—	1.7	1.8	1.5	1.5	1.3	1.2	0.9	0.9
Male	—	—	—	1.8	2.1	1.9	1.6	1.4	1.4	1.0	1.1
Female	—	—	—	1.5	1.4	1.2	1.3	1.1	1.0	0.8	0.5
White	—	—	—	1.7	1.7	1.5	1.5	1.2	1.0	0.7	0.7
Black or African American	—	—	—	0.4	0.4	0.8	0.7	0.4	0.7	0.5	0.6
All 8th graders	—	—	—	1.2	1.2	1.0	1.0	0.9	0.8	0.8	0.6
Male	—	—	—	1.1	1.3	0.9	1.0	0.7	0.9	0.8	0.6
Female	—	—	—	1.2	1.1	1.0	0.9	1.0	0.7	0.7	0.6
White	—	—	—	1.0	1.1	0.9	0.8	0.6	0.6	0.6	0.5
Black or African American	—	—	—	0.4	0.5	0.3	0.4	0.6	0.4	0.7	0.3
Inhalants											
All high school seniors	1.4	2.2	2.7	3.2	2.2	2.0	1.5	1.2	1.4	1.2	1.4
Male	1.8	2.8	3.5	3.9	2.9	2.4	1.5	1.5	1.6	1.2	2.1
Female	1.0	1.7	2.0	2.5	1.7	1.6	1.4	0.9	1.2	1.0	0.7
White	1.4	2.4	3.0	3.7	2.1	2.1	1.5	1.2	1.5	1.1	1.1
Black or African American	1.0	0.8	1.5	1.1	2.1	1.4	1.2	0.9	1.0	1.1	1.5
All 10th graders	—	—	—	3.5	2.6	2.2	2.3	2.5	2.1	2.2	2.0
Male	—	—	—	3.8	3.0	1.9	2.2	2.7	1.9	1.8	1.6
Female	—	—	—	3.2	2.2	2.5	2.4	2.4	2.3	2.6	2.4
White	—	—	—	3.9	2.8	2.2	2.4	2.6	1.6	1.9	1.7
Black or African American	—	—	—	1.2	1.5	1.4	1.8	1.5	1.9	1.3	1.8
All 8th graders	—	—	—	6.1	4.5	4.2	4.1	3.9	4.1	3.8	3.6
Male	—	—	—	5.6	4.1	3.1	3.6	3.4	2.9	3.3	2.8
Female	—	—	—	6.6	4.8	5.3	4.7	4.3	5.3	4.3	4.4
White	—	—	—	7.0	4.8	4.0	4.2	3.6	3.8	3.7	3.2
Black or African American	—	—	—	2.3	2.3	2.9	2.7	2.8	2.8	3.4	2.2

Table C-32. Use of Selected Substances Among High School Seniors, 10th Graders, and 8th Graders, by Sex and Race, Selected Years, 1980–2010—Continued

(Percent.)

Substance, grade in school, sex, and race	1980	1985	1990	1995	2000	2005	2006	2007	2008	2009	2010
MDMA (Ecstasy)											
All high school seniors	—	—	—	—	3.6	1.0	1.3	1.6	1.8	1.8	1.4
Male	—	—	—	—	4.1	1.0	1.5	1.5	2.3	2.4	1.5
Female	—	—	—	—	3.1	1.0	1.1	1.6	1.2	1.2	1.2
White	—	—	—	—	3.9	1.0	1.4	1.7	1.7	1.7	0.9
Black or African American	—	—	—	—	1.9	0.9	0.6	0.8	1.1	1.8	1.1
All 10th graders	—	—	—	—	2.6	1.0	1.2	1.2	1.1	1.3	1.9
Male	—	—	—	—	2.5	1.0	1.5	1.3	1.6	1.6	2.3
Female	—	—	—	—	2.5	0.9	0.8	1.1	0.7	1.0	1.5
White	—	—	—	—	2.5	1.0	1.3	1.4	1.0	1.0	1.5
Black or African American	—	—	—	—	1.8	0.3	1.0	0.4	0.1	0.6	1.1
All 8th graders	—	—	—	—	1.4	0.6	0.7	0.6	0.8	0.6	1.1
Male	—	—	—	—	1.6	0.8	0.5	0.7	0.7	0.5	1.2
Female	—	—	—	—	1.2	0.4	0.8	0.6	0.9	0.6	1.1
White	—	—	—	—	1.4	0.6	0.5	0.5	0.7	0.6	1.0
Black or African American	—	—	—	—	0.8	0.9	0.7	0.8	0.3	0.1	0.5
Alcohol[1]											
All high school seniors	72.0	65.9	57.1	51.3	50.0	47.0	45.3	44.4	43.1	43.5	41.2
Male	77.4	69.8	61.3	55.7	54.0	50.7	47.3	47.1	45.8	47.8	44.2
Female	66.8	62.1	52.3	47.0	46.1	43.3	43.0	41.4	40.9	38.9	37.9
White	75.8	70.2	62.2	54.8	55.3	52.2	49.1	49.4	47.8	46.6	44.1
Black or African American	47.7	43.6	32.9	37.4	29.3	28.8	29.5	27.9	29.3	32.2	30.8
All 10th graders	—	—	—	38.8	41.0	33.2	33.8	33.4	28.8	30.4	28.9
Male	—	—	—	39.7	43.3	32.8	33.8	33.4	28.6	31.0	30.1
Female	—	—	—	37.8	38.6	33.6	33.8	33.3	29.0	29.8	27.7
White	—	—	—	41.3	44.3	36.7	36.0	35.7	30.5	32.4	29.2
Black or African American	—	—	—	24.9	24.7	20.8	22.4	21.0	20.4	20.1	21.3
All 8th graders	—	—	—	24.6	22.4	17.1	17.2	15.9	15.9	14.9	13.8
Male	—	—	—	25.0	22.5	16.2	16.3	15.6	15.4	14.7	13.2
Female	—	—	—	24.0	22.0	17.9	17.6	16.0	16.4	14.9	14.3
White	—	—	—	25.4	23.9	17.3	16.5	14.7	15.8	15.1	12.8
Black or African American	—	—	—	17.3	15.1	13.9	12.4	12.3	13.5	11.1	12.7
Binge Drinking[2]											
All high school seniors	41.2	36.7	32.2	29.8	30.0	27.1	25.4	25.9	24.6	25.2	23.2
Male	52.1	45.3	39.1	36.9	36.7	32.6	28.9	30.7	28.4	30.5	28.0
Female	30.5	28.2	24.4	23.0	23.5	21.6	21.5	21.5	21.3	20.2	18.4
White	44.6	40.1	36.2	32.9	34.4	31.8	28.9	30.5	29.3	28.7	26.5
Black or African American	17.0	16.7	11.6	15.5	11.0	10.9	11.9	11.0	10.8	13.7	12.6
All 10th graders	—	—	—	22.0	24.1	19.0	19.9	19.6	16.0	17.5	16.3
Male	—	—	—	24.1	27.6	19.9	21.0	20.9	16.6	18.8	17.9
Female	—	—	—	19.7	20.6	17.9	18.9	18.3	15.4	16.1	14.6
White	—	—	—	24.1	26.6	21.5	21.8	21.7	17.4	18.4	16.0
Black or African American	—	—	—	9.6	10.6	8.4	9.9	10.0	9.6	10.0	11.5
All 8th graders	—	—	—	12.3	11.7	8.4	8.7	8.3	8.1	7.8	7.2
Male	—	—	—	12.5	11.7	8.2	8.6	8.2	8.1	7.8	6.5
Female	—	—	—	12.1	11.3	8.6	8.5	8.2	8.0	7.7	7.8
White	—	—	—	12.6	12.5	8.4	8.4	7.7	8.0	7.4	6.7
Black or African American	—	—	—	7.8	6.2	5.8	5.5	5.7	5.7	4.8	5.9

— = Data not available.
[1] In 1993, the alcohol question was changed to indicate that a drink meant more than a few sips.
[2] Five or more alcoholic drinks in a row at least once in the prior 2-week period.

AMBULATORY CARE

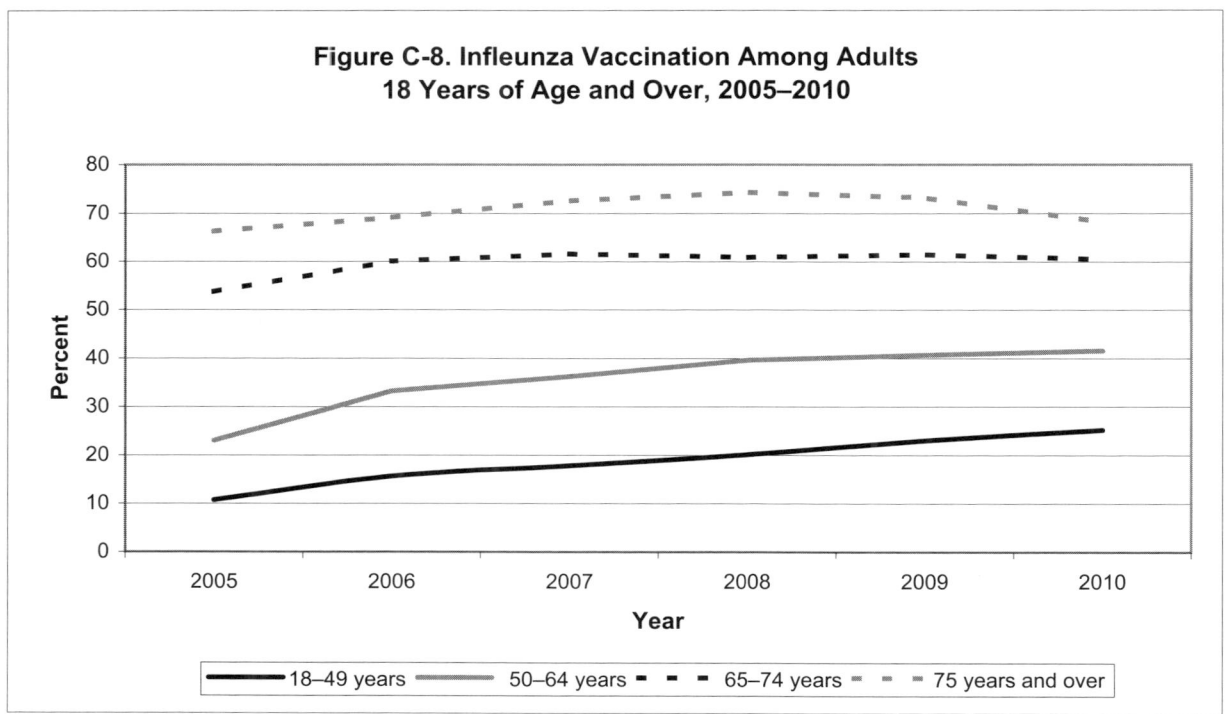

Figure C-8. Infleunza Vaccination Among Adults 18 Years of Age and Over, 2005–2010

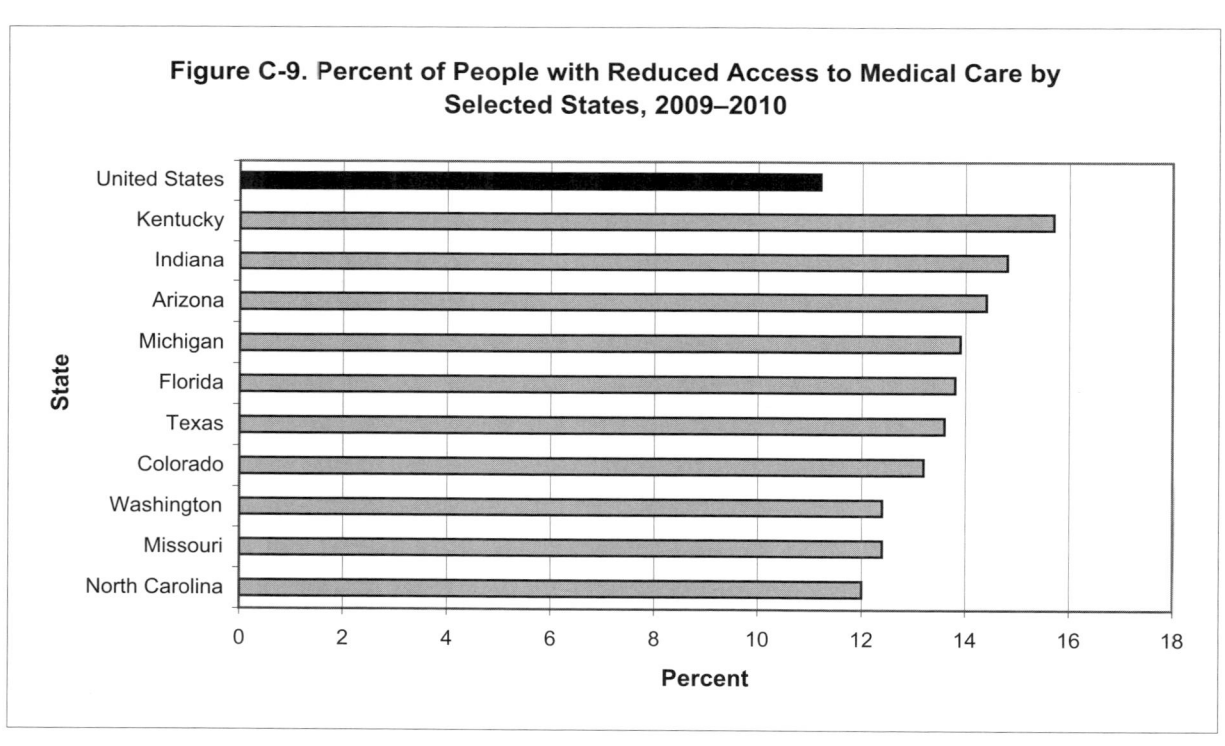

Figure C-9. Percent of People with Reduced Access to Medical Care by Selected States, 2009–2010

Table C-33. No Usual Source of Health Care[1] Among Children Under 18 Years of Age, by Selected Characteristics, Average Annual, Selected Years, 1993–1994 through 2009–2010

(Percent.)

Sex, grade level, race, and Hispanic origin	Under 18 years			Under 6 years			6–17 years		
	1993–1994[2]	1999–2000	2009–2010	1993–1994[2]	1999–2000	2009–2010	1993–1994[1]	1999–2000	2009–2010
ALL CHILDREN[3]	7.7	6.9	5.4	5.2	4.6	4.1	9.0	8.0	6.2
Sex									
Male	8.1	6.7	5.5	5.3	4.5	4.2	9.6	7.8	6.1
Female	7.3	7.1	5.4	5.0	4.7	4.0	8.5	8.2	6.2
Race[4]									
White only	7.0	6.3	5.3	4.7	4.4	3.8	8.3	7.2	6.1
Black or African American only	10.3	7.7	5.6	7.6	4.4	4.3	11.9	9.1	6.3
American Indian or Alaska Native only	*9.3	*9.4	*	*	*	*	*8.7	*9.4	*9.2
Asian only	9.7	10.0	6.1	*3.4	*5.8	*3.9	13.5	12.2	7.3
Native Hawaiian or Other Pacific Islander only	—	*	*	—	*	*	—	*	*
2 or more races	—	*4.9	4.6	—	*	*4.2	—	*7.2	*4.9
Hispanic Origin and Race[4]									
Hispanic or Latino	14.3	14.2	9.5	9.3	9.0	5.8	17.7	17.2	11.8
Not Hispanic or Latino	6.7	5.5	4.3	4.4	3.6	3.5	7.8	6.3	4.7
White only	5.7	4.7	3.8	3.7	3.3	2.9	6.7	5.4	4.1
Black or African American only	10.2	7.6	5.4	7.7	4.5	4.3	11.6	9.0	6.0
Percent of Poverty Level[5]									
Below 100%	13.9	13.1	8.3	9.4	7.6	6.6	16.8	16.2	9.3
100%–199%	9.8	10.6	7.5	6.7	7.5	4.8	11.6	12.2	9.0
200%–399%	3.7	4.8	4.7	1.9	3.2	*3.1	4.5	5.6	5.5
400% or more	3.7	2.6	2.1	*1.6	1.5	*1.9	5.0	3.0	2.2
Hispanic Origin and Race and Percent of Poverty Level[4,5]									
Hispanic or Latino									
Below 100%	19.6	19.4	10.7	12.7	11.6	7.1	24.8	24.5	13.4
100%–199%	15.3	17.1	10.6	9.9	11.3	6.3	18.9	20.4	13.2
200%–399%	5.2	8.3	8.5	*	*5.0	*4.1	6.7	10.1	10.9
400% or more	*	*3.8	*3.6	*	*	*	*	*5.0	*4.1
Not Hispanic or Latino									
White only									
Below 100%	10.2	10.7	6.1	6.5	*6.3	*5.0	12.7	13.1	*6.8
100%–199%	8.7	7.8	5.7	6.3	5.7	*4.0	10.1	8.8	6.6
200%–399%	3.3	4.0	3.7	1.6	2.7	*	4.0	4.6	4.2
400% or more	4.0	2.3	2.1	*1.7	*1.5	*1.9	5.4	2.6	2.1
Black or African American only									
Below 100%	13.7	9.4	6.3	10.9	*4.7	*6.2	15.5	11.8	6.4
100%–199%	9.1	9.7	6.2	*6.0	*6.4	*	10.8	11.2	8.1
200%–399%	5.0	5.0	5.1	*	*	*	6.2	5.7	5.4
400% or more	*	*3.5	*	*	*	*	*	*4.0	*
Health Insurance Status at the Time of Interview[6]									
Insured	5.0	3.9	3.4	3.3	2.6	2.8	5.9	4.5	3.7
Private	3.8	3.4	2.6	1.9	2.2	1.7	4.6	3.9	3.0
Medicaid	8.9	5.3	4.4	6.4	3.5	3.7	11.3	6.7	4.9
Uninsured	23.5	29.3	28.8	18.0	20.8	21.4	26.0	32.9	31.5
Health Insurance Status Prior to Interview[6]									
Insured continuously all 12 months	4.6	3.6	3.2	3.1	2.3	2.7	5.5	4.2	3.4
Uninsured for any period up to 12 months	15.3	15.0	11.7	10.9	12.5	10.4	18.1	16.4	12.4
Uninsured more than 12 months	27.6	35.8	36.2	21.4	26.8	27.5	30.0	39.1	38.5
Geographic Region									
Northeast	4.1	2.8	2.7	2.9	2.3	*2.6	4.8	3.0	2.7
Midwest	5.2	5.3	4.3	4.1	3.7	3.6	5.9	6.0	4.6
South	10.9	8.5	6.2	7.3	5.8	4.4	12.7	9.8	7.1
West	8.6	9.7	7.4	5.3	5.7	4.9	10.6	11.7	8.7
Location of Residence									
Within MSA[7]	7.7	6.8	5.5	5.0	4.7	4.2	9.2	7.8	6.2
Outside MSA[7]	7.8	7.4	5.0	6.0	4.2	3.3	8.7	8.7	5.8

* = Figure does not meet standards of reliability or precision.
— = Data not available.
[1]Persons who report the emergency department as their usual source of care are defined as having no usual source of care.
[2]Data prior to 1997 are not strictly comparable with data for later years due to the 1997 questionnaire redesign.
[3]Includes all other races not shown separately and unknown health insurance status.
[4]The race groups, White, Black, American Indian or Alaska Native, Asian, Native Hawaiian or Other Pacific Islander, and 2 or more races, include persons of Hispanic and non-Hispanic origin. Persons of Hispanic origin may be of any race.
[5]Percent of poverty level is based on family income and family size and composition using U.S. Census Bureau poverty thresholds.
[6]Health insurance categories are mutually exclusive. Persons who reported both Medicaid and private coverage are classified as having private coverage.
[7]MSA = metropolitan statistical area.

Table C-34. No Usual Source of Health Care Among Adults 18–64 Years of Age, by Selected Characteristics, Average Annual, Selected Years, 1993–1994 through 2009–2010

(Percent.)

Characteristic	1993–1994[1]	1995–1996[1]	1997–1998	1999–2000	2001–2002	2003–2004	2004–2005	2005–2006	2006–2007	2007–2008	2008–2009	2009–2010
PERCENT OF ADULTS WITHOUT A USUAL SOURCE OF HEALTH CARE[2]												
18–64 years	18.9	16.9	17.7	17.8	16.4	17.3	18.0	18.4	18.5	18.5	19.5	20.3
Age												
18–44 years	21.7	19.6	21.1	21.6	20.6	21.7	22.8	23.5	23.5	23.6	25.0	26.0
18–24 years	26.6	22.6	27.0	27.2	27.2	28.0	29.9	29.8	28.7	28.6	29.6	29.8
25–44 years	20.3	18.8	19.3	19.9	18.5	19.5	20.3	21.3	21.8	21.8	23.4	24.7
45–64 years	12.8	11.3	11.2	10.9	9.2	10.4	10.6	10.7	11.2	11.0	11.6	12.3
45–54 years	14.1	12.2	12.6	12.0	10.3	11.7	11.9	12.3	13.3	13.1	13.6	14.7
55–64 years	11.1	9.8	9.0	9.2	7.6	8.7	8.8	8.4	8.3	8.3	9.0	9.3
Sex												
Male	23.9	21.4	23.6	24.1	21.6	22.5	23.3	23.9	23.9	23.9	25.3	25.9
Female	14.1	12.6	12.0	11.8	11.4	12.4	12.9	13.0	13.3	13.1	13.8	14.8
Race[3]												
White only	18.4	16.5	17.0	16.7	15.4	17.0	17.7	18.1	18.3	18.0	18.9	19.7
Black or African American only	20.0	18.3	19.4	19.2	16.9	18.4	19.3	19.8	19.8	20.5	21.5	22.4
American Indian or Alaska Native only	19.7	16.5	21.3	19.2	16.3	21.5	22.8	21.9	24.4	24.4	24.8	26.7
Asian only	24.8	21.5	21.7	22.1	20.1	19.3	18.8	17.9	17.3	17.8	19.4	20.8
Native Hawaiian or Other Pacific Islander only	—	—	—	*	*	*	*	*	*	*	*	*
2 or more races	—	—	—	21.0	20.1	18.4	18.1	20.9	20.4	21.4	26.1	27.5
American Indian or Alaska Native; White	—	—	—	25.8	18.1	17.8	19.1	21.4	19.3	20.9	25.9	27.1
Hispanic Origin and Race[4]												
Hispanic or Latino	30.3	27.4	30.4	32.6	32.5	32.9	34.0	35.1	34.3	32.5	32.8	33.3
Mexican	32.4	29.8	35.9	36.5	36.5	36.4	37.8	39.3	39.0	36.6	36.1	35.7
Not Hispanic or Latino	17.7	15.7	16.2	15.8	14.0	14.9	15.4	15.6	15.9	16.0	17.1	17.9
White only	17.1	15.0	15.4	14.9	13.1	14.0	14.6	14.8	15.2	15.1	16.0	16.8
Black or African American only	19.7	18.1	19.3	19.2	16.8	18.1	19.0	19.2	18.9	20.2	21.4	22.2
Percent of Poverty Level[5]												
Below 100%	29.5	26.1	29.1	29.6	29.3	28.9	31.8	32.1	30.6	30.4	32.7	33.8
100%–199%	25.4	22.9	25.6	27.1	25.6	26.6	27.1	27.8	28.6	29.1	30.3	30.5
200%–399%	15.6	13.4	16.6	17.2	16.0	17.3	17.9	17.8	18.5	18.9	19.7	20.5
400% or more	13.4	13.8	11.6	11.6	9.6	10.1	10.3	10.4	10.4	10.2	10.6	10.8
Hispanic Origin and Race and Percent of Poverty Level[4,5]												
Hispanic or Latino												
Below 100%	40.0	34.3	42.8	44.4	46.3	42.8	44.5	46.7	46.7	43.7	44.1	45.5
100%–199%	36.9	32.9	35.4	40.6	40.0	39.7	40.7	41.8	42.1	40.6	40.7	39.7
200%–399%	20.7	19.5	23.6	26.9	27.9	28.2	30.1	31.2	29.5	28.0	27.9	29.1
400% or more	13.8	16.3	14.4	16.1	13.7	16.4	16.2	16.4	15.9	16.9	16.6	14.0
Not Hispanic or Latino												
White only:												
Below 100%	28.2	23.6	25.0	24.2	23.4	23.0	26.8	26.2	25.0	25.2	27.8	28.8
100%–199%	23.3	20.7	22.4	23.0	20.7	22.0	22.8	23.5	24.5	24.9	26.0	26.6
200%–399%	14.8	12.5	15.4	15.3	13.6	15.4	15.6	15.3	16.2	16.7	17.7	18.6
400% or more	13.4	13.7	11.3	11.2	9.1	9.4	9.6	9.8	10.0	9.5	9.9	10.3
Black or African American only												
Below 100%	24.7	21.9	23.9	23.7	22.8	24.3	28.3	29.5	26.5	27.1	29.4	30.1
100%–199%	22.3	22.1	25.3	24.4	20.4	22.8	22.1	22.6	23.4	25.7	27.6	28.5
200%–399%	16.5	14.5	17.6	18.2	16.2	16.3	16.6	16.2	18.0	19.7	19.9	20.1
400% or more	11.7	12.6	11.2	12.0	9.6	11.3	11.3	10.3	9.1	10.2	11.2	10.5
Health Insurance Status at the Time of Interview[6]												
Insured	13.3	11.4	11.4	10.9	9.1	9.4	9.7	9.7	9.9	10.1	10.4	10.6
Private	13.1	11.3	11.5	11.1	9.0	9.5	9.5	9.6	9.8	10.0	10.3	10.6
Medicaid	16.3	13.0	10.3	9.9	11.1	9.9	12.1	11.6	11.5	11.7	12.1	12.5
Uninsured	43.1	41.8	46.7	49.2	49.1	50.2	52.5	53.0	52.8	52.1	54.1	55.6
Health Insurance Status Prior to Interview[6]												
Insured continuously all 12 months	12.7	10.8	10.6	10.3	8.3	8.7	8.9	8.9	9.0	9.1	9.5	9.8
Uninsured for any period up to 12 months	30.9	29.6	30.7	31.2	33.3	32.1	34.0	33.4	33.6	35.1	36.7	36.5
Uninsured more than 12 months	46.9	44.8	51.4	54.8	54.6	55.0	57.4	58.0	57.9	56.1	57.2	59.5

Table C-34. No Usual Source of Health Care Among Adults 18–64 Years of Age, by Selected Characteristics, Average Annual, Selected Years, 1993–1994 through 2009–2010—*Continued*

(Percent.)

Characteristic	1993–1994[1]	1995–1996[1]	1997–1998	1999–2000	2001–2002	2003–2004	2004–2005	2005–2006	2006–2007	2007–2008	2008–2009	2009–2010
Disability Measure[7]												
Any basic actions difficulty or complex activity limitation	—	—	15.5	14.1	13.2	14.3	15.0	15.2	15.7	16.6	17.1	16.8
Any basic actions difficulty	—	—	15.7	14.1	13.1	14.5	15.2	15.4	15.8	16.5	17.1	16.7
Any complex activity limitation	—	—	13.1	11.6	10.4	10.7	11.5	11.1	12.6	13.6	13.8	13.5
No disability	—	—	18.2	18.8	17.5	18.2	18.8	19.4	19.5	19.1	20.3	21.5
Geographic Region												
Northeast	14.7	13.4	13.3	12.8	11.9	12.1	11.7	12.2	13.1	12.5	12.9	14.0
Midwest	16.2	14.7	15.1	17.0	14.1	14.7	15.4	15.8	16.2	16.6	17.3	17.5
South	21.8	18.7	20.7	19.7	18.3	19.7	21.0	21.4	21.4	21.4	22.5	23.5
West	21.1	19.9	20.2	20.1	19.9	21.0	21.2	21.1	20.5	20.0	21.8	22.9
Location of Residence												
Within MSA[8]	19.3	17.3	17.9	18.1	16.6	17.6	18.3	18.7	18.9	18.7	19.5	20.3
Outside MSA[8]	17.5	15.4	17.0	16.8	15.4	16.2	16.6	16.7	16.5	16.9	19.4	20.4

— =Data not available.
* = Figure does not meet standards of reliability or precision.
[1]Data prior to 1997 are not strictly comparable with data for later years due to the 1997 questionnaire redesign.
[2]Persons who report the emergency department as their usual source of care are defined as having no usual source of care.
[3]The race groups, White, Black, American Indian or Alaska Native, Asian, Native Hawaiian or Other Pacific Islander, and 2 or more races, include persons of Hispanic and non-Hispanic origin. Persons of Hispanic origin may be of any race.
[4]Persons of Hispanic origin may be of any race.
[5]Percent of poverty level is based on family income and family size and composition using U.S. Census Bureau poverty thresholds.
[6]Health insurance categories are mutually exclusive. Persons who reported both Medicaid and private coverage are classified as having private coverage. Medicaid includes other public assistance through 1996.
[7]Any basic actions difficulty or complex activity limitation is defined as having one or more of the following limitations or difficulties: movement difficulty, emotional difficulty, sensory (seeing or hearing) difficulty, cognitive difficulty, self-care (activities of daily living or instrumental activities of daily living) limitation, social limitation, or work limitation.
[8]MSA = metropolitan statistical area.

Table C-35. Reduced Access to Medical Care, Dental Care, and Prescription Drugs During the Past 12 Months Due to Cost, by Selected Characteristics, Selected Years, 1997–2010

(Percent.)

Characteristic	Did not get or delayed medical care due to cost[1]			Did not get prescription drugs due to cost[2]			Did not get dental care due to cost[3]		
	1997	2005	2010	1997	2005	2010	1997	2000	2010
TOTAL[4]	8.3	8.5	10.9	4.8	7.2	8.3	8.6	8.1	13.5
Age									
Under 19 years	4.5	4.3	4.5	2.1	3.0	2.8	6.0	6.2	6.6
Under 18 years	4.4	4.2	4.4	2.2	2.9	2.7	6.0	6.2	6.6
Under 6 years	3.3	3.3	3.7	1.6	2.5	2.5	3.9	4.1	3.9
6–17 years	4.9	4.7	4.8	2.4	3.1	2.8	6.8	6.8	7.5
18–64 years	10.7	11.0	14.7	6.3	9.4	11.2	10.6	9.7	17.3
18–44 years	11.0	11.3	14.5	6.9	9.8	11.2	11.7	10.7	17.9
18–24 years	10.2	11.3	13.5	6.7	9.6	9.7	11.6	11.7	17.4
25–34 years	11.4	11.8	15.3	6.9	10.2	12.0	12.3	10.8	18.3
35–44 years	11.0	10.8	14.4	7.1	9.6	11.3	11.2	10.1	17.8
45–64 years	10.1	10.6	14.9	5.1	8.7	11.3	8.4	7.9	16.5
45–54 years	10.6	10.8	15.0	5.6	9.2	11.5	9.4	9.0	17.8
55–64 years	9.3	10.4	14.6	4.2	8.0	11.0	7.0	6.2	14.9
65 years and over	4.6	4.6	5.0	2.8	5.1	4.7	3.5	3.4	6.9
65–74 years	5.0	5.4	6.3	3.4	6.4	6.3	4.2	4.6	9.0
75 years and over	4.1	3.7	3.4	2.0	3.6	2.8	2.6	1.9	4.3
18–64 YEARS									
Sex									
Male	9.3	10.0	13.5	5.1	7.2	8.8	8.8	8.2	15.2
Female	12.0	12.1	15.7	7.4	11.4	13.5	12.4	11.2	19.4
Race[5]									
White only	10.8	11.1	14.5	5.9	9.1	10.8	10.6	9.3	17.1
Black or African American only	10.8	12.0	17.4	9.5	11.6	15.6	10.8	10.1	20.7
American Indian or Alaska Native only	14.5	13.2	*15.7	*10.1	*14.1	18.6	18.8	*8.7	23.1
Asian only	6.3	5.0	8.0	*2.8	*3.5	4.2	7.8	5.5	8.7
Native Hawaiian or Other Pacific Islander only	—	*	*	—	*	*	—	*	*
2 or more races	—	19.9	24.0	—	22.9	16.6	—	15.2	25.6
Hispanic Origin and Race[5]									
Hispanic or Latino	10.5	11.5	15.4	6.7	11.2	13.0	11.5	9.8	21.6
Mexican	9.7	11.4	15.6	6.5	12.0	13.5	11.3	9.6	22.0
Not Hispanic or Latino	10.7	11.0	14.5	6.3	9.0	10.9	10.5	9.7	16.6
White only	10.9	11.1	14.3	5.9	8.7	10.3	10.5	9.8	16.2
Black or African American only	10.8	12.0	17.5	9.5	11.4	15.6	10.8	10.1	20.8
Education[6]									
No high school diploma or GED	16.2	16.2	20.6	11.5	16.4	18.1	14.5	13.9	26.3
High school diploma or GED	11.1	11.7	16.1	7.0	10.5	13.8	11.4	10.0	20.1
Some college or more	9.2	9.8	13.4	4.3	7.1	9.2	8.8	7.9	14.4
Percent of Poverty Level[7]									
Below 100%	19.6	20.0	23.4	14.8	19.5	21.5	19.4	18.7	30.4
100%–199%	17.9	18.9	24.0	11.6	16.3	18.4	18.3	16.7	29.2
200%–399%	10.5	11.8	15.2	5.5	9.5	11.4	10.2	10.6	17.3
400% or more	4.6	5.0	6.8	1.7	3.3	3.9	4.5	4.0	7.0
Hispanic Origin and Race and Percent of Poverty Level[5,7]									
Hispanic or Latino									
Below 100%	14.6	14.8	19.0	10.6	17.3	18.9	16.1	14.0	30.5
100%–199%	12.2	14.5	18.6	8.1	13.0	14.7	13.5	11.4	25.2
200%–399%	8.0	9.6	13.9	4.4	9.1	11.5	9.2	8.6	18.1
400% or more	5.1	6.2	7.7	*	*4.2	4.6	4.5	4.5	9.1
Not Hispanic or Latino									
White only:									
Below 100%	24.3	23.6	26.1	17.3	20.5	24.6	23.4	22.2	31.8
100%–199%	20.9	21.8	27.6	12.4	18.2	19.9	20.6	19.9	31.7
200%–399%	11.4	13.1	16.0	5.4	10.0	11.3	10.6	11.6	18.0
400% or more	4.6	5.0	6.9	1.7	3.2	3.8	4.5	4.0	6.9
Black or African American only									
Below 100%	16.1	20.1	24.4	14.9	21.7	21.1	14.8	17.3	29.7
100%–199%	14.3	16.2	22.9	13.9	14.3	21.3	16.4	12.6	28.2
200%–399%	8.8	9.2	14.6	7.0	7.9	13.7	8.6	8.6	16.1
400% or more	4.6	5.5	8.1	*2.9	*4.1	5.6	4.3	4.1	9.1

Table C-35. Reduced Access to Medical Care, Dental Care, and Prescription Drugs During the Past 12 Months Due to Cost, by Selected Characteristics, Selected Years, 1997–2010—Continued

(Percent.)

Characteristic	Did not get or delayed medical care due to cost[1]			Did not get prescription drugs due to cost[2]			Did not get dental care due to cost[3]		
	1997	2005	2010	1997	2005	2010	1997	2000	2010
Health Insurance Status at the Time of Interview[8]									
Insured	6.8	6.8	9.1	3.7	6.0	7.3	7.2	6.5	11.8
Private	6.0	5.9	8.2	2.9	4.7	6.0	6.2	5.6	9.2
Medicaid	11.9	12.0	12.5	11.1	14.0	13.5	14.8	15.6	24.2
Uninsured	27.6	29.5	34.5	18.0	23.1	25.7	26.1	24.0	37.7
Health Insurance Status Prior to Interview[8]									
Insured continuously all 12 months	5.5	5.5	7.6	2.8	5.0	6.2	6.0	5.4	10.5
Uninsured for any period up to 12 months	28.7	31.7	35.1	17.7	23.5	25.1	25.2	25.2	33.6
Uninsured more than 12 months	30.6	31.1	35.9	18.9	24.5	26.2	28.0	25.9	39.4
Disability Measure[9]									
Any basic actions difficulty or complex activity limitation	23.3	24.8	28.9	14.8	20.0	22.6	19.8	19.2	28.8
Any basic actions difficulty	24.2	26.1	28.9	15.3	20.5	23.3	20.1	19.7	29.2
Any complex activity limitation	25.7	26.9	30.8	19.4	25.3	27.3	23.2	21.8	33.7
No disability	9.0	9.8	13.2	3.4	5.7	7.0	7.5	6.8	13.1
Geographic Region									
Northeast	8.8	8.7	10.2	4.9	7.2	7.7	8.9	7.8	12.9
Midwest	10.5	10.6	14.8	5.9	9.0	11.6	9.7	8.3	16.0
South	11.8	12.6	16.5	7.3	11.3	13.5	10.9	10.7	19.6
West	10.8	11.1	15.1	6.3	8.2	10.0	13.1	11.6	18.4
Location of Residence									
Within MSA[10]	10.2	10.6	14.2	5.9	8.8	10.8	10.0	9.3	17.0
Outside MSA[10]	12.5	12.8	17.4	7.9	11.8	13.6	12.9	11.4	19.1

* = Figure does not meet standards of reliability or precision.
— = Data not available.
[1]Based on persons responding to the question, "During the past 12 months was there any time when person needed medical care but did not get it because person couldn't afford it?" and "During the past 12 months has medical care been delayed because of worry about the cost?"
[2]Based on persons responding to the question, "During the past 12 months was there any time when person needed prescription medicine but didn't get it because person couldn't afford it?"
[3]Based on persons responding to the question, "During the past 12 months was there any time when person needed dental care (including checkups) but didn't get it because person couldn't afford it?"
[4]Includes all other races not shown separately, unknown health insurance status, unknown education level, and unknown disability status.
[5]The race groups, White, Black, American Indian or Alaska Native, Asian, Native Hawaiian or Other Pacific Islander, and 2 or more races, include persons of Hispanic and non-Hispanic origin. Persons of Hispanic origin may be of any race.
[6]Estimates are for persons 25–64 years of age.
[7]Percent of poverty level is based on family income and family size and composition using U.S. Census Bureau poverty thresholds.
[8]For information on the health insurance categories.
[9]Any basic actions difficulty or complex activity limitation is defined as having one or more of the following limitations or difficulties: movement difficulty, emotional difficulty, sensory (seeing or hearing) difficulty, cognitive difficulty, self-care (activities of daily living or instrumental activities of daily living) limitation, social limitation, or work limitation.
[10]MSA = metropolitan statistical area.

Table C-36. Reduced Access to Medical Care During the Past 12 Months Due to Cost, by the 25 Largest States, Selected Annual Averages, 1997–1998 through 2009–2010

(Percent.)

State	Did not get or delayed medical care due to cost[1]				Did not get prescription drugs due to cost[2]				Did not get dental care[3]			
	1997–1998	2000–2001	2005–2006	2009–2010	1997–1998	2000–2001	2005–2006	2009–2010	1997–1998	2000–2001	2005–2006	2009–2010
United States	7.9	7.5	8.8	11.2	4.5	5.3	7.1	8.3	8.1	8.4	10.8	13.4
Alabama	7.6	7.7	9.8	10.8	6.8	8.3	13.8	10.5	8.7	10.3	13.3	12.9
Arizona	8.0	7.4	11.0	14.4	4.1	4.6	7.8	10.2	9.4	8.4	12.8	19.4
California	6.8	6.6	6.2	10.6	3.9	4.7	5.2	7.1	8.3	8.1	9.4	14.4
Colorado	6.4	8.1	10.7	13.2	3.1	5.5	5.6	6.5	8.9	11.5	14.5	13.7
Florida	9.8	9.6	11.2	13.8	4.8	5.8	7.7	10.3	7.2	8.4	12.9	18.7
Georgia	8.0	7.7	7.0	12.0	4.2	4.0	5.9	10.0	5.8	5.3	7.0	13.7
Illinois	6.1	6.5	7.0	8.8	3.0	4.2	5.3	6.4	5.7	6.8	9.0	10.9
Indiana	9.0	8.6	10.5	14.8	5.1	6.8	8.1	11.4	7.2	6.9	10.1	13.3
Kentucky	11.5	10.2	11.9	15.7	6.3	8.2	11.7	12.9	7.9	9.5	13.6	18.1
Maryland	8.0	7.4	6.2	8.1	5.8	5.2	5.8	7.3	9.8	7.8	8.8	9.5
Massachusetts	5.1	4.3	5.4	6.0	1.7	4.2	4.5	5.3	5.0	5.2	7.3	7.6
Michigan	7.2	7.0	9.3	13.9	3.8	5.1	6.9	10.7	7.5	7.9	10.7	15.5
Minnesota	8.1	7.0	8.5	11.4	3.6	3.9	6.5	7.3	8.7	8.3	11.7	11.0
Missouri	7.1	6.4	9.7	12.4	4.3	5.2	8.9	9.4	7.3	7.1	14.5	14.1
New Jersey	7.2	6.1	6.2	7.8	3.8	3.5	3.9	5.7	7.3	5.9	7.2	11.1
New York	6.4	5.8	5.6	6.9	2.8	3.8	5.3	5.2	5.6	7.5	7.3	7.6
North Carolina	7.8	7.9	8.3	12.0	4.0	5.8	5.4	9.1	8.2	7.9	6.9	11.1
Ohio	9.2	7.6	10.1	10.9	5.0	5.1	7.5	8.2	8.8	8.1	9.9	11.5
Pennsylvania	5.9	5.9	7.9	9.2	4.3	3.5	6.7	8.0	7.4	6.0	9.2	11.3
South Carolina	7.6	6.3	7.7	11.4	5.2	4.4	5.1	*9.3	*5.7	5.2	5.8	*13.2
Tennessee	10.0	8.6	9.7	11.9	8.0	8.5	8.1	11.5	10.5	10.4	9.4	16.3
Texas	7.9	8.1	12.4	13.6	4.7	6.6	11.1	10.7	8.8	10.4	17.0	17.8
Virginia	6.2	7.2	6.5	11.1	4.1	*5.2	5.1	6.5	8.3	7.4	7.0	9.8
Washington	8.6	9.2	11.0	12.4	4.8	6.8	6.5	7.2	11.6	11.9	12.9	16.8
Wisconsin	6.5	5.9	6.2	10.3	*3.0	4.0	4.8	6.3	5.5	6.6	9.1	10.4

* = Figure does not meet standards of reliability or precision.

[1] Based on persons responding to the question, "During the past 12 months was there any time when person needed medical care but did not get it because person couldn't afford it?" and "During the past 12 months has medical care been delayed because of worry about the cost?"

[2] Based on persons responding to the question, "During the past 12 months was there any time when you needed prescription medicine but didn't get it because you couldn't afford it?"

[3] Based on persons responding to the question, "During the past 12 months was there any time when you needed dental care (including check ups) but didn't get it because you couldn't afford it?"

Table C-37. No Health Care Visits[1] to an Office or Clinic Within the Past 12 Months Among Children Under 18 Years of Age, by Selected Characteristics, Selected Annual Averages, 1997–1998 through 2009–2010

(Percent.)

Characteristic	Under 18 years			Under 6 years			6-17 years		
	1997–1998	2005–2006	2009–2010	1997–1998	2005–2006	2009–2010	1997–1998	2005–2006	2009–2010
ALL CHILDREN[2]	12.8	11.7	9.6	5.7	6.1	4.9	16.3	14.4	12.1
Sex									
Male	12.9	12.0	9.8	4.9	6.2	5.0	16.8	14.7	12.4
Female	12.7	11.4	9.4	6.5	6.1	4.8	15.8	14.0	11.8
Race[3]									
White only	12.2	11.3	9.4	5.5	6.3	4.5	15.5	13.8	11.8
Black or African American only	14.3	11.7	10.1	6.5	4.6	6.4	18.1	15.1	12.1
American Indian or Alaska Native only	13.8	*15.7	*12.4	*	*	*	*17.6	*17.7	*14.7
Asian only	16.3	17.5	12.7	*5.6	10.5	*4.8	22.1	20.8	17.0
Native Hawaiian or Other Pacific Islander only	—	*	*	—	*	*	—	*	*
2 or more races	—	10.4	8.3	—	*	*5.7	—	14.8	10.1
Hispanic Origin and Race[3]									
Hispanic or Latino	19.3	17.4	13.5	9.7	9.6	7.7	25.3	21.9	17.2
Not Hispanic or Latino	11.6	10.3	8.5	4.8	5.1	4.0	14.9	12.6	10.7
White only	10.7	9.4	7.7	4.3	5.0	3.1	13.7	11.4	9.8
Black or African American only	14.5	11.7	10.3	6.5	*4.4	6.4	18.3	15.1	12.4
Percent of Poverty Level[4]									
Below 100%	17.6	14.2	12.4	8.1	7.7	6.9	23.6	18.2	16.0
100%–199%	16.2	14.9	12.7	7.2	8.4	6.4	20.8	18.2	16.2
200%–399%	11.7	11.1	9.0	4.9	6.1	4.2	14.8	13.4	11.4
400% or more	7.4	7.8	5.3	3.0	2.8	*2.3	9.5	10.0	6.7
Health Insurance Status at the Time of Interview[5]									
Insured	10.4	9.5	7.7	4.5	4.9	4.3	13.4	11.9	9.6
Private	10.4	9.4	7.0	4.3	4.4	3.5	13.1	11.6	8.6
Medicaid	10.1	9.5	8.8	5.0	5.8	5.3	14.4	12.2	11.1
Uninsured	28.8	31.7	31.0	14.6	20.6	14.4	34.9	35.6	37.3
Health Insurance Status Prior to Interview[5]									
Insured continuously all 12 months	10.3	9.5	7.4	4.4	4.9	4.1	13.2	11.9	9.2
Uninsured for any period up to 12 months	15.9	15.8	16.3	7.7	9.3	7.7	20.9	18.8	20.9
Uninsured more than 12 months	34.9	39.0	38.6	19.9	28.0	22.8	40.2	42.2	42.9
Geographic Region									
Northeast	7.0	6.8	5.6	3.1	4.0	3.3	8.9	8.1	6.7
Midwest	12.2	9.8	8.6	5.9	5.2	3.5	15.3	12.0	11.2
South	14.3	12.4	9.9	5.6	6.2	5.2	18.5	15.5	12.4
West	16.3	16.5	12.9	7.9	8.8	6.9	20.7	20.3	16.1
Location of Residence									
Within MSA[6]	12.3	11.4	9.4	5.4	5.9	4.7	15.9	14.1	11.9
Outside MSA[6]	14.6	12.9	10.8	6.9	7.4	6.0	17.9	15.4	13.1

* = Figure does not meet standards of reliability or precision.
— = Data not available.
[1]Respondents were asked how many times a doctor or other health care professional was seen in the past 12 months at a doctor's office, clinic, or some other place. Excluded are visits to emergency rooms, hospitalizations, home visits, and telephone calls. Starting with 2000 data, dental visits were also excluded.
[2]Includes all other races not shown separately and unknown health insurance status.
[3]The race groups, White, Black, American Indian or Alaska Native, Asian, Native Hawaiian or Other Pacific Islander, and 2 or more races, include persons of Hispanic and non-Hispanic origin. Persons of Hispanic origin may be of any race.
[4]Percent of poverty level is based on family income and family size and composition using U.S. Census Bureau poverty thresholds.
[5]Health insurance categories are mutually exclusive. Persons who reported both Medicaid and private coverage are classified as having private coverage.
[6]MSA = metropolitan statistical area.

Table C-38. Health Care Visits to Doctor Offices, Emergency Departments, and Home Visits Within the Past 12 Months, by Selected Characteristics, Selected Years, 2000–2010

(Percent.)

Characteristic	None 2000	None 2005	None 2010	1–3 visits 2000	1–3 visits 2005	1–3 visits 2010	4–9 visits 2000	4–9 visits 2005	4–9 visits 2010	10 or more visits 2000	10 or more visits 2005	10 or more visits 2010
Total, age-adjusted[1,2]	16.6	15.5	15.6	45.1	45.9	45.4	25.1	25.1	25.8	13.2	13.6	13.2
Total, crude[1]	16.7	15.4	15.4	45.2	45.9	45.2	25.0	25.1	26.0	13.1	13.6	13.5
Age												
Under 18 years	12.3	10.2	8.1	53.5	56.0	55.6	26.7	26.5	28.2	7.6	7.4	8.2
Under 6 years	6.2	5.1	3.7	44.0	47.4	48.9	38.7	38.0	36.8	11.0	9.5	10.6
6–17 years	15.1	12.6	10.4	57.9	60.1	59.1	21.0	20.9	23.6	5.9	6.3	6.9
18–44 years	23.4	22.9	24.2	44.9	45.8	43.9	19.6	19.2	20.6	12.1	12.0	11.3
18–24 years	24.5	24.2	25.9	45.0	44.4	43.4	19.4	19.6	21.1	11.1	11.8	9.6
25–44 years	23.0	22.5	23.6	44.9	46.3	44.1	19.6	19.1	20.5	12.5	12.1	11.9
45–64 years	14.9	14.0	14.8	43.1	42.9	42.8	26.2	26.8	26.1	15.8	16.3	16.4
45–54 years	16.3	15.8	17.6	44.9	44.8	43.5	24.3	24.3	23.9	14.5	15.0	15.0
55–64 years	12.7	11.4	11.1	40.4	40.2	41.9	29.2	30.3	28.8	17.7	18.2	18.2
65 years and over	7.4	5.6	5.3	31.8	30.7	33.8	37.3	37.5	36.7	23.5	26.2	24.2
65–74 years	8.9	5.9	6.3	34.2	34.4	36.1	35.1	35.8	35.7	21.9	23.9	21.9
75 years and over	5.7	5.2	4.1	29.0	26.4	31.0	39.9	39.5	38.0	25.5	28.8	27.0
Sex[2]												
Male	21.6	20.4	20.4	45.7	46.7	46.4	22.7	22.2	22.7	10.0	10.7	10.5
Female	11.8	10.7	10.9	44.4	45.1	44.4	27.5	27.9	28.8	16.2	16.3	15.9
Race[2,3]												
White only	16.0	15.1	15.3	44.8	45.6	44.9	25.7	25.4	26.1	13.6	13.9	13.7
Black or African American only	17.1	15.9	15.7	46.4	47.4	47.2	24.0	23.8	24.7	12.5	12.9	12.4
American Indian or Alaska Native only	21.2	20.4	19.4	42.8	36.4	40.3	20.3	29.8	28.1	15.7	13.4	12.2
Asian only	20.2	21.5	20.4	49.0	49.3	49.9	21.1	20.8	22.1	9.7	8.4	7.6
Native Hawaiian or Other Pacific Islander only	*	*	*	*	*	*	*	*	*	*	*	*
2 or more races	12.0	15.4	13.9	41.4	37.3	42.3	28.8	27.6	25.2	17.9	19.7	18.6
Hispanic Origin and Race[2,3]												
Hispanic or Latino	26.7	23.9	23.5	41.5	42.1	43.2	20.2	22.2	22.6	11.5	11.8	10.7
Mexican	30.9	26.6	25.2	40.6	41.5	43.3	18.2	20.8	21.4	10.3	11.1	10.1
Not Hispanic or Latino	15.1	13.9	14.0	45.6	46.5	45.8	25.8	25.7	26.5	13.6	13.9	13.7
White only	14.4	13.0	13.2	45.1	46.4	45.3	26.5	26.2	27.1	14.0	14.5	14.4
Black or African American only	17.0	15.9	15.6	46.5	47.4	47.3	24.0	23.8	24.9	12.5	12.9	12.2
Percent of Poverty Level[2,4]												
Below 100%	21.9	20.7	20.4	37.3	37.3	37.5	23.4	24.7	25.1	17.4	17.3	17.0
100%–199%	21.6	20.2	20.8	42.3	42.0	42.1	22.1	23.4	23.1	14.1	14.4	13.9
200%–399%	16.9	15.9	16.2	45.3	47.3	46.3	25.0	24.0	25.4	12.8	12.8	12.1
400% or more	12.3	11.0	10.2	48.1	49.2	49.4	27.3	27.0	27.6	12.4	12.8	12.7
Hispanic Origin and Race and Percent of Poverty Level[2,3,4]												
Hispanic or Latino												
Below 100%	32.3	27.9	28.7	33.3	37.2	36.5	19.2	20.2	22.5	15.1	14.6	12.3
100%–199%	30.5	27.6	27.7	40.6	38.8	42.7	17.6	22.6	19.9	11.3	11.1	9.8
200%–399%	24.2	22.7	21.6	45.5	44.9	45.0	19.9	23.1	23.1	10.3	9.2	10.3
400% or more	17.0	13.4	11.3	47.2	50.4	51.1	26.3	23.0	26.1	9.5	13.2	11.5
Not Hispanic or Latino												
White only												
Below 100%	18.0	16.4	15.0	36.9	36.1	37.0	25.3	28.0	27.4	19.8	19.5	20.6
100%–199%	18.5	17.5	18.4	41.5	41.8	40.4	24.1	24.0	24.7	15.9	16.8	16.5
200%–399%	15.3	13.8	14.7	44.6	47.3	46.0	26.1	24.7	26.3	13.9	14.2	13.0
400% or more	11.8	10.3	9.9	47.8	48.9	48.2	27.6	27.6	28.4	12.8	13.1	13.5
Black or African American only												
Below 100%	18.3	17.8	18.4	40.0	40.1	39.8	24.9	24.8	25.0	16.7	17.3	16.8
100%–199%	20.8	16.1	17.6	44.2	47.0	45.7	20.7	24.3	24.3	14.3	12.6	12.5
200%–399%	17.1	17.2	15.1	48.5	49.0	49.0	24.4	22.9	25.7	10.1	10.9	10.2
400% or more	11.3	12.1	10.0	52.2	52.0	58.2	24.8	24.7	22.5	11.7	11.2	9.3
Health Insurance Status at the Time of Interview[5,6]												
Under 65 years												
Insured	14.0	12.4	12.3	48.2	49.6	48.5	25.1	25.0	26.1	12.7	13.0	13.1
Private	14.3	12.8	12.4	49.9	51.5	51.0	24.8	24.5	25.5	11.0	11.2	11.1
Medicaid	10.4	9.9	10.9	32.4	37.8	38.2	27.6	26.8	28.0	29.6	25.5	23.0
Uninsured	36.8	37.5	37.2	41.9	42.0	42.2	14.1	14.7	15.2	7.2	5.8	5.4

Table C-38. Health Care Visits to Doctor Offices, Emergency Departments, and Home Visits within the Past 12 Months, by Selected Characteristics, Selected Years, 1997–2010—Continued

(Percent.)

Characteristic	None 2000	None 2005	None 2010	1–3 visits 2000	1–3 visits 2005	1–3 visits 2010	4–9 visits 2000	4–9 visits 2005	4–9 visits 2010	10 or more visits 2000	10 or more visits 2005	10 or more visits 2010
Health Insurance Status Prior to Interview[5,6]												
Under 65 years												
Insured continuously all 12 months	13.9	12.3	12.1	48.5	49.8	48.6	25.1	25.0	26.2	12.6	12.9	13.0
Uninsured for any period up to 12 months	20.4	18.9	18.5	44.1	44.9	47.8	21.5	22.5	22.0	13.9	13.7	11.6
Uninsured more than 12 months	43.1	43.5	43.8	39.5	40.0	39.7	12.3	12.3	12.6	5.1	4.2	3.9
Respondent-Assessed Health Status[2]												
Fair or poor	8.9	9.0	8.4	21.7	21.5	24.0	28.2	28.1	30.2	41.2	41.3	37.3
Good to excellent	17.2	16.1	16.3	47.3	48.2	47.5	25.0	24.8	25.5	10.5	10.8	10.7
Disability Measure Among Adults 18 Years of Age and Over[2,7]												
Any basic actions difficulty or complex activity limitation	10.8	9.6	11.5	28.0	29.7	30.9	30.1	29.6	29.3	31.1	31.1	28.3
Any basic actions difficulty	10.7	9.7	11.5	28.0	29.4	30.3	30.2	29.6	29.2	31.1	31.3	29.0
Any complex activity limitation	7.1	5.9	6.9	19.5	21.1	23.0	27.5	27.8	29.1	45.9	45.2	41.0
No disability	20.5	19.8	20.5	48.2	48.8	47.5	22.9	22.7	23.4	8.4	8.6	8.5
Geographic Region[2]												
Northeast	12.4	11.3	12.6	45.9	46.8	46.3	27.8	27.0	26.4	13.9	14.9	14.7
Midwest	14.3	13.8	13.4	45.8	47.2	46.8	26.1	25.2	26.4	13.8	13.9	13.3
South	18.4	16.0	16.1	44.4	45.7	44.2	24.5	25.1	26.6	12.8	13.3	13.2
West	20.2	20.0	19.1	44.6	44.2	45.2	22.5	23.3	23.5	12.7	12.5	12.2
Location of Residence[2]												
Within MSA[8]	16.6	15.5	15.6	45.5	46.2	45.8	24.9	24.9	25.6	13.0	13.3	13.0
Outside MSA[8]	16.7	15.3	15.9	43.3	44.5	42.7	26.0	25.6	27.0	14.1	14.6	14.4

— =Data not available.
* = Figure does not meet standards of reliability or precision.
[1] Includes all other races not shown separately, unknown health insurance status, and unknown disability status.
[2] Estimates are age-adjusted to the year 2000 standard population using six age groups: Under 18 years, 18–44 years, 45–54 years, 55–64 years, 65–74 years, and 75 years and over.
[3] The race groups, White, Black, American Indian or Alaska Native, Asian, Native Hawaiian or Other Pacific Islander, and 2 or more races, include persons of Hispanic and non-Hispanic origin. Persons of Hispanic origin may be of any race.
[4] Percent of poverty level is based on family income and family size and composition.
[5] Estimates for persons under 65 years of age are age-adjusted to the year 2000 standard population using four age groups: Under 18 years, 18–44 years, 45–54 years, and 55–64 years.
[6] Health insurance categories are mutually exclusive. Persons who reported both Medicaid and private coverage are classified as having private coverage.
[7] Any basic actions difficulty or complex activity limitation is defined as having one or more of the following limitations or difficulties: movement difficulty, emotional difficulty, sensory (seeing or hearing) difficulty, cognitive difficulty, self-care (activities of daily living or instrumental activities of daily living) limitation, social limitation, or work limitation.
[8] MSA = metropolitan statistical area.

Table C-39. Vaccination Coverage Among Children 19–35 Months of Age for Selected Diseases, by Race, Hispanic Origin, Poverty Level, and Location of Residence in Metropolitan Statistical Area, Selected Years, 1995–2009

(Percent.)

Vaccination and year	Race and Hispanic origin[1]								Poverty level		Location of residence		
	All	Not Hispanic or Latino						Hispanic or Latino	Below poverty level	At or above poverty level	Inside MSA[3]		Outside MSA
		White	Black or African American	American Indian or Alaska Native	Asian[2]	Native Hawaiian or Other Pacific Islander[2]	2 or more races				Central city	Remaining area	
Combined Series (4:3:1:4:3:1:4)[4]													
2009	44	45	40	—	39	—	41	46	41	46	45	45	42
Combined Series (4:3:1:3:3:1:4)[5]													
2007	67	67	62	75	69	*	66	67	65	67	67	68	63
2008	68	68	66	63	74	*	76	69	63	71	70	69	65
2009	64	64	58	—	55	—	57	67	61	65	—	—	—
Combined Series (4:3:1:3:3:1)[6]													
2002	66	66	62	—	74	—	61	66	62	66	64	68	61
2003	73	74	68	69	76	—	74	71	70	74	72	74	70
2004	76	77	71	67	80	—	77	76	73	77	75	78	74
2005	76	76	76	*	77	—	80	76	74	77	75	78	74
2006	77	78	74	75	76	—	75	77	73	78	77	78	75
2007	77	78	75	83	79	*	76	78	75	78	77	78	76
2008	76	75	73	77	82	*	79	78	72	78	77	76	74
2009	70	69	67	73	70	—	67	73	68	70	—	—	—
DTP/DT/DTaP (4 doses or more)[7]													
1995	78	80	74	71	84	—	—	75	71	81	77	79	78
1996	81	83	79	85	85	—	—	77	74	84	79	83	81
1997	82	84	77	80	80	—	—	78	76	84	80	83	81
1998	84	87	77	83	89	—	—	81	80	86	82	85	85
1999	83	86	79	80	87	—	—	80	79	85	82	84	83
2000	82	84	76	75	85	—	—	79	76	84	80	83	83
2001	82	84	76	77	84	—	—	83	77	84	81	83	82
2002	82	84	76	*	88	*	78	79	75	84	79	84	80
2003	85	88	80	80	89	*	84	82	80	87	84	86	83
2004	86	88	80	77	90	*	86	84	81	87	84	87	85
2005	86	87	84	*	89	*	86	84	82	87	85	87	85
2006	85	87	81	83	86	*	84	85	81	87	84	86	85
2007	85	85	82	86	88	*	84	84	81	86	85	85	83
2008	85	85	80	82	92	*	88	85	80	87	85	85	82
2009	84	86	79	82	87	93	82	83	80	86	84	84	84
Polio (3 doses or more):													
1995	88	89	84	86	90	—	—	87	85	89	87	88	89
1996	91	92	90	90	90	—	—	89	88	92	89	92	92
1997	91	92	89	90	89	—	—	90	89	92	90	91	92
1998	91	92	88	85	93	—	—	89	90	92	89	91	93
1999	90	90	87	88	90	—	—	89	87	91	89	90	90
2000	90	91	87	90	93	—	—	88	87	90	88	90	91
2001	89	90	85	88	90	—	—	91	87	90	88	90	91
2002	90	91	87	*	92	95	87	90	88	91	89	91	90
2003	92	93	89	91	91	90	91	90	89	93	91	92	92
2004	92	92	90	87	93	*	92	91	90	92	91	92	92
2005	92	91	91	*	93	*	94	92	90	92	91	93	92
2006	93	93	90	91	92	96	92	93	92	93	93	93	93
2007	93	93	91	95	95	87	92	93	92	93	92	93	94
2008	94	94	92	91	97	*	94	94	92	94	94	94	93
2009	93	93	91	92	94	97	93	93	92	93	94	92	92

Table C-39. Vaccination Coverage Among Children 19–35 Months of Age for Selected Diseases, by Race, Hispanic Origin, Poverty Level, and Location of Residence in Metropolitan Statistical Area, Selected Years, 1995–2009—*Continued*

(Percent.)

Vaccination and year	All	Race and Hispanic origin[1]							Poverty level		Location of residence		
		Not Hispanic or Latino						Hispanic or Latino	Below poverty level	At or above poverty level	Inside MSA[3]		Outside MSA
		White	Black or African American	American Indian or Alaska Native	Asian[2]	Native Hawaiian or Other Pacific Islander[2]	2 or more races				Central city	Remaining area	
Measles, Mumps, Rubella													
1995	90	91	87	88	95	—	—	88	86	91	90	90	89
1996	91	91	90	89	93	—	—	88	87	92	90	91	91
1997	90	91	89	92	90	—	—	88	86	92	90	91	91
1998	92	93	89	91	92	—	—	91	90	93	92	92	93
1999	92	92	90	92	93	—	—	90	90	92	91	92	90
2000	91	92	88	87	90	—	—	90	89	91	90	91	91
2001	91	92	89	94	90	—	—	92	89	92	91	92	91
2002	92	93	90	84	95	94	89	91	90	92	90	93	90
2003	93	93	92	92	96	*	94	93	92	93	93	93	92
2004	93	94	91	89	94	*	94	93	91	94	93	94	92
2005	92	91	92	90	92	90	94	91	89	92	92	92	90
2006	92	93	91	89	95	94	91	92	91	93	93	93	92
2007	92	92	92	96	94	88	95	93	91	93	92	93	92
2008	92	91	92	96	95	97	94	93	92	92	93	92	90
2009	90	91	88	95	91	97	89	89	89	91	91	89	89
Hib (3 doses or more)[8]													
1995	91	93	88	93	90	—	—	89	88	93	91	92	92
1996	91	93	89	91	92	—	—	89	87	93	90	93	92
1997	93	94	91	86	89	—	—	90	90	94	91	93	94
1998	93	95	90	90	92	—	—	92	91	95	92	94	94
1999	94	95	92	91	90	—	—	92	91	95	92	95	93
2000	93	95	93	90	92	—	—	91	90	95	92	94	95
2001	93	94	90	91	92	—	—	93	90	94	91	94	93
2002	93	94	92	*	95	93	90	92	90	94	92	94	93
2003	94	95	92	89	91	*	93	93	91	95	94	94	94
2004	94	95	91	90	92	*	96	93	92	94	93	94	94
2005	94	94	93	88	89	91	95	94	92	95	93	94	94
2006	93	94	91	94	90	96	91	94	91	94	93	94	92
2007	93	93	91	95	91	*	90	94	91	93	92	94	92
2008	91	91	89	89	93	96	90	92	88	92	91	92	89
Hib (Primary Series Plus Booster Dose)[8]													
2009	55	55	51	—	55	—	54	55	51	57	56	55	53
PERCENT OF CHILDREN 19-35 MONTHS OF AGE													
Hepatitis B (3 Doses or More)													
1995	68	68	66	52	80	—	—	70	65	69	69	71	59
1996	82	82	82	79	85	—	—	81	78	83	81	83	81
1997	84	85	82	83	88	—	—	81	81	85	82	85	85
1998	87	88	84	82	89	—	—	86	85	88	85	88	87
1999	88	89	87	*	88	—	—	87	87	89	87	89	88
2000	90	91	89	91	91	—	—	88	87	91	89	90	92
2001	89	90	85	86	90	—	—	90	87	90	88	90	89
2002	90	91	88	*	94	94	84	90	88	90	89	91	90
2003	92	93	92	90	94	*	93	91	91	93	92	93	93
2004	92	93	91	91	93	*	94	92	91	93	92	93	93
2005	93	93	93	90	93	*	94	93	91	94	92	94	93
2006	93	94	92	95	92	97	92	94	93	94	93	94	93
2007	93	93	91	97	94	*	92	94	92	93	92	93	94
2008	94	93	92	92	98	*	95	94	91	94	93	94	93
2009	92	92	92	93	93	96	93	93	92	93	93	92	92

Table C-39. Vaccination Coverage Among Children 19–35 Months of Age for Selected Diseases, by Race, Hispanic Origin, Poverty Level, and Location of Residence in Metropolitan Statistical Area, Selected Years, 1995–2009—Continued

(Percent.)

Vaccination and year	All	Race and Hispanic origin[1]						Poverty level		Location of residence		
		Not Hispanic or Latino					Hispanic or Latino	Below poverty level	At or above poverty level	Inside MSA[3]		Outside MSA
		White	Black or African American	American Indian or Alaska Native	Asian[2]	Native Hawaiian or Other Pacific Islander[2]	2 or more races				Central city	Remaining area	
Varicella[9]													
1997	26	28	21	20	36	—	—	22	17	29	26	29	17
1998	43	42	42	28	53	—	—	47	41	44	45	45	34
1999	58	56	58	*	64	—	—	61	55	58	59	61	47
2000	68	66	67	62	77	—	—	70	64	69	69	70	60
2001	76	75	75	69	82	—	—	80	74	77	78	78	68
2002	81	79	83	71	87	*	79	82	79	81	81	83	75
2003	85	84	85	81	91	*	86	86	84	85	86	86	80
2004	88	87	86	84	91	*	89	89	86	88	88	89	85
2005	88	86	91	82	92	*	90	89	87	88	88	88	86
2006	89	89	89	85	93	90	91	90	88	90	90	90	86
2007	90	89	90	95	94	89	92	91	89	90	90	90	89
2008	91	90	90	94	94	92	91	92	90	91	92	90	88
2009	90	89	88	89	90	98	91	91	89	90	91	89	89
PCV (4 Doses or More)[10]													
2005	54	57	46	*	56	*	54	51	45	57	52	58	48
2006	68	71	61	63	65	*	71	67	62	71	69	71	62
2007	75	77	70	80	75	*	74	75	73	76	75	77	71
2008	80	81	76	71	82	*	85	79	74	83	81	81	75
2009	80	83	73	76	73	—	73	81	75	83	80	82	82

Vaccination and year	Not Hispanic or Latino				Hispanic or Latino[1]	
	White		Black or African American			
	Below poverty level	At or above poverty level	Below poverty level	At or above poverty level	Below poverty level	At or above poverty level
Combined Series (4:3:1:4:3:1:4):[4]						
2009	43	46	38	44	44	49
Combined Series (4:3:1:3:3:1:4):[5]						
2007	60	68	60	64	69	66
2008	59	70	63	69	64	73
2009	62	65	55	63	66	68
Combined Series (4:3:1:3:3:1):[6]						
2002	59	67	59	62	66	66
2003	69	75	64	72	73	70
2004	72	78	68	75	75	78
2005	70	77	74	80	76	75
2006	69	79	72	77	76	78
2007	70	79	74	77	78	79
2008	68	77	70	75	75	81
2009	68	69	64	71	71	74

— = Data not available.
* = Figure does not meet standards of reliability or precision.
[1]Persons of Hispanic origin may be of any race.
[2]Prior to data year 2002, the category Asian included Native Hawaiian and Other Pacific Islander.
[3]MSA = metropolitan statistical area.
[4]The 4:3:1:4:3:1:4 combined series consists of 4 or more doses of diphtheria and tetanus toxoids and pertussis vaccine (DTP), diphtheria and tetanus toxoids (DT), or diphtheria and tetanus toxoids and acellular pertussis vaccine (DTaP); 3 or more doses of any poliovirus vaccine; 1 or more doses of a measles-containing vaccine (MCV); 3 or more doses of Haemophilus influenzae type b vaccine (Hib); 3 or more doses of hepatitis B vaccine; 1 or more doses of varicella vaccine; and 4 or more doses of pneumococcal conjugate vaccine (PCV).
[5]The 4:3:1:3:3:1:4 combined series consists of 4 or more doses of diphtheria and tetanus toxoids and pertussis vaccine (DTP), diphtheria and tetanus toxoids (DT), or diphtheria and tetanus toxoids and acellular pertussis vaccine (DTaP); 3 or more doses of any poliovirus vaccine; 1 or more doses of a measles-containing vaccine (MCV); 3 or more doses of Haemophilus influenzae type b vaccine (Hib); 3 or more doses of hepatitis B vaccine; 1 or more doses of varicella vaccine; and 4 or more doses of PCV.
[6]The 4:3:1:3:3:1 combined series consists of 4 or more doses of diphtheria and tetanus toxoids and pertussis vaccine (DTP), diphtheria and tetanus toxoids (DT), or diphtheria and tetanus toxoids and acellular pertussis vaccine (DTaP); 3 or more doses of any poliovirus vaccine; 1 or more doses of a measles-containing vaccine (MCV); 3 or more doses of Haemophilus influenzae type b vaccine (Hib); 3 or more doses of hepatitis B vaccine; and 1 or more doses of varicella vaccine.
[7]Diphtheria and tetanus toxoids and pertussis vaccine (DTP), diphtheria and tetanus toxoids (DT), and diphtheria and tetanus toxoids and acellular pertussis vaccine (DTaP).
[8]Haemophilus influenzae type b vaccine (Hib).
[9]Recommended in 1996. Data collection for varicella began in July 1996.
[10]PCV is pneumococcal conjugate vaccine. Recommended in 2000.

Table C-40. Vaccination Coverage Among Children 19–35 Months of Age, by State and Selected Urban Area, Selected Years, 2002–2009

(Percent.)

State and selected urban area	2002	2003	2004	2005	2006	2007	2008	2009
Percent of Children 19–35 Months of Age with 4:3:1:3:3:1 Combined Series[1]								
United States	66	73	76	76	77	77	76	70
Alabama	73	79	80	82	79	78	75	73
Jefferson County (Birmingham)	74	79	81	85	—	—	—	—
Alaska	56	73	66	68	67	70	69	64
Arizona	59	68	73	75	71	75	76	70
Maricopa County (Phoenix)	62	69	72	76	68	—	—	—
Arkansas	68	75	81	64	73	72	76	63
California	67	76	79	74	79	77	79	75
Alameda County	—	—	—	71	—	76	—	—
Fresno County	—	—	—	—	73	—	—	—
Los Angeles County (Los Angeles)	72	79	77	78	79	78	76	78
Northern California	—	—	—	—	71	—	69	—
Santa Clara County (Santa Clara)	75	77	80	—	78	—	81	—
Santa Bernadino County	—	—	—	63	—	70	—	—
San Diego County (San Diego)	71	75	74	—	80	—	—	—
Colorado	56	63	73	79	76	78	79	65
Denver	—	—	—	79	—	—	—	—
Connecticut	73	89	85	82	82	87	70	47
Delaware	70	66	80	82	80	80	72	65
District of Columbia	68	72	80	72	79	82	78	75
Florida	66	74	85	78	79	80	80	75
Dade County (Miami)	60	73	73	—	80	76	78	—
Duval County (Jacksonville)	70	75	69	77	76	—	—	—
Orange County	—	—	—	—	—	—	79	—
Georgia	77	75	82	82	81	80	72	69
Fulton/DeKalb Counties (Atlanta)	75	71	81	72	75	—	—	—
Hawaii	69	79	80	78	79	88	77	67
Idaho	53	61	70	68	68	66	60	52
Illinois	58	69	74	77	74	74	75	73
Chicago	58	71	71	70	77	71	78	72
Madison/St. Clair County	—	—	—	—	—	—	75	—
Indiana	59	62	68	70	76	74	76	66
Lake County	—	—	—	—	—	—	—	65
Marion County (Indianapolis)	62	66	74	—	77	71	—	72
Iowa	58	63	76	76	79	76	75	66
Kansas	55	63	66	72	70	76	77	77
Eastern Kansas	—	—	—	—	74	—	—	—
Kentucky	64	79	77	71	80	78	74	66
Louisiana	62	65	70	74	70	77	82	77
Orleans Parish (New Orleans)	53	68	68	—	—	—	—	—
Maine	62	69	74	76	76	73	74	53
Maryland	71	77	76	79	78	91	80	80
Baltimore City	69	74	80	77	72	—	75	63
Massachusetts	78	83	84	91	84	78	82	81
Boston	71	86	79	—	82	—	—	—
Michigan	72	79	79	81	78	79	75	71
Detroit	60	64	66	71	65	—	—	—
Minnesota	62	71	78	78	78	81	75	58
Twin Cities	—	—	—	—	—	—	75	—
Mississippi	64	78	80	79	73	77	76	73
Missouri	60	74	75	73	81	76	73	61
St. Louis County	—	—	—	74	—	—	—	—
Montana	49	65	65	65	66	65	59	55
Nebraska	64	68	73	84	75	83	72	60
Nevada	65	66	65	63	60	63	68	59
Clark County	—	—	—	59	—	—	—	—
New Hampshire	66	76	78	77	76	91	81	79
New Jersey	66	64	74	72	76	81	69	67
Newark	50	64	64	67	68	—	—	—
New Mexico	59	71	79	75	72	76	77	68
New York	67	73	78	74	77	78	73	69
New York City	71	69	77	71	72	76	75	72
North Carolina	70	77	78	82	82	77	71	56

Table C-40. Vaccination Coverage Among Children 19–35 Months of Age, by State and Selected Urban Area, Selected Years, 2002–2009—Continued

(Percent.)

State and selected urban area	2002	2003	2004	2005	2006	2007	2008	2009
North Dakota	56	63	71	79	80	77	70	56
Ohio	64	71	71	78	75	78	82	74
Cuyahoga County (Cleveland)	65	66	78	77	77	—	—	—
Franklin County (Columbus)	69	71	79	81	—	—	—	—
Oklahoma	60	67	71	72	78	79	72	70
Oregon	60	70	74	65	74	71	71	65
Pennsylvania	68	79	82	77	79	79	78	69
Allegheny County	—	—	—	—	74	—	—	—
Philadelphia	68	75	75	77	80	82	80	74
Rhode Island	81	80	82	80	81	76	78	51
South Carolina	74	80	77	76	81	80	78	67
South Dakota	62	60	73	80	74	77	77	75
Tennessee	67	74	79	80	77	79	81	74
Davidson County (Nashville)	67	76	88	81	—	—	—	—
Shelby County (Memphis)	61	69	71	74	73	—	—	—
Texas	65	70	69	77	75	77	78	74
Bexar County (San Antonio)	72	75	73	71	75	80	76	71
Dallas County (Dallas)	68	67	67	73	73	72	74	74
El Paso County (El Paso)	61	72	64	69	69	77	75	71
Houston	56	63	62	77	70	73	72	70
Utah	61	70	68	68	78	74	77	70
Vermont	58	65	67	63	75	67	65	65
Virginia	65	80	74	82	77	76	73	70
Washington	52	56	67	66	71	69	74	70
Eastern Washington	—	—	—	—	72	—	—	—
Eastern/Western Washington	—	—	—	—	—	—	76	67
King County (Seattle)	56	61	74	69	71	—	—	—
Western Washington	—	—	—	—	—	71	—	—
West Virginia	66	63	76	68	68	76	77	65
Wisconsin	68	73	78	77	81	77	80	59
Milwaukee County (Milwaukee)	60	71	73	74	78	—	—	—
Wyoming	54	57	64	67	63	70	65	62

— =Data not available.

[1]The 4:3:1:3:3:1 combined series consists of 4 or more doses of diphtheria and tetanus toxoids and pertussis vaccine (DTP), diphtheria and tetanus toxoids (DT), or diphtheria and tetanus toxoids and acellular pertussis vaccine (DTaP); 3 or more doses of any poliovirus vaccine; 1 or more doses of a measles-containing vaccine (MCV); 3 or more doses of Haemophilus influenzae type b vaccine (Hib) regardless of vaccine brand type; 3 or more doses of hepatitis B vaccine; and 1 or more doses of varicella vaccine.

Table C-41. Vaccination Coverage Among Adolescents 13–17 Years of Age for Selected Diseases, by Selected Characteristics, 2006–2009

(Percent.)

Vaccination coverage	2006[1]	2007[1]	2008	2009
Percent of Adolescents 13–17 Years				
Measles, mumps, rubella (2 doses or more)	86.9	88.9	89.3	89.1
Hepatitis B (3 doses or more)	81.3	87.6	87.9	89.9
History of varicella or received varicella vaccine (2 doses or more)[2]	—	—	73.5	75.7
Td or Tdap (1 dose or more)[3]	60.1	72.3	72.2	76.2
Tdap (1 dose or more)[3]	10.8	30.4	40.8	55.6
Meningococcal conjugate vaccine (MenACWY) (1 dose or more)[4]	11.7	32.4	41.8	53.6
Human papillomavirus (HPV) (1 dose or more)[5]	—	25.1	37.2	44.3
Human papillomavirus (HPV) (3 doses or more)[5]	—	—	17.9	26.7

| Vaccination and year | Race and Hispanic origin[6] | | | | | Poverty level[7] | | Location of residence | | |
| | Not Hispanic or Latino | | | | Hispanic or Latino | | | Inside MSA[8] | | |
	White	Black or African American	American Indian or Alaska Native	Asian		Below poverty level	At or above poverty level	Central city	Remaining area	Outside MSA
Measles, mumps, rubella (2 doses or more)	90.2	86.3	90.4	92.9	87.6	87.8	89.3	88.5	90.2	87.5
Hepatitis B (3 doses or more)	90.2	88.9	89.7	89.5	90.0	88.3	90.3	89.2	91.6	86.9
History of varicella or received varicella vaccine (2 doses or more)[2]	77.0	71.3	71.9	72.6	74.9	74.4	75.9	—	—	—
Td or Tdap (1 dose or more)[3]	76.5	72.5	78.0	84.5	76.7	71.8	77.0	79.7	77.3	64.4
Tdap (1 dose or more)[3]	55.8	52.7	59.3	64.3	55.6	52.8	56.1	60.1	55.0	46.3
Meningococcal conjugate vaccine (MenACWY) (1 dose or more)[4]	53.1	53.0	46.9	58.8	55.9	52.5	53.8	58.3	55.9	36.0
Human papillomavirus (HPV) (1 dose or more)[5]	43.9	44.6	52.3	41.5	45.5	51.9	42.5	49.4	42.5	37.5
Human papillomavirus (HPV) (3 doses or more)[5]	29.1	23.1	29.6	22.1	23.4	25.5	26.8	—	—	—

— =Data not available.
[1]For 2006 and 2007, data were only collected in the 4th quarter of the year. Starting with 2008, data were collected for the entire year.
[2]Varicella is chickenpox.
[3]Td or Tdap refers to tetanus toxoid-diphtheria vaccine (Td) or tetanus toxoid, reduced diphtheria toxoid, and acellular pertussis vaccine (Tdap) received since the age of 10 years.
[4]Includes persons receiving MenACWY or meningococcal-unknown type vaccine.
[5]Percentages reported among females.
[6]Persons of Hispanic origin may be of any race.
[7]Poverty level is based on family income and family size using U.S. Census Bureau poverty thresholds.
[8]MSA = metropolitan statistical area.

Table C-42. Influenza Vaccination[1] Among Adults 18 Years of Age and Over, by Selected Characteristics, Selected Years, 1989–2010

(Percent.)

Characteristic	1989	1995	2000	2005	2006	2007	2008	2009	2010
18 years and over, age-adjusted[2,3]	9.6	23.7	28.7	21.6	27.4	29.9	32.1	34.1	35.1
18 years and over, crude[3]	9.1	23.0	28.4	21.4	27.6	30.1	32.6	34.7	35.8
Age									
18–49 years	3.4	13.1	17.1	10.7	15.6	17.8	20.1	23.0	25.2
50 years and over	19.9	41.9	47.9	38.1	45.9	48.5	50.7	51.1	50.5
50–64 years	10.6	27.0	34.6	23.0	33.2	36.2	39.6	40.7	41.6
65 years and over	30.4	58.2	64.4	59.7	64.3	66.7	67.2	66.8	63.9
65–74 years	28.0	54.9	61.1	53.7	60.1	61.6	60.9	61.5	60.5
75 years and over	34.2	63.0	68.4	66.3	69.2	72.6	74.3	73.2	68.2
50 YEARS AND OVER									
Sex									
Male	19.2	40.2	45.9	34.7	43.2	45.6	47.6	49.2	47.4
Female	20.6	43.4	49.5	40.9	48.3	51.0	53.5	52.8	53.2
Race[4]									
White only	20.9	43.6	49.8	39.7	47.2	49.9	52.1	52.4	51.5
Black or African American only	12.5	28.2	33.2	26.9	34.9	38.2	41.1	41.7	40.4
American Indian or Alaska Native only	26.2	*	43.6	*22.9	56.3	45.8	49.3	42.8	54.7
Asian only	*9.2	35.6	43.3	30.6	44.8	45.3	47.1	50.4	55.9
Native Hawaiian or Other Pacific Islander only	—	—	*	*	*	*	*	*	*
2 or more races	—	—	50.7	30.4	40.2	44.8	46.3	47.7	49.8
Hispanic Origin and Race[4]									
Hispanic or Latino	13.2	33.8	34.4	24.7	31.7	35.5	38.0	40.3	40.6
Mexican	13.0	35.4	33.0	26.1	33.5	36.1	36.5	40.4	41.3
Not Hispanic or Latino	20.3	42.4	48.8	39.1	47.1	49.6	51.9	52.1	51.5
White only	21.3	44.3	50.6	41.0	48.6	51.3	53.6	53.7	52.7
Black or African American only	12.4	28.5	33.2	26.9	35.1	38.1	41.0	41.7	40.0
Percent of Poverty Level[5]									
Below 100%	19.6	39.7	44.1	35.8	42.1	44.8	44.4	45.2	37.5
100%–199%	24.0	43.2	50.7	41.2	47.5	47.9	52.0	49.4	47.6
200%–399%	20.5	43.7	51.5	42.1	48.0	50.7	51.8	52.6	51.2
400% or more	17.5	39.3	44.3	33.9	44.4	48.0	50.8	52.0	54.3
Hispanic Origin and Race and Percent of Poverty Level[4,5]									
Hispanic or Latino									
Below 100%	12.7	29.7	35.8	22.3	30.9	41.1	37.0	42.2	36.3
100%–199%	20.4	34.7	35.6	27.5	32.0	42.7	41.3	32.4	36.6
200%–399%	12.7	34.2	33.7	22.3	33.8	31.3	34.5	41.1	41.8
400% or more	*9.8	39.1	32.2	26.6	29.5	28.9	39.9	48.7	47.7
Not Hispanic or Latino									
White only									
Below 100%	22.5	44.4	48.6	42.2	47.8	47.4	49.3	49.8	38.7
100%–199%	26.1	46.7	54.8	46.1	51.7	50.8	57.0	54.3	51.1
200%–399%	21.6	45.4	54.6	46.4	50.8	54.3	54.6	55.0	53.4
400% or more	18.1	40.8	46.0	35.1	45.9	50.2	52.3	53.3	54.9
Black or African American only									
Below 100%	14.6	31.8	35.5	28.9	34.8	38.9	36.7	37.8	32.4
100%–199%	12.0	28.3	37.9	27.4	35.0	35.6	38.4	41.8	39.2
200%–399%	14.1	29.0	31.0	25.7	36.2	41.2	44.1	45.1	42.6
400% or more	*8.8	*20.0	28.7	26.2	34.6	36.2	42.9	41.0	44.4

Table C-42. Influenza Vaccination[1] Among Adults 18 Years of Age and Over, by Selected Characteristics, Selected Years, 1989–2010—Continued

(Percent.)

Characteristic	1989	1995	2000	2005	2006	2007	2008	2009	2010
Disability Measure[6]									
Any basic actions difficulty or complex activity limitation	—	—	55.2	46.5	53.4	55.8	57.2	56.9	54.5
Any basic actions difficulty	—	—	55.3	46.7	53.7	56.0	57.6	57.1	54.8
Any complex activity limitation	—	—	57.1	50.3	56.0	56.8	58.9	58.8	55.3
No disability	—	—	41.3	29.7	38.4	41.6	44.8	46.0	47.0
Geographic Region									
Northeast	17.9	39.7	45.9	38.4	44.1	49.0	52.7	52.0	52.4
Midwest	20.0	43.2	49.3	39.9	49.4	51.4	53.7	52.9	51.8
South	20.2	41.4	46.8	37.3	43.9	47.2	49.4	50.9	49.3
West	21.8	43.8	50.1	36.8	47.3	46.9	48.1	48.8	49.5
Location of Residence									
Within MSA[7]	18.9	41.6	47.1	37.2	44.9	47.1	50.2	51.0	50.8
Outside MSA[7]	23.3	42.9	50.2	41.0	49.7	53.7	53.0	51.6	49.3

* = Figure does not meet standards of reliability or precision.
— = Data not available.
[1] Questions concerning use of influenza vaccination differed slightly on the National Health Interview Survey across the years for which data are shown.
[2] Estimates are age-adjusted to the year 2000 standard population using four age groups: 18–49 years, 50–64 years, 65–74 years, and 75 years and over.
[3] Includes all other races not shown separately, unknown disability status, and unknown poverty level in 1989.
[4] The race groups, White, Black, American Indian or Alaska Native, Asian, Native Hawaiian or Other Pacific Islander, and 2 or more races, include persons of Hispanic and non-Hispanic origin. Persons of Hispanic origin may be of any race.
[5] Percent of poverty level is based on family income and family size and composition using U.S. Census Bureau poverty thresholds.
[6] Any basic actions difficulty or complex activity limitation is defined as having one or more of the following limitations or difficulties: movement difficulty, emotional difficulty, sensory (seeing or hearing) difficulty, cognitive difficulty, self-care (activities of daily living or instrumental activities of daily living) limitation, social limitation, or work limitation.
[7] MSA = metropolitan statistical area.

Table C-43. Pneumococcal Vaccination[1] Among Adults 18 Years of Age and Over, by Selected Characteristics, Selected Years, 1989–2010

(Percent.)

Characteristic	1989	1995	2000	2005	2006	2007	2008	2009	2010
18 years and over, age-adjusted[2,3]	4.6	12.0	15.4	16.7	17.0	16.7	18.3	19.0	19.0
18 years and over, crude[3]	4.4	11.7	15.1	16.5	17.0	16.7	18.5	19.3	19.6
Age									
18–49 years	2.1	6.5	5.4	5.8	5.7	5.3	6.8	7.5	7.3
50–64 years	4.4	10.0	14.7	17.1	18.2	17.3	18.5	19.2	21.0
65 years and over	14.1	34.0	53.1	56.2	57.1	57.7	60.0	60.6	59.7
65–74 years	13.1	31.4	48.2	49.4	52.0	51.8	52.5	54.6	54.6
75 years and over	15.7	37.8	59.1	63.9	63.0	64.4	68.7	68.0	66.0
High–Risk Group[4]									
Total, 18–64 years	—	—	18.3	22.6	23.1	24.4	24.9	17.4	18.3
18–49 years	—	—	12.2	15.0	13.5	16.0	16.0	11.2	10.6
50–64 years	—	—	26.0	30.6	32.5	32.2	33.9	28.2	30.8
65 YEARS AND OVER									
Sex									
Male	13.9	34.6	52.1	53.4	54.3	55.1	56.4	59.2	57.6
Female	14.3	33.6	53.9	58.4	59.2	59.6	62.8	61.7	61.3
Race[5]									
White only	14.8	35.3	55.6	58.4	60.0	60.1	62.5	63.1	61.6
Black or African American only	6.4	21.9	30.6	40.2	35.5	43.7	44.1	44.2	45.5
American Indian or Alaska Native only	31.2	*	70.1	*	*57.5	*	66.9	*	*48.5
Asian only	*	*23.4	40.9	35.0	35.6	33.4	45.7	44.8	47.9
Native Hawaiian or Other Pacific Islander only	—	—	*	*	*	*	*	*	*
2 or more races	—	—	55.6	64.8	63.6	55.8	*35.9	67.9	65.5
Hispanic Origin and Race[5]									
Hispanic or Latino	9.8	23.2	30.4	27.5	33.3	31.8	36.4	40.1	39.0
Mexican	12.9	*18.8	32.0	31.3	29.3	34.3	39.5	42.8	41.4
Not Hispanic or Latino	14.3	34.5	54.4	58.1	58.7	59.6	61.8	62.2	61.3
White only	15.0	35.9	56.8	60.6	62.0	62.2	64.5	64.8	63.5
Black or African American only	6.2	21.8	30.6	40.4	35.6	44.0	44.5	44.7	46.2
Percent of Poverty Level[6]									
Below 100%	11.2	28.7	40.6	46.7	45.4	48.7	46.5	48.5	42.6
100%–199%	15.1	30.7	51.4	54.5	55.8	55.6	59.5	60.6	57.2
200%–399%	15.1	36.1	55.8	60.8	59.9	59.8	61.4	62.9	62.2
400% or more	15.5	39.5	56.9	55.3	59.3	59.8	62.8	61.5	64.0
Hispanic Origin and Race and Percent of Poverty Level[5,6]									
Hispanic or Latino									
Below 100%	*	*14.1	23.8	20.9	24.5	*22.4	*25.7	32.6	30.2
100%–199%	*11.0	*15.6	32.3	26.9	30.9	37.9	32.9	41.8	36.9
200%–399%	*11.1	*34.4	37.6	35.2	42.3	29.6	44.8	40.0	45.8
400% or more	*	*55.1	*26.4	*25.2	*38.2	*33.7	42.4	49.1	43.0
Not Hispanic or Latino									
White only									
Below 100%	13.3	32.5	47.9	55.6	56.0	59.7	60.4	61.0	51.1
100%–199%	16.0	33.5	56.1	60.5	61.6	60.8	66.3	66.3	61.3
200%–399%	15.7	37.1	57.6	64.1	62.6	63.4	64.5	66.3	64.9
400% or more	15.9	39.3	59.5	57.4	63.0	62.4	64.1	62.9	66.0
Black or African American only									
Below 100%	*5.0	*22.6	28.8	42.3	38.4	40.7	37.6	33.8	34.9
100%–199%	7.8	*20.9	28.1	36.6	36.2	41.9	43.5	46.9	46.4
200%–399%	*5.9	*21.7	35.5	41.6	40.0	48.7	44.5	49.3	51.8
400% or more	*	*	*32.6	44.6	*24.7	43.6	56.5	45.8	50.1

PART C: HEALTH

Table C-43. Pneumococcal Vaccination[1] Among Adults 18 Years of Age and Over, by Selected Characteristics, Selected Years 1989–2010—*Continued*

(Percent.)

Characteristic	1989	1995	2000	2005	2006	2007	2008	2009	2010
Any Basic Actions Difficulty or Complex Activity Limitation[7]									
Any basic actions difficulty or complex activity limitation.....	—	—	56.6	61.6	61.4	64.2	64.9	65.9	63.9
Any basic actions difficulty................	—	—	56.8	61.6	61.6	64.4	65.1	66.0	64.2
Any complex activity limitation	—	—	58.0	63.3	61.6	63.9	67.0	67.8	65.2
No disability....................................	—	—	48.0	47.8	50.0	47.0	53.4	53.1	53.3
Geographic Region									
Northeast...	10.4	28.2	51.2	55.8	53.7	54.6	60.9	58.5	56.7
Midwest...	13.7	31.0	52.6	58.5	61.5	60.6	63.8	58.4	61.2
South...	14.9	35.9	51.3	57.4	55.7	58.5	59.8	61.9	60.9
West..	17.9	41.1	59.7	51.4	57.2	55.6	55.4	63.0	58.9
Location of Residence									
Within MSA[8]...................................	13.1	33.8	52.4	55.1	56.6	56.5	59.1	60.0	58.8
Outside MSA[8].................................	17.1	34.8	55.4	59.8	58.9	61.7	63.2	62.9	63.3

— =Data not available.
* = Figure does not meet standards of reliability or precision.
[1]Respondents were asked, "Have you ever had a pneumonia shot? This shot is usually given only once or twice in a person's lifetime and is different from the flu shot. It is also called the pneumococcal vaccine."
[2]Estimates are age-adjusted to the year 2000 standard population using four age groups: 18–49 years, 50–64 years, 65–74 years, and 75 years and over.
[3]Includes all other races not shown separately, unknown poverty level in 1989, and unknown disability status.
[4]High-risk group membership is based on recommendations of the Advisory Committee on Immunization Practices (ACIP). The high-risk group includes persons who reported diabetes, cancer, heart, lung, liver, or kidney disease.
[5]The race groups, White, Black, American Indian or Alaska Native, Asian, Native Hawaiian or Other Pacific Islander, and 2 or more races, include persons of Hispanic and non-Hispanic origin. Persons of Hispanic origin may be of any race.
[6]Percent of poverty level is based on family income and family size and composition using U.S. Census Bureau poverty thresholds.
[7]Any basic actions difficulty or complex activity limitation is defined as having one or more of the following limitations or difficulties: movement difficulty, emotional difficulty, sensory (seeing or hearing) difficulty, cognitive difficulty, self-care (activities of daily living or instrumental activities of daily living) limitation, social limitation, or work limitation.
[8]MSA = metropolitan statistical area.

Table C-44. Use of Mammography[1] Among Women 40 Years of Age and Over, by Selected Characteristics, Selected Years, 1987–2010

(Percent.)

Characteristic	1987	1990	1991	1993	1994	1998	1999	2000	2003	2005	2008	2010
40 years and over, age-adjusted[2,3]	29.0	51.7	54.7	59.7	61.0	67.0	70.3	70.4	69.5	66.6	67.1	66.5
40 years and over, crude[2]	28.7	51.4	54.6	59.7	60.9	66.9	70.3	70.4	69.7	66.8	67.6	67.1
50 years and over, age-adjusted[2,3]	27.3	49.8	54.3	59.7	60.9	69.0	72.1	73.7	72.4	68.2	70.3	68.8
50 years and over, crude[2]	27.4	49.7	54.1	59.7	60.6	68.9	71.9	73.6	72.4	68.4	70.5	69.2
Age												
40–49 years	31.9	55.1	55.6	59.9	61.3	63.4	67.2	64.3	64.4	63.5	61.5	62.3
50–64 years	31.7	56.0	60.3	65.1	66.5	73.7	76.5	78.7	76.2	71.8	74.2	72.6
65 years and over	22.8	43.4	48.1	54.2	55.0	63.8	66.8	67.9	67.7	63.8	65.5	64.4
65–74 years	26.6	48.7	55.7	64.2	63.0	69.4	73.9	74.0	74.6	72.5	72.6	71.9
75 years and over	17.3	35.8	37.8	41.0	44.6	57.2	58.9	61.3	60.6	54.7	57.9	55.7
Race[4]												
40 years and over, crude												
White only	29.6	52.2	55.6	60.0	60.6	67.4	70.6	71.4	70.1	67.4	67.9	67.4
Black or African American only	24.0	46.4	48.0	59.1	64.3	66.0	71.0	67.8	70.4	64.9	68.0	67.9
American Indian or Alaska Native only	*	43.2	54.5	49.8	65.8	45.2	63.0	47.4	63.1	72.8	62.7	71.2
Asian only	*	46.0	45.9	55.1	55.8	60.2	58.3	53.5	57.6	54.6	66.1	62.4
Native Hawaiian or Other Pacific Islander only	—	—	—	—	—	—	*	*	*	*	*	*
2 or more races	—	—	—	—	—	—	70.2	69.2	65.3	63.7	55.2	51.4
Hispanic Origin and Race[4]												
40 years and over, crude												
Hispanic or Latina	18.3	45.2	49.2	50.9	51.9	60.2	65.7	61.2	65.0	58.8	61.2	64.2
Not Hispanic or Latina	29.4	51.8	54.9	60.3	61.5	67.5	70.7	71.1	70.1	67.5	68.3	67.4
White only	30.3	52.7	56.0	60.6	61.3	68.0	71.1	72.2	70.5	68.3	68.7	67.8
Black or African American only	23.8	46.0	47.7	59.2	64.4	66.0	71.0	67.9	70.5	65.2	68.3	67.4
Age, Hispanic Origin, and Race[4]												
40–49 years												
Hispanic or Latina	*15.3	45.1	44.0	52.6	47.5	55.2	61.6	54.1	59.4	54.2	54.1	59.8
Not Hispanic or Latina												
White only	34.3	57.0	58.1	61.6	62.0	64.4	68.3	67.2	65.2	65.5	64.1	62.6
Black or African American only	27.8	48.4	48.0	55.6	67.2	65.0	69.2	60.9	68.2	62.1	59.5	63.5
50–64 years												
Hispanic or Latina	23.0	47.5	61.7	59.2	60.1	67.2	69.7	66.5	69.4	61.5	71.3	68.6
Not Hispanic or Latina												
White only	33.6	58.1	61.5	66.2	67.5	75.3	77.9	80.6	77.2	73.5	74.1	73.5
Black or African American only	26.4	48.4	52.4	65.5	63.6	71.2	75.0	77.7	76.2	71.6	76.7	74.0
65 years and over												
Hispanic or Latina	*	41.1	40.9	*35.7	48.0	59.0	67.2	68.3	69.5	63.8	59.0	65.2
Not Hispanic or Latina												
White only	24.0	43.8	49.1	54.7	54.9	64.3	66.8	68.3	68.1	64.7	66.1	65.0
Black or African American only	14.1	39.7	41.6	56.3	61.0	60.6	68.1	65.5	65.4	60.5	66.4	60.9
Age and Percent of Poverty Level[5]												
40 years and over, crude												
Below 100%	14.6	30.8	35.2	41.1	44.2	50.1	57.4	54.8	55.4	48.5	51.4	51.4
100%–199%	20.9	39.1	44.4	47.5	48.6	56.1	59.5	58.1	60.8	55.3	55.8	53.8
200%–399%	29.7	53.3	57.5	63.2	65.0	67.4	69.1	68.8	69.9	67.2	64.4	66.2
400% or more	42.9	68.7	69.8	74.1	74.1	76.8	79.8	81.5	77.7	76.6	79.0	78.1
40–49 years												
Below 100%	18.6	32.2	33.0	36.1	43.0	44.8	51.3	47.4	50.6	42.5	46.6	48.1
100%–199%	18.4	39.0	43.8	47.8	47.6	46.9	52.8	43.6	54.0	49.8	46.5	46.2
200%–399%	31.2	55.2	56.3	63.0	64.5	61.8	63.0	60.2	63.0	61.8	56.8	59.2
400% or more	44.1	68.9	69.6	69.6	69.9	72.7	77.4	75.8	71.6	73.6	72.5	73.6
50–64 years												
Below 100%	14.6	29.9	37.3	47.3	46.2	52.7	63.3	61.7	58.3	50.4	57.5	54.7
100%–199%	24.2	39.8	50.2	47.0	49.0	61.8	64.9	68.3	64.0	58.8	58.9	57.3
200%–399%	29.7	56.2	60.2	66.1	69.6	71.1	74.8	75.1	74.1	70.7	69.8	70.7
400% or more	44.7	71.6	72.6	78.7	78.0	83.4	83.4	86.9	84.9	80.6	84.3	82.8
65 years and over												
Below 100%	13.1	30.8	35.2	40.4	43.9	51.9	57.6	54.8	57.0	52.3	49.1	50.6
100%–199%	19.9	38.6	41.8	47.6	48.8	57.8	60.2	60.3	62.8	56.1	59.4	55.5
200%–399%	27.7	47.4	55.9	60.3	61.0	69.5	70.0	71.1	72.3	68.6	65.0	67.2
400% or more	34.7	61.2	63.0	71.3	73.0	71.1	76.7	81.9	73.0	72.6	78.3	74.5

Table C-44. Use of Mammography[1] Among Women 40 Years of Age and Over, by Selected Characteristics, Selected Years, 1987–2010—Continued

(Percent.)

Characteristic	1987	1990	1991	1993	1994	1998	1999	2000	2003	2005	2008	2010
Health Insurance Status at the Time of Interview[6]												
40–64 years												
Insured	—	—	—	66.2	68.3	72.3	75.5	76.0	75.1	72.5	73.4	74.1
Private	—	—	—	67.1	69.4	73.4	76.3	77.1	76.3	74.5	74.2	75.6
Medicaid	—	—	—	51.9	54.5	59.7	62.5	61.7	63.5	55.6	64.2	64.4
Uninsured	—	—	—	36.0	34.0	40.1	44.8	40.7	41.5	38.1	39.7	36.0
Health Insurance Status Prior to Interview[6]												
40–64 years												
Insured continuously all 12 months	—	—	—	66.6	68.6	73.0	76.1	76.8	75.6	73.1	74.1	74.7
Uninsured for any period up to 12 months	—	—	—	49.4	49.9	47.6	57.1	53.0	56.0	51.3	55.3	57.3
Uninsured more than 12 months	—	—	—	28.4	26.6	36.3	38.9	34.0	37.0	32.9	34.6	30.0
Age and Education[7]												
40 years and over, crude												
No high school diploma or GED	17.8	36.4	40.0	46.4	48.2	54.5	56.7	57.7	58.1	52.8	53.8	53.0
High school diploma or GED	31.3	52.7	55.8	59.0	61.0	66.7	69.2	69.7	67.8	64.9	65.2	64.4
Some college or more	37.7	62.8	65.2	69.5	69.7	72.8	77.3	76.2	75.1	72.7	73.4	72.1
40–49 years												
No high school diploma or GED	15.1	38.5	40.8	43.6	50.4	47.3	48.8	46.8	53.3	51.2	46.9	44.9
High school diploma or GED	32.6	53.1	52.0	56.6	55.8	59.1	60.8	59.0	60.8	58.8	57.2	58.4
Some college or more	39.2	62.3	63.7	66.1	68.7	68.3	74.4	70.6	68.1	68.3	66.3	66.5
50–64 years												
No high school diploma or GED	21.2	41.0	43.6	51.4	51.6	58.8	62.3	66.5	63.4	56.9	64.9	56.7
High school diploma or GED	33.8	56.5	60.8	62.4	67.8	73.3	77.2	76.6	71.8	70.1	70.4	69.9
Some college or more	40.5	68.0	72.7	78.5	74.7	79.8	81.2	84.2	82.7	77.0	78.5	77.0
65 years and over												
No high school diploma or GED	16.5	33.0	37.7	44.2	45.6	54.7	56.6	57.4	56.9	50.7	49.2	54.1
High school diploma or GED	25.9	47.5	54.0	57.4	59.1	66.8	68.4	71.8	69.7	64.3	65.7	62.5
Some college or more	32.3	56.7	57.9	64.8	64.3	71.3	77.1	74.1	75.1	73.0	75.6	70.9
Disability Measure[8]												
40 years and over, crude												
Any basic actions difficulty or complex activity limitation	—	—	—	—	—	65.8	67.6	67.8	67.2	63.5	63.9	63.3
Any basic actions difficulty	—	—	—	—	—	65.9	67.1	67.9	67.3	63.5	63.9	63.3
Any complex activity limitation	—	—	—	—	—	61.8	64.8	64.1	62.3	59.9	60.2	58.2
No disability	—	—	—	—	—	68.2	72.3	72.6	71.8	69.8	71.1	70.8

* = Figure does not meet standards of reliability or precision.
— =Data not available.
[1]Questions concerning use of mammography differed slightly on the National Health Interview Survey across the years for which data are shown.
[2]Includes all other races not shown separately, unknown poverty level in 1987, unknown health insurance status, unknown education level, and unknown disability status.
[3]Estimates for women 40 years of age and over are age-adjusted to the year 2000 standard population using four age groups: 40–49 years, 50–64 years, 65–74 years, and 75 years and over. Estimates for women 50 years of age and over are age-adjusted using three age groups.
[4]The race groups, White, Black, American Indian or Alaska Native, Asian, Native Hawaiian or Other Pacific Islander, and 2 or more races, include persons of Hispanic and non-Hispanic origin. Persons of Hispanic origin may be of any race.
[5]Percent of poverty level is based on family income and family size and composition using U.S. Census Bureau poverty thresholds.
[6]Health insurance categories are mutually exclusive. Persons who reported both Medicaid and private coverage are classified as having private coverage.
[7]Education categories shown are for 1998 and subsequent years.
[8]Any basic actions difficulty or complex activity limitation is defined as having one or more of the following limitations or difficulties: movement difficulty, emotional difficulty, sensory (seeing or hearing) difficulty, cognitive difficulty, self-care (activity of daily living or instrumental activities of daily living) limitation, social limitation, or work limitation.

Table C-45. Percent of Women 18 Years of Age and Over Who Have Had a Pap Smear[1] Within the Last Three Years, by Selected Characteristics, Selected Years, 1987–2010

(Percent.)

Characteristic	1987	1993	1994	1998	1999	2000	2003	2005	2008	2010
18 years and over, age–adjusted[2,3]	74.1	77.7	76.8	79.3	80.8	81.3	79.2	77.9	75.6	73.7
18 years and over, crude[2]	74.4	77.7	76.8	79.1	80.8	81.2	79.0	77.7	75.1	73.2
Age										
18–44 years	83.3	84.6	82.8	84.4	86.8	84.9	83.9	83.6	81.8	80.4
18–24 years	74.8	78.8	76.6	73.6	76.8	73.5	75.1	74.5	70.5	69.0
25–44 years	86.3	86.3	84.6	87.6	89.9	88.5	86.8	86.8	85.7	84.6
45–64 years	70.5	77.2	77.4	81.4	81.7	84.6	81.3	80.6	78.8	76.9
45–54 years	75.7	82.1	81.9	83.7	83.8	86.3	83.6	83.4	81.0	79.9
55–64 years	65.2	70.6	71.0	78.0	78.4	82.0	77.8	76.8	76.0	73.2
65 years and over	50.8	57.6	57.3	59.8	61.0	64.5	60.8	54.9	50.0	47.1
65–74 years	57.9	64.7	64.9	67.0	70.0	71.6	70.1	66.3	61.6	58.0
75 years and over	40.4	48.0	47.3	51.2	50.8	56.7	51.1	42.7	37.5	34.6
Race[4]										
18 years and over, crude										
White only	74.1	77.3	76.2	78.9	80.6	81.3	78.7	77.7	74.9	72.8
Black or African American only	80.7	82.7	83.5	84.2	85.7	85.1	84.0	81.1	80.1	77.9
American Indian or Alaska Native only	85.4	78.1	73.5	74.6	92.2	76.8	84.8	75.2	69.4	73.4
Asian only	51.9	68.8	66.4	68.5	64.4	66.4	68.3	64.1	65.1	68.0
Native Hawaiian or Other Pacific Islander only	—	—	—	—	*	*	*	*	*	*
2 or more races	—	—	—	—	86.9	80.0	81.6	86.2	77.1	70.8
Hispanic Origin and Race[4]										
18 years and over, crude										
Hispanic or Latina	67.6	77.2	74.4	75.2	76.3	77.0	75.4	75.5	75.4	73.6
Not Hispanic or Latina	74.9	77.8	77.0	79.6	81.3	81.7	79.5	78.0	75.1	73.1
White only	74.7	77.3	76.5	79.3	81.0	81.8	79.3	78.1	74.9	72.8
Black or African American only	80.9	82.7	83.8	84.2	86.0	85.1	83.8	81.2	80.0	77.4
Age, Hispanic Origin, and Race[4]										
18–44 years										
Hispanic or Latina	73.9	80.9	80.6	76.4	77.0	78.1	75.9	76.5	77.9	75.9
Not Hispanic or Latina										
White only	84.5	85.3	82.9	85.7	88.7	86.6	85.8	85.8	83.8	82.1
Black or African American only	89.1	88.0	89.1	88.9	90.8	88.5	88.6	86.4	83.5	84.2
45–64 years										
Hispanic or Latina	57.7	75.8	70.1	78.3	79.5	77.8	77.9	78.4	78.2	75.4
Not Hispanic or Latina										
White only	71.2	77.2	77.5	81.7	81.9	85.9	81.4	81.4	79.0	77.2
Black or African American only	76.2	80.3	82.2	84.1	84.6	85.7	84.7	80.5	82.1	78.2
65 years and over										
Hispanic or Latina	41.7	57.1	43.8	59.8	63.7	66.8	64.6	60.0	52.6	54.2
Not Hispanic or Latina										
White only	51.8	57.1	58.2	59.7	60.5	64.2	60.7	54.1	49.0	46.5
Black or African American only	44.8	61.2	59.5	61.7	64.5	67.2	59.6	60.1	58.7	48.0
Age and Percent of Poverty Level[5]										
18 years and over, crude										
Below 100%	64.3	70.3	68.8	69.8	73.6	72.0	70.5	68.7	68.9	65.1
100%–199%	68.2	71.2	68.8	70.6	72.5	73.4	71.4	69.0	65.0	64.3
200%–399%	77.6	80.6	80.1	79.7	80.6	80.2	78.6	77.9	72.5	71.3
400% or more	83.6	85.1	85.4	87.0	87.6	89.1	86.6	85.7	84.4	83.1
18–44 years										
Below 100%	77.1	77.0	78.9	77.1	79.7	77.1	77.1	76.2	76.5	73.0
100%–199%	80.4	81.9	78.2	79.2	84.0	79.4	79.5	78.1	75.5	75.7
200%–399%	84.8	86.6	84.5	85.3	86.7	86.1	84.0	85.5	82.6	79.8
400% or more	88.9	91.3	88.7	89.8	91.1	89.8	89.5	88.7	87.0	88.9
45–64 years										
Below 100%	53.6	66.5	62.0	67.6	73.1	73.6	66.0	65.9	66.2	61.7
100%–199%	60.4	64.8	66.2	69.9	70.4	76.1	71.4	69.6	65.6	63.2
200%–399%	71.0	79.5	80.3	79.7	79.9	80.0	80.8	79.3	75.3	75.2
400% or more	79.1	83.9	84.0	88.2	87.4	91.5	87.5	87.4	87.1	85.7
65 years and over										
Below 100%	33.2	47.4	44.0	48.2	51.9	53.7	52.6	44.4	41.6	35.1
100%–199%	50.4	55.7	51.5	55.1	54.7	61.0	55.4	49.5	43.5	40.7
200%–399%	58.0	59.7	63.7	64.2	64.0	65.1	62.4	56.8	45.8	47.1
400% or more	65.2	67.5	76.2	67.5	70.4	75.4	70.2	64.6	65.7	57.7

Table C-45. Percent of Women 18 Years of Age and Over Who Have Had a Pap Smear[1] Within the Last Three Years, by Selected Characteristics, Selected Years, 1987–2010—Continued

(Percent.)

Characteristic	1987	1993	1994	1998	1999	2000	2003	2005	2008	2010
Health Insurance Status at the Time of Interview[6]										
18–64 years, crude										
Insured	—	84.7	83.8	86.0	87.2	87.8	86.4	85.6	83.4	82.8
Private	—	84.8	83.6	86.5	87.5	88.0	87.0	86.5	84.2	84.2
Medicaid	—	82.7	86.2	83.0	84.2	85.8	82.8	80.9	80.3	78.0
Uninsured	—	69.4	68.6	69.6	73.3	70.4	66.6	67.7	67.1	61.9
Health Insurance Status Prior to Interview[6]										
18–64 years, crude										
Insured continuously all 12 months	—	84.8	83.7	86.3	87.3	88.0	86.6	85.8	83.7	83.2
Uninsured for any period up to 12 months	—	81.8	83.4	81.7	83.5	83.7	81.8	81.3	78.9	78.3
Uninsured more than 12 months	—	65.1	63.6	64.0	68.8	65.1	60.2	62.0	62.1	55.2
Age and Education[7]										
25 years and over, crude										
No high school diploma or GED	57.1	61.9	60.9	65.0	66.1	69.9	64.9	64.1	60.6	56.7
High school diploma or GED	76.4	78.2	76.0	77.4	79.3	79.8	75.9	73.8	69.5	66.8
Some college or more	84.0	84.4	85.2	86.9	87.8	88.0	86.2	84.6	82.6	80.7
25–44 years										
No high school diploma or GED	75.1	73.6	73.6	76.8	79.0	79.6	71.7	75.5	76.2	69.1
High school diploma or GED	85.6	85.4	82.4	83.9	87.6	86.2	84.3	83.1	80.0	79.0
Some college or more	90.1	89.8	89.1	91.5	93.0	91.4	90.8	90.5	89.3	89.0
45–64 years										
No high school diploma or GED	58.0	65.6	66.1	69.2	71.6	75.7	71.4	69.7	70.4	63.4
High school diploma or GED	72.3	77.6	75.9	81.0	79.8	81.8	77.6	79.0	73.9	72.4
Some college or more	80.1	83.0	84.7	85.5	85.7	89.1	86.2	84.1	83.0	81.5
65 years and over										
No high school diploma or GED	44.0	50.7	47.7	52.4	51.8	56.6	52.5	46.0	36.7	37.7
High school diploma or GED	55.4	61.6	61.2	60.7	63.7	66.9	61.2	52.5	49.3	42.6
Some college or more	59.4	62.3	66.5	67.9	68.8	69.8	67.8	63.8	59.0	54.9
Disability Measure[8]										
18 years and over, crude										
Any basic actions difficulty or complex activity limitation	—	—	—	72.7	74.4	75.4	72.7	69.1	66.1	63.8
Any basic actions difficulty	—	—	—	72.4	74.3	75.1	72.6	69.1	66.2	63.6
Any complex activity limitation	—	—	—	67.9	69.3	71.0	67.6	62.2	60.1	58.5
No disability	—	—	—	82.5	83.8	84.1	82.5	82.6	80.4	78.9

— = Data not available.
* = Figure does not meet standards of reliability or precision.
Data not shown have an RSE of greater than 30%.
[1]Questions concerning use of Pap smears differed slightly on the National Health Interview Survey across the years for which data are shown.
[2]Includes all other races not shown separately, unknown poverty level in 1987, unknown health insurance status, unknown education level, and unknown disability status.
[3]Estimates are age-adjusted to the year 2000 standard population using five age groups: 18–44 years, 45–54 years, 55–64 years, 65–74 years, and 75 years and over.
[4]The race groups, White, Black, American Indian or Alaska Native, Asian, Native Hawaiian or Other Pacific Islander, and 2 or more races, include persons of Hispanic and non-Hispanic origin. Persons of Hispanic origin may be of any race.
[5]Percent of poverty level is based on family income and family size and composition.
[6]Health insurance categories are mutually exclusive.
[7]Education categories shown are for 1998 and subsequent years.
[8]Any basic actions difficulty or complex activity limitation is defined as having one or more of the following limitations or difficulties: movement difficulty, emotional difficulty, sensory (seeing or hearing) difficulty, cognitive difficulty, self-care (activities of daily living or instrumental activities of daily living) limitation, social limitation, or work limitation.

Table C-46. Use of Colorectal Tests or Procedures Among Adults 50–75 Years of Age, by Selected Characteristics, Selected Years, 2000–2010

(Percent.)

Characteristic	Any colorectal test or procedure[1,2]					Colonoscopy[2,3]				
	2000	2003	2005	2008	2010	2000	2003	2005	2008	2010
All Adults 50–75 Years[4]	33.9	39.1	44.3	51.6	58.7	19.1	29.2	37.6	46.7	54.9
Sex										
Male	33.1	40.1	44.4	51.4	58.5	19.5	30.2	37.9	46.9	54.7
Female	34.5	38.1	44.2	51.9	58.8	18.8	28.4	37.4	46.6	55.1
Race[5]										
White only	34.9	39.8	45.6	52.8	59.8	19.7	30.0	38.9	47.8	56.0
Black or African American only	29.6	35.2	38.1	46.9	55.2	17.4	24.8	32.2	43.1	51.8
American Indian or Alaska Native only	*35.2	*37.9	*33.9	28.5	48.9	*	*	*	*26.7	46.7
Asian only	20.4	26.7	30.8	47.1	47.1	*8.6	20.0	24.4	39.3	43.6
Native Hawaiian or Other Pacific Islander only	*	*	*	*	*	*	*	*	*	*
2 or more races	37.5	40.7	33.8	38.4	51.9	*25.1	29.7	29.6	37.4	48.4
Hispanic Origin and Race[5]										
Hispanic or Latino	21.7	27.2	28.5	34.0	46.5	13.3	19.8	23.1	29.3	43.9
Mexican	19.3	22.4	24.6	27.5	44.6	11.2	14.2	18.2	21.2	41.3
Not Hispanic or Latino	34.7	40.0	45.6	53.3	59.9	19.5	30.0	38.9	48.4	56.0
White only	35.7	41.0	47.4	54.8	61.3	20.0	30.9	40.5	49.8	57.3
Black or African American only	29.7	35.3	38.0	47.4	55.3	17.5	25.0	32.0	43.5	52.0
Percent of Poverty Level[6]										
Below 100%	26.5	29.7	28.7	33.9	37.9	16.3	22.0	23.6	28.5	34.8
100%–199%	29.4	31.9	38.4	42.7	47.9	17.7	23.3	31.5	38.0	43.3
200%–399%	33.7	38.8	43.6	49.9	58.0	18.6	29.4	37.0	44.3	54.6
400% or more	37.1	43.8	49.6	58.9	67.3	20.5	32.7	42.8	54.5	63.6
Hispanic Origin and Race and Percent of Poverty Level[5,6]										
Hispanic or Latino										
Below 100%	15.3	21.4	19.3	21.1	33.7	*9.3	15.2	13.1	17.9	32.1
100%–199%	16.8	20.5	24.6	27.7	39.6	8.6	16.0	19.4	24.4	36.3
200%–399%	23.6	29.0	28.3	39.3	47.5	*13.7	20.7	21.6	33.8	46.0
400% or more	31.1	37.9	42.1	43.9	63.3	22.4	27.1	39.3	37.6	59.5
Not Hispanic or Latino										
White only										
Below 100%	29.6	33.9	30.6	39.8	40.4	19.3	26.8	26.8	33.2	36.4
100%–199%	32.1	34.7	42.4	46.0	50.0	19.7	25.7	35.0	40.7	44.5
200%–399%	35.2	40.3	47.3	51.6	59.7	19.3	31.0	40.2	45.8	56.3
400% or more	37.9	44.3	50.6	60.5	68.0	20.7	32.9	43.8	56.3	64.3
Black or African American only										
Below 100%	27.5	27.4	29.0	35.1	39.2	14.5	17.6	23.5	30.1	36.4
100%–199%	28.7	30.0	36.2	46.7	49.0	17.2	20.0	30.3	43.2	46.5
200%–399%	27.7	36.8	35.8	48.5	60.5	16.5	25.6	31.8	44.7	56.2
400% or more	33.9	43.5	48.9	54.3	68.1	20.7	33.3	40.2	50.6	64.6
Education										
No high school diploma or GED	25.9	28.9	34.5	36.2	44.6	14.9	21.2	29.0	31.8	41.5
High school diploma or GED	33.1	38.3	42.1	48.5	53.7	19.0	29.3	35.7	44.6	50.8
Some college or more	37.8	43.3	48.7	57.5	64.7	20.9	32.1	41.6	52.1	60.4

Table C-46. Use of Colorectal Tests or Procedures Among Adults 50–75 Years of Age, by Selected Characteristics, Selected Years, 2000–2010—*Continued*

(Percent.)

Characteristic	Any colorectal test or procedure[1,2]					Colonoscopy[2,3]				
	2000	2003	2005	2008	2010	2000	2003	2005	2008	2010
Disability Measure[7]										
Any basic actions difficulty or complex activity limitation	37.8	42.0	47.7	54.2	59.5	22.1	31.9	40.1	48.5	55.5
Any basic actions difficulty	38.1	41.9	47.9	54.6	59.7	22.5	31.9	40.6	48.9	55.8
Any complex activity limitation	37.4	41.5	48.1	52.4	59.4	22.6	31.3	39.7	46.7	55.1
No disability	30.9	36.9	41.6	50.0	58.5	16.6	27.1	35.6	45.8	54.9
Geographic Region										
Northeast	34.4	43.5	50.9	54.7	64.3	19.1	33.1	44.8	51.0	61.7
Midwest	35.2	40.4	43.5	52.5	58.4	19.8	30.6	36.6	47.8	55.2
South	32.5	36.7	43.9	51.6	57.4	20.0	28.5	38.1	47.4	54.4
West	34.1	37.0	39.6	48.2	56.3	16.3	24.3	31.3	41.1	49.7
Location of Residence										
Within MSA[8]	34.1	40.3	44.7	52.4	59.6	19.0	29.9	37.9	47.6	55.8
Outside MSA[8]	33.2	34.8	42.7	48.5	54.4	19.6	26.8	36.7	43.3	50.9

* = Figure does not meet standards of reliability or precision.

[1] Includes reports of home fecal occult blood test (FOBT) in the past year, sigmoidoscopy procedure in the past 5 years with FOBT in the past 3 years, or colonoscopy in the past 10 years. Colorectal procedures are performed for diagnostic and screening purposes.
[2] Questions differed slightly on the National Health Interview Survey across the years for which data are shown.
[3] Includes any colonoscopy in the past 10 years, alone or in addition to another type of colorectal test or procedure.
[4] Includes all other races not shown separately, unknown disability status, and unknown education level.
[5] The race groups White, Black, American Indian or Alaska Native, Asian, Native Hawaiian or Other Pacific Islander, and 2 or more races include persons of Hispanic and non–Hispanic origin. Persons of Hispanic origin may be of any race.
[6] Based on family income and family size and composition.
[7] Any basic actions difficulty or complex activity limitation is defined as having one or more of the following limitations or difficulties: movement difficulty, emotional difficulty, sensory (seeing or hearing) difficulty, cognitive difficulty, self–care (activities of daily living or instrumental activities of daily living) limitation, social limitation, or work limitation.
[8] MSA = metropolitan statistical area.

Table C-47. Emergency Department Visits Within the Past 12 Months Among Children Under 18 Years of Age, by Selected Characteristics, Selected Years, 1997–2010

(Percent.)

Characteristic	Under 18 years				Under 6 years				6–17 years			
	1997	2000	2005	2010	1997	2000	2005	2010	1997	2000	2005	2010
PERCENT OF CHILDREN WITH ONE OR MORE EMERGENCY DEPARTMENT VISITS												
All children[1]	19.9	20.3	20.5	22.1	24.3	25.7	26.8	27.8	17.7	17.6	17.4	19.1
Sex												
Male	21.5	21.5	21.7	23.3	25.2	27.7	27.6	29.3	19.6	18.6	18.8	20.1
Female	18.3	19.0	19.2	20.9	23.3	23.7	25.9	26.3	15.7	16.6	15.9	18.2
Race												
White only	19.4	19.9	19.8	21.2	22.6	24.8	25.3	26.6	17.8	17.6	17.1	18.4
Black or African American only	24.0	22.7	23.8	27.6	33.1	30.8	31.6	34.0	19.4	19.0	20.0	24.2
American Indian or Alaska Native only	*24.1	38.0	*32.1	20.9	*24.3	*	67.1	*35.4	*24.0	*39.0	*	*
Asian only	12.6	12.3	14.6	15.0	20.8	*16.7	20.2	18.4	8.6	9.8	12.3	13.3
Native Hawaiian or Other Pacific Islander only	—	*	*	*	—	*	*	*	—	*	*	*
2 or more races	—	24.2	24.8	27.2	—	31.7	38.3	34.9	—	18.3	17.1	21.6
Hispanic Origin and Race[2]												
Hispanic or Latino	21.1	18.6	19.5	23.6	25.7	23.9	28.0	30.2	18.1	15.6	14.5	19.4
Not Hispanic or Latino	19.7	20.6	20.7	21.7	24.0	26.2	26.5	27.0	17.6	18.0	18.0	19.0
White only	19.2	20.2	19.9	20.4	22.2	25.1	24.5	25.1	17.7	17.9	17.9	18.2
Black or African American only	23.6	22.7	23.8	27.2	32.7	30.9	31.8	34.4	19.2	19.0	20.0	23.3
Percent of Poverty Level[3]												
Below 100%	25.1	25.0	27.3	30.6	29.5	30.7	33.5	35.4	22.2	21.7	23.5	27.6
100%–199%	22.0	22.4	21.8	25.7	28.0	27.4	30.8	31.6	19.0	19.9	17.4	22.3
200%–399%	18.0	19.0	18.9	18.4	21.4	25.7	25.9	22.7	16.4	15.9	15.7	16.4
400% or more	16.3	17.0	16.8	15.9	19.1	20.3	19.1	21.7	15.1	15.6	15.8	13.3
Hispanic Origin and Race and Percent of Poverty Level[2,3]												
Hispanic or Latino												
Percent of poverty level												
Below 100%	21.9	19.9	21.8	27.0	25.0	25.7	28.4	32.0	19.6	16.4	17.4	23.4
100%–199%	20.8	18.2	17.8	23.3	28.8	20.8	26.1	31.6	15.6	16.6	13.1	18.0
200%–399%	21.4	17.9	20.2	19.5	24.6	26.1	31.7	25.2	19.6	13.3	14.3	16.1
400% or more	17.7	17.6	15.3	21.4	*20.2	*22.9	23.3	28.6	16.4	15.4	*11.5	18.0
Not Hispanic or Latino												
White only												
Percent of poverty level												
Below 100%	25.5	26.5	34.1	33.7	27.2	35.6	37.3	37.4	24.4	21.2	32.2	31.6
100%–199%	22.3	24.7	22.8	26.3	25.8	29.2	30.7	29.2	20.7	22.7	19.1	24.7
200%–399%	17.8	19.5	17.9	17.6	20.9	26.0	22.9	21.2	16.3	16.6	15.7	15.9
400% or more	16.5	16.9	16.8	15.5	19.0	18.5	18.7	21.0	15.4	16.2	16.0	13.2
Black or African American only												
Percent of poverty level												
Below 100%	29.3	27.8	27.1	32.4	39.5	28.9	34.8	41.6	23.0	27.3	22.6	26.6
100%–199%	22.5	20.8	24.1	27.5	31.7	35.3	33.3	34.5	18.5	13.8	20.3	23.7
200%–399%	18.5	19.6	22.6	22.3	23.9	28.3	33.3	24.6	16.3	16.2	17.8	21.4
400% or more	16.1	19.3	16.9	18.9	*18.8	32.8	*	*24.1	15.2	*13.9	17.4	16.1
Health Insurance Status at the Time of Interview[4]												
Insured	19.8	20.7	20.7	22.3	24.4	25.8	26.8	28.1	17.5	18.2	17.7	19.2
Private	17.5	18.4	17.4	17.1	20.9	22.8	21.7	21.8	15.9	16.5	15.5	14.9
Medicaid	28.2	28.6	28.5	30.0	33.0	33.2	35.5	35.5	24.1	25.5	23.6	26.4
Uninsured	20.2	17.2	18.4	19.4	23.0	24.5	26.6	24.0	18.9	13.9	15.4	17.6
Health Insurance Status Prior to Interview[4]												
Insured continuously all 12 months	19.6	20.2	20.5	22.2	24.1	25.3	26.7	28.1	17.3	17.8	17.3	19.1
Uninsured for any period up to 12 months	24.0	25.9	26.0	23.7	27.1	33.9	34.4	28.0	21.9	21.7	22.4	21.3
Uninsured more than 12 months	18.4	14.7	14.4	17.6	19.3	19.1	*15.7	*21.3	18.1	13.1	14.0	16.7
Geographic Region												
Northeast	18.5	19.7	20.9	22.3	20.7	21.6	26.3	27.8	17.4	18.8	18.5	19.6
Midwest	19.5	20.3	21.8	23.3	26.0	25.6	30.1	28.8	16.4	17.8	17.8	20.7
South	21.8	21.9	21.7	23.4	25.6	28.6	27.1	30.4	19.9	18.7	18.8	19.5
West	18.5	18.0	16.7	19.1	23.5	24.7	22.9	23.3	15.9	14.7	13.8	16.8
Location of Residence												
Within MSA[5]	19.7	19.9	20.0	21.8	23.9	24.5	25.7	27.7	17.4	17.6	17.2	18.6
Outside MSA[5]	20.8	21.9	22.4	24.2	26.2	31.3	31.8	28.6	18.6	17.8	18.2	22.1

Table C-47. Emergency Department Visits Within the Past 12 Months Among Children Under 18 Years of Age, by Selected Characteristics, Selected Years, 1997–2010—Continued

(Percent.)

Characteristic	Under 18 years				Under 6 years				6–17 years			
	1997	2000	2005	2010	1997	2000	2005	2010	1997	2000	2005	2010
PERCENT OF CHILDREN WITH TWO OR MORE EMERGENCY DEPARTMENT VISITS												
All children[1]	7.1	7.0	6.8	8.4	9.6	10.0	9.8	10.8	5.8	5.6	5.4	7.2
Sex												
Male	7.3	7.3	7.2	8.5	9.9	10.3	10.7	11.3	6.0	5.8	5.4	7.0
Female	6.9	6.7	6.5	8.3	9.4	9.6	8.9	10.3	5.7	5.3	5.3	7.3
Race[2]												
White only	6.6	6.4	6.3	7.6	8.4	8.7	9.1	10.1	5.7	5.4	4.9	6.3
Black or African American only	9.6	10.5	9.2	12.6	14.9	16.2	12.7	15.7	6.9	7.9	7.5	11.0
American Indian and Alaska Native only	*	*	*	*	*	*	*	*	*	*	*	*
Asian only	*5.7	*3.1	*4.6	7.3	*12.9	*	*	*	*	*	*3.9	*7.1
Native Hawaiian and Other Pacific Islander only	—	*	*	*	—	*	*	*	—	*	*	*
2 or more races	—	*8.7	*8.6	10.3	—	*14.3	*13.2	*11.7	—	*	*	*9.2
Hispanic Origin and Race[2]												
Hispanic or Latino	8.9	7.0	7.7	8.6	11.8	9.4	12.1	11.7	7.0	5.6	5.2	6.6
Not Hispanic or Latino	6.8	7.0	6.6	8.4	9.2	10.1	9.2	10.5	5.7	5.6	5.4	7.3
White only	6.2	6.3	5.9	7.4	7.8	8.6	8.2	9.3	5.5	5.2	4.9	6.4
Black or African American only	9.3	10.6	9.1	12.3	14.6	16.6	12.4	15.8	6.8	7.9	7.5	10.4
Percent of Poverty Level[3]												
Below 100%	11.1	11.9	11.2	13.4	14.5	16.4	15.9	15.3	8.9	9.4	8.4	12.1
100%–199%	8.3	8.0	7.9	10.3	12.2	11.8	12.7	13.4	6.3	6.1	5.5	8.4
200%–399%	6.2	5.6	5.7	6.3	7.4	8.0	7.6	7.3	5.6	4.5	4.8	5.9
400% or more	4.0	4.7	4.4	5.0	5.0	5.8	5.1	7.3	3.6	4.2	4.0	3.9
Hispanic Origin and Race and Percent of Poverty Level[2,3]												
Hispanic or Latino												
Percent of poverty level												
Below 100%	10.4	8.2	10.0	9.9	13.9	10.9	13.8	10.9	8.0	6.6	7.4	9.2
100%–199%	8.2	7.4	6.1	9.4	12.0	8.5	*8.7	15.4	5.7	6.7	*4.7	5.5
200%–399%	8.5	6.2	7.7	5.9	10.0	9.2	14.2	*8.0	*7.6	*4.5	*4.4	*4.6
400% or more	*5.0	*4.0	*5.4	*6.5	*	*	*	*	*	*	*	*5.2
Not Hispanic or Latino												
White only												
Percent of poverty level												
Below 100%	10.7	12.8	13.5	14.0	12.2	18.4	18.6	15.5	9.8	*9.5	10.4	13.1
100%–199%	8.0	8.0	8.2	10.4	11.2	11.8	13.7	12.3	6.4	6.3	*5.5	9.4
200%–399%	6.0	5.4	5.1	5.7	6.7	7.7	6.1	*6.5	5.6	4.4	4.6	5.4
400% or more	3.7	4.5	3.7	5.0	4.6	4.5	4.1	7.6	3.3	4.5	3.5	3.9
Black or African American only												
Percent of poverty level												
Below 100%	12.7	14.7	11.4	16.1	19.1	18.5	16.2	22.1	8.8	12.8	8.6	12.4
100%–199%	9.2	8.9	8.4	12.4	*13.5	17.5	*13.3	*14.6	*7.2	*4.8	*6.5	11.1
200%–399%	5.8	7.8	*7.6	9.9	*8.9	*12.5	*	*10.2	*4.5	*6.0	*7.5	*9.8
400% or more	*	*8.9	*7.2	*3.7	*	*17.8	*	*	*	*	*	*
Health Insurance Status at the Time of Interview[4]												
Insured	7.0	7.0	6.8	8.5	9.6	9.6	9.7	11.0	5.7	5.7	5.3	7.1
Private	5.2	5.2	5.0	5.5	6.8	7.1	6.2	7.4	4.5	4.5	4.4	4.6
Medicaid	13.1	13.1	11.1	12.8	16.2	15.9	15.8	15.3	10.4	11.2	7.7	11.2
Uninsured	7.7	6.6	7.0	8.0	9.8	11.3	11.5	*8.5	6.8	4.5	5.4	7.8

Table C-47. Emergency Department Visits Within the Past 12 Months Among Children Under 18 Years of Age, by Selected Characteristics, Selected Years, 1997–2010—Continued

(Percent.)

Characteristic	Under 18 years				Under 6 years				6–17 years			
	1997	2000	2005	2010	1997	2000	2005	2010	1997	2000	2005	2010
Health Insurance Status Prior to Interview[4]												
Insured continuously all 12 months	6.9	6.7	6.7	8.4	9.4	9.2	9.7	10.8	5.7	5.5	5.2	7.1
Uninsured for any period up to 12 months	8.5	10.6	8.9	10.1	11.5	16.0	13.6	13.3	6.6	7.7	6.9	8.4
Uninsured more than 12 months	6.8	5.8	5.5	7.8	*8.6	8.9	*	*	6.2	4.7	5.3	*7.9
Geographic Region												
Northeast	6.2	6.4	6.2	7.8	7.6	7.9	8.9	10.3	5.4	5.6	5.0	6.6
Midwest	6.6	6.6	6.9	9.1	10.4	9.0	9.6	11.4	4.8	5.5	5.5	8.0
South	8.0	8.5	7.9	9.1	10.1	12.6	10.8	12.9	6.9	6.6	6.3	7.1
West	7.1	5.4	5.5	7.2	10.0	8.5	9.1	7.6	5.6	3.9	3.9	7.0
Location of Residence												
Within MSA[5]	7.2	6.6	6.7	8.3	9.6	8.9	9.5	10.6	5.9	5.5	5.2	7.0
Outside MSA[5]	6.8	8.6	7.5	9.3	9.7	15.0	11.2	12.2	5.6	5.8	5.9	7.9

* = Figure does not meet standards of reliability or precision.
— = Data not available.
[1]Includes all other races not shown separately and unknown health insurance status.
[2]The race groups, White, Black, American Indian or Alaska Native, Asian, Native Hawaiian or Other Pacific Islander, and 2 or more races, include persons of Hispanic and non-Hispanic origin. Persons of Hispanic origin may be of any race.
[3]Percent of poverty level is based on family income and family size and composition using U.S. Census Bureau poverty thresholds.
[4]Health insurance categories are mutually exclusive. Persons who reported both Medicaid and private coverage are classified as having private coverage.
[5]MSA = metropolitan statistical area.

Table C-48. Emergency Department Visits[1] Within the Past 12 Months Among Adults 18 Years of Age and Over, by Selected Characteristics, Selected Years, 1997–2010

(Percent.)

Characteristic	One or more emergency department visits				Two or more emergency department visits			
	1997	2000	2005	2010	1997	2000	2005	2010
18 years and over, age-adjusted[2,3]	19.6	20.2	20.5	21.4	6.7	6.9	7.1	7.8
18 years and over, crude[2]	19.6	20.1	20.4	21.3	6.7	6.8	7.0	7.7
Age								
18–44 years	20.7	20.5	20.8	22.0	6.8	7.0	7.1	8.4
18–24 years	26.3	25.7	25.3	25.4	9.1	8.8	8.9	9.6
25–44 years	19.0	18.8	19.2	20.7	6.2	6.4	6.5	8.0
45–64 years	16.2	17.6	18.2	19.2	5.6	5.6	6.4	6.7
45–54 years	15.7	17.9	17.6	18.6	5.5	5.8	6.1	6.6
55–64 years	16.9	17.0	19.0	19.8	5.7	5.3	6.8	6.8
65 years and over	22.0	23.7	23.7	23.7	8.1	8.6	8.2	7.7
65–74 years	20.3	21.6	20.8	20.7	7.1	7.4	7.4	6.4
75 years and over	24.3	26.2	27.1	27.4	9.3	10.0	9.1	9.4
Sex[3]								
Male	19.1	18.7	18.6	18.5	5.9	5.7	5.9	6.0
Female	20.2	21.6	22.3	24.3	7.5	7.9	8.2	9.6
Race[3,4]								
White only	19.0	19.4	19.8	20.7	6.2	6.4	6.5	7.2
Black or African American only	25.9	26.5	26.3	28.6	11.1	10.8	11.9	12.6
American Indian or Alaska Native only	24.8	30.3	31.0	22.6	13.1	*12.6	*11.1	*11.8
Asian only	11.6	13.6	15.4	13.3	*2.9	*3.8	*3.8	3.3
Native Hawaiian or Other Pacific Islander only	—	*	*	*	—	*	*	*
2 or more races	—	32.5	25.7	29.7	—	11.3	12.8	11.1
American Indian or Alaska Native; White	—	33.9	29.3	31.1	—	*9.4	*15.3	*15.2
Hispanic Origin and Race[3,4]								
Hispanic or Latino	19.2	18.3	20.1	19.8	7.4	7.0	7.1	6.9
Mexican	17.8	17.4	17.2	18.1	6.4	7.1	5.8	6.1
Not Hispanic or Latino	19.7	20.6	20.7	21.9	6.7	6.9	7.1	8.1
White only	19.1	19.8	20.1	21.1	6.2	6.4	6.4	7.4
Black or African American only	25.9	26.5	26.2	29.0	11.0	10.8	11.9	12.7
Percent of Poverty Level[3,5]								
Below 100%	28.1	29.0	29.8	30.6	12.8	13.3	13.7	14.9
100%–199%	23.8	23.9	23.2	25.6	9.3	9.6	9.6	10.5
200%–399%	18.3	19.8	20.2	20.4	5.9	6.3	6.5	6.8
400% or more	15.9	16.8	16.9	17.0	3.9	4.5	4.5	4.7
Hispanic Origin and Race and Percent of Poverty Level[3,4,5]								
Hispanic or Latino								
Below 100%	22.1	22.4	24.0	23.6	9.8	9.7	9.2	11.5
100%–199%	19.2	18.1	18.7	19.9	8.1	6.7	7.1	6.3
200%–399%	18.5	17.3	18.9	18.1	6.0	7.4	5.9	5.2
400% or more	14.6	16.4	20.9	18.8	*3.8	*4.3	*6.9	*5.5
Not Hispanic or Latino								
White only								
Below 100%	29.5	30.1	30.8	33.3	13.0	13.9	13.7	15.5
100%–199%	24.3	25.5	24.3	26.8	9.1	10.4	9.8	11.2
200%–399%	18.1	20.1	20.7	20.3	5.8	6.3	6.4	6.5
400% or more	15.8	16.3	16.2	16.9	3.8	4.1	4.0	4.9
Black or African American only								
Below 100%	34.6	35.4	35.4	36.9	17.5	17.4	18.3	20.2
100%–199%	29.2	28.5	28.9	33.5	12.8	12.2	14.2	15.9
200%–399%	20.8	23.2	21.5	25.7	8.1	8.0	8.7	10.2
400% or more	18.2	22.6	22.6	18.8	5.9	8.8	*9.2	*4.0
Health Insurance Status at the Time of Interview[6,7]								
18–64 years								
Insured	18.8	19.5	20.0	20.8	6.1	6.4	6.6	7.5
Private	16.9	17.6	17.3	17.4	4.7	5.1	4.8	5.2
Medicaid	37.6	42.2	40.1	40.2	19.7	21.0	20.1	21.1
Uninsured	20.0	19.3	19.5	21.3	7.5	6.9	8.0	8.9

Table C-48. Emergency Department Visits[1] Within the Past 12 Months Among Adults 18 Years of Age and Over, by Selected Characteristics, Selected Years 1997–2010—Continued

(Percent.)

Characteristic	One or more emergency department visits				Two or more emergency department visits			
	1997	2000	2005	2010	1997	2000	2005	2010
Health Insurance Status Prior to Interview[6,7]								
18–64 years								
Insured continuously all 12 months	18.3	19.0	19.4	20.2	5.8	6.1	6.3	7.1
Uninsured for any period up to 12 months	25.5	28.2	28.0	26.0	9.4	10.3	12.4	12.5
Uninsured more than 12 months	18.9	17.3	18.0	20.6	7.1	6.4	7.0	8.1
Percent of Poverty Level and Health Insurance Status Prior to Interview[5,6,7]								
18–64 years								
Below 100%								
Insured continuously all 12 months	30.2	31.6	33.6	35.2	14.7	15.4	15.3	18.3
Uninsured for any period up to 12 months	34.1	43.7	39.1	34.2	16.1	18.1	21.5	16.5
Uninsured more than 12 months	20.8	20.5	20.5	23.4	8.1	9.1	8.5	11.7
100%–199%								
Insured continuously all 12 months	24.5	25.5	23.7	26.1	8.9	10.2	9.8	10.8
Uninsured for any period up to 12 months	28.7	27.7	28.4	29.7	12.3	11.7	12.7	15.6
Uninsured more than 12 months	19.0	17.4	18.5	21.2	8.3	6.4	7.7	7.8
200%–399%								
Insured continuously all 12 months	17.5	19.5	19.7	19.6	5.3	6.3	6.4	6.0
Uninsured for any period up to 12 months	21.6	24.6	26.8	25.4	6.6	7.3	10.6	12.2
Uninsured more than 12 months	16.8	15.6	14.7	17.6	5.9	4.5	4.5	5.7
400% or more								
Insured continuously all 12 months	14.9	15.5	15.6	15.9	3.7	3.7	3.6	4.5
Uninsured for any period up to 12 months	18.0	20.1	20.2	12.5	*3.1	6.4	7.2	*
Uninsured more than 12 months	19.1	15.8	17.9	19.4	*	*5.2	*7.4	*
Disability Measure[3,8]								
Any basic actions difficulty or complex activity limitation	30.8	32.0	34.4	34.9	13.5	14.6	15.6	16.8
Any basic actions difficulty	30.5	32.4	34.9	35.0	13.5	14.9	15.8	17.2
Any complex activity limitation	39.7	41.5	42.3	43.8	19.9	21.2	22.4	24.5
No disability	14.5	15.3	14.9	16.1	3.7	3.9	3.9	4.4
Geographic Region[3]								
Northeast	19.5	20.0	21.6	22.6	6.9	6.2	7.2	8.4
Midwest	19.3	20.1	21.6	22.3	6.2	6.9	7.2	8.2
South	20.9	21.2	20.7	22.1	7.3	7.6	7.6	8.0
West	17.7	18.6	17.8	18.9	6.0	6.3	6.0	6.7
Location of Residence[3]								
Within MSA[9]	19.1	19.6	20.1	20.8	6.4	6.6	6.8	7.5
Outside MSA[9]	21.5	22.5	22.3	25.5	7.8	7.8	8.1	9.8

* = Figure does not meet standards of reliability or precision.
— = Data not available.
[1] Starting with the 1997 National Health Interview survey, respondents were asked about the number of visits to hospital emergency rooms.
[2] Includes all other races not shown separately, unknown health insurance status, and unknown disability status.
[3] Estimates are for persons 18 years of age and over and are age-adjusted to the year 2000 standard population using five age groups: 18–44 years, 45–54 years, 55–64 years, 65–74 years, and 75 years and over.
[4] The race groups, White, Black, American Indian or Alaska Native, Asian, Native Hawaiian or Other Pacific Islander, and 2 or more races, include persons of Hispanic and non-Hispanic origin. Persons of Hispanic origin may be of any race.
[5] Percent of poverty level is based on family income and family size and composition using U.S. Census Bureau poverty thresholds.
[6] Estimates for persons 18–64 years of age are age-adjusted to the year 2000 standard population using three age groups: 18–44 years, 45–54 years, and 55–64 years.
[7] Health insurance categories are mutually exclusive. Persons who reported both Medicaid and private coverage are classified as having private coverage.
[8] Any basic actions difficulty or complex activity limitation is defined as having one or more of the following limitations or difficulties: movement difficulty, emotional difficulty, sensory (seeing or hearing) difficulty, cognitive difficulty, self-care (activities of daily living or instrumental activities of daily living) limitation, social limitation, or work limitation.
[9] MSA = metropolitan statistical area.

Table C-49. Initial Injury-Related Visits to Hospital Emergency Departments, by Sex, Age, and Intent and Mechanism of Injury, Selected Annual Averages, 2005–2006 and 2008–2009

(Number.)

Sex, age, and intent and mechanism of injury[1]	Initial injury-related visits in thousands			Initial injury-related visits per 10,000 persons		
	2005–2006	2007–2008	2008–2009	2005–2006	2007–2008[2]	2008–2009
Both Sexes						
All ages, age–adjusted[2,3]	31,706	28,699	31,328	1,076.4	960.9	1,040.8
All ages, crude[2]	31,706	28,699	31,328	1,068.6	951.3	1,029.4
Unintentional injuries[4]	25,658	23,670	25,725	864.7	784.6	845.3
Falls	8,100	8,144	8,900	273.0	270.0	292.4
Struck by or against objects or persons	2,935	2,746	2,916	98.9	91.0	95.8
Motor vehicle traffic	3,714	3,387	3,508	125.2	112.3	115.3
Cut or pierce	2,145	1,944	2,008	72.3	64.4	66.0
Intentional injuries	1,977	1,888	2,313	66.6	62.6	76.0
Male						
All ages, age–adjusted[2,3]	16,966	15,332	16,640	1,166.1	1,039.7	1,118.0
All ages, crude[2]	16,966	15,332	16,640	1,164.2	1,033.8	1,111.8
Unintentional injuries[4]	13,736	12,611	13,590	942.5	850.3	908.0
Falls	3,685	3,581	3,944	252.9	241.4	263.5
Struck by or against objects or persons	1,833	1,771	1,863	125.8	119.4	124.4
Motor vehicle traffic	1,733	1,693	1,734	118.9	114.2	115.8
Cut or pierce	1,392	1,270	1,263	95.5	85.7	84.4
Intentional injuries	1,135	1,020	1,266	77.8	68.8	84.6
Under 18 years[2]	5,072	4,602	5,132	1,346.6	1,216.8	1,351.1
Unintentional injuries[4]	4,391	3,995	4,509	1,165.8	1,056.3	1,187.1
Falls	1,362	1,305	1,512	361.5	345.0	398.1
Struck by or against objects or persons	816	850	909	216.6	224.6	239.2
Motor vehicle traffic	357	265	305	94.8	70.0	80.3
Cut or pierce	291	264	284	77.3	69.8	74.8
Intentional injuries	190	198	194	50.4	52.2	51.1
18–24 years[2]	2,552	2,305	2,562	1,729.5	1,547.4	1,695.5
Unintentional injuries[4]	1,985	1,788	1,947	1,345.4	1,200.6	1,288.6
Falls	318	309	366	215.2	207.7	242.4
Struck by or against objects or persons	290	280	283	196.9	188.0	187.4
Motor vehicle traffic	386	366	373	261.6	245.8	247.0
Cut or pierce	265	190	215	179.5	127.8	142.6
Intentional injuries	273	308	381	185.2	206.9	252.2
25–44 years[2]	5,199	4,471	4,611	1,243.6	1,072.7	1,109.5
Unintentional injuries[4]	4,001	3,531	3,540	957.1	847.0	851.8
Falls	763	677	703	182.4	162.5	169.2
Struck by or against objects or persons	472	384	401	112.9	92.1	96.4
Motor vehicle traffic	629	638	578	150.5	153.0	139.1
Cut or pierce	480	426	401	114.8	102.2	96.5
Intentional injuries	436	350	495	104.4	83.9	119.2
45–64 years[2]	2,842	2,707	2,996	790.0	718.3	780.7
Unintentional injuries[4]	2,275	2,223	2,437	632.5	590.0	635.1
Falls	599	651	669	166.6	172.8	174.2
Struck by or against objects or persons	208	205	216	57.9	54.3	56.4
Motor vehicle traffic	262	331	375	72.9	87.9	97.7
Cut or pierce	285	309	306	79.2	81.9	79.7
Intentional injuries	205	145	168	57.1	38.4	43.9
65 years and over[2]	1,301	1,247	1,340	837.5	768.6	805.1
Unintentional injuries[4]	1,082	1,073	1,157	696.8	661.7	695.2
Falls	644	638	694	414.5	393.2	416.7
Struck by or against objects or persons	46	*52	*54	29.8	*32.3	*32.2
Motor vehicle traffic	98	93	103	63.4	57.4	61.7
Cut or pierce	70	81	*57	45.3	50.0	*34.0
Intentional injuries	*	*	*	*	*	*
Female						
All ages, age–adjusted[2,3]	14,740	13,367	14,688	980.5	874.2	955.6
All ages, crude[2]	14,740	13,367	14,688	976.3	871.6	949.7
Unintentional injuries[4]	11,922	11,060	12,134	789.7	721.1	784.6
Falls	4,415	4,564	4,956	292.4	297.6	320.4
Struck by or against objects or persons	1,102	976	1,053	73.0	63.6	68.1
Motor vehicle traffic	1,981	1,695	1,774	131.2	110.5	114.7
Cut or pierce	753	673	745	49.9	43.9	48.2
Intentional injuries	843	867	1,048	55.8	56.5	67.7

Table C-49. Initial Injury-Related Visits to Hospital Emergency Departments, by Sex, Age, and Intent and Mechanism of Injury, Selected Annual Averages, 2005–2006 and 2008–2009—*Continued*

(Number.)

Sex, age, and intent and mechanism of injury[1]	Initial injury-related visits in thousands			Initial injury-related visits per 10,000 persons		
	2005–2006	2007–2008	2008–2009	2005–2006	2007–2008[2]	2008–2009
Under 18 years[2]	3,625	3,062	3,508	1,008.7	848.2	967.5
Unintentional injuries[4]	3,058	2,690	3,008	851.1	745.3	829.5
Falls	1,039	1,014	1,096	289.1	280.9	302.3
Struck by or against objects or persons	419	391	439	116.7	108.3	121.1
Motor vehicle traffic	367	282	249	102.1	78.2	68.6
Cut or pierce	160	145	154	44.4	40.1	42.4
Intentional injuries	188	163	222	52.3	45.1	61.4
18–24 years[2]	1,882	1,698	1,736	1,329.3	1,186.5	1,194.5
Unintentional injuries[4]	1,431	1,318	1,325	1,010.5	921.0	911.7
Falls	290	301	307	205.0	210.5	210.9
Struck by or against objects or persons	146	106	110	103.4	74.0	75.4
Motor vehicle traffic	397	378	360	280.6	264.5	247.5
Cut or pierce	116	89	77	82.2	61.9	53.2
Intentional injuries	176	209	232	124.2	145.8	159.7
25–44 years[2]	4,173	3,733	4,087	1,004.2	905.4	996.6
Unintentional injuries[4]	3,266	2,865	3,179	785.8	694.7	775.1
Falls	873	900	1,004	210.1	218.2	244.7
Struck by or against objects or persons	309	216	198	74.3	52.4	48.3
Motor vehicle traffic	719	572	621	173.1	138.8	151.3
Cut or pierce	269	214	270	64.7	51.8	65.9
Intentional injuries	313	345	396	75.4	83.6	96.5
45–64 years[2]	2,904	2,681	3,061	767.8	677.5	760.0
Unintentional injuries[4]	2,278	2,209	2,539	602.2	558.3	630.4
Falls	865	886	1,012	228.7	223.9	251.2
Struck by or against objects or persons	160	171	216	42.2	43.2	53.5
Motor vehicle traffic	359	345	399	94.8	87.3	99.0
Cut or pierce	158	163	190	41.7	41.1	47.2
Intentional injuries	149	130	161	39.4	32.9	39.9
65 years and over[2]	2,155	2,193	2,294	1,002.9	989.9	1,016.3
Unintentional injuries[4]	1,889	1,978	2,083	879.1	892.5	922.8
Falls	1,347	1,463	1,538	626.9	660.1	681.2
Struck by or against objects or persons	69	91	91	31.9	41.2	40.4
Motor vehicle traffic	139	116	146	64.5	52.5	64.7
Cut or pierce	*50	*64	*54	*23.3	*28.8	*23.9
Intentional injuries	*	*	*	*	*	*

* = Figure does not meet standards of reliability or precision.
[1]Intent and mechanism of injury are based on the first-listed external cause of injury code (E code). Intentional injuries include suicide attempts and assaults.
[2]Includes all injury-related visits not shown separately in table, including those with undetermined intent (1% in 2008–2009) and insufficient or no information to code cause of injury (9% in 2008–2009).
[3]Rates are age-adjusted to the year 2000 standard population using six age groups: under 18 years, 18–24 years, 25–44 years, 45–64 years, 65–74 years, and 75 years and over.
[4]Includes unintentional injury-related visits with mechanism of injury not shown in table.

Table C-50. Visits to Physician Offices, Hospital Outpatient Departments, and Hospital Emergency Departments, by Age, Sex, and Race, Selected Years, 1995–2009

(Number.)

Age, sex, and race	All places[1]			Physician offices			Hospital outpatient departments			Hospital emergency departments		
	1995	2000	2009	1995	2000	2009	1995	2000	2009	1995	2000	2009
NUMBER OF VISITS IN THOUSANDS												
Age												
Total	860,859	1,014,848	1,270,001	697,082	823,542	1,037,796	67,232	83,289	96,132	96,545	108,017	136,072
Under 18 years	194,644	212,165	239,590	150,351	163,459	183,999	17,636	21,076	22,418	26,657	27,630	33,173
18–44 years	285,184	315,774	341,209	219,065	243,011	257,890	24,299	26,947	29,535	41,820	45,816	53,784
45–64 years	188,320	255,894	374,775	159,531	216,783	316,395	14,811	20,772	29,083	13,978	18,339	29,297
45–54 years	104,891	142,233	190,701	88,266	119,474	158,120	8,029	11,558	15,310	8,595	11,201	17,271
55–64 years	83,429	113,661	184,074	71,264	97,309	158,275	6,782	9,214	13,774	5,383	7,138	12,026
65 years and over	192,712	231,014	314,428	168,135	200,289	279,514	10,486	14,494	15,096	14,090	16,232	19,818
65–74 years	102,605	116,505	153,884	90,544	102,447	137,452	6,004	7,515	8,036	6,057	6,543	8,396
75 years and over	90,106	114,510	160,544	77,591	97,842	142,062	4,482	6,979	7,060	8,033	9,690	11,423
Total, age-adjusted[2]	334	374	414	271	304	337	26	31	31	37	40	46
Total, crude	329	370	421	266	300	344	26	30	32	37	39	45
Under 18 years	275	293	322	213	226	247	25	29	30	38	38	45
18–44 years	264	291	309	203	224	234	22	25	27	39	42	49
45–64 years	364	422	475	309	358	401	29	34	37	27	30	37
45–54 years	339	385	431	286	323	358	26	31	35	28	30	39
55–64 years	401	481	532	343	412	457	33	39	40	26	30	35
65 years and over	612	706	829	534	612	737	33	44	40	45	50	52
65–74 years	560	656	749	494	577	669	33	42	39	33	37	41
75 years and over	683	766	923	588	654	817	34	47	41	61	65	66
Sex and Age												
Male, age-adjusted[2]	290	325	358	232	261	290	21	26	25	37	38	42
Male, crude	277	314	356	220	251	289	21	25	26	36	38	42
Under 18 years	273	302	334	209	231	257	25	29	30	40	41	46
18–44 years	190	203	201	139	148	145	14	17	16	37	38	40
45–54 years	275	316	361	229	260	296	20	26	28	26	30	36
55–64 years	351	428	473	300	367	403	26	32	35	25	30	34
65–74 years	508	614	731	445	539	654	29	38	37	34	36	40
75 years and over	711	771	907	616	670	807	34	42	37	61	59	63
Female, age-adjusted[2]	377	420	469	309	345	383	31	35	37	37	41	49
Female, crude	378	424	483	310	348	397	31	35	38	37	41	48
Under 18 years	277	285	310	217	221	237	25	29	30	35	35	43
18–44 years	336	377	416	265	298	322	31	33	38	40	46	57
45–54 years	400	451	499	339	384	417	32	36	41	29	31	42
55–64 years	446	529	586	382	453	507	38	45	44	26	31	35
65–74 years	603	692	764	534	609	681	36	46	41	32	37	42
75 years and over	666	763	934	571	645	823	34	49	43	61	69	68
Race and Age[3]												
White, age-adjusted[2]	339	380	421	282	315	351	23	28	29	34	37	41
White, crude	338	381	434	281	316	365	23	28	29	34	37	41
Under 18 years	295	306	339	237	243	269	23	27	29	35	36	40
18–44 years	267	301	312	211	239	244	20	23	24	36	39	43
45–54 years	334	386	432	286	330	369	23	28	30	25	28	34
55–64 years	397	480	531	345	416	466	28	36	34	24	28	30
65–74 years	557	641	752	496	568	678	29	38	35	32	35	38
75 years and over	689	764	936	598	658	835	31	44	36	60	63	64
Black or African American, age-adjusted[2]	309	353	459	204	239	314	48	51	59	58	62	85
Black or African American, crude	281	324	438	178	214	296	45	48	58	58	62	84
Under 18 years	193	264	315	100	167	198	39	40	42	53	57	75
18–44 years	260	257	373	158	149	228	38	40	50	64	68	94
45–54 years	387	383	486	281	269	329	55	61	74	51	53	83
55–64 years	414	495	645	294	373	478	73	70	91	47	52	76
65–74 years	553	656	821	429	512	667	*77	85	*81	47	59	73
75 years and over	534	745	908	395	568	718	66	85	*	73	92	95

* = Figure does not meet standards of reliability or precision.
[1] All places includes visits to physician offices and hospital outpatient and emergency departments.
[2] Estimates are age-adjusted to the year 2000 standard population using six age groups: under 18 years, 18–44 years, 45–54 years, 55–64 years, 65–74 years, and 75 years and over.
[3] Estimates by racial group should be used with caution because information on race was collected from medical records.

Table C-51. Visits to Primary Care Generalist and Specialist Physicians, by Selected Characteristics and Type of Physician, Selected Years, 1980–2009

(Percent.)

Age, sex, and race	Type of primary care generalist physician[1]											
	All primary care generalists				General and family practice				Internal medicine			
	1980	1990	2000	2009	1980	1990	2000	2009	1980	1990	2000	2009
Age												
Total	66.2	63.6	58.9	55.9	33.5	29.9	24.1	23.1	12.1	13.8	15.3	14.8
Under 18 years	77.8	79.5	79.7	78.8	26.1	26.5	19.9	16.3	2.0	2.9	*	*
18–44 years	65.3	65.2	62.1	61.5	34.3	31.9	28.2	29.7	8.6	11.8	12.7	11.0
45–64 years	60.2	55.5	51.2	48.6	36.3	32.1	26.4	25.5	19.5	18.6	20.1	18.0
45–54 years	60.2	55.6	52.3	50.9	37.4	32.0	27.8	27.5	17.1	17.1	18.7	17.1
55–64 years	60.2	55.5	49.9	46.4	35.4	32.1	24.7	23.5	21.8	20.0	21.7	19.0
65 years and over	61.6	52.6	46.5	43.9	37.5	28.1	20.2	18.8	22.7	23.3	24.5	23.5
65–74 years	61.2	52.7	46.6	41.9	37.4	28.1	19.7	19.9	22.1	23.0	24.5	20.0
75 years and over	62.3	52.4	46.4	45.9	37.6	28.0	20.8	17.7	23.5	23.7	24.5	26.9
Sex and Age												
Male												
Under 18 years	77.3	78.1	77.7	77.6	25.6	24.1	18.3	15.2	2.0	3.0	*	*
18–44 years	50.8	51.8	51.5	52.4	38.0	35.9	34.2	36.6	11.5	15.0	14.4	14.1
45–64 years	55.6	50.6	49.4	45.2	34.4	31.0	28.7	26.4	20.5	19.2	19.8	18.7
65 years and over	58.2	51.2	43.1	38.6	35.6	27.7	19.3	18.3	22.3	23.3	23.8	20.1
Female												
Under 18 years	78.5	81.1	82.0	80.2	26.6	29.1	21.7	17.6	2.0	2.8	*	*
18–44 years	72.1	71.3	67.2	65.6	32.5	30.0	25.3	26.6	7.3	10.3	11.9	9.6
45–64 years	63.4	58.8	52.5	51.1	37.7	32.8	24.9	24.9	18.9	18.2	20.2	17.6
65 years and over	63.9	53.5	48.9	47.8	38.7	28.3	20.9	19.2	22.9	23.3	25.0	26.0
Race and Age[2]												
White												
Under 18 years	77.6	79.2	78.5	78.1	26.4	27.1	21.2	16.3	2.0	2.3	*	*
18–44 years	64.8	64.4	61.4	60.4	34.5	31.9	29.2	30.3	8.6	10.6	11.0	10.1
45–64 years	59.6	54.2	49.3	47.6	36.0	31.5	27.3	25.9	19.2	17.6	17.1	17.0
65 years and over	61.4	51.9	45.1	43.2	36.6	27.5	20.3	18.7	23.3	23.1	23.0	22.9
Black or African American												
Under 18 years	79.9	85.5	87.3	80.8	23.7	20.2	*	*15.5	*2.2	9.8	*	*
18–44 years	68.5	68.3	65.0	64.4	31.7	31.9	22.0	26.6	9.0	18.1	20.9	*15.2
45–64 years	66.1	61.6	61.7	50.0	38.6	31.2	23.3	23.4	22.6	26.9	35.9	*21.4
65 years and over	64.6	58.6	52.8	45.7	49.0	28.9	*18.5	*15.8	14.2	28.7	33.4	*28.6

Age, sex, and race	Type of primary care generalist physician[1]											
	Obstetrics and gynecology				Pediatrics				Specialty care physicians			
	1980	1990	2000	2009	1980	1990	2000	2009	1980	1990	2000	2009
Age												
Total	9.6	8.7	7.8	7.0	10.9	11.2	11.7	11.1	33.8	36.4	41.1	44.1
Under 18 years	1.3	1.2	*1.1	0.8	48.5	48.9	57.3	60.5	22.2	20.5	20.3	21.2
18–44 years	21.7	20.8	20.4	19.8	0.7	0.7	*0.9	*1.1	34.7	34.8	37.9	38.5
45–64 years	4.2	4.6	4.5	4.9	*	*	*	*	39.8	44.5	48.8	51.4
45–54 years	5.6	6.3	5.6	6.0	*	*	*	*	39.8	44.4	47.7	49.1
55–64 years	2.9	3.1	3.3	3.8	*	*	*	*	39.8	44.5	50.1	53.6
65 years and over	1.4	1.1	1.5	*1.5	*	*	*	*	38.4	47.4	53.5	56.1
65–74 years	1.7	1.6	2.0	*1.8	*	*	*	*	38.8	47.3	53.4	58.1
75 years and over	1.0	*0.6	*1.0	*1.1	*	*	*	*	37.7	47.6	53.6	54.1
Sex and Age												
Male												
Under 18 years	X	X	X	X	49.4	50.7	58.0	61.2	22.7	21.9	22.3	22.4
18–44 years	X	X	X	X	1.0	0.7	*1.7	*1.8	49.2	48.2	48.5	47.6
45–64 years	X	X	X	X	*	*	*	*	44.4	49.4	50.6	54.8
65 years and over	X	X	X	X	*	*	*	*	41.8	48.8	56.9	61.4
Female												
Under 18 years	2.5	2.3	2.1	1.7	47.4	46.9	56.5	59.8	21.5	18.9	18.0	19.8
18–44 years	31.7	30.4	29.6	28.7	0.6	0.7	*	*	27.9	28.7	32.8	34.4
45–64 years	6.7	7.7	7.3	8.4	*	*	*	*	36.6	41.2	47.5	48.9
65 years and over	2.1	1.8	2.6	*2.5	*	*	*	*	36.1	46.5	51.1	52.2

Table C-51. Visits to Primary Care Generalist and Specialist Physicians, by Selected Characteristics and Type of Physician, Selected Years, 1980–2009—*Continued*

(Percent.)

Age, sex, and race	Type of primary care generalist physician[1]											
	Obstetrics and gynecology				Pediatrics				Specialty care physicians			
	1980	1990	2000	2009	1980	1990	2000	2009	1980	1990	2000	2009
Race and Age[2]												
White												
Under 18 years	1.1	1.0	*1.2	*0.7	48.2	48.8	54.7	60.1	22.4	20.8	21.5	21.9
18–44 years	21.0	21.1	20.4	18.8	0.7	0.7	*0.8	*1.2	35.2	35.6	38.6	39.6
45–64 years	4.1	4.8	4.7	4.5	*	*	*	*	40.4	45.8	50.7	52.4
65 years and over	1.4	1.2	1.5	*1.4	*	*	*	*	38.6	48.1	54.9	56.8
Black or African American												
Under 18 years	2.8	*3.4	*	*	51.2	52.1	75.0	62.7	20.1	14.5	*12.7	*19.2
18–44 years	27.1	17.9	20.7	22.1	*	*	*	*	31.5	31.7	35.0	35.6
45–64 years	4.8	3.5	*2.4	*5.1	*	*	*	*	33.9	38.4	38.3	50.0
65 years and over	*	*	*	*	*	*	*	*	35.4	41.4	47.2	54.3

* = Figure does not meet standards of reliability or precision.
X = Category not applicable.
[1]Type of physician is based on physician's self-designated primary area of practice.
[2]Estimates by racial group should be used with caution because information on race was collected from medical records.

Table C-52. Dental Visits in the Past Year, by Selected Characteristics, Selected Years, 1997–2010

(Percent.)

Characteristic	2 years and over			2–17 years			18–64 years			65 years and over[1]		
	1997	2000	2010	1997	2000	2010	1997	2000	2010	1997	2000	2010
TOTAL	65.1	66.2	64.7	72.7	74.1	78.9	64.1	65.1	61.1	54.8	56.6	57.7
Sex												
Male	62.9	63.5	61.7	72.3	73.7	78.3	60.4	60.7	56.8	55.4	56.1	56.2
Female	67.1	68.8	67.5	73.0	74.6	79.6	67.7	69.4	65.4	54.4	56.9	58.9
Race[2]												
White only	66.4	67.9	65.6	74.0	75.8	79.2	65.7	67.2	62.4	56.8	58.4	59.3
Black or African American only	58.9	59.5	58.8	68.8	70.0	79.0	57.0	57.1	53.1	35.4	38.2	40.6
American Indian or Alaska Native only	55.1	58.6	57.4	66.8	71.3	73.2	49.9	55.0	49.8	*	*	72.2
Asian only	62.5	67.1	66.5	69.9	72.8	74.8	60.3	65.6	64.6	53.9	60.6	61.9
Native Hawaiian or Other Pacific Islander only	—	*	*	—	*	*	—	*	*	—	*	*
2 or more races	—	65.1	65.2	—	71.4	77.9	—	60.5	54.7	—	57.4	48.1
Black or African American; White	—	63.5	72.5	—	65.7	78.4	—	60.7	62.1	—	*	*
American Indian or Alaska Native; White	—	61.7	54.7	—	63.4	70.0	—	61.6	49.0	—	*57.8	*54.5
Hispanic Origin and Race[3]												
Hispanic or Latino	54.0	52.3	56.5	61.0	60.6	74.8	50.8	48.6	48.5	47.8	44.5	42.1
Not Hispanic or Latino	66.4	68.2	66.2	74.7	76.8	80.1	65.7	67.5	63.4	55.2	57.2	59.0
White only	68.0	69.9	67.6	76.4	78.9	80.9	67.5	69.4	65.4	57.2	59.1	60.9
Black or African American only	58.8	59.4	58.7	68.8	70.0	79.2	56.9	57.2	53.1	35.3	38.0	40.5
Percent of Poverty Level[4]												
Below 100%	50.5	50.4	50.6	62.0	62.4	73.2	46.9	46.8	41.0	31.5	33.3	32.8
100%–199%	50.8	52.2	51.6	62.5	66.1	73.4	48.3	48.4	44.1	40.8	43.0	43.8
200%–399%	66.2	65.6	63.5	76.1	75.5	79.0	63.4	62.2	59.6	60.7	62.8	57.9
400% or more	78.9	79.5	79.3	85.7	85.9	88.0	77.7	78.5	77.5	74.7	73.8	77.2
Hispanic Origin and Race and Percent of Poverty Level[3,4]												
Hispanic or Latino												
Below 100%	45.7	43.4	50.8	55.9	54.2	74.3	39.2	36.8	34.7	33.6	31.3	32.4
100%–199%	47.2	45.5	50.8	53.8	56.9	71.1	43.5	39.2	40.2	47.9	42.9	39.5
200%–399%	61.2	57.2	59.1	70.5	65.6	76.5	57.5	53.7	54.1	57.0	54.8	46.0
400% or more	73.0	70.0	73.3	82.4	78.4	84.2	70.8	68.7	71.6	64.9	53.4	54.3
Not Hispanic or Latino												
White only												
Below 100%	51.7	53.6	49.3	64.4	65.0	69.1	50.6	53.3	44.4	32.0	37.2	36.4
100%–199%	52.4	53.8	52.7	66.1	69.7	75.3	50.4	51.7	47.2	42.2	43.4	45.4
200%–399%	67.5	67.6	64.7	77.1	78.3	79.6	65.0	64.4	61.4	61.9	63.9	59.8
400% or more	79.7	80.8	79.8	86.8	87.5	88.6	78.5	79.7	77.9	75.5	76.1	78.8
Black or African American only												
Below 100%	52.8	51.8	52.0	66.1	67.1	78.0	46.2	44.4	39.7	27.7	21.7	20.9
100%–199%	48.7	52.4	50.0	61.2	67.3	75.9	46.3	48.0	41.5	26.9	35.2	33.6
200%–399%	63.3	62.3	61.2	75.0	74.0	81.2	60.7	58.4	57.2	41.5	48.4	45.3
400% or more	74.6	72.8	77.2	81.8	74.2	87.2	73.4	73.3	75.9	66.1	60.5	69.8
Disability Measure[5]												
Any basic actions difficulty or complex activity limitation	X	X	X	X	X	X	55.1	57.3	53.5	49.0	50.7	50.7
Any basic actions difficulty	X	X	X	X	X	X	54.7	57.0	53.2	48.7	50.7	50.5
Any complex activity limitation	X	X	X	X	X	X	51.0	52.5	47.4	44.6	44.4	43.1
No disability	X	X	X	X	X	X	67.4	67.7	64.2	64.2	65.7	68.8
Geographic Region												
Northeast	69.6	72.3	70.1	77.5	81.1	83.8	69.6	72.1	67.9	55.5	58.1	61.5
Midwest	68.4	69.9	67.3	76.4	77.2	80.8	67.4	69.2	64.3	57.6	58.6	58.2
South	60.2	61.0	60.9	68.0	69.5	77.4	59.4	59.8	56.5	49.0	50.8	54.1
West	65.0	65.3	63.9	71.5	72.0	76.1	62.9	63.0	60.2	61.9	63.1	59.8
Location of Residence												
Within MSA[6]	66.7	67.5	65.9	73.6	74.3	79.3	65.7	66.5	62.4	57.6	58.9	59.4
Outside MSA[6]	59.1	61.2	58.4	69.3	73.3	76.4	58.0	59.7	53.8	46.1	49.3	51.3

* = Figure does not meet standards of reliability or precision.
— = Data not available.
X = Category not applicable.

[1] Based on the 1997–2010 National Health Interview Surveys, about 24%–30% of persons 65 years and over were edentulous (having lost all their natural teeth). In 1997–2010, about 69%–73% of older dentate persons, compared with 17%–21% of older edentate persons, had a dental visit in the past year.
[2] Includes all other races not shown separately and unknown disability status.
[3] The race groups, White, Black, American Indian or Alaska Native, Asian, Native Hawaiian or Other Pacific Islander, and 2 or more races, include persons of Hispanic and non-Hispanic origin. Persons of Hispanic origin may be of any race.
[4] Percent of poverty level is based on family income and family size and composition using U.S. Census Bureau poverty thresholds.
[5] Any basic actions difficulty or complex activity limitation is defined as having one or more of the following limitations or difficulties: movement difficulty, emotional difficulty, sensory (seeing or hearing) difficulty, cognitive difficulty, self-care (activities of daily living or instrumental activities of daily living) limitation, social limitation, or work limitation.
[6] MSA = metropolitan statistical area.

Table C-53. Prescription Drug Use in the Past 30 Days, by Sex, Age, Race and Hispanic Origin, Selected Years, 1988–1994 through 2005–2008

(Percent.)

Sex and age	All persons[1]			White only			Black or African American only			Mexican[2]		
	1988–1994	2001–2004	2005–2008	1988–1994	2001–2004	2005–2008	1988–1994	2001–2004	2005–2008	1988–1994	2001–2004	2005–2008
PERCENT OF POPULATION WITH AT LEAST ONE PRESCRIPTION DRUG IN PAST 30 DAYS												
Both Sexes, Age-Adjusted[3]	39.1	46.7	47.2	41.1	50.6	52.0	36.9	40.5	42.1	31.7	34.5	32.2
Male	32.7	41.6	41.8	34.2	45.0	46.1	31.1	36.2	37.2	27.5	28.8	28.8
Female	45.0	51.5	52.4	47.6	56.0	57.9	41.4	43.8	46.0	36.0	40.5	35.6
Both Sexes, Crude	37.8	46.5	47.9	41.4	52.6	55.0	31.2	36.5	39.5	24.0	25.4	24.5
Male	30.6	40.5	41.7	33.5	46.0	48.4	25.5	31.6	33.9	20.1	20.6	21.4
Female	44.6	52.2	53.9	48.9	59.0	61.5	36.2	40.7	44.4	28.1	30.6	27.9
Under 18 years	20.5	23.9	25.3	22.9	27.3	29.9	14.8	18.0	20.8	16.1	16.3	17.0
18–44 years	31.3	37.7	37.8	34.3	43.5	45.1	27.8	29.4	29.4	21.1	20.9	17.7
45–64 years	54.8	66.2	64.8	55.5	68.6	67.7	57.5	63.4	62.6	48.1	53.8	50.1
65 years and over	73.6	87.3	90.1	74.0	88.3	91.1	74.5	80.8	89.1	67.7	79.6	76.7
Male												
Under 18 years	20.4	25.3	25.3	22.3	29.4	29.2	15.5	18.8	23.4	16.3	16.9	17.3
18–44 years	21.5	29.2	27.5	23.5	33.4	33.3	21.1	22.6	20.9	14.9	14.1	14.2
45–64 years	47.2	58.7	59.3	48.1	60.8	62.3	48.2	58.0	54.7	43.8	42.7	46.0
65 years and over	67.2	83.6	89.7	67.4	84.8	91.6	64.4	75.9	85.1	61.3	74.4	67.8
Female												
Under 18 years	20.6	22.4	25.2	23.6	25.1	30.7	14.2	17.1	18.1	16.0	15.7	16.7
18–44 years	40.7	45.9	47.9	44.7	53.5	56.6	33.4	35.0	36.6	28.1	28.6	22.0
45–64 years	62.0	73.4	70.2	62.6	76.3	73.0	64.4	67.7	69.1	52.2	65.8	54.1
65 years and over	78.3	90.1	90.5	78.8	91.0	90.7	81.3	84.0	91.7	73.0	83.9	83.9
PERCENT OF POPULATION WITH THREE OR MORE PRESCRIPTION DRUGS IN PAST 30 DAYS												
Both Sexes, Age-Adjusted[3]	11.8	20.2	20.8	12.4	21.8	22.3	12.6	17.7	20.0	9.0	14.4	13.8
Male	9.4	17.3	18.3	9.9	18.7	19.5	10.2	15.1	17.5	7.0	12.1	11.6
Female	13.9	22.8	23.2	14.6	24.8	25.1	14.3	19.7	21.8	11.0	16.7	15.9
Both Sexes, Crude	11.0	19.9	21.4	12.5	23.6	25.3	9.2	14.7	17.5	4.8	7.9	7.8
Male	8.3	16.4	17.8	9.5	19.5	21.3	7.0	11.9	14.4	3.4	6.2	6.1
Female	13.6	23.4	24.8	15.4	27.6	29.1	11.1	17.1	20.2	6.4	9.8	9.7
Under 18 years	2.4	4.0	4.4	3.2	5.0	5.3	1.5	2.8	3.6	*1.2	2.0	2.7
18–44 years	5.7	10.2	9.8	6.3	12.2	12.1	5.4	8.1	7.3	3.0	4.3	2.7
45–64 years	20.0	34.2	34.1	20.9	35.6	35.6	21.9	33.7	34.5	16.0	27.5	24.5
65 years and over	35.3	59.8	65.0	35.0	62.0	65.7	41.2	50.1	67.0	31.3	47.8	52.5
Male												
Under 18 years	2.6	4.1	5.0	3.3	4.9	5.7	1.7	3.4	5.3	*0.9	*1.7	3.5
18–44 years	3.6	8.0	6.2	4.1	9.8	8.0	4.2	6.1	*4.9	*1.8	2.6	*1.5
45–64 years	15.1	28.3	28.6	15.8	29.1	29.4	18.7	28.2	29.0	11.6	23.8	19.7
65 years and over	31.3	54.2	64.6	30.9	56.4	66.3	31.7	44.0	61.5	27.6	42.0	45.0
Female												
Under 18 years	2.3	3.9	3.8	3.0	5.2	4.8	*1.2	2.1	*1.9	*1.5	2.4	1.8
18–44 years	7.6	12.3	13.3	8.5	14.7	16.1	6.4	9.7	9.4	4.3	*6.2	4.1
45–64 years	24.7	39.9	39.4	25.8	41.9	41.8	24.3	38.1	39.1	20.3	31.4	29.0
65 years and over	38.2	64.0	65.3	38.0	66.2	65.3	47.7	54.2	70.6	34.5	52.7	58.6

Table C-53. Prescription Drug Use in the Past 30 Days, by Sex, Age, Race and Hispanic Origin, Selected Years, 1988–1994 through 2005–2008—Continued

(Percent.)

Sex and age	All persons[1]			White only			Black or African American only			Mexican[2]		
	1988–1994	2001–2004	2005–2008	1988–1994	2001–2004	2005–2008	1988–1994	2001–2004	2005–2008	1988–1994	2001–2004	2005–2008
PERCENT OF POPULATION WITH FIVE OR MORE PRESCRIPTION DRUGS IN PAST 30 DAYS												
Both Sexes, Age-Adjusted[3]	4.0	9.2	10.2	4.2	9.8	10.7	3.8	8.7	11.2	2.9	6.1	6.9
Male	2.9	7.9	8.9	3.1	8.4	9.3	2.9	7.6	9.4	2.0	4.8	5.9
Female	4.9	10.4	11.5	5.1	11.1	12.1	4.5	9.5	12.6	3.7	7.6	7.9
Both Sexes, Crude	3.6	9.0	10.5	4.2	10.8	12.4	2.6	7.1	9.6	1.4	2.9	3.4
Male	2.5	7.3	8.6	2.9	8.8	10.3	1.8	5.9	7.6	0.9	2.1	2.6
Female	4.7	10.7	12.4	5.4	12.8	14.5	3.3	8.2	11.4	1.9	3.8	4.4
Under 18 years	*	0.8	1.0	*	*0.9	1.2	*	*0.7	*0.9	*	*	*0.5
18–44 years	1.2	3.3	3.4	1.4	3.8	4.2	1.0	4.1	2.8	*	*	*
45–64 years	7.4	15.7	17.0	7.8	16.3	17.4	7.1	16.8	20.6	5.4	12.4	11.5
65 years and over	13.8	33.3	38.3	13.9	35.4	38.6	14.3	25.4	42.0	11.6	23.4	31.1
Male												
Under 18 years	*	*0.8	*1.1	*	*	*	*	*	*	*	*	*
18–44 years	*0.8	2.6	*1.8	*	2.9	*2.4	*	*3.2	*	*	*	*
45–64 years	4.8	12.5	13.7	5.0	13.2	13.8	5.9	15.0	17.5	*3.5	*7.8	8.7
65 years and over	11.3	30.6	38.4	11.6	31.9	39.2	9.9	22.3	35.3	*8.7	20.7	28.9
Female												
Under 18 years	*	*0.7	*0.8	*	*0.9	*	*	*	*	*	*	*
18–44 years	1.7	3.9	5.0	1.8	4.6	6.0	1.2	4.7	3.6	*0.6	*	*
45–64 years	9.7	18.8	20.2	10.3	19.4	20.9	8.0	18.2	23.2	*7.2	17.2	14.2
65 years and over	15.6	35.4	38.3	15.7	38.0	38.2	17.4	27.5	46.4	14.0	25.6	32.9

* = Figure does not meet standards of reliability or precision.
[1]Includes persons of all races and Hispanic origins, not just those shown separately.
[2]Persons of Mexican origin may be of any race.
[3]Age-adjusted to the 2000 standard population using four age groups: Under 18 years, 18–44 years, 45–64 years, and 65 years and over.

Table C-54. Selected Prescription Drug Classes Used in the Past 30 Days, by Sex and Age, Selected Years, 1988–1994 through 2005–2008

(Percent.)

Age group and Multum Lexicon Plus therapeutic class[1] (primary indications for use)	Total			Male			Female		
	1988–1994	2001–2004	2005–2008	1988–1994	2001–2004	2005–2008	1988–1994	2001–2004	2005–2008
All Ages									
Antihyperlipidemic agents (high cholesterol)	1.7	7.8	11.4	1.5	8.7	12.0	1.8	7.0	10.8
Analgesics (pain relief)	7.2	11.1	9.0	5.4	8.8	7.7	9.0	13.3	10.2
Antidepressants (depression and related disorders)	1.8	7.8	8.9	1.2	5.4	5.0	2.3	10.0	12.7
Beta-adrenergic blocking agents (high blood pressure, heart disease)	3.1	5.4	7.3	2.7	5.2	6.8	3.5	5.5	7.6
Proton pump inhibitors (gastrointestinal reflux, ulcers)	*	5.0	6.3	*	4.6	5.6	*	5.4	6.9
ACE inhibitors (high blood pressure, heart disease)	2.4	5.2	5.9	2.4	5.4	6.3	2.4	5.1	5.6
Sex hormones (contraceptives, menopause, hot flashes)	X	X	X	X	X	X	9.9	13.3	9.7
Diuretics (high blood pressure, heart disease, kidney disease)	3.4	4.6	5.3	2.3	3.3	4.5	4.4	5.8	6.1
Thyroid drugs (hyper- and hypothyroidism)	2.3	4.5	5.2	0.8	1.7	1.7	3.7	7.1	8.5
Antidiabetic agents (diabetes)	2.6	4.3	5.2	2.5	4.1	4.8	2.6	4.4	5.5
Bronchodilators (asthma, breathing)	2.6	3.7	4.9	2.5	3.5	4.5	2.7	4.0	5.2
Anxiolytics, sedatives, and hypnotics (generalized anxiety and related disorders)	2.8	3.8	4.5	1.9	2.8	3.2	3.6	4.8	5.7
Antihypertensive combinations (high blood pressure)	2.4	3.5	4.1	1.4	2.8	3.0	3.3	4.1	5.1
Calcium channel blocking agents (high blood pressure, heart disease)	3.6	3.8	4.0	3.4	3.4	3.6	3.8	4.2	4.4
Antihistamines (allergies)	2.7	4.4	3.8	2.2	3.8	2.9	3.2	4.9	4.6
Under 18 Years									
Bronchodilators (asthma, breathing)	3.0	4.3	5.4	3.3	4.5	6.0	2.7	4.0	4.7
Penicillins (bacterial infections)	6.1	4.1	3.8	5.9	3.9	3.4	6.4	4.3	4.2
CNS stimulants (attention deficit disorder, hyperactivity)	*0.8	3.1	3.7	*1.2	4.8	4.8	*	1.3	2.6
Antihistamines (allergies)	2.0	4.0	2.9	2.1	4.1	3.0	1.9	4.0	2.7
Leukotriene modifiers (asthma, allergies)	X	1.1	2.9	X	1.2	3.3	X	*1.0	*2.4
Upper respiratory combinations (cough and cold, congestion)	2.3	2.6	1.8	2.6	2.7	1.6	2.0	2.4	1.9
Respiratory inhalant products (asthma, chronic obstructive pulmonary disease, and related disorders)	*0.7	1.3	1.8	*	1.3	2.4	*	1.3	1.3
Adrenal cortical steroids (anti-inflammatory)	*0.5	0.9	1.6	*	*0.9	2.1	*0.5	0.8	1.1
Antidepressants (depression and related disorders)	*	1.6	1.5	*	1.8	*1.5	*	*1.4	*1.6
Analgesics (pain relief)	1.2	1.7	1.4	*1.2	1.6	1.0	1.4	1.8	2.0
Cephalosporins (bacterial infections)	1.8	1.4	1.1	1.8	*1.7	1.1	1.8	*1.1	*1.2
Macrolide derivatives (bacterial infections)	1.0	1.1	*0.9	*0.7	1.3	*1.1	*1.3	*0.9	*
18–44 years									
Antidepressants (depression and related disorders)	1.6	7.3	7.8	*1.0	4.1	3.6	2.3	10.4	11.9
Analgesics (pain relief)	7.2	10.0	7.7	5.1	7.5	6.5	9.1	12.5	8.9
Sex hormones (contraceptives, menopause, hot flashes)	X	X	X	X	X	X	11.7	13.8	15.7
Proton pump inhibitors (gastrointestinal reflux, ulcers)	*	3.3	3.5	*	3.0	2.8	*	3.7	4.2
Bronchodilators (asthma, breathing)	1.4	2.4	3.3	*1.1	2.2	2.3	*1.8	2.6	4.2
Antihistamines (allergies)	2.5	4.0	3.2	1.8	3.9	*1.7	3.2	4.1	4.6
Anxiolytics, sedatives, and hypnotics (generalized anxiety and related disorders)	1.4	2.9	3.2	*1.0	2.2	2.1	1.9	3.7	4.3
Anticonvulsants (epilepsy, seizure, and related disorders)	0.8	2.2	2.9	*0.6	1.9	*2.0	1.0	2.5	3.8
Thyroid drugs (hyper- and hypothyroidism)	1.4	2.3	2.8	*	*	*	2.1	4.1	4.9
Antihyperlipidemic agents (high cholesterol)	*0.4	1.8	2.5	*	2.5	3.1	*	*1.2	*2.0
Antidiabetic agents (diabetes)	*1.0	1.8	2.1	*	1.6	1.7	*1.0	2.0	2.4
ACE inhibitors (high blood pressure, heart disease)	0.7	1.6	1.9	*0.9	2.1	1.7	*0.6	*1.2	2.0
Penicillins (bacterial infections)	3.1	2.1	1.8	2.3	*1.6	*1.1	3.8	2.7	2.5
Muscle relaxants (muscle spasm and related disorders)	1.0	1.7	1.6	*1.3	*1.5	*1.1	*0.7	1.9	2.0
Beta-adrenergic blocking agents (high blood pressure, heart disease)	1.1	1.4	1.4	*0.9	*1.5	*1.2	1.3	1.2	1.5
45–64 Years									
Antihyperlipidemic agents (high cholesterol)	4.3	15.3	19.6	4.4	18.7	21.2	4.2	12.1	18.0
Antidepressants (depression and related disorders)	3.5	14.1	15.3	*2.3	10.7	8.5	4.6	17.3	21.9
Analgesics (pain relief)	11.9	18.6	14.0	9.2	16.0	12.3	14.3	21.1	15.7
Beta-adrenergic blocking agents (high blood pressure, heart disease)	6.6	9.8	11.0	7.0	9.7	10.5	6.2	9.9	11.6
Proton pump inhibitors (gastrointestinal reflux, ulcers)	*	9.0	10.9	*	8.4	10.6	*	9.5	11.2
ACE inhibitors (high blood pressure, heart disease)	5.2	9.8	10.3	5.7	10.5	11.4	4.6	9.2	9.3
Antidiabetic agents (diabetes)	5.5	7.8	9.4	5.9	8.4	9.5	5.1	7.2	9.3
Thyroid drugs (hyper- and hypothyroidism)	4.7	8.2	8.5	*1.2	*3.1	*2.9	8.1	12.9	13.9
Sex hormones (contraceptives, menopause, hot flashes)	X	X	X	X	X	X	19.9	23.9	11.2
Antihypertensive combinations (high blood pressure)	5.3	6.9	8.1	3.3	6.6	6.3	7.1	7.3	9.7
Anxiolytics, sedatives, and hypnotics (generalized anxiety and related disorders)	6.0	6.8	7.8	4.3	*5.3	6.2	7.5	8.3	9.3
Diuretics (high blood pressure, heart disease, kidney disease)	6.1	7.2	6.7	4.8	4.8	6.0	7.3	9.6	7.5
Calcium channel blocking agents (high blood pressure, heart disease)	7.0	5.7	6.1	8.2	5.6	5.3	5.9	5.8	6.9
Anticonvulsants (epilepsy, seizure, and related disorders)	2.7	5.3	6.0	*2.5	4.5	5.0	2.9	6.0	7.0

Table C-54. Selected Prescription Drug Classes Used in the Past 30 Days, by Sex and Age, Selected Years, 1988–1994 through 2005–2008—Continued

(Percent.)

Age group and Multum Lexicon Plus therapeutic class[1] (primary indications for use)	Total			Male			Female		
	1988–1994	2001–2004	2005–2008	1988–1994	2001–2004	2005–2008	1988–1994	2001–2004	2005–2008
65 Years and Over									
Antihyperlipidemic agents (high cholesterol)	5.9	30.2	44.5	5.3	32.8	50.6	6.4	28.3	40.0
Beta-adrenergic blocking agents (high blood pressure, heart disease)	11.8	21.5	32.0	10.4	22.4	34.8	12.8	20.9	29.9
Diuretics (high blood pressure, heart disease, kidney disease)	16.2	21.4	24.5	12.2	18.3	24.6	19.1	23.7	24.4
ACE inhibitors (high blood pressure, heart disease)	9.5	19.7	21.0	9.8	21.1	25.1	9.3	18.6	18.1
Analgesics (pain relief)	13.8	20.8	18.1	11.4	16.8	17.8	15.6	23.7	18.3
Calcium channel blocking agents (high blood pressure, heart disease)	16.1	18.7	17.1	14.5	17.1	17.3	17.3	19.9	17.0
Proton pump inhibitors (gastrointestinal reflux, ulcers)	*	13.3	17.0	*	13.7	16.9	*	13.0	17.1
Antidiabetic agents (diabetes)	9.0	14.5	16.0	9.0	14.9	15.9	9.0	14.2	16.1
Thyroid drugs (hyper- and hypothyroidism)	7.1	14.5	15.5	3.5	8.2	6.2	9.8	19.2	22.4
Antidepressants (depression and related disorders)	3.0	10.4	14.2	*2.3	8.3	10.0	3.5	11.9	17.3
Antihypertensive combinations (high blood pressure)	9.6	11.9	13.2	6.0	8.6	9.6	12.2	14.4	15.8
Angiotensin II inhibitors (high blood pressure, heart disease)	X	7.5	10.7	X	6.6	9.7	X	8.2	11.5
Anxiolytics, sedatives, and hypnotics (generalized anxiety and related disorders)	7.8	8.6	9.8	6.1	5.9	7.1	9.1	10.5	11.8
Bisphosphonates (osteoporosis and related disorders)	*	7.1	8.4	*	*1.4	*	*	11.3	13.8
Antiadrenergic agents, peripherally acting (prostate conditions)[2]	X	X	X	2.8	14.4	15.9	X	X	X
65–74 Years									
Antihyperlipidemic agents (high cholesterol)	7.3	33.5	44.3	6.2	36.2	52.1	8.1	31.1	38.2
Beta-adrenergic blocking agents (high blood pressure, heart disease)	11.3	20.9	29.0	10.6	22.7	32.2	11.9	19.3	26.4
Diuretics (high blood pressure, heart disease, kidney disease)	14.2	16.8	21.0	10.8	15.0	19.6	17.0	18.3	22.1
ACE inhibitors (high blood pressure, heart disease)	9.6	19.6	19.5	10.6	22.4	24.2	8.9	17.2	15.8
Analgesics (pain relief)	13.0	21.8	18.6	10.5	17.8	16.5	15.0	25.3	20.3
Antidiabetic agents (diabetes)	8.8	16.0	17.8	8.0	16.6	18.2	9.4	15.4	17.5
Proton pump inhibitors (gastrointestinal reflux, ulcers)	*	13.6	16.9	*	14.2	17.0	*	13.0	16.8
Antidepressants (depression and related disorders)	2.8	10.4	15.0	*2.3	7.1	9.6	3.1	13.2	19.3
Calcium channel blocking agents (high blood pressure, heart disease)	15.0	16.7	14.0	14.0	16.5	15.5	15.8	16.8	12.9
Antihypertensive combinations (high blood pressure)	8.1	11.5	13.7	4.8	8.1	11.0	10.8	14.4	15.8
Thyroid drugs (hyper- and hypothyroidism)	6.6	12.9	13.1	*3.8	7.0	4.3	8.9	18.0	19.9
Angiotensin II inhibitors (high blood pressure, heart disease)	X	6.9	9.7	X	6.0	9.2	X	7.7	10.1
Anxiolytics, sedatives, and hypnotics (generalized anxiety and related disorders)	6.9	8.4	9.4	6.0	*5.7	6.8	7.6	10.7	11.4
Antiadrenergic agents, peripherally acting (prostate conditions)[2]	*	*	*	*2.6	14.9	13.1	*	*	*
Bisphosphonates (osteoporosis and related disorders)	*	6.2	7.2	*	*	*	*	10.8	12.5
Anticonvulsants (epilepsy, seizure, and related disorders)	3.0	6.0	7.1	*2.7	4.1	5.7	3.2	*7.6	8.2
75 Years and Over									
Antihyperlipidemic agents (high cholesterol)	3.8	26.5	44.8	*3.5	28.2	48.7	4.0	25.4	42.0
Beta-adrenergic blocking agents (high blood pressure, heart disease)	12.5	22.3	35.6	9.8	22.0	38.1	14.1	22.5	33.8
Diuretics (high blood pressure, heart disease, kidney disease)	19.2	26.7	28.7	14.7	22.9	31.1	21.9	29.1	27.0
ACE inhibitors (high blood pressure, heart disease)	9.3	19.8	22.9	8.5	19.3	26.2	9.8	20.1	20.6
Calcium channel blocking agents (high blood pressure, heart disease)	17.8	21.0	20.8	15.3	17.9	19.6	19.2	22.9	21.6
Thyroid drugs (hyper- and hypothyroidism)	8.0	16.4	18.5	3.0	9.9	8.7	10.9	20.5	25.2
Analgesics (pain relief)	15.1	19.5	17.5	13.0	15.3	19.5	16.3	22.2	16.1
Proton pump inhibitors (gastrointestinal reflux, ulcers)	*	13.0	17.3	*	13.0	16.8	*	12.9	17.6
Antidiabetic agents (diabetes)	9.3	12.8	13.9	10.7	12.4	12.9	8.5	13.0	14.5
Antidepressants (depression and related disorders)	3.4	10.4	13.3	*2.3	10.0	10.6	4.0	10.6	15.1
Antihypertensive combinations (high blood pressure)	11.9	12.4	12.6	8.3	9.2	7.8	14.0	14.4	15.9
Antiplatelet agents (blood thinning, reduce or prevent blood clots)	4.4	6.7	11.7	*4.2	9.1	14.6	4.6	5.2	9.7
Angiotensin II inhibitors (high blood pressure, heart disease)	X	8.2	11.9	X	7.4	10.2	X	8.7	13.0
Anticoagulants (blood thinning, reduce or prevent blood clots)	2.9	8.8	10.4	3.7	10.6	14.3	*2.4	7.7	7.7
Anxiolytics, sedatives, and hypnotics (generalized anxiety and related disorders)	9.2	8.8	10.3	6.3	6.2	7.5	10.9	10.3	12.3
Bisphosphonates (osteoporosis and related disorders)	*	8.1	10.0	*	*	*	*	11.8	15.4
Minerals and electrolytes mineral deficiencies	7.5	9.2	8.4	5.6	8.4	6.8	8.7	9.8	9.6
Antiadrenergic agents, peripherally acting (prostate conditions)[2]	X	X	X	X	*3.1	13.7	19.5	X	X

* = Figure does not meet standards of reliability or precision.
X = Category not applicable.
[1] The drug therapeutic class is based on Lexicon Plus, a proprietary database of Cerner Multum, Inc. Lexicon Plus is a comprehensive database of all prescription and some nonprescription drug products available in the U.S. drug market. Data on prescription drug use are collected by the National Health and Nutrition Examination Survey.
[2] Although some antiadrenergic agents are used to treat high blood pressure, they are generally used currently to treat prostate hyperplasia and related conditions.

Table C-55. Dietary Supplement Use Among Persons 20 Years of Age and Over, by Selected Characteristics, Selected Years, 1988–1994 through 2005–2008

(Percent.)

Characteristic	Any supplement use in past 30 days[1]			Any vitamin D supplement use in past 30 days[2]			Any folic acid supplement use in past 30 days[3]		
	1988–1994	2001–2004	2005–2008	1988–1994	2001–2004	2005–2008	1988–1994	2001–2004	2005–2008
20 YEARS AND OVER, AGE-ADJUSTED[4]									
Sex									
Both sexes	42.1	53.1	50.9	28.4	38.8	38.0	30.3	38.6	37.5
Male	35.7	47.0	44.4	24.3	33.3	32.2	26.2	34.7	32.9
Female	47.8	58.7	56.9	32.2	43.8	43.4	34.2	42.3	42.0
Race									
Not Hispanic or Latino									
White only, male	37.5	51.4	48.7	26.1	36.8	35.8	28.2	38.4	36.6
White only, female	50.9	64.5	61.3	35.4	49.9	47.7	37.7	48.5	46.1
Black or African American only, male	29.5	32.3	31.0	18.5	20.3	22.6	18.2	22.1	23.0
Black or African American only, female	38.2	38.3	43.0	22.7	25.2	30.5	23.7	25.2	30.3
Mexican male[5]	28.9	31.9	30.0	17.1	20.9	19.6	18.6	21.1	19.2
Mexican female[5]	36.8	43.8	41.5	21.9	30.8	28.1	23.3	28.0	26.5
Percent of Poverty Level[6]									
Below 100%	30.0	37.1	33.5	16.8	24.2	23.2	18.3	23.4	21.7
100%–199%	36.0	45.9	43.9	23.3	30.1	30.3	24.1	29.3	30.4
200%–399%	44.0	52.5	52.5	30.2	39.8	39.4	32.5	39.1	38.8
400% or more	51.0	63.9	60.8	35.8	48.8	47.7	38.5	49.3	47.3
20 YEARS AND OVER, CRUDE									
Sex									
Both sexes	41.8	52.7	51.3	28.4	38.6	38.3	30.3	38.4	37.8
Male	35.3	46.2	44.2	24.2	32.8	32.1	26.0	34.1	32.8
Female	47.7	58.8	57.8	32.2	43.9	44.1	34.3	42.4	42.5
Race									
White only, male	37.4	51.5	49.7	26.0	37.0	36.4	28.1	38.6	37.3
White only, female	51.1	65.5	63.3	35.4	50.5	49.1	37.7	48.9	47.2
Black or African American only, male	28.9	31.0	30.3	18.8	19.4	22.6	18.5	21.0	22.7
Black or African American only, female	37.0	37.6	42.4	22.9	24.7	30.4	23.9	24.8	30.1
Mexican male[5]	25.6	26.6	24.1	15.5	17.3	16.0	17.1	17.3	15.7
Mexican female[5]	34.9	39.1	37.6	21.9	27.1	26.5	23.1	25.8	25.8
Percent of Poverty Level[6]									
Below 100%	29.4	34.9	31.9	17.1	23.2	22.4	18.4	22.5	21.2
100%–199%	36.8	46.7	45.2	24.0	30.6	31.3	24.9	29.9	31.1
200%–399%	43.6	52.2	53.1	30.4	39.6	39.9	32.7	38.9	39.1
400% or more	50.8	63.7	61.0	36.0	48.6	47.6	38.7	49.1	47.3
Male									
20–34 years	31.0	34.7	31.2	21.9	24.2	22.9	23.5	24.9	23.0
35–44 years	36.8	43.2	38.4	26.3	31.1	29.2	28.5	32.5	29.6
45–54 years	32.8	47.9	47.0	23.6	35.3	32.4	25.3	36.1	33.9
55–64 years	42.9	55.9	56.6	28.1	41.5	42.1	30.2	43.2	43.0
65–74 years	39.4	64.4	60.0	24.4	43.8	43.7	26.3	46.6	44.3
75 years and over	40.9	64.0	64.0	23.0	41.7	44.7	24.1	44.4	45.1
Female									
20–34 years	43.6	47.9	44.4	33.1	36.3	35.6	35.5	37.1	35.6
35–44 years	46.5	52.0	49.7	32.2	38.7	37.9	34.8	37.9	38.2
45–54 years	47.8	62.7	60.3	32.3	45.6	44.9	33.7	44.5	43.2
55–64 years	52.3	72.6	70.2	33.4	55.7	53.8	35.8	51.3	52.0
65–74 years	52.9	69.3	75.5	30.0	51.6	57.7	31.2	46.8	52.1
75 years and over	54.0	72.2	71.1	29.8	53.1	50.6	30.7	48.6	44.8

[1]Respondents were asked "Have you used or taken any vitamins, minerals, herbals, or other dietary supplements in the past 30 days? Include prescription and non-prescription supplements." To facilitate their response, respondents were shown a card with some examples of different types of dietary supplements. The question wording differs slightly on the earlier, 1988–1994, survey.
[2]Includes supplements with vitamin D, cholecalciferol, calciferol, ergocalciferol, or calcitriol as an ingredient.
[3]Includes supplements with folic acid as an ingredient.
[4]Age-adjusted to the 2000 standard population using five age groups: 20–34 years, 35–44 years, 45–54 years, 55–64 years, and 65 years and over.
[5]Persons of Mexican origin may be of any race.
[6]Percent of poverty level is based on family income and family size.

INPATIENT CARE

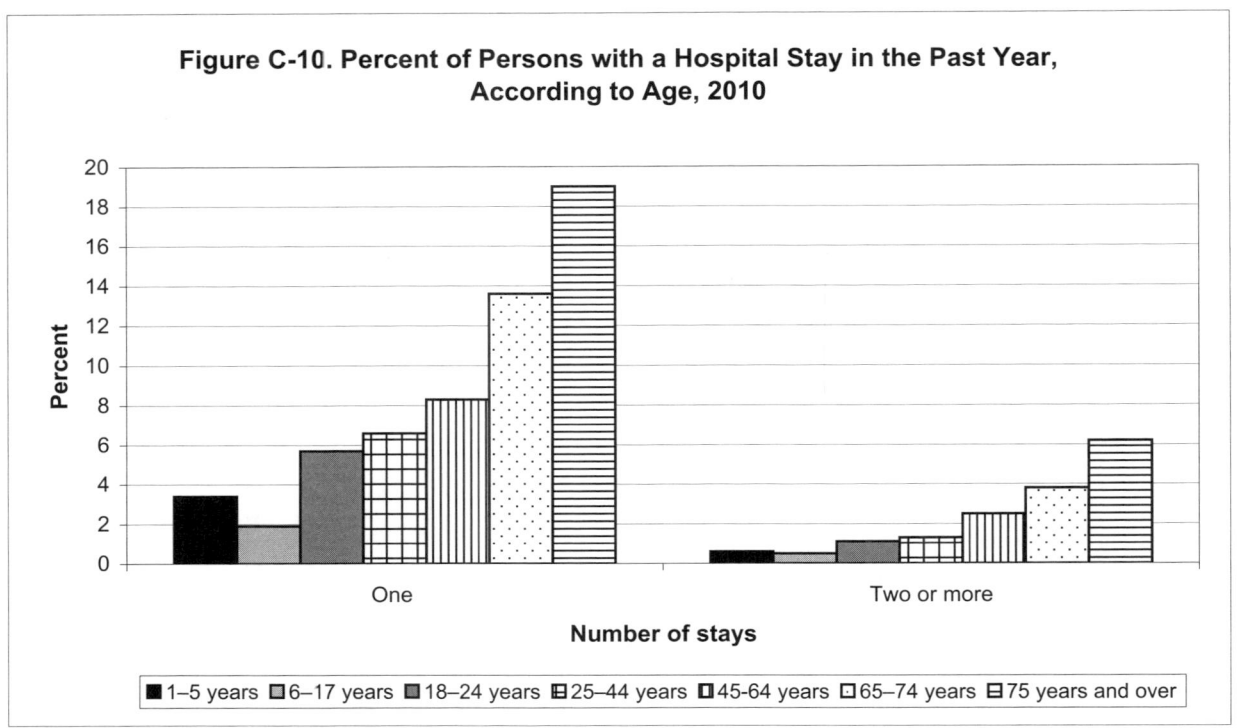

Figure C-10. Percent of Persons with a Hospital Stay in the Past Year, According to Age, 2010

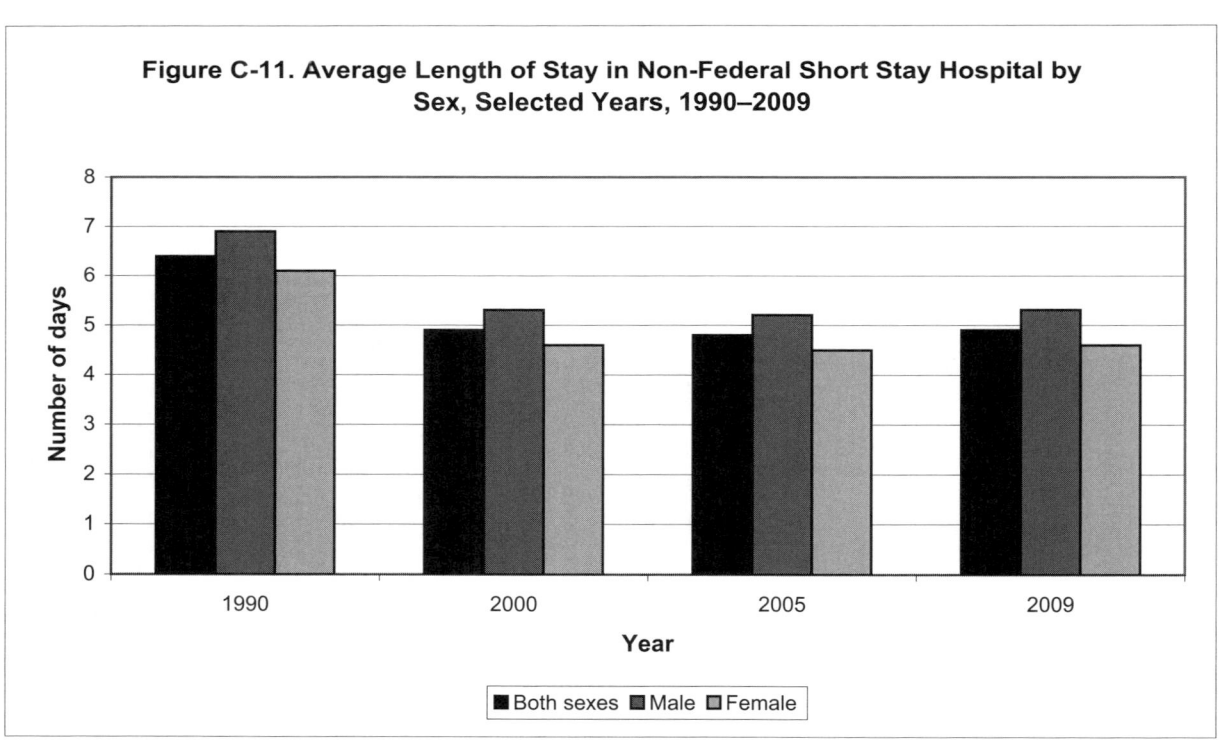

Figure C-11. Average Length of Stay in Non-Federal Short Stay Hospital by Sex, Selected Years, 1990–2009

Table C-56. Persons with Hospital Stays in the Past Year, by Selected Characteristics, Selected Years, 1997–2010

(Percent.)

Characteristic	One or more hospital stays[1]				Two or more hospital stays[1]			
	1997	2000	2005	2010	1997	2000	2005	2010
1 year and over, age-adjusted[2,3]	7.8	7.6	7.4	7.0	1.8	1.8	1.7	1.8
1 year and over, crude[2]	7.7	7.5	7.4	7.2	1.7	1.8	1.8	1.9
Age								
1–17 years	2.8	2.5	2.5	2.4	0.5	0.4	0.4	0.5
1–5 years	3.9	3.8	3.7	3.4	0.7	0.7	0.8	0.6
6–17 years	2.3	1.9	2.0	1.9	0.4	0.3	0.3	0.5
18–44 years	7.4	7.0	6.7	6.3	1.2	1.1	1.1	1.3
18–24 years	7.9	7.0	6.3	5.7	1.3	1.1	1.0	1.1
25–44 years	7.3	7.0	6.9	6.6	1.2	1.2	1.2	1.3
45–64 years	8.2	8.4	8.2	8.3	2.2	2.2	2.2	2.5
45–54 years	6.9	7.3	7.1	7.3	1.7	1.8	1.8	2.1
55–64 years	10.2	10.0	9.8	9.5	2.9	2.8	2.9	2.9
65 years and over	18.0	18.2	17.8	16.1	5.4	5.8	5.4	4.9
65–74 years	16.1	16.1	14.5	13.6	4.8	4.9	4.5	3.8
75 years and over	20.4	20.7	21.4	19.0	6.2	6.8	6.4	6.2
75–84 years	19.8	20.1	19.9	18.3	6.1	6.2	6.1	6.1
85 years and over	22.8	23.4	26.6	20.8	6.2	9.0	7.4	6.6
1–64 Years								
Total, 1–64 years[2,4]	6.3	6.1	5.9	5.7	1.3	1.2	1.2	1.3
Sex								
Male, crude	4.4	4.2	4.5	4.2	0.9	1.0	1.1	1.1
1–17 years	2.9	2.4	2.8	2.4	0.6	0.4	0.5	0.5
18–44 years	3.6	3.1	3.2	2.9	0.6	0.6	0.7	0.7
45–54 years	6.0	7.0	6.6	6.4	1.4	1.8	1.9	1.9
55–64 years	11.1	10.2	10.3	9.3	3.0	3.0	3.4	2.8
Female, crude	8.0	7.9	7.5	7.6	1.6	1.5	1.4	1.7
1–17 years	2.6	2.5	2.2	2.3	0.5	0.4	0.4	0.5
18–44 years	11.2	10.8	10.2	9.8	1.8	1.7	1.6	1.9
45–54 years	7.6	7.6	7.6	8.3	2.0	1.9	1.7	2.3
55–64 years	9.4	9.8	9.3	9.7	2.9	2.7	2.4	2.9
Race[4,5]								
White only	6.2	5.9	5.9	5.6	1.2	1.1	1.1	1.3
Black or African American only	7.6	7.4	6.6	6.7	1.9	1.9	1.8	1.9
American Indian or Alaska Native only	7.6	7.0	6.9	*7.6	*	*	*2.5	*2.4
Asian only	3.9	3.9	3.9	3.6	*0.5	*0.6	*0.5	*0.4
Native Hawaiian or Other Pacific Islander only	—	*	*	*	—	*	*	*
2 or more races	—	8.8	6.0	7.7	—	*1.6	*1.9	*2.4
Hispanic Origin and Race[4,5]								
Hispanic or Latino	6.8	5.5	5.4	5.2	1.3	0.9	1.2	1.1
Not Hispanic or Latino	6.2	6.1	6.0	5.8	1.3	1.3	1.2	1.4
White only	6.1	6.0	6.0	5.7	1.2	1.2	1.1	1.3
Black or African American only	7.5	7.4	6.6	6.7	1.9	1.9	1.7	1.9
Percent of Poverty Level[4,6]								
Below 100%	10.3	9.1	8.8	8.3	2.8	2.6	2.5	2.7
100%–199%	7.3	7.3	7.4	7.0	1.7	1.9	1.9	1.9
200%–399%	6.0	6.0	5.4	5.2	1.2	1.1	1.1	1.1
400% or more	4.7	5.0	4.8	4.5	0.7	0.8	0.8	0.8
Hispanic Origin and Race and Percent of Poverty Level[4,5,6]								
Hispanic or Latino								
Below 100%	9.1	7.4	7.6	7.3	2.0	1.6	2.0	2.0
100%–199%	5.9	5.4	5.9	4.8	1.0	0.8	1.4	1.1
200%–399%	5.9	4.6	4.4	4.3	1.1	0.7	0.8	0.7
400% or more	5.5	4.7	3.8	4.4	*1.1	*0.6	*0.6	*0.8
Not Hispanic or Latino								
White only:								
Below 100%	10.7	9.6	9.3	8.8	3.2	2.7	2.5	2.9
100%–199%	7.7	7.8	8.2	7.8	1.8	2.2	2.0	2.2
200%–399%	6.1	6.1	5.8	5.5	1.2	1.1	1.1	1.2
400% or more	4.7	5.0	4.9	4.6	0.7	0.8	0.7	0.8
Black or African American only								
Below 100%	11.4	10.8	9.4	9.4	3.3	3.4	3.1	3.1
100%–199%	8.0	8.5	7.7	7.7	2.1	2.3	2.0	2.3
200%–399%	6.2	6.1	5.2	5.3	1.5	1.3	1.3	1.4
400% or more	4.7	5.8	5.1	4.5	*0.9	*1.3	*1.2	*1.0

Table C-56. Persons with Hospital Stays in the Past Year, by Selected Characteristics, Selected Years, 1997–2010—Continued

(Percent.)

Characteristic	One or more hospital stays[1]				Two or more hospital stays[1]			
	1997	2000	2005	2010	1997	2000	2005	2010
Health Insurance Status at the Time of Interview[4,7]								
Insured	6.6	6.4	6.3	6.2	1.3	1.3	1.3	1.4
Private	5.6	5.5	5.2	5.0	1.0	1.0	0.9	0.9
Medicaid	16.1	15.9	14.6	12.7	4.9	4.7	4.1	4.5
Uninsured	4.8	4.5	4.4	4.0	1.0	0.9	0.9	0.9
Health Insurance Status Prior to Interview[4,7]								
Insured continuously all 12 months	6.5	6.3	6.1	6.0	1.3	1.2	1.2	1.4
Uninsured for any period up to 12 months	8.5	8.4	9.0	7.9	1.8	1.9	2.4	1.9
Uninsured more than 12 months	3.8	3.5	3.2	3.0	0.8	0.8	0.6	0.8
Disability Measure Among Adults 18–64 Years[4,8]								
Any basic actions difficulty or complex activity limitation	14.1	15.1	15.2	14.3	4.1	4.4	4.9	5.2
Any basic actions difficulty	13.9	15.1	15.1	14.2	4.1	4.4	4.9	5.1
Any complex activity limitation	21.5	22.6	23.2	21.2	7.7	8.8	8.6	8.6
No disability	5.8	5.6	5.4	5.4	0.6	0.7	0.6	0.8
Geographic Region[4]								
Northeast	6.0	5.5	5.8	5.2	1.2	1.0	1.1	1.2
Midwest	6.5	6.3	6.3	6.3	1.5	1.3	1.3	1.5
South	6.8	6.6	6.3	6.0	1.4	1.5	1.4	1.5
West	5.4	5.2	4.8	4.9	0.8	0.9	0.8	1.1
Location of Residence[4]								
Within MSA[9]	6.1	5.8	5.7	5.5	1.2	1.1	1.2	1.3
Outside MSA[9]	7.0	6.9	6.8	6.9	1.6	1.5	1.4	1.6
65 Years and Over								
Total 65 years and over[2,10]	18.1	18.3	17.8	16.2	5.4	5.8	5.4	4.9
65–74 years	16.1	16.1	14.5	13.6	4.8	4.9	4.5	3.8
75 years and over	20.4	20.7	21.4	19.0	6.2	6.8	6.4	6.2
Sex[10]								
Male	19.0	19.5	18.6	16.2	5.8	5.8	6.0	5.4
Female	17.5	17.4	17.3	16.2	5.1	5.7	4.9	4.6
Hispanic Origin and Race[5,10]								
Hispanic or Latino	17.3	16.6	17.7	13.9	6.2	6.4	5.7	5.0
Not Hispanic or Latino	18.2	18.4	17.9	16.4	5.4	5.8	5.4	4.9
White only	18.3	18.4	17.9	16.5	5.4	5.7	5.4	4.9
Black or African American only	18.9	19.8	19.0	16.9	5.5	7.5	6.3	5.5
Percent of Poverty Level[6,10]								
Below 100%	20.9	20.9	22.1	18.8	6.4	7.5	7.9	5.1
100%–199%	19.6	19.2	19.2	17.2	6.5	6.6	5.9	5.2
200%–399%	17.3	18.1	17.2	16.0	4.9	5.8	4.8	5.5
400% or more	16.6	16.0	16.1	15.0	4.7	4.2	5.1	4.1

Table C-56. Persons with Hospital Stays in the Past Year, by Selected Characteristics, Selected Years, 1997-2010—Continued

(Percent.)

Characteristic	One or more hospital stays[1]				Two or more hospital stays[1]			
	1997	2000	2005	2010	1997	2000	2005	2010
Disability Measure[8,10]								
Any basic actions difficulty or complex activity limitation	22.6	24.7	24.1	20.2	7.2	8.6	8.3	6.4
Any basic actions difficulty	22.7	24.7	24.2	20.4	7.2	8.7	8.5	6.6
Any complex activity limitation	29.0	31.5	29.3	25.4	10.8	12.2	11.1	9.2
No disability	7.8	9.7	8.3	10.6	1.1	1.9	*1.6	*1.6
Geographic Region[10]								
Northeast	17.2	16.6	16.1	16.5	5.1	4.5	4.5	6.1
Midwest	18.2	19.5	18.9	16.4	5.6	7.2	5.8	4.7
South	19.4	19.5	19.7	16.4	6.1	6.3	6.3	4.7
West	16.5	16.4	15.0	15.3	4.4	4.4	4.3	4.5
Location of Residence[10]								
Within MSA[9]	17.8	17.8	17.4	15.9	5.2	5.4	5.2	4.8
Outside MSA[9]	19.1	19.6	19.2	17.3	6.3	6.9	6.2	5.6

* = Figure does not meet standards of reliability or precision.
— = Data not available.
[1]These estimates exclude hospitalizations for institutionalized persons and those who died while hospitalized.
[2]Includes all other races not shown separately, unknown health insurance status, and unknown disability status.
[3]Estimates are for persons 1 year of age and over and are age-adjusted to the year 2000 standard population using six age groups: 1–17 years, 18–44 years, 45–54 years, 55–64 years, 65–74 years, and 75 years and over.
[4]Estimates are for persons 1–64 years of age and are age-adjusted to the year 2000 standard population using four age groups: 1–17 years, 18–44 years, 45–54 years, and 55–64 years. The disability measure is age-adjusted using the three adult age groups.
[5]The race groups, White, Black, American Indian or Alaska Native, Asian, Native Hawaiian or Other Pacific Islander, and 2 or more races, include persons of Hispanic and non-Hispanic origin. Persons of Hispanic origin may be of any race.
[6]Percent of poverty level is based on family income and family size and composition using U.S. Census Bureau poverty thresholds.
[7]Health insurance categories are mutually exclusive. Persons who reported both Medicaid and private coverage are classified as having private coverage.
[8]Any basic actions difficulty or complex activity limitation is defined as having one or more of the following limitations or difficulties: movement difficulty, emotional difficulty, sensory (seeing or hearing) difficulty, cognitive difficulty, self-care (activities of daily living or instrumental activities of daily living) limitation, social limitation, or work limitation.
[9]MSA = metropolitan statistical area.
[10]Estimates are for persons 65 years of age and over and are age-adjusted.

Table C-57. Discharges, Days of Care, and Average Length of Stay in Nonfederal Short-Stay Hospitals, by Selected Characteristics, Selected Years, 1980 through 2008–2009

(Number per 10,000 population, number.)

Characteristic	1980[1]	1985[1]	1990	1995	2000	2005	2006	2007	2008[2]	2009[2]	2008–2009[2]
DISCHARGES PER 10,000 POPULATION											
Total, age-adjusted[3]	1,744.5	1,522.3	1,252.4	1,180.2	1,132.8	1,162.4	1,153.1	1,124.0	1,150.3	1,149.3	1,149.8
Total, crude	1,676.8	1,484.1	1,222.7	1,157.4	1,128.3	1,174.4	1,168.7	1,143.9	1,178.6	1,181.2	1,179.9
Age											
Under 18 years	756.5	614.0	463.5	423.7	402.6	411.0	393.9	376.7	343.3	340.2	341.8
Under 1 year	2,317.6	2,137.9	1,915.3	1,977.6	2,027.6	1,949.3	1,818.4	1,639.3	1,657.5	1,550.7	1,604.5
1–4 years	864.6	650.2	466.9	457.1	458.0	429.7	418.8	389.9	337.1	335.2	336.1
5–17 years	609.3	477.4	334.1	290.2	268.6	286.5	276.0	271.5	238.2	244.9	241.6
18–44 years	1,578.8	1,301.2	1,026.6	914.3	849.4	898.0	906.7	888.8	884.6	886.7	885.7
18–24 years	1,570.3	1,297.8	1,065.3	928.9	854.1	862.4	870.4	846.1	817.0	811.8	814.4
25–44 years	1,582.8	1,302.5	1,013.8	909.9	847.9	910.3	919.3	903.8	908.6	914.0	911.3
25–34 years	1,682.9	1,416.9	1,140.3	1,015.0	942.5	1,007.8	1,011.2	1,003.5	1,003.8	998.1	1,001.0
35–44 years	1,438.3	1,153.1	868.8	808.0	764.8	821.5	834.6	810.4	817.4	830.2	823.7
45–64 years	1,947.6	1,707.8	1,354.5	1,185.4	1,114.2	1,147.0	1,161.2	1,143.9	1,197.6	1,221.3	1,209.6
45–54 years	1,750.2	1,470.7	1,123.9	984.7	920.8	964.3	970.5	959.3	1,033.3	1,021.8	1,027.6
55–64 years	2,153.6	1,948.0	1,632.6	1,483.4	1,415.0	1,402.4	1,422.1	1,391.2	1,413.8	1,476.6	1,445.7
65 years and over	3,836.9	3,698.0	3,341.2	3,477.4	3,533.6	3,595.6	3,507.9	3,395.1	3,576.5	3,521.5	3,548.8
65–74 years	3,158.4	2,972.6	2,616.3	2,600.0	2,546.0	2,628.9	2,533.6	2,439.9	2,531.3	2,554.9	2,543.3
75 years and over	4,893.0	4,756.1	4,340.3	4,590.7	4,619.6	4,588.4	4,512.6	4,392.4	4,698.4	4,591.7	4,645.0
75–84 years	4,638.6	4,464.2	3,957.0	4,155.7	4,124.4	4,131.7	4,025.9	3,983.3	4,213.1	4,068.0	4,140.2
85 years and over	5,764.6	5,728.9	5,606.3	5,925.1	6,050.9	5,758.1	5,711.4	5,358.9	5,803.2	5,814.6	5,808.9
Sex[3]											
Male	1,543.9	1,382.5	1,130.0	1,048.5	990.8	1,013.0	1,000.5	973.8	997.3	1,004.3	1,000.9
Female	1,951.9	1,675.6	1,389.5	1,317.3	1,277.3	1,319.6	1,312.3	1,280.6	1,311.8	1,303.4	1,307.6
Sex and Age											
Male, all ages	1,390.4	1,240.2	1,002.2	941.7	910.6	959.0	954.9	936.7	964.9	978.8	971.9
Under 18 years	762.6	626.4	463.1	431.3	408.6	412.2	401.5	385.6	353.1	348.0	350.5
18–44 years	950.9	776.9	579.2	507.2	450.0	471.1	476.8	460.8	439.3	456.0	447.6
45–64 years	1,953.1	1,775.6	1,402.7	1,212.0	1,127.4	1,148.8	1,175.7	1,156.6	1,214.1	1,235.4	1,224.8
65–74 years	3,474.1	3,255.2	2,877.6	2,762.2	2,649.1	2,742.6	2,584.3	2,559.3	2,601.6	2,678.2	2,640.6
75–84 years	5,093.5	5,031.8	4,417.3	4,361.1	4,294.1	4,388.1	4,220.3	4,162.6	4,498.4	4,242.3	4,369.0
85 years and over	6,372.3	6,406.9	6,420.9	6,387.9	6,166.6	5,984.1	5,983.5	5,440.6	6,003.9	6,425.5	6,210.0
Female, all ages	1,944.0	1,712.2	1,431.7	1,362.9	1,336.6	1,382.2	1,375.3	1,344.0	1,385.2	1,377.2	1,381.2
Under 18 years	750.2	601.0	464.1	415.7	396.2	409.8	385.9	367.3	333.1	332.0	332.5
18–44 years	2,180.2	1,808.3	1,468.0	1,318.0	1,248.1	1,330.9	1,343.5	1,324.5	1,338.7	1,326.4	1,332.5
45–64 years	1,942.5	1,645.9	1,309.7	1,160.5	1,101.7	1,145.3	1,147.3	1,131.7	1,182.0	1,207.8	1,195.0
65–74 years	2,916.6	2,754.8	2,411.2	2,469.4	2,461.0	2,533.1	2,490.7	2,338.4	2,471.3	2,449.3	2,460.1
75–84 years	4,370.4	4,130.4	3,678.9	4,024.1	4,013.5	3,957.7	3,893.0	3,859.8	4,015.1	3,944.7	3,979.9
85 years and over	5,500.3	5,458.0	5,289.6	5,743.7	6,003.3	5,654.4	5,584.1	5,320.0	5,706.2	5,531.7	5,619.1
Geographic Region[3]											
Northeast	1,622.9	1,428.7	1,332.2	1,335.3	1,274.8	1,245.9	1,261.4	1,274.6	1,283.7	1,361.0	1,322.5
Midwest	1,925.2	1,584.7	1,287.5	1,132.8	1,109.2	1,174.9	1,168.0	1,125.5	1,172.1	1,153.7	1,162.8
South	1,814.1	1,569.4	1,325.0	1,252.4	1,209.2	1,202.5	1,198.8	1,139.9	1,179.0	1,149.3	1,164.1
West	1,519.7	1,469.6	1,006.6	967.4	894.0	1,005.9	964.1	966.0	960.2	959.2	959.7
DAYS OF CARE PER 10,000 POPULATION											
Total, age-adjusted[3]	13,027.0	10,017.9	8,189.3	6,386.2	5,576.8	5,541.7	5,474.7	5,404.1	5,577.2	5,536.3	5,556.9
Total, crude	12,166.8	9,576.6	7,840.5	6,201.7	5,546.5	5,620.9	5,577.8	5,539.4	5,773.9	5,748.1	5,760.9
Age											
Under 18 years	3,415.1	2,812.3	2,263.1	1,846.7	1,789.7	1,918.3	1,857.6	1,785.0	1,482.8	1,491.6	1,487.2
Under 1 year	13,213.9	14,141.2	11,484.7	10,834.5	11,524.0	12,131.6	11,624.2	8,466.7	9,401.0	9,277.7	9,339.7
1–4 years	3,333.5	2,280.4	1,700.1	1,525.6	1,482.2	1,355.3	1,405.4	1,280.3	1,018.8	1,041.0	1,030.0
5–17 years	2,698.5	2,049.8	1,633.2	1,240.3	1,172.1	1,300.9	1,239.1	1,406.4	984.0	1,012.6	998.3
18–44 years	8,323.6	6,294.7	4,676.7	3,517.2	3,093.8	3,305.0	3,360.6	3,258.0	3,180.3	3,268.3	3,224.4
18–24 years	7,174.6	5,287.2	4,015.9	2,987.4	2,679.5	2,819.9	2,889.4	2,738.7	2,606.0	2,755.3	2,681.4
25–44 years	8,861.4	6,685.2	4,895.5	3,676.4	3,225.5	3,472.8	3,524.5	3,439.7	3,383.8	3,454.9	3,419.3
25–34 years	8,497.5	6,688.9	4,939.7	3,536.1	3,161.7	3,434.3	3,462.2	3,423.1	3,462.0	3,482.0	3,472.1
35–44 years	9,386.6	6,680.4	4,844.8	3,832.3	3,281.5	3,507.9	3,581.9	3,455.2	3,308.9	3,428.0	3,367.8
45–64 years	15,969.5	12,015.9	9,139.3	6,574.5	5,515.4	5,717.3	5,793.0	5,868.2	6,284.3	6,184.5	6,234.0
45–54 years	13,167.2	9,692.8	6,996.6	5,162.0	4,374.2	4,711.2	4,667.4	4,745.9	5,185.7	4,772.0	4,978.3
55–64 years	18,895.4	14,369.5	11,722.6	8,671.6	7,290.8	7,124.0	7,333.6	7,371.8	7,729.7	7,993.0	7,863.5
65 years and over	40,983.5	32,279.7	28,956.1	23,736.5	21,118.9	19,882.8	19,197.5	18,951.7	20,391.2	19,933.0	20,160.1
65–74 years	31,470.3	24,373.3	20,878.2	16,847.0	14,389.7	13,985.3	13,170.2	13,274.8	13,911.2	13,888.2	13,899.5
75 years and over	55,788.2	43,812.7	40,090.8	32,478.1	28,518.6	25,939.4	25,413.1	24,878.5	27,347.0	26,625.9	26,986.2
75–84 years	51,836.2	40,521.6	35,995.1	28,947.5	25,397.8	23,155.3	22,671.7	22,658.1	24,400.0	23,644.1	24,020.1
85 years and over	69,332.0	54,782.4	53,616.9	43,305.9	37,537.8	33,071.5	32,165.5	30,124.5	34,055.6	33,588.7	33,824.0

Table C-57. Discharges, Days of Care, and Average Length of Stay in Nonfederal Short-Stay Hospitals, by Selected Characteristics, Selected Years, 1980 through 2008-2009—*Continued*

(Number per 10,000 population, number.)

Characteristic	1980[1]	1985[1]	1990	1995	2000	2005	2006	2007	2008[2]	2009[2]	2008-2009[2]
Sex[3]											
Male	12,475.8	9,792.1	8,057.8	6,239.0	5,358.8	5,301.3	5,208.8	5,157.4	5,376.4	5,342.4	5,359.7
Female	13,662.9	10,340.4	8,404.5	6,548.8	5,809.7	5,828.7	5,764.2	5,685.1	5,832.4	5,784.1	5,808.2
Sex and Age											
Male, all ages	10,674.1	8,518.8	6,943.0	5,507.5	4,860.8	4,979.7	4,947.3	4,937.6	5,176.0	5,178.1	5,177.0
Under 18 years	3,473.1	2,942.7	2,335.7	1,998.0	1,955.7	2,006.2	1,968.0	1,858.1	1,646.9	1,526.4	1,586.4
18–44 years	6,102.4	4,746.6	3,517.4	2,729.7	2,175.0	2,282.7	2,375.6	2,241.8	2,045.7	2,203.9	2,124.9
45–64 years	15,894.9	12,290.1	9,434.2	6,822.7	5,704.4	5,773.5	6,004.3	6,103.5	6,553.3	6,443.8	6,498.1
65–74 years	33,697.6	26,220.5	22,515.5	17,697.4	14,897.4	14,502.6	13,262.1	13,666.7	14,473.2	14,915.8	14,698.4
75–84 years	54,723.3	44,087.4	38,257.8	29,642.6	26,616.7	25,106.9	23,972.7	23,894.6	26,208.6	24,959.5	25,577.6
85 years and over	77,013.1	58,609.5	60,347.3	45,263.6	37,765.3	35,179.0	32,604.0	31,480.6	37,292.7	37,649.7	37,467.3
Female, all ages	13,560.1	10,566.3	8,691.1	6,863.4	6,202.7	6,239.5	6,186.8	6,121.1	6,352.3	6,300.0	6,326.0
Under 18 years	3,354.5	2,675.5	2,186.8	1,687.9	1,615.1	1,826.1	1,741.8	1,708.3	1,310.9	1,455.1	1,383.3
18–44 years	10,450.7	7,792.0	5,820.3	4,297.9	4,010.8	4,341.8	4,361.5	4,292.3	4,337.0	4,354.8	4,345.9
45–64 years	16,037.1	11,765.5	8,865.1	6,341.7	5,336.4	5,663.9	5,592.2	5,644.3	6,028.1	5,937.5	5,982.4
65–74 years	29,764.7	22,949.2	19,592.7	16,162.0	13,971.3	13,549.0	13,092.4	12,942.1	13,431.6	13,007.9	13,216.5
75–84 years	50,133.3	38,424.7	34,628.3	28,502.5	24,601.0	21,830.1	21,782.1	21,806.2	23,144.7	22,713.5	22,928.9
85 years and over	65,990.5	53,253.6	51,000.5	42,538.6	37,444.4	32,103.5	31,960.3	29,479.5	32,492.0	31,707.4	32,100.2
Geographic Region[3]											
Northeast	14,024.4	11,143.1	10,266.8	8,389.7	7,185.9	6,636.5	6,608.5	7,284.4	7,055.4	7,512.7	7,285.5
Midwest	14,871.9	10,803.6	8,306.5	5,908.8	5,005.3	4,954.3	4,893.5	4,775.3	5,176.9	4,990.1	5,083.1
South	12,713.5	9,642.6	8,204.1	6,659.9	5,925.1	5,830.4	5,844.8	5,555.7	5,667.9	5,610.4	5,639.3
West	9,635.2	8,300.7	5,755.1	4,510.6	4,082.0	4,690.3	4,451.6	4,184.5	4,528.7	4,241.2	4,383.6
AVERAGE LENGTH OF STAY IN DAYS											
Total, age-adjusted[3]	7.5	6.6	6.5	5.4	4.9	4.8	4.7	4.8	4.8	4.8	4.8
Total, crude	7.3	6.5	6.4	5.4	4.9	4.8	4.8	4.8	4.9	4.9	4.9
Age											
Under 18 years	4.5	4.6	4.9	4.4	4.4	4.7	4.7	4.7	4.3	4.4	4.4
Under 1 year	5.7	6.6	6.0	5.5	5.7	6.2	6.4	5.2	5.7	6.0	5.8
1–4 years	3.9	3.5	3.6	3.3	3.2	3.2	3.4	3.3	3.0	3.1	3.1
5–17 years	4.4	4.3	4.9	4.3	4.4	4.5	4.5	5.2	4.1	4.1	4.1
18–44 years	5.3	4.8	4.6	3.8	3.6	3.7	3.7	3.7	3.6	3.7	3.6
18–24 years	4.6	4.1	3.8	3.2	3.1	3.3	3.3	3.2	3.2	3.4	3.3
25–44 years	5.6	5.1	4.8	4.0	3.8	3.8	3.8	3.8	3.7	3.8	3.8
25–34 years	5.0	4.7	4.3	3.5	3.4	3.4	3.4	3.4	3.4	3.5	3.5
35–44 years	6.5	5.8	5.6	4.7	4.3	4.3	4.3	4.3	4.0	4.1	4.1
45–64 years	8.2	7.0	6.7	5.5	5.0	5.0	5.0	5.1	5.2	5.1	5.2
45–54 years	7.5	6.6	6.2	5.2	4.8	4.9	4.8	4.9	5.0	4.7	4.8
55–64 years	8.8	7.4	7.2	5.8	5.2	5.1	5.2	5.3	5.5	5.4	5.4
65 years and over	10.7	8.7	8.7	6.8	6.0	5.5	5.5	5.6	5.7	5.7	5.7
65–74 years	10.0	8.2	8.0	6.5	5.7	5.3	5.2	5.4	5.5	5.4	5.5
75 years and over	11.4	9.2	9.2	7.1	6.2	5.7	5.6	5.7	5.8	5.8	5.8
75–84 years	11.2	9.1	9.1	7.0	6.2	5.6	5.6	5.7	5.8	5.8	5.8
85 years and over	12.0	9.6	9.6	7.3	6.2	5.7	5.6	5.6	5.9	5.8	5.8
Sex[3]											
Male	8.1	7.1	7.1	6.0	5.4	5.2	5.2	5.3	5.4	5.3	5.4
Female	7.0	6.2	6.0	5.0	4.5	4.4	4.4	4.4	4.4	4.4	4.4
Sex and Age											
Male, all ages	7.7	6.9	6.9	5.8	5.3	5.2	5.2	5.3	5.4	5.3	5.3
Under 18 years	4.6	4.7	5.0	4.6	4.8	4.9	4.9	4.8	4.7	4.4	4.5
18–44 years	6.4	6.1	6.1	5.4	4.8	4.8	5.0	4.9	4.7	4.8	4.7
45–64 years	8.1	6.9	6.7	5.6	5.1	5.0	5.1	5.3	5.4	5.2	5.3
65–74 years	9.7	8.1	7.8	6.4	5.6	5.3	5.1	5.3	5.6	5.6	5.6
75–84 years	10.7	8.8	8.7	6.8	6.2	5.7	5.7	5.7	5.8	5.9	5.9
85 years and over	12.1	9.1	9.4	7.1	6.1	5.9	5.4	5.8	6.2	5.9	6.0

Table C-57. Discharges, Days of Care, and Average Length of Stay in Nonfederal Short-Stay Hospitals, by Selected Characteristics, Selected Years, 1980 through 2008–2009—Continued

(Number per 10,000 population, number.)

Characteristic	1980[1]	1985[1]	1990	1995	2000	2005	2006	2007	2008[2]	2009[2]	2008–2009[2]
Female, all ages	7.0	6.2	6.1	5.0	4.6	4.5	4.5	4.6	4.6	4.6	4.6
Under 18 years	4.5	4.5	4.7	4.1	4.1	4.5	4.5	4.7	3.9	4.4	4.2
18–44 years	4.8	4.3	4.0	3.3	3.2	3.3	3.2	3.2	3.2	3.3	3.3
45–64 years	8.3	7.1	6.8	5.5	4.8	4.9	4.9	5.0	5.1	4.9	5.0
65–74 years	10.2	8.3	8.1	6.5	5.7	5.3	5.3	5.5	5.4	5.3	5.4
75–84 years	11.5	9.3	9.4	7.1	6.1	5.5	5.6	5.6	5.8	5.8	5.8
85 years and over	12.0	9.8	9.6	7.4	6.2	5.7	5.7	5.5	5.7	5.7	5.7
Geographic Region[3]											
Northeast	8.6	7.8	7.7	6.3	5.6	5.3	5.2	5.7	5.5	5.5	5.5
Midwest	7.7	6.8	6.5	5.2	4.5	4.2	4.2	4.2	4.4	4.3	4.4
South	7.0	6.1	6.2	5.3	4.9	4.8	4.9	4.9	4.8	4.9	4.8
West	6.3	5.6	5.7	4.7	4.6	4.7	4.6	4.3	4.7	4.4	4.6

[1]Comparisons of data from 1980–1985 with data from subsequent years should be made with caution because estimates of change may reflect improvements in the survey design rather than true changes in hospital use.
[2]Starting with 2008 data, the sample of nonfederal short-stay hospitals was cut in half. This smaller sample size has increased standard errors. Therefore, caution should be exercised in interpreting trends in these data.
[3]Estimates are age-adjusted to the year 2000 standard population using six age groups: under 18 years, 18–44 years, 45–54 years, 55–64 years, 65–74 years, and 75 years and over.

Table C-58. Discharges in Nonfederal Short-Stay Hospitals, by Sex, Age, and Selected First-Listed Diagnosis, Selected Years, 1990 through 2008–2009

(Number in thousands.)

Age and first-listed diagnosis	Both sexes			Male			Female		
	1990	1995	2009[1]	1990	1995	2009[1]	1990	1995	2009[1]
ALL AGES[2]	30,788	30,722	36,120	12,280	12,198	14,721	18,508	18,525	21,398
Under 18 Years[2]	3,072	3,002	*2,536	1,572	1,565	*1,327	1,500	1,437	*1,209
Dehydration	63	106	*73	32	59	*39	31	47	*34
Acute bronchitis and bronchiolitis	114	170	*109	67	109	*70	47	61	*40
Pneumonia	221	250	170	126	143	*86	95	107	*84
Asthma	182	227	*143	111	137	*92	71	90	*50
Appendicitis	83	69	*76	50	41	*47	34	28	29
Injury	329	286	161	210	171	*96	119	115	*65
Fracture	117	102	*67	76	66	*42	42	36	*25
Complications of care and adverse effects	41	46	*43	22	25	*23	19	*21	*20
18–44 Years[2]	11,138	9,996	9,963	3,120	2,761	2,588	8,018	7,235	7,375
HIV/AIDS	*20	88	23	*15	66	*17	*	22	*6
Cancer, all	181	150	113	64	47	*35	116	102	77
Childbirth							3,815	3,574	3,862
Uterine fibroids							110	115	81
Diabetes	105	102	159	61	52	79	44	50	80
Alcohol and drug	284	363	224	199	255	152	84	107	71
Schizophrenia, mood disorders, delusional disorders, nonorganic psychoses	384	551	544	184	262	268	200	289	276
Schizophrenia	145	*181	148	88	*118	88	57	63	*61
Mood disorders	211	324	359	83	121	160	128	203	199
Heart disease	236	265	239	163	157	144	73	108	95
Ischemic heart disease	129	130	72	95	90	48	34	39	*25
Pneumonia	136	149	126	69	74	59	67	75	67
Asthma	106	119	90	27	30	*28	79	89	62
Intervertebral disc disorders	222	157	105	138	94	53	84	62	52
Injury	935	688	555	641	465	359	294	223	196
Fracture	302	250	221	217	176	162	85	74	59
Poisoning and toxic effects	124	118	134	54	59	58	70	59	76
Complications of care and adverse effects	135	146	195	63	64	81	72	82	114
45–64 Years[2]	6,244	6,168	9,686	3,115	3,053	4,781	3,129	3,115	4,906
HIV/AIDS	*3	20	*16	*3	15	*12	*	*5	*4
Cancer, all	545	461	525	236	193	255	309	268	269
Colorectal cancer	59	29	66	33	17	32	26	13	34
Lung/bronchus/tracheal cancer	101	76	68	60	37	31	41	39	*37
Breast cancer[3]	X	X	X	X	X	X	69	61	48
Prostate cancer	X	X	X	19	32	*57	X	X	X
Uterine fibroids	X	X	X	X	X	X	70	74	93
Diabetes	134	172	256	65	86	124	70	86	132
Alcohol and drug	100	128	191	77	100	138	23	28	53
Schizophrenia, mood disorders, delusional disorders, nonorganic psychoses	152	194	384	56	75	177	95	118	207
Schizophrenia	47	*67	119	19	*	*66	28	36	54
Mood disorders	91	112	241	32	37	98	58	74	142
Heart disease	1,100	1,152	1,204	704	749	756	397	403	448
Ischemic heart disease	739	762	579	502	537	393	237	225	187
Heart attack	233	256	205	165	188	144	68	68	61
Arrhythmias	131	131	186	79	75	115	53	56	71
Heart failure	122	143	271	68	75	161	54	68	111
Hypertension	75	82	155	38	37	76	37	45	80
Stroke	162	182	275	91	96	149	72	86	126
Pneumonia	154	163	264	76	75	141	79	88	122
Chronic obstructive pulmonary disease	73	154	236	39	72	95	34	82	141
Asthma	86	87	132	26	21	40	59	66	93
Osteoarthritis	87	110	476	36	47	211	51	64	265
Intervertebral disc disorders	145	115	167	82	65	85	63	51	81
Injury	334	296	441	178	165	229	157	131	211
Fracture	149	147	211	74	74	109	75	72	102
Poisoning and toxic effects	29	30	101	10	13	44	19	17	57
Internal organ injury	36	38	64	23	27	36	14	11	*28
Complications of care and adverse effects	148	186	402	79	92	204	69	94	198

Table C-58. Discharges in Nonfederal Short-Stay Hospitals, by Sex, Age, and Selected First-Listed Diagnosis, Selected Years, 1990 through 2008-2009—Continued

(Number in thousands.)

Age and first-listed diagnosis	Both sexes			Male			Female		
	1990	1995	2009[1]	1990	1995	2009[1]	1990	1995	2009[1]
65-74 Years[2]	4,689	4,832	5,312	2,268	2,290	2,569	2,421	2,542	2,743
Septicemia	49	65	139	27	27	67	21	38	72
Cancer, all	436	416	326	222	203	178	214	212	147
Colorectal cancer	48	46	43	24	22	*23	24	24	*20
Lung/bronchus/tracheal cancer	77	73	61	50	44	*34	26	29	27
Breast cancer[3]	X	X	X	X	X	X	42	35	*21
Prostate cancer	X	X	X	40	41	*34	X	X	X
Diabetes	93	93	107	34	44	45	59	49	61
Schizophrenia, mood disorders, delusional disorders, nonorganic psychoses	59	80	*65	20	20	*26	39	60	*38
Dementia and Alzheimer's disease	10	18	*14	4	11	*	*6	7	*
Heart disease	1,000	1,115	888	547	618	514	453	497	375
Ischemic heart disease	576	614	389	331	365	241	245	250	148
Heart attack	185	210	138	110	129	83	75	82	54
Arrhythmias	124	153	176	67	74	97	57	79	79
Heart failure	188	233	209	93	126	114	95	107	95
Hypertension	39	42	*77	13	14	*32	26	28	*45
Stroke	222	250	225	108	141	125	114	109	100
Pneumonia	176	214	174	90	105	79	86	109	95
Chronic obstructive pulmonary disease	81	191	211	41	83	96	40	107	115
Gallstones	79	78	49	30	31	25	49	46	23
Kidney disease	18	31	121	9	16	65	9	15	56
Urinary tract infection	54	50	82	17	20	29	37	30	53
Hyperplasia of the prostate	X	X	X	113	62	*23	X	X	X
Osteoarthritis	122	154	308	44	53	115	78	101	193
Injury	193	176	201	71	67	80	122	109	121
Fracture	120	109	121	36	36	37	85	72	84
Hip fracture	48	44	40	12	15	12	36	29	*28
Complications of care and adverse effects	125	144	204	68	66	107	57	78	97
75-84 Years[2]	3,949	4,590	5,349	1,660	1,880	2,311	2,289	2,710	3,038
Septicemia	54	87	171	24	38	81	30	50	90
Cancer, all	300	281	236	158	131	108	142	150	128
Colorectal cancer	50	46	39	20	22	*15	29	24	24
Lung/bronchus/tracheal cancer	36	32	44	22	17	*21	*15	15	23
Breast cancer[3]	*	*	*	*	*	*	24	24	*10
Prostate cancer	*	*	*	37	18	*5	*	*	*
Diabetes	44	73	100	17	30	39	27	43	*60
Schizophrenia, mood disorders, delusional disorders, nonorganic psychoses	39	44	*	*10	10	*	28	35	*23
Dementia and Alzheimer's disease	20	46	53	9	19	*29	11	26	*25
Heart disease	865	1,057	1,025	377	471	480	488	585	545
Ischemic heart disease	382	479	358	177	228	189	205	251	169
Heart attack	156	188	165	83	91	79	73	97	86
Arrhythmias	133	175	241	58	83	99	76	92	143
Heart failure	261	290	296	108	116	132	153	174	164
Hypertension	23	31	64	*	*11	*21	19	20	43
Stroke	258	297	258	104	129	123	154	169	135
Pneumonia	224	282	234	112	142	109	112	140	124
Chronic obstructive pulmonary disease	55	143	181	34	63	86	22	80	94
Gallstones	48	55	51	20	22	20	28	33	*31
Kidney disease	24	28	143	10	17	70	*14	12	73
Urinary tract infection	86	99	158	25	35	46	61	64	112
Hyperplasia of the prostate	X	X	X	69	41	*21	X	X	X
Osteoarthritis	69	115	205	25	34	80	44	80	125
Injury	259	270	306	58	77	104	201	193	202
Fracture	195	208	211	35	53	60	161	154	151
Hip fracture	115	122	83	20	29	20	95	93	63
Complications of care and adverse effects	81	108	159	38	40	81	43	68	78

Table C-58. Discharges in Nonfederal Short-Stay Hospitals, by Sex, Age, and Selected First-Listed Diagnosis, Selected Years, 1990 through 2008–2009—Continued

(Number in thousands.)

Age and first-listed diagnosis	Both sexes			Male			Female		
	1990	1995	2009[1]	1990	1995	2009[1]	1990	1995	2009[1]
85 Years and Over[2]	1,694	2,134	3,274	543	648	1,145	1,151	1,486	2,129
Septicemia	41	57	134	12	17	52	29	40	82
Cancer, all	77	77	94	31	32	43	45	45	51
Colorectal cancer	14	17	*12	*5	*	*	9	11	*7
Lung/bronchus/tracheal cancer	*6	*4	*13	*	*2	*	*	*	*
Breast cancer[3]	X	X	X	X	X	X	*9	8	*
Prostate cancer	X	X	X	*7	X	X	X	X	X
Diabetes	16	22	*34	*5	*	*13	11	15	*21
Schizophrenia, mood disorders, delusional disorders, nonorganic psychoses	*8	16	*	*	*	*	*7	*12	*
Dementia and Alzheimer's disease	15	28	42	*2	*6	16	13	22	26
Heart disease	335	446	611	112	135	236	223	311	376
Ischemic heart disease	128	144	139	49	48	62	79	96	76
Heart attack	60	73	88	23	28	37	37	44	51
Arrhythmias	51	72	127	16	20	37	35	51	90
Heart failure	126	181	263	39	52	101	87	129	162
Hypertension	*5	8	37	*	*	*12	*4	*6	*25
Stroke	129	156	162	35	42	48	95	114	114
Pneumonia	151	194	207	64	73	74	88	121	134
Chronic obstructive pulmonary disease	13	39	81	*6	18	*28	*7	21	53
Gallstones	18	21	*24	*6	*7	*7	13	15	*17
Kidney disease	14	16	90	8	*8	36	*6	*9	54
Urinary tract infection	65	74	195	20	*18	46	45	56	149
Hyperplasia of the prostate	X	X	X	13	9	*6	*	*	*
Osteoarthritis	13	20	36	*	*6	*10	8	14	26
Injury	164	216	300	37	47	78	127	169	223
Fracture	133	172	227	28	32	54	104	140	173
Hip fracture	82	108	123	19	19	29	63	88	94
Complications of care and adverse effects	29	29	75	11	*10	*27	18	19	48

* = Figure does not meet standards of reliability or precision.
X = Category not applicable.
[1] Starting with 2008 data, the sample of nonfederal short-stay hospitals was cut in half. This smaller sample size has increased standard errors. Therefore, caution should be exercised in interpreting trends in these data.
[2] Includes discharges with first-listed diagnoses not shown in table.
[3] Shown for women only.

Table C-59. Discharge Rate in Nonfederal Short-Stay Hospitals, by Sex, Age, and Selected First-Listed Diagnosis, Selected Years, 1990 through 2008–2009

(Number per 10,000 population.)

Age and first-listed diagnosis	Both sexes			Male			Female		
	1990	2000	2008–2009[1]	1990	2000	2008–2009[1]	1990	2000	2008–2009[1]
All Ages, Age-Adjusted[2,3]	1,252.4	1,132.8	1,149.8	1,130.0	990.8	1,000.9	1,389.5	1,277.3	1,307.6
All Ages, Crude[3]	1,222.7	1,128.3	1,179.9	1,002.2	910.6	971.9	1,431.7	1,336.6	1,381.2
Under 18 Years[3]	463.5	402.6	*341.8	463.1	408.6	*350.5	464.1	396.2	*332.5
Dehydration	9.5	15.7	10.0	9.4	17.2	*10.6	9.7	14.2	9.3
Acute bronchitis and bronchiolitis	17.2	27.8	15.2	19.6	31.4	18.4	14.6	24.1	*11.8
Pneumonia	33.3	25.2	21.9	37.0	25.7	*23.8	29.5	24.6	19.8
Asthma	27.5	29.6	*18.6	32.7	34.8	*23.0	22.0	24.0	*14.0
Appendicitis	12.6	11.9	*11.2	14.6	13.0	*13.9	10.5	10.8	*8.4
Injury	49.7	33.6	24.7	62.0	42.0	*29.8	36.8	24.8	19.4
Fracture	17.7	13.8	10.2	22.3	18.3	13.5	12.9	9.0	*6.8
Complications of care and adverse effects	6.2	*7.3	*5.7	6.5	*7.9	*6.6	5.9	*6.6	*4.6
18–44 Years[3]	1,026.6	849.4	885.7	579.2	450.0	447.6	1,468.0	1,248.1	1,332.5
HIV/AIDS	*1.8	4.3	2.5	*2.8	5.8	3.4	*	2.8	*1.5
Cancer, all	16.6	10.5	10.3	11.9	7.3	7.2	21.3	13.7	13.5
Childbirth	*	*	*	*	*	*	698.6	645.2	707.4
Uterine fibroids	*	*	*	*	*	*	20.2	21.7	17.0
Diabetes	9.7	11.5	14.1	11.3	13.0	14.2	8.1	9.9	14.0
Alcohol and drug	26.2	29.7	18.5	37.0	39.1	23.9	15.5	*20.2	13.0
Schizophrenia, mood disorders, delusional disorders, nonorganic psychoses	35.4	*53.6	49.0	34.1	*53.2	46.8	36.7	*53.9	51.2
Schizophrenia	13.4	*14.4	13.4	16.4	*18.6	16.0	10.5	*10.1	10.8
Mood disorders	19.4	*35.9	32.8	15.4	*31.0	27.9	23.4	*40.9	37.9
Heart disease	21.7	21.8	22.2	30.2	26.6	26.6	13.4	17.0	17.8
Ischemic heart disease	11.9	9.9	7.3	17.7	14.2	9.5	6.3	5.6	5.2
Pneumonia	12.5	10.9	10.3	12.8	10.0	9.3	12.2	11.9	11.4
Asthma	9.8	9.0	7.9	5.1	5.4	4.5	14.4	12.6	11.3
Intervertebral disc disorders	20.5	12.5	10.3	25.6	14.5	9.9	15.4	10.4	10.7
Injury	86.2	45.8	50.3	119.0	62.3	66.9	53.8	29.4	33.4
Fracture	27.8	17.8	20.4	40.2	25.4	30.2	15.5	10.2	10.5
Poisoning and toxic effects	11.4	8.5	12.0	10.0	6.7	11.3	12.7	10.3	12.8
Complications of care and adverse effects	12.5	12.2	16.2	11.7	11.2	13.2	13.3	13.1	19.3
45–64 Years[3]	1,354.5	1,114.2	1,209.6	1,402.7	1,127.4	1,224.8	1,309.7	1,101.7	1,195.0
HIV/AIDS	*0.6	*3.2	2.8	*1.2	*4.9	3.4	*	*	*2.2
Cancer, all	118.3	62.9	66.5	106.3	62.1	66.4	129.5	63.6	66.6
Colorectal cancer	12.7	7.9	7.1	14.8	8.9	6.8	10.8	6.9	7.4
Lung/bronchus/tracheal cancer	21.8	6.9	8.3	26.8	8.6	8.3	17.2	5.2	8.3
Breast cancer[4]	X	X	X				29.0	14.2	10.4
Prostate cancer	X	X	X	8.5	9.6	13.8			
Uterine fibroids	X	X	X				29.3	35.6	24.8
Diabetes	29.1	33.1	29.8	29.1	37.4	31.9	29.2	29.0	27.7
Alcohol and drug	21.7	23.3	23.5	34.6	33.5	34.6	9.6	13.7	12.8
Schizophrenia, mood disorders, delusional disorders, nonorganic psychoses	32.9	42.7	49.7	25.4	*39.6	46.7	39.8	45.6	52.6
Schizophrenia	10.1	12.8	16.4	8.4	*14.4	18.2	11.7	11.3	14.8
Mood disorders	19.6	*26.9	30.8	14.5	*21.6	26.0	24.4	*32.0	35.3
Heart disease	238.7	203.6	153.4	316.8	264.0	199.3	166.1	146.4	109.7
Ischemic heart disease	160.3	126.4	74.6	226.1	177.3	104.7	99.2	78.2	46.0
Heart attack	50.6	38.8	26.9	74.4	58.7	38.9	28.4	19.9	15.6
Arrhythmias	28.5	25.1	25.8	35.5	31.8	33.0	22.1	18.7	18.9
Heart failure	26.4	31.4	31.6	30.7	33.5	38.3	22.4	29.3	25.3
Hypertension	16.3	19.0	19.8	16.9	17.6	19.9	15.6	20.3	19.8
Stroke	35.2	36.7	32.9	40.8	38.3	36.7	30.1	35.2	29.3
Pneumonia	33.5	35.3	32.9	34.0	34.2	34.7	33.0	36.4	31.2
Chronic obstructive pulmonary disease	15.8	30.8	28.4	17.4	30.8	24.0	14.3	30.8	32.6
Asthma	18.6	13.4	16.8	11.8	6.2	10.9	24.9	20.2	22.5
Osteoarthritis	18.9	24.0	55.3	16.3	20.8	49.5	21.2	27.0	60.7
Intervertebral disc disorders	31.5	21.2	20.7	36.8	22.5	21.2	26.5	20.0	20.1
Injury	72.5	47.9	57.4	79.9	51.2	65.1	65.6	44.7	50.0
Fracture	32.4	26.2	28.6	33.4	25.3	32.2	31.5	27.0	25.1
Poisoning and toxic effects	6.3	6.3	11.8	4.5	5.5	10.8	8.0	7.1	12.9
Internal organ injury	7.9	4.5	8.3	10.2	5.9	11.2	5.7	3.2	*5.6
Complications of care and adverse effects	32.0	34.5	48.8	35.6	36.3	50.2	28.7	32.7	47.5

Table C-59. Discharge Rate in Nonfederal Short-Stay Hospitals, by Sex, Age, and Selected First-Listed Diagnosis, Selected Years, 1990 through 2008–2009—Continued

(Number per 10,000 population.)

Age and first-listed diagnosis	Both sexes			Male			Female		
	1990	2000	2008–2009[1]	1990	2000	2008–2009[1]	1990	2000	2008–2009[1]
65–74 Years[3]	2,616.3	2,546.0	2,543.3	2,877.6	2,649.1	2,640.6	2,411.2	2,461.0	2,460.1
Septicemia	27.2	35.6	66.1	34.9	40.1	70.1	21.2	32.0	62.7
Cancer, all	243.1	159.0	151.2	281.4	176.4	175.1	213.0	144.7	130.8
Colorectal cancer	27.0	22.8	18.1	30.6	29.9	21.2	24.1	16.9	15.5
Lung/bronchus/tracheal cancer	42.9	26.1	27.4	63.9	28.2	30.3	26.4	24.5	24.8
Breast cancer[4]	X	X	X	X	X	X	42.3	31.2	18.9
Prostate cancer	X	X	X	50.6	37.1	31.6	X	X	X
Diabetes	51.8	46.4	49.8	43.6	46.8	47.3	58.3	46.2	52.0
Schizophrenia, mood disorders, delusional disorders, nonorganic psychoses	32.7	37.1	30.0	25.3	*34.2	24.3	38.6	39.6	*34.9
Dementia and Alzheimer's disease	5.6	*11.2	*7.0	4.9	*16.2	*7.4	*6.1	*7.0	*6.6
Heart disease	558.1	604.8	440.6	694.2	706.4	532.6	451.3	521.0	362.0
Ischemic heart disease	321.3	307.0	190.5	419.9	396.5	249.3	243.9	233.2	140.3
Heart attack	103.3	100.3	68.6	139.8	124.7	85.4	74.6	80.2	54.2
Arrhythmias	69.1	102.6	91.5	84.7	108.3	106.7	56.9	97.9	78.5
Heart failure	105.2	131.6	103.1	118.0	136.4	117.1	95.1	127.6	91.2
Hypertension	21.8	21.5	36.0	16.2	16.5	28.7	26.2	25.5	*42.2
Stroke	123.9	127.1	100.8	137.5	131.8	124.1	113.1	123.2	80.8
Pneumonia	98.1	121.3	88.0	113.6	127.7	90.9	85.9	116.1	85.5
Chronic obstructive pulmonary disease	45.3	102.3	98.6	52.6	102.6	92.1	39.6	102.0	104.2
Gallstones	44.2	33.4	27.2	38.2	30.2	29.9	48.9	36.0	24.9
Kidney disease	9.9	19.1	52.9	11.0	21.0	59.6	9.0	17.5	47.1
Urinary tract infection	30.2	25.5	39.4	21.7	19.7	28.2	36.9	30.3	48.9
Hyperplasia of the prostate	X	X	X	143.5	53.6	25.2	X	X	X
Osteoarthritis	68.0	101.4	148.4	55.2	103.1	125.8	78.0	100.1	167.8
Injury	107.7	101.5	97.7	90.7	83.8	87.5	121.1	116.2	106.4
Fracture	67.2	63.3	60.7	45.2	46.8	43.7	84.4	76.9	75.3
Hip fracture	26.7	26.4	21.0	15.3	*20.0	16.1	35.7	31.7	25.2
Complications of care and adverse effects	69.7	80.0	101.3	85.7	95.7	109.1	57.2	67.1	94.6
75–84 Years[3]	3,957.0	4,124.4	4,140.2	4,417.3	4,294.1	4,369.0	3,678.9	4,013.5	3,979.9
Septicemia	53.9	68.3	136.5	63.8	78.1	156.3	47.9	61.9	122.6
Cancer, all	300.3	194.0	189.7	420.8	211.0	221.3	227.6	182.9	167.5
Colorectal cancer	49.8	33.0	31.1	54.0	37.5	33.2	47.3	30.1	29.6
Lung/bronchus/tracheal cancer	36.5	27.0	34.7	57.2	32.2	43.2	*24.0	23.6	28.7
Breast cancer[4]	X	X	X	X	X	X	38.7	30.8	13.6
Prostate cancer	X	X	X	99.2	27.4	*15.2	X	X	X
Diabetes	44.3	63.4	71.4	44.8	68.1	68.8	44.0	60.3	73.3
Schizophrenia, mood disorders, delusional disorders, nonorganic psychoses	38.8	41.4	*	*27.3	*30.6	*	45.7	48.5	*32.2
Dementia and Alzheimer's disease	20.0	36.5	41.3	22.8	36.8	47.7	18.3	36.3	36.8
Heart disease	866.6	954.8	774.3	1,003.8	1,062.5	885.7	783.7	884.3	696.2
Ischemic heart disease	382.4	416.7	268.8	470.5	528.5	337.6	329.1	343.6	220.6
Heart attack	155.9	166.9	123.3	220.9	212.8	138.9	116.7	136.9	112.3
Arrhythmias	133.4	176.8	181.0	153.3	174.4	189.0	121.4	178.3	175.3
Heart failure	261.4	263.1	220.8	286.2	271.0	246.5	246.4	257.9	202.8
Hypertension	22.6	39.7	42.4	*	*28.4	*32.9	30.7	47.1	49.0
Stroke	259.0	255.5	208.0	277.7	278.4	230.8	247.7	240.6	191.9
Pneumonia	224.6	263.5	199.9	297.8	310.8	221.7	180.4	232.6	184.6
Chronic obstructive pulmonary disease	55.4	146.2	143.8	89.4	179.6	160.0	34.8	124.3	132.4
Gallstones	47.6	39.6	39.4	51.9	41.4	41.2	45.0	38.5	38.1
Kidney disease	24.5	37.6	104.8	27.6	48.7	132.0	*22.6	30.4	85.8
Urinary tract infection	86.0	85.6	120.7	66.6	72.5	86.2	97.8	94.2	144.8
Hyperplasia of the prostate	*	*	*	183.3	67.2	33.1	X	X	X
Osteoarthritis	68.6	100.6	153.8	65.2	76.5	145.4	70.7	116.4	159.7
Injury	259.1	229.1	229.6	153.4	171.7	180.6	323.0	266.6	264.0
Fracture	195.8	170.2	161.7	92.6	116.4	111.4	258.1	205.4	197.0
Hip fracture	115.2	99.0	66.6	53.7	68.6	43.7	152.4	118.8	82.7
Complications of care and adverse effects	81.5	101.4	122.4	101.4	136.0	153.1	69.4	78.8	100.9

Table C-59. Discharge Rate in Nonfederal Short-Stay Hospitals, by Sex, Age, and Selected First-Listed Diagnosis, Selected Years, 1990 through 2008–2009—*Continued*

(Number per 10,000 population.)

Age and first-listed diagnosis	Both sexes			Male			Female		
	1990	2000	2008–2009[1]	1990	2000	2008–2009[1]	1990	2000	2008–2009[1]
85 Years and Over[3]	5,606.3	6,050.9	5,808.9	6,420.9	6,166.6	6,210.0	5,289.6	6,003.3	5,619.1
Septicemia	135.6	153.9	253.9	139.0	207.3	278.8	134.3	131.9	242.2
Cancer, all	254.0	194.5	159.1	370.6	250.5	215.4	208.7	171.5	132.4
Colorectal cancer	47.6	49.7	25.6	*59.1	*58.8	*29.6	43.2	45.9	*23.7
Lung/bronchus/tracheal cancer	*19.1	12.1	*16.2	*	*20.9	*24.2	*	*8.5	*
Breast cancer[4]	X	X	X	X	X	X	*41.7	*20.5	*14.9
Prostate cancer	X	X	X	*87.8	*49.3	*20.0	X	X	X
Diabetes	53.0	65.6	60.5	*53.5	*54.2	*65.3	52.8	70.3	*58.3
Schizophrenia, mood disorders, delusional disorders, nonorganic psychoses	*27.9	*37.3	*30.6	*	*	*45.9	*30.7	*43.0	*23.3
Dementia and Alzheimer's disease	49.7	107.0	85.3	*28.9	94.3	102.0	57.7	112.2	77.4
Heart disease	1,107.0	1,298.2	1,079.2	1,320.3	1,407.4	1,277.5	1,024.1	1,253.4	985.4
Ischemic heart disease	423.0	427.2	259.4	581.6	534.4	368.8	361.3	383.2	207.6
Heart attack	199.8	251.1	160.9	274.2	296.0	206.9	170.9	232.7	139.2
Arrhythmias	167.2	232.4	224.3	189.6	247.1	209.3	158.5	226.4	231.4
Heart failure	416.7	480.4	454.0	460.5	455.7	530.1	399.7	490.5	418.1
Hypertension	*17.9	41.1	67.0	*	*18.3	*55.6	*19.3	50.4	72.3
Stroke	427.2	373.8	289.6	408.2	396.7	302.3	434.6	364.3	283.6
Pneumonia	501.0	514.9	370.1	753.7	607.8	448.3	402.8	476.8	333.0
Chronic obstructive pulmonary disease	44.1	130.9	147.6	*72.9	150.4	167.4	*32.9	123.0	138.3
Gallstones	60.7	39.2	38.9	*68.2	*29.7	39.1	57.8	*43.1	38.8
Kidney disease	47.1	49.5	157.5	92.4	*68.1	189.3	*29.4	*41.9	142.5
Urinary tract infection	216.5	191.5	289.6	239.3	153.1	194.4	207.6	207.2	334.6
Hyperplasia of the prostate	X	X	X	158.6	*69.0	*45.9	X	X	X
Osteoarthritis	44.5	56.0	70.3	*	*	*48.0	35.8	57.3	80.9
Injury	542.0	545.5	535.8	435.4	355.6	401.7	583.4	623.5	599.3
Fracture	439.0	450.9	412.7	335.7	252.4	286.0	479.2	532.4	472.7
Hip fracture	272.3	275.1	223.7	224.4	146.5	167.4	291.0	327.9	250.3
Complications of care and adverse effects	96.6	79.1	126.5	132.3	90.5	151.5	82.7	74.4	114.7

* = Figure does not meet standards of reliability or precision.
X = Category not applicable.
[1]Starting with 2008 data, the sample of nonfederal short-stay hospitals was cut in half. This smaller sample size has increased standard errors. Therefore, caution should be exercised in interpreting trends in these data.
[2]Estimates are age-adjusted to the year 2000 standard population using six age groups: under 18 years, 18–44 years, 45–54 years, 55–64 years, 65–74 years, and 75 years and over.
[3]Includes discharges with first-listed diagnoses not shown in table.
[4]Shown for women only.

Table C-60. Average Length of Stay[1] in Nonfederal Short-Stay Hospitals, by Sex, Age, and Selected First-Listed Diagnosis, Selected Years, 1990 through 2009

(Number of days.)

Age and first-listed diagnosis	Both sexes				Male				Female			
	1990	2000	2005	2009[2]	1990	2000	2005	2009[2]	1990	2000	2005	2009[2]
All Ages, Crude[3]	6.4	4.9	4.8	4.9	6.9	5.3	5.2	5.3	6.1	4.6	4.5	4.6
Under 18 Years[3]	4.9	4.4	4.7	4.4	5.0	4.8	4.9	4.4	4.7	4.1	4.5	4.4
Dehydration	3.0	2.2	2.0	2.1	2.9	2.2	2.1	2.0	3.0	2.1	2.0	2.3
Acute bronchitis and bronchiolitis	3.7	3.1	2.9	3.4	3.6	3.0	3.0	3.4	3.8	*3.3	2.9	3.3
Pneumonia	4.6	3.6	3.2	3.4	4.6	3.4	3.1	3.5	4.7	3.9	3.3	3.4
Asthma	2.9	2.2	2.3	2.5	2.8	2.1	2.3	2.3	3.1	2.3	2.2	2.7
Appendicitis	4.0	3.2	3.4	3.1	3.9	2.9	3.6	3.1	4.0	3.5	*3.1	3.2
Injury	4.1	3.8	*4.2	3.2	4.2	4.1	*4.8	2.9	3.8	*3.2	3.0	3.6
Fracture	4.5	3.5	3.5	3.1	4.2	3.9	*3.8	2.9	5.0	2.5	3.0	3.3
Complications of care and adverse effects	*5.3	*5.7	5.9	5.9	*6.0	*5.5	5.5	*7.1	*4.5	*5.9	*6.1	*4.7
18–44 Years[3]	4.6	3.6	3.7	3.7	6.1	4.8	4.8	4.8	4.0	3.2	3.3	3.3
HIV/AIDS	*10.7	*8.8	*8.8	8.5	*10.6	*9.4	7.5	8.9	*	*7.5	*	7.4
Cancer, all	7.8	6.3	6.9	6.6	8.4	7.9	7.5	*9.4	7.5	5.4	*6.6	5.4
Childbirth	X	X	X	X	X	X	X	X	2.8	2.5	2.6	2.7
Uterine fibroids	X	X	X	X	X	X	X	X	4.2	2.5	2.7	2.4
Diabetes	5.8	3.9	3.8	3.7	6.2	3.7	3.7	3.7	5.2	4.3	3.9	3.6
Alcohol and drug	9.0	*5.0	4.8	3.5	8.9	4.8	4.6	3.6	9.1	*5.3	*5.1	3.4
Schizophrenia, mood disorders, delusional disorders, nonorganic psychoses	14.3	*7.9	*7.4	7.7	13.8	*8.2	*8.3	7.8	14.8	*7.6	*6.7	7.5
Schizophrenia	15.4	*11.0	*10.2	10.7	15.3	*10.6	*10.7	10.0	15.6	*11.9	9.4	11.8
Mood disorders	14.3	*6.6	*6.3	6.4	*13.2	*6.6	*6.7	6.9	15.0	*6.5	*6.0	6.0
Heart disease	5.4	3.6	4.0	4.2	5.4	3.5	3.8	3.9	5.4	3.7	4.4	4.7
Ischemic heart disease	4.6	3.0	3.1	3.4	4.8	2.8	3.3	3.8	4.1	3.6	2.8	2.7
Pneumonia	6.9	5.1	5.0	4.1	7.8	5.0	5.7	4.4	6.0	5.2	4.5	3.9
Asthma	4.4	2.9	2.7	3.8	3.8	2.5	2.4	2.2	4.6	3.1	2.8	*4.5
Intervertebral disc disorders	4.4	2.3	2.3	2.5	4.2	2.2	2.3	2.1	4.7	2.3	2.2	3.0
Injury	5.1	4.3	4.3	4.2	5.0	4.5	4.4	4.6	5.3	4.1	4.1	3.4
Fracture	6.0	4.9	5.1	4.5	5.6	5.0	5.0	4.4	6.9	4.4	5.4	4.5
Poisoning and toxic effects	2.7	2.5	2.9	2.5	2.7	2.8	3.5	2.6	2.7	2.4	2.3	2.4
Complications of care and adverse effects	5.6	4.7	5.1	5.2	5.3	4.9	5.4	5.8	*5.9	4.6	4.9	4.8
45–64 Years[3]	6.7	5.0	5.0	5.1	6.7	5.1	5.0	5.2	6.8	4.8	4.9	4.9
HIV/AIDS	*	*	*9.9	8.6	*	*	10.4	8.3	*	*	*	*9.5
Cancer, all	8.8	6.2	6.4	5.9	9.3	6.8	6.6	6.0	8.4	5.6	6.1	5.7
Colorectal cancer	13.3	7.4	7.3	7.5	*13.0	7.4	7.9	7.7	*13.6	7.4	6.7	7.3
Lung/bronchus/tracheal cancer	7.7	6.2	6.8	6.5	7.1	6.0	7.3	6.6	8.6	6.4	6.3	6.5
Breast cancer[4]	X	X	X	X	X	X	X	X	4.3	2.0	2.5	2.3
Prostate cancer	X	X	X	X	7.3	3.2	3.1	1.4	X	X	X	*
Uterine fibroids	X	X	X	X	X	X	X	X	4.5	2.8	3.0	2.2
Diabetes	8.1	5.6	5.1	5.8	7.3	6.0	5.3	6.8	8.9	5.2	4.9	4.8
Alcohol and drug	8.5	4.8	4.7	4.7	8.6	4.6	4.8	5.0	8.3	*5.0	4.4	4.1
Schizophrenia, mood disorders, delusional disorders, nonorganic psychoses	14.3	*7.9	*7.4	7.7	13.8	*8.2	*8.3	7.8	14.8	*7.6	*6.7	7.5
Schizophrenia	15.6	*11.9	10.9	11.0	14.2	*11.4	10.1	11.0	16.5	*12.5	11.6	11.0
Mood disorders	14.7	*7.9	7.8	7.2	13.4	*7.3	8.1	7.0	15.4	*8.3	7.6	7.3
Heart disease	5.9	3.9	4.1	4.1	5.8	3.8	3.8	3.8	6.1	4.1	4.7	4.5
Ischemic heart disease	5.7	3.7	3.8	3.7	5.7	3.6	3.5	3.4	5.8	3.8	*4.5	4.2
Heart attack	7.5	4.8	4.9	4.6	7.5	4.7	4.6	4.5	7.6	5.0	5.6	5.0
Arrhythmias	4.6	2.9	2.9	3.0	4.6	2.8	2.7	3.2	4.6	2.9	3.2	2.8
Heart failure	7.0	4.9	5.2	5.0	6.9	5.2	4.9	4.9	7.3	4.7	5.6	5.1
Hypertension	3.9	2.2	2.1	2.2	*4.3	2.0	2.1	2.1	3.6	2.4	2.0	2.2
Stroke	10.3	5.3	5.6	4.6	10.0	5.2	5.9	4.5	10.7	5.5	5.4	4.8
Pneumonia	8.0	5.8	5.5	4.9	8.0	6.0	5.7	4.9	7.9	5.7	5.3	5.0
Chronic obstructive pulmonary disease	6.5	4.7	4.1	5.7	6.8	5.0	3.6	4.3	6.2	4.4	4.5	*6.7
Asthma	5.2	3.9	3.9	4.1	5.3	*3.2	3.4	*4.5	5.2	4.0	4.1	4.0
Osteoarthritis	7.4	3.9	3.5	3.4	7.1	3.6	3.4	3.2	7.5	4.1	3.6	3.6
Intervertebral disc disorders	5.2	2.8	2.9	3.5	5.0	2.6	2.5	*3.8	5.4	3.1	3.2	3.1
Injury	6.5	5.1	5.0	4.8	6.6	5.5	5.0	4.7	6.4	4.6	4.9	4.9
Fracture	7.6	5.6	5.3	5.4	7.2	6.4	5.6	5.2	7.9	4.9	5.0	5.6
Poisoning and toxic effects	4.9	3.0	3.4	3.3	*	*2.9	3.4	2.8	4.3	3.1	3.3	3.6
Internal organ injury	*8.3	7.6	6.7	5.9	*	8.3	7.3	5.9	*8.1	*	*5.6	6.1
Complications of care and adverse effects	7.9	6.1	6.0	6.1	8.4	5.9	6.2	6.2	7.4	6.4	5.8	6.0

Table C-60. Average Length of Stay[1] in Nonfederal Short-Stay Hospitals, by Sex, Age, and Selected First-Listed Diagnosis, Selected Years, 1990 through 2009—Continued

(Number of days.)

Age and first-listed diagnosis	Both sexes				Male				Female			
	1990	2000	2005	2009[2]	1990	2000	2005	2009[2]	1990	2000	2005	2009[2]
65–74 Years[3]	8.0	5.7	5.3	5.4	7.8	5.6	5.3	5.6	8.1	5.7	5.3	5.3
Septicemia	*15.9	8.6	8.1	8.7	*	8.5	8.1	7.9	14.4	8.8	8.1	9.5
Cancer, all	9.4	7.0	6.7	6.7	9.9	6.9	6.8	6.8	9.0	7.1	6.5	6.5
Colorectal cancer	12.9	9.1	7.7	7.2	11.3	9.2	7.9	8.1	14.5	9.0	7.5	6.1
Lung/bronchus/tracheal cancer	9.2	7.0	7.3	6.1	8.7	6.8	7.6	6.3	10.2	*7.1	7.1	5.9
Breast cancer[4]	X	X	X	X	X	X	X	X	4.4	*	*3.2	2.0
Prostate cancer	X	X	X	X	6.5	3.8	*3.3	2.0	X	X	X	X
Diabetes	8.4	5.9	5.2	4.9	9.1	6.2	5.6	5.0	8.0	5.6	4.8	4.8
Schizophrenia, mood disorders, delusional disorders, nonorganic psychoses	16.6	11.7	10.7	11.9	17.4	*11.7	10.0	12.8	16.3	11.7	11.1	11.3
Dementia and Alzheimer's disease	*12.6	*9.3	*8.4	*7.8	*10.4	*9.6	*8.1	*8.6	*14.0	*8.9	*8.6	*7.1
Heart disease	7.0	4.8	4.4	4.7	7.0	4.7	4.4	4.5	7.0	4.9	4.4	4.9
Ischemic heart disease	6.6	4.6	4.2	4.1	6.8	4.3	4.3	4.0	6.3	4.9	4.0	4.3
Heart attack	8.4	5.9	5.8	4.9	8.8	5.3	6.1	4.7	7.8	6.6	5.3	5.1
Arrhythmias	5.7	3.8	3.3	3.5	5.6	3.8	3.4	3.1	5.8	3.7	3.2	4.1
Heart failure	8.4	5.5	4.9	5.4	7.9	5.7	4.9	5.1	8.8	5.4	4.9	5.7
Hypertension	4.3	2.6	2.3	2.1	*4.6	*2.7	2.4	2.0	4.1	2.4	2.3	2.2
Stroke	8.4	4.7	4.5	4.9	8.3	4.5	4.6	4.6	8.5	4.8	4.3	5.3
Pneumonia	9.5	6.4	5.3	5.6	9.5	6.4	5.1	5.7	9.5	6.3	5.6	5.5
Chronic obstructive pulmonary disease	8.2	4.8	4.8	4.4	8.6	4.5	4.8	4.2	7.7	5.0	4.8	4.6
Gallstones	6.6	4.4	4.2	5.4	6.9	*5.2	4.3	5.1	6.5	3.9	4.2	5.8
Kidney disease	10.4	7.6	6.9	6.5	8.4	6.9	7.2	6.8	*12.4	8.2	6.6	6.1
Urinary tract infection	8.0	4.8	4.4	4.4	7.2	5.1	5.1	4.6	8.4	4.7	4.1	4.2
Hyperplasia of the prostate					4.5	2.8	2.4	2.1				
Osteoarthritis	9.3	4.7	3.8	3.5	8.8	4.7	3.8	3.4	9.5	4.7	3.8	3.6
Injury	9.2	5.6	5.8	6.0	8.4	5.7	6.4	6.9	9.7	5.6	5.4	5.4
Fracture	11.1	5.9	5.5	6.4	10.2	6.4	5.6	*7.8	11.5	5.7	5.5	5.7
Hip fracture	*15.5	7.1	7.1	*7.6	*11.8	*7.9	*7.2	*	*16.7	6.7	7.0	5.9
Complications of care and adverse effects	7.8	6.4	6.5	5.6	7.3	6.1	6.0	5.7	8.5	6.8	7.1	5.4
75–84 Years[3]	9.1	6.2	5.6	5.8	8.7	6.2	5.7	5.9	9.4	6.1	5.5	5.8
Septicemia	12.1	7.9	8.0	8.8	12.9	7.4	8.1	9.1	11.5	8.4	7.8	8.6
Cancer, all	10.4	7.2	7.3	6.3	9.3	7.2	7.2	6.4	11.7	7.2	7.4	6.2
Colorectal cancer	12.9	9.0	9.3	7.8	12.5	*9.3	9.1	8.3	13.2	8.8	9.4	7.4
Lung/bronchus/tracheal cancer	9.5	6.5	6.9	6.4	9.6	6.2	6.9	6.7	*9.4	6.9	6.9	6.2
Breast cancer[4]	X	X	X	X	X	X	X	X	5.7	*3.2	*	2.1
Prostate cancer	X	X	X	X	6.6	*5.1	*5.7	2.9	X	X	X	X
Diabetes	12.5	6.0	5.6	*6.3	11.7	6.4	7.1	*6.3	13.1	5.6	4.6	*6.2
Schizophrenia, mood disorders, delusional disorders, nonorganic psychoses	15.8	10.8	9.3	*11.7	*15.7	*11.6	*9.7	*11.6	15.8	10.4	9.1	11.7
Dementia and Alzheimer's disease	*15.3	8.2	8.5	8.8	*12.8	7.6	7.2	6.8	*	8.6	*9.2	11.0
Heart disease	8.0	5.3	4.7	5.1	8.1	5.4	4.7	5.2	7.8	5.3	4.7	5.0
Ischemic heart disease	7.9	5.1	4.6	4.8	8.5	5.2	4.8	5.2	7.4	5.1	4.4	4.4
Heart attack	9.7	6.2	6.2	5.6	10.1	5.8	6.6	6.0	9.3	6.6	5.8	5.3
Arrhythmias	6.6	4.2	3.4	4.8	6.5	4.3	3.2	5.2	6.7	4.1	3.6	4.6
Heart failure	8.0	5.9	5.1	5.3	7.7	6.1	5.1	4.9	8.2	5.8	5.1	5.6
Hypertension	6.0	2.6	2.7	3.1	*	*2.1	2.7	2.3	*5.6	2.8	2.6	*3.5
Stroke	10.4	5.9	5.1	4.6	10.0	5.7	5.6	4.6	10.6	6.0	4.7	4.6
Pneumonia	10.4	6.3	5.9	6.1	9.8	6.4	5.8	6.5	11.0	6.3	5.9	5.8
Chronic obstructive pulmonary disease	8.0	4.9	5.4	4.7	6.6	4.8	*5.9	4.6	*10.1	4.9	4.9	4.7
Gallstones	8.5	5.3	4.9	5.0	8.0	5.6	4.5	5.6	8.8	5.1	5.3	4.6
Kidney disease	10.5	7.4	6.7	6.3	11.0	8.2	6.6	5.7	*10.1	6.6	6.8	6.9
Urinary tract infection	11.0	5.2	4.6	5.2	8.1	5.5	5.2	5.2	12.3	5.1	4.4	5.2
Hyperplasia of the prostate	X	X	X	X	6.0	3.1	*3.0	*	X	X	X	X
Osteoarthritis	10.1	4.6	3.9	3.7	9.9	4.4	3.8	3.4	10.2	4.7	3.9	3.9
Injury	10.1	6.8	5.5	6.0	8.9	*8.2	6.3	7.7	10.4	6.3	5.2	5.2
Fracture	11.0	7.4	5.7	6.0	10.0	*	6.8	7.6	11.2	6.7	5.4	5.4
Hip fracture	12.1	7.7	6.7	6.3	10.4	7.8	7.7	7.4	12.5	7.6	6.3	6.0
Complications of care and adverse effects	12.5	7.1	6.1	6.1	14.0	8.1	5.9	6.2	11.2	6.0	6.4	6.1

Table C-60. Average Length of Stay[1] in Nonfederal Short-Stay Hospitals, by Sex, Age, and Selected First-Listed Diagnosis, Selected Years, 1990 through 2009—Continued

(Number of days.)

Age and first-listed diagnosis	Both sexes				Male				Female			
	1990	2000	2005	2009[2]	1990	2000	2005	2009[2]	1990	2000	2005	2009[2]
85 Years and Over[3]	9.6	6.2	5.7	5.8	9.4	6.1	5.9	5.9	9.6	6.2	5.7	5.7
Septicemia	12.6	6.9	7.1	8.5	*11.8	6.7	7.7	10.2	12.9	6.9	6.8	7.4
Cancer, all	12.1	7.5	6.8	6.6	13.4	8.6	6.6	6.0	11.3	6.8	6.9	7.0
Colorectal cancer	22.4	*10.1	9.4	8.7	*	*	*	8.0	*21.1	8.2	8.9	9.2
Lung/bronchus/tracheal cancer	*	*8.0	7.0	5.3	*	*5.9	*	3.2	*	*	*6.8	6.7
Breast cancer[4]	X	X	X	X	X	X	X	X	*5.3	X	X	*2.4
Prostate cancer	X	X	X	X	*7.5	X	X	*5.5	*	X	X	X
Diabetes	9.1	5.5	5.4	4.9	*	*	*5.3	*6.9	9.2	4.9	*5.5	3.8
Schizophrenia, mood disorders, delusional disorders, nonorganic psychoses	*	*10.5	*11.4	*9.5	*	*	*	8.4	*	*10.8	*12.0	*10.5
Dementia and Alzheimer's disease	11.4	7.9	*7.6	6.5	*	*8.8	*7.3	5.7	*11.0	*7.6	*7.7	7.0
Heart disease	8.1	5.2	4.9	5.0	7.8	5.1	4.9	5.3	8.2	5.3	4.9	4.8
Ischemic heart disease	7.5	5.4	4.9	4.6	6.8	5.4	5.2	5.2	7.9	5.4	4.6	4.2
Heart attack	9.8	6.7	5.8	5.5	8.9	6.4	6.4	6.6	10.3	6.9	5.5	4.7
Arrhythmias	8.3	4.4	4.2	4.4	*9.6	4.3	3.7	5.0	7.7	4.4	4.4	4.2
Heart failure	8.6	5.3	5.3	5.4	8.0	4.9	5.0	5.6	8.8	5.5	5.4	5.2
Hypertension	*	*4.2	2.8	2.8	*	*	*	2.9	*	*	2.6	2.8
Stroke	9.6	5.3	5.3	*	9.6	5.6	5.1	6.3	9.5	5.1	5.5	*
Pneumonia	10.9	7.0	5.9	6.2	11.1	6.1	6.0	5.6	10.7	7.5	5.9	6.5
Chronic obstructive pulmonary disease	*9.0	5.7	5.0	4.7	*7.8	5.5	4.7	5.3	*	5.7	5.3	4.4
Gallstones	10.3	5.8	6.1	5.6	*9.3	*5.6	*	5.7	10.7	*5.9	6.4	5.6
Kidney disease	*12.6	8.5	5.7	6.3	*	*9.0	*6.1	5.8	*13.8	*8.2	5.5	6.6
Urinary tract infection	10.2	5.6	5.0	4.9	9.3	5.7	4.7	5.5	10.7	5.5	5.1	4.7
Hyperplasia of the prostate	X	X	X	X	6.6	*3.7	*4.3	3.8	X	X	X	X
Osteoarthritis	10.5	4.7	4.2	3.7	*	*	*4.0	3.4	*9.6	4.4	4.3	3.9
Injury	10.5	5.9	5.5	5.2	11.0	6.4	6.2	5.8	10.3	5.8	5.3	5.0
Fracture	11.1	6.1	5.7	5.3	11.2	6.4	*6.9	5.7	11.1	6.0	5.4	5.2
Hip fracture	12.7	6.5	5.8	5.8	12.6	6.8	6.1	5.8	12.7	6.5	5.7	5.7
Complications of care and adverse effects	*11.7	*8.2	6.1	6.1	*10.7	*6.4	*6.2	7.0	*12.3	*9.1	6.0	5.6

* = Figure does not meet standards of reliability or precision.
X = Category not applicable.
[1] Average length of stay is calculated by dividing days of care by number of discharges.
[2] Starting with 2008 data, the sample of nonfederal short-stay hospitals was cut in half. This smaller sample size has increased standard errors. Therefore, caution should be exercised in interpreting trends in these data.
[3] Includes discharges with first-listed diagnoses not shown in table.
[4] Shown for women only.

Table C-61. Discharges with at Least One Procedure in Nonfederal Short-Stay Hospitals, by Sex, Age, and Selected Procedures, Selected Years, 1990 through 2009

(Percent.)

Age and procedure (any listed)	Both sexes				Male				Female			
	1990	2000	2005	2009[1]	1990	2000	2005	2009[1]	1990	2000	2005	2009[1]
18 Years and Over												
Hospital discharges with at least one procedure, crude[2]	67.4	62.1	62.6	63.3	65.2	59.2	59.4	60.0	68.7	63.9	64.7	65.5
Hospital discharges with at least one procedure, age-adjusted[2,3]	1,020.1	859.9	893.5	908.8	882.2	701.4	722.0	733.7	1,176.4	1,026.2	1,078.1	1,098.0
Hospital discharges with at least one procedure, crude[2]	1,006.4	856.8	893.8	920.0	788.1	648.4	683.9	716.3	1,205.9	1,049.8	1,090.9	1,112.3
Operations on vessels of heart	28.3	41.2	41.2	36.0	41.9	56.9	58.5	50.2	15.8	26.7	25.0	22.6
Coronary angioplasty or arthrectomy	14.0	26.2	28.5	25.6	20.5	34.9	40.5	34.8	8.0	18.1	17.3	17.0
Coronary artery stent insertion	X	21.7	27.0	22.6	X	28.7	38.5	30.4	X	15.3	16.2	15.2
Drug-eluting stent insertion	X	X	23.9	15.8	X	X	34.1	21.0	X	X	14.4	10.9
Coronary artery bypass graft (CABG)	14.1	15.0	11.8	10.5	21.2	21.8	16.6	15.6	7.7	8.7	7.2	5.7
Cardiac catheterization	52.1	57.8	53.9	46.1	68.3	72.1	68.5	55.1	37.4	44.6	40.2	37.5
Pacemaker	8.6	8.5	9.6	9.2	10.1	8.5	10.5	9.0	7.1	8.5	8.8	9.4
Carotid (neck arteries) endarterectomy	3.6	5.9	4.6	4.0	4.1	6.6	5.7	4.6	3.1	5.3	3.6	3.5
Endoscopy of small intestine	40.8	42.5	45.8	45.7	38.6	39.1	42.3	42.3	42.8	45.6	49.1	48.9
Endoscopy of large intestine	27.9	25.0	24.0	21.9	22.5	20.2	19.7	19.1	32.8	29.4	28.0	24.4
Gall bladder removal	27.9	19.6	17.7	18.4	16.5	13.3	13.2	14.5	38.2	25.5	21.9	22.2
Laparoscopic gall bladder removal	X	14.8	13.5	14.7	X	9.2	8.8	10.4	20.1	17.9	18.7	
Treatment of intra-abdominal scar tissue	17.0	14.4	15.3	15.1	6.5	5.7	6.5	7.8	26.6	22.4	23.5	22.0
Reduction of fracture	27.6	24.9	23.2	22.8	27.3	22.0	21.1	20.5	27.8	27.7	25.2	25.0
Excision of intervertebral disc and spinal fusion	18.7	18.2	18.4	22.3	22.3	20.0	18.8	22.5	15.4	16.4	18.0	22.2
Total hip replacement	6.4	7.3	10.5	13.8	5.4	6.8	10.1	14.0	7.3	7.7	10.9	13.5
Partial hip replacement	4.8	5.0	10.2	13.3	2.0	2.3	7.8	*11.3	7.3	7.6	12.3	15.2
Total knee replacement	6.7	13.8	23.1	28.0	4.9	11.0	16.4	20.2	8.4	16.4	29.3	35.4
CT scan	68.4	29.2	27.9	*17.1	68.6	27.4	26.1	16.0	68.2	30.9	29.7	*18.1
Arteriography and angiocardiography with contrast	59.7	63.0	59.9	56.4	75.6	76.2	72.1	64.9	45.2	50.7	48.5	48.3
Diagnostic ultrasound	72.3	36.9	36.0	34.7	62.1	33.1	35.2	34.0	81.7	40.4	36.7	35.4
Magnetic resonance imaging	9.5	9.2	11.2	*10.1	9.4	8.2	10.3	*9.4	9.6	10.2	12.1	*10.7
Mechanical ventilation	17.6	23.0	27.0	32.9	18.8	23.9	29.5	34.9	16.4	22.1	24.7	31.1
18–44 Years												
Hospital discharges with at least one procedure[2]	73.0	71.7	71.7	71.9	62.6	55.9	54.0	53.6	77.0	77.4	78.1	78.4
Hospital discharges with at least one procedure[2]	749.3	609.1	644.0	638.0	362.8	251.6	254.4	244.3	1,130.6	965.9	1,039.0	1,039.7
Operations on vessels of heart	3.0	3.9	4.1	*3.1	4.9	5.5	5.7	4.5	*1.2	2.3	2.4	*
Coronary angioplasty or arthrectomy	1.9	3.0	3.0	*2.5	3.0	4.3	4.3	*3.5	*0.8	1.6	*1.7	*
Coronary artery stent insertion	X	2.5	3.1	*2.3	X	3.6	4.3	*3.1	X	1.4	*1.8	*
Drug-eluting stent insertion	X	X	2.6	*	X	X	3.4	*	X		*1.8	*
Coronary artery bypass graft (CABG)	1.0	0.9	0.8	*	*1.8	1.1	*1.1	*	*	*0.7	*	*
Cardiac catheterization	9.0	8.5	7.6	7.1	12.5	11.0	9.6	8.7	5.5	5.9	5.6	5.5
Endoscopy of small intestine	13.1	10.3	13.3	15.7	13.2	10.4	11.7	12.2	13.0	10.2	14.9	19.3
Endoscopy of large intestine	6.9	5.5	6.5	7.2	5.6	4.7	5.5	*6.2	8.1	6.3	7.5	8.3
Gall bladder removal	18.7	11.9	11.5	13.5	6.2	4.3	5.1	6.5	31.0	19.4	17.9	20.6
Laparoscopic gall bladder removal	X	9.9	9.9	11.0		3.0	4.1	4.5		16.8	15.8	17.7
Treatment of intra-abdominal scar tissue	14.1	10.8	11.7	11.1	2.0	1.5	*1.8	*2.9	26.0	20.1	21.7	19.4
Hysterectomy	X	X	X	X	X	X	X	X	63.3	55.7	51.2	37.4
Abdominal hysterectomy	X	X	X	X	X	X	X	X	47.1	34.6	31.5	22.8
Vaginal hysterectomy	X	X	X	X	X	X	X	X	15.8	19.1	15.6	*10.6
Forceps, vacuum, and breech delivery	X	X	X	X	X	X	X	X	77.5	59.9	51.1	*45.0
Episiotomy	X	X	X	X	X	X	X	X	293.3	160.8	90.9	52.3
Other procedures inducing or assisting delivery	X	X	X	X	X	X	X	X	387.9	384.2	396.7	418.5
Medical induction of labor	X	X	X	X	X	X	X	X	41.1	77.7	107.5	120.5
Cesarean section	X	X	X	X	X	X	X	X	167.1	149.5	220.7	232.5
Reduction of fracture	19.1	13.7	13.2	12.0	27.9	19.0	18.9	17.2	10.4	8.4	7.5	6.8
Excision of intervertebral disc and spinal fusion	17.0	14.1	11.7	11.9	21.5	16.2	13.1	11.7	12.6	12.1	10.3	12.1
CT scan	27.5	10.6	12.6	*6.5	32.3	11.0	12.3	5.8	22.7	10.3	12.8	*7.2
Arteriography and angiocardiography with contrast	12.5	10.3	10.5	9.7	17.4	12.9	12.2	9.7	7.6	7.7	8.7	9.7
Diagnostic ultrasound	34.2	11.6	12.3	9.8	19.3	8.3	9.5	*7.3	48.9	14.9	15.1	12.3
Magnetic resonance imaging	4.9	3.8	4.3	*4.4	4.9	3.6	3.8	*	4.9	*4.0	4.8	*5.6
Mechanical ventilation	4.6	7.0	8.8	11.0	5.4	8.2	10.1	11.9	3.8	5.8	7.5	10.1

Table C-61. Discharges with at Least One Procedure in Nonfederal Short-Stay Hospitals, by Sex, Age, and Selected Procedures, Selected Years, 1990 through 2009—Continued

(Percent.)

Age and procedure (any listed)	Both sexes				Male				Female			
	1990	2000	2005	2009[1]	1990	2000	2005	2009[1]	1990	2000	2005	2009[1]
45–64 Years												
Hospital discharges with at least one procedure[2]	68.2	62.3	62.6	63.2	68.9	63.4	63.3	63.5	67.6	61.3	61.8	62.9
Hospital discharges with at least one procedure[2]	924.2	694.6	717.4	771.7	965.9	714.4	727.3	784.1	885.4	675.9	708.1	759.9
Operations on vessels of heart	53.0	57.7	53.5	42.5	83.2	88.5	83.5	62.8	24.8	28.4	24.9	23.1
Coronary angioplasty or arthrectomy	29.4	37.5	38.4	31.2	45.3	55.9	59.4	46.1	14.5	20.0	18.3	17.1
Coronary artery stent insertion	X	31.1	36.7	26.9	X	46.5	57.7	39.9	X	16.5	16.7	14.6
Drug-eluting stent insertion	X	X	33.0	18.7	X	X	51.8	28.1	X	X	15.1	*9.8
Coronary artery bypass graft (CABG)	23.4	20.3	14.0	11.5	37.5	32.5	21.9	17.1	10.3	8.6	6.4	*6.1
Cardiac catheterization	98.2	83.0	69.7	56.6	136.8	113.9	95.6	75.7	62.3	53.7	45.1	38.4
Pacemaker	7.8	4.0	3.9	3.2	10.9	5.2	4.6	*4.5	*4.9	2.8	3.2	*2.0
Carotid (neck arteries) endarterectomy	4.0	5.2	2.9	2.6	5.2	5.2	3.7	*3.1	3.0	*5.2	2.2	*2.1
Endoscopy of small intestine	45.0	36.4	42.5	43.5	46.3	40.7	44.7	45.3	43.8	32.3	40.3	41.9
Endoscopy of large intestine	28.5	19.3	19.4	18.9	25.4	18.1	17.4	16.7	31.4	20.4	21.2	21.0
Gall bladder removal	36.4	20.6	17.6	18.4	22.3	16.3	14.0	15.6	49.5	24.6	20.9	21.0
Laparoscopic gall bladder removal	X	15.3	13.0	15.0	X	12.1	9.0	11.8	X	18.5	16.8	18.0
Treatment of intra-abdominal scar tissue	17.1	15.0	15.6	14.6	9.5	7.0	6.2	8.5	24.2	22.6	24.5	20.4
Removal of prostate	X	X	X	X	35.8	15.6	14.4	*17.9	X	X	X	X
Transurethral prostatectomy	X	X	X	X	30.4	7.0	4.6	*2.7	X	X	X	X
Hysterectomy	X	X	X	X	X	X	X	X	76.4	78.2	63.8	54.5
Abdominal hysterectomy	X	X	X	X	X	X	X	X	58.4	53.2	39.7	33.9
Vaginal hysterectomy	X	X	X	X	X	X	X	X	17.6	21.6	19.3	14.4
Reduction of fracture	20.3	18.5	16.5	17.0	19.5	17.6	17.9	16.7	21.0	19.3	15.3	17.3
Excision of intervertebral disc and spinal fusion	26.1	25.7	26.9	31.1	29.4	27.1	27.0	30.6	23.1	24.4	26.8	31.7
Total hip replacement	6.2	8.1	10.9	18.3	5.7	9.1	12.3	20.8	6.5	7.2	9.6	15.8
Partial hip replacement	*	*1.3	9.1	*14.0	*	*0.8	8.8	*14.1	*	*1.7	9.5	*13.9
Total knee replacement	6.7	12.7	25.4	36.5	5.8	8.7	17.7	27.0	*7.4	16.4	32.7	45.5
Mastectomy	X	X	X	X	X	X	X	X	21.2	10.6	8.1	8.5
CT scan	65.4	25.2	26.1	17.0	69.9	25.9	26.7	18.0	61.2	24.5	25.5	*16.1
Arteriography and angiocardiography with contrast	105.4	85.3	73.2	66.3	138.5	111.4	94.6	86.7	74.6	60.7	52.8	46.9
Diagnostic ultrasound	69.5	34.3	33.5	30.9	73.8	38.0	39.4	35.9	65.5	30.9	27.9	26.2
Magnetic resonance imaging	10.9	8.9	11.6	8.9	10.7	9.4	12.4	9.2	11.0	8.4	11.0	*8.6
Mechanical ventilation	17.6	21.2	24.7	32.2	18.6	22.9	28.0	33.5	16.7	19.6	21.6	30.8
65–74 Years												
Hospital discharges with at least one procedure[2]	66.5	61.3	62.9	63.9	69.3	63.9	65.0	64.4	63.8	58.9	60.9	63.4
Hospital discharges with at least one procedure[2]	1,739.4	1,559.8	1,653.0	1,632.6	1,994.1	1,692.3	1,783.2	1,725.0	1,539.4	1,450.6	1,543.1	1,553.5
Operations on vessels of heart	97.0	139.8	142.1	117.4	148.9	195.3	211.0	165.8	56.3	94.1	84.0	75.9
Coronary angioplasty or arthrectomy	44.1	86.3	91.2	83.2	64.9	116.0	138.2	113.2	27.8	61.9	51.5	57.4
Coronary artery stent insertion	X	71.7	86.2	73.6	X	94.9	129.4	97.3	X	52.5	49.8	53.2
Drug-eluting stent insertion	X	X	76.8	53.5	X	X	115.7	69.1	X	X	44.0	*40.2
Coronary artery bypass graft (CABG)	52.1	53.9	47.4	34.4	83.1	79.7	68.1	52.9	27.7	32.6	30.0	*18.6
Cardiac catheterization	164.0	174.2	170.3	130.9	213.8	222.7	230.4	159.3	124.9	134.2	119.6	106.6
Pacemaker	24.6	22.5	23.7	19.6	32.1	22.8	29.0	*17.3	18.7	22.3	19.1	*21.5
Carotid (neck arteries) endarterectomy	14.6	24.1	24.0	*17.8	18.0	29.5	31.2	*21.8	11.9	19.6	18.0	*14.3
Endoscopy of small intestine	92.8	106.6	102.5	99.4	91.5	102.4	102.6	106.7	93.7	110.0	102.4	93.2
Endoscopy of large intestine	70.3	64.8	58.3	45.7	62.5	59.7	52.1	44.9	76.5	69.0	63.6	46.4
Gall bladder removal	45.0	42.1	34.4	31.3	42.0	37.9	34.0	33.7	47.4	45.5	34.8	29.3
Laparoscopic gall bladder removal	X	29.5	23.6	21.9	X	24.4	22.4	*20.3	X	33.7	24.6	23.2
Treatment of intra-abdominal scar tissue	23.1	21.4	23.5	27.4	17.1	14.5	19.6	*20.5	27.7	27.1	26.8	*33.2
Removal of prostate	X	X	X	X	201.1	83.7	65.3	56.9	X	X	X	X
Transurethral prostatectomy	X	X	X	X	180.9	59.4	39.5	*23.7	X	X	X	X
Hysterectomy	X	X	X	X	X	X	X	X	37.4	35.9	28.0	*29.3
Abdominal hysterectomy	X	X	X	X	X	X	X	X	20.8	20.5	12.8	*12.2
Vaginal hysterectomy	X	X	X	X	X	X	X	X	16.5	14.7	14.1	*15.0
Reduction of fracture	36.2	36.4	38.0	34.8	24.3	26.2	25.8	19.0	45.5	44.8	48.3	48.3
Excision of intervertebral disc and spinal fusion	16.3	21.1	31.1	41.7	14.2	22.5	27.6	*45.9	18.0	20.0	34.1	*38.0
Total hip replacement	24.0	25.4	36.6	37.4	23.0	26.4	36.2	34.6	24.9	24.5	37.0	39.9
Partial hip replacement	8.9	7.6	20.1	*24.7	*4.0	*	15.4	*20.8	*12.7	10.5	24.1	*27.9
Total knee replacement	33.2	65.4	99.5	104.6	26.4	64.5	71.8	76.2	38.6	66.0	122.8	128.9
Mastectomy	X	X	X	X	X	X	X	X	30.7	22.7	*11.5	*15.5
CT scan	153.7	64.3	53.7	*30.9	163.4	65.7	53.6	*32.6	146.1	63.1	53.7	*29.5
Arteriography and angiocardiography with contrast	184.5	186.2	180.8	153.6	239.0	231.9	233.2	191.5	141.7	148.5	136.6	121.2
Diagnostic ultrasound	155.2	92.7	80.9	82.7	165.2	94.1	87.0	*93.0	147.4	91.6	75.8	73.9
Magnetic resonance imaging	20.6	17.2	24.4	*18.1	19.2	*14.6	19.9	*19.2	21.7	*19.3	28.3	*
Mechanical ventilation	48.6	60.0	70.1	79.5	58.7	70.3	83.0	86.0	40.6	51.6	59.3	73.9

Table C-61. Discharges with at Least One Procedure in Nonfederal Short-Stay Hospitals, by Sex, Age, and Selected Procedures, Selected Years, 1990 through 2009—Continued

(Percent.)

Age and procedure (any listed)	Both sexes				Male				Female			
	1990	2000	2005	2009[1]	1990	2000	2005	2009[1]	1990	2000	2005	2009[1]
75–84 Years												
Hospital discharges with at least one procedure[2]	59.0	53.6	54.9	57.1	61.7	56.3	58.1	59.6	57.0	51.8	52.5	55.2
Hospital discharges with at least one procedure[2]	2,332.9	2,212.3	2,269.1	2,322.2	2,723.9	2,416.5	2,549.4	2,528.1	2,096.7	2,078.8	2,078.7	2,176.6
Operations on vessels of heart	69.1	143.2	142.3	138.6	107.6	202.5	199.6	208.3	45.8	104.5	103.4	89.2
Coronary angioplasty or arthrectomy	22.4	84.7	97.3	87.3	33.7	109.3	134.8	121.2	15.7	68.7	71.9	63.3
Coronary artery stent insertion	X	69.8	88.2	79.6	X	86.5	122.2	111.4	X	58.8	65.2	57.1
Drug-eluting stent insertion	X	X	75.5	55.6	X	X	104.9	77.5	X	X	55.6	*40.2
Coronary artery bypass graft (CABG)	47.0	57.7	44.4	*50.7	74.7	90.5	62.6	*86.2	30.3	36.2	32.0	*25.7
Cardiac catheterization	116.6	190.2	183.9	159.3	166.0	236.9	238.1	179.6	86.8	159.6	147.1	144.8
Pacemaker	50.8	58.1	67.9	59.9	70.6	72.2	91.0	79.6	38.8	48.9	52.2	46.0
Carotid (neck arteries) endarterectomy	19.8	32.8	24.4	23.3	24.2	45.5	34.1	31.6	*17.1	24.5	17.7	*17.5
Endoscopy of small intestine	171.4	189.7	182.2	167.4	188.9	193.8	202.0	162.5	160.8	187.0	168.7	170.9
Endoscopy of large intestine	131.1	123.7	106.4	93.7	126.1	113.8	109.3	89.5	134.1	130.1	104.3	96.7
Gall bladder removal	51.8	43.4	43.3	38.2	64.4	46.7	48.9	50.7	44.2	41.3	39.4	29.3
Laparoscopic gall bladder removal	X	28.9	30.5	32.3		29.6	30.4	40.7	X	28.5	30.5	26.4
Treatment of intra-abdominal scar tissue	34.0	28.6	27.9	28.1	28.2	26.3	*34.5	*30.0	37.5	30.2	23.4	26.7
Removal of prostate	X	X	X	X	273.5	98.0	65.4	*47.0	X	X	X	X
Transurethral prostatectomy	X	X	X	X	257.5	89.0	58.6	*44.0	X	X	X	X
Hysterectomy	X	X	X	X	X	X	X	X	28.5	25.5	16.1	*23.2
Abdominal hysterectomy	X	X	X	X	X	X	X	X	18.8	16.2	8.6	*14.7
Vaginal hysterectomy	X	X	X	X	X	X	X	X	*9.4	8.1	7.1	*
Reduction of fracture	86.2	80.1	70.7	61.9	43.4	57.2	41.5	*41.9	112.1	95.0	90.6	76.0
Excision of intervertebral disc and spinal fusion	12.0	17.4	16.4	36.1	*13.2	*20.4	14.3	*42.8	11.3	15.3	17.8	31.3
Total hip replacement	30.7	26.3	44.4	47.3	*26.9	*21.3	36.6	*44.4	33.1	29.6	49.7	49.4
Partial hip replacement	43.6	36.6	39.9	41.2	*14.3	20.0	27.4	*29.9	61.2	47.5	48.3	49.1
Total knee replacement	28.4	59.3	90.4	89.8	*19.5	48.7	83.6	80.4	33.9	66.3	95.0	96.5
Mastectomy	X	X	X	X	X	X	X	X	29.2	22.0	16.2	*8.7
CT scan	279.7	119.2	95.8	*56.8	307.2	127.9	92.3	*58.3	263.0	113.5	98.1	*55.8
Arteriography and angiocardiography with contrast	141.0	219.2	212.4	198.1	192.3	287.9	269.9	219.0	109.9	174.3	173.3	183.4
Diagnostic ultrasound	273.5	134.1	133.0	122.4	315.7	142.8	148.3	135.8	248.0	128.4	122.6	113.0
Magnetic resonance imaging	30.5	*37.3	38.4	*38.5	43.0	*33.6	41.3	*47.9	*23.0	*39.8	36.5	*31.9
Mechanical ventilation	79.8	91.1	102.6	105.3	110.3	106.5	119.4	139.7	61.3	80.9	91.1	81.1
85 Years and Over												
Hospital discharges with at least one procedure[2]	49.3	44.6	45.4	47.0	52.4	45.4	47.7	51.4	47.8	44.3	44.2	44.6
Hospital discharges with at least one procedure[2]	2,762.1	2,700.5	2,612.5	2,731.1	3,367.3	2,797.9	2,857.1	3,301.9	2,526.8	2,660.6	2,500.2	2,466.7
Operations on vessels of heart	*14.0	51.1	53.9	60.9	*	83.0	86.2	*124.2	*	38.0	39.1	*31.6
Coronary angioplasty or arthrectomy	*	36.3	45.0	*51.7	*	*52.9	*64.6	*101.8	*	29.5	35.9	*28.4
Coronary artery stent insertion	X	31.6	43.2	45.5	X	*48.9	*62.3	*83.9	X	*24.4	34.4	*27.7
Drug-eluting stent insertion	X	X	38.4	*27.2	X	X	*55.8	*	X	X	30.4	*19.6
Coronary artery bypass graft (CABG)	*	*15.1	*	*	*	*30.1	*	*	*	*9.0	*3.0	*
Cardiac catheterization	*23.7	87.7	88.8	*96.7	*	122.8	122.5	*145.1	*19.0	73.2	73.3	*74.4
Pacemaker	79.5	82.9	92.7	105.3	120.4	104.3	122.7	*121.0	63.5	74.2	78.9	*98.0
Carotid (neck arteries) endarterectomy	*	*12.0	*9.2	*	*	*	*	*	*	*4.8	*	*
Endoscopy of small intestine	228.8	262.4	251.8	192.1	288.7	245.1	217.8	224.3	205.5	269.5	267.3	177.2
Endoscopy of large intestine	180.8	158.1	139.4	99.2	188.0	133.3	104.3	131.1	178.0	168.3	155.6	84.4
Gall bladder removal	46.4	40.9	29.1	*24.7	*68.4	*42.9	*48.4	*	37.8	*40.1	20.3	*22.7
Laparoscopic gall bladder removal	X	*30.4	18.6	*15.6	X	*	*28.2	*	X	*30.5	*14.2	*13.5
Treatment of intra-abdominal scar tissue	29.6	24.3	29.0	*28.9	*	*16.4	*20.6	*	33.7	*27.5	*32.8	*35.2
Removal of prostate	X	X	X	X	257.1	*113.0	73.0	*39.7	X	X	X	X
Transurethral prostatectomy	X	X	X	X	247.1	*110.0	67.1	*39.7	X	X	X	X
Hysterectomy	X	X	X	X	X	X	X	X	*	*	*5.9	*
Abdominal hysterectomy	X	X	X	X	X	X	X	X	*	*	*4.3	*
Vaginal hysterectomy	X	X	X	X	X	X	X	X	*	*	*	*
Reduction of fracture	196.2	200.5	160.6	182.9	150.6	93.8	75.4	147.5	213.9	244.3	199.7	199.4
Excision of intervertebral disc and spinal fusion	*	*2.3	*	*	*	*	*	*	*	*	*	*
Total hip replacement	*27.8	*20.7	*24.8	*31.6	*	*	*	*	*23.2	*26.3	*23.6	*
Partial hip replacement	67.4	82.2	71.2	78.1	*52.9	*44.1	56.4	67.0	73.1	97.9	78.0	83.3
Total knee replacement	*12.4	*22.9	*30.2	*26.7	*	*	*27.0	*	*	*16.2	*31.7	*31.1
Mastectomy									*28.9	*15.7	*	*
CT scan	378.4	158.7	123.7	*86.2	401.2	141.4	*131.8	*79.2	369.5	165.9	119.9	*
Arteriography and angiocardiography with contrast	50.6	120.8	126.6	156.8	*87.6	164.4	175.2	197.2	36.2	102.8	104.3	138.2
Diagnostic ultrasound	327.7	208.5	179.3	203.3	394.5	181.4	200.7	215.6	301.7	219.6	169.6	*197.6
Magnetic resonance imaging	*18.5	*40.4	40.5	*	*	*	*40.8	*	*16.2	*	*40.5	*
Mechanical ventilation	91.5	106.0	110.0	139.1	97.9	116.5	166.1	199.1	89.1	101.7	84.3	111.3

X = Category not applicable.
* = Figure does not meet standards of reliability or precision.
[1]Starting with 2008 data, the sample of nonfederal short-stay hospitals was cut in half. This smaller sample size has increased standard errors. Therefore, caution should be exercised in interpreting trends in these data.
[2]Includes discharges for procedures not shown separately.
[3]Estimates are age-adjusted to the year 2000 standard population using five age groups: 18-44 years, 45-54 years, 55-64 years, 65-74 years, and 75 years and over.

Table C-62. Certified Intermediate Care Facilities and Specialty Hospitals, Number of Facilities and Beds, by State, Selected Years, 1995–2010

(Number.)

State	Facilities											
	ICF/MR[1]		Hospitals									
			Long-term		Psychiatric		Rehabilitation		Children's		Critcial Access Hospital	
	1995	2010	1995	2010	1995	2010	1995	2010	1995	2010	1995	2010
United States	7,106	6,424	175	438	689	508	190	233	70	76	X	1,325
Alabama	8	5	2	7	10	11	5	7	1	2	X	3
Alaska	6	0	0	1	3	2	0	0	0	0	X	13
Arizona	12	12	3	8	11	8	4	7	1	2	X	14
Arkansas	40	40	0	8	9	9	6	8	1	1	X	29
California	687	1,164	8	20	64	32	12	5	7	10	X	31
Colorado	7	16	5	8	9	9	5	3	2	1	X	29
Connecticut	145	115	5	3	10	6	1	1	1	1	X	0
Delaware	6	2	0	1	3	4	1	0	1	1	X	0
District of Columbia	122	81	0	2	2	3	1	1	1	1	X	0
Florida	110	101	10	19	43	25	13	13	2	2	X	13
Georgia	12	9	5	15	28	15	2	3	1	2	X	34
Hawaii	15	18	1	1	1	1	1	1	1	1	X	9
Idaho	48	67	0	3	6	5	1	1	0	0	X	27
Illinois	315	309	4	6	19	14	3	4	2	2	X	51
Indiana	578	529	5	14	30	23	6	6	0	0	X	35
Iowa	116	141	0	2	4	4	0	0	0	0	X	82
Kansas	47	32	2	5	10	4	4	4	0	1	X	83
Kentucky	9	14	0	6	13	11	4	5	0	0	X	30
Louisiana	454	534	13	39	40	39	9	21	1	1	X	27
Maine	42	17	0	0	4	4	1	1	0	0	X	16
Maryland	5	3	4	4	14	9	3	2	2	2	X	0
Massachusetts	8	6	21	16	18	14	5	8	2	2	X	3
Michigan	503	1	2	19	15	11	4	4	1	1	X	36
Minnesota	348	215	1	2	6	8	0	0	3	3	X	79
Mississippi	12	14	1	10	4	5	1	0	0	0	X	28
Missouri	26	17	3	12	17	13	2	5	3	3	X	36
Montana	3	1	0	1	2	2	0	0	0	0	X	48
Nebraska	4	3	1	2	5	3	1	1	2	2	X	65
Nevada	14	9	2	6	5	7	2	3	0	0	X	11
New Hampshire	7	1	0	0	3	2	2	2	0	0	X	13
New Jersey	10	8	3	7	14	17	8	8	1	2	X	0
New Mexico	32	42	2	3	6	2	5	5	1	0	X	7
New York	892	569	7	4	35	28	4	0	2	1	X	13
North Carolina	320	332	2	9	15	10	1	2	0	0	X	23
North Dakota	65	66	1	2	1	3	1	0	0	0	X	36
Ohio	416	429	5	25	19	14	0	3	8	6	X	34
Oklahoma	37	86	4	13	18	10	3	2	2	2	X	34
Oregon	2	1	0	1	4	3	0	0	0	0	X	25
Pennsylvania	252	199	5	23	31	24	17	16	5	5	X	13
Rhode Island	55	5	2	1	3	2	1	1	0	0	X	0
South Carolina	174	85	1	6	9	8	3	6	0	0	X	5
South Dakota	10	1	0	1	2	1	0	0	0	1	X	38
Tennessee	74	113	2	9	16	11	5	6	3	2	X	17
Texas	879	860	35	77	52	37	28	49	7	8	X	78
Utah	14	15	1	3	7	3	1	1	1	1	X	11
Vermont	6	1	0	0	2	1	0	0	0	0	X	8
Virginia	20	41	3	5	19	9	4	9	2	3	X	7
Washington	28	14	2	2	4	5	1	1	2	2	X	38
West Virginia	63	66	0	2	5	4	6	5	0	0	X	18
Wisconsin	44	14	1	5	17	11	2	2	1	2	X	59
Wyoming	4	1	1	0	2	2	1	1	0	0	X	16

Table C-62. Certified Intermediate Care Facilities and Specialty Hospitals, Number of Facilities and Beds, by State, Selected Years, 1995–2010—*Continued*

(Number.)

State	ICF/MR[1]		Hospitals								Critical Access Hospital	
			Long-term		Psychiatric		Rehabilitation		Children's			
	1995	2010	1995	2010	1995	2010	1995	2010	1995	2010	1995	2010
United States	159,557	108,427	21,373	29,388	105,165	68,531	13,731	14,999	12,719	13,204	X	32,844
Alabama	981	281	341	429	1,760	1,056	289	392	225	434	X	75
Alaska	121	0	0	60	244	205	0	0	0	0	X	217
Arizona	690	242	203	557	955	874	211	396	15	250	X	299
Arkansas	1,802	1,590	0	283	730	919	446	463	280	280	X	763
California	14,334	10,998	1,477	1,825	7,737	4,922	838	367	1,346	1,980	X	1,054
Colorado	382	188	1,264	430	1,375	943	271	226	378	253	X	600
Connecticut	1,350	1,134	796	715	1,990	1,032	60	60	98	129	X	0
Delaware	405	170	0	35	514	483	60	0	97	180	X	0
District of Columbia	797	492	0	171	583	800	160	160	279	279	X	0
Florida	3,495	2,955	745	1,119	5,385	2,925	833	1,042	376	467	X	344
Georgia	2,240	1,647	372	713	4,103	2,797	108	168	235	483	X	857
Hawaii	207	91	13	9	88	88	100	100	232	207	X	88
Idaho	541	555	0	140	221	263	54	56	0	0	X	555
Illinois	13,001	10,413	1,385	805	3,172	2,321	371	448	351	339	X	1,190
Indiana	7,387	4,129	265	649	2,213	1,555	388	316	0	0	X	946
Iowa	3,679	3,127	0	74	522	287	0	0	0	0	X	2,401
Kansas	2,233	994	54	167	1,717	718	217	257	0	34	X	1,928
Kentucky	1,203	930	0	546	2,086	1,695	225	288	0	0	X	737
Louisiana	6,847	6,347	797	1,852	3,868	2,098	435	549	188	201	X	685
Maine	555	192	0	0	551	392	80	100	0	0	X	398
Maryland	1,042	238	465	465	3,846	1,788	352	131	165	150	X	0
Massachusetts	2,707	1,674	4,218	3,561	2,137	1,449	636	1,064	458	421	X	69
Michigan	3,556	272	249	1,012	3,280	1,308	340	240	260	228	X	836
Minnesota	5,162	1,871	264	356	1,432	458	0	0	329	339	X	2,190
Mississippi	2,131	2,739	25	393	316	1,741	110	0	0	0	X	800
Missouri	1,659	1,020	317	675	1,969	1,792	120	297	592	432	X	867
Montana	188	56	0	40	54	194	0	0	0	0	X	998
Nebraska	761	261	192	148	767	488	60	72	142	200	X	1,418
Nevada	229	121	79	413	407	644	122	189	0	0	X	231
New Hampshire	78	25	0	0	423	341	152	152	0	0	X	316
New Jersey	4,637	3,622	476	442	3,486	3,249	848	783	60	120	X	0
New Mexico	604	272	86	106	397	124	194	212	37	0	X	174
New York	15,379	8,860	1,351	1,010	14,199	6,327	428	0	404	92	X	301
North Carolina	5,294	5,173	182	490	2,941	3,435	80	213	0	0	X	775
North Dakota	721	635	68	72	328	303	88	0	0	0	X	795
Ohio	8,936	7,268	683	1,693	3,079	1,448	0	199	2,535	1,356	X	840
Oklahoma	3,132	2,078	194	636	1,726	638	219	107	168	160	X	777
Oregon	546	76	0	28	670	742	0	0	0	0	X	830
Pennsylvania	7,412	4,536	369	1,355	7,334	3,472	1,574	1,395	721	1,103	X	337
Rhode Island	297	51	1,062	495	371	177	82	82	0	0	X	0
South Carolina	3,550	1,828	166	308	1,089	1,093	213	355	0	0	X	125
South Dakota	558	240	0	24	145	320	0	0	0	114	X	766
Tennessee	2,590	1,247	125	335	1,721	1,215	350	370	395	200	X	395
Texas	15,868	12,659	1,803	4,068	6,561	4,299	1,838	2,769	1,447	1,631	X	1,746
Utah	965	855	34	111	741	486	50	84	194	232	X	236
Vermont	36	6	0	0	164	149	0	0	0	0	X	194
Virginia	2,758	1,715	892	236	1,677	1,345	231	353	250	296	X	175
Washington	1,482	940	97	73	1,541	1,417	102	102	276	276	X	1,130
West Virginia	782	511	0	60	564	485	246	280	0	0	X	722
Wisconsin	4,083	961	34	204	1,720	1,133	135	121	186	338	X	1,321
Wyoming	164	142	230	0	266	98	15	41	0	0	X	343

X = Category not applicable.
[1] ICF/MR is intermediate care facilities for persons with mental retardation.

PART C: HEALTH

HEALTH PERSONNEL

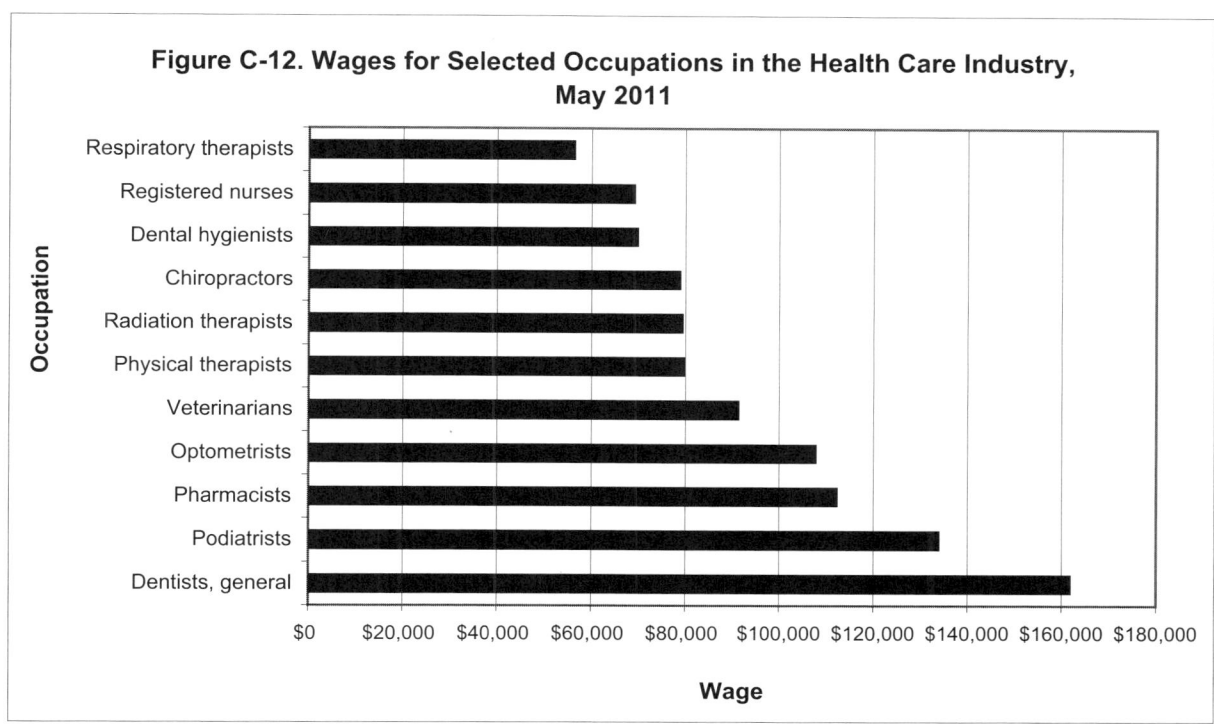

Figure C-12. Wages for Selected Occupations in the Health Care Industry, May 2011

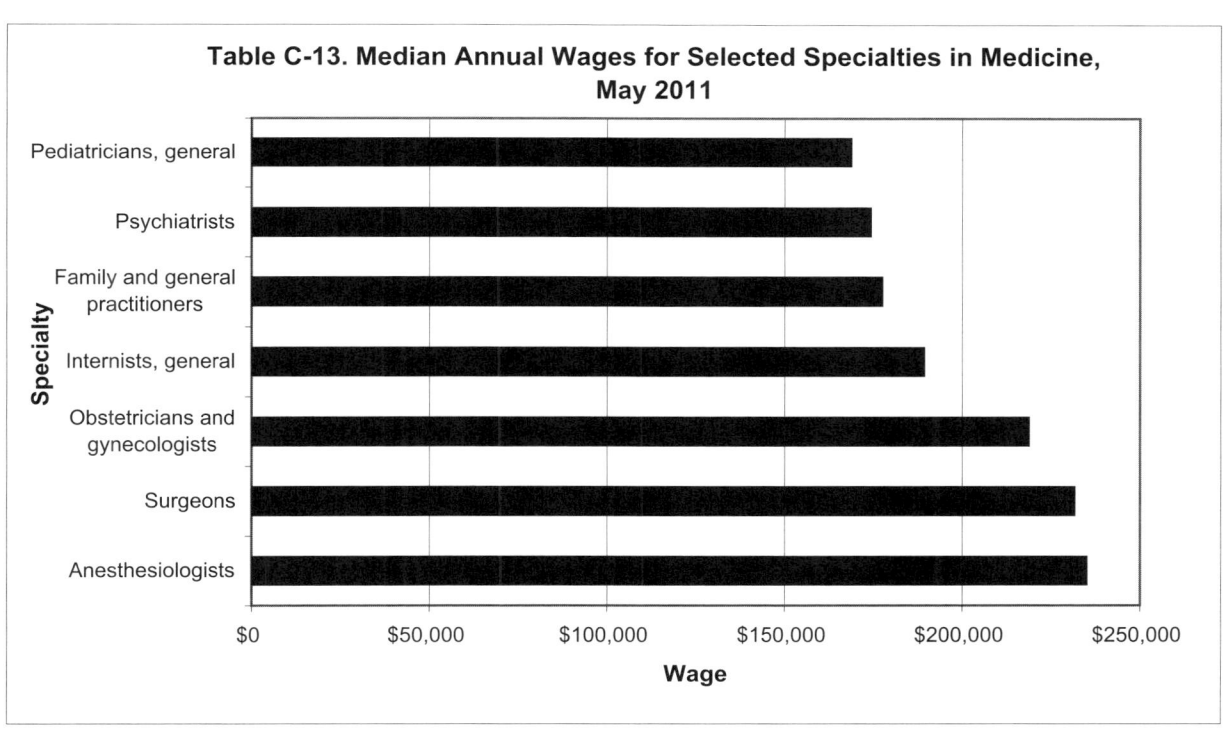

Table C-13. Median Annual Wages for Selected Specialties in Medicine, May 2011

Table C-63. Health Care Employment[1] and Wages, by Selected Occupations, Selected Years, 2001–2010

(Number.)

Occupation title	Employment						Mean hourly wage[2]					
	2001	2005	2008	2009	2010	Average annual percent change, 2001–2010	2001	2005	2008	2009	2010	Average annual percent change, 2001–2010
Health Care Practitioners and Technical Occupations												
Audiologists	11,040	10,030	12,480	12,590	12,860	1.7	$23.89	$27.72	$31.49	$32.14	$33.58	3.9
Cardiovascular technologists and technicians	40,990	43,560	48,040	48,070	48,720	1.9	17.55	19.99	23.38	23.91	24.38	3.7
Dental hygienists	149,880	161,140	173,090	173,900	177,520	1.9	27.30	29.15	32.19	32.63	33.02	2.1
Diagnostic medical sonographers	32,990	43,590	48,920	51,630	53,010	5.4	23.08	26.65	30.12	30.60	31.20	3.4
Dietetic technicians	28,940	23,780	24,620	24,510	23,890	-2.1	11.23	12.20	13.26	13.72	13.86	2.4
Dietitians and nutritionists	43,200	48,850	53,630	53,220	53,510	2.4	19.74	22.09	24.75	25.59	26.13	3.2
Emergency medical technicians and paramedics	170,690	196,880	207,610	217,920	221,760	3.0	12.24	13.68	15.38	15.88	16.01	3.0
Licensed practical and licensed vocational nurses	683,790	710,020	730,500	728,670	730,290	0.7	15.14	17.41	19.28	19.66	19.88	3.1
Nuclear medicine technologists	17,360	18,280	21,200	21,670	21,600	2.5	24.65	29.10	32.44	32.91	33.20	3.4
Occupational therapists	77,080	87,430	94,800	97,840	100,300	3.0	25.10	28.41	32.65	33.98	35.28	3.9
Opticians, dispensing	63,120	70,090	59,470	60,840	62,200	-0.2	13.49	14.80	16.85	16.73	16.73	2.4
Pharmacists	223,630	229,740	266,410	267,860	268,030	2.0	35.02	42.62	50.13	51.27	52.59	4.6
Pharmacy technicians	207,140	266,790	324,110	331,890	333,500	5.4	10.82	12.19	13.70	13.92	14.10	3.0
Physical therapists	126,450	151,280	167,300	174,490	180,280	4.0	28.43	31.42	35.77	36.64	37.50	3.1
Physician assistants	56,200	63,350	71,950	76,900	81,420	4.2	30.00	34.17	39.24	40.78	41.89	3.8
Psychiatric technicians	59,750	62,040	54,800	70,730	72,650	2.2	12.94	14.04	15.48	14.77	15.15	1.8
Radiation therapists	13,460	14,120	14,850	15,570	16,590	2.4	25.71	30.59	36.28	37.18	37.64	4.3
Radiologic technologists and technicians	168,240	184,580	208,570	213,560	216,730	2.9	18.68	22.60	25.59	26.05	26.80	4.1
Recreational therapists	26,830	23,260	22,510	21,960	20,830	-2.8	14.92	16.90	19.20	19.84	19.92	3.3
Registered nurses	2,217,990	2,368,070	2,542,760	2,583,770	2,655,020	2.0	23.19	27.35	31.31	31.99	32.56	3.8
Respiratory therapists	82,930	95,320	103,870	107,270	109,270	3.1	19.17	22.24	25.55	26.06	26.54	3.7
Respiratory therapy technicians	28,700	22,060	16,210	15,100	13,570	-8.0	16.93	18.57	21.00	21.96	22.28	3.1
Speech-language pathologists	83,110	94,660	107,340	111,640	112,530	3.4	24.20	27.89	31.80	32.86	33.60	3.7
Health Care Support Occupations												
Dental assistants	267,840	270,720	293,090	294,020	294,030	1.2	13.29	14.41	15.95	16.35	16.41	2.7
Home health aides	560,190	663,280	892,410	955,220	982,840	7.3	8.90	9.34	10.31	10.39	10.46	2.0
Massage therapists	26,440	37,670	51,250	55,920	60,040	10.8	15.93	19.33	19.16	19.13	19.12	2.3
Medical assistants	345,930	382,720	475,950	495,970	523,260	5.3	11.71	12.58	13.97	14.16	14.31	2.5
Medical equipment preparers	33,540	41,790	44,340	47,070	47,310	4.4	11.29	12.42	14.08	14.32	14.59	3.3
Medical transcriptionists	94,090	90,380	86,200	82,810	78,780	-2.2	12.99	14.36	15.84	16.03	16.12	2.7
Nursing aides, orderlies, and attendants	1,307,600	1,391,430	1,422,720	1,438,010	1,451,090	1.3	9.54	10.67	11.84	12.01	12.09	3.0
Occupational therapy aides	7,560	6,220	7,410	8,040	7,180	-0.6	11.70	13.20	14.22	13.89	14.95	3.1
Occupational therapy assistants	17,520	22,160	25,610	26,680	27,720	5.9	17.39	19.13	23.29	24.44	24.66	4.5
Pharmacy aides	58,130	46,610	53,190	52,230	49,580	-2.0	9.22	9.76	10.34	10.74	10.98	2.2
Physical therapist aides	35,250	41,930	44,410	44,160	45,900	3.4	10.45	11.01	11.91	12.01	12.02	1.8
Physical therapist assistants	47,810	58,670	61,820	63,750	65,960	4.1	17.18	18.98	22.26	23.36	23.95	4.2
Psychiatric aides	59,640	56,150	59,050	62,610	64,730	1.0	11.42	11.47	13.10	13.19	12.84	1.5

[1]Employment is the number of filled positions. This table includes both full-time and part-time wage and salary positions. Estimates do not include business establishments where persons are self-employed, owners and partners in unincorporated firms, household workers, or unpaid family workers and were rounded to the nearest 10.
[2]The mean hourly wage rate for an occupation is the total wages that all workers in the occupation earn in an hour divided by the total employment of the occupation.

Table C-64. Employment and Wages in the Health Care Industry by Occupation, May 2011

(Number, dollar.)

Occupation	Employment	Employment per 1,000 jobs	Median hourly wage	Mean hourly wage	Annual mean wage
Healthcare Practitioners and Technical Occupations	7,514,980	58.583	$28.64	$34.97	$72,730
Chiropractors	27,510	0.214	$31.76	$37.88	$78,780
Dentists, General	90,950	0.709	$68.62	$77.76	$161,750
Oral and Maxillofacial Surgeons	5,800	0.045	(1)	$104.51	$217,380
Orthodontists	5,040	0.039	(1)	$98.40	$204,670
Prosthodontists	560	0.004	$52.55	$62.89	$130,820
Dentists, All Other Specialists	4,850	0.038	$78.01	$80.77	$168,000
Dietitians and Nutritionists	56,130	0.438	$26.19	$26.66	$55,460
Optometrists	27,950	0.218	$45.53	$51.79	$107,720
Pharmacists	272,320	2.123	$54.51	$53.92	$112,160
Anesthesiologists	33,310	0.26	(1)	$112.96	$234,950
Family and General Practitioners	101,800	0.794	$80.29	$85.26	$177,330
Internists, General	46,740	0.364	$88.06	$90.97	$189,210
Obstetricians and Gynecologists	20,540	0.16	(1)	$105.10	$218,610
Pediatricians, General	29,640	0.231	$76.04	$81.08	$168,650
Psychiatrists	23,140	0.18	$81.90	$83.73	$174,170
Surgeons	42,340	0.33	(1)	$111.32	$231,550
Physicians and Surgeons, All Other	305,590	2.382	(1)	$88.78	$184,650
Physician Assistants	83,540	0.651	$42.62	$43.01	$89,470
Podiatrists	9,210	0.072	$57.33	$64.36	$133,870
Registered Nurses	2,724,570	21.24	$31.71	$33.23	$69,110
Occupational Therapists	103,570	0.807	$35.49	$36.05	$74,970
Physical Therapists	185,440	1.446	$37.63	$38.38	$79,830
Radiation Therapists	18,380	0.143	$36.84	$38.14	$79,340
Recreational Therapists	19,650	0.153	$19.74	$20.65	$42,940
Respiratory Therapists	113,980	0.889	$26.56	$27.05	$56,260
Speech-Language Pathologists	117,210	0.914	$33.22	$34.61	$72,000
Therapists, All Other	15,720	0.123	$23.61	$25.43	$52,890
Veterinarians	55,410	0.432	$39.86	$43.87	$91,250
Audiologists	12,490	0.097	$32.88	$34.13	$71,000
Health Diagnosing and Treating Practitioners, All Other	32,300	0.252	$33.98	$40.24	$83,710
Medical and Clinical Laboratory Technologists	165,220	1.288	$27.41	$27.94	$58,120
Medical and Clinical Laboratory Technicians	156,860	1.223	$17.76	$18.73	$38,960
Dental Hygienists	184,110	1.435	$33.31	$33.54	$69,760
Cardiovascular Technologists and Technicians	50,410	0.393	$24.53	$25.08	$52,160
Diagnostic Medical Sonographers	54,760	0.427	$31.35	$31.63	$65,800
Nuclear Medicine Technologists	21,200	0.165	$33.39	$33.64	$69,960
Radiologic Technologists and Technicians	220,540	1.719	$26.50	$27.29	$56,760
Emergency Medical Technicians and Paramedics	229,340	1.788	$14.77	$16.36	$34,030
Dietetic Technicians	23,490	0.183	$12.85	$14.04	$29,200
Pharmacy Technicians	343,550	2.678	$13.91	$14.43	$30,020
Psychiatric Technicians	69,840	0.544	$13.69	$15.08	$31,370
Respiratory Therapy Technicians	13,940	0.109	$22.28	$22.76	$47,330
Surgical Technologists	94,490	0.737	$19.69	$20.41	$42,460
Veterinary Technologists and Technicians	78,800	0.614	$14.49	$15.18	$31,570
Licensed Practical and Licensed Vocational Nurses	729,140	5.684	$19.79	$20.21	$42,040
Medical Records and Health Information Technicians	180,280	1.405	$16.01	$17.27	$35,920
Opticians, Dispensing	60,680	0.473	$15.91	$16.70	$34,750
Orthotists and Prosthetists	6,860	0.053	$31.37	$34.13	$71,000
Health Technologists and Technicians, All Other	103,120	0.804	$18.31	$20.11	$41,830
Occupational Health and Safety Specialists	57,950	0.452	$31.86	$32.37	$67,340
Occupational Health and Safety Technicians	11,090	0.086	$22.13	$23.19	$48,240
Athletic Trainers	18,240	0.142	—	—	$44,640
Healthcare Practitioners and Technical Workers, All Other	55,450	0.432	$21.61	$25.64	$53,330

Table C-64. Employment and Wages in the Health Care Industry by Occupation, May 2011—Continued

(Number, dollar.)

Occupation	Employment	Employment per 1,000 jobs	Median hourly wage	Mean hourly wage	Annual mean wage
Healthcare Support Occupations	3,954,070	30.824	$12.08	$13.16	$27,370
Home Health Aides	924,650	7.208	$9.91	$10.49	$21,820
Nursing Aides, Orderlies, and Attendants	1,466,700	11.434	$11.63	$12.22	$25,420
Psychiatric Aides	71,570	0.558	$12.10	$13.11	$27,270
Occupational Therapy Assistants	29,130	0.227	$25.02	$25.07	$52,150
Occupational Therapy Aides	7,090	0.055	$13.56	$15.28	$31,770
Physical Therapist Assistants	67,550	0.527	$24.54	$24.57	$51,110
Physical Therapist Aides	47,640	0.371	$11.39	$12.11	$25,190
Massage Therapists	63,810	0.497	$17.23	$19.19	$39,920
Dental Assistants	296,810	2.314	$16.42	$16.70	$34,740
Medical Assistants	539,220	4.204	$13.99	$14.51	$30,170
Medical Equipment Preparers	49,560	0.386	$14.45	$14.99	$31,180
Medical Transcriptionists	76,570	0.597	$16.10	$16.37	$34,050
Pharmacy Aides	45,130	0.352	$10.56	$11.23	$23,350
Veterinary Assistants and Laboratory Animal Caretakers	72,530	0.565	$10.98	$11.75	$24,430
Healthcare Support Workers, All Other	196,100	1.529	$14.80	$15.50	$32,240

— =Data not available.
[1]Represents a wage above $90 per hour.

Table C-65 Employment and Wages for the Highest and Lowest Paying Occupations, May 2011

(Dollar, number.)

Occupation title	Median wage[1]	Employment
Anesthesiologists	(2)	33,310
Surgeons	(2)	42,340
Obstetricians and Gynecologists	(3)	20,540
Oral and Maxillofacial Surgeons	(3)	5,800
Orthodontists	(3)	5,040
Physicians and Surgeons, All Other	(3)	305,590
Internists, General	$183,170	46,740
Psychiatrists	$170,350	23,140
Family and General Practitioners	$167,000	101,800
Chief Executives	$166,910	267,370
Dentists, All Other Specialists	$162,260	4,850
Pediatricians, General	$158,170	29,640
Dentists, General	$142,740	90,950
Petroleum Engineers	$122,280	30,880
Architectural and Engineering Managers	$122,190	184,530
Judges, Magistrate Judges, and Magistrates	$120,130	26,570
Podiatrists	$119,250	9,210
Computer and Information Systems Managers	$118,010	300,830
Marketing Managers	$116,010	168,410
Natural Sciences Managers	$114,770	47,510

[1]The median wage is the wage where half the workers in the occupation earn more and half earn less. The OES program can not estimate percentile wages above $187,200.
[2]At least 75 percent of workers in this occupaiton have wages above $187,200 per year.
[3]At least 50 percent of workers in this occuapiton have wages above $187,200 per year.

Table C-66. Industries with the Highest Levels of Employment and Highest Concentration of Employment in Health Care and Practitioner and Technical Occupations, May 2011

(Number, percent, dollar.)

Industry	Employment[1]	Percent of industry employment	Hourly mean wage	Annual mean wage[2]
Industries with the Highest Levels of Employment in Health Care and Practitioner and Technical Occupations				
General Medical and Surgical Hospitals	2,828,590	54.46	$32.37	$67,320
Offices of Physicians	973,370	41.52	$55.54	$115,510
Nursing Care Facilities	416,290	24.94	$24.80	$51,590
Health and Personal Care Stores	340,630	34.41	$29.20	$60,730
Home Health Care Services	283,520	25.19	$29.97	$62,340
Industries with the Highest Concentration of Employment in Health Care and Practitioner and Technical Occupations				
Other Ambulatory Health Care Services	142,770	55.66	$17.91	$37,250
General Medical and Surgical Hospitals	2,828,590	54.46	$32.37	$67,320
Specialty (except Psychiatric and Substance Abuse) Hospitals	109,420	49.63	$34.09	$70,910
Offices of Physicians	973,370	41.52	$55.54	$115,510
Medical and Diagnostic Laboratories	92,790	40.43	$30.13	$62,680

[1] Estimates for detailed occupations do not sum to the totals because the totals include occupations not shown separately. Estimates do not include self-employed workers.
[2] Annual wages have been calculated by multiplying the hourly mean wage by a "year-round, full-time" hours figure of 2,080 hours; for those occupations where there is not an hourly mean wage published, the annual wage has been directly calculated from the reported survey data.

Table C-67. States with the Highest Level of Employment and Highest Concentration of Jobs in Health Care Practitioner and Technical Occupations, May 2011

(Number, dollar.)

State	Employment[1]	Employment per thousand jobs	Location quotient[2]	Hourly mean wage	Annual mean wage[3]
States with the Highest Employment Level in this Occupation					
California	703,190	50.09	0.86	$41.95	$87,260
Texas	555,780	53.94	0.92	$32.85	$68,330
New York	489,900	58.13	0.99	$38.88	$80,870
Florida	444,830	62.2	1.06	$33.31	$69,290
Pennsylvania	350,850	63.23	1.08	$33.57	$69,820
States with the Highest Concentration of Jobs and Location Quotients in this Occupation					
West Virginia	51,430	73.44	1.25	$28.72	$59,730
Massachusetts	227,900	72.19	1.23	$39.55	$82,270
Mississippi	73,960	68.93	1.18	$28.42	$59,120
Rhode Island	30,920	68.56	1.17	$37.57	$78,150
Maine	39,320	68.31	1.17	$35.58	$74,010

[1] Estimates for detailed occupations do not sum to the totals because the totals include occupations not shown separately. Estimates do not include self-employed workers.
[2] The location quotient is the ratio of the area concentration of occupational employment to the national average concentration. A location quotient greater than one indicates the occupation has a higher share of employment than average, and a location quotient less than one indicates the occupation is less prevalent in the area than average.
[3] Annual wages have been calculated by multiplying the hourly mean wage by a "year-round, full-time" hours figure of 2,080 hours; for those occupations where there is not an hourly mean wage published, the annual wage has been directly calculated from the reported survey data.

Table C-68. Top Paying Metropolitan Area for Health Care Practitioner and Technical Occupations, May 2011

(Number, dollar.)

Metropolitan area	Employment[1]	Employment per thousand jobs	Location quotient[2]	Hourly mean wage	Annual mean wage[3]
San Jose-Sunnyvale-Santa Clara, CA	34,720	39.61	0.68	$51.13	$106,350
Napa, CA	4,310	69.81	1.19	$51.05	$106,170
Vallejo-Fairfield, CA	7,810	66.47	1.13	$48.17	$100,200
Oakland-Fremont-Hayward, CA Metropolitan Division	57,130	60.00	1.02	$47.89	$99,600
San Francisco-San Mateo-Redwood City, CA Metropolitan Division	44,150	46.00	0.79	$46.88	$97,510
Sacramento–Arden-Arcade–Roseville, CA	43,380	53.88	0.92	$45.01	$93,630
Salinas, CA	6,610	43.52	0.74	$44.89	$93,360
Bethesda-Rockville-Frederick, MD Metropolitan Division	37,980	68.34	1.17	$44.42	$92,400
Anchorage, AK	9,220	54.84	0.94	$43.83	$91,170
Carson City, NV	1,580	59.28	1.01	$43.49	$90,470

[1]Estimates for detailed occupations do not sum to the totals because the totals include occupations not shown separately. Estimates do not include self-employed workers.
[2]The location quotient is the ratio of the area concentration of occupational employment to the national average concentration. A location quotient greater than one indicates the occupation has a higher share of employment than average, and a location quotient less than one indicates the occupation is less prevalent in the area than average.
[3]Annual wages have been calculated by multiplying the hourly mean wage by a "year-round, full-time" hours figure of 2,080 hours; for those occupations where there is not an hourly mean wage published, the annual wage has been directly calculated from the reported survey data.

Table C-69. Employers' Costs Per Employee-Hour Worked for Total Compensation, Wages and Salaries, and Health Insurance, by Selected Characteristics, Selected Years, 1991–2011

(Dollar, percent.)

Characteristic	1991	1995	2000	2005	2006	2007	2008	2009	2010	2011
TOTAL COMPENSATION PER EMPLOYEE-HOUR WORKED										
State and local government	$22.31	$24.86	$29.05	$35.50	$36.96	$38.66	$37.84	$39.51	$39.81	$40.54
Total private industry	15.40	17.10	19.85	24.17	25.09	25.91	26.76	27.46	27.73	28.10
Industry										
Goods producing	18.48	20.75	23.55	28.48	29.36	30.12	31.38	32.29	32.42	32.91
Service providing	14.31	15.88	18.72	23.11	24.05	24.84	25.63	26.37	26.77	27.11
Occupational Group[1]										
White collar	18.15	20.50	24.19	—	—	—	—	—	—	—
Blue collar	15.15	16.69	18.73	—	—	—	—	—	—	—
Service	7.82	8.39	9.72	—	—	—	—	—	—	—
Management, professional, and related	—	—	—	42.09	44.32	46.05	47.55	48.82	48.80	50.08
Sales and office	—	—	—	19.30	19.93	20.55	21.15	21.40	21.77	22.02
Service	—	—	—	12.07	12.30	12.87	13.27	13.53	13.71	13.98
Natural resources, construction, and maintenance	—	—	—	27.26	28.07	28.96	30.13	30.97	31.10	30.93
Production, transportation, and material moving	—	—	—	20.82	21.19	22.22	23.07	23.28	23.72	23.70
Census Region										
Northeast	17.56	20.09	22.67	27.09	28.75	29.56	30.56	31.73	32.13	32.16
Midwest	15.05	15.89	19.22	24.23	24.65	25.16	25.98	26.44	26.75	27.47
South	13.68	15.31	17.81	21.36	22.35	23.17	23.90	24.45	24.72	24.93
West	15.97	18.35	20.88	25.98	26.56	27.77	28.70	29.53	29.52	29.95
Union Status										
Union	19.76	22.40	25.88	33.17	34.07	35.27	36.28	36.59	37.16	37.68
Nonunion	14.56	16.26	19.07	23.09	24.03	24.82	25.64	26.39	26.67	27.08
Establishment Employment Size										
1–99 employees	13.38	14.58	17.16	20.22	20.43	21.29	22.23	22.56	22.84	23.21
100 or more	17.34	19.44	22.81	28.94	30.34	30.86	31.68	32.83	33.33	33.69
100–499	14.31	16.30	19.30	24.44	25.91	26.31	26.80	28.19	28.55	28.69
500 or more	20.60	22.85	26.93	34.59	35.94	36.48	37.60	38.71	39.76	40.53
WAGES AND SALARIES AS A PERCENT OF TOTAL COMPENSATION										
State and local government	69.6	69.6	70.8	68.3	67.6	67.0	65.9	65.7	65.9	65.5
Total private industry	72.3	71.6	73.0	71.0	70.7	70.8	70.6	70.8	70.6	70.7
Industry										
Goods producing	68.7	67.3	69.0	65.5	66.2	66.8	66.7	66.9	66.7	66.5
Service providing	74.0	73.5	74.5	72.6	72.0	72.0	71.8	71.9	71.6	71.7
Occupational Group[1]										
White collar	73.8	73.0	74.0	—	—	—	—	—	—	—
Blue collar	68.4	67.6	69.4	—	—	—	—	—	—	—
Service	76.3	75.7	77.9	—	—	—	—	—	—	—
Management, professional, and related	—	—	—	71.5	70.9	71.1	71.0	71.1	70.7	70.8
Sales and office	—	—	—	72.6	72.2	72.1	72.0	71.8	71.6	71.6
Service	—	—	—	75.7	75.3	75.0	74.8	75.3	75.4	75.4
Natural resources, construction, and maintenance	—	—	—	68.0	68.0	68.3	68.3	68.2	68.0	68.3
Production, transportation, and material moving	—	—	—	66.2	66.7	66.8	66.6	67.0	66.8	66.7
Census Region										
Northeast	72.1	70.9	72.2	70.4	70.0	69.7	69.8	69.6	69.0	69.5
Midwest	71.1	70.8	72.4	70.1	69.4	69.9	69.8	70.3	70.0	69.8
South	73.3	72.1	73.5	72.1	72.1	72.0	71.8	71.9	71.8	71.9
West	72.8	73.0	74.0	70.9	71.0	71.0	70.8	71.1	71.1	71.0
Union Status										
Union	65.9	64.3	65.2	62.6	62.3	62.2	61.9	62.2	61.6	61.1
Nonunion	74.0	73.2	74.4	72.4	72.1	72.2	72.1	72.2	72.0	72.1
Establishment Employment Size										
1–99 employees	74.7	74.1	75.5	73.9	73.7	73.8	73.8	74.0	73.6	74.0
100 or more	70.5	69.9	71.0	68.5	68.4	68.5	68.2	68.4	68.2	68.0
100–499	72.1	71.3	72.8	70.2	70.0	70.1	69.8	70.0	70.0	69.9
500 or more	69.3	68.8	69.4	67.0	66.9	67.1	66.9	67.0	66.5	66.2

Table C-69. Employers' Costs Per Employee-Hour Worked for Total Compensation, Wages and Salaries, and Health Insurance, by Selected Characteristics, Selected Years, 1991–2011—*Continued*

(Dollar, percent.)

Characteristic	1991	1995	2000	2005	2006	2007	2008	2009	2010	2011
HEALTH INSURANCE AS A PERCENT OF TOTAL COMPENSATION										
State and local government	6.9	7.8	7.8	10.2	10.6	10.9	11.0	10.9	11.4	11.7
Total private industry	6.0	6.2	5.5	6.8	6.9	7.1	7.2	7.3	7.5	7.5
Industry										
Goods producing	6.9	7.4	6.9	8.0	8.4	8.4	8.5	8.7	8.9	8.9
Service providing	5.5	5.7	4.9	6.4	6.4	6.7	6.8	6.9	7.2	7.2
Occupational Group[1]										
White collar	5.6	5.7	5.0	—	—	—	—	—	—	—
Blue collar	7.0	7.5	6.8	—	—	—	—	—	—	—
Service	4.6	5.1	4.3	—	—	—	—	—	—	—
Management, professional, and related	—	—	—	5.5	5.6	5.8	5.8	6.0	6.2	6.3
Sales and office	—	—	—	7.5	7.5	7.8	7.9	8.3	8.6	8.6
Service	—	—	—	6.1	6.2	6.7	6.8	6.7	6.7	6.5
Natural resources, construction, and maintenance	—	—	—	7.5	7.7	7.6	7.6	7.9	8.0	8.0
Production, transportation, and material moving	—	—	—	8.9	9.0	9.3	9.6	9.7	9.9	10.1
Census Region										
Northeast	6.2	6.4	5.6	6.8	6.7	6.9	6.9	7.2	7.5	7.8
Midwest	6.3	6.7	5.8	7.3	7.6	7.8	7.9	8.1	8.3	8.3
South	5.5	6.0	5.4	6.6	6.7	6.9	6.9	7.0	7.2	7.2
West	5.8	5.6	5.0	6.3	6.4	6.7	6.9	6.9	7.1	7.1
Union Status										
Union	8.2	9.3	8.4	10.3	10.3	10.8	10.9	11.4	11.8	12.3
Nonunion	5.4	5.5	5.0	6.2	6.3	6.4	6.5	6.6	6.8	6.8
Establishment Employment Size										
1–99 employees	5.1	5.3	4.8	5.9	6.0	6.1	6.1	6.3	6.4	6.3
100 or more	6.6	6.9	6.0	7.5	7.5	7.8	8.0	8.1	8.4	8.6
100–499	6.3	6.5	5.6	7.5	7.4	7.7	7.9	7.9	8.3	8.4
500 or more	6.8	7.2	6.4	7.6	7.6	7.9	8.0	8.2	8.5	8.7

— =Data not available.

[1]Starting with 2004 data, sample establishments were classified by industry categories based on the North American Industry Classification System (NAICS), as defined by the U.S. Office of Management and Budget. Within a sample establishment, specific job categories were selected and classified into about 840 occupational classifications according to the 2000 Standard Occupational Classification (SOC) system.

HEALTH EXPENDITURES

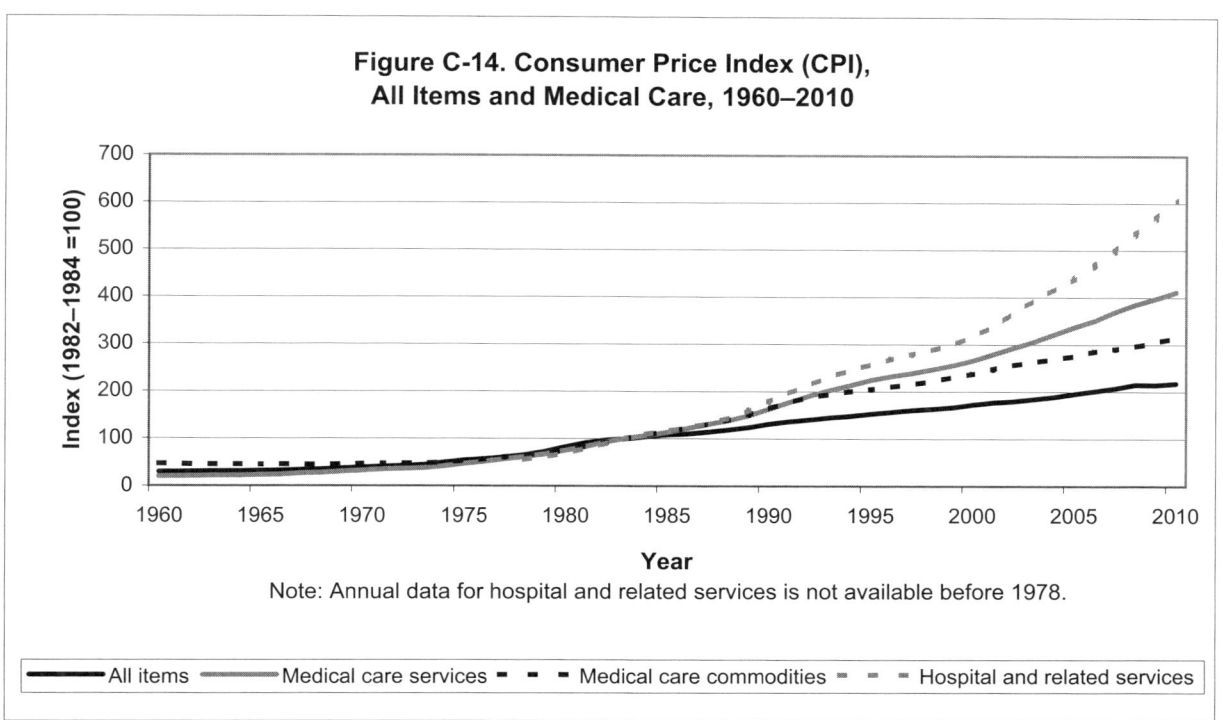

Figure C-14. Consumer Price Index (CPI), All Items and Medical Care, 1960–2010

Note: Annual data for hospital and related services is not available before 1978.

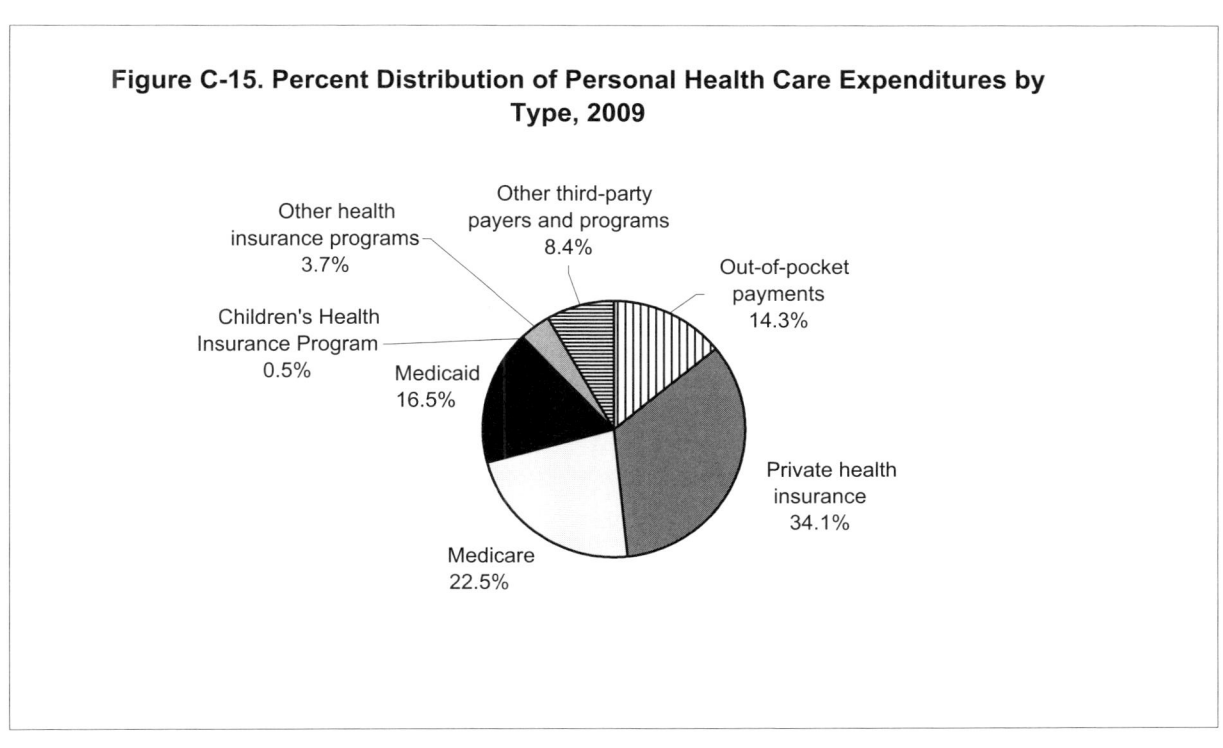

Figure C-15. Percent Distribution of Personal Health Care Expenditures by Type, 2009

Table C-70. Gross Domestic Product, National Health Expenditures, Per Capita Amounts, Percent Distribution, and Average Annual Percent Change, Selected Years, 1960–2009

(Dollars, percent.)

Gross domestic product and national health expenditures	1960	1970	1980	1990	2000	2005	2008	2009
Amount in Billions								
Gross domestic product (GDP)	$526	$1,038	$2,788	$5,801	$9,952	$12,638	$14,369	$14,119
Implicit price deflator for GDP[1] (2005 =100.0)	18.6	24.3	47.8	72.2	88.6	100.0	108.6	109.6
National health expenditures	$27.3	$74.8	$255.7	$724.0	$1,378.0	$2,021.0	$2,391.4	$2,486.3
Health consumption expenditures	24.8	67.0	235.6	675.3	1,288.5	1,890.3	2,234.2	2,330.1
Personal health care	23.3	63.1	217.1	616.6	1,164.4	1,692.6	1,997.2	2,089.9
Administration and net cost of private health insurance	1.1	2.6	12.0	38.7	81.1	141.6	164.0	163.0
Public health	0.4	1.4	6.4	20.0	43.0	56.2	72.9	77.2
Investment[1]	2.6	7.8	20.1	48.7	89.6	130.7	157.2	156.2
Per Capita Amount in Dollars								
National health expenditures	$147	$356	$1,110	$2,853	$4,878	$6,827	$7,845	$8,086
Health consumption expenditures	133	319	1,022	2,661	4,561	6,385	7,329	7,578
Personal health care	125	300	942	2,430	4,122	5,717	6,552	6,797
Administration and net cost of private health insurance	6	12	52	153	287	478	538	530
Public health	2	6	28	79	152	190	239	251
Investment[1]	14	37	87	192	317	441	516	508
National health expenditures as percent of GDP	5.2	7.2	9.2	12.5	13.8	16.0	16.6	17.6
Percent Distribution								
National health expenditures	100.0	100.0	100.0	100.0	100.0	100.0	100.0	100.0
Health consumption expenditures	90.6	89.6	92.1	93.3	93.5	93.5	93.4	93.7
Personal health care	85.4	84.3	84.9	85.2	84.5	83.7	83.5	84.1
Administration and net cost of private health insurance	3.9	3.5	4.7	5.4	5.9	7.0	6.9	6.6
Public health	1.4	1.8	2.5	2.8	3.1	2.8	3.1	3.1
Investment[1]	9.4	10.4	7.9	6.7	6.5	6.5	6.6	6.3
Average Annual Percent Change from Previous Year Shown								
GDP	X	7.0	10.4	7.6	5.5	4.9	4.4	-1.7
National health expenditures	X	10.6	13.1	11.0	6.6	8.0	5.8	4.0
Health consumption expenditures	X	10.5	13.4	11.1	6.7	8.0	5.7	4.3
Personal health care	X	10.4	13.2	11.0	6.6	7.8	5.7	4.6
Administration and net cost of private health insurance	X	9.4	16.4	12.4	7.7	11.8	5.0	-0.6
Public health	X	13.8	16.9	12.0	8.0	5.5	9.1	5.9
Investment[1]	X	11.7	10.0	9.2	6.3	7.9	6.3	-0.6
National health expenditures, per capita	X	9.3	12.0	9.9	5.5	7.0	4.7	3.1
Health consumption expenditures	X	9.1	12.4	10.0	5.5	7.0	4.7	3.4
Personal health care	X	9.1	12.1	9.9	5.4	6.8	4.6	3.7
Administration and net cost of private health insurance	X	8.1	15.4	11.3	6.5	10.8	4.0	-1.5
Public health	X	12.5	15.8	10.9	6.8	4.5	8.0	4.9
Investment[1]	X	10.4	8.9	8.2	5.2	6.8	5.3	-1.5

X = Category not applicable.

[1]Investment consists of research and structures and equipment.

Table C-71. Consumer Price Index and Average Annual Percent Change for All Items, Selected Items, and Medical Care Components, Selected Years, 1960–2010

(Percent change.)

Items and medical care components	1960	1970	1980	1990	1995	2000	2005	2007	2008	2009	2010
Consumer Price Index (CPI)											
All items	29.6	38.8	82.4	130.7	152.4	172.2	195.3	207.3	215.3	214.5	218.1
All items less medical care	30.2	39.2	82.8	128.8	148.6	167.3	188.7	200.1	207.8	206.6	209.7
Services	24.1	35.0	77.9	139.2	168.7	195.3	230.1	246.8	255.5	259.2	261.3
Food	30.0	39.2	86.8	132.4	148.4	167.8	190.7	202.9	214.1	218.0	219.6
Apparel	45.7	59.2	90.9	124.1	132.0	129.6	119.5	119.0	118.9	120.1	119.5
Housing	—	36.4	81.1	128.5	148.5	169.6	195.7	209.6	216.3	217.1	216.3
Energy	22.4	25.5	86.0	102.1	105.2	124.6	177.1	207.7	236.7	193.1	211.4
Medical care	22.3	34.0	74.9	162.8	220.5	260.8	323.2	351.1	364.1	375.6	388.4
Components of Medical Care											
Medical care services	19.5	32.3	74.8	162.7	224.2	266.0	336.7	369.3	384.9	397.3	411.2
Professional services	—	37.0	77.9	156.1	201.0	237.7	281.7	300.8	311.0	319.4	328.2
Physicians' services	21.9	34.5	76.5	160.8	208.8	244.7	287.5	303.2	311.3	320.8	331.3
Dental services	27.0	39.2	78.9	155.8	206.8	258.5	324.0	358.4	376.9	388.1	398.8
Eyeglasses and eye care[1]	—	—	—	117.3	137.0	149.7	163.2	171.6	174.1	175.5	176.7
Services by other medical professionals[1]	—	—	—	120.2	143.9	161.9	186.8	197.4	205.5	209.8	214.4
Hospital and related services	—	—	69.2	178.0	257.8	317.3	439.9	498.9	534.0	567.9	607.7
Hospital services[2]	—	—	—	—	—	115.9	161.6	183.6	197.2	210.7	227.2
Inpatient hospital services[2,3]	—	—	—	—	—	113.8	156.6	178.1	190.8	203.6	221.5
Outpatient hospital services[1,3]	—	—	—	138.7	204.6	263.8	373.0	424.2	456.8	490.6	520.6
Hospital rooms	9.3	23.6	68.0	175.4	251.2	—	—	—	—	—	—
Other inpatient services[1]	—	—	—	142.7	206.8	—	—	—	—	—	—
Nursing homes and adult day care[2]	—	—	—	—	—	117.0	145.0	159.6	165.3	171.6	177.0
Health insurance[4]	—	—	—	—	—	—	—	113.5	114.2	110.5	106.6
Medical care commodities	46.9	46.5	75.4	163.4	204.5	238.1	276.0	290.0	296.0	305.1	314.7
Medicinal drugs[5]	—	—	—	—	—	—	—	—	—	—	102.3
Prescription drugs[6]	54.0	47.4	72.5	181.7	235.0	285.4	349.0	369.2	378.3	391.1	407.8
Nonprescription drugs[5]	—	—	—	—	—	—	—	—	—	—	100.0
Medical equipment and supplies[5]	—	—	—	—	—	—	—	—	—	—	99.1
Nonprescription drugs and medical supplies[1,7]	—	—	—	120.6	140.5	149.5	151.7	156.8	158.3	161.4	—
Internal and respiratory over-the-counter drugs[8]	—	42.3	74.9	145.9	167.0	176.9	179.7	186.4	188.7	193.0	—
Nonprescription medical equipment and supplies[9]	—	—	79.2	138.0	166.3	178.1	180.6	185.1	185.6	188.2	—
Average Annual Percent Change from Previous Year Shown											
All items	X	2.7	7.8	4.7	3.1	2.5	2.5	3.0	3.8	2.4	1.6
All items less medical care	X	2.6	7.8	4.5	2.9	2.4	2.4	3.0	3.8	2.3	1.5
Services	X	3.8	8.3	6.0	3.9	3.0	3.3	3.6	3.5	3.0	0.8
Food	X	2.7	8.3	4.3	2.3	2.5	2.6	3.1	5.5	3.4	0.8
Apparel	X	2.6	4.4	3.2	1.2	-0.4	-1.6	-0.2	-0.1	0.1	-0.5
Housing	X	—	8.3	4.7	2.9	2.7	2.9	3.5	3.2	2.6	-0.4
Energy	X	1.3	12.9	1.7	0.6	3.4	7.3	8.3	13.9	2.2	9.5
Medical care	X	4.3	8.2	8.1	6.3	3.4	4.4	4.2	3.7	3.8	3.4

Table C-71. Consumer Price Index and Average Annual Percent Change for All Items, Selected Items, and Medical Care Components, Selected Years, 1960–2010—Continued

(Percent change.)

Items and medical care components	1960	1970	1980	1990	1995	2000	2005	2007	2008	2009	2010
Components of Medical Care											
Medical care services	X	5.2	8.8	8.1	6.6	3.5	4.8	4.7	4.2	4.2	3.5
Professional services	X	—	7.7	7.2	5.2	3.4	3.5	3.3	3.4	3.2	2.8
Physicians' services	X	4.6	8.3	7.7	5.4	3.2	3.3	2.7	2.7	2.8	3.3
Dental services	X	3.8	7.2	7.0	5.8	4.6	4.6	5.2	5.1	4.6	2.7
Eyeglasses and eye care[1]	X	—	—	—	3.2	1.8	1.7	2.5	1.4	1.8	0.7
Services by other medical professionals[1]	X	—	—	—	3.7	2.4	2.9	2.8	4.1	2.9	2.2
Hospital and related services	X	—	—	9.9	7.7	4.2	6.8	6.5	7.0	6.6	7.0
Hospital services[2]	X	—	—	—	—	—	6.9	6.6	7.4	6.9	7.8
Inpatient hospital services[2,3]	X	—	—	—	—	—	6.6	6.6	7.1	6.8	8.8
Outpatient hospital services[1,3]	X	—	—	—	8.1	5.2	7.2	6.6	7.7	7.1	6.1
Hospital rooms	X	9.8	11.2	9.9	7.4	—	—	—	—	—	—
Other inpatient services[1]	X	—	—	—	7.7	—	—	—	—	—	—
Nursing homes and adult day care[2]	X	—	—	—	—	—	4.4	4.9	3.6	4.3	3.1
Health insurance[4]	X	—	—	—	—	—	—	—	0.6	—	-3.5
Medical care commodities	X	-0.1	5.0	8.0	4.6	3.1	3.0	2.5	2.1	2.5	3.1
Medicinal drugs[5]	X	—	—	—	—	—	—	—	—	—	—
Prescription drugs[6]	X	-1.3	4.3	9.6	5.3	4.0	4.1	2.9	2.5	2.9	4.3
Nonprescription drugs[5]	X	—	—	—	—	—	—	—	—	—	—
Medical equipment and supplies[5]	X	—	—	—	—	—	—	—	—	—	—
Nonprescription drugs and medical supplies[1,7]	X	—	—	—	3.1	1.2	0.3	1.7	0.9	1.6	—
Internal and respiratory over-the-counter drugs[8]	X	—	5.9	6.9	2.7	1.2	0.3	1.8	1.2	1.8	—
Nonprescription medical equipment and supplies[9]	X	—	—	5.7	3.8	1.4	0.3	1.2	0.3	1.0	—

— = Data not available.
X = Category not applicable.
[1]December 1986 = 100.
[2]December 1996 = 100.
[3]Special index based on a substantially smaller sample.
[4]December 2005 = 100.
[5]December 2009 = 100.
[6]Prior to 2006, this category included medical supplies.
[7]Starting with 2010 updates, this index series will no longer be published.
[8]Starting with 2010 updates, replaced by the series, nonprescription drugs.
[9]Starting with 2010 updates, replaced by the series, medical equipment and supplies.

Table C-72. **Growth in Personal Health Care Expenditures and Percent Distribution of Factors Affecting Growth, 1960–2009**

(Percent.)

Period	Average annual percent increase	Factors affecting growth				
		Percent distribution[1]				
		All factors	Inflation[1]		Population growth	Intensity growth[4]
			Economy-wide inflation[2]	Excess medical price inflation[3]		
		Percent distribution of factors affecting growth[5]				
1960–2009	9.6	100	39	13	11	36
1960–1965	8.3	100	17	9	18	56
1965–1970	12.7	100	33	11	8	47
1970–1975	12.4	100	55	0	8	37
1975–1980	13.9	100	54	12	7	27
1980–1985	11.7	100	46	30	9	15
1985–1990	10.4	100	32	21	10	37
1990–1995	7.2	100	35	17	16	32
1995–2000	5.9	100	29	10	17	43
1995–1996	5.6	100	35	5	18	42
1996–1997	5.7	100	31	1	19	49
1997–1998	5.5	100	21	17	19	43
1998–1999	5.9	100	26	17	17	40
1999–2000	6.9	100	32	11	14	43
2000–2005	7.8	100	32	11	13	44
2000–2001	8.6	100	27	17	12	44
2001–2002	8.5	100	20	17	12	52
2002–2003	7.8	100	28	11	12	49
2003–2004	7.2	100	40	10	14	36
2004–2005	6.8	100	50	-4	14	40
2005–2006	6.3	100	53	-3	16	34
2006–2007	5.9	100	51	7	18	24
2007–2008	4.9	100	45	9	19	26
2008–2009	4.6	100	20	40	19	21

[1]Two measures of inflation are presented: economy-wide and excess medical inflation (changes in medical-specific prices in excess of those included in economy-wide inflation).
[2]Economy-wide inflation is calculated using the implicit price deflator (IDP) for gross domestic product (GDP). The IDP is a broad measure of the prices of the goods and services that the U.S. produces.
[3]Excess medical price inflation is the measured amount of medical price growth above general economy-wide price growth. This excess rate captures if medical prices have tended to rise more or less quickly than general economy-wide prices.
[4]Intensity is the residual percentage of growth that cannot be attributed to inflation or population growth. It includes changes in the use or kinds of services and supplies and captures any errors in measuring prices or total spending.
[5]Percents may not sum to 100 due to rounding.

Table C-73. National Health Expenditures for Mental Health Services, Average Annual Percent Change and Percent Distribution, by Type of Expenditure, Selected Years, 1986–2005

(Dollar, percent.)

Type of expenditure	1986	1990	1995	2000	2001	2002	2003	2004	2005
Amount in Millions									
Total expenditures	$31,764	$45,200	$60,602	$79,295	$86,984	$93,637	$100,302	$106,910	$112,787
Total, all service providers	27,860	39,130	50,927	57,528	61,017	63,805	67,045	70,624	74,429
General nonspecialty hospitals	5,345	7,377	10,380	12,444	13,304	14,268	14,960	15,919	16,750
General hospital specialty units	3,026	6,015	7,251	9,131	9,617	10,187	10,831	11,197	11,540
General hospital nonspecialty units	2,320	1,362	3,129	3,313	3,687	4,081	4,129	4,723	5,210
Specialty hospitals	8,251	11,069	11,473	10,999	11,482	11,966	12,449	12,932	13,416
All physicians	3,814	5,887	8,971	11,193	12,010	12,776	13,736	14,903	16,266
Psychiatrists	2,755	4,361	6,473	8,100	8,547	8,734	9,332	10,400	11,403
Nonpsychiatric physicians	1,058	1,525	2,498	3,093	3,464	4,042	4,405	4,502	4,864
Other professionals	1,519	2,770	3,956	4,765	5,198	5,071	5,364	5,541	5,812
Freestanding nursing homes	4,903	5,658	5,294	5,313	5,733	5,957	6,266	6,535	6,855
Freestanding home health	112	221	592	609	673	740	832	944	1,070
Specialty mental health centers	3,916	6,148	10,260	12,205	12,616	13,027	13,438	13,849	14,259
Retail prescription drug	2,362	3,718	5,958	16,697	20,109	23,242	25,826	28,398	29,974
Insurance administration	1,542	2,353	3,717	5,071	5,858	6,590	7,430	7,888	8,384
Amount in Inflation-Adjusted Millions									
Total expenditures, inflation-adjusted dollars	$50,470	$62,604	$74,326	$89,450	$95,956	$101,649	$106,590	$110,478	$112,787
GDP implicit price deflator (2005 = 1.00)[1]	0.63	0.72	0.82	0.89	0.91	0.92	0.94	0.97	1.00
Average Annual Percent Change from Previous Year Shown									
Total expenditures	X	9.2	6.0	5.5	—	—	—	7.8	5.5
Total, all service providers	X	8.9	5.4	2.5	—	—	—	5.3	5.4
General nonspecialty hospitals	X	8.4	7.1	3.7	—	—	—	6.4	5.2
General hospital specialty units	X	18.7	3.8	4.7	—	—	—	5.2	3.1
General hospital nonspecialty units	X	-12.5	18.1	1.1	—	—	—	9.3	10.3
Specialty hospitals	X	7.6	0.7	-0.8	—	—	—	4.1	3.7
All physicians	X	11.5	8.8	4.5	—	—	—	7.4	9.1
Psychiatrists	X	12.2	8.2	4.6	—	—	—	6.4	9.6
Nonpsychiatric physicians	X	9.6	10.4	4.4	—	—	—	9.8	8.0
Other professionals	X	16.2	7.4	3.8	—	—	—	3.8	4.9
Freestanding nursing homes	X	3.6	-1.3	0.1	—	—	—	5.3	4.9
Freestanding home health	X	18.5	21.8	0.6	—	—	—	11.6	13.3
Specialty mental health centers	X	11.9	10.8	3.5	—	—	—	3.2	3.0
Retail prescription drug	X	12.0	9.9	22.9	—	—	—	14.2	5.5
Insurance administration	X	11.1	9.6	6.4	—	—	—	11.7	6.3
Percent Distribution									
Total expenditures	100.0	100.0	100.0	100.0	100.0	100.0	100.0	100.0	100.0
Total, all service providers	87.7	86.6	84.0	72.5	70.1	68.1	66.8	66.1	66.0
General nonspecialty hospitals	16.8	16.3	17.1	15.7	15.3	15.2	14.9	14.9	14.9
General hospital specialty units	9.5	13.3	12.0	11.5	11.1	10.9	10.8	10.5	10.2
General hospital nonspecialty units	7.3	3.0	5.2	4.2	4.2	4.4	4.1	4.4	4.6
Specialty hospitals	26.0	24.5	18.9	13.9	13.2	12.8	12.4	12.1	11.9
All physicians	12.0	13.0	14.8	14.1	13.8	13.6	13.7	13.9	14.4
Psychiatrists	8.7	9.6	10.7	10.2	9.8	9.3	9.3	9.7	10.1
Nonpsychiatric physicians	3.3	3.4	4.1	3.9	4.0	4.3	4.4	4.2	4.3
Other professionals	4.8	6.1	6.5	6.0	6.0	5.4	5.3	5.2	5.2
Freestanding nursing homes	15.4	12.5	8.7	6.7	6.6	6.4	6.2	6.1	6.1
Freestanding home health	0.4	0.5	1.0	0.8	0.8	0.8	0.8	0.9	0.9
Specialty mental health centers	12.3	13.6	16.9	15.4	14.5	13.9	13.4	13.0	12.6
Retail prescription drug	7.4	8.2	9.8	21.1	23.1	24.8	25.7	26.6	26.6
Insurance administration	4.9	5.2	6.1	6.4	6.7	7.0	7.4	7.4	7.4

— = Data not available.
X = Category not applicable.
[1] Gross Domestic Product (GDP) implicit price deflator developed by the U.S. Department of Commerce, Bureau of Economic Analysis.

Table C-74 National Health Expenditures for Substance Abuse Treatment, Average Annual Percent Change and Percent Distribution, by Type of Expenditure, Selected Years, 1986–2005

(Dollar, percent.)

Type of expenditure	1986	1990	1995	2000	2001	2002	2003	2004	2005
Amount in Millions									
Total expenditures	$9,147	$11,718	$15,369	$16,756	$18,116	$19,134	$20,078	$20,849	$22,175
Total, all service providers	8,634	11,109	14,464	15,779	16,960	17,886	18,722	19,401	20,557
General nonspecialty hospitals	3,254	3,333	3,942	3,436	3,683	3,841	4,116	4,186	4,343
General hospital specialty units	2,505	2,275	3,236	2,592	2,690	2,785	2,896	2,846	2,842
General hospital nonspecialty units	748	1,058	706	844	992	1,057	1,220	1,340	1,502
Specialty hospitals	1,409	1,346	1,315	1,000	1,061	1,123	1,144	1,187	1,214
All physicians	1,091	1,090	1,156	1,287	1,320	1,312	1,369	1,355	1,391
Psychiatrists	237	294	435	434	385	370	444	441	482
Nonpsychiatric physicians	854	796	722	853	935	942	925	914	909
Other professionals	651	1,056	1,242	1,378	1,460	1,438	1,581	1,648	1,760
Freestanding nursing homes	114	134	177	248	263	265	262	257	273
Freestanding home health	2	3	15	10	10	3	3	3	4
Specialty mental health centers	325	657	1,012	1,570	1,647	1,723	1,799	1,875	1,951
Specialty substance abuse centers	1,788	3,490	5,605	6,851	7,516	8,182	8,449	8,889	9,621
Retail prescription drug	6	9	12	21	24	32	35	69	141
Insurance administration	507	599	893	956	1,132	1,216	1,322	1,378	1,477
Amount in Inflation-Adjusted Millions									
Total expenditures, inflation-adjusted dollars	$14,533	$16,230	$18,849	$18,902	$19,984	$20,771	$21,337	$21,544	$22,175
GDP implicit price deflator (2005 = 1.00)[1]	0.63	0.72	0.82	0.89	0.91	0.92	0.94	0.97	1.00
Average Annual Percent Change from Previous Year Shown									
Total expenditures	X	6.4	5.6	1.7	—	—	—	5.6	6.4
Total, all service providers	X	6.5	5.4	1.8	—	—	—	5.3	6.0
General nonspecialty hospitals	X	0.6	3.4	-2.7	—	—	—	5.1	3.7
General hospital specialty units	X	-2.4	7.3	-4.3	—	—	—	2.4	-0.1
General hospital nonspecialty units	X	9.0	-7.8	3.6	—	—	—	12.3	12.0
Specialty hospitals	X	-1.1	-0.5	-5.3	—	—	—	4.4	2.2
All physicians	X	0.0	1.2	2.2	—	—	—	1.3	2.6
Psychiatrists	X	5.5	8.1	0.0	—	—	—	0.4	9.4
Nonpsychiatric physicians	X	-1.7	-2.0	3.4	—	—	—	1.7	-0.6
Other professionals	X	12.9	3.3	2.1	—	—	—	4.6	6.8
Freestanding nursing homes	X	4.1	5.7	6.9	—	—	—	0.9	6.0
Freestanding home health	X	15.9	35.9	-9.0	—	—	—	-23.2	8.0
Specialty mental health centers	X	19.3	9.0	9.2	—	—	—	4.5	4.1
Specialty substance abuse centers	X	18.2	9.9	4.1	—	—	—	6.7	8.2
Retail prescription drug	X	11.1	6.0	11.6	—	—	—	34.1	104.8
Insurance administration	X	4.3	8.3	1.4	—	—	—	9.6	7.2
Percent Distribution									
Total expenditures	100.0	100.0	100.0	100.0	100.0	100.0	100.0	100.0	100.0
Total, all service providers	94.4	94.8	94.1	94.2	93.6	93.5	93.2	93.1	92.7
General nonspecialty hospitals	35.6	28.4	25.6	20.5	20.3	20.1	20.5	20.1	19.6
General hospital specialty units	27.4	19.4	21.1	15.5	14.9	14.6	14.4	13.7	12.8
General hospital nonspecialty units	8.2	9.0	4.6	5.0	5.5	5.5	6.1	6.4	6.8
Specialty hospitals	15.4	11.5	8.6	6.0	5.9	5.9	5.7	5.7	5.5
All physicians	11.9	9.3	7.5	7.7	7.3	6.9	6.8	6.5	6.3
Psychiatrists	2.6	2.5	2.8	2.6	2.1	1.9	2.2	2.1	2.2
Nonpsychiatric physicians	9.3	6.8	4.7	5.1	5.2	4.9	4.6	4.4	4.1
Other professionals	7.1	9.0	8.1	8.2	8.1	7.5	7.9	7.9	7.9
Freestanding nursing homes	1.3	1.1	1.2	1.5	1.5	1.4	1.3	1.2	1.2
Freestanding home health	0.0	0.0	0.1	0.1	0.1	0.0	0.0	0.0	0.0
Specialty mental health centers	3.6	5.6	6.6	9.4	9.1	9.0	9.0	9.0	8.8
Specialty substance abuse centers	19.5	29.8	36.5	40.9	41.5	42.8	42.1	42.6	43.4
Retail prescription drug	0.1	0.1	0.1	0.1	0.1	0.2	0.2	0.3	0.6
Insurance administration	5.5	5.1	5.8	5.7	6.2	6.4	6.6	6.6	6.7

— = Data not available.
X = Category not applicable.
0.0 = Quantity more than zero but less than 0.05.
[1] Gross Domestic Product (GDP) implicit price deflator developed by the U.S. Department of Commerce, Bureau of Economic Analysis.

Table C-75. National Health Expenditures, Average Annual Percent Change, and Percent Distribution, by Type of Expenditure, Selected Years, 1960–2009

(Number, percent.)

Type of national health expenditure	1960	1970	1980	1990	2000	2005	2006	2007	2008	2009
Amount in Billions										
National health expenditures	$27.3	$74.8	$255.7	$724.0	$1,378.0	$2,021.0	$2,152.1	$2,283.5	$2,391.4	$2,486.3
Health consumption expenditures	24.8	67.0	235.6	675.3	1,288.5	1,890.3	2,016.9	2,135.1	2,234.2	2,330.1
Personal health care	23.3	63.1	217.1	616.6	1,164.4	1,692.6	1,798.8	1,904.3	1,997.2	2,089.9
Hospital care	9.0	27.2	100.5	250.4	415.5	606.5	648.3	686.8	722.1	759.1
Professional services	8.0	19.7	64.5	207.9	389.0	559.4	588.4	619.4	652.2	674.9
Physician and clinical services	5.6	14.3	47.7	158.9	290.0	419.6	441.6	462.6	486.5	505.9
Other professional services	0.4	0.7	3.5	17.4	37.0	53.1	55.4	59.5	63.4	66.8
Dental services	2.0	4.7	13.3	31.5	62.0	86.8	91.4	97.3	102.3	102.2
Other health, residential, and personal care	0.5	1.3	8.5	24.3	64.7	96.5	102.1	108.3	113.3	122.6
Home health care[1]	0.1	0.2	2.4	12.6	32.4	48.7	52.6	57.8	62.1	68.3
Nursing care facilities and continuing care retirement communities[1]	0.8	4.0	15.3	44.9	85.1	112.1	117.0	126.5	132.8	137.0
Retail outlet sales of medical products	5.0	10.6	25.9	76.5	177.6	269.3	290.4	305.6	314.7	328.0
Prescription drugs	2.7	5.5	12.0	40.3	120.9	201.7	219.8	230.2	237.2	249.9
Durable medical equipment	0.7	1.7	4.1	13.8	25.1	30.4	31.9	34.4	35.1	34.9
Other nondurable medical products	1.6	3.3	9.8	22.4	31.6	37.2	38.7	41.1	42.3	43.3
Government administration[2]	0.1	0.3	2.5	6.2	17.1	26.8	28.3	29.2	29.2	29.8
Net cost of health insurance[3]	1.0	2.0	9.5	32.5	64.0	114.7	127.2	132.8	134.8	133.2
Government public health activities[4]	0.4	1.4	6.4	20.0	43.0	56.2	62.6	68.8	72.9	77.2
Investment	2.6	7.8	20.1	48.7	89.6	130.7	135.2	148.4	157.2	156.2
Research[5]	0.7	2.0	5.4	12.7	25.5	40.3	41.4	41.9	43.2	45.3
Structures and equipment	1.9	5.8	14.7	36.0	64.1	90.4	93.8	106.4	114.0	110.9
Average Annual Percent Change from Previous Year Shown										
National health expenditures	X	10.6	13.1	11.0	6.6	8.0	6.5	6.1	4.7	4.0
Health consumption expenditures	X	10.5	13.4	11.1	6.7	8.0	6.7	5.9	4.6	4.3
Personal health care	X	10.4	13.2	11.0	6.6	7.8	6.3	5.9	4.9	4.6
Hospital care	X	11.7	14.0	9.6	5.2	7.9	6.9	5.9	5.2	5.1
Professional services	X	9.5	12.6	12.4	6.5	7.5	5.2	5.3	5.3	3.5
Physician and clinical services	X	9.8	12.8	12.8	6.2	7.7	5.3	4.8	5.2	4.0
Other professional services	X	6.3	17.0	17.5	7.8	7.5	4.4	7.4	6.6	5.3
Dental services	X	9.1	11.1	9.0	7.0	7.0	5.3	6.5	5.1	-0.1
Other health, residential, and personal care	X	11.4	20.4	11.1	10.3	8.3	5.8	6.1	4.6	8.3
Home health care[1]	X	14.5	26.9	18.1	9.9	8.5	8.0	9.9	7.5	10.0
Nursing care facilities and continuing care retirement communities[1]	X	17.4	14.2	11.4	6.6	5.7	4.3	8.1	5.0	3.1
Retail outlet sales of medical products	X	7.7	9.4	11.4	8.8	8.7	7.8	5.2	3.0	4.2
Prescription drugs	X	7.5	8.2	12.8	11.6	10.8	9.0	4.7	3.1	5.3
Durable medical equipment	X	9.0	8.8	13.0	6.2	3.9	5.2	7.6	2.3	-0.8
Other nondurable medical products	X	7.4	11.4	8.6	3.5	3.4	4.0	6.0	3.1	2.2
Government administration[2]	X	16.7	25.9	9.5	10.6	9.4	5.6	3.1	0.1	2.0
Net cost of health insurance[3]	X	6.9	17.0	13.1	7.0	12.4	10.9	4.4	1.5	-1.2
Government public health activities[4]	X	13.8	16.9	12.0	8.0	5.5	11.4	9.9	6.0	5.9
Investment	X	11.7	10.0	9.2	6.3	7.9	3.4	9.8	6.0	-0.6
Research[5]	X	10.9	10.8	8.9	7.2	9.6	2.6	1.3	3.1	4.8
Structures and equipment	X	12.0	9.7	9.4	5.9	7.1	3.7	13.5	7.1	-2.7

Table C-75. National Health Expenditures, Average Annual Percent Change, and Percent Distribution, by Type of Expenditure, Selected Years, 1960–2009—Continued

(Number, percent.)

Type of national health expenditure	1960	1970	1980	1990	2000	2005	2006	2007	2008	2009
Percent Distribution										
National health expenditures	100.0	100.0	100.0	100.0	100.0	100.0	100.0	100.0	100.0	100.0
Health consumption expenditures	90.6	89.6	92.1	93.3	93.5	93.5	93.7	93.5	93.4	93.7
Personal health care	85.4	84.3	84.9	85.2	84.5	83.7	83.6	83.4	83.5	84.1
Hospital care	32.9	36.3	39.3	34.6	30.2	30.0	30.1	30.1	30.2	30.5
Professional services	29.2	26.4	25.2	28.7	28.2	27.7	27.3	27.1	27.3	27.1
Physician and clinical services	20.6	19.2	18.7	22.0	21.0	20.8	20.5	20.3	20.3	20.3
Other professional services	1.4	1.0	1.4	2.4	2.7	2.6	2.6	2.6	2.7	2.7
Dental services	7.2	6.2	5.2	4.4	4.5	4.3	4.2	4.3	4.3	4.1
Other health, residential, and personal care	1.6	1.8	3.3	3.4	4.7	4.8	4.7	4.7	4.7	4.9
Home health care[1]	0.2	0.3	0.9	1.7	2.4	2.4	2.4	2.5	2.6	2.7
Nursing care facilities and continuing care retirement communities[1]	3.0	5.4	6.0	6.2	6.2	5.5	5.4	5.5	5.6	5.5
Retail outlet sales of medical products	18.4	14.1	10.1	10.6	12.9	13.3	13.5	13.4	13.2	13.2
Prescription drugs	9.8	7.3	4.7	5.6	8.8	10.0	10.2	10.1	9.9	10.1
Durable medical equipment	2.7	2.3	1.6	1.9	1.8	1.5	1.5	1.5	1.5	1.4
Other nondurable medical products	5.9	4.4	3.8	3.1	2.3	1.8	1.8	1.8	1.8	1.7
Government administration[2]	0.2	0.3	1.0	0.9	1.2	1.3	1.3	1.3	1.2	1.2
Net cost of health insurance[3]	3.7	2.6	3.7	4.5	4.6	5.7	5.9	5.8	5.6	5.4
Government public health activities[4]	1.4	1.8	2.5	2.8	3.1	2.8	2.9	3.0	3.1	3.1
Investment	9.4	10.4	7.9	6.7	6.5	6.5	6.3	6.5	6.6	6.3
Research[5]	2.5	2.6	2.1	1.8	1.8	2.0	1.9	1.8	1.8	1.8
Structures and equipment	6.8	7.8	5.7	5.0	4.7	4.5	4.4	4.7	4.8	4.5

X = Category not applicable.
[1] Includes expenditures for care in freestanding facilities only. Additional services of this type are provided in hospital-based facilities and are considered hospital care.
[2] Includes all administrative costs (federal and state and local employees' salaries, contracted employees including fiscal intermediaries, rent and building costs, computer systems and programs, other materials and supplies, and other miscellaneous expenses) associated with insuring individuals enrolled in the following health insurance programs: Medicare, Medicaid, Children's Health Insurance Program, Department of Defense, Department of Veterans Affairs, Indian Health Service, workers' compensation, maternal and child health, vocational rehabilitation, Substance Abuse and Mental Health Services Administration, and other federal programs.
[3] Net cost of health insurance is calculated as the difference between calendar year incurred premiums earned and benefits paid for private health insurance.
[4] Includes personal care services delivered by government public health agencies.
[5] Research and development expenditures of drug companies and other manufacturers and providers of medical equipment and supplies are excluded. They are included in the expenditure class in which the product falls because such expenditures are covered by the payment received for that product.

Table C-76. Personal Health Care Expenditures, by Source of Funds and Type of Expenditure, Selected Years, 1960–2009

(Number, percent.)

Type of personal health care expenditures and source of funds	1960	1970	1980	1990	2000	2005	2006	2007	2008	2009
Amount										
Per capita	$125	$300	$942	$2,430	$4,122	$5,717	$6,016	$6,305	$6,552	$6,797
Amount in Billions										
All personal health care expenditures[1]	$23.3	$63.1	$217.1	$616.6	$1,164.4	$1,692.6	$1,798.8	$1,904.3	$1,997.2	$2,089.9
Out-of-pocket payments	13.0	25.0	58.4	138.8	202.1	263.8	272.1	289.4	298.2	299.3
Health insurance	6.6	29.6	131.9	403.0	843.5	1,278.3	1,367.6	1,444.7	1,528.1	1,615.0
Private health insurance	4.9	14.0	61.4	204.8	405.8	603.8	636.4	663.8	692.7	712.2
Medicare	X	7.3	36.3	107.3	215.9	326.4	381.7	407.4	440.8	471.3
Medicaid	X	5.0	24.7	69.7	186.9	287.7	283.7	302.5	315.5	345.7
Federal	X	2.7	13.7	40.3	109.3	165.5	161.7	172.7	187.4	230.2
State and local	X	2.3	11.0	29.4	77.6	122.2	122.0	129.8	129.0	115.4
CHIP[2]	X	X	X	X	2.5	6.4	7.0	7.6	8.7	9.5
Other health insurance programs[3]	1.7	3.3	9.6	21.2	32.3	54.0	58.9	63.4	69.5	76.3
Other third-party payers and programs[4]	3.7	8.5	26.7	74.8	118.8	150.5	159.1	170.3	170.9	175.6
Personal health care implicit price deflator[5] (2005 = 100.0)	10.1	14.7	31.4	63.1	85.0	100.0	103.0	106.5	109.3	112.2
Percent Distribution										
All sources of funds	100.0	100.0	100.0	100.0	100.0	100.0	100.0	100.0	100.0	100.0
Out-of-pocket payments	55.9	39.6	26.9	22.5	17.4	15.6	15.1	15.2	14.9	14.3
Health insurance	28.3	46.9	60.8	65.4	72.4	75.5	76.0	75.9	76.5	77.3
Private health insurance	21.1	22.2	28.3	33.2	34.9	35.7	35.4	34.9	34.7	34.1
Medicare	X	11.5	16.7	17.4	18.5	19.3	21.2	21.4	22.1	22.5
Medicaid	X	8.0	11.4	11.3	16.1	17.0	15.8	15.9	15.8	16.5
Federal	X	4.3	6.3	6.5	9.4	9.8	9.0	9.1	9.4	11.0
State and local	X	3.7	5.1	4.8	6.7	7.2	6.8	6.8	6.5	5.5
CHIP[2]	X	X	X	X	0.2	0.4	0.4	0.4	0.4	0.5
Other health insurance programs[3]	7.2	5.2	4.4	3.4	2.8	3.2	3.3	3.3	3.5	3.7
Other third-party payers and programs[4]	15.8	13.5	12.3	12.1	10.2	8.9	8.8	8.9	8.6	8.4
Amount in Billions										
Hospital expenditures[6]	$9.0	$27.2	$100.5	$250.4	$415.5	$606.5	$648.3	$686.8	$722.1	$759.1
Percent Distribution										
All sources of funds	100.0	100.0	100.0	100.0	100.0	100.0	100.0	100.0	100.0	100.0
Out-of-pocket payments	20.6	9.0	5.4	4.5	3.2	3.1	3.1	3.2	3.2	3.2
Health insurance	50.7	71.4	79.7	82.6	86.2	87.7	87.5	87.2	87.8	88.2
Private health insurance	35.6	32.5	36.6	38.6	33.9	35.4	36.1	35.7	35.8	35.0
Medicare	X	19.7	26.2	27.1	29.9	29.5	28.9	28.4	28.8	29.0
Medicaid	X	9.7	9.2	10.6	17.1	17.3	17.0	17.4	17.1	17.9
Federal	X	5.2	5.0	6.3	10.3	10.1	9.7	10.0	10.1	11.9
State and local	X	4.5	4.2	4.3	6.8	7.2	7.3	7.4	7.0	6.1
CHIP[2]	X	X	X	X	0.2	0.4	0.4	0.4	0.4	0.4
Other health insurance programs[3]	15.1	9.5	7.7	6.3	5.0	5.1	5.2	5.3	5.6	5.8
Other third-party payers and programs[4]	28.7	19.5	15.0	12.9	10.5	9.1	9.4	9.7	9.0	8.6
Amount in Billions										
Physician and clinical expenditures	$5.6	$14.3	$47.7	$158.9	$290.0	$419.6	$441.6	$462.6	$486.5	$505.9
Percent Distribution										
All sources of funds	100.0	100.0	100.0	100.0	100.0	100.0	100.0	100.0	100.0	100.0
Out-of-pocket payments	60.2	45.1	30.0	19.0	11.2	10.3	10.2	10.2	10.0	9.5
Health insurance	32.6	48.8	59.7	67.7	76.4	79.1	79.3	79.3	80.0	80.5
Private health insurance	28.2	29.4	35.0	42.3	47.5	48.8	48.5	48.2	48.0	47.0
Medicare	X	11.5	17.2	18.9	20.0	20.2	20.4	20.4	21.0	21.6
Medicaid	X	4.5	5.1	4.4	6.6	7.1	7.2	7.2	7.3	7.9
Federal	X	2.4	2.9	2.6	3.9	4.2	4.3	4.2	4.5	5.5
State and local	X	2.1	2.2	1.8	2.7	2.9	2.9	2.9	2.8	2.4
CHIP[2]	X	X	X	X	0.3	0.4	0.5	0.5	0.5	0.6
Other health insurance programs[3]	4.3	3.4	2.4	2.1	2.1	2.6	2.7	3.0	3.2	3.4
Other third-party payers and programs[4]	7.3	6.1	10.3	13.4	12.4	10.7	10.5	10.5	10.1	10.0
Amount in Billions										
Nursing care facilities and continuing care retirement communities expenditures[7]	$0.8	$4.0	$15.3	$44.9	$85.1	$112.1	$117.0	$126.5	$132.8	$137.0

Table C-76. Personal Health Care Expenditures, by Source of Funds and Type of Expenditure, Selected Years, 1960–2009—Continued

(Number, percent.)

Type of personal health care expenditures and source of funds	1960	1970	1980	1990	2000	2005	2006	2007	2008	2009
Percent Distribution										
All sources of funds	100.0	100.0	100.0	100.0	100.0	100.0	100.0	100.0	100.0	100.0
Out-of-pocket payments	74.8	49.5	40.7	40.3	32.5	30.5	30.0	30.4	30.4	29.1
Health insurance	0.0	28.5	51.9	48.8	60.5	62.9	63.1	61.6	62.6	63.9
Private health insurance	0.0	0.2	1.3	6.2	8.9	6.7	7.4	7.3	7.5	7.7
Medicare	X	3.5	2.0	3.8	11.9	17.0	18.0	18.5	19.6	20.4
Medicaid	X	23.3	46.2	36.6	37.4	36.7	35.3	33.3	32.8	32.8
Federal	X	12.5	26.1	20.6	21.7	20.7	19.9	18.8	19.3	21.9
State and local	X	10.8	20.1	16.0	15.7	16.0	15.4	14.5	13.6	10.9
CHIP[2]	X	X	X	X	0.0	0.0	0.0	0.0	0.0	0.0
Other health insurance programs[3]	0.0	1.5	2.4	2.2	2.2	2.5	2.4	2.6	2.8	2.9
Other third-party payers and programs[4]	25.2	21.9	7.4	10.9	7.0	6.6	6.9	7.9	6.9	7.1
Amount in Billions										
Home health care expenditures	$0.1	$0.2	$2.4	$12.6	$32.4	$48.7	$52.6	$57.8	$62.1	$68.3
Percent Distribution										
All sources of funds	100.0	100.0	100.0	100.0	100.0	100.0	100.0	100.0	100.0	100.0
Out-of-pocket payments	12.5	9.4	15.2	17.9	19.6	12.8	11.3	9.5	8.7	8.8
Health insurance	5.6	37.9	53.7	66.2	71.4	81.6	84.0	86.3	87.6	87.5
Private health insurance	2.5	3.0	14.7	22.9	23.8	12.6	10.7	8.9	7.7	7.4
Medicare	X	26.7	26.8	26.0	26.4	37.4	40.0	41.9	43.3	43.7
Medicaid	X	6.7	11.7	17.1	20.9	31.0	32.7	34.8	35.8	35.6
Federal	X	3.3	6.2	9.1	11.3	16.7	17.7	18.8	20.3	23.1
State and local	X	3.4	5.4	7.9	9.6	14.3	15.0	16.0	15.6	12.5
CHIP[2]	X	X	X	X	0.0	0.0	0.0	0.0	0.0	0.0
Other health insurance programs[3]	3.1	1.4	0.5	0.3	0.3	0.5	0.5	0.6	0.7	0.9
Other third-party payers and programs[4]	81.9	52.7	31.1	16.0	9.0	5.6	4.8	4.3	3.7	3.7
Amount in Billions										
Prescription drug expenditures	$2.7	$5.5	$12.0	$40.3	$120.9	$201.7	$219.8	$230.2	$237.2	$249.9
Percent Distribution										
All sources of funds	100.0	100.0	100.0	100.0	100.0	100.0	100.0	100.0	100.0	100.0
Out-of-pocket payments	96.0	82.4	71.3	56.7	28.1	25.1	22.7	22.8	21.9	21.2
Health insurance	1.5	16.5	26.9	40.2	70.0	73.0	75.4	75.5	76.6	77.4
Private health insurance	1.3	8.8	15.0	27.0	50.2	49.4	45.1	44.1	43.6	43.4
Medicare	X	0.0	0.0	0.5	1.7	2.0	18.0	19.9	21.2	21.9
Medicaid	X	7.6	11.7	12.6	16.3	18.0	8.6	7.9	8.0	8.0
Federal	X	4.1	6.8	7.2	9.3	10.3	4.9	4.5	4.7	5.3
State and local	X	3.5	4.9	5.4	7.0	7.7	3.7	3.4	3.2	2.7
CHIP[2]	X	X	X	X	0.3	0.5	0.5	0.5	0.5	0.6
Other health insurance programs[3]	0.1	0.1	0.2	0.2	1.5	3.1	3.2	3.2	3.3	3.4
Other third-party payers and programs[4]	2.5	1.1	1.8	3.0	1.9	1.9	1.8	1.6	1.5	1.4
Dental services expenditures	$2.0	$4.7	$13.3	$31.5	$62.0	$86.8	$91.4	$97.3	$102.3	$102.2
All sources of funds	100.0	100.0	100.0	100.0	100.0	100.0	100.0	100.0	100.0	100.0
Out-of-pocket payments	95.9	89.9	65.8	48.4	44.4	44.1	44.1	43.9	43.9	41.6
Health insurance	3.3	9.6	33.4	51.1	55.0	55.5	55.6	55.7	55.7	58.0
Private health insurance	1.9	4.5	28.4	47.8	50.3	49.4	49.4	49.2	48.0	48.9
Medicare	X	0.0	0.0	0.0	0.1	0.1	0.1	0.2	0.2	0.3
Medicaid	X	3.5	3.8	2.4	3.7	4.9	4.8	4.9	5.7	7.0
Federal	X	1.9	2.1	1.3	2.1	2.8	2.8	2.8	3.4	4.7
State and local	X	1.6	1.7	1.0	1.6	2.1	2.0	2.1	2.3	2.3
CHIP[2]	X	X	X	X	0.4	0.5	0.5	0.7	0.7	0.7
Other health insurance programs[3]	1.3	1.6	1.2	0.9	0.5	0.6	0.7	0.9	1.0	1.1
Other third-party payers and programs[4]	0.8	0.4	0.8	0.6	0.6	0.4	0.4	0.4	0.4	0.5

Table C-76. Personal Health Care Expenditures, by Source of Funds and Type of Expenditure, Selected Years, 1960–2009—Continued

(Number, percent.)

Type of personal health care expenditures and source of funds	1960	1970	1980	1990	2000	2005	2006	2007	2008	2009
Amount in Billions										
All other personal health care expenditures[8]	$3.2	$7.1	$25.8	$77.9	$158.4	$217.1	$228.1	$243.2	$254.2	$267.5
Percent Distribution										
All sources of funds	100.0	100.0	100.0	100.0	100.0	100.0	100.0	100.0	100.0	100.0
Out-of-pocket payments	84.8	74.5	57.2	50.1	38.3	33.3	33.1	33.5	33.0	32.0
Health insurance	3.5	8.3	25.0	33.4	44.3	50.1	50.6	50.5	50.7	51.8
Private health insurance	2.0	3.4	6.7	12.2	12.7	13.1	13.0	13.1	13.1	12.9
Medicare	X	1.0	2.8	5.5	8.0	9.8	10.0	10.0	10.7	10.7
Medicaid	X	2.9	14.7	14.9	22.6	25.9	26.3	26.5	26.2	27.4
Federal	X	1.6	8.1	8.5	12.9	14.7	14.9	15.0	15.4	18.1
State and local	X	1.4	6.7	6.4	9.7	11.2	11.4	11.5	10.8	9.2
CHIP[2]	X	X	X	X	0.2	0.3	0.4	0.3	0.4	0.4
Other health insurance programs[3]	1.4	0.9	0.8	0.9	0.8	1.0	0.9	0.6	0.3	0.4
Other third-party payers and programs[4]	11.7	17.2	17.7	16.5	17.4	16.6	16.3	16.0	16.3	16.2

X = Category not applicable.
0.0 = Quantity more than zero but less than 0.05.
[1]Includes all expenditures for specified health services and supplies other than expenses for government administration, net cost of health insurance, public health activities, research, and structures and equipment.
[2]Children's Health Insurance Program (CHIP). Medicaid CHIP expansions are included.
[3]Includes Department of Defense and Department of Veterans Affairs.
[4]Includes worksite health care, other private revenues, Indian Health Service, workers' compensation, general assistance, maternal and child health, vocational rehabilitation, other federal programs, Substance Abuse and Mental Health Services Administration, other state and local programs, and school health.
[5]Constructed from the Producer Price Indexes for hospitals, offices of physicians, medical and diagnostic laboratories, home health care services, and nursing care facilities; and Consumer Price Indices specific to each of the remaining personal health care components.
[6]Includes expenditures for hospital-based nursing home and home health agency care.
[7]Includes expenditures for care in freestanding nursing homes. Expenditures for care in hospital-based nursing homes are included with hospital care.
[8]Includes expenditures for other professional services, other nondurable medical products, durable medical equipment, and other health, residential, and personal care, not shown separately.

Table C-77. Cost of Hospital Discharges with Common Hospital Operating Room Procedures in Nonfederal Community Hospitals, by Age and Selected Principal Procedure, Selected Years, 2000–2009

(Dollar.)

Age and principal operating room procedure[1]	Mean inflation-adjusted cost per hospitalization: 2009 dollars[2]			Number of discharges with operating room principal procedure			Total inflation-adjusted national costs: 2009 dollars (in millions of dollars)		
	2000	2005	2009	2000	2005	2009	2000	2005	2009
All Ages									
Hospital discharges with an operating room principal procedure[3]	$12,858	$15,375	$16,175	9,022,288	10,285,810	10,275,152	$115,295	$158,291	$166,312
Laminectomy (back surgery)	7,916	8,923	9,842	294,345	255,955	210,788	2,340	2,286	2,076
Heart valve procedures	41,564	50,759	48,661	82,826	96,715	118,623	3,437	4,929	5,781
Coronary artery bypass graft (CABG)	30,295	36,770	35,864	349,967	227,774	209,382	10,642	8,389	7,513
Percutaneous coronary angioplasty (PTCA) (balloon angioplasty of heart)	14,512	17,826	17,234	601,832	749,572	638,113	8,735	13,368	11,000
Insertion, revision, replacement, removal of cardiac pacemaker or cardioverter/defibrillator	26,822	34,163	32,798	68,723	165,619	159,013	1,858	5,651	5,215
Colorectal resection (removal of part of the bowel)	18,869	21,872	22,058	261,519	283,453	282,162	5,036	6,207	6,220
Appendectomy	7,100	8,205	8,444	277,029	308,634	298,273	1,945	2,532	2,518
Cholecystectomy (gall bladder removal)	10,078	11,675	11,765	400,818	388,252	406,329	4,005	4,534	4,783
Hysterectomy	6,334	7,017	7,965	596,889	567,964	459,954	3,752	3,993	3,669
Cesarean section	5,268	5,289	5,351	927,397	1,301,770	1,378,721	4,770	6,888	7,381
Treatment, fracture or dislocation of hip and femur	12,193	14,744	15,571	244,706	259,071	254,382	3,034	3,817	3,964
Arthroplasty knee (knee replacement)	13,375	15,068	15,254	328,118	549,867	679,260	4,363	8,289	10,361
Hip replacement	14,508	16,494	16,370	304,709	381,318	435,926	4,475	6,283	7,133
Spinal fusion	16,890	23,940	26,026	210,677	331,912	432,406	3,475	7,954	11,258
Under 18 Years									
Hospital discharges with an operating room principal procedure[3]	12,892	18,645	17,603	394,504	551,952	382,434	4,917	10,249	6,772
Incision and excision of CNS (a type of brain surgery)	27,959	33,814	35,191	6,581	11,786	7,751	177	399	273
Tonsillectomy and/or adenoidectomy	4,267	5,517	5,457	12,524	16,842	11,444	56	93	63
Small bowel resection (removal of part of the small bowel)	35,082	48,773	43,225	1,769	3,075	1,914	61	148	82
Appendectomy	6,371	7,833	7,734	77,676	88,563	78,996	482	694	612
Cesarean section	5,847	5,552	5,587	24,419	29,549	28,116	129	165	157
Spinal fusion	28,351	44,452	48,772	7,704	13,305	9,227	215	586	450
18–44 Years									
Hospital discharges with an operating room principal procedure[3]	8,498	9,573	10,172	2,894,835	3,202,648	3,079,014	24,070	30,692	31,369
Incision and excision of CNS (a type of brain surgery)	24,678	29,462	32,678	20,221	18,779	19,465	480	556	636
Laminectomy	7,122	8,310	8,970	98,649	69,320	46,182	707	577	414
Appendectomy	6,540	7,467	7,774	137,667	140,028	135,219	888	1,046	1,051
Cholecystectomy	8,256	9,084	9,382	136,587	133,060	149,542	1,083	1,209	1,405
Oophorectomy (removal of one or both ovaries)	6,153	7,135	7,879	39,388	34,430	27,381	245	246	216
Ligation of fallopian tubes ("tying" of fallopian tubes)	4,557	4,392	4,783	77,428	77,073	52,555	333	339	251
Hysterectomy	5,871	6,371	7,172	299,858	262,861	199,340	1,736	1,677	1,431
Cesarean section	5,250	5,278	5,342	900,964	1,267,786	1,345,340	4,629	6,696	7,190
Treatment, fracture or dislocation of lower extremity (other than hip or femur)	9,047	11,426	12,296	70,112	61,369	58,209	623	700	715
Spinal fusion	15,875	22,161	24,255	75,502	89,893	92,222	1,159	1,993	2,239
45–64 Years									
Hospital discharges with an operating room principal procedure[3]	14,064	16,859	18,204	2,513,848	3,001,674	3,208,533	35,198	50,676	58,465
Laminectomy	7,984	8,808	9,977	111,022	98,847	81,411	888	871	813
Heart valve procedures	39,047	46,496	46,981	23,731	27,467	34,437	921	1,284	1,621
Coronary artery bypass graft (CABG)	28,302	33,674	33,939	144,812	97,449	90,787	4,119	3,289	3,082
Percutaneous coronary angioplasty (PTCA)	14,045	17,211	16,941	261,110	328,248	284,284	3,661	5,654	4,818
Insertion, revision, replacement, removal of cardiac pacemaker or cardioverter/defibrillator	32,824	37,069	34,805	16,558	45,357	45,860	540	1,680	1,597
Colorectal resection	16,977	19,482	20,140	78,937	98,142	105,593	1,367	1,915	2,127
Cholecystectomy	9,504	11,238	11,477	120,985	121,446	128,619	1,150	1,367	1,476
Oophorectomy	7,371	8,388	9,215	21,888	23,172	18,588	161	194	171
Hysterectomy	6,461	7,155	8,142	238,417	249,676	211,505	1,538	1,790	1,724
Arthroplasty knee (knee replacement)	13,683	15,121	15,328	98,691	205,869	278,621	1,343	3,113	4,270
Hip replacement	15,074	16,728	16,294	67,121	108,449	143,104	1,019	1,811	2,330
Spinal fusion	16,210	22,246	24,740	90,101	154,618	212,111	1,422	3,443	5,247

Table C-77. Cost of Hospital Discharges with Common Hospital Operating Room Procedures in Nonfederal Community Hospitals, by Age and Selected Principal Procedure, Selected Years, 2000–2009—Continued

(Dollar.)

Age and principal operating room procedure[1]	Mean inflation-adjusted cost per hospitalization: 2009 dollars[2]			Number of discharges with operating room principal procedure			Total inflation-adjusted national costs: 2009 dollars (in millions of dollars)		
	2000	2005	2009	2000	2005	2009	2000	2005	2009
65–74 Years									
Hospital discharges with an operating room principal procedure[3]	15,757	18,771	19,466	1,559,874	1,653,945	1,773,788	24,709	31,095	34,528
Laminectomy	8,368	8,895	9,675	47,332	47,031	43,981	396	418	426
Heart valve procedures	42,531	51,641	48,709	24,127	25,535	32,650	1,018	1,322	1,593
Coronary artery bypass graft (CABG)	30,830	37,503	36,144	116,648	72,447	69,216	3,595	2,719	2,503
Percutaneous coronary angioplasty (PTCA)	14,450	17,659	17,086	172,403	202,718	170,259	2,487	3,582	2,909
Insertion, revision, replacement, removal of cardiac pacemaker or cardioverter/defibrillator	29,298	35,256	34,162	19,805	46,292	43,646	583	1,630	1,491
Endarterectomy (plaque removal from artery lining of brain, head, neck)	8,428	9,003	9,223	52,875	41,903	40,638	457	379	376
Colorectal resection	18,967	22,151	22,289	65,640	64,326	65,169	1,283	1,428	1,449
Cholecystectomy	11,142	13,326	13,972	67,897	57,382	56,178	769	765	786
Arthroplasty knee	13,625	15,023	15,129	114,150	182,838	228,078	1,540	2,749	3,451
Hip replacement	14,452	16,224	16,086	74,103	89,657	105,649	1,087	1,454	1,699
Spinal fusion	17,862	25,714	27,734	24,143	48,299	79,402	430	1,242	2,202
75–84 Years									
Hospital discharges with an operating room principal procedure[3]	15,996	19,411	19,798	1,263,420	1,405,406	1,336,418	20,504	27,313	26,444
Laminectomy	9,031	9,764	10,119	31,988	32,853	30,263	292	320	307
Heart valve procedures	43,868	54,396	50,711	21,844	25,893	33,181	969	1,415	1,684
Coronary artery bypass graft (CABG)	33,424	41,690	39,271	71,235	46,557	38,995	2,400	1,942	1,533
Percutaneous coronary angioplasty (PTCA)	15,297	18,875	17,800	115,128	149,285	121,029	1,773	2,818	2,156
Insertion, revision, replacement, removal of cardiac pacemaker or cardioverter/defibrillator	24,042	33,138	32,541	20,711	50,092	44,201	508	1,657	1,438
Endarterectomy (plaque removal from artery lining of brain, head, neck)	8,754	9,338	9,630	46,719	39,208	34,965	422	368	337
Colorectal resection	20,687	24,575	25,275	63,982	63,255	54,308	1,359	1,555	1,369
Cholecystectomy	12,755	15,703	15,960	54,014	51,443	46,298	703	807	738
Treatment, fracture or dislocation of hip and femur	11,480	13,740	14,511	75,452	75,221	71,552	891	1,035	1,039
Arthroplasty knee	13,618	15,117	15,181	81,404	125,729	136,235	1,110	1,901	2,069
Hip replacement	14,278	16,366	16,552	95,401	108,919	108,377	1,384	1,781	1,793
Spinal fusion	18,600	26,826	28,246	12,139	23,530	35,562	224	631	1,006
85 Years and Over									
Hospital discharges with an operating room principal procedure[3]	14,668	17,881	17,883	394,256	450,122	477,971	5,873	8,056	8,546
Heart valve procedures	46,148	58,334	49,523	3,114	4,088	6,614	144	238	328
Coronary artery bypass graft (CABG)	37,608	48,038	44,790	5,483	4,315	3,867	204	209	173
Percutaneous coronary angioplasty (PTCA)	17,370	21,050	18,566	17,268	29,810	29,715	297	627	552
Insertion, revision, replacement, removal of cardiac pacemaker or cardioverter/defibrillator	14,274	24,156	24,347	7,301	14,121	15,422	106	340	375
Colorectal resection	22,365	26,306	25,718	21,347	21,140	19,773	488	556	508
Cholecystectomy	15,540	17,445	16,787	16,163	17,286	17,749	254	301	298
Treatment, fracture or dislocation of hip and femur	11,177	13,196	13,949	79,202	80,284	79,574	911	1,061	1,112
Arthroplasty knee	13,810	15,878	15,809	10,414	16,274	18,992	145	258	300
Hip replacement	13,891	16,432	16,560	51,469	55,699	59,883	727	914	992
Amputation of lower extremity (amputation of leg, foot or toe)	12,826	16,603	15,964	13,260	10,403	9,224	173	173	148

[1]Data are based on valid operating room procedures.
[2]Charges (the amount billed by the hospital) were converted to costs using cost-charge ratios from the Centers for Medicare & Medicaid ServicesCosts are for the entire hospitalization including the principal procedure.
[3]Includes discharges for operating room principal procedures not shown separately.

PART C: HEALTH

Table C-78. Expenses[1] for Health Care by Selected Population Characteristics, Selected Years, 1987–2008

(Number, percent, dollar.)

Characteristic	Population in millions[2]				Percent of persons with expense				Mean annual expense per person with expense[3]			
	1997	2000	2005	2008	1987	2000	2005	2008	1987	2000	2005	2008
All Ages	271.3	278.4	296.2	304.4	84.5	83.5	84.7	84.4	$2,960	$3,376	$4,500	$4,470
Under 65 Years												
Total	237.1	243.6	258.7	264.6	83.2	81.8	82.9	82.6	2,305	2,659	3,571	3,571
Under 6 years	23.8	24.1	23.8	24.7	88.9	86.7	88.9	88.8	1,958	1,405	1,711	2,049
6–17 years	48.1	48.4	49.7	49.6	80.2	80.0	83.0	82.5	1,291	1,397	1,807	1,699
18–44 years	108.9	109.0	111.1	111.0	81.5	77.7	77.1	76.5	2,026	2,382	3,175	2,974
45–64 years	56.3	62.1	74.1	79.4	87.0	88.5	89.7	89.1	3,923	4,454	5,769	5,843
Sex												
Male	118.0	120.9	129.2	132.2	78.8	76.6	77.5	77.5	2,174	2,546	3,225	3,299
Female	119.1	122.7	129.6	132.4	87.5	87.0	88.4	87.6	2,416	2,758	3,874	3,811
Hispanic Origin and Race[4]												
Hispanic or Latino	29.4	32.0	41.1	45.0	71.0	69.0	69.3	69.9	1,838	1,812	2,425	2,472
Not Hispanic or Latino:												
White	166.2	169.2	166.5	167.3	86.9	86.6	88.1	87.6	2,312	2,782	3,873	3,936
Black or African American	31.3	32.1	32.8	33.5	72.2	71.3	76.4	75.7	2,788	2,824	3,637	3,268
Asian[5]	X	X	11.3	11.7	X	X	75.5	78.1	X	X	2,205	1,871
American Indian, Alaska Native, Native Hawaiian, Other Pacific Islander, and Multiple Race[5]	10.2	10.2	7.0	7.1	72.8	76.0	82.0	83.7	1,529	2,267	3,291	4,312
Insurance Status[6]												
Any private insurance	174.0	181.6	180.1	178.2	86.5	85.9	87.9	88.1	2,210	2,533	3,597	3,613
Public insurance only	29.8	29.7	42.2	45.8	82.4	83.6	84.2	85.0	3,707	4,037	4,342	4,391
Uninsured all year	33.3	32.3	36.4	40.7	61.8	57.3	56.8	55.7	1,440	1,875	2,046	1,870
65 Years and Over												
Total	34.2	34.8	37.5	39.7	93.7	95.5	96.7	96.6	7,312	7,677	10,003	9,585
Sex												
Male	14.6	15.0	16.0	17.2	92.0	93.4	95.9	95.7	7,482	8,232	9,788	9,433
Female	19.6	19.8	21.5	22.6	94.9	97.1	97.2	97.3	7,192	7,273	10,161	9,698
Hispanic Origin and Race[4]												
Hispanic or Latino	1.7	1.9	2.4	2.8	82.5	92.5	92.0	93.3	6,963	6,889	8,659	9,437
Not Hispanic or Latino:												
White	28.8	28.9	30.0	31.5	94.9	95.9	97.3	97.5	7,198	7,793	10,118	9,603
Black or African American	2.8	2.9	3.1	3.5	88.5	94.0	94.9	93.8	8,813	7,383	11,985	10,414
Asian[5]	X	X	1.3	1.3	X	X	94.4	94.9	X	X	5,875	6,037
American Indian, Alaska Native, Native Hawaiian, Other Pacific Islander, and Multiple Race[5]	*	*	*	*	*	*	*	*	*	*	*	*
Insurance Status[7]												
Medicare only	8.8	12.0	10.9	15.8	85.9	94.8	96.2	95.8	5,760	6,592	9,673	8,886
Medicare and private insurance	21.7	19.2	20.7	18.6	95.4	96.0	97.8	98.2	7,234	7,872	9,610	9,425
Medicare and other public coverage	3.2	3.2	5.5	4.8	94.4	96.3	95.5	96.4	11,235	10,534	12,290	12,486

X = Category not applicable.
* = Figure does not meet standards of reliability or precision.
[1]Includes expenses for inpatient hospital and physician services, ambulatory physician and nonphysician services, prescribed medicines, home health services, dental services, and other medical equipment, supplies, and services that were purchased or rented during the year.
[2]Includes persons in the civilian noninstitutionalized population for all or part of the year. Expenditures for persons in this population for only part of the year are restricted to those incurred during periods of eligibility (e.g., expenses incurred during periods of institutionalization and military service are not included in estimates).
[3]Estimates of expenses were converted to 2008 dollars using the Consumer Price Index (all items).
[4]Persons of Hispanic origin may be of any race.
[5]Starting with 2002 data, MEPS respondents were allowed to report as non-Hispanic Asian-only. Prior to 2002, Asian respondents were reported with the American Indian, Alaska Native, Native Hawaiian, Other Pacific Islander, and Multiple Race category.
[6]Any private insurance includes individuals with insurance that provided coverage for hospital and physician care at any time during the year, other than Medicare, Medicaid, or other public coverage for hospital or physician services. Public insurance only includes individuals who were not covered by private insurance at any time during the year but were covered by Medicare, Medicaid, other public coverage for hospital or physician services, and/or CHAMPUS/CHAMPVA (TRICARE) at any point during the year.
[7]Populations do not add to total because uninsured persons and persons with unknown insurance status were excluded.

Table C-79. Percent Distribution of Payment for Health Care, by Selected Population Characteristics, Selected Years, 1987–2008

(Percent.)

Characteristic	All sources	Out of pocket			Private insurance[1]			Public sources[2]			Other[3]		
		1987	2000	2008	1987	2000	2008	1987	2000	2008	1987	2000	2008
All Ages	100.0	24.8	19.4	16.7	36.6	40.3	41.1	34.1	35.4	37.2	4.5	5.0	5.0
Under 65 Years													
Total	100.0	26.2	20.3	17.7	46.6	52.5	53.9	21.3	21.3	22.9	6.0		
Under 6 years	100.0	18.5	10.3	7.3	39.5	51.2	37.2	35.8	33.6	47.7	6.2	6.0	5.6
6–17 years	100.0	35.7	27.7	23.2	47.3	48.8	48.8	11.8	20.1	25.8	5.2	4.9	*7.8
18–44 years	100.0	27.4	19.9	19.4	46.8	51.2	55.7	19.4	21.1	18.9	6.4	3.4	2.1
45–64 years	100.0	24.0	20.2	16.8	47.8	54.5	55.5	22.4	20.2	22.2	5.8	7.8	6.1
												5.2	5.5
Sex													
Male	100.0	24.5	18.1	17.1	44.6	52.2	52.5	23.9	23.5	23.7	7.1	6.3	6.7
Female	100.0	27.5	22.1	18.1	48.1	52.7	54.9	19.2	19.5	22.3	5.2	5.7	4.7
Hispanic Origin and Race[4]													
Hispanic or Latino	100.0	22.0	20.5	15.1	36.1	45.8	39.0	35.8	27.5	33.0	6.0	6.2	9.4
Not Hispanic or Latino													
White	100.0	28.2	21.7	18.9	50.1	55.1	57.7	15.9	18.0	19.1	5.8	5.2	4.4
Black or African American	100.0	15.5	11.8	11.6	30.0	40.5	39.0	47.2	38.8	40.2	7.3	8.8	9.2
Asian[5]	100.0	X	X	24.1	X	X	60.1	X	X	11.8	X	X	4.0
American Indian, Alaska Native, Native Hawaiian, Other Pacific Islander, and Multiple Race[5]	100.0	27.2	17.0	12.0	46.7	51.2	48.0	21.0	19.0	30.1	5.1	*12.8	*10.0
Insurance Status													
Any private insurance[6]	100.0	29.0	21.2	18.9	60.0	70.2	74.0	6.2	5.3	4.8	4.8	3.3	2.4
Public insurance only[7]	100.0	8.9	9.8	6.6	X	X	X	87.2	84.4	86.4	3.9	5.8	7.0
Uninsured all year[8]	100.0	40.6	40.4	46.0	X	X	X	28.6	*21.2	*9.5	30.9	38.4	44.5
Under 65 Years	100.0	22.0	17.5	14.6	15.8	14.9	14.1	60.8	64.7	67.5	1.5	2.9	3.8
Sex													
Male	100.0	21.7	14.2	13.6	17.6	16.8	15.9	58.8	66.9	67.2	*1.9	2.2	3.3
Female	100.0	22.2	20.2	15.3	14.4	13.3	12.7	62.3	63.0	67.8	1.1	3.5	4.2
Hispanic Origin and Race[2]													
Hispanic or Latino	100.0	*13.5	13.9	8.9	*4.7	8.4	*12.3	80.2	75.6	76.1	*1.6	*2.2	2.7
Not Hispanic or Latino													
White	100.0	23.7	18.3	15.8	16.7	15.2	14.8	58.0	64.1	65.4	1.6	2.4	3.9
Black or African American	100.0	11.2	13.6	8.4	*11.9	9.3	9.2	76.3	68.3	77.7	0.6	*8.9	*4.7
Asian[5]	100.0	X	X	16.6	X	X	10.9	X	X	70.9	X	X	*1.5
American Indian, Alaska Native, Native Hawaiian, Other Pacific Islander, and Multiple Race[5]	100.0	*	*	*	*	*	*	*	*	*	*	*	*
Insurance Status													
Medicare only	100.0	29.8	22.2	16.9	X	X	X	68.8	72.2	74.5	1.4	5.7	8.6
Medicare and private insurance	100.0	23.4	17.0	16.2	18.9	25.3	28.9	56.1	57.1	54.7	1.6	*0.6	*0.3
Medicare and other public coverage	100.0	*6.2	9.1	4.2	X	X	X	92.9	87.3	93.4	1.0	*3.6	*2.0

* = Figure does not meet standards of reliability or precision.
X = Category not applicable.
[1]Private insurance includes any type of private insurance payments reported for people with private health insurance coverage during the year.
[2]Public sources include payments made by Medicare, Medicaid, the Department of Veterans Affairs, other federal sources (e.g., Indian Health Service, military treatment facilities, and other care provided by the federal government), CHAMPUS/CHAMPVA (TRICARE), and various state and local sources (e.g., community and neighborhood clinics, state and local health departments, and state programs other than Medicaid).
[3]Other sources includes Workers' Compensation, unclassified sources (automobile, home, or liability insurance, and other miscellaneous or unknown sources), Medicaid payments reported for people who were not enrolled in the program at any time during the year, and any type of private insurance payments reported for people without private health insurance coverage during the year.
[4]Persons of Hispanic origin may be of any race.
[5]Starting with 2002 data, MEPS respondents were allowed to report as non-Hispanic Asian-only. Prior to 2002, Asian respondents were reported with the American Indian, Alaska Native, Native Hawaiian, Other Pacific Islander, and Multiple Race category.
[6]Includes individuals with insurance that provided coverage for hospital and physician care at any time during the year, other than Medicare, Medicaid, or other public coverage for hospital or physician services.
[7]Includes individuals who were not covered by private insurance at any time during the year but were covered by Medicare, Medicaid, other public coverage for hospital or physician services, and/or CHAMPUS/CHAMPVA (TRICARE) at any point during the year.
[8]Includes individuals not covered by either private or public insurance throughout the entire year or period of eligibility for the survey. However, some expenses for the uninsured were paid by sources that were not defined as health insurance coverage, such as the Department of Veterans Affairs, community and Compensation, and other unclassified sources (e.g., automobile, home, or liability insurance).

PART C: HEALTH

Table C-80. Out-of-Pocket Health Care Expenses Among Persons with Medical Expenses, by Age, Selected Years, 1987–2008

(Percent.)

Age and year	Percent of persons with expenses	Amount paid out of pocket among persons with expenses[1]					
		Total	$0	$1–99	$100–499	$500–999	$1,000–1,999	$2,000+
All Ages								
1987	84.5	100.0	10.4	19.9	36.6	15.3	10.0	7.7
1997	84.1	100.0	8.5	26.1	35.1	14.3	9.4	6.6
1998	83.8	100.0	7.7	26.6	35.6	14.0	9.5	6.5
1999	84.3	100.0	7.4	27.1	34.2	14.5	9.5	7.3
2000	83.5	100.0	6.9	26.6	34.4	14.4	9.8	7.8
2001	85.4	100.0	7.1	24.6	33.8	14.6	11.0	8.8
2002	85.2	100.0	7.8	23.4	32.5	15.1	11.9	9.4
2003	85.6	100.0	7.6	21.9	32.1	15.8	12.1	10.4
2004	84.7	100.0	8.8	22.1	31.2	14.9	12.0	11.1
2005	84.7	100.0	8.7	21.2	31.5	15.8	11.9	10.8
2006	84.6	100.0	8.7	21.4	31.6	15.8	12.2	10.2
2007	84.9	100.0	9.8	22.6	31.6	15.3	11.5	9.2
2008	84.4	100.0	9.9	22.9	32.1	14.8	11.2	9.1
Under 6 Years								
1987	88.9	100.0	19.2	28.0	39.8	8.5	2.5	2.0
1997	88.0	100.0	20.0	44.5	28.7	4.0	2.2	0.7
1998	87.6	100.0	17.4	48.0	28.7	4.0	1.5	0.3
1999	87.9	100.0	17.7	50.7	26.0	4.2	0.7	0.7
2000	86.7	100.0	16.7	51.4	25.9	4.1	1.4	0.5
2001	88.8	100.0	18.5	49.0	27.9	3.0	1.3	0.3
2002	88.8	100.0	21.5	42.8	28.8	4.9	1.4	0.5
2003	91.3	100.0	20.6	42.4	29.6	5.4	1.4	0.6
2004	90.0	100.0	26.0	40.5	26.0	4.8	2.1	0.7
2005	88.9	100.0	27.2	36.6	27.5	6.1	1.9	0.7
2006	89.2	100.0	27.1	39.3	26.4	4.3	1.9	1.0
2007	88.7	100.0	30.2	36.5	24.7	5.1	2.0	1.4
2008	88.8	100.0	31.4	36.1	25.9	3.9	1.9	0.8
6–17 Years								
1987	80.2	100.0	15.5	27.4	37.4	9.0	5.7	5.0
1997	81.7	100.0	16.5	36.2	32.1	7.5	3.6	4.1
1998	80.6	100.0	16.3	36.3	32.7	7.9	3.9	3.0
1999	81.5	100.0	15.0	38.0	31.6	7.9	3.8	3.8
2000	80.0	100.0	14.7	37.2	33.0	6.5	4.1	4.5
2001	83.2	100.0	15.0	36.5	32.3	7.3	3.8	5.2
2002	83.6	100.0	16.6	35.8	31.8	7.9	3.7	4.3
2003	84.1	100.0	16.1	32.8	33.1	8.9	5.4	3.8
2004	83.9	100.0	18.7	33.8	30.2	8.3	4.7	4.4
2005	83.0	100.0	18.6	32.4	31.1	9.2	4.6	4.0
2006	83.6	100.0	19.2	32.8	29.9	8.7	4.1	5.3
2007	84.0	100.0	21.6	33.0	29.4	7.6	4.2	4.1
2008	82.5	100.0	22.4	33.0	28.3	7.4	4.0	4.9

Table C-80. Out-of-Pocket Health Care Expenses Among Persons with Medical Expenses, by Age, Selected Years, 1987–2008—Continued

(Percent.)

Age and year	Percent of persons with expenses	Amount paid out of pocket among persons with expenses[1]						
		Total	$0	$1–99	$100–499	$500–999	$1,000–1,999	$2,000+
18–44 Years								
1987	81.5	100.0	10.1	22.0	39.4	14.9	8.3	5.4
1997	78.3	100.0	7.3	28.4	39.4	14.0	6.9	3.9
1998	78.0	100.0	6.4	29.1	40.3	13.1	7.0	4.1
1999	78.9	100.0	6.4	29.6	39.2	13.3	7.1	4.4
2000	77.7	100.0	5.8	29.4	39.8	13.8	6.9	4.4
2001	79.3	100.0	6.0	26.4	39.7	15.1	8.4	4.5
2002	78.5	100.0	6.7	26.3	38.3	14.6	8.8	5.3
2003	79.0	100.0	6.4	24.5	38.8	15.4	9.2	5.7
2004	77.0	100.0	7.2	24.8	37.6	14.8	9.4	6.2
2005	77.1	100.0	7.0	24.8	37.9	15.0	9.0	6.2
2006	76.9	100.0	6.8	24.2	38.3	15.2	8.9	6.5
2007	77.3	100.0	7.7	26.7	37.1	14.2	8.8	5.5
2008	76.5	100.0	7.9	27.1	36.6	14.0	8.3	6.1
45–64 Years								
1987	87.0	100.0	5.7	12.5	35.7	20.9	14.7	10.5
1997	89.2	100.0	3.4	16.8	36.3	19.6	14.8	9.2
1998	89.2	100.0	2.9	17.2	36.3	19.7	14.5	9.5
1999	88.9	100.0	2.7	16.6	35.9	20.2	14.7	9.9
2000	88.5	100.0	2.6	15.7	35.2	20.4	15.1	11.0
2001	89.9	100.0	2.4	14.3	33.8	19.9	17.2	12.4
2002	90.0	100.0	2.3	14.0	31.2	21.1	18.3	13.1
2003	89.6	100.0	2.4	12.9	29.9	21.2	18.1	15.6
2004	88.9	100.0	2.7	13.1	30.8	20.8	17.3	15.2
2005	89.7	100.0	2.4	12.9	29.5	21.7	18.5	14.8
2006	89.2	100.0	2.7	12.9	30.4	21.1	17.9	15.0
2007	89.2	100.0	2.9	14.3	30.6	21.2	17.0	14.1
2008	89.1	100.0	2.8	15.2	33.2	20.0	16.4	12.3
65–74 Years								
1987	92.8	100.0	5.3	10.0	27.3	21.8	19.4	16.2
1997	94.6	100.0	3.2	10.7	31.6	23.6	17.0	14.0
1998	94.3	100.0	2.0	9.8	33.6	21.6	19.5	13.6
1999	95.3	100.0	1.4	10.0	27.4	23.8	19.4	17.9
2000	94.7	100.0	1.5	10.0	27.2	22.1	21.0	18.3
2001	95.6	100.0	1.5	9.9	27.0	21.5	20.5	19.5
2002	96.1	100.0	1.8	6.3	25.4	21.4	24.1	21.1
2003	95.3	100.0	1.7	6.5	21.0	23.8	23.3	23.8
2004	96.6	100.0	1.5	8.0	23.2	19.3	20.5	27.3
2005	95.9	100.0	1.7	6.5	24.8	20.8	21.5	24.6
2006	95.7	100.0	1.7	7.3	23.7	22.0	25.5	19.7
2007	95.8	100.0	2.7	8.8	28.9	23.0	20.3	15.9
2008	95.8	100.0	1.5	9.6	28.8	22.0	20.4	17.7

Table C-80. Out-of-Pocket Health Care Expenses Among Persons with Medical Expenses, by Age, Selected Years, 1987–2008—*Continued*

(Percent.)

Age and year	Percent of persons with expenses	Amount paid out of pocket among persons with expenses[1]						
		Total	$0	$1–99	$100–499	$500–999	$1,000–1,999	$2,000+
75 Years and Over								
1987	95.1	100.0	5.6	7.6	24.7	20.0	19.7	22.4
1997	95.8	100.0	2.4	9.8	27.5	19.5	21.2	19.7
1998	96.3	100.0	3.0	9.6	26.6	20.3	21.0	19.4
1999	95.3	100.0	2.7	8.9	26.3	22.4	19.7	20.0
2000	96.5	100.0	2.6	10.0	25.2	21.5	19.8	20.9
2001	97.0	100.0	1.7	7.0	22.1	19.5	23.0	26.7
2002	96.5	100.0	2.2	6.2	20.1	18.5	24.9	28.2
2003	97.5	100.0	1.9	6.2	19.0	19.5	23.5	29.9
2004	97.7	100.0	1.8	6.1	19.2	16.9	24.8	31.1
2005	97.4	100.0	1.6	6.3	21.2	19.7	19.7	31.4
2006	97.6	100.0	1.7	6.8	22.1	22.8	24.0	22.6
2007	97.3	100.0	1.9	8.7	25.9	19.8	21.8	21.9
2008	97.6	100.0	1.9	10.0	25.9	20.5	22.0	19.7

[1] Estimates of expenses were converted to 2008 dollars using the Consumer Price Index (all items).

Table C-81. Expenditures for Health Services and Supplies and Percent Distribution, by Sponsor, Selected Years, 1987–2009

(Dollars, percent.)

Type of sponsor	1987	1990	1995	2000	2003	2004	2005	2006	2007	2008	2009
NATIONAL HEALTH EXPENDITURES (AMOUNT IN BILLIONS)	$518.9	$724.0	$1,027.3	$1,378.0	$1,772.2	$1,894.7	$2,021.0	$2,152.1	$2,283.5	$2,391.4	$2,486.3
Business, Households and Other Private Revenues	353.9	488.0	642.2	889.5	1,085.0	1,147.6	1,219.4	1,283.8	1,358.8	1,406.0	1,403.1
Private business	122.2	178.1	243.6	345.5	427.4	451.9	478.3	492.0	511.4	521.0	518.3
Employer contribution to private health insurance premiums[1]	84.2	129.4	176.2	254.1	325.8	345.1	367.3	376.3	390.6	395.9	397.5
Employer contribution to Medicare hospital insurance trust fund	24.6	29.4	43.1	62.3	64.6	68.7	72.6	77.3	81.7	82.7	77.7
Workers compensation and temporary disability insurance and worksite health care	13.4	19.3	24.2	29.1	37.1	38.0	38.4	38.4	39.1	42.4	43.1
Household	189.9	253.0	319.0	434.2	528.2	559.7	595.5	634.9	671.2	707.2	708.4
Employee contribution to private health insurance premiums and individual policy premiums[2]	43.9	68.4	100.3	133.1	183.0	194.6	205.9	218.9	228.1	247.1	247.6
Employee and self-employment contributions and voluntary premiums paid to Medicare hospital insurance trust fund[3]	29.5	35.6	56.0	82.6	86.3	91.5	96.5	103.6	109.3	112.3	108.5
Premiums paid by individuals to Medicare supplementary medical insurance trust fund	6.2	10.2	16.4	16.4	21.8	24.8	29.3	40.3	44.5	49.6	53.0
Out-of-pocket health spending	110.3	138.8	146.4	202.1	237.1	248.8	263.8	272.1	289.4	298.2	299.3
Other private revenues	41.9	56.9	79.6	109.9	129.3	135.9	145.7	156.9	176.2	177.8	176.4
Governments	164.9	236.0	385.1	488.5	687.2	747.1	801.6	868.2	924.7	935.4	1,083.2
Federal government	86.1	125.3	217.2	261.1	389.3	425.9	452.6	494.6	525.0	575.5	678.4
Employer contributions to private health insurance premiums	4.9	9.9	11.4	14.3	19.7	21.6	23.1	24.3	24.6	25.1	26.8
Employer contributions to Medicare hospital insurance trust fund	1.7	2.0	2.3	2.7	3.1	3.3	3.3	3.4	3.6	3.7	3.9
Adjusted Medicare[4]	17.4	27.7	57.6	48.8	92.4	107.4	120.5	157.5	168.6	192.3	233.1
Medicaid[5]	28.2	43.3	87.9	119.3	164.4	176.5	182.4	179.6	192.0	208.8	254.3
Other programs[6]	33.9	42.5	58.1	76.0	109.7	117.2	123.2	129.8	136.2	145.6	160.3
State and local government	78.9	110.7	167.8	227.4	297.9	321.3	349.0	373.6	399.7	410.0	404.8
Employer contributions to private health insurance premiums	16.0	26.3	38.9	56.6	83.8	92.4	100.9	110.3	116.6	118.6	123.4
Employer contributions to Medicare hospital insurance trust fund	3.1	4.1	5.6	7.5	8.7	9.0	9.4	10.0	10.6	11.3	11.6
Medicaid[5]	22.7	31.5	60.3	85.3	110.6	121.3	135.4	137.0	145.1	145.0	130.5
Other programs[7]	37.1	48.7	63.0	78.0	94.9	98.5	103.3	116.5	127.3	135.0	139.3
PERCENT DISTRIBUTION											
NATIONAL HEALTH EXPENDITURES	100.0	100.0	100.0	100.0	100.0	100.0	100.0	100.0	100.0	100.0	100.0
Business, Households and Other Private Revenues	68.2	67.4	62.5	64.6	61.2	60.6	60.3	59.7	59.5	58.8	56.4
Private business	23.5	24.6	23.7	25.1	24.1	23.9	23.7	22.9	22.4	21.8	20.8
Employer contribution to private health insurance premiums[1]	16.2	17.9	17.2	18.4	18.4	18.2	18.2	17.5	17.1	16.6	16.0
Employer contribution to Medicare hospital insurance trust fund	4.7	4.1	4.2	4.5	3.6	3.6	3.6	3.6	3.6	3.5	3.1
Workers compensation and temporary disability insurance and worksite health care	2.6	2.7	2.4	2.1	2.1	2.0	1.9	1.8	1.7	1.8	1.7
Household	36.6	34.9	31.1	31.5	29.8	29.5	29.5	29.5	29.4	29.6	28.5
Employer contribution to private health insurance premiums[2]	8.5	9.4	9.8	9.7	10.3	10.3	10.2	10.2	10.0	10.3	10.0
Employee and self-employment contributions and voluntary premiums paid to Medicare hospital insurance trust fund[3]	5.7	4.9	5.4	6.0	4.9	4.8	4.8	4.8	4.8	4.7	4.4
Premiums paid by individuals to Medicare supplementary medical insurance trust fund	1.2	1.4	1.6	1.2	1.2	1.3	1.4	1.9	1.9	2.1	2.1
Out-of-pocket health spending	21.3	19.2	14.3	14.7	13.4	13.1	13.1	12.6	12.7	12.5	12.0
Other private revenues	8.1	7.9	7.7	8.0	7.3	7.2	7.2	7.3	7.7	7.4	7.1
Governments	31.8	32.6	37.5	35.4	38.8	39.4	39.7	40.3	40.5	41.2	43.6
Federal government	16.6	17.3	21.1	18.9	22.0	22.5	22.4	23.0	23.0	24.1	27.3
Employer contributions to private health insurance premiums	0.9	1.4	1.1	1.0	1.1	1.1	1.1	1.1	1.1	1.1	1.1
Employer contributions to Medicare hospital insurance trust fund	3.3	2.8	2.2	2.0	1.8	1.7	1.6	1.6	1.6	1.6	1.6
Adjusted Medicare[4]	3.4	3.8	5.6	3.5	5.2	5.7	6.0	7.3	7.4	8.0	9.4
Medicaid[5]	5.4	6.0	8.6	8.7	9.3	9.3	9.0	8.3	8.4	8.7	10.2
Other programs[6]	6.5	5.9	5.7	5.5	6.2	6.2	6.1	6.0	6.0	5.1	6.4
State and local government	15.2	15.3	16.3	16.5	16.8	17.0	17.3	17.4	17.5	17.1	16.3
Employer contributions to private health insurance premiums	3.1	3.6	3.8	4.1	4.7	4.9	5.0	5.1	5.1	5.0	5.0
Employer contributions to Medicare hospital insurance trust fund	0.6	0.6	0.5	0.5	0.5	0.5	0.5	0.5	0.5	0.5	0.5
Medicaid[5]	4.4	4.4	5.9	6.2	6.2	6.4	6.7	6.4	6.4	6.1	5.2
Other programs[7]	7.1	6.7	6.1	5.7	5.4	5.2	5.1	5.4	5.6	5.6	5.6

[1]Estimates for 2006–2009 exclude Retiree Drug Subsidy (RDS) payments.
[2]Estimates for 2009 exclude subsidized Consolidated Omnibus Budget Reconciliation Act (COBRA) payments.
[3]Includes one-half of self-employment contribution to Medicare hospital insurance trust fund and taxation of Social Security benefits.
[4]Excludes Medicaid buy-in premiums for Medicare. Estimates for 2006–2009, include RDS payments to private and state and local plans.
[5]Includes Medicaid buy-in premiums for Medicare.
[6]Includes maternal and child health, vocational rehabilitation, Substance Abuse and Mental Health Services Administration, Indian Health Service, federal workers' miscellaneous general hospital and medical programs, public health activities, Department of Defense, Department of Veterans Affairs, and Children's Health Insurance Program (CHIP).
[7]Includes other public and general assistance, maternal and child health, vocational rehabilitation, public health activities, hospital subsidies, and state phase-down payments and investment (research, structures, and equipment).

Table C-82. Department of Veterans Affairs Health Care Expenditures and Use, and Persons Treated, by Selected Characteristics, Selected Fiscal Years, 1970–2010

(Number, percent.)

Type of expenditure and use	1970	1980	1985	1990	1995	2000	2005[1]	2006[1]	2007[1]	2008[1]	2009[1]	2010[1]
All Expenditures (Amount in Millions)[2]	$1,689	$5,981	$8,936	$11,500	$16,126	$19,327	$30,291	$31,909	$34,025	$38,282	$42,955	$47,280
Percent Distribution												
All services	100.0	100.0	100.0	100.0	100.0	100.0	100.0	100.0	100.0	100.0	100.0	100.0
Inpatient hospital	71.3	64.3	60.3	57.5	49.0	37.3	24.3	24.0	24.0	23.5	22.7	21.4
Outpatient care	14.0	19.1	18.9	25.3	30.2	45.7	53.4	55.2	53.5	53.2	53.5	52.5
Nursing home care	5.5	7.1	5.4	9.5	10.0	8.2	8.4	8.2	8.3	8.1	7.8	7.4
All other[3]	9.1	9.6	12.4	7.7	10.8	8.8	13.9	12.6	14.2	15.2	16.0	18.8
Health Care Use												
Inpatient hospital discharges[4,5]	787	1,248	1,306	1,029	879	579	614	601	607	622	640	656
Outpatient visits[6]	7,312	17,971	19,601	22,602	27,527	38,370	57,169	59,132	62,234	66,484	73,969	79,457
Nursing home discharges[5,7]	47	57	73	75	79	91	61	59	63	64	65	67
Inpatients[8]	—	—	—	598	527	417	488	467	477	492	512	532
Percent Distribution												
Total	—	—	—	100.0	100.0	100.0	100.0	100.0	100.0	100.0	100.0	100.0
Veterans with service-connected disability	—	—	—	38.9	39.3	34.4	37.6	38.8	39.9	41.1	42.6	43.5
Veterans without service-connected disability	—	—	—	60.3	59.9	64.7	61.5	60.2	59.1	58.0	56.4	55.6
Low income	—	—	—	54.8	56.2	41.7	39.9	37.9	36.9	35.4	34.8	34.6
Veterans receiving aid and attendance or housebound benefits or who are catastrophically disabled[9]	—	—	—	—	—	16.0	12.1	11.6	11.3	11.1	10.5	10.1
Veterans receiving medical care subject to copayments[10]	—	—	—	2.8	2.8	5.2	8.6	9.7	9.8	10.0	9.5	9.3
Other and unknown[11]	—	—	—	2.7	0.9	1.8	1.0	1.0	1.0	1.6	1.6	1.6
Nonveterans	—	—	—	0.8	0.8	0.9	0.9	0.9	0.9	0.9	1.0	0.9
Outpatients[8]	—	—	—	2,564	2,790	3,657	5,077	5,180	5,221	5,291	5,439	5,631
Percent Distribution												
Total	—	—	—	100.0	100.0	100.0	100.0	100.0	100.0	100.0	100.0	100.0
Veterans with service-connected disability	—	—	—	38.3	37.5	30.7	31.6	32.4	33.8	34.7	37.1	38.6
Veterans without service-connected disability	—	—	—	49.8	50.5	60.8	62.7	62.0	60.8	59.7	57.2	56.4
Low income	—	—	—	41.1	42.2	37.6	31.8	30.3	28.9	27.2	25.9	25.7
Veterans receiving aid and attendance or housebound benefits or who are catastrophically disabled[9]	—	—	—	—	—	3.8	3.5	3.4	3.5	3.5	3.4	3.4
Veterans receiving medical care subject to copayments[10]	—	—	—	3.6	4.2	15.4	25.4	25.7	25.5	25.2	23.8	23.0
Other and unknown[11]	—	—	—	5.1	4.1	4.0	2.0	2.6	3.0	3.8	4.0	4.3
Nonveterans	—	—	—	11.8	12.0	8.5	5.7	5.6	5.4	5.7	5.7	5.1

— =Data not available.

[1]Starting with FY2005, the cost report data are taken from a different report than earlier years.
[2]Health care expenditures exclude construction, medical administration, and miscellaneous operating expenses at Department of Veterans Affairs headquarters.
[3]Includes miscellaneous benefits and services, contract hospitals, education and training, subsidies to state veterans hospitals, nursing homes and residential rehabilitation treatment programs (formerly domiciliaries), and the Civilian Health and Medical Program of the Department of Veterans Affairs.
[4]Discharges from medicine, surgery, psychiatry, rehabilitation medicine, spinal cord, and neurology units. Starting with FY2005 data, includes domiciliary care. Does not include long-term stays. One-day dialysis patients were included in 1980. Interfacility transfers were included starting with 1990 data.
[5]Until FY2004, includes Department of Veterans Affairs nursing home and residential rehabilitation treatment programs (formerly domiciliary) stays, and community nursing home care stays.
[6]Hospital outpatient care. Includes the following services: physicians, laboratory tests, home-based primary care, or outpatient fee-basis care.
[7]Includes state nursing home veteran patients.
[8]Individuals receiving services. Individuals with multiple discharges or visits are only counted once in the inpatient or outpatient category.
[9]Includes veterans who are receiving aid and attendance or housebound benefit and veterans who have been determined by the Department of Veterans Affairs to be catastrophically disabled.
[10]Includes veterans who receive medical care subject to copayments according to income level, based on financial means testing.
[11]Includes expenditures for services for veterans who were prisoners of war, exposed to Agent Orange, and other. Prior to FY1994, veterans who reported exposure to Agent Orange were classified as having a service-connected disability.

HEALTH INSURANCE

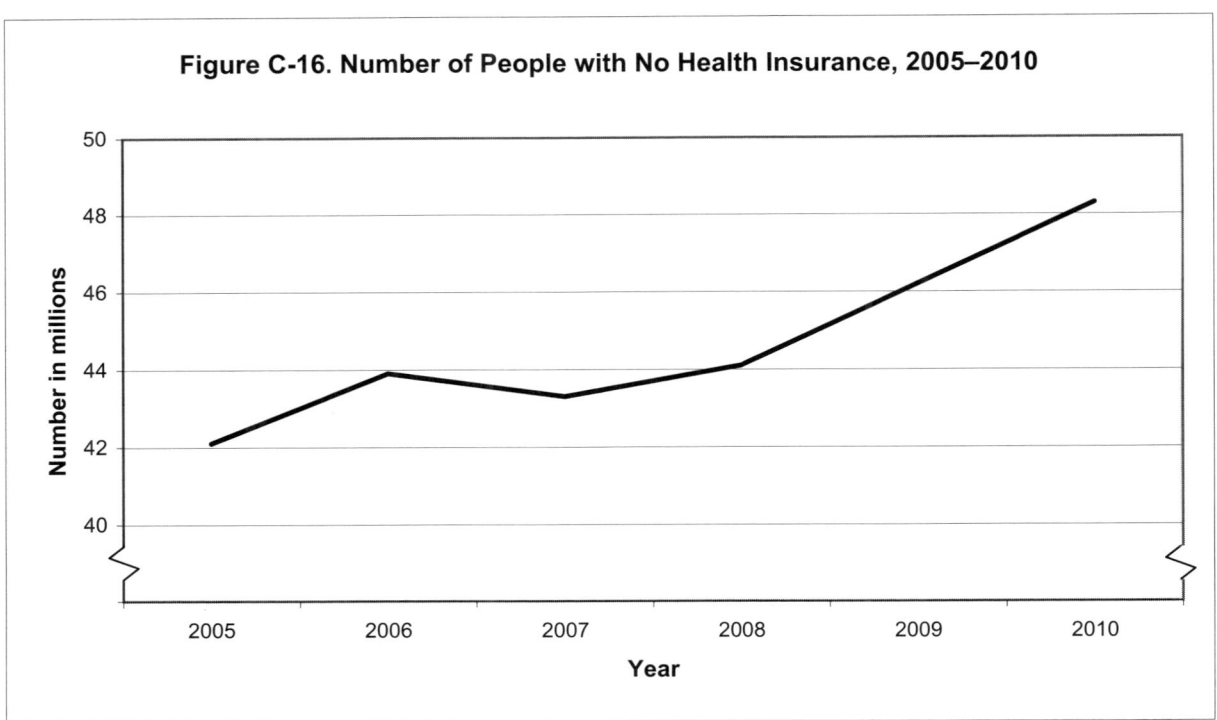

Figure C-16. Number of People with No Health Insurance, 2005–2010

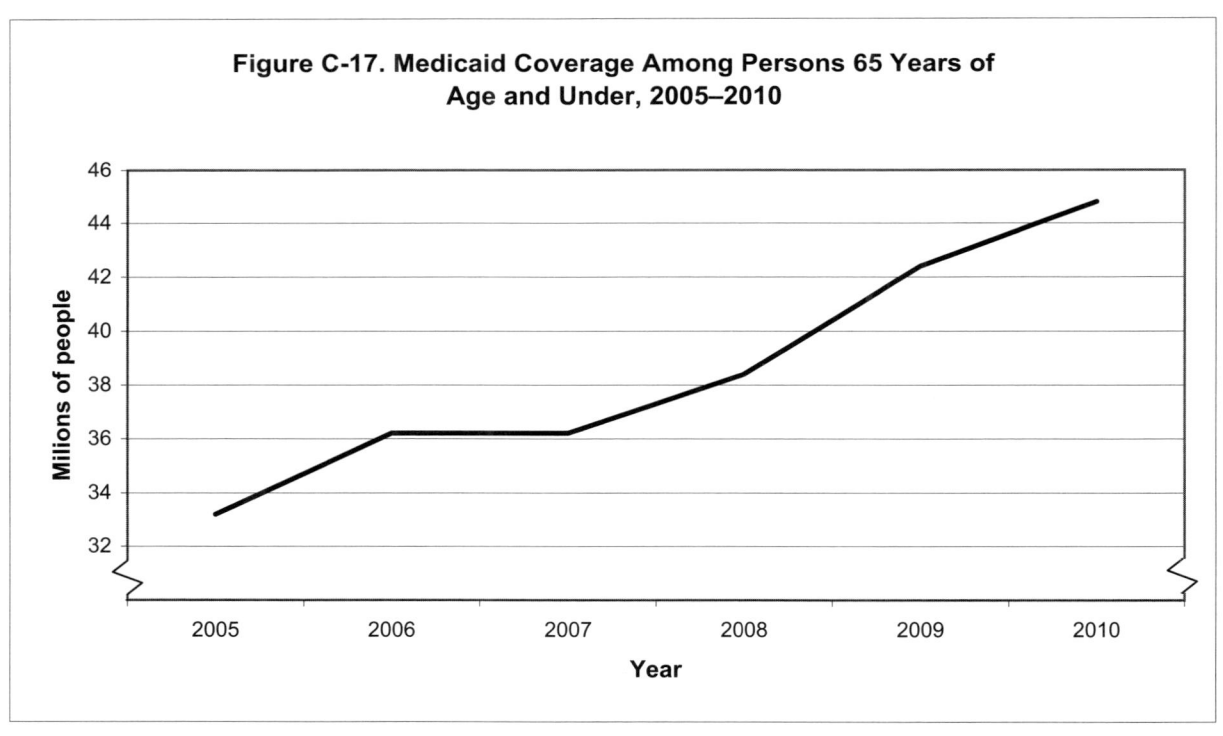

Figure C-17. Medicaid Coverage Among Persons 65 Years of Age and Under, 2005–2010

Table C-83. Private Health Insurance[1] Coverage Obtained Through the Workplace Among Persons Under 65 Years of Age, by Selected Characteristics, Selected Years, 1984–2010

(Number, percent.)

Characteristic	1984[2]	1989[2]	1995[2]	2000[3]	2005	2006	2007	2008	2009	2010
Total (number in millions)[4]	141.8	146.3	150.7	160.8	160.1	155.8	157.9	155.6	150.2	147.6
Total (percent of population)[4]	69.1	68.3	65.4	67.1	63.6	61.5	61.6	60.5	58.0	56.6
Age										
Under 19 years	66.4	65.6	60.5	63.1	58.7	55.6	55.8	54.5	52.0	50.9
Under 6 years	62.1	62.3	55.1	58.9	53.4	50.8	50.8	49.6	46.3	44.9
6–18 years	68.4	67.3	63.1	64.9	61.1	57.8	58.1	56.9	54.8	53.8
Under 18 years	66.5	65.8	60.4	63.0	58.6	55.5	55.8	54.4	51.8	50.7
6–17 years	68.7	67.7	63.3	65.0	61.1	57.8	58.3	56.9	54.7	53.8
18–64 years	70.3	69.4	67.6	68.8	65.7	63.9	63.9	62.9	60.4	58.9
18–44 years	69.6	68.4	65.3	66.5	62.2	60.6	60.3	59.4	56.6	54.6
18–24 years	58.7	55.3	53.5	55.5	52.1	51.7	52.3	49.5	47.4	45.3
19–25 years	59.0	55.0	53.0	54.2	50.6	50.7	51.4	48.9	45.9	44.1
25–34 years	71.2	69.5	65.0	66.4	61.1	59.3	59.0	58.4	55.5	53.3
35–44 years	77.4	76.2	72.7	73.2	69.9	67.5	67.0	67.0	64.3	62.8
45–64 years	71.8	71.6	72.2	72.9	70.9	68.9	69.2	68.0	65.7	64.8
45–54 years	74.6	74.4	74.7	75.6	72.6	70.2	70.4	69.5	67.1	65.9
55–64 years	69.0	68.3	68.4	68.6	68.6	67.2	67.7	66.2	64.0	63.4
Sex										
Male	69.8	68.7	65.9	67.3	63.6	61.2	61.3	60.3	57.6	56.1
Female	68.4	67.9	64.9	66.9	63.6	61.8	61.9	60.8	58.4	57.1
Sex and Marital Status[5]										
Male										
Married	77.9	76.9	74.9	77.5	75.3	73.3	73.3	72.7	70.6	70.1
Divorced, separated, widowed	58.0	57.3	56.4	57.4	51.9	51.0	50.8	51.0	48.0	45.3
Never married	61.5	58.8	58.2	58.8	54.9	52.6	53.5	51.9	48.8	46.2
Female										
Married	76.1	75.5	73.2	76.3	74.2	73.1	72.7	72.2	70.7	69.8
Divorced, separated, widowed	51.9	54.9	54.6	57.8	54.3	51.5	51.3	51.4	48.6	48.1
Never married	63.5	60.9	59.2	60.1	56.3	54.2	55.1	53.0	50.6	48.2
Race[6]										
White only	72.0	71.2	68.4	71.0	66.1	64.0	64.2	63.0	60.6	59.3
Black or African American only	52.4	52.8	49.3	53.4	50.6	48.5	49.1	47.7	45.3	42.3
American Indian or Alaska Native only	45.8	40.9	40.2	41.7	39.9	33.7	35.1	29.4	33.6	*29.4
Asian only	59.0	61.1	59.6	65.8	64.4	64.5	64.6	66.2	62.5	60.6
Native Hawaiian or Other Pacific Islander only	—	—	—	*	*	*	*	*	*	*
2 or more races	—	—	—	59.8	54.8	50.6	49.7	54.3	45.0	49.5
Hispanic Origin and Race[6]										
Hispanic or Latino	52.0	47.3	43.4	45.3	40.0	37.7	38.8	37.6	34.9	34.6
Mexican	50.5	44.2	40.9	43.6	37.6	34.9	35.7	35.2	32.6	31.6
Puerto Rican	45.9	42.3	44.5	49.4	46.2	43.5	51.2	45.9	42.9	43.6
Cuban	57.4	56.5	54.0	53.6	53.5	56.9	54.7	49.2	46.4	47.4
Other Hispanic or Latino	57.4	54.7	46.7	47.3	42.6	40.9	40.8	39.8	36.9	37.8
Not Hispanic or Latino	70.7	70.5	68.2	70.6	68.0	66.0	66.1	65.2	62.8	61.3
White only	74.0	74.1	72.1	74.5	71.9	69.9	70.2	69.0	66.8	65.7
Black or African American only	52.5	52.8	49.8	53.6	50.9	49.5	49.5	48.2	45.9	42.6
Age and Percent of Poverty Level[7]										
Under 65 years:										
Below 100%	24.1	19.8	17.5	21.0	17.8	17.6	17.4	15.5	11.9	12.4
100%–199%	61.7	56.1	49.3	45.4	40.1	38.3	35.5	33.8	33.3	30.2
100%–133%	50.0	44.3	36.0	35.0	31.3	30.0	25.3	23.8	22.6	20.6
134%–199%	66.9	61.5	56.6	50.5	44.8	42.9	40.7	39.1	39.0	35.3
200%–399%	82.8	82.2	80.5	73.4	69.8	69.7	67.7	66.8	64.7	65.3
400% or more	88.8	87.8	86.7	87.9	86.1	84.7	85.5	84.6	84.1	84.2
Under 19 years:										
Below 100%	23.6	18.6	15.1	17.1	13.3	12.7	12.1	11.3	7.9	8.2
100%–199%	67.0	62.1	50.5	45.8	38.3	35.5	32.7	31.4	31.9	28.8
100%–133%	56.1	49.9	37.4	33.6	29.1	27.0	22.4	21.0	19.8	17.9
134%–199%	72.3	67.9	58.8	52.2	43.7	41.0	38.6	37.1	38.9	35.1
200%–399%	85.7	86.0	83.9	76.9	72.4	72.5	71.2	68.3	67.7	68.7
400% or more	90.8	90.3	87.5	89.5	88.3	86.3	87.5	86.9	86.0	86.5

Table C-83. Private Health Insurance[1] Coverage Obtained Through the Workplace Among Persons Under 65 Years of Age, by Selected Characteristics, Selected Years, 1984–2010—*Continued*

(Number, percent.)

Characteristic	1984[2]	1989[2]	1995[2]	2000[3]	2005	2006	2007	2008	2009	2010
Under 18 years:										
Below 100%	23.0	17.5	13.6	16.6	12.5	11.8	11.2	10.3	7.5	7.8
100%–199%	67.5	62.5	50.9	45.8	38.2	35.4	32.7	31.4	32.0	28.8
100%–133%	56.3	50.3	37.2	33.5	28.6	27.1	22.5	21.0	19.8	17.8
134%–199%	72.8	68.4	59.6	52.4	43.9	40.8	38.5	37.1	38.9	35.2
200%–399%	85.9	86.4	84.1	77.1	72.4	72.7	71.5	68.4	67.6	68.7
400% or more	90.7	90.5	87.1	89.7	88.5	86.4	87.7	87.1	86.0	86.6
18-64 years:										
Below 100%	24.8	21.8	20.5	24.0	21.2	21.3	21.2	18.7	14.8	15.4
100%–199%	58.3	52.3	48.4	45.2	41.1	39.9	37.0	35.1	34.0	30.9
100%–133%	46.0	40.4	35.3	35.9	32.9	31.8	27.0	25.5	24.2	22.1
134%–199%	63.6	57.5	55.0	49.5	45.3	43.9	41.8	40.1	39.0	35.3
200%–399%	81.4	80.2	78.8	71.7	68.7	68.4	66.2	66.1	63.6	63.9
400% or more	88.5	87.5	86.7	87.5	85.4	84.3	84.9	83.9	83.6	83.6
Disability Measure Among Adults 18-64 Years[8]										
Any basic actions difficulty or complex activity limitation	—	—	—	58.5	53.3	52.0	51.5	49.1	46.7	48.0
Any basic actions difficulty	—	—	—	59.1	54.0	52.6	52.1	49.9	47.4	48.9
Any complex activity limitation	—	—	—	43.5	38.9	37.2	35.4	33.5	31.1	32.8
No disability	—	—	—	72.5	68.5	67.3	67.1	67.5	64.8	63.5
Geographic Region										
Northeast	74.0	75.0	69.8	72.5	70.6	67.5	68.2	68.0	65.3	64.4
Midwest	72.0	73.3	71.2	74.9	70.1	67.0	68.0	64.7	62.0	61.8
South	66.2	63.6	61.8	62.5	58.0	57.2	57.2	56.7	54.1	52.2
West	64.7	63.9	60.4	61.1	59.7	58.1	57.3	56.8	54.5	52.7
Location of Residence										
Within MSA[9]	70.9	69.6	66.6	68.2	64.5	62.7	62.7	61.5	59.3	57.9
Outside MSA[9]	65.3	63.5	60.7	62.6	59.6	55.4	55.7	55.1	50.8	49.4

— = Data not available.
* = Figure does not meet standards of reliability or precision.
[1]Any private insurance at the time of interview that was originally obtained through a present or former employer or union, or, starting with 1997 data, through the workplace, self-employment, or a professional association; includes those who also had another type of coverage.
[2]Data prior to 1997 are not strictly comparable with data for later years due to the 1997 questionnaire redesign.
[3]Estimates for 2000–2002 were calculated using 2000-based sample weights and may differ from estimates in other reports that used 1990-based sample weights for 2000–2002 estimates.
[4]Includes all other races not shown separately, those with unknown marital status, unknown disability status, and, in 1984 and 1989, persons with unknown poverty level.
[5]Includes persons 14–64 years of age.
[6]The race groups, White, Black, American Indian or Alaska Native, Asian, Native Hawaiian or Other Pacific Islander, and 2 or more races, include persons of Hispanic and non-Hispanic origin. Persons of Hispanic origin may be of any race.
[7]Percent of poverty level is based on family income and family size and composition using U.S. Census Bureau poverty thresholds.
[8]Any basic actions difficulty or complex activity limitation is defined as having one or more of the following limitations or difficulties: movement difficulty, emotional difficulty, sensory (seeing or hearing) difficulty, cognitive difficulty, self-care (activities of daily living or instrumental activities of daily living) limitation, social limitation, or work limitation.
[9]MSA = metropolitan statistical area.

Table C-84. Private Health Insurance[1] Coverage Among Persons Under 65 Years of Age, by Selected Characteristics, Selected Years, 1984–2010

(Percent.)

Characteristic	1984[2]	1995[2]	2000[3]	2005	2006	2007	2008	2009	2010
TOTAL[4]	157.5	164.2	174.0	174.7	171.2	174.1	171.9	166.7	163.9
Percent of Population									
Total[4]	76.8	71.3	71.5	68.2	66.3	66.8	65.6	63.3	61.7
Age									
Under 19 years	72.6	65.4	66.7	62.3	59.5	59.9	58.6	56.1	54.3
Under 6 years	68.1	59.5	62.7	56.6	54.7	54.1	53.2	50.1	48.3
6–18 years	74.8	68.3	68.5	64.9	61.7	62.6	61.1	59.0	57.2
Under 18 years	72.6	65.2	66.6	62.1	59.4	59.8	58.4	55.8	54.1
6–17 years	74.9	68.3	68.5	64.7	61.7	62.6	61.1	58.8	57.2
18–64 years	78.6	73.9	73.5	70.7	69.1	69.5	68.5	66.2	64.7
18–44 years	76.5	70.9	70.5	66.6	65.0	65.5	64.4	61.7	60.0
18–24 years	67.4	60.8	60.3	58.0	57.0	59.0	56.2	54.4	52.3
19–25 years	67.4	60.1	59.1	56.3	56.1	57.9	55.8	53.0	51.8
25–34 years	77.4	70.1	70.1	65.1	63.0	63.5	62.7	60.0	58.7
35–44 years	83.9	77.7	77.0	73.7	72.0	71.7	71.7	68.4	66.9
45–64 years	83.3	80.1	78.7	76.9	75.2	75.5	74.3	72.6	71.3
45–54 years	83.3	80.9	80.0	77.4	75.1	75.4	74.8	72.6	70.9
55–64 years	83.3	79.0	76.7	76.2	75.4	75.5	73.6	72.6	71.8
Sex									
Male	77.3	71.6	71.6	68.0	65.9	66.4	65.3	62.9	61.1
Female	76.2	70.9	71.3	68.4	66.7	67.1	65.9	63.7	62.4
Sex and Marital Status[5]									
Male									
Married	85.0	80.2	81.5	79.6	78.1	78.1	77.7	75.8	75.1
Divorced, separated, widowed	65.5	62.4	62.2	56.7	55.4	55.8	56.0	52.9	50.6
Never married	71.3	65.4	63.8	60.2	57.8	59.8	57.9	54.9	52.5
Female									
Married	83.8	79.3	81.0	79.3	78.6	78.4	77.7	76.7	75.6
Divorced, separated, widowed	63.1	61.7	63.2	59.9	56.3	57.0	56.3	54.2	53.9
Never married	72.2	66.2	64.2	61.5	59.0	60.8	58.8	56.4	54.1
Race[6]									
White only	79.9	74.5	75.7	70.9	69.1	69.7	68.5	66.3	64.9
Black or African American only	58.1	53.0	55.9	52.9	51.3	51.8	50.0	47.4	44.8
American Indian or Alaska Native only	49.1	45.3	43.7	43.0	36.3	36.4	30.7	35.9	31.7
Asian only	69.9	68.4	72.1	72.2	72.1	73.2	74.3	71.3	68.1
Native Hawaiian or Other Pacific Islander only	—	—	*	*	*	*	*	*	*
2 or more races	—	—	61.4	57.6	54.0	52.7	58.0	47.8	52.4
Hispanic Origin and Race[6]									
Hispanic or Latino	55.7	46.4	47.8	42.4	40.0	41.7	39.9	37.3	36.8
Mexican	53.3	42.6	45.4	39.7	36.5	37.9	36.8	34.7	33.4
Puerto Rican	48.4	47.6	51.1	48.5	46.1	54.2	48.2	46.2	46.0
Cuban	72.5	63.6	63.9	58.1	63.4	64.8	57.9	54.3	53.8
Other Hispanic or Latino	61.6	51.4	50.7	45.6	44.3	44.3	43.5	39.7	40.9
Not Hispanic or Latino	78.7	74.4	75.2	73.0	71.3	71.7	70.8	68.6	67.0
White only	82.4	78.6	79.5	77.3	75.6	76.2	75.3	73.3	72.0
Black or African American only	58.2	53.4	56.0	53.1	52.2	52.3	50.6	48.0	45.1
Age and Percent of Poverty Level[7]									
Under 65 years									
Below 100%	32.2	22.6	25.2	21.4	21.4	21.4	19.2	15.3	16.0
100%–199%	70.3	55.3	50.1	44.7	42.8	40.0	38.1	37.4	34.8
100%–133%	59.4	41.7	39.3	36.0	33.6	29.5	27.3	26.1	24.4
134%–199%	75.2	62.7	55.3	49.4	47.8	45.4	43.7	43.3	40.3
200%–399%	89.3	86.4	78.1	74.8	74.9	73.2	72.3	70.6	70.7
400% or more	95.4	93.2	91.9	90.6	89.8	91.0	90.1	90.2	89.9
Under 19 years									
Below 100%	29.6	19.0	20.3	15.0	15.0	14.1	12.4	9.7	9.8
100%–199%	73.6	55.8	49.5	41.6	38.5	35.7	34.1	34.0	31.5
100%–133%	63.8	42.5	37.1	32.6	29.0	25.4	23.2	21.3	20.1
134%–199%	78.4	64.4	56.1	47.0	44.6	41.7	40.1	41.3	38.1
200%–399%	91.1	89.1	80.8	76.6	77.1	75.8	73.7	73.2	72.6
400% or more	96.2	93.3	93.0	92.5	91.4	93.2	92.0	91.8	91.2

Table C-84. Private Health Insurance[1] Coverage Among Persons Under 65 Years of Age, by Selected Characteristics, Selected Years, 1984–2010—Continued

(Percent.)

Characteristic	1984[2]	1995[2]	2000[3]	2005	2006	2007	2008	2009	2010
Under 18 years									
Below 100%	28.5	16.9	19.5	14.2	14.0	12.7	11.3	9.3	9.2
100%–199%	73.9	56.1	49.4	41.4	38.3	35.6	34.1	34.0	31.5
100%–133%	63.9	42.3	36.8	32.0	29.0	25.4	23.2	21.1	19.9
134%–199%	78.6	64.9	56.2	47.0	44.4	41.5	40.1	41.3	38.3
200%–399%	91.3	89.2	81.1	76.6	77.3	76.0	73.8	73.0	72.6
400% or more	96.1	93.1	93.1	92.5	91.6	93.4	92.2	91.8	91.4
18–64 years									
Below 100%	35.0	27.0	29.1	25.9	26.1	26.8	24.0	19.2	20.4
100%–199%	68.3	54.8	50.5	46.5	45.1	42.5	40.2	39.1	36.4
100%–133%	56.6	41.4	40.9	38.3	36.4	32.1	29.6	28.8	26.9
134%–199%	73.3	61.5	54.9	50.7	49.4	47.5	45.7	44.3	41.3
200%–399%	88.3	85.0	76.7	74.0	73.9	72.0	71.7	69.6	70.0
400% or more	95.2	93.2	91.6	90.1	89.3	90.4	89.6	89.8	89.5
Disability Measure Among Adults 18–64 Years[8]									
Any basic actions difficulty or complex activity limitation	—	—	63.1	58.1	56.4	56.4	53.2	51.6	53.0
Any basic actions difficulty	—	—	63.9	58.8	57.1	56.9	54.3	52.3	53.8
Any complex activity limitation	—	—	48.4	44.0	41.7	40.3	37.0	36.0	38.6
No disability	—	—	77.2	73.7	72.5	72.9	73.3	70.4	69.3
Geographic Region									
Northeast	80.5	75.4	76.3	74.0	70.8	72.2	71.3	69.7	68.2
Midwest	80.6	77.3	78.8	74.6	71.7	72.0	69.9	67.5	66.7
South	74.3	66.9	66.8	62.5	61.8	62.6	62.1	59.3	57.5
West	71.9	67.5	66.5	65.6	64.6	64.0	62.8	60.6	58.9
Location of Residence									
Within MSA[9]	77.5	72.1	72.3	69.0	67.5	67.8	66.5	64.6	62.9
Outside MSA[9]	75.2	67.9	67.8	64.6	60.3	61.0	61.1	56.2	55.1

— = Data not available.
* = Figure does not meet standards of reliability or precision.
[1]Any private health insurance coverage (both individual and insurance obtained through the workplace) at the time of interview; includes those who also had another type of coverage.
[2]Data prior to 1997 are not strictly comparable with data for later years due to the 1997 questionnaire redesign.
[3]Estimates for 2000–2002 were calculated using 2000-based sample weights and may differ from estimates in other reports that used 1990-based sample weights for 2000–2002 estimates.
[4]Includes all other races not shown separately, those with unknown marital status, unknown disability status, and, in 1984 and 1989, persons with unknown poverty level.
[5]Includes persons 14–64 years of age.
[6]The race groups, White, Black, American Indian or Alaska Native, Asian, Native Hawaiian or Other Pacific Islander, and 2 or more races, include persons of Hispanic and non-Hispanic origin. Persons of Hispanic origin may be of any race.
[7]Percent of poverty level is based on family income and family size and composition using U.S. Census Bureau poverty thresholds.
[8]Any basic actions difficulty or complex activity limitation is defined as having one or more of the following limitations or difficulties: movement difficulty, emotional difficulty, sensory (seeing or hearing) difficulty, cognitive difficulty, self-care (activities of daily living or instrumental activities of daily living) limitation, social limitation, or work limitation.
[9]MSA = metropolitan statistical area.

Table C-85. No Health Insurance Coverage Among Persons Under 65 Years of Age, by Selected Characteristics, Selected Years, 1984–2010

(Number, percent.)

Characteristic	1984[1]	1989[1]	1995[1]	2000[2]	2005[3]	2006[3]	2007[3]	2008[3]	2009[3]	2010[3]
Total (number in millions)[4]	29.8	33.4	37.1	41.4	42.1	43.9	43.3	44.1	46.2	48.3
Total (percent of population)[4]	14.5	15.6	16.1	17.0	16.4	17.0	16.6	16.8	17.5	18.2
Age										
Under 19 years	14.1	15.0	13.7	12.9	9.7	9.8	9.4	9.5	8.5	8.3
Under 6 years	14.9	15.1	11.8	11.8	7.7	7.5	7.3	7.6	6.6	6.3
6–18 years	13.8	15.0	14.6	13.4	10.6	10.9	10.4	10.5	9.4	9.2
Under 18 years	13.9	14.7	13.4	12.6	9.3	9.5	9.0	9.0	8.2	7.8
6–17 years	13.4	14.5	14.3	13.0	10.1	10.5	9.9	9.8	9.0	8.6
18–64 years	14.8	16.0	17.3	18.9	19.3	20.0	19.6	19.9	21.2	22.3
18–44 years	17.1	18.4	20.4	22.4	23.5	24.6	23.9	24.4	25.9	27.1
18–24 years	25.0	27.1	28.0	30.4	29.1	29.9	27.9	29.0	29.6	31.4
19–25 years	25.1	27.9	28.8	32.3	31.7	32.4	30.5	31.1	32.8	33.8
25–34 years	16.2	18.3	21.1	23.3	25.6	27.2	26.1	26.6	27.8	28.3
35–44 years	11.2	12.3	15.1	16.9	17.9	18.8	19.1	19.1	21.4	22.6
45–64 years	9.6	10.5	10.9	12.6	12.9	13.2	13.5	13.6	14.6	15.7
45–54 years	10.5	11.0	11.6	12.8	14.2	15.0	14.9	14.9	16.5	17.9
55–64 years	8.7	10.0	9.9	12.4	11.1	10.8	11.6	11.8	12.2	12.8
Sex										
Male	15.3	16.8	17.4	18.1	17.9	18.8	18.2	18.3	19.4	20.3
Female	13.8	14.4	14.8	15.9	15.0	15.3	15.1	15.4	15.7	16.1
Sex and Marital Status[5]										
Male										
Married	11.1	12.5	15.0	14.1	14.4	15.3	15.3	15.4	16.3	17.2
Divorced, separated, widowed	24.9	25.0	24.0	25.8	28.6	29.1	28.1	27.0	29.8	31.4
Never married	22.4	25.0	25.6	27.2	27.6	28.6	27.0	27.6	29.4	31.1
Female										
Married	11.2	11.8	13.6	13.3	13.0	13.5	13.5	13.5	14.2	14.7
Divorced, separated, widowed	19.2	19.1	18.1	21.3	22.1	23.0	22.6	22.1	22.8	23.6
Never married	16.3	18.0	17.5	21.1	20.0	20.4	19.5	20.7	21.0	21.9
Race[6]										
White only	13.6	14.5	15.5	15.4	15.9	16.7	16.3	16.7	17.1	17.6
Black or African American only	19.9	21.6	18.0	19.5	18.4	18.1	17.0	18.0	18.9	20.6
American Indian or Alaska Native only	22.5	28.4	34.3	38.4	32.2	38.0	38.8	28.4	32.5	44.0
Asian only	18.5	16.9	18.6	17.6	17.1	15.0	15.4	13.9	16.2	17.1
Native Hawaiian or Other Pacific Islander only	—	—	—	*	*	*	*	*	*	*
2 or more races	—	—	—	16.8	16.5	18.4	15.0	15.8	18.2	15.8
Hispanic Origin and Race[6]										
Hispanic or Latino	29.5	33.7	31.4	35.6	33.0	35.0	31.8	33.3	32.9	32.0
Mexican	33.8	39.9	35.6	39.9	36.0	38.6	34.7	36.1	35.0	34.8
Puerto Rican	18.3	24.7	17.6	16.4	16.3	16.8	12.8	16.8	17.8	13.7
Cuban	21.6	20.6	22.3	25.4	23.2	22.8	20.7	28.1	27.8	26.5
Other Hispanic or Latino	27.4	25.8	30.2	33.4	32.6	33.2	32.7	32.5	33.4	32.4
Not Hispanic or Latino	13.2	13.7	14.2	14.0	13.4	13.6	13.7	13.5	14.4	15.2
White only	11.9	12.1	13.0	12.5	12.0	12.5	12.6	12.5	13.2	13.7
Black or African American only	19.7	21.5	17.9	19.5	18.3	17.5	16.8	17.9	18.8	20.7
Age and Percent of Poverty Level[7]										
Under 65 years										
Below 100%	33.9	35.2	29.6	34.2	30.6	30.2	28.4	29.0	30.4	30.3
100%–199%	21.8	25.6	28.3	31.0	28.6	29.6	30.0	30.6	29.8	32.4
100%–133%	28.8	32.3	34.1	35.7	30.1	31.3	32.0	32.8	30.1	34.9
134%–199%	18.7	22.6	25.1	28.7	27.8	28.7	29.0	29.5	29.6	31.0
200%–399%	7.6	8.3	10.0	15.4	15.7	15.5	16.9	16.6	17.8	17.4
400% or more	3.2	4.2	5.4	5.9	6.3	6.5	5.6	6.2	5.8	5.6
Under 19 years										
Below 100%	29.0	31.7	20.4	22.6	15.2	14.2	12.7	14.0	12.2	11.3
100%–199%	18.0	20.7	22.6	22.1	15.6	16.4	16.4	16.3	13.0	13.5
100%–133%	24.4	27.6	26.4	26.5	15.6	17.9	17.4	17.3	12.9	15.9
134%–199%	14.9	17.4	20.1	19.7	15.6	15.5	15.9	15.8	13.1	12.0
200%–399%	5.1	4.9	6.7	9.6	8.2	7.8	8.5	8.0	8.0	7.4
400% or more	1.8	2.1	4.4	3.5	3.3	3.4	2.3	2.8	2.4	2.3

Table C-85. No Health Insurance Coverage Among Persons Under 65 Years of Age, by Selected Characteristics, Selected Years, 1984–2010—Continued

(Number, percent.)

Characteristic	1984[1]	1989[1]	1995[1]	2000[2]	2005[3]	2006[3]	2007[3]	2008[3]	2009[3]	2010[3]
Under 18 years										
Below 100%	28.9	31.6	20.0	22.0	14.3	13.9	11.9	13.3	11.8	10.6
100%–199%	17.5	20.2	22.0	21.7	15.0	16.0	15.7	15.5	12.3	12.7
100%–133%	24.0	27.1	26.1	26.4	15.1	17.5	16.5	16.4	11.8	15.1
134%–199%	14.4	16.9	19.5	19.1	15.0	15.1	15.3	15.0	12.6	11.3
200%–399%	4.9	4.7	6.6	9.3	7.8	7.4	8.2	7.5	7.8	7.0
400% or more	1.8	1.9	4.6	3.3	3.2	3.1	2.2	2.7	2.3	2.1
18–64 years										
Below 100%	37.6	38.2	37.0	42.4	40.9	40.7	38.6	38.6	42.5	42.7
100%–199%	24.4	28.8	32.0	36.4	35.9	36.7	37.9	38.9	38.9	42.1
100%–133%	31.9	35.6	39.7	41.7	38.9	39.8	41.7	42.1	40.4	45.7
134%–199%	21.1	25.9	28.2	34.0	34.4	35.1	36.1	37.3	38.1	40.3
200%–399%	8.9	10.0	11.7	18.2	19.0	18.8	20.5	20.2	21.7	21.3
400% or more	3.4	4.4	5.5	6.6	7.1	7.4	6.5	7.1	6.7	6.5
Disability Measure Among Adults 18–64 Years[8]										
Any basic actions difficulty or complex activity limitation	—	—	—	17.6	19.6	20.0	19.6	19.5	21.4	20.8
Any basic actions difficulty	—	—	—	17.6	19.8	20.0	19.6	19.4	21.2	20.9
Any complex activity limitation	—	—	—	16.1	16.9	17.3	18.3	15.8	19.2	17.2
No disability	—	—	—	18.5	19.5	20.5	19.9	19.8	21.2	21.6
Geographic Region										
Northeast	10.2	10.9	13.3	12.2	11.3	11.2	11.0	11.4	11.4	12.4
Midwest	11.3	10.7	12.2	12.3	11.9	13.4	13.0	13.9	14.6	14.1
South	17.7	19.7	19.4	20.5	21.0	21.1	20.1	20.1	21.2	21.9
West	18.2	18.8	17.9	20.7	18.4	18.8	18.9	18.8	19.4	20.6
Location of Residence										
Within MSA[9]	13.6	15.2	15.5	16.6	16.1	16.6	16.1	16.4	17.1	17.8
Outside MSA[9]	16.6	17.0	18.6	18.6	17.8	19.3	19.4	19.1	20.2	20.4

— = Data not available.
* = Figure does not meet standards of reliability or precision.
[1] Data prior to 1997 are not strictly comparable with data for later years due to the 1997 questionnaire redesign.
[2] Estimates for 2000–2002 were calculated using 2000-based sample weights and may differ from estimates in other reports that used 1990-based sample weights for 2000–2002 estimates.
[3] Beginning in quarter 3 of the 2004 NHIS, persons under 65 years of age with no reported coverage were asked explicitly about Medicaid coverage.
[4] Includes all other races not shown separately, those with unknown marital status, unknown disability status, and, in 1984 and 1989, persons with unknown poverty level.
[5] Includes persons 14–64 years of age.
[6] The race groups, White, Black, American Indian or Alaska Native, Asian, Native Hawaiian or Other Pacific Islander, and 2 or more races, include persons of Hispanic and non-Hispanic origin. Persons of Hispanic origin may be of any race.
[7] Percent of poverty level is based on family income and family size and composition using U.S. Census Bureau poverty thresholds.
[8] Any basic actions difficulty or complex activity limitation is defined as having one or more of the following limitations or difficulties: movement difficulty, emotional difficulty, sensory (seeing or hearing) difficulty, cognitive difficulty, self-care (activities of daily living or instrumental activities of daily living) limitation, social limitation, or work limitation.
[9] MSA= metropolitan statistical area.

Table C-86. Health Insurance Coverage of Medicare Beneficiaries 65 Years of Age and Over, by Type of Coverage and Selected Characteristics, Selected Years, 1992–2008

(Number, percent.)

Characteristic	Medicare Risk Health Maintenance Organization[1]					Medicaid[2]				
	1992	1995	2000	2005	2008	1992	1995	2000	2005	2008
Age										
65 years and over (number in millions)	1.1	2.6	5.9	4.6	8.1	2.7	2.8	2.7	3.2	3.2
65 years and over (percent of population)	3.9	8.9	19.3	14.5	22.1	9.4	9.6	9.0	10.1	8.8
65–74 years	4.2	9.5	20.6	13.9	22.9	7.9	8.8	8.5	9.9	8.2
75–84 years	3.7	8.3	18.5	15.3	23.0	10.6	9.6	8.9	9.9	9.1
85 years and over	*	7.3	16.3	13.9	16.5	16.6	13.6	11.2	11.9	10.3
Sex										
Male	4.6	9.2	19.3	13.5	23.6	6.3	6.2	6.3	7.2	5.8
Female	3.4	8.6	19.3	15.2	20.9	11.6	12.0	10.9	12.3	11.2
Race and Hispanic Origin										
White, not Hispanic or Latino	3.6	8.4	18.4	13.2	20.2	5.6	5.4	5.1	6.1	5.4
Black, not Hispanic or Latino	*	7.9	20.7	17.1	28.5	28.5	30.3	23.6	23.6	20.0
Hispanic	*	15.5	27.5	27.2	37.5	39.0	40.5	28.7	29.2	21.1
Percent of Poverty Level[3]										
Below 100%	3.6	7.7	18.4	—	—	22.3	17.2	15.9	—	—
100%–less than 200%	3.7	9.5	23.4	—	—	6.7	6.3	8.4	—	—
200% or more	4.2	10.1	18.0	—	—	*	*	*	—	—
Marital Status										
Married	4.6	9.5	18.7	13.8	24.2	4.0	4.3	4.3	5.4	4.0
Widowed	2.3	7.7	19.4	15.0	17.1	14.9	15.0	13.6	14.9	13.9
Divorced	*	9.7	24.4	17.1	25.5	23.4	24.5	20.2	20.0	16.8
Never married	*	*	15.8	13.9	20.7	19.2	19.0	17.0	21.3	18.2

Characteristic	Employer-sponsored plan[4]					Medigap[5]				
	1992	1995	2000	2005	2008	1992	1995	2000	2005	2008
Age										
65 years and over (number in millions)	12.5	11.3	10.7	11.6	12.0	9.9	9.5	7.6	8.2	7.9
65 years and over (percent of population)	42.8	38.6	35.2	36.4	32.7	33.9	32.5	25.0	25.7	21.5
65–74 years	46.9	41.1	36.6	38.1	34.0	31.4	29.9	21.7	23.2	19.6
75–84 years	38.2	37.1	35.0	35.5	31.2	37.5	35.2	27.8	27.3	22.7
85 years and over	31.6	30.2	29.4	31.8	31.1	38.3	37.6	31.1	30.8	26.3
Sex										
Male	46.3	42.1	37.7	39.4	35.3	30.6	30.0	23.4	23.8	20.1
Female	40.4	36.0	33.4	34.2	30.7	36.2	34.4	26.2	27.1	22.7
Race and Hispanic Origin										
White, not Hispanic or Latino	45.9	41.3	38.6	39.5	35.4	37.2	36.2	28.3	29.1	24.9
Black, not Hispanic or Latino	25.9	26.7	22.0	27.9	23.2	13.6	10.2	7.5	9.5	6.5
Hispanic	20.7	16.9	15.8	18.6	19.7	15.8	10.1	11.3	11.1	7.8
Percent of Poverty Level[3]										
Below 100%	29.0	32.1	28.1	—	—	30.8	29.8	22.6	—	—
100%–less than 200%	37.5	32.0	27.0	—	—	39.3	39.1	28.4	—	—
200% or more	58.4	52.8	49.0	—	—	32.8	32.2	26.2	—	—
Marital Status										
Married	49.9	44.6	41.0	41.7	38.3	33.0	32.6	25.6	27.0	21.4
Widowed	34.1	30.3	28.7	30.4	27.6	37.5	35.2	26.7	26.2	23.6
Divorced	27.3	26.6	22.4	25.1	19.3	27.9	24.1	16.9	19.8	18.5
Never married	38.0	35.1	28.5	29.1	28.9	29.1	26.2	21.9	15.4	14.6

Table C-86. **Health Insurance Coverage of Medicare Beneficiaries 65 Years of Age and Over, by Type of Coverage and Selected Characteristics, Selected Years, 1992–2008**—*Continued*

(Number, percent.)

Characteristic	Medicare fee-for-service only or other[6]				
	1992	1995	2000	2005	2008
Age					
65 years and over (number in millions)	2.9	3.1	3.5	4.3	5.5
65 years and over (percent of population)	9.9	10.5	11.5	13.3	14.9
65–74 years	9.7	10.7	12.6	14.9	15.2
75–84 years	10.1	9.9	9.9	11.9	14.0
85 years and over	10.8	11.3	12.1	11.6	15.8
Sex					
Male	12.2	12.6	13.3	16.2	15.1
Female	8.3	8.9	10.2	11.2	14.7
Race and Hispanic Origin					
White, not Hispanic or Latino	7.7	8.7	9.6	12.2	14.1
Black, not Hispanic or Latino	26.7	25.0	26.1	21.9	21.7
Hispanic	18.3	17.1	16.7	13.9	13.9
Percent of Poverty Level[3]					
Below 100%	14.3	13.3	15.1	—	—
100%–less than 200%	12.9	13.1	12.7	—	—
200% or more	4.0	4.5	6.3	—	—
Marital Status					
Married	8.5	9.0	10.5	12.1	12.1
Widowed	11.2	11.9	11.6	13.5	17.7
Divorced	15.7	15.1	16.1	17.9	20.0
Never married	*	13.1	16.8	20.4	17.7

* = Figure does not meet standards of reliability or precision.
—= Data not available.
[1]Enrollee has Medicare risk Health Maintenance Organization (HMO) regardless of other insurance.
[2]Enrolled in Medicaid and not enrolled in a Medicare risk HMO.
[3]Percent of poverty level is based on family income and family size and composition using U.S. Census Bureau poverty thresholds.
[4]Private insurance plans purchased through employers (own, current, or former employer, family business, union, or former employer or union of spouse) and not enrolled in a Medicare risk HMO or Medicaid.
[5]Supplemental insurance purchased privately or through organizations such as American Association of Retired Persons or professional organizations, and not enrolled in a Medicare risk HMO, Medicaid, or employer-sponsored plan.
[6]Medicare fee-for-service only or other public plans (except Medicaid).

Table C-87. Persons Without Health Insurance Coverage, by State, Average Annual, Selected Years, 1995–1997 through 2007–2009

(Percent.)

State	1995–1997	1998–2000	2001–2003	2004–2006[1]	2005–2007[1]	2006–2008	2007–2009
United States	15.7	14.4	15.1	15.3	15.4	15.5	15.8
Alabama	14.0	14.2	13.3	14.1	13.9	13.0	13.6
Alaska	14.7	18.1	17.8	16.7	17.3	18.2	18.6
Arizona	23.0	19.5	17.3	19.0	19.6	19.6	19.1
Arkansas	21.3	15.3	16.6	17.5	17.5	17.6	17.7
California	20.7	19.2	18.7	18.5	18.6	18.5	18.9
Colorado	15.5	14.1	16.3	16.6	16.7	16.5	15.9
Connecticut	10.6	9.5	10.4	10.4	9.9	9.6	10.5
Delaware	14.1	11.2	10.1	12.5	11.8	11.4	11.8
District of Columbia	16.1	14.5	13.3	12.4	11.4	10.4	10.6
Florida	18.9	17.2	17.6	20.3	20.5	20.5	20.9
Georgia	17.8	15.2	16.4	17.6	17.8	17.7	18.6
Hawaii	8.3	9.8	9.9	8.6	8.3	8.1	7.8
Idaho	16.1	16.5	17.5	14.9	14.7	15.0	14.9
Illinois	11.6	13.3	14.0	13.6	13.7	13.4	13.7
Indiana	11.5	11.3	12.9	13.1	12.3	11.8	12.6
Iowa	11.6	8.2	9.5	9.3	9.4	9.8	10.0
Kansas	11.8	11.0	10.9	11.1	11.8	12.4	12.7
Kentucky	15.0	13.1	13.3	13.8	13.8	15.0	15.3
Louisiana	18.8	19.5	19.4	18.5	19.4	20.1	18.2
Maine	13.5	11.5	10.7	9.5	9.5	9.5	9.8
Maryland	13.4	11.9	13.2	13.5	13.6	13.2	13.2
Massachusetts	12.0	9.2	9.6	10.3	8.3	7.1	5.1
Michigan	10.1	10.6	11.0	10.6	10.8	11.3	12.4
Minnesota	9.1	8.2	8.2	8.5	8.5	8.7	8.6
Mississippi	19.4	15.7	17.0	18.1	18.8	19.1	18.1
Missouri	13.5	9.0	10.9	12.3	12.5	12.8	13.5
Montana	15.3	18.3	16.1	17.0	16.1	16.3	15.7
Nebraska	10.4	9.5	10.3	11.1	12.0	12.5	12.2
Nevada	17.3	17.5	18.3	18.3	17.9	18.5	18.9
New Hampshire	10.4	8.6	9.9	10.4	10.5	10.7	10.4
New Jersey	15.8	12.9	13.7	14.6	15.2	15.1	15.2
New Mexico	23.5	22.6	21.3	21.0	21.9	23.0	22.6
New York	16.6	15.3	15.5	13.2	13.4	13.8	14.0
North Carolina	15.3	13.7	16.1	16.0	16.6	16.6	16.6
North Dakota	11.1	12.1	10.5	11.1	11.1	11.4	10.8
Ohio	11.6	10.2	11.7	10.7	11.0	11.1	12.5
Oklahoma	18.0	17.7	18.7	18.7	18.2	16.9	16.6
Oregon	13.7	13.7	14.8	16.6	16.8	17.0	16.9
Pennsylvania	9.8	8.3	10.7	10.2	9.8	9.8	10.3
Rhode Island	11.0	6.9	9.3	10.2	10.3	10.4	11.6
South Carolina	16.2	13.8	13.1	16.0	16.5	16.1	16.4
South Dakota	10.2	12.0	11.0	11.6	11.2	11.5	12.0
Tennessee	14.5	10.8	11.8	13.4	13.9	14.4	14.9
Texas	24.4	22.2	24.6	24.1	24.4	24.9	25.5
Utah	12.4	13.2	13.6	15.7	15.6	14.5	13.6
Vermont	11.3	10.3	9.9	10.8	11.0	10.2	10.1
Virginia	12.9	12.9	12.5	13.2	13.6	13.5	13.4
Washington	12.4	12.8	14.3	12.5	12.1	11.8	12.2
West Virginia	15.8	15.2	14.8	15.5	14.9	14.2	14.4
Wisconsin	7.9	9.3	9.5	9.4	8.8	8.9	9.1
Wyoming	15.0	15.1	16.5	14.0	14.3	13.9	14.3

Table C-88. Change in the Number and Percent of People Without Health Insurance During First Year After a Recession

(Number in thousands.)

Recession[1]	Year in which the recession ended		First calendar year after the recession ended		Change during first calendar year after the recession ended[2]	
	Number	Percent	Number	Percent	Number	Percent
July 1990 to March 1991	35,445	14.1	38,641	15.0	3,196	0.9
March 2001 to November 2001	38,023	13.5	39,776	13.9	1,753	0.4
December 2007 to June 2009	48,985	16.1	49,904	16.3	919	0.2

[1]Business cycle peaks and troughs used to delineate the beginning and end of recessions are determined by the National Bureau of Economic Research, a private research organization.
[2]Details may not sum to totals because of rounding.

Table C-89. Medicaid Coverage Among Persons Under 65 Years of Age, by Selected Characteristics, Selected Years, 1984–2010

(Percent.)

Characteristic	1984[1]	1989[1]	1995[1]	2000[2]	2005[3]	2006[3]	2007[3]	2008[3]	2009[3]	2010[3]
Total (Number in Millions)[4]	14.0	15.4	26.6	23.2	33.2	36.2	36.2	38.4	42.4	44.8
Total (Percent of Population)[4]	6.8	7.2	11.5	9.5	12.9	14.0	13.9	14.7	16.1	16.9
Age										
Under 19 years	11.7	12.2	21.1	19.2	26.6	29.4	29.3	30.6	33.9	35.7
Under 6 years	15.5	15.7	29.3	24.7	34.0	36.6	36.6	38.1	41.4	43.7
6–18 years	9.8	10.5	17.0	16.8	23.3	26.1	25.9	27.1	30.3	31.8
Under 18 years	11.9	12.6	21.5	19.6	27.2	29.9	29.8	31.3	34.5	36.4
6–17 years	10.1	10.9	17.4	17.2	23.9	26.7	26.4	27.9	30.9	32.5
18–64 years	4.5	4.9	7.1	5.2	7.2	7.7	7.5	8.1	8.9	9.2
18–44 years	5.1	5.2	7.8	5.6	8.3	8.6	8.7	9.2	10.3	10.9
18–24 years	6.4	6.8	10.4	8.1	11.3	11.4	11.4	12.2	14.0	14.5
19–25 years	6.3	6.6	10.2	7.3	10.3	9.7	9.9	10.6	12.2	12.6
25–34 years	5.3	5.2	8.2	5.5	8.0	8.3	8.5	9.3	10.1	11.1
35–44 years	3.5	4.0	5.9	4.3	6.6	7.1	7.0	7.1	7.7	8.1
45–64 years	3.4	4.3	5.6	4.5	5.5	6.3	5.9	6.4	6.9	6.8
45–54 years	3.2	3.8	5.1	4.2	5.2	6.4	6.0	6.2	7.0	7.0
55–64 years	3.6	4.9	6.4	4.9	5.8	6.1	5.7	6.8	6.8	6.6
Sex										
Male	5.4	5.7	9.6	8.2	11.6	12.6	12.5	13.4	14.4	15.2
Female	8.1	8.6	13.4	10.8	14.3	15.5	15.2	15.9	17.8	18.5
Sex and Marital Status[5]										
Male										
Married	1.9	1.8	2.9	2.2	3.5	3.7	3.5	3.6	4.1	4.0
Divorced, separated, widowed	4.9	5.4	7.7	6.1	7.0	7.9	7.8	8.1	8.3	9.3
Never married	4.8	5.6	8.1	7.2	10.4	11.6	11.3	12.1	13.1	13.5
Female										
Married	2.6	3.0	5.2	3.1	4.7	4.6	4.7	5.2	5.3	5.7
Divorced, separated, widowed	16.0	16.1	19.0	12.7	14.6	16.2	16.3	17.2	18.7	17.6
Never married	10.7	11.9	16.5	13.2	17.3	19.0	18.1	18.7	20.9	22.2
Race[6]										
White only	4.6	5.1	8.9	7.1	11.0	11.8	11.4	12.1	13.7	14.5
Black or African American only	20.5	19.0	28.5	21.2	24.9	26.6	27.7	28.3	29.5	30.4
American Indian or Alaska Native only	*28.2	29.7	19.0	15.1	24.2	24.3	21.2	37.0	29.7	21.6
Asian only	*8.7	*8.8	10.5	7.5	8.2	9.7	8.7	9.2	9.9	12.0
Native Hawaiian or Other Pacific Islander only	—	—	—	*	*	*	*	*	*	*
2 or more races	—	—	—	19.1	22.0	24.0	27.9	24.7	30.1	27.4
Hispanic Origin and Race[6]										
Hispanic or Latino	13.3	13.5	21.9	15.5	22.9	23.1	24.7	24.9	27.6	28.6
Mexican	12.2	12.4	21.6	14.0	23.0	23.0	25.9	25.4	28.4	29.5
Puerto Rican	31.5	27.3	33.4	29.4	31.9	35.7	28.0	31.0	32.1	35.7
Cuban	*4.8	*7.7	13.4	9.2	17.7	*11.3	13.3	13.0	16.7	17.3
Other Hispanic or Latino	7.9	11.1	18.2	14.5	19.7	20.2	21.4	22.3	24.6	24.5
Not Hispanic or Latino	6.2	6.5	10.2	8.5	11.1	12.3	11.7	12.6	13.7	14.4
White only	3.7	4.1	7.1	6.1	8.5	9.5	8.5	9.2	10.4	11.0
Black or African American only	20.7	19.0	28.1	21.0	24.8	26.2	27.3	27.9	29.1	30.0
Age and Percent of Poverty Level[7]										
Under 65 years										
Below 100%	33.0	37.6	48.4	38.4	45.7	45.8	47.6	49.1	51.2	50.8
100%–199%	5.3	7.5	14.4	16.2	23.4	23.8	26.1	27.4	29.0	28.5
100%–133%	8.7	11.9	23.1	22.4	30.6	30.8	34.8	36.1	39.3	36.3
134%–199%	3.7	5.6	9.7	13.1	19.5	20.0	21.7	22.9	23.6	24.4
200%–399%	0.8	1.3	2.3	4.0	6.6	7.0	6.8	7.8	8.0	8.4
400% or more	0.2	0.5	0.4	0.9	1.5	1.7	1.5	1.6	1.7	2.0
Under 19 years										
Below 100%	42.0	45.8	63.5	56.9	69.4	70.4	72.7	73.4	77.5	78.4
100%–199%	6.5	8.6	21.3	27.8	41.7	44.1	47.2	48.5	52.7	53.5
100%–133%	10.3	13.4	32.4	36.4	51.0	51.3	57.5	60.0	65.6	63.5
134%–199%	4.7	6.3	14.3	23.3	36.2	39.4	41.3	42.3	45.3	47.7
200%–399%	1.0	1.7	3.5	7.6	13.0	13.5	13.3	16.4	16.4	17.7
400% or more	*	*1.2	*	2.1	2.9	3.5	3.0	3.5	3.6	4.3

Table C-89. Medicaid Coverage Among Persons Under 65 Years of Age, by Selected Characteristics, Selected Years, 1984–2010—Continued

(Percent.)

Characteristic	1984[1]	1989[1]	1995[1]	2000[2]	2005[3]	2006[3]	2007[3]	2008[3]	2009[3]	2010[3]
Under 18 years										
Below 100%	43.3	47.8	66.0	58.5	71.2	72.0	75.0	75.3	78.3	79.8
100%–199%	6.6	8.7	21.6	28.4	42.5	44.7	48.1	49.5	53.5	54.3
100%–133%	10.4	13.5	32.9	36.9	52.0	51.7	58.4	61.1	66.9	64.6
134%–199%	4.8	6.4	14.4	23.8	36.9	40.1	42.2	43.2	45.9	48.2
200%–399%	1.0	1.7	3.5	7.6	13.3	13.8	13.3	16.8	16.8	18.0
400% or more	*	*1.1	*	2.2	2.9	3.4	3.0	3.6	3.7	4.3
18–64 years										
Below 100%	25.3	29.1	34.8	24.9	29.6	28.9	30.6	33.0	33.6	32.4
100%–199%	4.5	6.8	10.2	9.1	13.1	13.0	14.0	15.3	16.2	15.7
100%–133%	7.6	10.8	16.3	13.2	17.9	17.8	20.2	21.9	23.7	21.0
134%–199%	3.1	5.1	7.2	7.2	10.7	10.5	11.0	11.8	12.4	13.0
200%–399%	0.7	1.1	1.7	2.4	3.8	4.2	4.0	4.1	4.6	4.8
400% or more	0.2	0.4	0.4	0.6	1.1	1.2	1.1	1.1	1.2	1.3
Disability Measure Among Adults 18–64 Years[8]										
Any basic actions difficulty or complex activity limitation	—	—	—	12.8	16.4	16.2	16.5	18.6	18.2	17.8
Any basic actions difficulty	—	—	—	12.2	15.5	15.3	15.9	17.7	17.8	16.7
Any complex activity limitation	—	—	—	23.2	28.5	28.7	28.7	31.0	30.2	30.0
No disability	—	—	—	3.0	4.9	5.1	5.2	4.9	6.4	6.8
Geographic Region										
Northeast	8.6	6.6	11.7	10.6	13.3	16.8	15.4	16.1	17.3	17.9
Midwest	7.4	7.6	10.5	8.0	12.3	13.9	13.7	14.5	16.4	17.3
South	5.1	6.5	11.3	9.4	12.7	12.9	12.9	13.5	14.8	16.0
West	7.0	8.5	12.9	10.4	13.8	13.8	14.5	15.7	16.8	17.1
Location of Residence										
Within MSA[9]	7.1	7.0	11.3	8.9	12.4	13.3	13.3	14.2	15.2	16.1
Outside MSA[9]	6.1	7.9	12.3	11.9	15.5	17.7	17.1	17.2	20.8	21.4

— = Data not available.
* = Figure does not meet standards of reliability or precision.
[1]Data prior to 1997 are not strictly comparable with data for later years due to the 1997 questionnaire redesign.
[2]Estimates for 2000–2002 were calculated using 2000-based sample weights and may differ from estimates in other reports that used 1990-based sample weights for 2000–2002 estimates.
[3]Beginning in quarter 3 of the 2004 NHIS, persons under 65 years of age with no reported coverage were asked explicitly about Medicaid coverage.
[4]Includes all other races not shown separately, those with unknown marital status, unknown disability status, and, in 1984 and 1989, persons with unknown poverty level.
[5]Includes persons 14–64 years of age.
[6]The race groups, White, Black, American Indian or Alaska Native, Asian, Native Hawaiian or Other Pacific Islander, and 2 or more races, include persons of Hispanic and non-Hispanic origin. Persons of Hispanic origin may be of any race.
[7]Percent of poverty level is based on family income and family size and composition using U.S. Census Bureau poverty thresholds.
[8]Any basic actions difficulty or complex activity limitation is defined as having one or more of the following limitations or difficulties: movement difficulty, emotional difficulty, sensory (seeing or hearing) difficulty, cognitive difficulty, self-care (activities of daily living or instrumental activities of daily living) limitation, social limitation, or work limitation.
[9]MSA = metropolitan statistical area.

Table C-90. Medicaid Beneficiaries and Payments, by Basis of Eligibility, and Race and Hispanic Origin, Selected Fiscal Years, 1999–2009

(Number, percent, dollar.)

Characteristic	1999	2000	2001	2002	2003	2004	2005	2006	2007	2008	2009
Beneficiaries (Number in Millions)[1]											
All beneficiaries	40.1	42.8	46.2	49.3	52.0	55.6	57.7	57.8	56.8	58.8	56.0
Percent of Beneficiaries											
Basis of eligibility											
Aged (65 years and over)	9.4	8.7	8.3	7.9	7.8	7.8	7.6	7.6	7.1	7.1	6.5
Blind and disabled	16.7	16.1	15.4	15.0	14.8	14.6	14.2	14.4	14.8	14.8	14.0
Adults in families with dependent children[2]	18.7	20.5	21.2	22.8	22.5	22.5	21.5	21.9	21.8	21.8	22.6
Children under age 21[3]	46.9	46.1	45.7	47.1	47.8	47.8	47.5	48.0	48.4	48.0	48.4
Other Title XIX[4]	8.4	8.6	9.4	7.2	7.2	7.3	9.1	8.1	7.8	8.4	8.5
Race and Hispanic Origin[5]											
White	—	—	40.1	40.9	41.2	41.1	39.3	39.1	38.6	38.1	36.5
Black or African American	—	—	23.0	22.8	22.4	22.1	21.5	21.8	21.6	21.1	21.1
American Indian or Alaska Native	—	—	1.3	1.3	1.4	1.3	1.2	1.2	1.2	1.3	1.3
Asian or Pacific Islander	—	—	3.3	3.4	3.3	3.3	3.5	3.5	3.5	3.5	3.5
Asian	—	—	—	2.2	2.4	2.4	2.5	2.6	2.6	2.6	2.6
Pacific Islander	—	—	—	1.2	0.9	0.9	0.9	0.9	0.9	0.9	0.8
Hispanic or Latino	—	—	17.9	19.0	19.3	19.4	20.6	21.0	21.6	21.7	23.6
Multiple race or unknown	—	—	14.5	12.6	12.5	12.7	13.9	13.3	13.5	14.3	14.1
Payments (Number in Billions)[6]											
All payments	$153.5	$168.3	$186.9	$213.5	$233.2	$257.7	$274.9	$269.0	$276.2	$294.2	$287.1
Percent	100.0	100.0	100.0	100.0	100.0	100.0	100.0	100.0	100.0	100.0	100.0
Basis of Eligibility											
Aged (65 years and over)	27.7	26.4	25.9	24.4	23.7	23.1	23.1	21.6	20.7	20.6	19.2
Blind and disabled	42.9	43.2	43.1	43.3	43.7	43.3	43.4	43.3	43.3	43.5	43.5
Adults in families with dependent children[2]	10.3	10.6	10.8	11.0	11.5	12.0	11.7	12.3	12.4	12.6	13.9
Children under age 21[3]	15.7	15.9	16.3	16.8	17.1	17.2	17.3	18.8	19.4	19.4	19.9
Other Title XIX[4]	3.4	3.9	3.9	4.5	4.0	4.5	4.6	3.9	4.2	4.0	3.5
Race and Hispanic Origin[5]											
White	—	—	54.3	54.1	53.8	53.4	53.0	52.1	50.7	50.2	48.6
Black or African American	—	—	19.8	19.6	19.7	19.8	19.8	20.4	20.8	20.6	21.3
American Indian or Alaska Native	—	—	1.1	1.1	1.2	1.2	1.2	1.2	1.2	1.3	1.3
Asian or Pacific Islander	—	—	2.6	2.8	2.4	2.5	2.7	2.8	2.8	2.9	3.0
Asian	—	—	—	1.5	1.6	1.7	1.9	2.0	2.0	2.1	2.2
Pacific Islander	—	—	—	1.4	0.8	0.8	0.8	0.8	0.8	0.8	0.8
Hispanic or Latino	—	—	9.4	9.7	10.6	10.7	12.2	12.8	13.1	13.7	15.2
Multiple race or unknown	—	—	12.8	12.6	12.2	12.3	11.1	10.8	11.4	11.4	10.5
Payments per Beneficiary[6]											
All beneficiaries	$3,819	$3,936	$4,049	$4,328	$4,487	$4,639	$4,768	$4,657	$4,862	$5,051	$5,122
Basis of eligibility											
Aged (65 years and over)	11,268	11,929	12,705	13,370	13,677	13,687	14,427	13,276	14,141	14,742	15,141
Blind and disabled	9,832	10,559	11,308	12,470	13,303	13,714	14,531	13,982	14,194	14,843	15,921
Adults in families with dependent children[2]	2,104	2,030	2,057	2,093	2,292	2,471	2,587	2,622	2,753	2,917	3,156
Children under age 21[3]	1,282	1,358	1,447	1,545	1,606	1,664	1,735	1,825	1,951	2,038	2,107
Other Title XIX[4]	1,532	1,778	1,689	2,718	2,474	2,896	2,380	2,255	2,622	2,407	2,087
Race and Hispanic Origin[5]											
White	—	—	5,483	5,721	5,870	6,026	6,422	6,199	6,390	6,657	6,832
Black or African American	—	—	3,479	3,733	3,944	4,158	4,397	4,358	4,669	4,928	5,184
American Indian or Alaska Native	—	—	3,451	3,774	4,001	4,320	4,626	4,489	4,826	5,218	5,439
Asian or Pacific Islander	—	—	3,255	3,562	3,327	3,513	3,710	3,696	3,863	4,133	4,445
Asian	—	—	—	2,836	2,993	3,198	3,624	3,657	3,847	4,123	4,389
Pacific Islander	—	—	—	4,919	4,223	4,366	3,947	3,799	3,907	4,161	4,619
Hispanic or Latino	—	—	2,127	2,215	2,463	2,563	2,822	2,831	2,960	3,175	3,298
Multiple race or unknown	—	—	3,586	4,338	4,396	4,493	3,816	3,770	4,106	4,014	3,804

— = Data not available.
[1]Beneficiaries include those who received services through Medicaid.
[2]Includes adults who meet the requirements for the Aid to Families with Dependent Children (AFDC) program that were in effect in their state on July 16, 1996, or, at state option, more liberal criteria (with some exceptions). Includes adults in the Temporary Assistance for Needy Families (TANF) program.
[3]Includes children (including those in the foster care system) in the TANF program.
[4]Includes some participants in the Supplemental Security Income program and other people deemed medically needy in participating states. Prior to 2001, includes unemployed adults. Excludes foster care children and includes unknown eligibility.
[5]Race and Hispanic origin are as determined on initial Medicaid application. Categories are mutually exclusive.
[6]Medicaid payments exclude disproportionate share hospital (DSH) payments ($14.7 billion in FY2009) and DSH mental health facility payments ($3.1 billion in FY2009).

Table C-91. Medicaid Beneficiaries and Payments, by Type of Service, Selected Fiscal Years, 1999–2009

(Number, percent.)

Type of service	1999	2000	2001	2002	2003	2004	2005	2006	2007	2008	2009
All Beneficiaries[1]	40.2	42.8	46.0	49.3	52.0	55.6	57.7	57.5	56.8	58.8	56.0
Percent											
Inpatient hospital	11.2	11.5	10.6	10.2	10.0	9.8	9.5	10.9	9.0	8.9	9.0
Mental health facility	0.2	0.2	0.2	0.2	0.2	0.2	0.2	0.2	0.2	0.2	0.2
Intermediate care facility for the mentally retarded	0.3	0.3	0.3	0.2	0.2	0.2	0.2	0.2	0.2	0.2	0.2
Nursing facility	4.0	4.0	3.7	3.6	3.3	3.1	3.0	3.0	2.9	2.7	2.6
Physician	45.7	44.7	43.5	44.7	44.0	43.1	42.0	40.2	38.8	36.9	38.2
Dental	14.0	13.8	15.3	16.0	16.4	16.2	16.2	16.4	16.8	16.7	17.8
Other practitioner	9.9	11.1	11.1	11.3	11.1	10.7	10.2	10.1	9.5	8.8	8.9
Outpatient hospital	30.9	30.9	29.8	30.1	29.8	28.7	28.2	27.6	26.2	25.2	27.0
Clinic	16.8	17.9	18.4	19.2	19.6	20.0	20.7	20.5	20.6	20.2	20.3
Laboratory and radiological	25.4	26.6	26.8	28.5	28.3	28.9	27.7	28.0	27.8	26.6	26.4
Home health	2.0	2.3	2.2	2.2	2.3	2.1	2.1	2.1	2.1	1.9	1.8
Prescribed drugs	49.4	48.0	47.6	49.4	50.2	50.3	49.2	47.1	42.1	41.8	43.1
Capitated care	51.5	49.7	50.5	51.7	53.1	54.2	58.1	61.0	64.5	64.9	64.7
Primary care case management	9.7	13.0	13.9	14.6	14.5	15.4	15.1	14.8	12.5	14.9	14.0
Personal support	10.1	10.6	10.8	11.5	11.6	11.3	11.8	11.8	11.6	10.8	11.2
Other care[2]	21.6	21.4	21.5	22.6	23.1	22.9	21.9	21.6	21.5	21.3	21.1
Payments in Billions[3]											
All payments	$153.5	$168.3	$186.3	$213.5	$233.2	$257.7	$274.9	$267.4	$276.2	$294.2	$287.1
Percent Distribution	100.0	100.0	100.0	100.0	100.0	100.0	100.0	100.0	100.0	100.0	100.0
Inpatient hospital	14.5	14.4	13.9	13.6	13.5	13.5	12.8	13.5	13.4	12.5	12.4
Mental health facility	1.1	1.1	1.1	1.0	0.9	0.9	0.8	0.9	0.9	0.8	0.8
Intermediate care facility for the mentally retarded	6.1	5.6	5.2	5.0	4.7	4.3	4.3	4.4	4.3	4.2	4.0
Nursing facility	21.7	20.5	20.0	18.4	17.3	16.3	16.3	17.0	16.8	16.1	14.5
Physician	4.3	4.0	4.0	3.9	3.9	4.0	4.1	3.9	3.6	3.5	3.8
Dental	0.8	0.8	1.0	1.1	1.1	1.1	1.1	1.2	1.2	1.3	1.5
Other practitioner	0.3	0.4	0.4	0.4	0.4	0.4	0.4	0.4	0.3	0.3	0.3
Outpatient hospital	4.0	4.2	4.0	4.0	4.0	4.0	3.6	3.8	3.7	3.7	3.8
Clinic	3.8	3.7	3.0	3.1	3.1	3.2	3.2	3.2	3.1	3.1	3.2
Laboratory and radiological	0.8	0.8	0.9	1.0	1.0	1.0	1.1	1.1	1.1	1.0	1.0
Home health	1.9	1.9	1.9	1.8	1.9	1.8	2.0	2.2	2.3	2.2	2.1
Prescribed drugs	10.8	11.9	12.7	13.3	14.5	15.3	15.6	10.4	8.0	7.9	8.0
Capitated care	14.0	14.5	15.7	15.8	16.0	16.5	16.9	18.8	21.2	23.0	23.7
Primary care case management	0.3	0.1	0.1	0.1	0.1	0.2	0.1	0.1	0.1	0.1	0.1
Personal support	6.9	6.9	7.0	7.2	7.4	7.2	7.5	8.0	8.4	8.3	8.6
Other care[2]	8.6	8.8	9.2	10.3	10.2	10.3	10.2	11.1	11.6	12.0	12.2
Payments per Beneficiary[3]											
Total payment per beneficiary	$3,819	$3,936	$4,053	$4,328	$4,487	$4,639	$4,768	$4,654	$4,862	$5,051	$5,122
Inpatient hospital	4,943	4,919	5,313	5,771	6,047	6,424	6,411	5,781	7,191	7,083	7,047
Mental health facility	18,094	17,800	21,482	21,377	20,503	19,928	19,252	17,156	21,407	21,975	22,172
Intermediate care facility for the mentally retarded	76,443	79,330	83,227	91,588	95,287	97,497	107,028	110,340	113,735	123,053	125,236
Nursing facility	20,568	20,220	21,894	22,326	23,882	24,475	26,185	26,531	28,282	29,533	29,070
Physician	357	356	371	378	403	426	465	456	457	485	506
Dental	214	238	270	293	305	318	326	329	340	389	423
Other practitioner	118	139	149	151	154	160	200	196	170	171	174
Outpatient hospital	491	533	546	571	596	639	617	642	695	736	713
Clinic	860	805	662	706	720	750	749	731	741	772	808
Laboratory and radiological	114	113	131	154	161	168	183	185	185	188	194
Home health	3,571	3,135	3,478	3,689	3,720	3,978	4,487	4,977	5,334	5,789	5,823
Prescribed drugs	837	975	1,083	1,165	1,293	1,411	1,509	1,030	926	957	950
Capitated care	1,040	1,148	1,257	1,318	1,357	1,415	1,386	1,431	1,598	1,786	1,879
Primary care case management	119	30	29	28	28	58	27	29	33	32	41
Personal support	2,583	2,543	2,639	2,704	2,864	2,946	3,035	3,160	3,534	3,852	3,961
Other care[2]	1,508	1,600	1,734	1,963	1,975	2,086	2,228	2,388	2,611	2,856	2,967

[1] Beneficiaries include those who received services through Medicaid.
[2] Unknown services (0.3% of beneficiaries and 0.3% of payments in 2009) are included with other care.
[3] Medicaid payments exclude disproportionate share hospital (DSH) payments ($14.7 billion in FY2009) and DSH mental health facility payments ($3.1 billion in FY2009).

PART C: HEALTH 419

Table C-92. Medicaid Beneficiaries, Beneficiaries in Managed Care, Payments per Beneficiary, and Beneficiaries per 100 Persons Below the Poverty Level, by State, Selected Fiscal Years, 2000–2009

(Number.)

State	Beneficiaries in thousands[1]		Percent of beneficiaries in managed care[2]		Payments per beneficiary[3]		Beneficiaries per 100 persons below the poverty level	
	2000	2009	2000	2009	2000	2009	1999–2000	2008–2009
United States	42,763	56,041	56	71	$3,936	$5,122	131	138
Alabama	619	877	60	67	3,860	4,135	88	118
Alaska	96	119	-	-	4,876	8,990	180	175
Arizona	681	1,588	92	90	3,100	5,426	113	117
Arkansas	489	825	57	79	3,086	4,338	113	170
California	7,915	11,519	50	52	2,155	3,058	162	201
Colorado	381	678	90	95	4,747	4,852	107	113
Connecticut	420	558	72	75	6,762	9,475	184	191
Delaware	115	209	79	74	4,584	6,052	147	204
District of Columbia	139	175	66	98	5,715	11,077	179	168
Florida	2,360	3,261	60	66	3,114	4,310	136	122
Georgia	1,290	1,805	96	92	2,774	4,087	136	108
Hawaii	204	—	74	97	2,626	—	83	—
Idaho	131	253	30	84	4,530	5,345	75	123
Illinois	1,516	2,626	10	55	5,150	4,483	115	152
Indiana	705	1,109	67	74	4,224	4,858	148	116
Iowa	314	482	90	83	4,707	5,974	149	162
Kansas	263	355	56	87	4,670	6,528	94	98
Kentucky	771	942	81	83	3,780	5,326	158	126
Louisiana	761	1,184	6	69	3,456	4,585	95	164
Maine	192	315	35	64	6,820	4,704	155	203
Maryland	665	846	81	79	5,396	7,480	170	156
Massachusetts	1,047	—	64	60	5,153	—	153	—
Michigan	1,352	1,890	100	89	3,611	5,381	135	139
Minnesota	559	802	63	63	5,857	8,766	178	145
Mississippi	605	932	39	76	2,987	3,432	139	134
Missouri	890	—	40	99	3,673	—	157	—
Montana	104	113	61	67	4,173	6,344	73	88
Nebraska	229	256	77	84	4,185	6,218	136	139
Nevada	138	281	39	84	3,733	4,259	70	85
New Hampshire	97	141	6	78	6,712	7,037	119	140
New Jersey	822	1,151	59	75	5,724	7,208	128	139
New Mexico	376	562	64	74	3,325	5,185	110	140
New York	3,420	4,985	25	66	7,646	9,004	128	171
North Carolina	1,209	1,782	68	70	3,996	5,423	122	125
North Dakota	61	77	55	68	5,852	7,643	87	106
Ohio	1,305	2,238	21	70	5,434	6,243	103	139
Oklahoma	507	809	69	88	3,163	4,419	106	165
Oregon	542	564	83	88	3,135	4,957	132	115
Pennsylvania	1,492	—	73	82	4,266	—	141	—
Rhode Island	179	203	69	62	5,982	7,654	187	153
South Carolina	685	906	6	100	3,900	5,199	157	143
South Dakota	102	141	93	80	3,935	5,188	155	128
Tennessee	1,568	1,479	100	100	2,226	4,910	211	151
Texas	2,603	4,283	34	65	3,487	4,330	85	102
Utah	224	—	90	86	4,277	—	132	—
Vermont	139	171	47	88	3,451	5,684	208	294
Virginia	627	917	59	64	3,960	6,053	115	108
Washington	895	1,177	100	86	2,717	4,872	155	162
West Virginia	335	386	35	46	4,154	6,699	129	140
Wisconsin	577	—	44	60	5,039	—	113	—
Wyoming	46	72	-	-	4,609	7,635	84	136

- =Quantity zero.
— =Data not available.
[1]Beneficiaries include those who received services through Medicaid.
[2]Medicaid managed care enrollment data include individuals in state health care reform programs that expand eligibility beyond traditional Medicaid eligibility standards. The managed care enrollment data include enrollees receiving comprehensive and limited benefits. Managed care enrollment as of June 30 of year shown.
[3]Medicaid payments exclude disproportionate share hospital (DSH) payments ($14.7 billion in FY2009) and DSH mental health facility payments ($3.1 billion in FY2009).

Table C-93. Medicare Enrollees and Expenditures and Percent Distribution, by Medicare Program and Type of Service, Selected Years, 1970–2010

(Number, percent.)

Medicare program and type of service	1970	1980	1990	1995	2000	2005	2006	2007	2008	2009[1]	2010[1]
Enrollees											
Total Medicare[2]	20.4	28.4	34.3	37.6	39.7	42.6	43.4	44.4	45.5	46.6	47.5
Hospital insurance	20.1	28.0	33.7	37.2	39.3	42.2	43.1	44.0	45.1	46.2	47.1
Supplementary medical insurance (SMI)[3]	19.5	27.3	32.6	35.6	37.3	—	—	—	—	—	—
Part B	19.5	27.3	32.6	35.6	37.3	39.8	40.4	41.1	42.0	42.9	43.8
Part D[4]	—	—	—	—	—	1.8	30.5	31.2	32.4	33.5	34.5
Expenditures											
Total Medicare	$7.5	$36.8	$111.0	$184.2	$221.8	$336.4	$408.3	$431.7	$468.1	$509.0	$522.8
Total hospital insurance (HI)	5.3	25.6	67.0	117.6	131.1	182.9	191.9	203.1	235.6	242.5	247.9
HI payments to managed care organizations[5]	—	0.0	2.7	6.7	21.4	24.9	32.9	39.0	50.6	59.4	60.7
HI payments for fee-for-service utilization	5.1	25.0	63.4	109.5	105.1	156.6	159.6	163.4	172.8	179.5	183.3
Inpatient hospital	4.8	24.1	56.9	82.3	87.1	123.3	124.1	124.1	130.2	134.0	136.1
Skilled nursing facility	0.2	0.4	2.5	9.1	11.1	19.3	20.3	22.6	24.6	26.3	26.9
Home health agency	0.1	0.5	3.7	16.2	4.0	6.0	5.9	6.3	6.7	7.0	7.0
Hospice	—	—	0.3	1.9	2.9	8.0	9.3	10.5	11.3	12.2	13.2
Other[6]	—	—	—	—	—	—	—	—	—	—	0.1
Home health agency transfer[7]	—	—	—	—	1.7	—	—	—	—	—	—
Medicare Advantage premiums[8]	—	—	—	—	—	—	0.0	0.1	0.1	0.1	0.2
Accounting error (CY 2005–2008)[9]	—	—	—	—	—	-1.9	-3.9	-2.7	8.5	—	—
Administrative expenses[10]	0.2	0.5	0.9	1.4	2.9	3.3	3.3	3.2	3.6	3.5	3.8
Total supplementary medical insurance (SMI)[3]	2.2	11.2	44.0	66.6	90.7	153.5	216.4	228.6	232.6	266.5	274.9
Total Part B	2.2	11.2	44.0	66.6	90.7	152.4	169.0	178.9	183.3	205.7	212.9
Part B payments to managed care organizations[5]	—	0.0	0.2	2.8	6.6	18.4	22.0	31.5	38.9	48.1	53.4	55.2
Part B payments for fee-for-service utilization[11]	1.9	10.4	39.6	58.4	72.2	125.0	130.2	134.6	140.5	149.0	154.3
Physician/supplies[12]	1.8	8.2	29.6	—	—	—	—	—	—	—	—
Outpatient hospital[13]	0.1	1.9	8.5	—	—	—	—	—	—	—	—
Independent laboratory[14]	0.0	0.1	1.5	—	—	—	—	—	—	—	—
Physician fee schedule	—	—	—	31.7	37.0	57.7	58.1	58.8	60.6	62.4	64.5
Durable medical equipment	—	—	—	3.7	4.7	8.0	8.3	8.2	8.6	8.0	8.3
Laboratory[15]	—	—	—	4.3	4.0	6.3	6.6	7.1	7.2	8.1	8.4
Other[16]	—	—	—	9.9	13.6	26.7	27.9	28.8	29.6	31.9	32.6
Hospital[17]	—	—	—	8.7	8.4	19.3	21.4	22.6	24.2	27.0	28.4
Home health agency	0.0	0.2	0.1	0.2	4.5	7.1	7.8	9.2	10.3	11.6	12.1
Home health agency transfer[7]	—	—	—	—	-1.7	—	—	—	—	—	—
Medicare Advantage premiums[8]	—	—	—	—	—	—	0.0	0.1	0.1	0.1	0.2
Accounting error (CY 2005–2008)[9]	—	—	—	—	—	1.9	3.9	2.7	-8.5	—	—
Administrative expenses[10]	0.2	0.6	1.5	1.6	1.8	2.8	3.1	2.7	3.1	3.2	3.2
Part D start-up costs[18]	—	—	—	—	—	0.7	0.2	0.0	0.0	—	—
Total Part D[4]	—	—	—	—	—	1.1	47.4	49.7	49.3	60.8	62.0
Percent Distribution of Expenditures											
Total hospital insurance (HI)	100.0	100.0	100.0	100.0	100.0	100.0	100.0	100.0	100.0	100.0	100.0
HI payments to managed care organizations[5]	—	0.0	4.0	5.7	16.3	13.6	17.1	19.2	21.5	24.5	24.5
HI payments for fee-for-service utilization	96.2	97.7	94.6	93.1	80.2	85.6	83.2	80.5	73.3	74.0	73.9
Inpatient hospital	90.6	94.1	84.9	70.0	66.4	67.4	64.7	61.1	55.3	55.3	54.9
Skilled nursing facility	3.8	1.6	3.7	7.7	8.5	10.6	10.6	11.1	10.4	10.8	10.9
Home health agency	1.9	2.0	5.5	13.8	3.1	3.3	3.1	3.1	2.8	2.9	2.8
Hospice	—	—	0.4	1.6	2.2	4.4	4.8	5.2	4.8	5.0	5.3
Other	—	—	—	—	—	—	—	—	—	—	0.0
Home health agency transfer[7]	—	—	—	—	1.3	—	—	—	—	—	—
Medicare Advantage premiums[8]	—	—	—	—	—	—	0.0	0.0	0.0	0.0	0.1
Accounting error (CY 2005-2008)[9]	—	—	—	—	—	-1.0	-2.0	-1.3	3.6	—	—
Administrative expenses[10]	3.8	2.0	1.3	1.2	2.2	1.8	1.7	1.6	1.5	1.4	1.5
Total supplementary medical insurance (SMI)[3]	100.0	100.0	100.0	100.0	100.0	100.0	100.0	100.0	100.0	100.0	100.0

PART C: HEALTH

Table C-93. Medicare Enrollees and Expenditures and Percent Distribution, by Medicare Program and Type of Service, Selected Years, 1970–2010—*Continued*

(Number, percent.)

Medicare program and type of service	1970	1980	1990	1995	2000	2005	2006	2007	2008	2009[1]	2010[1]
Total Part B	100.0	100.0	100.0	100.0	100.0	99.3	78.1	78.3	78.8	77.2	77.4
Part B payments to managed care organizations[5]	1.2	1.8	6.4	9.9	20.2	14.3	14.5	17.0	20.7	20.0	20.1
Part B payments for fee-for-service utilization[11]	88.1	92.8	90.1	87.6	79.6	81.5	60.2	58.9	60.4	55.9	56.1
Physician/supplies[12]	80.9	72.8	67.3	—	—	—	—	—	—	—	—
Outpatient hospital[13]	5.2	16.9	19.3	—	—	—	—	—	—	—	—
Independent laboratory[14]	0.5	1.0	3.4	—	—	—	—	—	—	—	—
Physician fee schedule	—	—	—	47.5	40.8	37.6	26.9	25.7	26.0	23.4	23.5
Durable medical equipment	—	—	—	5.5	5.2	5.2	3.8	3.6	3.7	3.0	3.0
Laboratory[15]	—	—	—	6.4	4.4	4.1	3.1	3.1	3.1	3.0	3.1
Other[16]	—	—	—	14.8	15.0	17.4	12.9	12.6	12.7	12.0	11.8
Hospital[17]	—	—	—	13.0	9.3	12.5	9.9	9.9	10.4	10.1	10.3
Home health agency	1.5	2.1	0.2	0.3	4.9	4.6	3.6	4.0	4.4	4.4	4.4
Home health agency transfer[7]	—	—	—	—	-1.9	—	—	—	—	—	—
Medicare Advantage premiums[8]	—	—	—	—	—	—	0.0	0.0	0.0	0.0	0.1
Accounting error (CY 2005–2008)[9]	—	—	—	—	—	1.2	1.8	1.2	-3.6	—	—
Administrative expenses[10]	10.7	5.4	3.5	2.4	2.0	1.8	1.4	1.2	1.3	1.2	1.2
Part D start-up costs[18]	—	—	—	—	—	0.4	0.1	0.0	0.0	—	—
Total Part D[4]	—	—	—	—	—	0.7	21.9	21.7	21.2	22.8	22.6

— =Category not applicable or data not available.
0.0 = Quantity more than zero but less than 0.05.
[1]Preliminary estimates.
[2]Average number enrolled in the hospital insurance (HI) and/or supplementary medical insurance (SMI) programs for the period.
[3]Starting with 2004 data, the SMI trust fund consists of two separate accounts: Part B (which pays for a portion of the costs of physicians' services, outpatient hospital services, and other related medical and health services for voluntarily enrolled individuals) and Part D (Medicare Prescription Drug Account, which pays private plans to provide prescription drug coverage).
[4]The Medicare Modernization Act, enacted on December 8, 2003, established within SMI two Part D accounts related to prescription drug benefits: the Medicare Prescription Drug Account and the Transitional Assistance Account.
[5]Medicare-approved managed care organizations.
[6]Reflects Community Based Care Transition Program ($25 million in 2010) and Electronic Health Records Incentive Program ($113 million in 2010).
[7]For 1998 to 2003 data, reflects annual home health HI to SMI transfer amounts.
[8]When a beneficiary chooses a Medicare Advantage plan whose monthly premium exceeds the benchmark amount, the additional premiums (that is, amounts beyond those paid by Medicare to the plan) are the responsibility of the beneficiary.
[9]Represents misallocation of benefit payments between the HI trust fund and the Part B account of the SMI trust fund from May 2005 to September 2007, and the transfer made in June 2008 to correct the misallocation.
[10]Includes expenditures for research, experiments and demonstration projects, peer review activity (performed by Peer Review Organizations from 1983 to 2001 and by Quality Review Organizations from 2002 to present), and to combat and prevent fraud and abuse.
[11]Type-of-service reporting categories for fee-for-service reimbursement differ before and after 1991.
[12]Includes payment for physicians, practitioners, durable medical equipment, and all suppliers other than independent laboratory through 1990. Starting with 1991 data, physician services subject to the physician fee schedule are shown. Payments for laboratory services paid under the laboratory fee schedule and performed in a physician office are included under Laboratory beginning in 1991.
[13]Includes payments for hospital outpatient department services, skilled nursing facility outpatient services, Part B services received as an inpatient in a hospital or skilled nursing facility setting, and other types of outpatient facilities.
[14]Starting with 1991 data, those independent laboratory services that were paid under the laboratory fee schedule (most of the independent laboratory category) are included in the Laboratory line; the remaining services are included in the Physician fee schedule and other lines.
[15]Payments for laboratory services paid under the laboratory fee schedule performed in a physician office, independent laboratory, or in a hospital outpatient department.
[16]Includes payments for physician-administered drugs; freestanding ambulatory surgical center facility services; ambulance services;supplies; freestanding end-stage renal disease (ESRD) dialysis facility services; rural health clinics; outpatient rehabilitation facilities; psychiatric hospitals; and federally qualified health centers.
[17]Includes the hospital facility costs for Medicare Part B services that are predominantly in the outpatient department, with the exception of hospital outpatient laboratory services, which are included on the Laboratory line. Physician reimbursement is included on the Physician fee schedule line.
[18]Part D start-up costs were funded through the SMI Part B account in 2004–2008.

Table C-94. Medicare Enrollees[1] and Program Payments Among Fee-for-Service Medicare Beneficiaries, by Sex and Age, Selected Years, 1994–2009

(Dollar, percent.)

Sex and age	1994	1995	2000	2005	2006	2007	2008	2009
FEE-FOR-SERVICE ENROLLEES IN THOUSANDS								
Total	34,076	34,062	32,740	36,685	35,847	35,490	35,320	35,360
Sex								
Male	14,533	14,563	14,195	16,251	15,958	15,879	15,890	15,968
Female	19,543	19,499	18,545	20,433	19,890	19,611	19,430	19,392
Age								
Under 65 years	4,031	4,239	4,907	6,286	6,225	6,318	6,359	6,435
65–74 years	16,713	16,373	14,230	15,587	15,179	15,041	15,182	15,336
75–84 years	9,845	9,911	9,919	10,689	10,298	9,947	9,592	9,335
85 years and over	3,486	3,540	3,684	4,123	4,146	4,184	4,187	4,254
FEE-FOR-SERVICE PROGRAM PAYMENTS IN BILLIONS								
Total	$146.6	$159.0	$174.3	$274.1	$280.7	$288.5	$301.1	$318.0
Sex								
Male	63.9	68.8	76.2	121.0	123.6	126.5	131.5	139.1
Female	82.6	90.2	98.0	153.2	157.0	162.1	169.7	178.9
Age								
Under 65 years	18.8	21.0	25.8	46.7	48.4	50.9	54.2	59.7
65–74 years	55.1	58.1	57.5	86.6	87.4	89.1	92.9	98.1
75–84 years	50.7	55.3	62.7	95.2	96.2	96.4	97.9	100.2
85 years and over	21.8	24.6	28.3	45.6	48.7	52.1	56.1	60.0
PERCENT DISTRIBUTION OF FEE-FOR-SERVICE PROGRAM PAYMENTS								
Total	100.0	100.0	100.0	100.0	100.0	100.0	100.0	100.0
Sex								
Male	43.6	43.2	43.7	44.1	44.0	43.8	43.7	43.7
Female	56.4	56.8	56.3	55.9	56.0	56.2	56.3	56.3
Age								
Under 65 years	12.9	13.2	14.8	17.0	17.2	17.6	18.0	18.8
65–74 years	37.6	36.5	33.0	31.6	31.1	30.9	30.9	30.9
75–84 years	34.6	34.8	36.0	34.7	34.3	33.4	32.5	31.5
85 years and over	14.9	15.5	16.2	16.6	17.3	18.0	18.6	18.9
AVERAGE FEE-FOR-SERVICE PAYMENT PER ENROLLEE								
Total	$4,301	$4,667	$5,323	$7,473	$7,830	$8,129	$8,526	$8,993
Sex								
Male	4,397	4,721	5,370	7,443	7,747	7,964	8,274	8,711
Female	4,229	4,627	5,286	7,497	7,896	8,263	8,732	9,226
Age								
Under 65 years	4,673	4,960	5,252	7,435	7,774	8,058	8,530	9,280
65–74 years	3,300	3,548	4,040	5,558	5,756	5,924	6,119	6,398
75–84 years	5,152	5,576	6,320	8,904	9,345	9,696	10,206	10,731
85 years and over	6,267	6,950	7,684	11,061	11,742	12,440	13,396	14,103

[1] Medicare enrollees in managed care plans are not included in the denominator used to calculate average payments.

Table C-95. Medicare Beneficiaries, by Race, Hispanic Origin, and Selected Characteristics, Selected Years, 1992–2007

(Number, percent.)

Characteristic	All			White			Black			Hispanic or Latino		
	1992	2000	2007	1992	2000	2007	1992	2000	2007	1992	2000	2007
All Medicare beneficiaries (number in millions)	36.8	40.6	45.0	30.9	32.4	35.2	3.3	3.7	4.1	1.9	2.8	3.5
All Medicare beneficiaries (percent distribution)	100.0	100.0	100.0	84.2	80.1	78.3	8.9	9.1	9.0	5.2	7.0	7.8
Medical Care Use												
All Medicare beneficiaries:												
Long–term care facility stay	7.7	9.3	9.0	8.0	9.7	9.7	6.2	8.8	7.7	4.2	6.0	5.6
Community–only residents												
Inpatient hospital	17.9	19.2	16.6	18.1	19.2	16.4	18.4	22.8	19.2	16.6	16.2	16.6
Outpatient hospital	57.9	69.8	74.4	57.8	70.7	75.0	61.1	69.0	74.4	53.1	63.7	69.2
Physician/supplier[1]	92.4	94.9	97.2	93.0	95.4	97.6	89.1	92.8	96.3	87.9	92.9	95.2
Dental	40.4	43.5	46.1	43.1	46.9	50.1	23.5	24.1	24.4	29.1	33.9	36.3
Prescription medicine	85.2	91.1	94.6	85.5	91.5	94.7	83.1	89.5	95.9	84.6	90.1	93.2
Expenditures												
All Medicare beneficiaries												
Total health care[2]	$6,716	$10,490	$15,636	$6,816	$10,475	$15,460	$7,043	$12,328	$16,891	$5,784	$9,089	$17,019
Long–term care facility[3]	1,581	2,310	2,785	1,674	2,406	2,969	1,255	2,438	2,924	*758	1,799	1,374
Community–only residents												
Total personal health care	5,054	7,911	11,431	4,988	7,814	11,033	5,530	9,419	13,060	4,938	6,934	13,470
Inpatient hospital	2,098	2,664	2,468	2,058	2,605	2,339	2,493	3,465	3,089	1,999	2,133	2,844
Outpatient hospital	504	875	1,315	478	796	1,230	668	1,523	1,709	511	915	2,370
Physician/supplier[1]	1,524	2,491	3,124	1,525	2,503	3,163	1,398	2,621	3,078	1,587	2,234	3,194
Dental	142	258	379	153	278	412	70	101	206	97	193	367
Prescription medicine	468	1,163	2,652	481	1,182	2,589	417	1,135	2,860	389	1,014	3,190
Long–term care facility[4]	23,054	32,442	43,253	23,177	31,795	42,207	21,272	36,132	50,810	*25,026	*39,057	*48,911
Sex												
Both sexes	100.0	100.0	100.0	100.0	100.0	100.0	100.0	100.0	100.0	100.0	100.0	100.0
Male	42.9	43.4	44.6	42.7	43.3	44.6	42.0	40.0	43.2	46.7	46.9	45.4
Female	57.1	56.6	55.4	57.3	56.7	55.4	58.0	60.0	56.8	53.3	53.1	54.6
Eligibility Criteria and Age												
All Medicare beneficiaries[5]	100.0	100.0	100.0	100.0	100.0	100.0	100.0	100.0	100.0	100.0	100.0	100.0
Disabled	10.2	13.6	16.0	8.6	11.5	13.9	19.1	23.3	30.5	16.5	21.7	20.9
Under 45 years	3.5	3.9	3.8	2.9	3.2	3.1	7.6	7.5	7.6	6.9	5.5	5.7
45–64 years	6.5	9.8	12.2	5.8	8.3	10.8	11.5	15.8	22.9	9.6	16.3	15.2
Aged	89.8	86.4	84.0	91.4	88.5	86.1	81.0	76.7	69.5	83.5	78.3	79.1
65–74 years	51.5	45.4	44.2	52.0	46.7	43.9	48.0	41.7	39.7	49.4	45.5	47.1
75–84 years	28.8	30.0	28.3	29.5	31.4	29.8	24.0	25.9	22.0	27.1	22.9	22.4
85 years and over	9.7	10.9	11.5	9.9	11.5	12.4	9.0	9.0	7.8	6.9	9.9	9.6
Living Arrangement												
All living arrangements	100.0	100.0	100.0	100.0	100.0	100.0	100.0	100.0	100.0	100.0	100.0	100.0
Alone	27.0	29.3	29.7	27.5	29.8	30.2	27.7	32.5	32.9	20.2	22.9	24.2
With spouse	51.2	49.0	47.3	53.3	51.0	49.6	33.3	30.0	28.3	50.4	49.2	43.2
With children	9.1	9.5	10.3	7.7	7.6	8.3	16.8	18.6	18.3	16.6	14.8	18.6
With others	7.6	7.1	7.8	6.2	6.2	6.5	18.1	13.7	15.2	10.8	9.9	11.6
Long–term care facility	5.1	5.1	5.0	5.3	5.4	5.4	4.0	5.2	5.4	*2.0	*3.3	*2.5

Table C-95. Medicare Beneficiaries, by Race, Hispanic Origin, and Selected Characteristics, Selected Years, 1992–2007—Continued

(Number, percent.)

Characteristic	All			White			Black			Hispanic or Latino		
	1992	2000	2007	1992	2000	2007	1992	2000	2007	1992	2000	2007
Age and Limitation of Activity[6]												
Disabled, under age 65	100.0	100.0	100.0	100.0	100.0	100.0	100.0	100.0	100.0	100.0	100.0	100.0
None	22.7	27.3	29.1	21.8	25.2	28.7	26.2	35.7	36.0	21.2	30.1	19.1
IADL only	39.0	35.1	36.7	38.9	35.5	38.1	35.8	33.2	33.0	46.1	37.3	37.8
1 or 2 ADL	21.2	21.8	21.1	21.5	23.2	20.3	21.2	17.7	19.8	*20.9	*16.8	*26.7
3–5 ADL	17.2	15.9	13.1	17.9	16.1	12.9	*16.8	*13.5	*11.1	*11.9	*15.8	*16.4
65–74 years	100.0	100.0	100.0	100.0	100.0	100.0	100.0	100.0	100.0	100.0	100.0	100.0
None	67.0	71.5	71.6	68.7	72.6	74.1	55.1	64.8	66.9	59.2	69.4	58.9
IADL only	17.8	15.4	16.4	17.0	15.1	15.4	22.9	18.0	16.5	*20.9	*13.6	20.5
1 or 2 ADL	10.4	8.6	8.4	9.6	8.2	7.8	14.4	10.8	*9.9	*15.7	*13.2	*12.0
3–5 ADL	4.8	4.5	3.6	4.6	4.2	2.7	*7.6	*6.3	*6.7	*4.2	*4.0	*8.6
75–84 years	100.0	100.0	100.0	100.0	100.0	100.0	100.0	100.0	100.0	100.0	100.0	100.0
None	46.6	52.2	55.3	47.5	53.1	56.5	42.0	46.2	47.4	44.3	48.3	51.8
IADL only	23.9	23.0	22.2	23.6	22.7	22.3	26.7	20.9	19.3	*27.8	29.9	22.6
1 or 2 ADL	16.5	14.3	12.6	16.8	13.8	12.3	15.3	17.7	*13.3	*14.9	*18.6	*13.8
3–5 ADL	13.0	10.6	9.9	12.2	10.4	8.9	*15.9	15.2	20.0	*13.0	*8.2	*11.7
85 years and over	100.0	100.0	100.0	100.0	100.0	100.0	100.0	100.0	100.0	100.0	100.0	100.0
None	19.9	24.9	28.0	20.2	25.1	29.3	*19.6	*25.9	*22.0	*19.7	*23.4	*19.7
IADL only	20.9	22.6	26.5	20.2	22.4	26.2	*22.1	*19.7	*27.4	*24.7	*24.7	*29.8
1 or 2 ADL	23.5	22.2	19.0	23.5	22.3	19.2	*24.3	*19.3	*21.6	*23.7	*28.1	*15.1
3–5 ADL	35.8	30.4	26.5	36.1	30.2	25.3	*34.0	35.1	*29.0	*31.8	*23.8	*35.4

* = Figure does not meet standards of reliability or precision.
[1]Physician/supplier services include medical and osteopathic doctor and health practitioner visits, diagnostic laboratory and radiology services, medical and surgical services, and durable medical equipment and nondurable medical supplies.
[2]Total health care expenditures by Medicare beneficiaries, including expenses paid by Medicare and all other sources of payment for the following services: inpatient hospital, outpatient hospital, physician/supplier, dental, prescription medicine, home health, and hospice and long-term care facility care. Does not include health insurance premiums.
[3]Expenditures for long-term care in facilities for all beneficiaries include facility room and board expenses for beneficiaries who resided in a facility for the full year, for beneficiaries who resided in a facility for part of the year and in the community for part of the year, and expenditures for short-term facility stays for full-year or part-year community residents.
[4]Expenditures for facility-based long-term care for facility-based beneficiaries include facility room and board expenses for beneficiaries who resided in a facility for the full year and for beneficiaries who resided in a facility for part of the year and in the community for part of the year. They do not include expenditures for short-term facility stays for full-year community residents.
[5]Medicare beneficiaries with end-stage renal disease (ESRD) are included within the subgroups Aged and Disabled. In 2007, less than 1% of Medicare beneficiaries qualified because of ESRD.
[6]IADL is instrumental activities of daily living; ADL is activities of daily living. Includes data for both community and long-term care facility residents.

Table C-96. Medicare Enrollees, Enrollees in Managed Care, Payment per Enrollee, and Short-Stay Hospital Utilization, by State, Selected Years, 1995–2009

(Number, percent.)

State	Enrollment in thousands[1]		Percent of enrollees in managed care[2]		Payment per fee-for-service enrollee		Discharges per 1,000 enrollees[3]		Average length of stay in days[3]	
	1995	2009	1995	2009	1995	2009	1995	2009	1995	2009
United States[4]	36,789	45,467	9.5	23.7	$4,750	$9,121	351	335	7.0	5.5
Alabama	642	828	1.9	22.1	4,895	8,496	413	384	6.5	5.5
Alaska	34	63	0.5	1.5	4,775	7,744	283	221	6.3	5.2
Arizona	598	899	28.8	36.8	4,269	8,405	320	294	5.5	4.9
Arkansas	422	520	0.3	13.9	4,026	7,847	370	328	6.6	5.4
California	3,653	4,620	33.9	34.8	5,651	9,411	384	285	5.8	5.6
Colorado	425	602	20.3	33.4	4,354	7,998	309	272	5.6	4.8
Connecticut	504	558	2.8	17.1	5,034	9,968	290	338	7.3	5.8
Delaware	102	145	1.3	5.0	4,154	9,139	315	319	7.4	5.7
District of Columbia	80	77	4.8	10.5	5,828	10,910	360	380	8.5	6.5
Florida	2,633	3,289	16.6	28.9	5,477	10,894	333	355	6.6	5.5
Georgia	841	1,194	0.5	15.2	4,784	8,320	377	320	6.6	5.5
Hawaii	151	200	30.1	39.7	3,419	5,802	308	194	9.3	6.7
Idaho	151	222	2.7	28.0	3,341	6,929	273	206	5.0	4.5
Illinois	1,620	1,806	6.1	10.0	4,693	9,367	372	381	6.8	5.3
Indiana	817	985	2.6	15.4	4,281	8,650	342	335	6.5	5.3
Iowa	473	512	3.3	13.0	3,315	7,257	332	271	6.1	5.2
Kansas	382	425	2.9	10.9	4,274	8,071	352	302	6.2	5.1
Kentucky	589	743	2.3	15.4	4,141	8,517	391	378	6.6	5.3
Louisiana	581	671	4.3	22.9	6,119	10,338	421	370	6.8	5.6
Maine	202	259	0.1	10.7	3,547	7,264	321	267	6.7	5.2
Maryland	606	764	2.1	7.7	5,351	10,322	369	392	7.0	5.0
Massachusetts	935	1,039	9.4	19.3	6,070	9,988	354	358	6.8	5.2
Michigan	1,347	1,615	0.8	25.3	4,813	10,085	339	383	7.1	5.4
Minnesota	631	767	18.7	37.3	3,731	8,647	338	347	5.5	4.6
Mississippi	398	488	0.1	9.7	4,750	9,479	432	381	7.0	5.8
Missouri	827	985	4.3	20.2	4,451	8,528	359	360	6.7	5.2
Montana	130	165	0.5	17.5	3,532	6,576	312	222	5.5	4.9
Nebraska	250	276	2.3	11.8	3,303	7,906	290	276	5.9	5.1
Nevada	197	343	23.0	30.7	4,440	8,619	310	291	6.4	5.7
New Hampshire	155	217	0.6	7.1	3,619	7,951	277	242	7.2	5.4
New Jersey	1,171	1,304	3.9	12.3	4,815	10,327	357	362	9.3	6.0
New Mexico	211	304	14.8	24.7	3,548	6,782	308	255	5.8	4.9
New York	2,623	2,937	7.8	29.1	5,322	10,014	344	363	10.4	6.8
North Carolina	1,025	1,448	0.5	17.8	3,943	8,433	331	323	7.3	5.5
North Dakota	102	108	0.6	8.2	3,460	6,453	320	244	6.2	4.8
Ohio	1,670	1,870	2.9	26.9	4,320	9,202	354	377	6.6	5.2
Oklahoma	487	592	3.5	14.7	4,625	8,826	353	365	6.6	5.2
Oregon	475	602	31.3	41.8	3,724	6,561	330	212	4.9	4.8
Pennsylvania	2,072	2,252	6.2	38.5	4,987	9,036	383	374	7.3	5.6
Rhode Island	167	180	7.4	36.2	4,644	8,650	328	327	7.2	5.7
South Carolina	510	749	0.2	15.2	3,944	8,453	329	319	7.4	5.7
South Dakota	116	134	0.1	7.7	3,399	6,927	348	258	5.9	5.0
Tennessee	770	1,031	0.4	23.0	4,859	8,642	376	372	6.6	5.3
Texas	2,079	2,900	6.8	18.7	5,416	10,413	344	334	6.7	5.5
Utah	187	274	9.9	31.7	3,996	7,352	250	237	5.1	4.5
Vermont	83	108	0.8	4.3	3,751	7,338	288	197	7.4	5.3
Virginia	824	1,110	2.1	14.2	4,021	7,744	344	317	7.0	5.4
Washington	691	938	15.4	24.3	3,779	7,376	275	248	5.2	4.8
West Virginia	330	377	7.9	23.8	4,224	8,200	419	363	6.7	5.7
Wisconsin	758	892	2.0	27.6	3,581	7,815	311	287	6.3	5.0
Wyoming	60	78	3.2	6.1	3,980	6,774	327	254	5.7	4.5

[1]Total persons enrolled in hospital insurance, supplementary medical insurance, or both, as of July 1. Includes fee-for-service and managed care enrollees.
[2]Includes enrollees in Medicare-approved managed care organizations.
[3]Data are for fee-for-service enrollees only.
[4]Includes residents of any of the 50 states and the District of Columbia.

Table C-97. Medicare-Certified Providers and Suppliers, Selected Years, 1975–2009

(Number.)

Providers or suppliers	1975	1980	1985	1990	2000	2005	2006	2007	2008	2009
Skilled nursing facilities	—	5,052	6,451	8,937	14,841	15,006	15,028	15,054	15,032	15,071
Home health agencies	2,242	2,924	5,679	5,730	7,857	8,090	8,618	9,024	9,407	10,184
Clinical Laboratory Improvement Amendments facilities	—	—	—	—	171,018	196,296	199,817	206,065	210,872	218,139
End-stage renal disease facilities	—	999	1,393	1,937	3,787	4,755	4,892	5,095	5,317	5,476
Outpatient physical therapy	117	419	854	1,195	2,867	2,962	3,009	2,915	2,781	2,640
Portable X-ray	132	216	308	443	666	553	549	550	547	546
Rural health clinics	—	391	428	551	3,453	3,661	3,723	3,781	3,757	3,752
Comprehensive outpatient rehabilitation facilities	—	—	72	186	522	634	589	539	476	406
Ambulatory surgical centers	—	—	336	1,197	2,894	4,445	4,707	4,964	5,174	5,260
Hospices	—	—	164	825	2,326	2,872	3,071	3,255	3,346	3,405

— =Data not available.

NOTES AND DEFINITIONS

SOURCES OF DATA

The principal source for data presented in this part is from *Health, United States, 2011: With Special Feature on Socioeconomic Status and Health,* an annual report on trends in health statistics compiled by the National Center of Health Statistics (NCHS), a component of the Centers for Disease Control and Prevention (CDC). For more detailed information see: National Center for Health Statistics. *Health, United States, 2011: With Special Feature on Medical Technology.* Hyattsville, MD: 2012.

The data for Tables C-64 through C-69 are from the Bureau of Labor Statistics (BLS), Occupational Employment Statistics Program. For more detailed information, see Occupational Employment and Wages news release (USDL-12-0548).

Table C-88 is from the U.S. Census Bureau. For more detailed information see: DeNavas-Walt, Carmen, Bernadette D. Proctor, and Jessica C. Smith, U.S. Census Bureau, U.S. Department of Commerce, Current Population Reports, P60-239, *Income, Poverty, and Health Insurance Coverage in the United States: 2010.* U.S. Government Printing Office, Washington, DC, 2011.

CONCEPTS AND DEFINITIONS

Age-adjustment—used to compare risks of two or more populations at one point in time or one population at two or more points in time. Age-adjusted rates are computed by the direct method by applying age-specific rates in a population of interest to a standardized age distribution, to eliminate differences in observed rates that result from age differences in population composition. Age-adjusted rates should be viewed as relative indexes rather than actual measures of risk.

Body mass index (BMI)—a measure that adjusts body-weight for height. It is calculated as weight in kilograms divided by height in meters squared. Overweight for children and adolescents is defined as BMI at or above the sex- and age-specific 95th percentile BMI cut points from the 2000 CDC Growth Charts. Healthy weight for adults is defined as a BMI of 18.5 to less than 25; overweight, as greater than or equal to a BMI of 25; and obesity, as greater than or equal to a BMI of 30.

Cholesterol, serum—a measure of the total blood cholesterol. Elevated total blood cholesterol—a combination of high-density lipoproteins (HDL), low-density lipoproteins (LDL), and very-low density lipoproteins (VLDL)—is a risk factor for cardiovascular disease. According to the National Cholesterol Education Program, high serum cholesterol is defined as greater than or equal to 240 mg/dL (6.20 mmol/L). Borderline high serum cholesterol is defined as greater than or equal to 200 mg/dL and less than 240 mg/dL. Assessments of the components of total cholesterol or lower thresholds for high total cholesterol may be used for individuals with other risk factors for cardiovascular disease.

Condition—A health condition is a departure from a state of physical or mental well-being. In the National Health Interview Survey, each condition reported as a cause of an individual's activity limitation has been classified as chronic, not chronic, or unknown if chronic, based on the nature and duration of the condition.

Consumer Price Index (CPI)—prepared by the U.S. Bureau of Labor Statistics. It is a monthly measure of the average change in the prices paid by urban consumers for a fixed market basket of goods and services. The medical care component of CPI shows trends in medical care prices based on specific indicators of hospital, medical, dental, and drug prices. A revision of the definition of CPI has been in use since January 1988.

Dental caries—evidence of tooth decay on any surface of the tooth. Untreated dental caries are determined by an oral examination conducted by a trained dentist.

Diagnosis—the act or process of identifying or determining the nature and cause of a disease or injury through evaluation of patient history, examination, and review of laboratory data.

Gross domestic product (GDP)—the market value of the goods and services produced by labor and property located in the United States. As long as the labor and property are located in the United States, the suppliers (i.e., the workers and, for property, the owners) may be U.S. residents or residents of other countries.

Health expenditures, national—estimated by the Centers for Medicare & Medicaid Services (CMS) it measures spending for health care in the United States by type of service delivered (e.g., hospital care, physician services, nursing home care) and source of funding for those services (e.g., private health insurance, Medicare, Medicaid, out-of-pocket spending). CMS produces both historical and projected estimates of health expenditures by category.

Health insurance coverage—broadly defined to include both public and private payers who cover medical expenditures incurred by a defined population in a variety of settings.

Health maintenance organization (HMO)—a health care system that assumes or shares both the financial risks and the delivery risks associated with providing comprehensive medical services to a voluntarily enrolled population in a particular geographic area, usually in return for a fixed, prepaid fee. Pure HMO enrollees use only the prepaid capitated health services of the HMO panel of medical care providers. Open-ended HMO enrollees use the prepaid HMO health services but, in addition, may receive medical care from providers who are not part of the HMO panel. There is usually a substantial deductible, *co-payment*, or co-insurance associated with use of non-panel providers.

Hispanic origin—includes persons of Mexican, Puerto Rican, Cuban, Central and South American, and other or unknown Latin American or Spanish origins. Persons of Hispanic origin may be of any race.

Hypertension—elevated blood pressure or hypertension is defined as having an average systolic blood pressure reading of at least 140 mmHg or diastolic pressure of at least 90 mmHg, which is consistent with the Seventh Report of the Joint National Committee on Prevention, Detection, Evaluation, and Treatment of High Blood Pressure. People are also considered to have hypertension if they report that they are taking a prescription medicine for high blood pressure, even if their blood pressure readings are within normal range.

Incidence—the number of cases of disease having their onset during a prescribed period of time. It is often expressed as a rate (e.g., the incidence of measles per 1,000 children 5–15 years of age during a specified year). Incidence is a measure of morbidity or other events that occur within a specified period of time. Measuring incidence may be complicated because the population at risk for the disease may change during the period of interest, for example, due to births, deaths, or migration. In addition, determining that a case is new—that is, that its onset occurred during the prescribed period of time—may be difficult. Because of these difficulties in measuring incidence, many health statistics are measured using prevalence.

Instrumental activities of daily living (IADL)—activities related to independent living and include preparing meals, managing money, shopping for groceries or personal items, performing light or heavy housework, and using a telephone. In the National Health Interview Survey (NHIS) respondents are asked whether they or family members 18 years of age and over need the help of another person for handling routine IADL needs because of a physical, mental, or emotional problem. Persons are considered to have an IADL limitation in the NHIS if any causal condition is chronic.

Limitation of activity—may be defined different ways, depending on the conceptual framework. In the National Health Interview Survey, limitation of activity refers to a long-term reduction in a person's capacity to perform the usual kind or amount of activities associated with his or her age group as a result of a chronic condition. Limitation of activity is assessed by asking persons a series of questions about limitations in their or household members' ability to perform activities usual for their age group because of a physical, mental, or emotional problem. Persons are asked about limitations in activities of daily living, instrumental activities of daily living, play, school, work, difficulty walking or remembering, and any other activity limitations. For reported limitations, the causal health conditions are determined, and persons are considered limited if one or more of these conditions is chronic.

Children under 18 years of age who receive special education or early intervention services are considered to have a limitation of activity.

Mammography—an x-ray image of the breast used to detect irregularities of the breast tissue.

Managed care—a term originally used to refer to the pre-paid health care sector (health maintenance organizations or HMOs) where care is provided under a fixed budget and costs are therein capable of being managed. Increasingly, the term is being used to include preferred provider organizations (PPOs) and even forms of indemnity.

Medicare—the federal program which helps pay health care costs for people 65 and older and for certain people under 65 with long-term disabilities.

Medicaid—a program authorized by the Social Security Act in 1965 as a jointly funded cooperative venture between the federal and state governments to assist states in the provision of adequate medical care to eligible needy persons. Families with dependent children, the aged, blind, and disabled who are in financial need are eligible for Medicaid.

Notifiable disease—a disease, that when diagnosed, health providers are required, usually by law, to report to state or local public health officials. Notifiable diseases are those of public interest by reason of their contagiousness, severity, or frequency.

Pap smear—a microscopic examination of cells scraped from the cervix that is used to detect cancerous or precancerous conditions of the cervix or other medical conditions.

Physical activity, leisure-time—starting with 1998 data, leisure-time physical activity has been assessed in the National Health Interview Survey by asking adults a series of questions about how often they do vigorous or light/moderate physical activity of at least 10 minutes duration and for about how long these sessions generally last. Vigorous physical activity is described as causing heavy sweating or a large increase in breathing or heart rate and light/moderate as causing light sweating or a slight to moderate increase in breathing or heart rate. Adults classified as inactive did not report any sessions of light/moderate or vigorous leisure-time physical activity of at least 10 minutes duration or reported they were unable to perform leisure-time physical activity. Adults classified with some leisure-time activity reported at least one session of light/moderate or vigorous activity of at least 10 minutes duration but did not meet the requirement for regular leisure-time activity. Adults classified with regular leisure-time activity reported at least three sessions per week of vigorous leisure-time physical activity lasting at least 20 minutes in duration or at least five sessions per week of light/moderate physical activity lasting at least 30 minutes in duration.

Estimates have recently changed to reflect the federal 2008 *Physical Activity Guidelines for Americans.*

Poverty—based on definitions originally developed by the Social Security Administration. These include a set of money income thresholds that vary by family size and composition. Families or individuals with income below their appropriate thresholds are classified as below poverty. These thresholds are updated annually by the U.S. Census Bureau to reflect changes in the Consumer Price Index for all urban consumers (CPI-U). For example, the average poverty threshold for a family of four was $22,314 in 2010, $17,603 in 2000, and $13,359 in 1990.

Preferred provider organization (PPO)—a type of medical plan where coverage is provided to participants through a network of selected health care providers (such as hospitals and physicians). The enrollees may go outside the network, but they would pay a greater percentage of the cost of coverage than within the network.

Prevalence—the number of cases of a disease, infected persons, or persons with some other attribute present during a particular interval of time. It is often expressed as a rate (e.g., the prevalence of diabetes per 1,000 persons during a year).

Short-stay hospital—hospitals that provide general (rather than specialized) care and have an average length of stay of less than 30 days.

Specialty hospital—hospitals that provide a particular type of service to the majority of their patients such as psychiatric, tuberculosis, chronic disease, rehabilitation, maternity, and alcoholic or narcotic.

State Children's Health Insurance Program (SCHIP)—Title XXI of the Social Security Act, known as the State Children's Health Insurance Program (SCHIP) or more simply as the Children's Health Insurance Program (CHIP), is a program initiated by the Balanced Budget Act of 1997 (BBA). SCHIP provides more federal funds for states to provide health care coverage to low-income, uninsured children. SCHIP gives states broad flexibility in program design while protecting beneficiaries through federal standards. Funds from SCHIP may be used to expand Medicaid or to provide medical assistance to children during a presumptive eligibility period for Medicaid. This is one of several options from which states may select to provide health care coverage for more children, as prescribed within the BBA's Title XXI program.

Substance use—the use of selected substances including alcohol, tobacco products, drugs, inhalants, and other substances that can be consumed, inhaled, injected, or otherwise absorbed into the body with possible detrimental effects.

Suicidal ideation—having thoughts of suicide or of taking action to end one's own life. Suicidal ideation includes all thoughts of suicide, both when the thoughts include a plan to commit suicide and when they do not include a plan. Suicidal ideation is measured in the Youth Risk Behavior Survey by the question "During the past 12 months, did you ever seriously consider attempting suicide?"

Uninsured—in the Current Population Survey (CPS) persons are considered uninsured if they do not have coverage through private health insurance, Medicare, Medicaid, State Children's Health Insurance Program, military or Veterans coverage, another government program, a plan of someone outside the household, or other insurance. Persons with only Indian Health Service coverage are considered uninsured. In addition, if the respondent has missing Medicaid information but has income from certain low-income public programs, then Medicaid coverage is imputed. The questions on health insurance are administered in March and refer to the previous calendar year.

INDEX

A
ABNORMAL CONDITIONS
Newborns, by age and race of mother, 95, 96
ACCIDENTS
Injury deaths, generally, 166
Leading causes of death, 115, 168, 172
Number of deaths from selected causes, 119–156
ADDICTIVE SUBSTANCES
Alcohol
heavier drinking and drinking five or more drinks a day, 303
Cigarette smoking
age-adjusted prevalence of smoking among adults 25 and over, 305
current smoking among adults, 305–308
Illicit drug use
death rates for opioid drug poisoning, selected characteristics, 211
use of selected substances among persons 12 years and over, 301
use of selected substances among students, 310
ADOLESCENTS
Birth and fertility rates for mothers 15 to 19, 24, 25
Birth rates for mothers 10 to 19, by race and Hispanic origin, 28
Never-married females
response to statement "if you got pregnant now," 27
Obesity among children and adolescents 2 to 19 years of age, 294
Vaccination coverage among adolescents 13 to 17 years of age, 327
AEROBICS
Physical activity among adults, 288
AGE
AIDS cases, by age, 245
Alcohol, drinking five or more drinks a day among adults, 303
Asthma, children under 18 who suffer from, 283
Basic actions difficulty and complex activity limitation, 272
Birth rates
age and race of father, 40
age of father, 37
age of mother, by state and territory, 38
age of mother and live-birth order, 5, 7, 39
mothers aged 10 to 19, by race and Hispanic origin, 28
mothers under 20 years of age, by state and territory, 9
probability of a first birth, ages 15 through 24 26
selected demographic characteristics, 18, 53
teenagers 15 to 19 years of age, 24, 25
women under age 20, by race and Hispanic origin, 8
Cancer rates, by age, 201–206, 247
Cholesterol among persons 20 years of age and over, 285
Cigarette smoking, by age, 305–308
Colorectal tests or procedures, use among adults, 336
Congenital anomalies of newborns, by age of mother, 95, 96
Contraception use, individuals aged 15 to 19, 87–90
Deaths and death rates
abridged life table for total population, 108
adjusted death rates, 15 leading causes of death, 115
adjusted death rates, by race and sex, 102, 150–163
all causes, 190
cancer deaths, 201–206
cerebrovascular disease death rates, 197
fatal occupational injuries, 177
firearm-related injuries, 224
heart disease death rates, 194
HIV death rates, 209
homicide, 218
leading causes of death, 115, 172
life expectancy at birth, 110, 113
life expectancy at selected ages, 112, 113
motor vehicle-related injuries, 214
number of deaths, by age 104–107
number of deaths from selected causes, by age, 119–156
state death rates, by age-adjusted, 184
suicide, 221
years of potential life lost before age 75, 181
Dental caries, by age, 295
Dental visits in past year, by age, 348
Diabetes rates, among adults, 261
Disability and health status, by age, 278
Discharge rate in nonfederal short-stay hospitals, by age, 358–370
Educational attainment of mothers, by age and race, 92
Energy and macronutrient intake, persons 20 years of age and over, 287
Fathers
birth rates by age and race of father, 40
Fertility rates
age, live-birth order, and race of mother, 42–51
Health care, no usual source of, by age, 313
Health care, percent distribution of payment for, 398
Health care expenses, by age, 397
Health care visits, by selected characteristics, 320, 338–345
Health care visits, lack of by children, 319
Health insurance
coverage among persons under 65, 405, 407
no health coverage among persons under 65, 409
Health-related behaviors of children 6 to 11 years of age, 296
Hospital stays in the past year, by age, 355
Hypertension among persons 20 years of age and over, 284
Joint pain among adults 18 years and over, 268
Live births
by age of mother, 6, 33, 34
mothers under 20 years of age, by state and territory, 9

plurality of birth and ratios, by age, 81
risk factors during pregnancy, 65, 67
Mammography, use of among women, 334
Mean age of mother, by live-birth order and race, 29
Medicaid coverage, persons under 65, 415
Medical care, reduced access to, by age, 316
Medicare beneficiaries, by age, 411, 422
Occupational injuries and diseases
    deaths from selected diseases among persons 15 years and over, 174
    fatal occupational injuries, 177
Out-of-pocket health care expenses, by age, 399
Overweight, obesity, and healthy weight, 291, 294
Pap smears, use of among women, 334
Physical activity among adults, 288
Prenatal care
    month began, by age and race of mother, 93
Prescription drug classes used in past 30 days, by age, 351
Prescription drug use in past 30 days, by age, 349
Psychological distress among adults, 282
Renal disease, end-stage patients, 263
Smoking during pregnancy, 87
Substance abuse
    death rates for opioid drug poisoning, by age, 211
    students, 310
    use of selected substances by persons 12 years of age and over, 301
Unmarried women
    number and percentage of births to, 11, 56-59
Vaccination coverage, 322–330

AIDS
Cases, by year of diagnosis and selected characteristics, 245
Death rates, 209
Number of deaths from selected causes, 119–156

ALCOHOL
Heavier drinking and drinking five or more drinks a day, 303
Use of selected substances among persons 12 years and over, 301
Use of selected substances among students, 310

ALZHEIMER'S DISEASE
Leading causes of death, 115, 168
Number of deaths from selected causes, 119–156

AMBULATORY CARE
Colorectal tests or procedures, use among adults, 336
Dental visits in past year, 349
Dietary supplement use among persons 20 years and over, 353
Doctor office visits, 320, 345
Emergency department visits, 320, 338–345
Health care visits, by selected characteristics, 320
Home visits, 320
Hospital outpatient visits, 345
Injury-related visits to hospital emergency departments, 343
Mammography among women 40 years and over, 332
No health care visits to an office among children under 18, 319

No usual source of health care among adults 18 to 64 years of age, 314
No usual source of health care among children under 18, 313
Pap smears among women 18 years and over, 334
Physician office visits, 320, 345
Prescription drug classes used in past 30 days, 351
Prescription drug use in the past 30 days, by selected characteristics, 349
Primary care visits, 346
Reduced access to medical care due to cost, 316, 318
Specialist care visits, 346
Vaccination coverage among adolescents 13 to 17 years of age, 327
Vaccination coverage among adults for influenza, 328
Vaccination coverage among adults for pneumococcal disease, 330
Vaccination coverage among children 19 to 35 months of age, 322, 325
Vitamin use among persons 20 years and over, 353

AMERICAN INDIAN OR ALASKA NATIVE
AIDS cases, by race, 245
Alcohol, drinking five or more drinks a day among adults, 303
Birth rates
    age of mother and live-birth order, 7, 39
    by race, 4, 5, 30
    demographic characteristics of births by race, 53
    mothers aged 10 to 19, 28
    percentage of births with selected medical or health characteristics, 60, 61
    selected characteristics, 4, 13
    teenagers 15 to 19 years of age, 24
    women under age 20, 8
Colorectal tests or procedures, use among adults, 336
Deaths and death rates
    age-adjusted death rates, 102, 150–163
    all causes, 190
    fatal occupational injuries, 177
    firearm-related injuries, 224
    number of deaths, 104–107
Dental visits in past year, by race, 348
Fertility rates by race, 30
Health care, no usual source of, by race, 313, 314
Health care, percent distribution of payment for, 398
Health care expenses, by race, 397
Health care visits, by selected characteristics, 320, 338–345
Health care visits, lack of by children, 319
Health insurance
    coverage among persons under 65, 405, 407
    no health coverage among persons under 65, 409
Hospital stays in the past year, by race, 355
Live births
    age and race of mother, 6, 33
    by race, 12, 30, 35
    risk factors during pregnancy, 65, 67
Mammography, use of among women, 332
Mean age of mother, by live-birth order and race, 29
Medicaid coverage, by race, 415, 417

Medical care, reduced access to, by race, 316
Order of birth, by race, 20
Pap smears, use of among women, 334
Physical activity among adults, 288
Substance abuse
death rates for opioid drug poisoning, by race, 209
use of selected substances among persons 12 years and over, 301
Total number of births, selected demographic characteristics, 18, 53
Unmarried women
number and percentage of births to, 56-59
Vaccination coverage, 322–330

ANEMIA
Number of deaths from selected causes, 119–156
ANESTHESIOLOGISTS
Wages, 377
ARCHITECTURAL MANAGERS
Wages, 378
ASIAN OR PACIFIC ISLANDER
AIDS cases, by race, 245
Alcohol, drinking five or more drinks a day among adults, 303
Birth rates
age of mother and live-birth order, 7, 39
by race, 4, 5, 30
demographic characteristics of births by race, 53
mothers aged 10 to 19, 28
percentage of births with selected medical or health characteristics, 60, 61
selected characteristics, 4, 13
teenagers 15 to 19 years of age, 24
women under age 20, 8
Colorectal tests or procedures, use among adults, 336
Death and death rates
age-adjusted death rates, 102, 150–163
all causes, 190
fatal occupational injuries, 177
firearm-related injuries, 224
number of deaths, 104–107
Dental visits in past year, by race, 348
Fertility rates by race, 30
Health care, no usual source of, by race, 313, 314
Health care, percent distribution of payment for, 398
Health care expenses, by race, 397
Health care visits, by selected characteristics, 320, 338–345
Health care visits, lack of by children, 319
Health insurance
coverage among persons under 65, 405, 407
no health coverage among persons under 65, 409
Hospital stays in the past year, by race, 355
Live births
age and race of mother, 6, 33
by race, 12, 30, 35
risk factors during pregnancy, 65, 67
Mammography, use of among women, 332
Mean age of mother, by live-birth order and race, 29
Medicaid coverage, by race, 415, 417
Medical care, reduced access to, by race, 316

Order of birth, by race, 20
Pap smears, use of among women, 334
Physical activity among adults, 288
Substance abuse
death rates for opioid drug poisoning, by race, 211
use of selected substances among persons 12 years and over, 301
Total number of births, selected demographic characteristics, 18, 53
Unmarried women
number and percentage of births to, 56–59
Vaccination coverage, 322–330
ASTHMA
Children under 18 who suffer from asthma, 283
ATHLETIC TRAINERS
Wages, 377
ATTENDANTS
Number of live births by attendant, place of delivery, and race, 91
AUDIOLOGISTS
Wages, 376, 377

B
BACTERIAL SEPSIS
Leading causes of death, 172
BIRTH DEFECTS
Congenital anomalies of newborns, by age and race of mother, 95, 96
BIRTH RATES
Age, live-birth order, and race of mother, 4, 5, 42–51
Age and race of father, 40
Age of father, 37
Age of mother, by state and territory, 38
Age of mother and live-birth order, 5, 7, 39
Cesarean deliveries, 13, 17, 68–71
Demographics
total number of births and rates by demographic characteristics, 53, 60
Fathers
rates by age and race of father, 40
Gestation periods, 72, 86
Live births
see **LIVE BIRTHS**
Low and very low birthweight rates, 14, 72–80
Medical or health characteristics, percentage of births by, 60, 61
Mothers
aged 10 to 19, by race and Hispanic origin, 28
under 20 years of age, by state and territory, 9
Observed birth rates, 53
Order of birth, by race and Hispanic origin, 20
Plurality of births and ratios, 81
Preterm birth rates, 15, 16, 74–78
Probability of a first birth, ages 15 through 24, 26
Race and Hispanic origin of mother, by state and territory, 12, 35, 36
Rates by Hispanic or non-Hispanic origin, 31
Rates by race, 30
Risk factors, births to mothers with, 65, 67
Seasonally adjusted rates, 53

Selected characteristics by race and Hispanic origin, 4, 13
Teenagers 15 to 19 years of age, 24, 25
Total number of births, selected demographic characteristics, 18, 53
Twins, triplets, and multiple births, 81–86
Unmarried women
   number and percentage of births to, 11, 54–59
   rates of births by state and territory, 22, 62
Weight gain, number of live births by, 63
Women under age 20, by race and Hispanic origin, 8

BIRTH RECORDS
Total count of records and completeness of preliminary file, 23

BIRTHS
Age, race, and Hispanic origin of mother, 4, 5
Birth rates
   see **BIRTH RATES**
Birthweight distribution in 500 gram intervals, 75
Cesarean delivery rates, 13, 17, 68–71
Contraception
   use among individuals aged 15 to 19, 87–90
Day of week, births by, 53
Demographics
   total number of births and rates by demographic characteristics, 53, 60
Educational attainment and race of mothers, 94
Fertility rates
   see **FERTILITY RATES**
Forceps or vacuum extraction, deliveries by, 68
Gestation periods, 72, 86
Live births
   see **LIVE BIRTHS**
Low and very low birthweight rates, 14, 72–80
Medical or health characteristics, percentage of births by, 60, 61
Method of delivery, occurrence by, 53
Mothers
   aged 10 to 19, by race and Hispanic origin, 28
   mean age of mother, by live-birth order and race, 29
   teenagers 15 to 19 years of age, 24, 25
   under 20 years of age, by state and territory, 9
Never-married females
   response to statement "if you got pregnant now," 27
Number of births by Hispanic or non-Hispanic origin, 31
Number of live births by attendant, place of delivery, and race, 91
Plurality of births and ratios, 81
Preterm birth rates, 15, 16, 74–78
Probability of a first birth, ages 15 through 24, 26
Risk factors, births to mothers with, 65, 67
Smoking during pregnancy, 87
Total number of births, selected demographic characteristics, 18, 53
Twins, triplets, and multiple births, 81–86
Unmarried women
   number and percentage of births to, 11, 54–59
   rates of births by state and territory, 22, 62

BLACK RACE
Generally
   see **RACE**

BREAST CANCER
Death rates, 204
Mammograms, use of among women 40 years and over, 332

C
CANCER
Death rates from, 201–206
Five-year relative survival rates, 253
Health, determinants and measures of
   age-adjusted cancer incidence rates, 247
   five-year relative survival rates, 253
   respondent-reported prevalence among adults, 255
Leading causes of death, 115, 168, 172
Number of deaths from selected causes, 119–156

CARDIOVASCULAR TECHNOLOGISTS
Wages, 376, 377

CAVITIES
Untreated dental caries, by selected characteristics, 295

CEREBROVASCULAR DISEASES
Death rates from, 197

CESAREAN DELIVERIES
Delivery rates, by selected characteristics, 13, 17, 68–71
Low birthweights and preterm births, 72–80
Percentage of births with selected medical or health characteristics, 60, 61
Risk factors, births to mothers with, 67

CHIEF EXECUTIVES
Wages, 378

CHILDREN
AIDS cases, by age, 245
Health care, no usual source of, 313
Health-related behaviors of children 6 to 11 years of age, 296
Infant, neonatal, and postneonatal mortality rates, 228–234
Overweight children 2 to 19 years of age, 294
Vaccination coverage among children 19 to 35 months of age, 322, 325

CHIROPRACTORS
Wages, 377

CHLAMYDIA
Number of new cases, 243

CHOLESTEROL
Health conditions and risk factors, selected years, 297
High cholesterol among persons 20 years of age and over, 285

CIGARETTE SMOKING
Age-adjusted prevalence of smoking among adults 25 years and over, 305
Smoking among adults, 305–308
Smoking during pregnancy, 87
Use of selected substances among persons 12 years and over, 301
Use of selected substances among students, 310

CLINICS
Medicaid beneficiaries and payments, 418

COCAINE
Use of selected substances among students, 310

COLITIS
Number of deaths from selected causes, 119–156

COLORECTAL TESTS
  Use among adults 50 to 75 years of age, 336
COMPUTER MANAGERS
  Wages, 380
CONDOMS
  Contraception use, individuals aged 15 to 19, 87–90
CONGENITAL ANOMALIES
  Leading causes of death, 172
  Newborns, by age and race of mother, 95, 96
  Risk factors, births to mothers with, 65, 67
CONSUMER PRICE INDEX (CPI)
  Health expenditures, 387
CONTRACEPTION
  Use among individuals aged 15 to 19, 87–90
CONTROLLED SUBSTANCES
  Death rates for opioid drug poisoning, selected characteristics, 211
  Use of selected substances among persons 12 years and over, 301
  Use of selected substances among students, 310
CUTTING OR PIERCING
  Injury deaths, 166

D
DEATHS AND DEATH RATES
  Abridged life table for total population, 108
  Age
    age-adjusted death rates, 102, 150–163
    all causes, 190
    cancer deaths, 201–206
    cerebrovascular disease death rates, 197
    fatal occupational injuries, 177
    firearms injuries, 224
    heart disease death rates, 194
    HIV death rates, 209
    homicide, 218
    leading causes of death, 172
    life expectancy at birth, 110, 113
    life expectancy at selected ages, 112, 113
    motor vehicle-related injuries, 214
    number of deaths, by age, 104–107
    number of deaths from selected causes, by age, 119–156
    suicide, 221
    years of potential life lost before age 75, 181
  AIDS death rates, 209
  All causes, 190
  Cancer death rates, 201–206
  Firearm-related injuries, 224
  Heart disease, 194
  Hispanic origin
    age-adjusted death rates, 102, 150–163
    all causes, 190
    cancer deaths, 201–206
    cerebrovascular disease death rates, 197
    fatal occupational injuries, 177
    firearms injuries, 224
    heart disease death rates, 194
    HIV death rates, 209
    homicide, 218
    life expectancy at birth, 110, 113
    life expectancy at selected ages, 112, 113
    motor vehicle-related injuries, 214
    number of deaths, 104–107
    number of deaths from selected causes, 119–156
    suicide, 221
    years of potential life lost before age 75, 181
  HIV death rates, 209
  Homicide, 218
  Hospice care patients, 235, 236
  Industry
    fatal occupational injuries, 177
  Infant, neonatal, and postneonatal mortality rates, 228–234
  Injury deaths, generally, 166
  Leading causes of death, 168, 172
  Life expectancy at birth, 110, 113
  Life expectancy at selected ages, 112, 113
  Motor vehicle-related injuries, 213, 214
  Number of deaths, selected years, 102, 150–163
  Number of deaths from selected causes, 119–156
  Occupational injuries and diseases, 174–180
  Occupational injuries and diseases
    fatal occupational injuries, 177
  Race
    age-adjusted death rates, 102, 150–163
    all causes, 190
    cancer deaths, 201–206
    cerebrovascular disease death rates, 197
    fatal occupational injuries, 177
    firearms injuries, 224
    heart disease death rates, 194
    HIV death rates, 209
    homicide, 218
    life expectancy at birth, 110, 113
    life expectancy at selected ages, 112, 113
    motor vehicle-related injuries, 214
    number of deaths, 104–107
    number of deaths from selected causes, 119–156
    suicide, 221
    years of potential life lost before age 75, 181
  Sex
    age-adjusted death rates. 102, 150–163
    all causes, 190
    cancer deaths, 201–206
    cerebrovascular disease death rates, 197
    fatal occupational injuries, 177
    firearms injuries, 224
    heart disease death rates, 194
    HIV death rates, 209
    homicide, 218
    life expectancy at birth, 110, 113
    life expectancy at selected ages, 112, 113
    motor vehicle-related injuries, 214
    number of deaths, 104–107
    number of deaths from selected causes, 119–156
    suicide, 221
    years of potential life lost before age 75, 181
  States and territories
    fatal work injuries, 180
    major causes of death by state, 184

Stroke, 197
Suicide, 221
DELIVERY METHODS
  Live births by method of delivery, 68
DEMOGRAPHICS
  Births
    total number of births and rates by demographic characteristics, 53, 60
DENTAL ASSISTANTS
  Wages, 376, 377
DENTAL CARIES
  Health conditions and risk factors, selected years, 297
  Untreated dental caries, by selected characteristics, 295
DENTAL HYGIENISTS
  Wages, 376, 377
DENTAL VISITS
  Percentages of persons with a visit in past year, 348
DENTISTS
  Medicaid beneficiaries and payments, 418
  Wages, 376, 378
DIABETES
  Adults 20 years of age and over, 261
  Health conditions and risk factors, selected years, 297
  Leading causes of death, 115, 168
  Number of deaths from selected causes, 119–156
  Percentage of births with selected medical or health characteristics, 60, 61
  Risk factors, births to mothers with, 67
DIAGNOSTIC MEDICAL SONOGRAPHERS
  Wages, 376, 377
DIETARY SUPPLEMENTS
  Use among persons 20 years and over, 353
DIETICIANS AND DIETETIC TECHNICIANS
  Wages, 376, 377
DIPHTHERIA
  Number of new cases, 243
DISABILITY
  Selected measures of disability and health status among adults, 278
DISEASE
  Health, determinants and measures of
    selected notifiable rates and numbers of new cases, 243
  Infant mortality rates, 228–234
  Leading causes of death, 115, 168, 172
  Number of deaths from selected causes, 119–156
  Occupational injuries and diseases, 174–180
  Percentage or births with selected medical or health characteristics, 60, 61
DOCTORS' OFFICES
  Health care visits to, 320, 345
DROWNING
  Injury deaths, 166
DRUG ABUSE
  Death rates for opioid drug poisoning, selected characteristics, 211
  Use of selected substances among persons 12 years and over, 301
  Use of selected substances among students, 310

E
ECSTASY (MDMA)
  Use of selected substances among students, 310
EDUCATIONAL ATTAINMENT
  Births, by education and race of mother, 94
  Cigarette smoking by education level, 305, 306
  Mothers, by age and race, 92
  Physical activity, by educational attainment, 288
EMERGENCY MEDICAL TECHNICIANS
  Wages, 376, 377
EMERGENCY ROOMS
  Health care visits to, 320, 338–345
EMPLOYMENT
  Health personnel
    see HEALTH PERSONNEL
ENCEPHALITIS
  Number of deaths from selected causes, 119–156
ENERGY AND MACRONUTRIENT INTAKE
  Persons 20 years of age and over, 287
ENGINEERING MANAGERS
  Wages, 378
ENTERITIS
  Number of deaths from selected causes, 119–156
ENVIRONMENT
  Injury deaths, 166
EXERCISE
  Leisure-time physical activity among adults 18 and over, 288
EXPENDITURES
    see HEALTH EXPENDITURES
EYESIGHT
  Vision limitations, adults 18 and over, 274

F
FALLS
  Injury deaths, 166
FATAL OCCUPATIONAL INJURIES
  Comparison of 2010 preliminary and final figures, 176
  Industry, sex, age, race, and Hispanic origin, 177
  Most frequent type, 179
  Number, by state, 180
  Number and rate, by industry sector and occupation, 179
FATHERS
  Birth rates by age and race of father, 37, 40
FEDERAL, STATE, AND LOCAL GOVERNMENT EXPENDITURES
  Health expenditures, 384, 402
FEMALE CONDOMS
  Contraception use, individuals aged 15 to 19, 87–90
FERTILITY RATES
  Age, live-birth order, and race of mother, 42–51
  Live births and fertility rates, by state, 12
  Mothers aged 10 to 19, by race and Hispanic origin, 28
  Observed fertility rates, 53
  Race and Hispanic origin of mother, 4, 51
  Rates by Hispanic or non-Hispanic origin, 31
  Rates by race, 30
  Seasonally adjusted rates, 53

Teenagers 15 to 19 years of age, 24, 25
Total number of births, selected demographic characteristics, 18, 53
FINGER PAIN
Joint pain among adults 18 years and over, 268
FIREARM-RELATED INJURIES
Deaths and death rates, 224
Injury deaths, 166
FIRES
Injury deaths, 166
FIRST BIRTHS
Probability of a first birth, ages 15 through 24, 26
FORCEPS
Deliveries by, 68

G
GESTATION PERIODS
Age and birthweight characteristics by plurality, 86
Birthweight figures, 72, 86
Leading causes of death, 172
Percent distribution of gestational age, 86
Weight gain, number of live births by gestation period, 63
GLYCEMIC CONTROL
Diabetes rates among adults, 261
GONORRHEA
Number of deaths from selected causes, 119–156
Number of new cases, 243
GROSS DOMESTIC PRODUCT
Health expenditures, 384
GYNECOLOGISTS
Wages, 377, 378

H
HANDGUNS
Deaths and death rates, 224
HEADACHE OR MIGRAINE
Adults 18 and over, 266
HEALTH
Addictive substances
  see **ADDICTIVE SUBSTANCES**
Ambulatory care
  see **AMBULATORY CARE**
Inpatient care
  see **INPATIENT CARE**
Insurance
  see **HEALTH INSURANCE**
HEALTH, DETERMINANTS AND MEASURES OF
AIDS
  cases by year of diagnosis and selected characteristics, 245
Asthma, children under 18 who suffer from, 283
Basic actions difficulty and complex activity limitation, 272
Cancer
  age-adjusted cancer incidence rates, 247
  five-year relative survival rates, 253
  respondent-reported prevalence among adults, 255

Cholesterol
  high cholesterol among persons 20 years of age and over, 285
Dental caries, by selected characteristics, 295
Diabetes
  adults 20 years of age and over, 261
Disability, selected measures of, 278
Disease
  selected notifiable rates and numbers of new cases, 243
Energy and macronutrient intake, persons 20 years of age and over, 287
Headache or migraine
  adults 18 and over, 266
Health conditions and risk factors, selected years, 297
Health-related behaviors of children 6 to 11 years of age, 296
Health risk behaviors among students in grades 9 to 12, 298
Health status, selected measures of, 278
Hearing limitations
  adults 18 and over, 274
Heart disease
  respondent-reported prevalence among adults, 255
Hypertension
  persons 20 years of age and over, 284
Joint pain
  adults 18 years and over, 268
Low back pain
  adults 18 and over, 266
Neck pain
  adults 18 and over, 266
Occupational diseases and injuries
  nonfatal, with days away from work, 242
Overweight, obesity, and healthy weight
  children and adolescents 2 to 19 years of age, 294
  persons 20 years of age and over, 291
Physical activity
  leisure-time activity among adults 18 and over, 288
Psychological distress
  adults 18 and over, 282
Renal disease
  end-stage renal disease patients, 263
Respondent-assessed health status, 276
Stroke
  respondent-reported prevalence among adults, 255
Vision limitations
  adults 18 and over, 274
HEALTH CARE
Adults, no usual source of health care, 314
Children, no health care visits in past 12 months, 319
Children, no usual source of health care, 313
Reduced access to medical care due to cost, 316, 318
HEALTH EXPENDITURES
Average annual percent changes, 384–390
Consumer Price Index, 385
Gross domestic product, 384
Growth in personal health care expenditures, 387, 392
Health services and supplies and percent distribution, 402

Hospital discharges with common operating room procedures, 395
Mental health services, 388
National health expenditures, 388–390
Out-of-pocket health care expenses, 399
Per capita amounts of expenditures, 384
Percent distribution of payment for health care, by population, 398
Personal health care expenditures, 387, 392
Selected population characteristics, 397
Substance abuse treatment, 389
Veterans Affairs health care expenditures and use, and persons treated, 403

HEALTH INSURANCE
Medicaid
    basis of eligibility, and race and Hispanic origin, 417
    coverage among persons under 65, selected characteristics, 415
    managed care beneficiaries, 419
    type of service, 418
Medicare
    beneficiaries by race, Hispanic origin, and selected characteristics, 423
    certified providers and suppliers, 426
    coverage of beneficiaries 65 and over, selected characteristics, 411
    enrollees and expenditures, by program and type of service, 420
    enrollees and expenditures, fee-for-service beneficiaries, 422
    managed care beneficiaries, 425
    short-stay hospital utilization, 425
No health insurance coverage
    change in number and percent during first year after a recession, 414
    persons under 65, selected characteristics, 409
    persons without coverage, by state, 413
Private health insurance
    coverage among persons under 65, selected characteristics, 407
    obtained through the workplace, persons under 65, 405

HEALTH PERSONNEL
Employers' costs per employee-hour worked, 381
Highest and lowest paying occupations, 378
Industries with the highest levels and concentration of employment, 379
States with the highest levels and concentration of employment, 379
Top paying metropolitan areas for health care, 380
Wages, selected occupations, 376, 377

HEALTH PROBLEMS
Leading causes of death, 168
Number of deaths from selected causes, 119–156
Percentage of births with selected medical or health characteristics, 60, 61
Risk factors, births to mothers with, 65, 67
Smoking during pregnancy, 87

HEARING LIMITATIONS
Adults 18 and over, 274

HEART DISEASE
Death rates from, 194
Health, determinants and measures of respondent-reported prevalence among adults, 255
Leading causes of death, 115, 168, 172
Number of deaths from selected causes, 119–156

HEPATITIS
Number of deaths from selected causes, 119–156
Number of new cases, 243

HIGH SCHOOL STUDENTS
Substance abuse, by sex and race, 310

HIP PAIN
Joint pain among adults 18 years and over, 268

HISPANIC ORIGIN
AIDS cases, by Hispanic origin, 247
Alcohol, drinking five or more drinks a day among adults, 303
Asthma, children under 18 who suffer from, 283
Basic actions difficulty and complex activity limitation, 272
Birth rates
    age, live-birth order, and Hispanic origin of mother, 7, 39–51
    by Hispanic origin, 4, 5, 31
    demographic characteristics of births, 53
    mothers aged 10 to 19, 28
    number of births by Hispanic and non-Hispanic origin, 31
    selected characteristics, 4, 13
    teenagers 15 to 19 years of age, 24
    very low birthweight births, 80
    women under age 20, 8
Cancer
    five-year relative survival rates, 253
    rates, by Hispanic origin, 201–206, 247
Cesarean deliveries
    low birthweights and preterm births, 72–80
    selected criteria, 68–71
Cholesterol among persons 20 years of age and over, 285
Cigarette smoking among adults, 306
Colorectal tests or procedures, use among adults, 336
Congenital anomalies of newborns, by Hispanic origin of mother, 95, 96
Contraception use, individuals aged 15 to 19, 87–90
Deaths and death rates
    age-adjusted death rates, 102, 150–163
    all causes, 190
    cancer deaths, 201–206
    cerebrovascular disease death rates, 197
    fatal occupational injuries, 177
    firearm-related injuries, 224
    heart disease death rates, 194
    HIV death rates, 209
    homicide, 218
    infant mortality rates, 228–234
    leading causes of death, 168
    life expectancy at birth, 110, 113
    life expectancy at selected ages, 112, 113
    motor vehicle-related injuries, 214
    number of deaths, 104–107
    number of deaths from selected causes, 119–156
    suicide, 221
    years of potential life lost before age 75, 181

Dental caries, by Hispanic origin, 295
Dental visits in past year, by Hispanic origin, 348
Diabetes rates, by Hispanic origin, 261
Disability and health status, by Hispanic origin, 278
Educational attainment of mothers, by age and race, 92, 94
Fertility rates by Hispanic origin, 31, 51
Firearm-related injuries, 224
Health care, no usual source of, by Hispanic origin, 313, 314
Health care, percent distribution of payment for, 398
Health care expenses, by Hispanic origin, 397
Health care visits, by selected characteristics, 320, 338–345
Health care visits, lack of by children, 319
Health insurance
    coverage among persons under 65, 405, 407
    no health coverage among persons under 65, 409
Health-related behaviors of children 6 to 11 years of age, 296
Health risk behaviors among students in grades 9 to 12, 298
Hospital stays in the past year, by Hispanic origin, 355
Hypertension among persons 20 years of age and over, 284
Joint pain among adults 18 years and over, 268
Live births
    by age and Hispanic origin of mother, 6
    by Hispanic origin, 31
    by mother and state and territory, 12, 35, 36
    by plurality of birth and ratios, 81
    number of births by attendant and place of delivery, 91
    preterm birth rates, 74–78
    risk factors during pregnancy, 65, 67
Mammography, use of among women, 332
Mean age of mother, by live-birth order and Hispanic origin, 29
Medicaid coverage, by Hispanic origin, 415, 417
Medical care, reduced access to, by Hispanic origin, 316
Medical or health characteristics, percentage of births by, 60, 61
Medicare beneficiaries, by Hispanic origin, 411, 423
Occupational injuries and diseases
    fatal occupational injuries, 177
Order of birth, by Hispanic origin, 20
Overweight, obesity, and healthy weight, 291, 294
Pap smears, use of among women, 334
Physical activity among adults, 288
Prenatal care
    month began, by age and race of mother, 93
Prescription drug use in past 30 days, by Hispanic origin, 349
Psychological distress among adults, 282
Renal disease, end-stage patients, 263
Smoking during pregnancy, 87
Substance abuse
    death rates for opioid drug poisoning, by Hispanic origin, 211
    students, 310
    use of selected substances among persons 12 years and over, 301

Total number of births, selected demographic characteristics, 18, 53
Twins, triplets, and multiple births, 82
Unmarried women
    number and percentage of births to, 54–59, 62
Vaccination coverage, 322–330
Weight gain, live births by, 63

HIV
Cases, by year of diagnosis and selected characteristics, 245
Death rates, 209
Number of deaths from selected causes, 119–156

HOME HEALTH AIDES
Wages, 376, 377

HOME HEALTH SERVICES
Medicaid beneficiaries and payments, 418

HOMICIDE
Deaths and death rates, 218
Injury deaths, 166
Leading causes of death, 115, 168, 172
Number of deaths from selected causes, 119–156

HOSPICE CARE PATIENTS
Drugs prescribed to patients in last week of life, 236
Primary admission diagnosis of discharged patients, 235
Selected characteristics of discharged patients, 235
Services offered to patients' family or friends, 235
Symptoms of patients at last care visit before death, 236

HOSPITAL EMERGENCY DEPARTMENTS
Health care visits to, 320, 338–345

HOSPITAL OUTPATIENT DEPARTMENTS
Visits to, 345

HOSPITALS
Ambulatory care
    see **AMBULATORY CARE**
Average length of stay in nonfederal short-stay hospitals, 358, 367
Cost of hospital discharges with common operating room procedures, 395
Days of care in nonfederal short-stay hospitals, 358
Discharge rate in nonfederal short-stay hospitals, 358–370
Discharges with at least one procedure, 370
Intermediate care facilities, by state, 373
Persons with hospital stays in the past year, 355
Specialty hospitals, by state, 373

HYPERTENSION
Health conditions and risk factors, selected years, 297
Leading causes of death, 115, 168
Number of deaths from selected causes, 119–156
Persons 20 years of age and over, 284
Risk factors, births to mothers with, 67

I

INDUSTRY
Deaths and death rates
    fatal occupational injuries, 177

INFANT, NEONATAL, AND POSTNEONATAL MORTALITY RATES
Causes of death, rates for 130 selected causes, 231
Race, state and territory, rates by, 234
Race and sex, rates by, 228

INFLUENZA
Leading causes of death, 115, 168, 172
Number of deaths from selected causes, 119–156
INFLUENZA VACCINATIONS
Adults 18 years and over, 328
INFORMATION SYSTEMS MANAGERS
Wages, 378
INHALANTS
Use of selected substances among students, 310
INJURY DEATHS
Number of deaths and death rates for injury deaths, 166
INPATIENT CARE
Average length of stay in nonfederal short-stay hospitals, 358, 367
Certified intermediate care facilities and specialty hospitals, 373
Days of care in nonfederal short-stay hospitals, 358
Discharge rate in nonfederal short-stay hospitals, 358–370
Discharges with at least one procedure, 370
Medicaid beneficiaries and payments, 418
Persons with hospital stays in the past year, 355
INSURANCE
see **HEALTH INSURANCE**
INTERMEDIATE CARE FACILITIES
Certified care facilities and specialty hospitals, by state, 373
Medicaid beneficiaries and payments, 418
INTERNISTS
Wages, 377, 378

J
JOINT PAIN
Adults 18 years and over, 268
JUDGES
Wages, 378

K
KIDNEY DISEASE
see **RENAL DISEASE**
KNEE PAIN
Joint pain among adults 18 years and over, 268

L
LATINO ORIGIN
see **HISPANIC ORIGIN**
LEADING CAUSES OF DEATH
Number of deaths from selected causes, 119–156
LICENSED PRACTICAL NURSES
Wages, 376
LIFE EXPECTANCY
Abridged life table for total population, 108
Leading causes of death, 168, 172
Life expectancy at birth, 110, 113
Life expectancy at selected ages, 112, 113
LIVE BIRTHS
Age, live-birth order, and race of mother, 6, 33, 34, 39–51
Birth rates
see **BIRTH RATES**
Birth records
total count of records and completeness of preliminary file, 23
Births
see **BIRTHS**
Birthweight figures, 72, 86
Cesarean delivery rates, 68–71
Day of week, births by, 53
Deaths from selected causes, 119–156
Fertility rates and live-birth order, 28–38
Forceps or vacuum extraction, deliveries by, 68
Gestation periods, 72, 86
Low and very low birthweight rates, 14, 72–80
Mean age of mother, by live-birth order and race, 29
Method of delivery, occurrence by, 53
Mothers under 20 years of age, by state and territory, 9
Number of live births by attendant, place of delivery, and race, 91
Observed live births, by month, 53
Order of birth, by race and Hispanic origin, 20
Plurality of births and ratios, 81
Preterm birth rates, 15, 16, 74–78
Race and Hispanic origin of mother, by state and territory, 12, 35, 36
Rates by Hispanic or non-Hispanic origin, 31
Rates by race, 30
Risk factors, births to mothers with, 65, 67
Seasonally adjusted rates, 53
Teenagers 15 to 19 years of age, 24, 25
Twins, triplets, and multiple births, 81–86
Unmarried mothers, rates of births by state and territory, 22, 62
Weight gain, live births by, 63
LIVER DISEASE
Leading causes of death, 115, 168
Number of deaths from selected causes, 119–156
LOCAL GOVERNMENT
Health expenditures, 384, 402
LOW AND VERY LOW BIRTHWEIGHT BIRTHS
Gestational age and birthweight characteristics by plurality, 86
Percentage of births with selected medical or health characteristics, 60, 61
Percentages by race and Hispanic origin, 13, 72–80
Rates by state and territory, 14, 80
LOW BACK PAIN
Adults 18 and over, 268
LUNG CANCER
Death rates, 206
LYME DISEASE
Number of new cases, 243

M
MACHINERY
Injury deaths, 166
MAGISTRATES
Wages, 378
MALARIA
Number of deaths from selected causes, 119–156
MALIGNANT NEOPLASMS
see **CANCER**

MALNUTRITION
  Number of deaths from selected causes, 119–156
MAMMOGRAMS
  Use of mammography among women 40 years and over, 332
MANAGED CARE
  Medicaid beneficiaries, 419
MARIJUANA
  Use of selected substances among persons 12 years and over, 301
  Use of selected substances among students, 310
MARITAL STATUS
  Medicaid coverage, by marital status, 415
  Medicare beneficiaries, by marital status, 411
MARKETING MANAGERS
  Wages, 378
MASSAGE THERAPISTS
  Wages, 376, 377
MDMA (ECSTASY)
  Use of selected substances among students, 310
MEASLES
  Number of deaths from selected causes, 119–156
  Number of new cases, 243
MEDICAID
  Basis of eligibility, by race and Hispanic origin, 417
  Coverage among persons under 65, selected characteristics, 415
  Managed care beneficiaries, 419
  Type of service, 418
MEDICAL ASSISTANTS
  Wages, 376, 377
MEDICAL CARE
  Adults, no usual source of health care, 314
  Children, no health care visits in past 12 months, 319
  Children, no usual source of health care, 313
  Reduced access to medical care due to cost, 316, 318
MEDICAL EXPENSES
  see HEALTH EXPENDITURES
MEDICAL PROBLEMS
  Percentage of births with selected medical or health characteristics, 60
  Risk factors, births to mothers with, 65, 67
MEDICAL TRANSCRIPTIONISTS
  Wages, 376, 377
MEDICARE
  Certified providers and suppliers, 426
  Coverage of beneficiaries 65 and over, by type of coverage, 411
  Enrollees and expenditures
    by program and type of service, 420
    by race, Hispanic origin, and selected characteristics, 423
    fee-for-service beneficiaries, 422
MEN
  see SEX
MENINGITIS
  Number of deaths from selected causes, 119–156
  Number of new cases, 243
MENTAL HEALTH SERVICES
  Health expenditures, 388
  Medicaid beneficiaries and payments, 418

MIDWIVES
  Number of live births by attendant, place of delivery, and race, 91
MIGRAINE OR HEADACHE
  Adults 18 and over, 266
MORTALITY
  Deaths and death rates
    see DEATHS AND DEATH RATES
MOTHERS
  Birth rates
    age of mother, 5, 7
    probability of a first birth, ages 15 through 24, 26
    states and territories, 38
    teenagers aged 15 to 19, by state, 25
    under 20 years of age, by state and territory, 9
    women aged 10 to 19, by race and Hispanic origin, 28
  Educational attainment, by age and race, 92
  Fertility rates by age, live-birth order, and race of mother, 42–51
  Gestation periods, 72, 86
  Live births by race and Hispanic origin of mother, 12, 35, 36
  Low birthweight births, 72–80
  Mean age of mother, by live-birth order and race, 29
  Medical or health characteristics, percentage of births by, 60
  Prenatal care
    month began, by age and race of mother, 93
  Preterm birth rates, 15, 16, 74–78
  Probability of a first birth, ages 15 through 24, 26
  Risk factors, births to mothers with, 65, 67
  Smoking during pregnancy, 87
  Total number of births, selected demographic characteristics, 18, 53
  Twins, triplets, and multiple births, 81–86
  Weight gain, live births by, 63
MOTOR VEHICLE-RELATED INJURIES
  Deaths and death rates, 214
  Injury deaths, 166
  Unintentional deaths, by state, 213
MULTIPLE BIRTHS
  Twins, triplets, and multiple births, 81–86
MUMPS
  Number of new cases, 243

N
NATURAL SCIENCES MANAGERS
  Wages, 378
NECK PAIN
  Adults 18 and over, 266
NEPHRITIS
  Leading causes of death, 115, 168
  Number of deaths from selected causes, 119–156
NEVER-MARRIED FEMALES
  Contraception use, individuals aged 15 to 19, 87–90
  Response to statement "if you got pregnant now," 27
NUCLEAR MEDICINE TECHNOLOGISTS
  Wages, 376, 377
NURSES
  Medicaid beneficiaries and payments, 418
  Wages, 376, 377

NURSING AIDES AND ORDERLIES
  Wages, 376
NUTRITIONISTS
  Wages, 376

O

OBESITY
  Children and adolescents 2 to 19 years of age, 294
  Health conditions and risk factors, selected years, 297
  Persons 20 years of age and over, 291
OBSTETRICIANS
  Wages, 377, 378
OBSTETRIC PROCEDURES
  Risk factors, births to mothers with, 65, 67
OCCUPATIONAL INJURIES AND DISEASES
  Age
    deaths from selected diseases among persons 15 years and over, 174
  Deaths and death rates, 174–180
  Fatal occupational injuries
    comparison of 2010 preliminary and final figures, 176
    industry, sex, age, race, and Hispanic origin, 177
    most frequent type, 179
    number and rate, by industry sector and occupation, 179
    number of, by state, 180
  Nonfatal occupational injuries, with days away from work, 242
OCCUPATIONAL THERAPISTS
  Wages, 376, 377
OPIOID DRUGS
  Death rates for opioid drug poisoning, selected characteristics, 211
OPTICIANS
  Wages, 376, 377
OPTOMETRISTS
  Wages, 377
ORAL SURGEONS
  Wages, 377, 378
ORTHODONTISTS
  Wages, 377, 378
OUTPATIENT HOSPITALS
  Medicaid beneficiaries and payments, 418
OVERWEIGHT, OBESITY, AND HEALTHY WEIGHT
  Children and adolescents 2 to 19 years of age, 294
  Health conditions and risk factors, selected years, 297
  Persons 20 years of age and over, 291

P

PAP SMEARS
  Use of Pap smears among women 18 years and over, 334
PARAMEDICS
  Wages, 376, 377
PARKINSON'S DISEASE
  Leading causes of death, 115, 168
PEDIATRICIANS
  Wages, 377, 378

PETROLEUM ENGINEERS
  Wages, 378
PHARMACISTS
  Wages, 376, 377
PHARMACY TECHNICIANS
  Wages, 376, 377
PHYSICAL ACTIVITY
  Leisure-time physical activity among adults 18 and over, 288
PHYSICAL THERAPISTS
  Wages, 376, 377
PHYSICIANS
  Medicaid beneficiaries and payments, 418
  Number of live births by attendant, place of delivery, and race, 91
  Wages, 377, 378
PHYSICIANS' OFFICES
  Health care visits to, 320, 345
PLACE OF DELIVERY
  Number of live births by attendant, place of delivery, and race, 91
PNEUMOCOCCAL VACCINATIONS
  Adults 18 years and over, 330
PNEUMONIA
  Leading causes of death, 115, 168, 172
  Number of deaths from selected causes, 119–156
PODIATRISTS
  Wages, 377, 378
POISONING
  Death rates for opioid drug poisoning, 211
  Injury deaths, 166
POLIOMYELITIS
  Number of deaths from selected causes, 119–156
  Number of new cases, 243
PREGNANCY
  Leading causes of death, 172
  Never-married females
    response to statement "if you got pregnant now," 27
  Risk factors, births to mothers with, 65, 67
  Weight gain of mother during pregnancy, 63
PRENATAL CARE
  Month care began, by age and race of mother, 93
PRESCRIPTION DRUGS
  Death rates for opioid drug poisoning, selected characteristics, 211
  Hospice care patients, drugs prescribed in last week of life, 236
  Medicaid beneficiaries and payments, 418
  Reduced access to prescription drugs due to cost, 316
  Selected drug classes used in past 30 days, 351
  Use in the past 30 days, by selected characteristics, 349
  Use of selected substances among persons 12 years and over, 301
PRETERM BIRTHS
  Gestational age and birthweight characteristics by plurality, 86
  Live birth rates, 15, 16, 74–78
  Live births preterm by race and Hispanic origin, 13, 74–78

Percentage of births with selected medical or health characteristics, 60, 61

PRIMARY CARE GENERALISTS
Health care visits to, 346

PSYCHIATRIC TECHNICIANS
Wages, 376, 377

PSYCHIATRISTS
Wages, 377, 378

PSYCOLOGICAL DISTRESS
Adults 18 and over, 282

R

RACE
AIDS cases, by race, 245
Alcohol, drinking five or more drinks a day among adults, 303
Asthma, children under 18 who suffer from, 283
Basic actions difficulty and complex activity limitation, 272
Birth rates
    age, live-birth order, and race of mother, 7, 39–51
    age and race of father, 40
    by race, 4, 5, 30
    demographic characteristics of births by race, 53
    mothers aged 10 to 19, 28
    number of births by Hispanic and non-Hispanic origin, 31
    selected characteristics, 4, 13
    teenagers 15 to 19 years of age, 24
    very low birthweight births, 80
    women under age 20, 8
Cancer
    five-year relative survival rates, 253
    rates, by race, 201–206, 247
Cesarean deliveries
    low birthweights and preterm births, 72–80
    selected criteria, 68–71
Cholesterol among persons 20 years of age and over, 285
Cigarette smoking, by race, 305–308
Colorectal tests or procedures, use among adults, 336
Congenital anomalies of newborns, by race of mother, 95, 96
Contraception use, individuals aged 15 to 19, 87–90
Deaths and death rates
    age-adjusted death rates, 102, 150–163
    all causes, 190
    cancer deaths, 201–206
    cerebrovascular disease death rates, 197
    fatal occupational injuries, 177
    firearm-related injuries, 224
    heart disease death rates, 194
    HIV death rates, 209
    homicide, 218
    infant mortality rates, 228–234
    leading causes of death, 168
    life expectancy at birth, 110, 113
    life expectancy at selected ages, 112, 113
    motor vehicle-related injuries, 215
    number of deaths, 104–107
    number of deaths from selected causes, 119–156
    suicide, 221
    years of potential life lost before age 75, 181
Dental caries, by race, 295
Dental visits in past year, by race, 348
Diabetes rates, by race, 261
Disability and health status, by race, 278
Educational attainment of mothers, by age and race, 92, 94
Fathers
    birth rates by age and race of father, 40
Fertility rates by age, live-birth order, and race of mother, 30, 42–51
Firearm-related injuries, 224
Health care, no usual source of, by race, 313, 314
Health care, percent distribution of payment for, 398
Health care expenses, by race, 397
Health care visits, by selected characteristics, 320, 338–345
Health care visits, lack of by children, 319
Health insurance
    coverage among persons under 65, 405, 407
    no health coverage among persons under 65, 409
Health-related behaviors of children 6 to 11 years of age, 296
Health risk behaviors among students in grades 9 to 12, by race, 298
Hospital stays in the past year, by race, 355
Hypertension among persons 20 years of age and over, 284
Joint pain among adults 18 years and over, 268
Live births
    by age and race of mother, 6, 33, 34
    by mother and state and territory, 12, 35, 36
    by plurality of birth and ratios, 81
    by race, 30
    number of live births by attendant and place of delivery, 91
    preterm birth rates, 74–78
    risk factors during pregnancy, 65, 67
Mammography, use of among women, 332
Mean age of mother, by live-birth order and race, 29
Medicaid coverage, by race, 415, 417
Medical care, reduced access to, by race, 316
Medical or health characteristics, percentage of births by, 60, 61
Medicare beneficiaries, by race, 411, 423
Order of birth, by race, 20
Overweight, obesity, and healthy weight, 291, 294
Pap smears, use of among women, 334
Physical activity among adults, 288
Prenatal care
    month began, by age and race of mother, 93
Prescription drug use in past 30 days, by race, 349
Psychological distress among adults, 282
Renal disease, end-stage patients, 263
Smoking during pregnancy, 87
Substance abuse
    death rates for opioid drug poisoning, by race, 211
    students, 312

use of selected substances among persons 12 years and over, 301
Total number of births, selected demographic characteristics, 18, 53
Twins, triplets, and multiple births, 82
Unmarried women, number and percentage of births to, 54–59, 62
Vaccination coverage, 322–330
Weight gain, live births by, 63

RADIATION THERAPISTS
Wages, 376, 377

RADIOLOGIC TECHNICIANS
Wages, 376, 377

RECESSION
Health insurance
people without insurance during first year after a recession, 414

RECREATIONAL THERAPISTS
Wages, 376, 377

REGISTERED NURSES
Wages, 376, 377

RENAL DISEASE
End-stage renal disease patients, 263
Leading causes of death, 168
Number of deaths from selected causes, 119–156

RESPIRATORY DISEASES
Leading causes of death, 115, 168
Number of deaths from selected causes, 119–156

RESPIRATORY DISTRESS SYNDROME
Leading causes of death, 172

RESPIRATORY THERAPISTS
Wages, 376, 377

RISK FACTORS
Births to mothers with, 65, 67
Medical or health characteristics, births by, 60, 61
Smoking during pregnancy, 87

ROCKY MOUNTAIN SPOTTED FEVER
Number of new cases, 243

S

SALARIES
see **WAGES**

SALMONELLA
Number of deaths from selected causes, 119–156
Number of new cases, 243

SCARLET FEVER
Number of deaths from selected causes, 119–156

SEPTICEMIA
Leading causes of death, 115, 168
Number of deaths from selected causes, 119–156

SEX
AIDS cases, by sex, 245
Alcohol, drinking five or more drinks a day among adults, 303
Asthma, children under 18 who suffer from, 283
Basic actions difficulty and complex activity limitation, 272
Cancer
five-year survival rates, by sex, 253
rates, by sex, 201–206, 247
Cholesterol among persons 20 years of age and over, 285
Cigarette smoking, by sex, 305–308
Colorectal tests or procedures, use among adults, 336
Deaths and death rates
age-adjusted death rates. 102, 150–163
all causes, 190
cancer deaths, 201–206
cerebrovascular disease death rates, 197
fatal occupational injuries, 177
firearm-related injuries, 224
heart disease death rates, 194
HIV death rates, 209
homicide, 218
infant mortality rates, 228
leading causes of death, 168
life expectancy at birth, 110, 113
life expectancy at selected ages, 112, 113
motor vehicle-related injuries, by sex, 214
number of deaths, 104–107
number of deaths from selected causes, 119–156
suicide, 221
years of potential life lost before age 75, 181
Dental caries, by sex, 295
Dental visits in past year, by sex, 348
Diabetes rates, by sex, 261
Disability and health status, by sex, 278
Discharge rate in nonfederal short-stay hospitals, by sex, 358–370
Energy and macronutrient intake, by sex, 287
Firearm-related injuries, 224
Health care, no usual source of, by sex, 313, 314
Health care, percent distribution of payment for, 398
Health care expenses, by sex, 397
Health care visits, by selected characteristics, 320, 338–345
Health care visits, lack of by children, 319
Health insurance
coverage among persons under 65, 405, 407
no health coverage among persons under 65, 409
Health-related behaviors of children 6 to 11 years of age, 296
Health risk behaviors among students in grades 9 to 12, by sex, 298
Hospital stays in the past year, by sex, 355
Hypertension among persons 20 years of age and over, 284
Joint pain among adults 18 years and over, 268
Mammography, use of among women, 332
Medicaid coverage, by sex, 415
Medical care, reduced access to, by sex, 316
Medicare beneficiaries, by sex, 411, 422
Occupational injuries and diseases
fatal occupational injuries, 177
Overweight, obesity, and healthy weight, 291, 294
Pap smears, use of among women, 334
Physical activity among adults, by sex, 288
Prescription drug classes used in past 30 days, by sex, 351
Prescription drug use in past 30 days, by sex, 349
Psychological distress among adults, by sex, 282

Renal disease, end-stage patients, 263
Substance abuse
    death rates for opioid drug poisoning, by sex, 211
    students, 310
    use of selected substances among persons 12 years and over, 301
Vaccination coverage, 322–330

SEXUALLY TRANSMITTED DISEASES
Number of new cases, 243

SHIGELLOSIS
Number of new cases, 243

SHOULDER PAIN
Joint paint among adults 18 years and over, 268

SMOKING
    see **CIGARETTE SMOKING**

SPECIALIST PHYSICIANS
Health care visits to, 346

SPEECH-LANGUAGE PATHOLOGISTS
Wages, 376, 377

STATES AND TERRITORIES
Birth rates
    age of mothers, 38
    mothers under 20 years of age, by state and territory, 9
    teenagers 15 to 19 years of age, 25
    unmarried mothers, 22, 62
Birth records
    total count of records and completeness of preliminary file, 23
Births
    educational attainment of mothers, by state, 94
Cesarean delivery rates, 17, 71
Deaths and death rates
    fatal work injuries, 180
    infant mortality rates, 233
    major causes of death by state, 184
Educational attainment of mothers, by age and race, 92
Health expenditures, 384, 402
Health insurance
    persons without coverage, by state, 413
Health personnel
    highest levels and concentrations of employment, 379
Hospitals
    certified intermediate care facilities and specialty hospitals, 373
Live births
    mothers under 20 years of age, by state and territory, 9
    race and Hispanic origin of mother, 12, 35, 36
Low birthweight birth rates, 14, 80
Medicaid beneficiaries, by state, 419
Medical care, reduced access to, by states, 318
Medicare enrollees, by state, 425
Mothers smoking during pregnancy, 87
Motor vehicle deaths, unintentional, by state, 213
Occupational injuries and diseases
    number of fatal work injuries, by state, 180
Preterm birth rates, 16
Teenage birth rates, 24, 25
Twin, triplets, and multiple births, 85
Unmarried mothers, rates, 22, 62

STROKE
Death rates for cerebrovascular disease, 197
Health, determinants and measures of respondent-reported prevalence among adults, 255
Leading causes of death, 115, 168

STUDENTS
Health risk behaviors among students in grades 9 to 12, 298
Use of selected substances among students, 310

SUBSTANCE ABUSE
Death rates for opioid drug poisoning, selected characteristics, 211
Health expenditures for treatment, 389
Use of selected substances among persons 12 years and over, 301

SUDDEN INFANT DEATH SYNDROME
Leading causes of death, 172

SUFFOCATION
Injury deaths, 166

SUICIDE
Deaths and death rates, 220
Injury deaths, 166
Leading causes of death, 115, 168

SURGEONS
Wages, 377, 378

SYPHILIS
Number of deaths from selected causes, 119–156
Number of new cases, 243

T
TEENAGERS
    see **ADOLESCENTS**

TERRITORIES
    see **STATES AND TERRITORIES**

THROAT CANCER
Death rates, 206

TOBACCO USE
    see **CIGARETTE SMOKING**

TRANSPORTATION
Injury deaths, 166

TUBERCULOSIS
Number of deaths from selected causes, 119–156
Number of new cases, 243

TWINS, TRIPLETS, AND MULTIPLE BIRTHS
Numbers and rates, 81–86

U
UNINTENTIONAL INJURIES
Leading causes of death, 168, 172

UNMARRIED WOMEN
Births to unmarried mothers, by state and territory, 22, 62
Number and percentage of births to, 11, 54–59, 62

V
VACCINATIONS
Coverage among adolescents 13 to 17 years of age, 327

Coverage among children 19 to 35 months of age, 322, 325
Influenza vaccinations among adults, 328
Pneumococcal vaccinations among adults, 330

VACUUM EXTRACTION
Deliveries by, 68

VETERANS AFFAIRS, DEPARTMENT OF
Health care expenditures and use, and persons treated, 403

VETERINARIANS
Wages, 377

VISION LIMITATIONS
Adults 18 and over, 274

VITAMINS
Use among persons 20 years and over, 353

W

WAGES
Anesthesiologists, 377
Athletic trainers, 377
Audiologists, 376, 377
Cardiovascular technologists, 376, 377
Chiropractors, 377
Dental assistants, 376, 377
Dental hygienists, 376, 377
Dentists, 377
Diagnostic medical sonographers, 376, 377
Dietetic technicians, 376, 377
Emergency medical technicians, 376, 377
Gynecologists, 377
Home health aides, 376, 377
Massage therapists, 376, 377
Medical assistants, 376, 377
Medical transcriptionists, 376, 377
Nuclear medicine technologists, 376, 377
Nurses, 376, 377
Nursing aides and orderlies, 376, 377
Nutritionists, 376, 377
Obstetricians, 377
Occupational therapists, 376, 377
Opticians, 376, 377
Optometrists, 377
Orthodontists, 377
Paramedics, 376, 377
Pediatricians, 377
Pharmacists, 376, 377
Pharmacy technicians, 376, 377
Physical therapists, 376, 377
Physician assistants, 376, 377
Physicians, 377
Podiatrists, 377
Psychiatric technicians, 376, 377
Psychiatrists, 377
Radiation therapists, 376, 377
Radiologic technicians, 376, 377
Recreational therapists, 376, 377
Registered nurses, 376, 377
Respiratory therapists, 376, 377
Speech-language pathologists, 376, 377
Surgeons, 377
Veterinarians, 377

WAR
Number of deaths from selected causes, 119–156

WEAPONS
Deaths and death rates, 224

WEIGHT
Overweight, obesity, and healthy weight
children and adolescents 2 to 19 years of age, 294
health conditions and risk factors, selected years, 297
persons 20 years of age and over, 291

WEIGHT GAIN
Live births by weight gain of mother, 63

WHITE RACE
Generally
see **RACE**

WHOOPING COUGH
Number of deaths from selected causes, 119–156
Number of new cases, 243

WOMEN
see **SEX**

WORK INJURIES
see **OCCUPATIONAL INJURIES AND DISEASES**